Community Health
NURSING

Community Health NURSING

Volume 1

Third Edition

BT Basavanthappa MSc(N) PhD

Principal
Rajarajeshwari College of Nursing
Bengaluru, Karnataka, India

Professor and Principal (Rtd)
Government College of Nursing
Bengaluru, Karnataka, India

PhD Guide for Research Work
Ex-Member
Faculty of Nursing, RGUHS, Karnataka, India
Academic Council, RGUHS, Karnataka, India

Examiner
UG, PG and Doctoral Degree Courses on Nursing in various universities

Ex-program In-Charge
IGNOU, BSc Nursing Course, Karnataka and Goa, India

Life Member
Nursing Research Society of India, New Delhi, India
Trained Nurses Association of India, New Delhi, India

President
RGUHS Nursing Teachers Association, Karnataka, India

Winner
Bharat Excellence Award and Gold Medal
Vikas Rattan Gold Award
UWA Lifetime Achievement Award
Shree Veeranjaneya 'Shrujanashri' Award

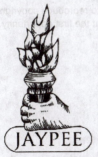

JAYPEE The Health Sciences Publisher

New Delhi | London | Philadelphia | Panama

Jaypee Brothers Medical Publishers (P) Ltd

Headquarters
Jaypee Brothers Medical Publishers (P) Ltd
4838/24, Ansari Road, Daryaganj
New Delhi 110 002, India
Phone: +91-11-43574357
Fax: +91-11-43574314
Email: jaypee@jaypeebrothers.com

Overseas Offices

J.P. Medical Ltd
83 Victoria Street, London
SW1H 0HW (UK)
Phone: +44 20 3170 8910
Fax: +44 (0)20 3008 6180
Email: info@jpmedpub.com

Jaypee-Highlights Medical Publishers Inc
City of Knowledge, Bld. 237, Clayton
Panama City, Panama
Phone: +1 507-301-0496
Fax: +1 507-301-0499
Email: cservice@jphmedical.com

Jaypee Medical Inc
325 Chestnut Street
Suite 412, Philadelphia, PA 19106, USA
Phone: +1 267-519-9789
Email: jpmed.us@gmail.com

Jaypee Brothers Medical Publishers (P) Ltd
17/1-B Babar Road, Block-B, Shaymali
Mohammadpur, Dhaka-1207
Bangladesh
Phone: +08801912003485
Email: jaypeedhaka@gmail.com

Jaypee Brothers Medical Publishers (P) Ltd
Bhotahity, Kathmandu, Nepal
Phone: +977-9741283608
Email: kathmandu@jaypeebrothers.com

Website: www.jaypeebrothers.com
Website: www.jaypeedigital.com

© 2016, BT Basavanthappa

The views and opinions expressed in this book are solely those of the original contributor(s)/author(s) and do not necessarily represent those of editor(s) of the book.

All rights reserved. No part of this publication may be reproduced, stored or transmitted in any form or by any means, electronic, mechanical, photocopying, recording or otherwise, without the prior permission in writing of the publishers.

All brand names and product names used in this book are trade names, service marks, trademarks or registered trademarks of their respective owners. The publisher is not associated with any product or vendor mentioned in this book.

Medical knowledge and practice change constantly. This book is designed to provide accurate, authoritative information about the subject matter in question. However, readers are advised to check the most current information available on procedures included and check information from the manufacturer of each product to be administered, to verify the recommended dose, formula, method and duration of administration, adverse effects and contraindications. It is the responsibility of the practitioner to take all appropriate safety precautions. Neither the publisher nor the author(s)/editor(s) assume any liability for any injury and/or damage to persons or property arising from or related to use of material in this book.

This book is sold on the understanding that the publisher is not engaged in providing professional medical services. If such advice or services are required, the services of a competent medical professional should be sought.

Every effort has been made where necessary to contact holders of copyright to obtain permission to reproduce copyright material. If any have been inadvertently overlooked, the publisher will be pleased to make the necessary arrangements at the first opportunity.

Inquiries for bulk sales may be solicited at: jaypee@jaypeebrothers.com

Community Health Nursing (Volume 1)

First Edition: 1998
Reprints: 1999, 2001, 2003, 2005, 2006
Second Edition: 2008
Third Edition: **2016**

ISBN 978-93-5152-918-7

Printed at Sanat Printers

Dedicated to

My parents
Late Shri Thukkappa
&
Smt Hanumanthamma
and also
My dear students of nursing profession

Preface to the Third Edition

It gives me a great pleasure with professional satisfaction to introduce third edition of my title *Community Health Nursing*. In offering this textbook, I remain grateful to all those who have given support to all my titles in 'nursing' and have provided constructive feedbacks as well as encouraging comments.

A development in health care that has been growing through the last several decades was brought about by consumer awareness and activity. Now people are interested in self-care, improving their own health rather than having the healthcare system to take care of their health. Aims of nursing include promoting wellness, preventing illness, restoring health and facilitating coping. These become overwhelmed by the demand placed on the nurse's knowledge, technical competence, interpersonal skills and commitment. Therefore, much care has been taken in selection of both the content of this edition and the manner of its presentation.

Today, there is a need of student-friendly, knowledge-oriented, clinical competence-oriented, as well as informative textbooks. This has compelled me to write and compile this book, which is organized into 16 sections, with 85 chapters. Many changes are made in response to feedback of the respective readers, suggestions and constructive comments from faculty and students using my previous titles and also according to curriculum prescribed by the statutory bodies.

The features of each section include the following:

1. Section 1 comprises Chapters 1 to 5, which describes the concepts/dimensions of community health and nursing, and also promotion of health and its maintenance.
2. Section 2 comprises Chapters 6 to 26 (divided into Parts I and II), which presents the determinants of health. Part I describes the eugenics as determinant of health. Part II describes the environment as determinant of health, which includes physical (water, air, light, ventilation, noise, radiation, climate, housing, sanitation, etc.), biological (forestation, bacterial/viral agents, food, etc.) and sociocultural environment (customs, taboos, family, lifestyle, hygiene, physical activity, etc.).
3. Section 3 comprises Chapter 27, which presents the concepts of epidemiology related to community health and the community health nursing.
4. Section 4 comprises Chapters 28 to 35, which describes the communicable diseases and their nursing management; including respiratory infections, intestinal infection, arthropod infestations, zoonoses, surface infections and sexually transmitted diseases.
5. Section 5 comprises Chapters 36 to 45, which describes the prevailing non-communicable diseases and conditions; including malnutrition, obesity, cardiovascular diseases, cancer, accidents, diabetes mellitus, mental illness, epilepsy and fluorosis.
6. Section 6 comprises Chapters 46 and 47, which focuses on demography, population explosion and its control at community level.
7. Section 7 comprises Chapters 48 and 49, which discusses the concepts, scope and historical development (in brief) of community health and the community health nursing.
8. Section 8 comprises Chapters 50 to 54, which describes the health planning, policies and health problems; including health planning, planning commission, health in five-year plans, committees and commissions of health and family welfare, National Health Policy and health problems in India.
9. Section 9 comprises Chapters 55 to 58, which discusses the delivery of community health services; including healthcare system, planning, budgeting, and material management, rural and urban health services.
10. Section 10 comprises Chapters 59 to 66, which discusses the components of health services; including environmental sanitation, health education, vital statistics, maternal and child health services, family welfare, school health services, occupational health services and mental health services.
11. Section 11 comprises Chapters 67 to 71, which describes the community health nursing approaches; including nursing theories, nursing process, problem-solving and epidemiological approaches, and also primary health care, millennium development goals and proposed sustainable development goals.
12. Section 12 comprises Chapters 72 to 77, which describes the roles and responsibilities of community health nursing personnel; including roles, functions and responsibilities of community health nurse, family health services,

information, education and communication, management information system, training and supervision of health services and biomedical waste management.
13. Section 13 comprises Chapters 78 to 82, which discusses the job responsibilities of community health nursing personnel; including home visits, job descriptions, treatment of minor ailments, empowering people, monitoring procedures of need in the community.
14. Section 14 comprises Chapter 83, which focuses on social issues affecting health; including women empowerment, women abuse, child abuse, abuse of elders, female feticide, commercial sex workers, food adulteration and substance abuse.
15. Section 15 comprises Chapter 84, which describes the important national health programs launched and existed in India, and some of them that were in operation.
16. Section 16 comprises Chapter 85, which describes the health agencies of national and international importance that supports the health of population/community.

So this textbook is organized into 16 sections with 85 chapters ideally and the text is followed sequentially, but every effort has been made to respect the differing needs of diverse curricula and students. Here, each chapter stands on its own merit and may be read independently of others.

I am aware that for manifold reasons, errors might have crept in and shall feel obliged, if such errors are brought to my notice. I sincerely welcome constructive comments and suggestions.

BT Basavanthappa

Preface to the First Edition

I have a great pleasure in presenting the book *Community Health Nursing* to nursing community. I conceived the idea of writing this book due to lack of nursing books, written by Indian authors in the context of Indian situation.

Now we are witnessing so much changes taking place in healthcare system. To meet the demands of a constantly changing system, nurses must become increasingly futuristic in developing roles and responsibilities. For this, nursing personnel must know the importance of many factors associated with community health nursing, which includes principles of community health and nursing, the current and evolving characteristics of the healthcare system, a heightened awareness of the roles and responsibilities of the nurses, for placing health on the hands of the people.

The text has been written in simple language and style in well-organized and systematized way, and utmost care has been taken to cover the entire prescribed course material for nursing students. It may be a comprehensive source book that offers valuable base for designing community health nursing strategies for the individuals, families, groups and communities.

It is hoped that this book will offer the nursing students enough exposure to the subject matter and enable to equip them in their success. I am sure that students would come out with flying colors if they strictly and sincerely make use of this book.

It is a sense of honor and pride to place on record my sincere thanks and deep sense of gratitude to my well-wisher and guide Dr (Mrs) Manjula K Vasundhra, former Professor and Head, Department of Preventive and Social Medicine, Bangalore Medical College, Bengaluru.

I wish to express sincere appreciation to my wife Smt Lalitha and lovely children BB Mahesh and BB Ganashree, who bore with patience throughout my work of this text.

I express my deep appreciation to M/s Jaypee Brothers Medical Publishers (P) Ltd, New Delhi, for their interest, hard work and sincere labor for publication of this book.

BT Basavanthappa

Acknowledgments

I owe a great deal of thanks to many who supported me with their time and encouragement throughout:
- Shri G Basavannappa, former Minister of Karnataka State, for initiating and supporting me to take up this Noble Nursing Profession as my career.
- Dr (Mrs) Manjula K Vasundhra, former Professor and Head, Department of Community Medicine, Bangalore Medical College and Research Institute, Bengaluru, Karnataka, India, who continuously encouraged me to write textbooks in the field of nursing, since nursing is a major force in medical and health services.
- My father Shri Thukkappa, who continuously blessed for the progress of my career and all-round development of my personality for the welfare of the community.
- My mother Smt Hanumanthamma, who continues to be a bright spot in the lives of all who knew her and whose grace gave me strength to progress in my life.
- My wife Smt Lalitha, who gives meaning to my life in so many ways. She is the one whose encouragement keeps me motivated, whose support gives me strength and whose gentleness gives me comfort.
- My lovely children BB Mahesh and BB Ganashree, for all the joy they provided me and all the hope that they instilled in me and who bore with patience throughout my works of the nursing textbooks. They keep me young at heart.
- Finally, my warmest appreciation goes to Shri Jitendar P Vij (Group Chairman), Mr Ankit Vij (Group President), Mr Tarun Duneja (Director–Publishing) and staff of Bengaluru Production Unit/Bengaluru Branch of M/s Jaypee Brothers Medical Publishers (P) Ltd, New Delhi, India, for sharing my vision for this book and giving me the chance to turn my vision into reality.

Contents

VOLUME 1

SECTION 1: CONCEPTS OF COMMUNITY, HEALTH AND NURSING

1. **Concepts of Community**   3
   - Functions of Community   5
   - Characteristics of Community   5
   - Dimension of Community   7
   - Health and the Community Systems   8

2. **Concepts and Dimensions of Health**   11
   - Expert Views on Health   11
   - Models of Health   14
   - Dimension of Health   15

3. **Concepts of Nursing**   17
   - Purposes of Nursing Care   20
   - Settings of Nursing Care   21
   - Standards of Nursing Care   22

4. **Promotion of Health**   26
   - Principles   28
   - Health Promotion Model   28
   - Nurse's Role in Health Promotion   32
   - Individual Health Promotion   34

5. **Maintenance of Health**   37
   - Health Promotion   37
   - Specific Protection   40
   - Types of Health Promotion Programs   42
   - Sites for Health Promotion Activities   43
   - Nurse's Role in Health Promotion and its Maintenance   44

SECTION 2: DETERMINANTS OF HEALTH

Part I: Eugenics as Determinant of Health

6. **Eugenics**   49
   - Genetics   49
   - Mechanism of Inheritance   52
   - Eugenics   54
   - Early Diagnosis and Treatment   56
   - Euthenics   56
   - Genetic Counseling   57
   - Role of Nurses in Genetic Counseling   59

Part II: Environment as Determinant of Health
A. Physical Environment

7. **Water as a Determinant of Health**   63
   - Physical Environment   64
   - Water   64
   - Water Pollution and its Hazards   68
   - Purification of Water   70
   - Guidelines for Potable Water by WHO   78
   - Surveillance of Drinking Water Quality   85
   - Hardness of Water   87
   - Water Act (Prevention and Control of Pollution), 1974   91

8. **Air as a Determinant of Health**   94
   - Changes in Air During Occupancy   95
   - Thermal Comfort   96
   - Air Pollution   97
   - Role of Nurses in Prevention and Control of Air Pollution   105

9. **Light as a Determinant of Health**   108
   - Light   108
   - Methods to Improve Lighting   110

10. **Ventilation as a Determinant of Health**   114
    - Standards of Ventilation   114
    - Types of Ventilation   115

11. **Noise as a Determinant of Health**   119
    - Noise   119

12. **Radiation Exposure as a Determinant of Health**   124
    - Radiation   124
    - Types of Radiation   126
    - Non-ionizing Radiation   126
    - Ionizing Radiation   128
    - Radiation Measurements   129
    - Protective Measures and Radiation   130
    - Prevention and Control of Radiation Hazards   130

13. **Climate as a Determinant of Health**   132
    Atmospheric Pressure 132
    Air, Temperature and its Tool for Measurement 134
    Humidity 138
    Rain 139
    Wind 139
    Clouds and Weather 139
    Climate Change and its Impact on Health 139
    Global Warming 140
    Containment Measures 141

14. **Housing as a Determinant of Health**   143
    Physical Needs of House 143
    Housing 143
    Town Planning 147
    Overcrowding in the House 147
    Indicators of Housing 148
    Housing Problem 148

15. **Sanitation: Disposal of Waste**   150
    Waste and Refuse 150
    Public Education and Expenditure in Disposal 154
    Human Excreta Disposal 155
    Disposal of Dead Bodies 171
    Problem of Sanitation in India 173
    Sanitation Problems Affects the Public Health 174
    Fairs, Festivals and Traffic Sanitation, and Measures 174
    Role of Nurses in Environmental Health 175

16. **Communication, Infrastructure Facilities and Linkages**   176
    Communication Process 176
    Types of Communication 176
    Barriers of Communication 178
    Present Trend in Communication 178
    Infrastructure Facilities and Linkages 179
    Current Problems 183
    Linkages 184

B. Biological Environment

17. **Forestation**   189
    Biological Environment 189
    Importance of Forests 189
    Afforestation 190
    Deforestation 190
    Sustaining the Forest System 191
    Management of Forests 191
    Plans and Policies for Forestation, and Prevention for Deforestation 192
    Acts Regulating the Environment National Pollution Control Board 193
    Action Taken by the Government of India 195
    Environment Protection Act 196
    Air Prevention and Control of Pollution Act (1981) 198
    Water Act or the Water (Prevention and Control of Pollution) Act (1974) 198
    Central and State Pollution Control Boards 199
    Noise Pollution and Legislative Measures 200
    What to Do to Seek Redressal? 201
    How Can We Seek Redressal? 201

18. **Bacterial and Viral Agents: Host and Immunity**   203
    Agent 203
    Bacteria 204
    Viruses 205
    Host 206
    Immunity 208
    Immunization and Immunizing Agents 210

19. **Arthropods**   215
    Classification of Arthropods 215
    Diseases Caused by Arthropods 216
    Mechanism of Transmission of Disease 216
    Classes of Arthropods 217
    Bugs 231
    Control of Ticks and Mites 233

20. **Rodents**   240
    Classification 240
    Rats 240

21. **Food Hygiene**   245
    Food Additives 246
    Food Preservation 249
    Food Processing (Preparation) 253
    Methods of Food Preparation 253
    Safe Food Handling 255
    Personnel Hygiene of Food Handler 256
    Sanitation of Food Establishments (Restaurants, Eating Houses) 257
    Conservation of Nutrients 259
    Food Adulteration 261
    Milk Hygiene 269
    Meat Hygiene 271
    Fish Hygiene 271
    Food Allergy 272

C. Sociocultural Environment

22. Sociocultural Determinants — 275
- Customs and Taboos 275
- Marriage System 278
- Family Structure 281
- Status of Special Groups 284

23. Introduction to Lifestyle — 289
- Importance of Lifestyle 289
- Lifestyle Risks and Habits 290
- Lifestyle and Behavioral Changes 290
- Nurses Role in Lifestyle Issues 291
- Lifestyle/Health Risk Assessment 291

24. Lifestyle: Hygiene — 293
- Type of Hygiene 293
- Objectives 294
- Principles Relevant to Hygiene 294
- Factors Affecting Hygienic Practices 294
- Habit 294
- Maintaining Personal Hygiene 298

25. Lifestyle: Physical Activity — 309
- Benefits of Physical Activity 309
- Exercise 310
- Sleep and Rest 313
- Sexual Life as a Form of Activity 320
- Spiritual Life 323
- Self-reliance 324
- Dietary Pattern 325
- Education 334
- Occupation 337

26. Financial Management — 345
- Objectives 346
- Scope 346
- Elements 346
- Functions 346
- Income 347
- Purchasing Power 347
- Finance Security 348

SECTION 3: CONCEPTS OF EPIDEMIOLOGY

27. Epidemiology — 353
- Aims of Epidemiology 354
- Objectives of Epidemiology 354
- Epidemiological Approach 355
- Uses of Epidemiology 356
- Scope of Epidemiology 356
- Advantages of Using Epidemiology in Community Health Nursing Practice 356
- Epidemiological Process 358
- Importance of Epidemiological Process/Surveillance 363
- Natural Life History of Disease 364
- Implications of Epidemiology in Community Health Nursing 371
- Dynamics of Disease Transmission 385
- Immunity 388
- Dynamics of Infectious Disease Transmission 390

SECTION 4: COMMUNICABLE DISEASES

28. Respiratory Infections — 399
- Smallpox (Variola) 399
- Chickenpox (Varicella) 403
- Mumps 405
- Measles (Rubella) 408
- Rubella (German Measles) 413
- Influenza 414
- Acute Respiratory Infections 417
- Diphtheria 421
- Pertussis (Whooping Cough) 425
- Meningococcal Meningitis 429
- Tuberculosis 432
- Severe Acute Respiratory Syndrome 446
- Avian Flu 449

29. Intestinal Infections — 458
- Poliomyelitis 458
- Viral Hepatitis 467
- Cholera 468
- Typhoid Fever 472
- Diarrheal Diseases 478
- Bacillary Dysentery 483
- Amebiasis (Amebic Dysentery) 487
- Worm Infestations 491
- Roundworm Infestation (Ascariasis) 491
- Pinworm Infestation 493
- Hookworm Infestation 495
- Tapeworm Infestation 497
- Dracunculiasis 500
- Food Allergy 502
- Food Poisoning 502

30. Arthropod Infestations — 506
- Dengue Fever 506
- Chikungunya Fever (Epidemic Polyarthritis) 511

Malaria 515
Kala-azar 526
Filariasis 529

31. Zoonoses: Viral — 535
Rabies 535
Arboviral Diseases 541

32. Zoonoses: Bacterial — 554
Brucellosis 554
Plague 558
Human Salmonellosis 563
Anthrax 566
Leptospirosis 569

33. Zoonoses: Rickettsial — 574
Epidemic Typhus 574
Endemic Typhus 576
Scrub Typhus 576
Murine Typhus 577
Tick Typhus 578
Indian Tick Typhus 578
Rocky Mountain Spotted Fever 579
Rickettsialpox 579
Trench Fever 579
Q Fever 579

34. Zoonoses: Parasitic — 582
Teniasis 582
Hydatid Disease 585
Leishmaniasis 588

35. Important Surface Infections and Sexually Transmitted Diseases — 592
Trachoma 592
Tetanus 595
Leprosy 599
Sexually Transmitted Diseases 609
Yaws 623
Gas Gangrene 626

SECTION 5: NON-COMMUNICABLE DISEASES

36. An Introduction to Non-communicable Diseases — 631
Magnitude of Problem of NCDs 631
Hypertension 632
Rheumatic Heart Disease 632
Cardiovascular Diseases 632
Diabetes 632
Injuries 632
Mental Disorders 632
Cancer 633
Orodental Problems 633
Blindness 633

37. Malnutrition — 637
Protein-Energy Malnutrition 637
Assessment of Nutritional Status 643
Nutritional Requirement 645
Vitamin Deficiency Diseases 649
Mineral Deficiency Diseases 651

38. Obesity — 657
Indicators of Obesity 657
Risk Factors of Obesity 659
Prevention and Control Measures 661
Nursing Management of Obese Clients/Patients 664

39. Cardiovascular Diseases — 665
Classification of Heart Diseases 665
Angina Pectoris 667
Cardiac Arrhythmias 667
Congestive Heart Failure 668
Coronary Artery Disease 669
Congenital Heart Diseases 671
Rheumatic Heart Disease 672
Hypertension 674
Cerebrovascular Accident (Stroke) 678

40. Cancer — 681
Magnitude of Problem 681
Problems in India 681
Etiology of Cancer 682
Epidemiological Features 683
Pathophysiology of Cancer Cells 684
Clinical Features 684
Lung Cancer: Sputum Cytology 684
Nurse's Role in Cancer Prevention 685
National Cancer Control Program 686
Tobacco-related Health Problems and Education 687
Gutka and Oral Cancer 688
Projects for Control of Cervical Cancer 688
Cancer of Gallbladder 688
Breast Cancer 689
Operational Research to Control Cancer 689

Contents

41. Accidents — 690
  Accidents in India 690
  Domestic Accidents 694
  Suicide 697

42. Diabetes Mellitus — 700
  Magnitude of Diabetes Mellitus 700
  Epidemiology 700
  Types of Diabetes Mellitus 701
  Classification 701
  Etiology 702
  Pathophysiology 703
  Clinical Features 704
  Complications 705
  Prevention 705
  Nursing Management 706

43. Mental Illness — 709
  Significance of Problem 709
  Etiology 710
  Types of Mental Health Disorders 711
  Prevention and Control of Mental Illness 712

44. Epilepsy — 715
  Classification 715
  Etiology 715
  Pathophysiology 716
  Clinical Manifestation 716
  Management 717

45. Fluorosis — 720
  Etiology 720
  Clinical Manifestation 720
  Prevention and Control 721

SECTION 6: DEMOGRAPHY

46. Demography — 725
  Demographic Process 725
  Demographic Cycle 725
  Demographic Trends in the World 726
  Demographic Trends in India 727
  Scope of Demography 729
  Demographic Rates and Ratios 734

47. Population and its Control — 738
  Problems of Overpopulation in India 738
  Population Explosion 739
  Population Stabilization 741
  Family Planning 752

VOLUME 2

SECTION 7: CONCEPTS OF COMMUNITY HEALTH AND COMMUNITY HEALTH NURSING

48. Concepts and Scope of Community Health and Community Health Nursing — 765
  Review of Community 765
  Concepts of Community Health 766
  Purpose of Community Health 766
  Scope of Community Health 766
  Objectives of Community Health 768
  Determinants of Community Health 768
  Elements of Community Health Practice 768
  Concept of Community Health Nursing 770
  Philosophy of Community Health Nursing 770
  Nature of Community Health Nursing 771
  Assumptions and Beliefs of Community Health Nursing 773
  Visions and Commitments 777
  Scope of Community Health Nursing 778

49. Historical Developments of Community Health and Community Health Nursing — 781
  Brief History of Community Health in India 781

SECTION 8: HEALTH PLANNING, POLICIES AND PROBLEMS

50. Introduction to Health Planning — 793
  Health Planning 793
  Planning Commission 796
  Health in Five-year Plans 797

51. Health in Five-year Plans — 799
  Five-year Plans 799
  First Five-year Plan (1951–1956) 800
  Second Five-year Plan (1956–1961) 801
  Third Five-year Plan (1961–1966) 801
  Annual Plans (1966–1969) 801
  Fourth Five-year Plan (1969–1974) 802
  Achievements from First FYP to Fourth FYP 802
  Fifth Five-year Plan (1974–1979) 802
  Rolling Plan (1978–1980) 803
  Sixth Five-year Plan (1980–1985) 803
  Seventh Five-year Plan (1985–1989) 804
  Annual Plans (1990–1991) 804
  Eighth Five-year Plan (1991–1995) 805
  Ninth Five-year Plan (1997–2002) 805

Tenth Five-year Plan (2002–2007) 806
Eleventh Five-year Plan (2007–2012) 806
Twelfth Five-year Plan 808

52. Committees and Commissions of Health, and Family Welfare 813
Principles of Community
  Health Administration 813
Objectives of Community Health Planning 814
Community Health Planning and Policy 814
National Health Committees in India 815
Central Council of Health 832

53. National Health Policy 833
National Health Policy (1983) 833
National Health Policy (2002) 840
Current Scenario 843
Policy Prescriptions (2002) 851
National Population Policy (2000) 858

54. Health Problems in India 866
Demographic Profile 866
Mortality Profile 866
Health Problems 867

SECTION 9: DELIVERY OF COMMUNITY HEALTH SERVICES

55. Healthcare System 873
Healthcare System 873

56. Planning, Budgeting and Material Management 881
Planning 881
Budget 885
Material Management 889

57. Rural Health Services 895
Village Level 895
Primary Health Center 900
Community Health Center 903
Hospitals 905
Health Insurance 906
Other Agencies of Healthcare Services 907
Indigenous Systems of Medicine 907
Traditional Systems of Medicine
  in Public Health 908
Organization of Health Services in India 909

58. Urban Health Services 917
Criteria for Urban Area 917

SECTION 10: COMPONENTS OF HEALTH SERVICES

59. Environmental Sanitation 923
Sanitation 923
Disposal of Wastes 924

60. Health Education 934
Aims and Objectives of Health Education 934
Health Education Approaches 934
Steps in Carrying Out a Health
  Education Program 937
Common Topics of Health Education 941
Methods of Health Education 943
Administration of Health Education
  in India 945
Planning for Health Education Program 946
Tips for Health Teaching 946

61. Vital Statistics 947
Sources of Vital Statistics 948
Health Statistics of India 952
National Health Programs 953

62. Maternal and Child Health Services 954
Policy Guidelines 955
Maternal and Child Health Problems 956
Goals of MCH Services 960
Need for MCH Services 961
Maternal Health Services 962
Child Health Services 965
Activities of Nursing Personnel
  in MCH Services 971
Medical Termination of
  Pregnancy Act (1971) 972
Prenatal Diagnostics Techniques Act (1996) 973
Child Adoption Act 976

63. Family Welfare 979
Family Planning 979
Family Welfare Program 980
Hazards of the Large and
  Unplanned Family 981
Family Planning Methods 983
Role of Nurses in Family Welfare Program 991
Concept of Family Welfare 992
New Focus of Family Welfare Program 993
Activities at Subcenter and
  Public Health Centers 994

64. School Health Services 996
School Health Program 996

65. Occupational Health Services — 1004
Aims of Occupational Health Program 1004
Objectives of the Occupational Health Program 1004
Occupational Hazards 1005
Measures for Health Protection of Workers 1005
Prevention of Occupational Diseases 1007
Occupational Health Nursing 1011
Role of Nurse in Occupational Health Program 1012
Functions of Occupational Health Nursing 1012
Occupational Health in India 1016
Rajiv Gandhi Shramik Kalyan Yojna 1017

66. Mental Health Services: Community Mental Health Nursing Program — 1018
Criteria of Good Mental Health 1018
Mental Health Nursing 1019
Intervention/Prevention 1021
Promotion of Mental Health through Lifespan 1024
Nurse and Community Mental Health 1031
National Mental Health Program 1034

SECTION 11: COMMUNITY HEALTH NURSING APPROACHES

67. Nursing Theories — 1039
Theory and Community Health Nursing 1039
Hierarchy of Component 1039
General Systems Theory 1041
Theorist Views 1043
Theoretical Thinking for Nurses 1044
Nursing Diagnosis 1051
Nursing Process 1052

68. Nursing Process — 1054
Nature of Nursing Process 1054
Importance of Nursing Process 1054
Advantages of Nursing Process 1055
Nursing Process in Community Health 1055
Components of Nursing Process 1056
Assessment 1056
Community Health Diagnosis 1057
Nursing Diagnosis 1058
Planning 1062
Implementation 1064
Evaluation 1065

69. Problem-solving Approach — 1067
Trial and Error 1067
Intuitive Problem Solving 1067
Experimentation 1068
Scientific Method 1068
Modified Scientific Method (Problem-solving Process) 1068
Decision-making 1068

70. Epidemiological Approach — 1072
Epidemiological Triangle 1072
Types of Studies 1074
Levels of Preventive Interventions 1074
Applications of Epidemiology in Community Health Nursing 1077
Evidence-based Approach 1084

71. Concepts of Primary Health Care — 1089
Evolution of Primary Health Care 1089
Characteristics of Primary Health Care 1091
Principles of Primary Health Care 1092
Elements of Primary Health Care 1093
Role of Nurses in Primary Health Care in India 1094
Millennium Development Goals 1101
Sustainable Development Goals 1104

SECTION 12: ROLES AND RESPONSIBILITIES OF COMMUNITY HEALTH NURSING PERSONNEL

72. Roles, Functions and Responsibilities of Community Health Nurse — 1109
Roles of Community Health Nurse 1109
Functions of Community Health Nursing Personnel 1112
Responsibilities of Community Health Nurses 1115

73. Family Health Service — 1124
Family Health Care 1124
Family Health Nursing 1125
Genograms 1135
Ecomap 1135
Family Experiencing a Health Crisis 1136

74. Information, Education and Communication — 1139
Need for Information, Education and Communication 1139

IEC in Leprosy 1146
IEC in Reproductive and
  Child Health Program 1146

**75. Management Information System,
Maintenance of Records and Reports** 1148

*Advantages of Management
  Information System* 1148
Need for Information System 1148
Information System 1150
Management Information System 1151
Types of Information System 1153
*Records and Reports to be Maintained
  at Subcenter and Primary Health
  Center Levels* 1156

**76. Training and Supervision of
Health Services** 1161

Training Methods 1161
Need for Training in Health 1162
Essential Components of Training 1162
Staff Development Activities 1163
*Educational Approaches in
  Continuing Nursing Education* 1164
Supervision of Health Workers 1167
Objectives and Areas of Training Programs 1171
Planning of Education/Training Programs 1171

**77. Waste Management and Biomedical
Waste Management** 1174

Waste Management 1174
Methods of Disposal of Waste 1175
Biomedical Waste Management 1176
Terminologies for Biomedical Wastes 1177
Classification of Biomedical Waste 1177
Sources of Healthcare Waste 1181
Surveys on Healthcare Waste 1182
Sources of Biomedical Waste 1182
Problems of Biomedical Waste 1183
*Health Hazards of Biomedical Waste
  and its Management* 1185
*World Health Organization Healthcare
  Waste Policy, 2005* 1188
*Biomedical Waste (Management
  and Handling) (Second Amendment
  Rules, 2000)* 1189

SECTION 13: JOB RESPONSIBILITIES OF COMMUNITY HEALTH NURSING PERSONNEL

78. Home Visit 1197

Importance of Home Visit 1197
Purpose 1197
Advantages and Disadvantages 1198
Principles of Home Visit 1198
Process of Home Visit 1199
*Problems of Home Visit and
  Possible Solutions* 1203
Nursing Responsibilities in Home Visits 1203
Establishing Relationship 1205
Procedures Used in CHN Practice 1205
Community Health Nursing Procedures 1208

**79. Job Description of Community
Health Personnel** 1209

Qualities of Community Health Nurse 1209
*Job Description of Community
  Health Personnel* 1209
Job Responsibilities of Computer Assistant 1226
Activities of Health Guide 1226
Activities of Dai 1228
Activities of Anganwadi Worker 1228
*Job Descriptions of Public Health
  Nurse (District)* 1229

80. Treatment of Minor Ailments 1231

Common Ailments 1231

81. Empowering People to Care for Themselves 1242

Empowering Families 1242
*Client Empowerment and
  Health Education* 1242

82. Monitoring Growth and Development 1245

Growth and Development 1245
Taking Anthropometric Measurements 1249
Social Development 1250
*Taking Temperature, Pulse
  and Respiration* 1257
Teaching Breast Self-examination 1262
Teaching Testicular Self-examination 1264
Blood Pressure Measurement 1269

SECTION 14: HEALTH AND SOCIAL ISSUES

83. Social Issues Affecting Health   1273

Women Empowerment 1273
Women and Child Abuse 1275
Abuse of Elders 1284
Female Feticide 1291
Commercial Sex Workers 1293
Food Adulteration 1296
Substance Abuse 1297

SECTION 15: NATIONAL HEALTH PROGRAMS

84. National Health Programs   1303

National Acute Respiratory Infections Control Program 1303
Revised National Tuberculosis Control Program 1305
National Antimalarial Program 1308
Urban Malaria Scheme 1311
National Filaria Control Program 1313
National Kala-azar Control Program 1314
National Japanese Encephalitis Control Program 1315
National Dengue Fever/Dengue Hemorrhagic Fever Control Program 1315
Chikungunya Fever 1316
National Vector Borne Disease Control Program 1316
National Guinea Worm Eradication Program 1319
National Leprosy Eradication Program 1320
National AIDs Control Program 1324
National Iodine Deficiency Disorders Control Program 1328
National Program for the Control of Blindness 1329
Universal Immunization Program 1332
National Poliomyelitis Eradication Program 1344
National Diarrheal Diseases Control Program 1347
National Water Supply and Sanitation Program 1350
National Family Welfare Program 1351
New Focus of Family Welfare Program 1352
Reproductive and Child Health Program 1361
Janani Suraksha Yojana 1368
Vande Mataram Scheme 1369
Safe Abortion Services 1369
Village Health and Nutrition Day 1369
Maternal Death Review 1370
Pregnancy Tracking 1370
Janani Shishu Suraksha Karyakram 1370
Navjat Shishu Suraksha Karyakram 1373
Minimum Needs Program 1374
Twenty Point Program 1374
Integrated Child Development Services 1375
Nutrition Program 1376
National Cancer Control Program 1379
National Diabetes Control Program 1379
National Program on Prevention and Control for Diabetes, Cardiovascular Diseases and Stroke 1380
Yaws Eradication Program 1383
National Mental Health Program 1383
National Program for Control and Treatment of Occupational Disease 1385
Health Insurance 1386
National Rural Health Mission 1392

SECTION 16: HEALTH AGENCIES

85. Health Agencies   1399

International Health Agencies 1399
Objectives of WHO 1399
National Health Agencies 1413

APPENDICES

Appendix I: Objectives and Activities of Rural-Urban Field Experience for Students 1425
Appendix II: Guidelines for Students to Write Report of the Community Field Experience 1425
Appendix III: Guidelines for Students to Assess PHC Activities 1426
Appendix IV: Criteria for the Evaluation of Nursing Student's Performance in the Field 1428
Appendix V: Important Definitions Used in Community Health Nursing 1429
Appendix VI: Maternal and Child Health Calculations and Estimation 1431
Appendix VII: Terms Used in Community Health Nursing 1432

Index   Ii-Ixii

Abbreviations

ABER	Annual blood examination rate	CDSCO	Central Drugs Standard Control Organization
ACD	Active case detection		
ACT	Artemisinin-based combined therapy	CGHS	Central government health services
ADB	Asian Development Bank	CHC	Community health center
ADLA	Acute dermatolymphangioadenitis	CHW	Community health worker
AEFI	Adverse event following immunization	CMO	Chief Medical Officer
AES	Acute encephalitis syndrome	CNS	Central nervous system
AFB	Acid-fast bacilli	COPD	Chronic obstructive pulmonary disease
AFP	Acute flaccid paralysis	CPCB	Central Pollution Control Board
AIDS	Acquired immunodeficiency syndrome	CPM	Critical path method
AIMS	All India Institute of Medical Sciences	CPR	Couple protection rate
ALRI	Acute lower respiratory tract infection	CRY	Child Rights and You
ANC	Antenatal care	CSF	Cerebrospinal fluid
ANCDR	Annual new case detection rate	CSSM	Child survival and safe motherhood
ANM	Auxiliary Nurse Midwife	CVD	Cardiovascular disease
API	Annual parasite incidence	DALY	Disability-adjusted life year
AR	Attributable risk	DANIDA	Danish International Development Agency
ARC	AIDS-related complex		
ARI	Acute respiratory infection	DBCS	District Blindness Control Society
ART	Antiretroviral therapy	DDC	Drug distribution center
ART	Antiretroviral treatment	DEC	Diethylcarbamazine
ASFR	Age-specific fertility rate	DES	Diethylstilboestrol
ASHA	Accredited Social Health Activist	DFWO	District Family Welfare Officer
ASMFR	Age-specific marital fertility rate	DGHS	Director General of Health Services
AURI	Acute upper respiratory tract infection	DHF	Dengue hemorrhagic fever
AUWSP	Accelerated Urban Water Supply Program	DHO/DMO	District Health Officer/District Medical Officer
AWC	Anganwadi center	DHS	Directorate of Health Services
AWW	Anganwadi worker	DM	Diabetes mellitus
AYUSH	Ayurveda, Unani, Siddha and Homeopathy system of medicine	DMC	Designated microscopy center
		DOTS	Directly observed therapy short course
B cells	Bone marrow-derived lymphocytes	DPT	Diphtheria, pertussis and tetanus vaccine
BCC	Behavior change communication	DSS	Dengue shock syndrome
BCG	Bacillus Calmette-Guérin	DT	Diphtheria-tetanus toxoid
BDO	Block Development Officer	DTa	Diphtheria-tetanus adult type
BEE	Block Extension Educator	DTC	District tuberculosis center
BEO	Block Extension Officer	DTP	District Tuberculosis Program
BFHI	Baby-friendly hospital initiatives	DTPa	Diphtheria, tetanus, acellular pertussis
BLAC	Block Leprosy Awareness Campaign	DTPw	Diphtheria, tetanus, whole-cell pertussis
BMI	Body mass index		
BPL	Below poverty line	%E	Percentage of total energy
CABG	Coronary artery bypass grafting	EAA	Essential amino acids
CARE	Cooperative assistance and relief everywhere	EAG	Empowered action group
		EFA	Essential fatty acids
CBR	Crude birth rate	EMCP	Enhanced Malaria Control Project
CDPO	Child Development Project Officer	EPI	Expanded program on immunization

EQA	External quality assessment	IPHS	Indian Public Health Standards
ESI scheme	Employees state insurance scheme	IPPI	Intensified pulse polio immunization
ETEC	Enterotoxin *Escherichia coli*	IPV	Inactivated polio vaccine
FAO	Food and Agriculture Organization	IRC	International Red Cross
F-IMNCI	Facility-based IMNCI	IRLs	Intermediate reference laboratories
FLEP	Focused Leprosy Elimination Plan	IRS	Indoor residual spray
FRUs	First referral units	ISM	Indian system of medicine
FSW	Female sex worker	ITN	Insecticide-treated bed nets
FTD	Fever treatment depot	IUCD	Intrauterine contraceptive device
GDP	Gross domestic product	IUD	Intrauterine device
GFR	General fertility rate	JE	Japanese encephalitis
GMFR	General marital fertility rate	JSSK	Janani Shishu Suraksha Karyakram
GNL	Gross national income	JSY	Janani Suraksha Yojana
GNP	Gross national product	KFD	Kyasanur forest disease
HAV	Hepatitis A virus	LBW	Low birth weight
HBIG	Hepatitis B immunoglobulin	LDL	Low-density lipoproteins
HBNC	Home-based newborn care	LECs	Leprosy Elimination Campaigns
HBV	Hepatitis B virus	LEM	Leprosy elimination monitoring
HCV	Hepatitis C virus	LHVs	Lady health visitors
HDL	High-density lipoproteins	LLIN	Long-lasting insecticidal nets
HDV	Hepatitis D virus	LPS	Low performing states
HEV	Hepatitis E virus	LSD	Lysergic acid diethylamide
HFA	Health for all	MAP	Malaria action plan
Hib vaccine	*Haemophilus influenzae* type B vaccine	MCH	Maternal and child health
HIV	Human immunodeficiency virus	MDA	Mass drug administration
HPS	High performing states	MDGs	Millennium development goals
HPV	Human papillomavirus	MDMP	Mid-day Meal Program
HRD	Human resource development	MDR-TB	Multidrug-resistant tuberculosis
HW (F)	Health worker (female)	MDT	Mulidrugs therapy
HW (M)	Health worker (male)	Mf	Microfilaria
ICDS	Integrated child development service	MLEC	Modified leprosy elimination campaign
ICMR	Indian Council of Medical Research	MMr	Maternal mortality ratio
ICTC	Integrated Counseling and Testing Center	MNP	Minimum need program
IDD	Iodine deficiency disorder	MO	Medical Officer
IDDM	Insulin-dependent diabetes mellitus	MOPHC	Medical Officer of Primary Health Center
IDSP	Integrated Disease Surveillance Program	MOU	Memorandum of understanding
IDUS	Intravenous drug users	MPO	Modified plan of operation
IEC	Information, education and communication	MPW	Multipurpose worker
IFA	Iron and folic acid	MRFIT	Multiple risk factor intervention trial
IHD	Ischemic heart disease	MSM	Men having sex with men
IHR	International Health Regulations	MTCT	Mother-to-child transmission
ILO	International Labor Organization	MTP	Medical termination of pregnancy
IMCI	Integrated management of childhood illness	MUFA	Monounsaturated fatty acids
		MVA	Manual vacuum aspiration
IMR	Infant mortality rate	NACO	National AIDS Control Organization
INH	Isoniazid	NAMP	National Antimalaria Program
IMNCI	Integrated management of neonatal and childhood infections	NBCC	Newborn care corner
		NBSU	Newborn stabilization unit
IOL	Intraocular lens	NCCP	National Cancer Control Program
		NCD	Non-communicable disease

Abbreviations

NCDs	Non-communicable diseases	PTCA	Percutaneous transluminal coronary angiography
NFHS	National Family Health Survey		
NGO	Non-government organization	PTCT	Parent-to-child transmission
NHP	National Health Policy	PUFA	Polyunsaturated fatty acids
NID	National immunization day	PWB	Patient-wise boxes
NIMH	National Institute for Mentally Handicapped	RBM	Roll back malaria
		RCA	Research-cum-action projects
NLCP	National Leprosy Control Program	RCH	Reproductive and child health
NLEP	National Leprosy Eradication Program	RCT	Randomized controlled trials
NMEP	National Malaria Eradication Program	RDT	Rapid diagnostic test
NMHP	National Mental Health Program	RF	Rheumatic fever
NNMR	Neonatal mortality rate	RHME	Representative, resampled, routine household interview of mortality with medical evaluation
NNR	Net reproduction rate		
NORAD	Norwegian Agency for Development Cooperation		
		RLF	Retrolental fibroplasia
NPAC	National Plan of Action for Children	RMP	Rifampicin
NPSU	National Polio Surveillance Unit	RNTCP	Revised National Tuberculosis Control Program
NPU	Net protein utilization		
NRCS	Nutritional rehabilitation centers	RR	Relative risk
NRHM	National Rural Health Mission	RTI	Reproductive tract infection
NSI	Nutrition Society of India	SAARC	South Asian Association for Regional Cooperation
NTCP	National Tuberculosis Control Program		
NVBDCP	National Vector Borne Disease Control Program	SACS	State AIDS Control Society
		SAPEL	Special Action Project for Elimination of Leprosy
OPV	Oral polio vaccine		
ORS	Oral rehydration salts	SAR	Secondary attack rate
ORT	Oral rehydration therapy	SARS	Severe acute respiratory syndrome
PCD	Passive case detection	SC	Subcenter
PCV7	Pneumococcal conjugate vaccine	SEAR	South-East Asian Region
PEM	Protein-energy malnutrition	SEARO	South-East Asian Regional Office
PERT	Program evaluation and review technique	SFD	Small-for-date baby
		SIA	Supplemental immunization activities
PFA	Prevention of Food Adulteration Act	SIDA	Swedish International Development Agency
PHAs	Polynuclear aromatic hydrocarbons		
PHC	Primary health care/center	SMR	Standard mortality ratio
PHFI	Public Health Foundation of India	SNCU	Special newborn care unit
PHI	Peripheral health institutions	SNID	Sub-national immunization day
PLHA	People living with HIV/AIDS	SRS	Sample registration system
PMDT	Programmatic management of drug-resistant TB	STDs	Sexually transmitted diseases
		STIs	Sexually transmitted infections
PNDT	Prenatal Diagnostic Technique Act	TB	Tuberculosis
PPBS	Planning programming budgeting system	TBA	Trained birth attendant
PPD	Purified protein derivative	TFR	Total fertility rate
PPP	Purchasing power parity	TG	Triglycerides
PPSV23	Pneumococcal polysaccharide vaccine containing 23 serotypes	T cells	Thymus-derived lymphocytes
		TMFR	Total marital fertility rate
PPTCT	Prevention of parent-to-child transmission	TORCH agents	*Toxoplasma gondii*, rubella virus, cytomegalovirus and herpesvirus
PRAI	Planning, Research and Action Institute	TT	Tetanus toxoid
PTB	Pulmonary tuberculosis	TU	Tuberculosis unit

UCI	Universal child immunization	VDPV	Vaccine-derived poliovirus
UHC	Urban health center	VHAI	Voluntary Health Association of India
UIP	Universal Immunization Program	VLDL	Very low-density lipoproteins
UN	United Nations	VPD	Vaccine preventable disease
UNDP	United Nations Development Program	VVM	Vaccine vial monitor
UNESCO	United Nations Educational, Scientific and Cultural Organization	WB	World Bank
		WHO	World Health Organization
UNFPA	United Nations Population Fund	WPV1	Wild poliovirus type 1
UNICEF	United Nations Children's Fund	WPV2	Wild poliovirus type 2
USAID	United States Agency for International Development	WPV3	Wild poliovirus type 3
		WTO	World Trade Organization
UT	Union Territory	XDR-TB	Extensively drug-resistant tuberculosis
VCTC	Voluntary counseling and testing center	ZDV	Zidovudine

SECTION 1

Concepts of Community, Health and Nursing

- Concepts of Community
- Concepts and Dimensions of Health
- Concepts of Nursing
- Promotion of Health
- Maintenance of Health

Concepts of Community

CHAPTER 1

INTRODUCTION

The community has been described as one of the most fruitful areas of improving the health of the people. It is a fact that social, physical and cultural aspects of the community have a major influence on an individual's health status. The social environment is important since social problems and social supports are directly related to physical and mental illness. Similarly, physical environment is important since physical problems such as air, water and soil pollution lead to various diseases in human beings. Likewise, the cultural environment, which includes food patterns and lifestyles also has major implications for health. Nurses and all health professionals must actively consider the influence of the community on the health status of the patient. More importantly, nurses need to become involved in influencing the structure and functioning of systems within the community. A focus on preserving and promoting health and preventing illness for all people in the community will not only have an impact on the health of the identified client but also will reach the lives of numerous people, who are not in the healthcare system. So, it is important to review the community once again to get acquainted with its concepts.

MEANING OF COMMUNITY

The word 'community' is used in a variety of contexts and by the people with different perspectives. The term 'community' suggests a shared pattern of feelings, behaviors and lifestyles together with close, and frequent personal relationship with others. —*Little Wood, 1985*

The knowledge, values, beliefs and behaviors of given groups have a major implication for well-being, morbidity and mortality.

Man has lived in communities since the dawn of human histories. In fact, grouping very similar to human communities exist among animals and even among plants. The term 'community' has been used very loosely, but experts have sought to give it a more exact connotation. They agree concerning some of its basic things, which the term should denote.

The word 'community' has been derived from two Latin words namely, 'com' and 'munis'. In English 'com' means together and 'munis' means to serve. Thus, community means to 'serve together'. It means 'community' is an organization of human beings framed for the purposes of serving together. A community is a collection of interdependent people with residential ties to a particular locality. The territorial boundaries differentiate it from other groups, because most of the other groups are not tied to specific localities.

Communities are spatially specific, but otherwise are unrestricted. They are unlike groups and organizations that have special interests and touch only a narrow part of their participants' level. Communities encompass major portions of the lives and roles of their members. The term 'community' denotes almost uniformly and permanently shared lives of people over a definite region. It may be considered as a permanent local aggregation of people having diversified as well as common interests and served by a constellation of institutions.

DEFINITIONS OF COMMUNITY

The term 'community' has been defined in various ways. Some of the definitions are as follows:

1. "Community is a group of people who live together, who belong together, so that they share, not ties or that particular interest, but as a whole set of interests, wide enough and complete enough to include their lives. He included in 'community' small aggregations such as villages and large ones such as cities, and tribes and nations." —*MacIver*

2. "Community is the smallest territorial group that can embrace all aspects of social life." —*Kingsley Davis*
3. "Community is a local area over which people are using the same language, conforming to the same norms, feeling more or less the same sentiments and acting upon the same attitudes."
   —*Robert E Park and Ernest W Burgess*
4. "A society that inhabit is a definite geographical area is known as community." —*Manzer MC*
5. "By community, I mean a complex of social life; a complex including a number of human beings living together under conditions of social relationship bound together by a common behavior, changing stock of conventions, customs and traditions, and conscious to some extent of common social objects and interests."
   —*Childe CF*
6. "A community may be defined as a permanent local aggregation of people having diversified as well as common interests and served by a constellation of institutions." —*Lumbi*
7. "A community is a unit of territory within which is distributed a population, which possessed the basic institutions in their simple and more specialized from by means of which a common life is made possible."
   —*Dawson and Gettys*
8. "Community is a living population within a limited geographical area carrying on a common interest."
   —*Lundberg*
9. "A community is an organic, natural kind of social group whose members are bound together by a sense of belonging, created out of everyday contacts covering the whole orange of human activities."
   —*Ferdinand Tonnies*
10. "A community may be defined as a group of collection of groups that inhabit a delimited geographical area and whose members live together in such a way that they share the basic conditions of common life."
    —*Talcott Parsons*

The definitions quoted above, emphasize the structural and sociological aspects of the community. But it is not less important to note that community is a separated part of society viewed in its ecologically permanent state wherein the impulses, precisely spoken of as community sentiments play their diverse, but at the same time unifying role.

The mark of a community is that one's life may be lived wholly within it. One cannot live wholly within a tribe or a city. The basic criterion of community then is that all of one's social relationships may be found within it.

Sutherland defines 'community' as a local area over which people using the same language, conforming to the same feelings, more or less the same sentiments and acting upon the same attitudes. This means community is a social group of any size whose members resides in a specific locality, share a government and have a common cultural and historical heritage.

Community in Sander's View

Sanders viewed community in three ways—as a place, as a social system and as a collection of people:
1. It is a place, where the environment, housing, transportation, etc. are all related to geographical locations, as are population composition and distribution, health services, resources and facilities.
2. It is a social system, because community is a combination of all the social units and systems, which have been developed to carry out its major functions with its patterns of interactions.
3. It is a collection of people, where the health workers will find both individuals who are well (healthy) and who are ill (unhealthy). The statistical data of the people will help the health authorities to plan and implement health schemes to attain health of its citizens.

Definition of Community by WHO

World Health Organization (WHO) defines 'community' as a social group determined by geographical boundaries and/or common values and interests. Its members know and interact with each other. It functions within a particular social structure and exhibits, and creates certain norms, values and social institutions.

A community may be defined, as "group of inhabitants living together in a somewhat localized area under the same general regulations and having common interests, functions, needs and organization." It goes beyond city, village and people defined by relationships between people as well as physical contours. Now, the community is seen as a social unit, wherein finds transactions of a common life among people who compose the unit. According to above definition, the whole country may be viewed as 'community'.

FUNCTIONS OF COMMUNITY

The basic functions of the community might be summarized in the following order:
- To determine the use of space for living and other purposes
- To make available that means of production and distribution of necessary goods and services
- To protect and conserve the health, life, resources and property of individuals
- To educate and acculturate newcomers, i.e. children and immigrants
- To transmit information, ideas and beliefs
- To provide opportunities for interaction between individuals and groups.

The community is basically the medium for the development of its inhabitants. It provides the means whereby the society imposes its expectations on people. The environment of the home or neighborhood is influenced by the character of the community and in turn, influences the community. Ultimately, a community is judged by the kind of people it produces. Whether it expands, grows or dries up and wither away will be determined by many factors.

The shifting of nursing focus from the individual to the community requires some different perspectives and different skills. The view of the community as an aggregate implies the need for skills in assessment of structural characteristics and functioning of the system. It requires identification of strengths, problems and high-risk populations. It requires a scientific base of knowledge and program planning skills in order to set goals and priorities, while collaborating with community members. The aggregate focus also involves implementation strategies at the individual group and environmental level. This approach enhances the likelihood of the nursing role and activities will be based on population needs and will be implemented on a rational basis and evaluated in the light of community's functioning and the health outcomes and the population.

CHARACTERISTICS OF COMMUNITY

In the past, communities used to be self-sufficient, because then the people lived a very simple life and many complications had till then not arisen. But today, character of the community is very complex and politically, socially or economically, no community can be self-sufficient in any way. Therefore, one character of a community is that it cannot be self-sufficient these days. MacIver has said, "No civilized community has walls around it to cut it off completely from a larger one, whatever 'iron curtains' may be drawn by the rulers of the nation or that communities exist within the greater communities, the town within a region, the region within a nation and nation within the world community, which perhaps, is in the process of development". The basic characteristics of a community are given as follows.

Territorial Character

A community is always considered in relation to a physical environment of a territory. As MacIver and Page have stated, "The community possesses a distinctively territorial character. This characteristics is most marked in the case of primitive communities, which consisted of small clearly defined group of individuals relatively dependent of the other communities for the goods required by the prevailing standards of life and also territorial distinction of such communities was very marked". Even in this era of rapid migration, locality as a factor in the settlement of a community still holds its importance. The habitation of human beings in cities and villages, the relatively thin and dense distribution of population over geographical regions, and the characteristics modes of their life in their respective settlements strike to use when we think of a community.

Home Instinct of Special Attachment

Home instinct is very powerful instinct and in a sense it lays the foundation of our attachment to a particular house, community or nation itself. Whenever people live together for some time, uniformity in the modes of their lives take place by their daily interaction. These intercourses bring into play those social impulses, which manifest themselves and get in course of time related to the community environment and then determine its external structure.

Common Life

Common life has been maintained that the life of the people in a community is near about the same. There is no epochal difference between the ways of life of the individuals. Due to their inhabitation on a particular geographical area, they develop a kind of emotional and cultural uniformity. This is also because of the fact that community is never formed with a particular aim, but they are the outcome of the social uniformity among the individuals. If they are formed with any particular aim they would cease being a community and will be known as association.

Community Feeling

The external structure of a community is mainly the expression of social impulse, which are particularly locality sets into play. Thus, the psychological feelings of a community are more important than they appear. The life of a man is mostly lived in a community, though it may not be a self-sufficient whole. "Whenever human beings are thrown together, separated in whole or in part from the world outside, so that they must live their lives in one another's company; the effects of these social impulses, which bring men into communities. In other words, the formation of 'community sentiment'. This separation of group of people or a whole, lot of them may not be only physical factors. Psychological factors such as identical hopes, aspirations and destinies may also become important demarking factors.

Community sentiment is developed by the socialization process itself, by education in the largest sense, working, through prescription and authority, social esteem or disfavor, until habits, and conformities become the ground of loyalties and convictions. For the individual, when once his/her early training period is passed, community sentiment is not an outer compulsion, but an inner necessity always a part of his/her own individual. Even when he/she revolts against some of its code, as he/she often does, in fact, he/she still belongs in feeling to some community. He/She cannot escape the impact of a socializing experience found wherever man has built a common life.

The psychological sentiment of a community is a complex of various attitudes and emotions of this complex of community sentiment is formulated, and developed by the process of socialization and as though at first acts by ways of compulsion, by when the initial period of an individual is over, the community feelings become a part of his/her integrated personality and community sentiments become a part of his/her emotional build up.

Feeling of Oneness

The collective participation in the affair and prevalent mode of life in the community grows a sense of mutual identification of the hopes and aspirations of his/her members. This gives rise to a feeling of oneness within a particular community, which may be expressed as 'we-feeling.' This 'we-feeling' is the foundation upon which the upper super structure of the whole community sentiment is build up.

Role Feeling

One dominant characteristic of human nature is the sense of satisfaction in life. People want to play a definite role in the reciprocal exchange of the community. Generally, this process of role finding involves a subordination of our personal interests and aims, if not completely, to those of the community as a whole. This factor helps the functional harmony of the community and at the same time weaves the personality of the members into a mutually balancing system.

Dependency Feeling

Human beings feel a sense of dependency right from their birth. The dependency feeling involves both a physical dependency and psychological dependency for his/her material needs as well as emotional needs.

Spontaneous Growth

No community ever comes into existence with the making by a certain group or some committee, but every community grows itself spontaneously. A kind of natural automatic force acts behind the origin and development of communities. Various factors such as customs, conventions and religious beliefs bind the individuals together.

Permanence

Communities are never formed with any particular aim and object as associations are formed. Associations vanquish after achieving the object, but community still prevails. It is durable, because it has developed itself. The proof of this assertion lies in the existence of age-old communities in the modern era.

Particular Name

Society is nameless, but not the community, because community is the group of people living at some particular place with common culture. Community is always known with a particular name, their immediate bases of origin give such a community with particular name.

Wider Ends

In communities the people associate not for the fulfillment of a particular end. The ends of a community are wider, these are natural and not artificial.

No Legal Status

A community is not a legal body. It cannot sue, nor can it be sued. In the eyes of law, it has no rights and duties.

DIMENSION OF COMMUNITY

Community may be geographically or socially found, categorized as emotional, structural or functional or defined in terms of relational and territorial bonds. The operational definition of community considering the following three factors (Fig. 1.1):
1. 'Who', includes people factors.
2. 'Where and when', such as space and time factors.
3. 'Why and how', specifies for what purpose.

Thus, a community is a group of people with a common identity or perspective, occupying space during a given period of time and functioning through a social system to meet the needs within a larger social environment.

It is useful to envision the community as the 'what?' And then to consider the dimension of 'who?', 'where and when?' And 'why and how?'. This simple, straight forward approach emphasizes the interdependence of the three major dimensions. It has been believed that an adequate definition should take into account the following factors. The perspective of the individual, the system of people, organizations, agencies and institution, and the temporal spatial aspect. Thus, a community is 'people and the relationship that energic among them as they develop and use in common some agencies and institution, and a physical environment'.

The 'dimension of whom or the people factors' is the heart of the operational definition. The community health nurse can collect information about the socioeconomic and demographic variable that fall under this rubric. Data are available about the risk factors shared by the aggregates, as they are about ethnocultural characteristics, values and ideals. Commonly used labels such as special interest groups [best is scheduled caste (SC), scheduled tribe (ST), vulnerable] face-to-face communities and ethnocultural groups, refer primarily to the 'who' dimension.

The 'people factors' coexists within a time-space framework or the where and when dimension of the definition. As such, population characteristics are influenced by the passage of time and by the space within which they exist. The community health nurse can identity geopolitical boundaries.

Function as a Dimension of Community

The why and how dimension 'addresses the function of the community'. Warren (1987) defines community as 'a complex, interrelated structure of interaction patterns on the basis of which certain relevant function are performed'. The function of the community as described by Warren are:
- Production—distribution—consumption
- Socialization
- Social control
- Social participation
- Mutual support.

The 'why and how dimension' accounts for the network of associations and the dynamic interplay of such forces as communications, power and authority.

Production, distribution, consumption of goods and services: It provides for the economic needs of the members of the community. It includes not only the supplying of food and clothing but also the provision of water, electricity, police and fire protection and the disposal of refuse. In this function, a community is usually interdependent with other communities and with business and organizations outside its boundaries.

Socialization: It is the process of transmitting values, knowledge, culture and skills to others. Communities usually contain a number of established institutions for socialization—families, temples, churches, mosques, schools, media, voluntary and social organizations, and so on.

Social interparticipation or community participation: It refers to community activities that are designed to meet people's need for companionship. Families and temples have traditionally met this need; however, many public and private organizations also serve this function.

Mutual support: It refers to community ability to provide resources at a time of illness or disaster. Although the family is usually relied on to fulfil this function, health and social services may be necessary to augment the family's assistance, if help is required over an extended period.

When the nurses are identifying the problems in the community, each of the dimensions of the operational

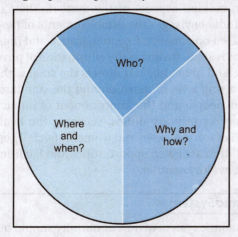

Figure 1.1: Interdependent of dimensions of community

definitions—who, where, when, why, how—carefully explicated contains variables for which data can be collected and analyzed. An operational definition of community is also important in planning health promotion programs for high-risk groups. In such programs, the high-risk groups are visualized as the community. So, a community can refer to the context or arena in which change operates or social factors viewed as less than desirable. A community, therefore, becomes the target for help. In the other hand, since a community contains some of the requisite elements for modifying present conditions, it can be seen as a vehicle for change.

A community health nurse need to know about a community of importance is the composition, character, role and capabilities of population group and agencies that exist in the community. The community health nurse needs to have a development perspective on the community—the trends, patterns of change and a problem orientation in which the needs, and demands of groups are viewed against the real and potential resources available to address the needs and demand.

HEALTH AND THE COMMUNITY SYSTEMS

Health is human's greatest possession, for it lays a solid foundation for his/her happiness. Good health is very essential to economic and technological development. A healthy community is the infrastructure upon which is built an economically viable society. Good health is a prerequisite to human productivity and development.

The community itself is composed of a number of subsystems such as a living organism. It has a shape and form of a skeleton, so as to speak of streets, city limits/village limits, blocks, buildings. Also, community has a life that of its people circulating in, through and around those features, which constitute is skeleton. As stated earlier, the community is a social system with its own pattern of interaction and results from the interrelationships of many systems within the community. In the community, the individuals with certain status, role and position, function together in an attempt to achieve certain goals of the system. Communication and information processing, boundary maintenance, and linkage with other systems are components that fit well with the system as whole. The subsystem of the community will include sociocultural system, the political system, economical system, educational system, recreational system, environmental system and healthcare delivery systems, but equally important to assess the operations of the other subsystems in the community. It is better to examine the concept of subsystem of the community in brief and their influence on community health.

Sociocultural System

The sociocultural system incorporates the traditions, value, norms and sanctions that are accepted and reinforced by the people. The sociocultural system influence the lifestyles and priorities placed on various elements of life. The prevailing attitudes and values about health and illness, and about traditional medicines are directly associated with the community's health. Some cultural factors promote the acceptance of certain illness, for example, due to bad deeds in life, a person gets disease, e.g. leprosy. Some cultural factors promote the acceptance of certain risk factors, for example, due to some traditions, the pregnant woman may face some high risks in antenatal period. Some cultural groups tend to have an over dependence on health personnel. For simple ailments they approach the doctors and specialists. Some of them tend to show mistrust and suspicion toward health personnel regarding getting tablets, injections, etc. They feel drugs might kill them, doctor might give them wrong medication, etc. In some cultures there is a lack of understanding regarding personal cleanliness and other healthy habits, which leads to many health hazards within them.

Political System

The democratic form of government provides for the expression of various groups within the community. There is a great need for a strong political will at all levels for promotion of health and health development must be considered as a positive investment for socioeconomic development. The political system provides the framework for potential representation of interest groups with a mechanism for changing structure and influencing decisions in the community knowing the legislative and decision-making aspects of the system. The Constitution of India envisages the establishments of new social order based on equality, freedom, justice and the dignity of the individual. It aims at the elimination of poverty, ignorance and ill health, and directs the state with regard to the raising level of nutrition and the standard of living of its people and the improvement of public health as among its primary duties, securing the health and strength of workers, men and women, specially ensuring that children are given opportunities and facilities to develop in healthy manner.

Economic System

The economic system of the community should be sound to attain and maintain good health. The people of the community should produce suitable food grains, cash crops and other goods and services. Health of the community sometimes depend upon the economic system of the country. India has a large dependency ratio about 39% of the population are in the age group of below 15 years and only 38% of the population constitute the working force. Barely 14.41% of the working population comprises of female workers. Being predominantly an agriculture country, about 51% of the employment generated is from the agricultural sector. The per capita availability of food grains is 178 kg per annum. Using a caloric consumption as a criterion, it is estimated that about 37% of the population lives below poverty line. Certain disadvantage groups in the society such as the SC and ST continue to suffer from social disabilities and poor economic status. Therefore, because of low-economic status, malnutrition and other related ill-health conditions are is still prevailing in our country.

Educational System

Educational system provides several important functions in the community including the learning and preparations of adult roles. Education is the main tool for changing or modifying the health practice in improved form in the community. In India, the literacy rate is still very low only—63.8% of males and 39.4% of the females are literate. In rural areas, female literacy rate is still lower. This coupled with highly dependent status of the woman, acts as barrier to communication and destroy their initiative, and enthusiasm for any social change. People in general, particularly in rural areas and urban slums are not knowledgeable about health matters such as, what are the prevailing health problems in the community? And how to prevent and control these? What are the needs for maintenance and promotion of health? What are the resources available? And how and when to utilize these?, etc. Socioeconomics backwardness, ignorance, traditions and superstitions due to low-educational status of the people of the community, blocking the progressive thinking, development and the concept of positive health. As per 2001 census, total literacy rate 65.4%, 75.9% in males, 54.2% in females.

Religious System

The religious system in any community may be homogeneous or heterogeneous. The practices in some religious bodies such as stream rituals may expose individuals to certain water-borne disease. Nutritional pattern leads to conditions of malnutritious and related hazards, e.g. in some cultures nutritious food is restricted to pregnant woman. This leads to nutritional anemia. Practice of eating raw mutton or raw pork increases the risk of acquiring trichinosis.

The religious system may also be a source of health promotion, the beliefs and values of some religious bodies emphasizes techniques and practices related to smoking, dietary intake, use of alcohol and prohibition of extramarital relations, etc. This type of active participation of religious bodies in the values and attitudes influence the lifestyles and health activities.

Environmental System

Environmental system is one of the intersecting system in the community. When environmental conditions are not suitable to community, air and water pollution may arise in it and the pollutants affect the food one eats, the air one breaths and the water one drinks. The control of the environment is thought to be a major avenue for protecting the health of the entire population, otherwise many health hazards will emerge in the human environment. In India only 31% of rural population has access to portable water supply and 0.5% enjoys basic sanitation. Our country has 80% of villages and some percentage of urban slums among 20% of urban area. In urban slum, majority have only one living room in which kitchen is attached. In rural areas most the houses were attached to cattle sheds, using firewood and cow dung as fuel. There are no proper ventilation, lighting and drainage systems.

Environmental pollution leads to various diseases. The woman who are exposed to fumes of firewood and dried cow dung and also kerosene are often attacked by pulmonary artery diseases. Non-availability of safe drinking water and improper disposal of human excreta leads to so many water-borne diseases.

Communication and Transport System

Transport system is needed for people to move from place of residence to other places such as shopping, school, work place, etc. So, there should be good roads and related facilities such as vehicle and other means of transportation. Language plays a very important role in the communication of ideas from person to person and also helps in spreading the health messages to the community. Thus, the transport and communication helps in organizing information, communication and education activities for motivating people for adopting positive health practices and small family norms.

Healthcare delivery system exists to provide services and resources for better health. This system includes hospitals, clinics, health centers, nursing homes and special health programs in schools, industries and community. The location, utilization, staffing and the facilities provided in the health centers are important to note, while taking care of the community as a whole in relation to health matters. The healthcare system is enhanced through linkages that bring together various subsystems to provide an array of resources, technologies and skills. Cost of services, duplication of services, gaps in services, continuity and comprehensiveness are results of incomplete linkages. So, strengthening of multisectoral approach should be maintained in the community to achieve health for all.

CONCLUSION

Community refers to a collection of people who can share some attribution to their lives. Community healthcare system those provides health-related services within the contest of people's daily lives, i.e. in places where people spend their time in the community.

Concepts and Dimensions of Health

CHAPTER 2

INTRODUCTION

Nursing in the minds of many people is associated with medicine and hospitals, because most nurses work for hospitals caring sick people. The major purpose of the hospital is to support the medical regimen in treating disease and dysfunction. The public image of what nursing is and what nurses do has been influenced by medical definition of health as a 'absence of disease'. The association of nursing with disease and sickness is at the heart of traditional characterization of the nurse as the physician handmaiden care of the disease is the major purpose of medicine, but healthcare delivery aimed predominantly at cure of disease is wasteful of resources and very costly. Increasingly, the public is becoming aware of the need to prevent illness and promote well-being. Both laypersons and health professionals often define good health as the absence of the clinical signs of disease.

EXPERT VIEWS ON HEALTH

Good health is prerequisite of human productivity and the development process. It is essential to economic and technological development. Health has been viewed by different experts according to their own field of interest. Broadly, these views are discussed below:

1. Biomedical scientist stress on the germ theory, i.e. disease organisms. The individual was considered to be healthy only, if person was free from diseases. This concept has been rejected by other scientists because it will not help to solve some of the major health problems, which were primarily not due to disease-causing organisms such as malnutrition, chronic diseases, accidents, drug abuse, mental illness, environmental pollution, population explosion, etc.
2. Ecologists views health as a harmonious equilibrium between man and environmental, and disease as a maladjustment of the human organisms to the environment. This environment includes air, water and other necessary things needed by human beings for their life. Environmental pollution leads to health problems.
3. Sociologists visualize health not only as a biomedical phenomenon, but also that it is influenced by various factors such as social, psychological, cultural, economical and political. These factors are essential in defining and measuring health. All these factors help to determine and maintain health status of the population.
4. Holistic view is a synthesis of the views of the above experts. According to this concept of health is viewed as a multidimensional process involving the well-being of the whole person in the context of the environment.
5. Health is essential for leading a socioeconomically productive life. The provision of health should be considered a fundamental human right.

DEFINITIONS OF HEALTH

Health is a state of well-being of individual and community. So, it can be examined at individual or community level. For individual the term 'health' refers to the optimal functioning of the individual, absence of disease, illness, impairment or injury. In the context of the community it refers to various objective measures of health, health status or health indices such as incidence of and prevalence of disease applied to different segments of population. Defining good health is difficult because each person has personal concept of health.

The definition of health range on a continuum from the absence of diseases of the optimal functioning to utopian ideals of complete state of physical, mental, emotional, spiritual and social well-being.

About 500 BC, Pericles defined health as "This state of moral, mental and physical well-being, which enables a person to face any crisis in life with the utmost grace (of God) and facility."

Hayman HS defines health as "A state of feeling sound in body, mind and spirit, with a sense of reserve power". This perception, if health is based on normal functioning of the body's physiological process, understanding the principles of healthful living and attitude that regards health not only as a means of survival, and self-fulfillment in itself, but as means of to a creative social adjustment and a richer, fuller life as measured in constructive service to mankind.

Blum H defines health as "The person's capacity to function in a way to maximize potential, to maintain a balance appropriate to age and social needs, to be reasonably free of gross dissatisfaction, discomfort, disease or disability, and to behave in ways that promote survival as well as self-fulfillment or enjoyment."

1. Health is the condition of being sound in body, mind or spirit especially freedom from physical disease or pain. —*Webber*
2. Health refers to a 'soundness of body or mind' that condition in which its functions are duly and efficiently discharged. —*Oxford English Dictionary*
3. Health is a condition or quality of the human organisms expressing the adequate functioning of the organisms in the given, genetic and environmental conditions.
4. Health is a modus vivendi enabling imperfect men to achieve a rewarding and not too painful existence, while they cope with an imperfect world.

Dubois R views 'Health' as adaptation, a function of adjustment. He believes an (WHO's) utopian state of health can never be reached because the person can never be so perfectly adapted to the environment that life will not involve struggle, failure and suffering. Humans can adapt the environmental conditions or change the environment, but each new adaptation produces new problems that demand new solution.

"Health is the achievement of a state of harmony between man's internal and external milieu."
 —*Liverpool School of Tropical Medicine*

Rathbone EF formulate "Health as a wholeness of function, movement toward self-actualization, relating of experiences and coordination of attitudinal, physiological, and behavioral adaptations."

Imogene King defined 'Health' as a "dynamic state in the life cycle of an organism that implies continuous adaptation to stresses in the internal and external environment through optimum use of one's resources to achieve maximum potential for daily living."

According to Perkin S "Health is a state of relative equilibrium of body form and functions, which results from its successful, dynamic adjustment to forces tending to disturb it." It is not passive interplay between body substance and forces infringing upon it, but an active response of the body forces working toward adjustment.

Health is wellness of an individual. According to Dunn 'high-level wellness' implies well-being in degree or level. High-level wellness for the individual is defined as an integrated method of functioning, which is oriented towards maximizing the potential of which the individual maintains a continuous balance and purposeful direction within the environment whereby he/she is functioning.

Duhl equates the state of health within an individual and ability to control his/she environment, and defines health "as a state of competence of emotional, mental and physical strength enabling (a person) to set goals, investigate alternatives, make decisions and take actions to control environment."

Terris M, a famous epidemiologist believes the WHO definition should be reworded as "health is a state of physical, mental and social well-being and ability to function and not merely the absence of illness and excluding 'complete' as health is not an absolute. The addition of and ability to function is necessary, as a definition of health requires both objective and subjective components. The objective components being the 'ability to function', the subjective being feeling of well-being."

A singular definition and one, which returns more to Pericles version is that of the Liverpool School of Tropical Medicine, "health is the achievement of a state of harmony between man's internal and external milieu." However, WHO's definition has the following characteristics that promotes a more positive concepts of health:

1. A concern for the individual as a total system.
2. A view of health that identifies internal and external environment.
3. An acknowledgment of the importance of an individual's role in life.

Planning Commission of India states that "health is fundamental to the nation's progress in any sphere. In terms of resources for the development of economy, nothing can be considered of higher importance than health of the people, which is a measure of their energy and capacity as well as the potential man-hours for productive work in relation to the total number of persons maintained by the nation. For the efficiency of industry and agriculture, the health of the worker is an essential consideration."

CHAPTER 2 — Concepts and Dimensions of Health

And also defines health "as a positive state of well-being in which harmonious development of mental and physical capacities of the individual leads to the enjoyment of a rich and full life. It implies adjustment of the individual to his/her total environment—physical and social".

Seal SC defines health as "a flexible state of body and mind, which may be described in terms of range within which a person may sway from the condition wherein he/she is at the peak of enjoyment of physical, mental and emotional experience, having regard to environment, age, sex and other biological characteristics due to operations of internal and/or external stimuli and can regain without outside aid."

Health in its broadest sense is a dynamic state in which the individual adapts to change in internal and external environment includes many factors that influence health, including genetic and psychological variables, intellectual and spiritual dimensions, and disease processes. The external environment includes factors outside the person that may influence health including the physical environment, social relationships and economic variables. Because both environments continuously change, the person must adapt to maintain a state of well-being.

Bauer WW defines "health as a state of feeling well in body, mind and spirit together with a sense of reserve organs of the body on normal functioning of tissues and the physical and psychological environment, together with our attitude, which regards health is not an end in itself, but a means to a richer life as measured in constructive service of mankind. Thus good health is based upon the capacity of an individual, physical, mental and emotional and takes into what the individual does during his life."

Health is a changing, evolving concept that is basic to nursing. For centuries, the concept of disease was the yardstick by which health was measured. Now, there has been an increasing emphasizes on health. Health is very difficult to define. There is no consensus about any definition of health. There is no consensus about any definitions of health. There is knowledge of how to attain a certain level of health, but health itself cannot be measured.

Health is described in various sources as a value judgment, a subjective state, a relative concept, a spectrum, a cycle, a process and as an abstraction that cannot be measure objectively. In many definitions physiological and psychological components that might be included in definitions of health include environmental and social influences (economical or financial), freedom of pain or disease, optimum capability, ability to adapt, purposeful direction, and meaning of life and harmony, balance or sense of well-being.

Historically, health and illness were viewed as extremes on a continuum, with the absence of clinically recognizable disease being equated with the presence of health. In 1974, WHO defines health in terms of total well-being and discouraged the conceptualization of health as simply the absence of diseases. At the time, some considered this definition impractical; some viewed it as a possible goal for all people, while others consider complete well-being unattainable. However this definition of health includes three characteristics of basic to a positive concept of health:

- It refers concern for the individual as a total person rather than a merely the sum of various parts
- It places health in the context of environment
- It equates health with productive and creative living
- The harmonious balance of the state of physical, mental, social and spiritual well-being of the human individual integrated into his/her health and constitutes health.

The state of health of positive health implies the notion of 'perfect functioning' of the body and mind. It conceptualize health biologically as a state in which every cell and every organ in functioning at optimum capacity, and in perfect harmony with the rest of the body; psychologically, as a state in which the individuals feels a sense of perfect well-being and mastery over his/her environment; socially, as a state in which the individual, capacity for participation in the social system are optional and spiritually, as state in which the individual, which reaches out, and strives for meaning and purpose in life.

Perception of health and illness, nurses can provide more meaningful assistance to help clients regain or attain a state of health. The following questions can help nurses to develop a personal definition of health:

1. Is a person more than a biophysiological system?
2. Is health more than the absence of disease symptoms?
3. Is health solely the result of the interaction between host, agent and environment?
4. Is health, the ability of an individual to perform work?
5. Is health the ability of an individual adapt the environment?
6. Is health a condition of a person's actualization?
7. Is health a state or a process?
8. Is health the effective functioning of self-care activities?
9. Is health static or changing?
10. Are health and wellness the same?
11. Are diseases and illness separate entities or points along a continuum?
12. Is health socially determined?
13. How do you rate your health and why?

MODELS OF HEALTH

Health is such a complex concept, various researcher have developed models or paradigms to explain health in some instances its relationship to illness or injury. A model or paradigm is an abstract outline or theoretical depiction of a complex phenomenon.

Smith (1981) presents four models of health that can be viewed as forming scale—a progressive expansion of the idea of health:
1. Clinical model.
2. Role performance model.
3. Adaptive model.
4. Eudemonistic model.

Clinical Model

The clinical model views health as the absence of physiological disease or the absence of disequilibrium. Persons with clinical symptoms of disease are not considered healthy from this perspective. People are viewed as physiological system with related functions and symptoms or disease, or injury. To laypersons it is considered the state of not being 'sick'. In this model, the opposite of health is disease or injury. Dunn describes this model as a relatively passive state of freedom from illness, a condition of relative's homeostasis. Health is identified as the absence of signs and symptoms of disease or disability as identified by medical science. Many medical practitioners use the clinical model. The focus of many medical practices are the relief of signs and symptoms of disease, and the elimination of malfunctioning; and pain when the signs and symptoms of disease are no longer present in a person, the medical practitioner often considers that the individual's health is resorted.

In the clinical model, the opposite end of continuum from health is disease. In this model health is motivated by the absence of diagnosable disease. Here client statement may be "if I eat better I can avoid getting a heart attack." Nursing response is to conduct routine health screen to foster early detection of disease. Stress on health-promoting behavior that may prevent the onset of disease.

Role Performance Model

Role performance model adds social and psychological standards to the concept of health. Health is defined in terms of the individual ability to fulfill social roles, i.e. to perform work. This critical criterion of health is the person's ability to fulfill his/her roles in society with the maximum (e.g. best, highest) expected performances. If a person is unable to perform his/her expected roles, it can mean illness even if he/she appeared clinically healthy. For example, a man who works all day at his/her job as expected to be healthy even though an film X-ray of his/her lung indicates a tumor.

Parson (1972) views health in this light. Health also been defined as 'the state of optimum capacity of an individual for the effective performance of his/her roles and tasks'. An emphasis in this definition is the capacity of the individual rather than a commitment to roles and tasks.

The role performance model of health, views health as the ability to perform social roles. Illness is determined by the capacity to function and performs ones daily activities. It assumed that sickness is the inability to perform ones work. A problem of this model is the assumption that a person's most important roles is the work role. People usually fulfill several roles, i.e. mother, father, daughter, son, friend and certain individual may consider non-work roles paramount in their lives.

In this model health is motivated by being able to fulfill responsibilities at work, play, home, community. Accordingly client statement will be "as long as I can work and fulfill obligations to my family and my job, I consider myself healthy. Nursing response here is the reinforce influence of health promotion and risk-reduction behaviors on ability to fulfill role expectations."

For example, of this type of definitions is somatic health is the state of optimum capacity for the elective performance of valued tasks. In the role performance model of health, the opposite end of the continuum from health in sickness.

Adaptive Model

The focus of the adaptive model is adaptation. Incorporating the clinical and role performance model is the adaptive model. This model is derived from the writings of Dubos who views health as a creative process. Individual are actively, continually adapting to their environments. Accordingly the individuals must have sufficient knowledge to make informed choices about their health and also the income, and resources to act on choices. They believe that complete well-being is unobtainable.

Health is perceived as a condition in which the person can engage in effective interaction with the physical and social environment. There is an indication of growth and change in this model, i.e. health is state of well-being in which the person is able use purposeful, adaptive responses and processes, physically, mentally, emotionally, spiritually, socially in responses to internal, and external stimuli (stressor) in order to maintain relative stability and comfort; and to strive for personal objectives and cultural goals. The adaptive model of health defines health as the ability to interact effectively within the physical and social environment. The disease state thus represents a failure in adaptation and ineffective coping with environmental changes. The aim of treatment is to restore the ability of their person to adapt, i.e. to cope ascending to this model, extreme good health is flexible adaptation to the environment and interaction with the environment to maximum advantage. The focus of this model is stability, although there is an element of growth and change.

Siegel (1973) describes health as "an outcome of interplay between the internal environment and external multi environments." In the adaptive model health, the opposite end of the continuum from health is illness.

Accordingly, health is motivated by altering oneself or the risks in the environment as situations changes, i.e. engaging in stress reduction, dietary or exercise program, community, recycling or reducing exposure to environmental hazards. The client statement may be "I get sick when I am no longer able to cope with the stresses in my environments." The nursing responses is here to explore with client lifestyle or environment changes that can be made to protect health and reduce the risk of illness.

Eudemonistic Model

Eudemonistic is a term derived from the Greek word eudemon meaning 'fortunate' or 'happy'. The eudemonistic perspective defines health as the realization of ones potential for completed development. The eudemonistic models incorporated the most comprehensive view of health. Health is seen as a condition of actualization or realization of a person's potential for complete development. The eudemonistic model incorporates the most comprehensive view of health. Health is seen as a condition of actualization or realization of a person's potential. Actualization is the apex of the fully developed personality. In this model the highest aspiration of people is fulfillment and complete development, i.e. actualization. In the words of Dubos (1978), health is primarily "measures of each person's ability to do what he/she wants to do and become what he/she wants to become." It is the same as high-level wellness. Illness, in this model, is a condition that prevents self-actualization.

Pender includes, stabilizing and actualizing tendencies in her definition of health, "health is the actualization of inherent and acquired human potential through satisfying relationships with others, while adjustments are made as needed to maintain structural integrity and harmony with environment."

Accordingly to eudemonistic model health is motivated by joy and self-fulfillment, client statement will be 'to be healthy is to realize my full potential'. The nursing response is to explore with client health promoting behavior such as diet, exercises or recreational activities that foster self-esteem and a sense of personal accomplishment.

DIMENSIONS OF HEALTH

Nurses need to clarify their understanding of health and weakness because their definitions largely determine the scope and nature of nursing practice. Individual's health belief also influences their health problems. As per the definition of WHO, there are three dimensions of health:
- Physical
- Mental
- Social.

As the knowledge grows in the minds of people, some other dimension are adding to it, which includes spiritual, emotional, vocational and others (Fig. 2.1).

Physical Dimension

Physical dimension implies perfect functioning of body, which health is a biological state in which every cell and organ in function at optimum level, harmoniously. Here the person has the ability to carry out daily tasks, achieve fitness, maintain adequate nutrition and proper body fat, avoid abusing drugs and alcohol or using tobacco products, and generally to practice positive lifestyle habits The signs of physical health will be good complexion of a clean skin, bright eyes, lustrous hair, well-built with firm flesh, good breath, a good appetite and sound sleep. Normal bowel and bladder activities, and coordination movements. This dimension of health can be assessed by history, physical or other related factors.

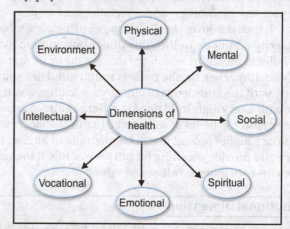

Figure 2.1: Dimensions of health

Mental Dimension

Mental dimension is a state of balance between the individual and the surrounding world, a state of harmony between oneself and others; a coexistence between realities of the self and that of other people, and that of the environment. An individual is said to be mentally healthy, when he/she is having a perfect state of balance with the surrounding world, having harmonious relations with others; the intelligence and memory, learning capacity, judgment are normal not having any internal conflict, accepts criticism sportively has good self-control emotionally, solves this problems intelligently has full self-confidence is well-adjusted with others and is satisfied with what they possesses. They are cheerful and calm. This dimension of health can be assessed by their behavior and attitude.

Social Dimension

Social dimension implies the person's ability to interact successfully with people and within the environment of which each person is a part to develops, and maintain intimacy with significant others; and to develops respect and tolerance for those with different opinions, and beliefs. The person is said to be socially healthy when he/she accepted, respected and loved by all in the family, by their friends, relatives, neighbors, colleagues, and others. This dimension of health includes the level of social skills, one possesses, social functioning and ability to see oneself in a member of a larger society.

Spiritual Dimension

Spiritually means in touch with deeper self and exploring the purpose of life. As people believe in some force than transcends physiology and psychology of human beings. It includes love, charity, purpose, principles, ethics, integrity and hope in life. This dimension in proponent of holistic health in which person is said to be spiritually healthy, when he/she possess sound mind in a sound body with the knowledge of philosophy, leading a simple life with a very high-level thinking. Here as already stated the person has belief in some force (nature, science, religion or a higher power) that serves to unite in human beings and provide meaning for purpose of life. It includes persons own morals, values and ethics.

Emotional Dimension

Emotional dimension of health relates to feeling in which person has the ability to manage stress and to express emotions appropriately. Emotional health involves the ability to recognize, accept and express feelings to accept one's limitations. An emotionally healthy person has positive thinking and is capable of coping, adjusting self, and also adopts according to the circumstances. Also participates in all the activities, which are related to the personal growth and to his/her self-esteem.

Vocational Dimension

A vocational dimension of health has an important role in mainstream physical, social, emotional and spiritual health. So a person is said to be called healthy, he/she is capable of earning sufficiently to lead the life successfully. For which individual work in fully adapted to his/her goals. When an individual has an inability to utilize interest and skills on job will cause disturbance in emotional dimension, which leads to boredom frustrations, and negative feelings.

Intellectual Dimension

In this dimension of health, the person has the ability to learn and use information effectively for personal, family, and career development. Intellectual health involves striving for continued growth and learning to deal with new challenges effectively.

Environmental Dimension

Environmental dimension is the external factors present around person and has got influence on health of human being. So health is a state of dynamics equilibrium between man and his/her environment and when the equilibrium is disturbed, ill-health occurs. In this, the person has an ability to promote health measures that improve the standards of living and quality of life in the community. This includes influences such as food, water and air; and there is an internal environment, i.e. within the individual about genetic influence on health for parents can transmit disease through attached to chromosome to the offspring.

CONCLUSION

Health is the state of well-being of individual and community. It is the balance of the person both within one is being, physical, mental, social and spiritual in the outside world—natural, communal and metaphysical. Health behaviors are the actions of a person takes to understand his/her health state, maintain an optimal state of belief, prevent illness and injury, and reach his/her maximum physical and mental potential.

Concepts of Nursing

CHAPTER 3

INTRODUCTION

Nursing has been called oldest of the art and youngest of the professions. The term 'nurse' evolved from the Latin word nutrix, which means 'nourishing'. The roots of medicines in nursing are intertwined and found in mythology, ancient cultures religion, and reasoned thinking.

Historically, the term nursing most often has been used as a verb signifying 'to do'. The word 'nourish' means to supply that which is necessary to life. Nurse means to foster or cherish, i.e. to nurse one's egg; to bring up, train or nurse, to clasp or handle carefully or fondly (i.e. to nurse a moment to preserve and to nurse a drink), so the term 'nurse' suggests attendance and service. Its antonym is 'neglect'. When nursing is perceived as a science, the term nursing becomes a noun signifying 'a body of abstract knowledge'.

Today nursing emerged as a learned profession, i.e. both a science and art. Science is observation, identification, description, experimental investigations and theoretical explanation of natural phenomena. It is a body of knowledge. Knowledge is an awareness or perception of reality, which is acquired through learning or investigation. Science is defined as both an unified body of knowledge concerned with specific subject matter and the skills, and methodology necessary to provide such knowledge. Therefore, nursing science is that knowledge of germane to the discipline or nursing plus the processes and methodologies used to gain that knowledge. Goal of science is identification of truths or facts about the subject matter of discipline ascertaining that what, where, when, who and how phenomena of interest to the discipline.

According to Jean Watson (1979), nursing is both scientific and artistic. I seek to combine science with humanism. Nursing is therapeutic interpersonal process. Nursing is a scientific discipline that derives its practical base from scientific research.

Modern nursing involves many activities, concepts and skills related to basic sciences, social sciences, growth and development, contemporary issues, and other areas of nursing. Nursing as profession is unique because it addresses the responses of the individuals and families to actual or potential health problems in a humanist, and holistic manner. Now nurses have many roles, such as caretakers, decision-makers, advocates and teachers, and they often assume several roles at the same time. Because of the diversity of nursing role, nurses need a philosophy of nursing to guide their practice.

Nursing has a fascinating history that parallels the history of humankind. For a long as there has been life, so there has been the need to seek care and comfort from illness, and injury. From the dawn of civilization, evidence prevails to support the premise that nursing has been essential for the preservation of life. Survival of the human race, therefore, inextricably intertwined with the development of nursing.

Nursing is an art. Art is the application of knowledge and skill to bring about desired results. Art is an individualized action. Nursing art is carried out by the nurse in a one-to-one relationship with the patient and constitutes the nurse's conscious responses to specific, and the patient's immediate situation. The art of clinical nursing is directed toward achievement of the four main goals:

1. Understanding of the patient and his/her condition or situation, and need.
2. Enhancement of the patient's capability.
3. Improvement of his/her condition or situation within framework of medical plan for his/her cares.
4. Prevention of the recurrence of his/her problem or development of a new one, which may cause anxiety, disability or distress.

Nursing art involves three initial operations, i.e. stimulus, preconception and interpretation. Nurse's action may be rational, reactionary or deliberative.

Nursing is the art and science of assisting individuals in learning to care for themselves whenever possible and of caring for them, when they are unable to their own needs. Nursing has developed into a scientific profession from an unorganized way of caring for the ill, resulting in change from mystical beliefs to sophisticated technology and caring. Nursing uses caring behaviors, critical thinking skills and scientific knowledge. Nursing focuses on the client response to illness rather than on the illness. Nursing promotes health and assists client's move to a higher level of wellness, including assistance during a terminal illness with the maintenance of comfort, and dignity during the final stage of life.

Florence Nightingale (1876) viewed that nursing has been limited to signify little more than the administration of medicine and the application of poultice. It ought to signify the proper use of fresh air, light, warmth, cleanliness, quiet and the proper to the patient. As stated earlier, nursing has been called oldest arts and the youngest of the professions. As such, it has gone through may stages and has been an integral part of social movements. Nursing has been involved in the existing culture shaped by it and helping development.

Nursing means the care and nurturing of healthy and ill people, individually or in groups and communities. Nurses, provide care for people in the midst of health, pain, loss, fear, disfigurement, death, grieving, challenge, growth, birth and transition on intimate front-line basis. Expert nurses call this 'privileged place of nursing'.

DEFINITIONS OF NURSING

According to International Council of Nurses

International Council of Nurses (ICN) 1973, defined nursing according to the belief of Virginia Henderson (1966), "the unique function of the nurse is to assist the individual, sick or well in the performance of those activities contributing to health or its recovery (or peaceful death) that he would perform unaided, if he had the necessary strength, will or knowledge."

Now nursing throughout the universe has changed. Because advance in health care have altered the type of care required by clients. Nurses have taken on expanded roles and there is renewed interest in providing care outside the hospital. Keeping in view of these changes, the ICN (2003) defines the nursing as follows; 'Nursing encompasses autonomous and collaborative care of individuals of all ages, families, groups and communities, sick or well, and in all setting. Nursing includes the promotion of health, prevention of illness and the care of ill, disabled, and dying people. Advocacy, promotion of safety environment, research, participation in shaping health policy, inpatient and health system management, and education are also key nursing roles'.

According to American Nurses Association

American Nurses Association (ANA) 1980, defined nursing as "the diagnosis and treatment of human responses to actual and potential health and treatment of human responses to actual and potential health problems." Since nurses are a heterogeneous group of people with varying skills.

World Health Organization (WHO) performs activities designed to provide care ranging from basic to complex in a growing number of settings. It is very difficult to describe the professional boundaries. So, in 2003 ANA acknowledged six essential features of professional nursing:

1. Provision of caring relationship that facilities health and healing.
2. Attention of the range of human experience and responses to health and illness within the physical and social environments.
3. Integration of objective data with knowledge gained from and appreciation of the patient or groups subjective experience.
4. Application of scientific knowledge to the processes of diagnosis and treatment through the use of judgment, and critical thinking.
5. Advancement of professional nursing knowledge through scholarly inquiry.
6. Influence of social and public policy to promote social justice.

Keeping in view of the above essential features, the ANA (2004) redefined professional nursing as "the protection, promotion, and optimization of health and abilities, prevention of illness and injury alleviating of suffering through the diagnosis and treatment through the human responses, and advocacy in the care of individuals, families, communities and populations."

It will never be possible to defines, precisely and in great details, which activities are inside and which are outside the boundaries of nursing. This is partly because of the 'state of the art' of health care and nursing are changing so rapidly that such lists become outdated almost before they are completed, and partly because the file has become far too complex to be reduced to lists of tasks and procedures. As the nursing profession matures and the body of nursing knowledge expands, it will become easier to clearly desirable the principles, models and functions that are the basis of nursing [Canadian Nurses Association (CNA), 1993].

CHAPTER 3 Concepts of Nursing

Expert's Views on Nursing

Definitions of the nurse and nursing are based on this word origin to describe the nurse as a person, who nourishes, fosters and protects; a person prepared to take care of the sick, injured and aged people. Defining nursing is a difficult task, since nursing is not static, but is always responding to new advances, increased knowledge and consumer needs. However, the expanding roles and function of a nurse in present days have made anyone definition too limited. In the decades, since Nightingale thought about, preached, wrote about the transformed nursing and others have attempted to distill into one definition the essence of nursing. So, it is better to review the number of definitions of nursing that evolved over the years with its themes and goals.

Florence Nightingale (1859)

Nursing ought to signify the proper use of fresh air, warmth, cleanliness, quiet and the proper selection and administration of diet all at the least expense of vital power of the patient. Nurse means any person in charge of the personal health of another. Nursing means to have charge of the personal health of somebody and what nursing has to do is put the patient in the least condition of nature to act upon him/her. The theme of this definition is that the 'nurses' center of concern is patient. Nature, a healthful restful environment are nurses allies. The goal of nursing is to facilitate body's reparative process by manipulating environments include appropriate nursing, nutrition, hygiene, light comfort, socialization and hope. In brief, health maintenance and restoration are the nurses' goals.

Shaw (1907)

Nursing is an art. It properly includes as well as the execution of specific orders, the administration of food and medicine, the personal care of the patient. To fill such a position requires certain physical and mental attributes as well as special training. The theme of this definition is that more than knowledge and skills needed by nurse, the attribute of personal caring is also needed.

Harmer (1922)

Nursing is rooted in the needs of the humanity. It is object, which is not only to cure the sick, but to bring health and ease, rest, and comfort to mind and body. Its object is to prevent disease and to preserve health. The theme here is disease prevention and health promotion.

Harmer and Henderson (1943)

Nursing may be defined as 'that service to individual that helps him/her to attain or maintain a health state of mind or body. The definition tells that nursing deals with the health of body psyche (mind and body).

Mother Olivia Gowan (1943)

Nursing is both an art and science involving the patient, as promoting spiritual, mental and physical health, stressing health education and health preservation, ministering to sick, caring for the patients, environment and giving health service to the family, community and to the individual.

Hildegard E Peplau (1952)

Nursing is a significant, therapeutic, interpersonal process. It functions cooperatively with other human processes that make health possible for individuals in community. Nursing is an educative instrument that aims to promote forward movement of personality in the direction of creative, constructive, productive, personal and community living. The definition tells that effective nursing results from a therapeutic relationship between nurse and patient. Accordingly, the goal of nursing is to develop interaction between nurse and client. Nurses participate in structuring healthcare systems to facilitate natural ongoing tendencies of humans to develop interpersonal relationship.

Virginia Henderson (1955)

The unique function of the nurse is to assist the individual, sick or well, in the performance of those activities contributing to health (its recovery or to a peaceful death) that he/she would perform unaided, if he had the necessary strength, will or knowledge, to do this in such a way as to help him gain independence as rapidly as possible.

Henderson translates this unique function as (the nurse) in temporarily the conscious or the unconscious; the love of life for the suicidal; the leg for the amputee; the eyes for the newly blind; a means of locomotion for the infant; knowledge and confidence for the younger mother; the voice for those who are too week or withdrawn to speak; she also urges that in these activities nurse should be an independent practitioner. The main theme of this definition is either well or ill people are the focus of nursing. Responsibility for care is shared by nurse and patient. The goal of nursing to work independently with other healthcare workers assisting client to gain independence as quickly as possible, to help client gain lacking strength.

Faye Glenn Abdellah (1960)

Nursing is a helping profession. Nursing care is doing something to or for the person, for providing information to the person with goal of meeting needs, increasing or restoring self-help ability or alleviating an impairment. Abdellah concept of 21 problems is the main focus of nursing. The nurse is a problem solver and decision-maker. The goal of nursing is to provide services to the individuals, families and society. A nurse should not only be kind and caring, but also intelligent, competent and technically well-prepared to provide this service.

Dorothea E Orem (1960)

Nursing is described as the giving of direct assistance to a person, as required, because of the person's specific inabilities in self-care resulting from a situation of personal health. This tells nursing is doing for a person what he/she cannot do at this time due to health-related limitations. The goal of nursing is to care for and help client attain total self-care or return to self-care is the goal (1971). Nursing care becomes necessary where client is unable to fulfill biological, psychological, developmental or social needs (1985), as nursing is giving assistance to persons who are unable to meet their own needs.

Ida Jean Orlando (1961)

The function of professional nursing is conceptualized as finding out and meeting the patient's immediate need for help. Orlando viewed three dimensions, i.e. client behavior, nurse's reactions and nurse action, compose nursing situation. The goal of nursing is to respond to client behavior in terms of immediate needs. To interact with client to meet immediate needs by identifying client behavior, reaction of nurse and nursing action to be taken.

Lydia E Hall (1962)

Nursing can and should be professional. The professional nurse functions most therapeutically, when patients have entered the second stage of their hospital stay (the second stay in the recuperating or non-acute phase of illness).

Hall viewed that client is composed of the overlapping parts, i.e. person pathological stage (core), treatment (cure), and body (care). Nurse is a caretaker. The goal of nursing to provide care and comfort to client during disease process.

Ernestine Wiedenbach (1964)

Nursing is a service, helping art, a goal-directed activity. The purpose (goal) of clinical nursing is to facilitate the efforts of the individual to overcome the obstacles, which currently interfere with the ability to response capably to demand made of him/her by their conditions, environment situation and time.

Nursing is a practice, which is related to individuals who need help because of behavioral stimulus. Clinical nursing has four interlocking components, i.e. philosophy (way), purpose (why), practice (what) and art (how).

Myra Estrin Levine (1966)

Nursing is a human interaction. Nursing intervention is based on four conservation principles of nursing, i.e. conservative energy, conservation of structural integrity, conservation of personal integrity and conservation of social integrity. The goal of nursing is to use conservation activities aimed at optimum use of client resources.

Dorothy E Johnson (1968)

Nursing is an external force acting to preserve the organization of patient behavior, while the patient is under stress by means of imposing regulatory mechanism or by providing resources. Nursing is an art and science; it supplies external assistance both before and during system balance disturbances, and therefore requires knowledge of order, disorder and control. The goal of nursing is to reduce stress so that client can move more easily, through recovery process.

Martha E Rogers (1970)

Nursing is a humanistic science dedicated to compassionate concern for maintaining and promoting health, preventing illness and caring for and rehabilitating the sick and disabled. Her unitary man evolves along life process. Client continuously changes and coexists with environment. Accordingly each person has a personal maximal health potential.

PURPOSES OF NURSING CARE

Nurses provide care to achieve the goals of health promotion, illness prevention, health restoration and end-of-life care. Together these aspects of care represent a range of services that cover the spectrum from complete well-being to death.

CHAPTER 3 — Concepts of Nursing

Health Promotion

The WHO defines health as "a state of complete physical, mental and social well-being, and not merely the absence of disease or infirmity." This inclusive definition can be applied to individuals, groups, families or communities. Health promotion activities are any activities that foster the highest state of well-being of the recipient of the activities. For example, might counsel a pregnant client about the importance of adequate prenatal nutrition to promote health at the individual level. Group and family-level health promotion activities might include teaching about nutrition during pregnancy in prenatal classes and in family education programs. On a community level the nursing activities would be focused on reaching a larger number of people. For example, could advocate for prominent billboards highlighting the importance of prenatal care and nutrition, post signs in grocery stores recommending food sources for pregnant women, and lobby for labeling of substances that should be avoided in pregnancy.

Illness Prevention

Illness prevention focuses on avoidance of disease. Activities are targeted to decrease the risk of developing an illness or to minimize the risk of exposure to disease. To avoid disease, people must know the causes of disease and the route of disease transmission. For example, pneumonia causes many deaths every year. Those affected are society's most vulnerable, i.e. the very young, old and ill. Some nursing activities to decrease the risk of pneumonia include:
- Teaching the importance of handwashing to decrease the transmission of infection
- Advocating for and administering pneumonia immunizations to those at high risk.

Health Restoration

Health restoration encompasses activities that foster a return to health for those already ill. To restore health, the nurse provides direct care to ill individuals, groups, families or communities. This aspect of care is what most people think of when they envision the nursing role. Recall that health has physical, mental and social dimensions. When one engage in health restoration activities, your care should address each of these dimensions. Health restoration activities include the following:
- Providing hygiene and nutrition for someone unable to do so independently
- Assessing an ill client's health status
- Performing diagnostic tests on a client
- Administering medications or treatments
- Counseling individuals or groups
- Tracking clients with a communicable disease to ensure that they receive appropriate therapy
- Lobbying for community changes to decrease the prevalence of disease within a community.

End-of-life Care

Not all nursing activities can be directed toward promoting or restoring health or preventing disease. Death is an inevitable consequence of life. Nurses have been active in promoting the respectful care of those who are terminally ill or dying. Nursing activities for dying are designed to promote comfort, maintain quality of life, provide culturally relevant spiritual care and ease the emotional burden of death. Nurses work with dying individuals, their family members and support persons and with organizations that focus on the needs of the terminally ill.

SETTINGS OF NURSING CARE

As nurses will have an opportunity to work in a variety of settings. During their education, nurses will be placed in many settings and clinical units that will allow them to see some of the possible options available upon graduation. Approximately, 60% of nurses work in hospitals. The remaining 40% work in extended facilities, ambulatory care and community or home health settings.

Hospitals provide services to clients who require round-the-clock nursing care. This type of care is frequently referred to as acute care. Length of stay is limited to the amount of time that the client requires 24-hour observation.

Extended care facilities provide care for clients to an extended period of time, usually longer than 1 month. These facilities include skilled nursing facilities (SNF) also known as begin receiving care at these sites directly or may be transferred there for ongoing care after hospitalization.

Ambulatory care is synonymous with outpatient care. Clients reside at home or in non-hospital settings and come to the site for care. Ambulatory care sites include private health and medical offices, clinics and outpatient therapy centers.

Home care is provided to clients who are homebound or unable to get themselves to ambulatory care centers for services. Services are usually coordinated by a home health or visiting nurse service and include nursing care as well as various therapies, and home assistance programs. Home care services may also be employed when the client or family decides that home is the preferred site of care particularly when the client is terminally ill. Home care is also appropriate when clients still requiring skilled care are discharged from the hospital because of their reimbursable length of stay has expired.

Community health deals with provision care for the community at large. Community health nurses provide services to at-risk populations and devise strategies to improve the health status of the surrounding community. Examples of community health programs include health care for the homeless and school-based programs designed to decrease the incidence of teen pregnancies.

STANDARDS OF NURSING CARE

The standards of nursing practice in clinical setting are given in Table 3.1.

NURSING

Competency refers to the quality or extent being competent. Competent means having the necessary ability or knowledge to do something successfully. The term competence used to describe a person's decision-making ability. Competence is the ability to adequately fulfill one's role and handle one's affairs. Competence usually describes a status and ability to make all or no decisions for oneself. Increasingly nurses encounter clients who are in need of care for their health, so they should develop and have competency in dealing with their health, so they should develop and have competency in dealing with their clients. The client may be an individual, family or the community.

Need for Competency in Nursing

Competency in nursing is the one of major factors in the accelerating pace of nursing movement toward professional status in the growth of its theoretical and conceptual base for practice. It is the growth that allows the nurses to be truly accountable in this technological and scientific era. Theoretical-based knowledge is now available in other as the result of nursing research and existing literature:

1. As nursing has come closure to being the true profession, it is expected that its concern with accountability has always been acknowledged as one of the hallmarks of a profession.
2. Competence in nursing practice determined and maintained by various credentialing methods such as licensure, certification and accreditation that protect the public welfare and safety.
3. Competent practice is major legal safeguard for nurses. Nurses need to provide care, i.e. within the legal boundaries of their practice and within the boundaries of agencies policies and procedures. Nurses therefore must be familiar with their various job descriptions. Every nurse is responsible for ensuring that his/her education and experience are adequate to meet the responsibilities delineated in the job description.
4. Competency also involves care that protects the client from harm. Nurses need to anticipate sources of client injury, educate clients about hazards and implement measures to prevent injury.

Competency in Nursing Practice

One attribute, i.e. always been expected of the professional nurse, it is that he/she is competent in her/his practice. Just what that practice encompasses has been a matter of discussion and dissension at various times, and just what the 'professional' before the word 'nurse' really means hotly contended. But everyone on all sides of these issues has always agreed that whatever it is that any type of nurse does, it must be done well. Currently many level of nurses reflected in the makeup of the healthcare term, it is imperative that each level have clear idea of the scope of practice at the level and responsibilities perform to the maximum limit of the level. The nurse's accountability may be called into question, if he/she is functioning beyond the limits of her particular level.

The key to expertise in practice lies both in the knowledge and the skills area, a somewhat artificial distinction that nevertheless allows for more clarity in this discussion. Nursing has always a strong manual skill competent and to the extent that the nurse is in a role, which contains that kind of activity, gentleness, quickness and accuracy remain hallmarks of excellence. Where the skills required are in communication, teaching, leadership and research, the matter of expertise is no less pressing. Underlying all skills in excellence in terms of the nurse's command of 'nursing knowledge'. Nurses can never expect to contribute significantly to health care in this planning, implementation and evaluation aspects, if they do whatever they do in a mediocre manner. Competence is an absolute prerequisite of accountability.

Need of Competency in Community Health Nursing

1. Community health nursing refers to a synthesis of both public health science and nursing science is

CHAPTER 3 — Concepts of Nursing

Table 3.1: Standards of clinical nursing practice

Standards	Feature	Role of nurse
Standards of care		
Standard 1	Assessment	The registered nurse collects comprehensive data pertinent to the patient's health or the situation
Standard 2	Diagnosis	The registered nurse analyzes the assessment data to determine the diagnoses of issues
Standard 3	Outcome identification	The registered nurse identifies expected outcomes for a plan individualized to the patient or situation
Standard 4	Planning	The registered nurse develops a plan that describes strategies and to attain expected outcomes
Standard 5	Implementation	The registered nurse implements the identified plan
Standard 5A	Coordination of care	The registered nurse coordinates care delivery
Standard 5B	Health teaching and health promotion	The registered nurse employs strategies to promote health and a safe environment
Standard 5C	Consultation	The advanced practice registered nurse and the nursing role specialist provide consultations to influence the identified plan, enhance the abilities of others, and effect change
Standard 5D	Prescriptive authority and treatment	The advanced practice registered nurse uses prescriptive authority, procedures, referrals, treatments and therapies in accordance with state, and federal laws and regulations
Standard 6	Evaluation	The registered nurse evaluates progress toward attainment of outcomes
Standard of professional performance		
Standard 7	Quality of practice	The registered nurse systematically enhances the quality and effectiveness of nursing practice
Standard 8	Education	The registered nurse attains knowledge and competency that reflects current nursing practice
Standard 9	Professional practice evaluation	The registered nurse evaluates one's own nursing practice in relation to professional practice standards and guidelines, relevant statutes, rules and regulation
Standard 10	Collegiality	The registered nurse interacts with and contributes to the professional development of peers and colleagues
Standard 11	Collaboration	The registered nurse collaborates with patient, family and others in the conduct of nursing practice
Standard 12	Ethics	The registered nurse integrates ethical provisions in all areas of practice
Standard 13	Research	The registered nurse integrates research findings into practice
Standard 14	Resource utilization	The registered nurse considers factors related to safety, effectiveness, cost and impact on practice in the planning, and delivery of nursing services
Standard 15	Leadership	The registered nurse provides leadership in the professional practice setting and the profession

theoretically responsive to our prevailing ideas of social justice and methods of distributing healthcare resources as chosen by the community (Archer SE, 1982).
2. Community health nursing is a learned practice discipline with ultimate goal of contributing, as an individual and in collaboration with other, to the promotion of the client's optimum level of functioning through teaching and delivery of care.

   Since the community health nurses re accountable to their services in their respective areas should have to show their competency for following reasons.
3. As consumers become more knowledgeable through formal education and informal education provide by vast array of mixed media, they know more about the professions are supposed to be doing. They also able to demand more effectively and more visibly. Nursing must be aware of consumers increased knowledge and sophistication, and be prepared to respond to it in an equally knowledgeable and sophisticated manner, the nurse able to demonstrate clearly those principles and concepts on which practice is based.
4. As a knowledgeable professional, the nurse should ultimately accountable for healthcare delivery nationally, when she/he seeks to blame others (such as physician, administrator or politician) for the state of healthcare delivery system or constantly looks to others for improvement of this system, he/she weakens his/her positions and his/her power base. By accepting an appropriate degree of responsibility for current situations and actively pursuing methods of improving it, the nurse act on a more professional level stakes his/her claim to a piece of healthcare pie.
5. As accountable to public in guarding ill prepared coworkers being certified to give nursing care under the guide of a new category of healthcare worker, a nurse by any other name is still a nurse, so they should be properly trained to be oriented to practice properly.

Competencies Required for Future Community Health Nursing

The competencies required for community health nurses include the following (De Tornyay R, 1992):
- Care for community's health
- Expand access to effective care
- Provide contemporary clinical care
- Emphasizing primary care
- Participate in coordinate care
- Ensure cost effective and appropriate care
- Practice prevention.

Clients' optimum level of functioning through teaching and delivery of care (Margaret J Jacobson). Now primary health care is the key component of community health nursing. Community health care is almost similar to primary healthcare provides health-related services in place, where people's spend their time homes, in shelters, in long term residence at work place, in schools, old age homes and soon or in other words nurses providing community based care.

An approaches are emerging to address community-based care will include an integrated healthcare system, community initiatives, community coalitions, managed care, case management and outreach programs using lay health workers. To practice community-based healthcare system nurses need knowledge and competencies such as:
- Determinants of a healthy community
- Primary and secondary preventive strategies
- Health promotion strategies
- Collaborative and interdisciplinary term work
- Determinants of an accessible, cost-effective healthcare system
- A decision-making process that involves consumer and information management
- Education in public health policies and strategies to influence, and effect change are essential.

The scope of community health nursing practice in very broad and involves the delivery of continuum of preventive health service aimed at enhancing the health of the individuals, families, groups and community, community health nurses places priority on delivery of primary prevention services believing that the most effective ways to address community health problems to prevent them occurring when providing preventive services to individual. Community health nurses views these services within the context of the family and the community. Community health nurses recognize that the health of the individual can affect the health of the families and community. Family as seen as a significant entry point from which to identify community strengths, needs and resources related to the delivery healthcare services. The healthcare services are:
- Involve clients in decision-making processes
- Provide healthy lifestyles
- Access and use technology appropriately
- Improve healthcare system
- Manage information
- Understand the role of physical environment
- Practice counseling on ethical issues
- Accommodate expanded accountability
- Participate in racially and culturally diverse society
- Continue to learn.

CONCLUSION

Today nursing emerged as a learned profession than a science, art and discipline. Nurses provide a unique preoperative on the healthcare system because of their constant present in a varieties of settings and then contest both with consumers, who receive the benefit of the system's most complex services and with those who have problem with the systems insufficiencies. Since the nurses are accountable to their client, public, profession, self and employing agency, the need is expressed for ground work to be laid for the nurse to act in accountable manner along with specific areas to be covered during educational process by developing competencies in respective areas to be covered during educational process by developing competencies in respective areas of nursing. For which educational system will prepare its members most satisfactorily for practice and the level of entry into the professional practice.

Promotion of Health

CHAPTER 4

INTRODUCTION

Health is a state of being free from illness or injury, or a person's mental or physical condition. Health promotion is an activity than support or encouraging the person being healthy.

Good health is a prerequisite of human productivity and development process. It is essential for the economic and technological development. Health as defined by Pericles (500 BC) is that 'it is a state of moral, mental and physical well-being, which enables a person to face any crisis in life with utmost grace (of God) and facility. WHO (1958), reflected a holistic perspective in its classical definition of health as a state of complete physical, mental and sound well-being, not merely the absence of disease and infirmity'. Terries (1975) considered with the definition to be 'vague and imprecise with utopian aura'. So, Terries (epidemiologist) expanded the definition that health is a state of physical, mental and social well-being, and ability to function and not merely absence of illness, and infirmity by deleting the word 'complete' and adding ability to function, and made WHO definition, which was placed in a more realistic context, providing a useful framework for health promotion.

More contemporary definitions of health have emphasized the relationship between health and wellness and health promotion. Although health may be viewed as a static state of being at any given point in time, wellness is the process of moving toward integrating human functioning and maximizing human potential. Health promotion is the process of helping people enhance their well-being and maximize their human potential. The focus of health promotion is on changing patterns of behavior or environmental structures to promote health rather than simply to avoid illness. The goal of health promotion is to enable people to exercise control over their well-being and ultimately improve their health, focusing on people and population as a whole and not solely on people who are at risk for specific disease. Health promotion combines education, organizational involvement, economics and political influences to bring about changes in behaviors of individuals and groups, or changes in environmental structures related to improved health and well-being. This classic definition of health promotion remains pertinent, and today the terms 'wellness' and 'health promotion' are frequently used interchangeably, with both terms having elements of physical, mental and social well-being for both the individual and the community.

DEFINITIONS

1. Activities directed toward increasing the level of well-being and actualizing the potential of individuals, families and groups; a category separate from primary prevention.

   — *Pender, 1987*

2. Maintaining or improving the general level of health of individuals, families and groups; part of primary prevention.

   —*Leavell and Clark, 1965*

3. Individual and community activities to promote healthful lifestyles.

   —*Julius Richmond, 1979*

4. Positive health promotion is the process of enabling people to increase control over and improve their own health; aimed primarily at improving health potential and maintaining health balance.

   —*Amelia Mangay-Maglacas, Chief Nurse WHO, 1988*

Pender (1987) considers health promotion separate from primary prevention. She defines health promotion as 'activities directed toward increasing the level of well-being', and primary prevention as 'activities directed toward decreasing the probability of specific illnesses'. In this instance, health promotion is considered to be an approach behavior, whereas primary prevention is considered avoidance behavior. Health promotion is not disease oriented, i.e. no specific problem is being avoided. By contrast, primary prevention activities are geared toward avoiding specific problems. Having analyzed the terms used in the health promotion literature (Brubaker, 1983) agrees with Pender's definition and further argues that even dictionary definitions support differences between the terms 'health promotion' and 'primary or illness prevention'. Brubaker notes that promotion is geared to 'helping and encouraging to flourish', whereas to prevent is defined as 'to keep from occurring'. For example, a 40-year-old male may begin a program of walking 3 miles each day. If the goal of his program is to 'decrease the risk of heart disease', then the activity would be considered prevention. By contrast, if his walking regimen is instituted to 'increase his overall health and feeling of well-being', then the activity would be considered health promotion behavior. Most authors do not take health promotion to mean simply the avoidance of risk factors or the maintenance of stability. Rather, health promotion is seen as being directed toward self-development, growth and a high level of wellness (Brubaker, 1983).

In a document of 1979 called Healthy People, the Surgeon General of the United States differentiates health promotion, health protection and preventive health services. He outlines specific activities for each category as detailed below.

Health promotion: Individual and community activities to promote healthful lifestyles. Examples of health promotion activities include improving nutrition, preventing alcohol and drug misuse, maintaining fitness and exercising.

Health protection: Actions by government and industry to minimize environmental health threats. Health protection relates to activities such as maintaining occupational safety, controlling radiation and toxic agents, and preventing infectious diseases and accidents.

Preventive health services: Actions of healthcare providers to prevent health problems. These services include control of high blood pressure, control of sexually transmitted disease, immunization, family planning and health care during pregnancy and infancy.

The Chief Scientist for nursing from the World Health Organization (WHO), Amelia Mangay-Maglacas, uses the terms positive health and positive health promotion, and presents them in a broader context. According to Maglacas, positive health for all does not mean the eradication of every disease or the healing of every body part. Rather, health should be considered in the context of its contribution to social and economic development, so that all people have the necessary social and economic support to lead satisfying lives (1988). Positive health promotion is the process of enabling people to improve and to increase their control over their own health. The goal of positive health is attained by caring for ourselves and for others, by controlling life's making, and by ensuring that conditions in society allow people to attain health.

Health promotion is an important component of nursing practice and also it is an accepted aim of nursing practice, although it is rarely defined, and is not often differentiated from disease prevention or health maintenance. In narrow sense, prevention means avoiding the development of disease in the future and in broader sense, it consists of all interventions to limit progression of a disease. The levels of prevention occur at various points of a course of disease progression.

Leavell and Clark (1965) strongly influenced the evolution of health promotion and disease prevention strategies through their classic definitions of primary, secondary and tertiary levels of promotion that were rooted in the biomedical model of health and epidemiology. The applications of preventive measures, according to them corresponds to the natural history or stages of disease. Classic definitions of primary, secondary and tertiary levels of promotions are:

1. Primary prevention: Focuses on health promotion and protection against specific health problems. So, primary prevention measures are directed toward 'well' individuals in the prepathogenesis period to promote their health and to provide specific protection from diseases [e.g. immunization against diseases such as diphtheria, tetanus, pertussis (DTP) and polio]. The purposes of primary prevention are to decrease the risk or exposure of the individual or community to disease.
2. Secondary prevention: Focuses on early identification of health problems and prompts intervention to alleviate health problems. Its goal is to identify individuals in an early stage of a disease process and to limit future disability. So, here secondary preventive measures are applied to diagnose or treat individuals in the period of pathogenesis.
3. Tertiary prevention: Focuses on restoration and rehabilitation with the goals of returning the individual to an optimum level of functioning. So, the tertiary prevention addresses rehabilitation and the return of people with chronic illness to a maximal ability to function.

The three levels of prevention may overlap in practice. For example, person may experience heart attack and the goal of secondary prevention is to limit the disability. The teaching of lifestyle changes for that person's rehabilitation will be health education activities of primary prevention in which primary prevention has no distinct component of health promotions and specific protection. Health promotion focuses on positive measures such as education for healthy living and prevention of promotion of favorable environmental conditions as well as periodic selective examinations, e.g. assessment of health education. Specific protection includes measures to reduce the threat of specific diseases such as hygiene and the elimination of workplace hazards. Both components are not the same; the term health promotion is linked to a positive view of health, e.g. health habits, whereas specific protection is linked to the negative view of absence of disease, e.g. disease prevention.

Health promotion is considered as primary prevention and is directed towards modifying the human behavior to adopt positive health practices. So, health promotion is a behavior directed toward achieving a greater level of health illness prevention, reducing the threat of illness or disease; and health maintenance is directed toward keeping a current state of health. Some feels that health promotion has to be different from health protection or illness prevention, and stated that health promotion is a behavior motivated by the desire to increase well-being and actualize human health potential; and health promotion or illness prevention as a 'behavior motivated by a desire to actively avoid illness, detect early or maintain functioning within the constraints of illness'.

Now the public has become increasingly aware of and interested in health promotion, and there is an increasing trend towards improving the quality of life rather than the traditional approach of disease control in the field of health. Many persons are aware of the relationships between lifestyle and illness, and are developing health-promoting habits such as getting adequate exercise, rest, relaxation, maintaining good nutrition, and controlling the use of tobacco, alcohol and other drugs.

PRINCIPLES

World Health Organization describes health promotion as the process of enabling people to increase control over and improve their health (WHO, 1984). Accordingly, the five principles, which are basis of health promotion includes:

1. It involves the population as a whole in the context of their everyday life, rather than focusing on people at risk in specific disease.
2. It is directed toward action on the determination of health.
3. It combines diverse, but complimentary methods or approaches including communication, education, legislation, fiscal measures, organizational change, community developmental and spontaneous local activities against health hazards.
4. It aims at effective and concrete public participations.
5. It is basically an activity in health and social field, and not medical service health professionals, particularly in primary health care have a vital role in nurturing and enabling health promotion.

According to Ottawa Charter (1986), health promotion combines both individual and community level strategies including 'building healthy public, creating supportive environments, strengthening community action, developing personal skills and reorienting health services'. Health is a source of daily living. For individuals or communities to realize physical, mental and social well-being, they must become aware of; learn to use the social and personal resources available within their environment.

According to Bangkok Charter (2005), for health, promotion in the universe requires certain actions, which includes:

1. Advocating for health benefit based on human rights and solidarity.
2. Investing in sustainable policies, action and infrastructures to address determination of health.
3. Building capacity for policy development, leadership, health promotion practices, knowledge transfer and research, and health literacy.
4. Regulating the legislate to ensure high level of protection from harm, and enable equal opportunity for health and well-being for all people.
5. Partner and build alliance with public, nongovernmental, international organization, and civil society to create sustainable actions.

Health promotional activities need to be carried out for target people. According to the WHO, target people includes workers at workplace, adolescents, elderly people, women and children:

1. Health promotion activities at workplace are that there should be facilities for health assessment, stress, management, prevention of accidents, prohibiting smoking, provide nutritional education and facilities for exercise and fitness, and recreation. If provided, it helps to reduce the burden of employees by reducing rising cost of health, develops caring image, decrease absenteeism and increased productivity.
2. Health promotion activities for adolescents are required to reduce behavioral and lifestyle problems, and to prevent risk-taking behavior such as reckless driving, and including sexual activities, etc.

HEALTH PROMOTION MODEL

The initial version of the Health Promotion Model (HPM) appeared in the nursing literature in the early 1980s and focused on health-promoting behaviors rather than health protection or illness prevention behaviors. The initial

CHAPTER 4 — Promotion of Health

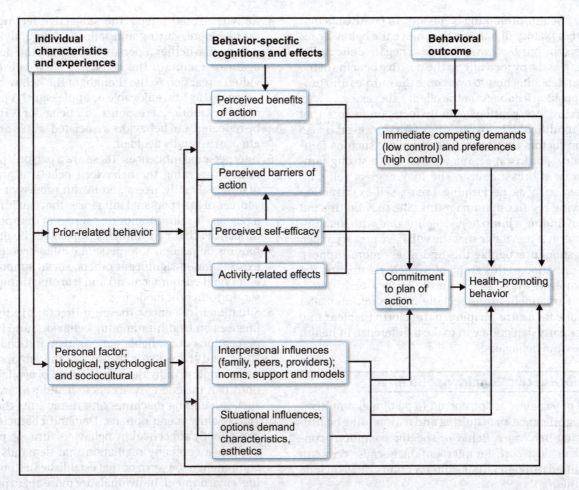

Figure 4.1: Health promotion model

model has recently been replaced by the HPM (revised) as shown in Figure 4.1. The HPM is a competence- or approach-oriented model that depicts the multidimensional nature of persons interacting with their interpersonal and physical environments as they pursue health. The assumptions of HPM are the variables in the revised HPM and their interrelationships that are described as follows:

1. Persons seek to create living through which they can express their unique human health potential.
2. Persons have the capacity for reflective self-awareness, including assessment of their own competencies. Person's value growth in directions viewed as positive and attempt a personally acceptable balance between change and stability.
3. Individuals seek to actively regulate their own behavior.
4. Individuals in all their biopsychosocial complexity interact with the environment, progressively transforming the environment and being transformed over time. Health professionals constitute a part of the interpersonal environment, which exerts influence on persons throughout their life span.
5. Self-initiated reconfiguration of person-environment interactive patterns is essential to change behavior.

Individual Characteristics and Experiences

The importance of an individual's unique personal factors or characteristics and experiences will depend on the target behavior for health promotion. There is flexibility in the HPM to select those characteristics that are relevant to the particular health behavior. Personal factors are categorized as biological (e.g. age, strength, balance), psychological (e.g. self-esteem, self-motivation) and sociocultural (e.g. race, ethnicity, education and socioeconomic status). Some personal factors can influence health behaviors, while others such as age, cannot be changed. Prior-related behavior includes previous health-promoting behavior and received a positive benefit; as a result, it will engage in future health-promoting behaviors. In contrast, a person with a history of barriers to achieve the behavior remembers the hurdles, which creates a negative effect. The nurse can assist by focusing on the positive benefits of the behavior, teaching how to overcome the hurdles and providing positive feedback for the client's successes.

Nursing interventions usually focus on factors that can be modified. It is just as important, however, it also focus on factors that cannot be changed, such as family history. For instance, if a woman has a strong family history of breast cancer, she may neglect self-care practices such as performing breast self-examination and having regular mammograms. She may do this out of fear of finding a lump or just feeling that with her family history, it is inevitable that she will have breast cancer. Nurses should recognize this and direct more support, and information to this group of women, reinforcing the idea that even with a strong family history, early detection and treatment are especially important, and offer more hope for a cure. Helping to transform that fear into hope for early detection can make a difference in health attitudes and behaviors.

Behavior-specific Cognitions and Affect

The set of variables is considered to be of major motivational significance for acquiring and maintaining health-promoting behaviors. Behavior-specific cognitions constitute a critical 'core' for intervention, because they can be modified through nursing interventions. They include the following:

1. Perceived benefits of action-anticipated benefits or outcomes (e.g. physical fitness, stress reduction) affect the person's plan to participate in health-promoting behaviors and may facilitate continued practice. Prior positive experience with the behavior or observations of others engaged in the behavior is a motivational factor.
2. Perceived barriers to action: A person's perceptions about available time, inconvenience, expense and difficulty performing the activity may act as barriers (imagined or real). Perceived barriers to action affect health-promoting behaviors by decreasing the individual's commitment to a plan of action.
3. Perceived self-efficacy: This concept refers to the conviction that a person can successfully carry out the behavior necessary to achieve a desired outcome, such as maintaining an exercise program to lose weight. Often people who have serious doubts about their capabilities, decrease their efforts and give up; whereas those with a strong sense of efficacy exert greater effort to master problems or challenges.
4. Activity-related affect: The subjective feelings that occur before, during and following an activity can influence whether a person will repeat the behavior again or maintain the behavior. What is the individual's reaction to the thought of the behavior? It is perceived as fun, enjoyable or unpleasant? A positive affect or emotional response to a behavior is likely to be repeated and behaviors associated with a negative affect are usually avoided.
5. Interpersonal influences: These are a person's perceptions concerning the behaviors, beliefs or attitudes of others. Family, peers and health professionals are sources of interpersonal influences that can influence a person's health-promoting sources of interpersonal influences that can influence a person's health-promoting behaviors. Interpersonal influences include expectation of significant others, social support (e.g. emotional encouragement) and learning through observing others or modeling.
6. Situational influences: These are direct and indirect influences on health-promoting behaviors, and include perceptions of available options, demand characteristics, and the esthetic features of the environment. An example of individual's perception of available options can include easy access to healthy alternatives such as vending machines and restaurants that provide healthy menu options. Demand characteristics can directly affect healthy behaviors through policies such as a company regulation that demands safety equipment to be worn or that establishes as 'no smoking' environment. Individuals are more apt to perform health-promotion behaviors, if they are comfortable in the environment versus feeling alienated. Environments are considered safe as well as interesting and also include desirable esthetic features that facilitate health-promoting behaviors.

Commitment to a Plan of Action

Commitment to a plan of action involves two processes; one is commitment and the other is identifying specific strategies for carrying out and reinforcing the behavior. Strategies are important because commitment alone often results in 'good intentions' and not actual performance of the behavior.

Immediate Competing Demands and Preferences

Competing demands are those behaviors over which an individual has a low level of control. For example, an unexpected work or family responsibility may compete with a planned visit to the health club and not responding to this responsibility may cause a more negative outcome than missing the exercise routine. Competing preferences are behaviors over which an individual has a high level of control; however, this control depends on the individual's ability to be self-regulating or not to 'give in'. For example, a person who chooses a high-fat food over a low-fat food, because it tastes better, has 'given in' to an urge based on a competing preference.

Behavioral Outcome

Health-promoting behavior, the outcome of the health promotion model is directed toward attaining positive health outcomes for the client. Health-promoting behaviors should result in improved health, enhanced functional ability and better quality of life at all stages of development.

Health behavior change is a cyclic phenomenon in which people progress through several stages. In the first stage, the person does not think seriously about changing behavior; by the time, the person reaches the final stage, he/she is successfully maintaining the change in behavior. Several behavioral change models have been proposed. The stage model proposed by Prochaska, Norcross and DiClemente (1994) is discussed here. As shown in Figure 4.2, the stages are:

1. Precontemplation.
2. Contemplation.
3. Preparation.
4. Action.
5. Maintenance.
6. Termination.

If the person does not succeed in changing behavior, relapse occurs.

Precontemplation Stage

In the precontemplation stage, the person typically denies having a problem, views other as having a problem, and therefore, wants others to change their behavior. They do not think about changing behavior, nor are they interested in information about the behavior. Some people believe that behaviors are not under their control and may become defensive when confronted with information, because they believe the situation is hopeless.

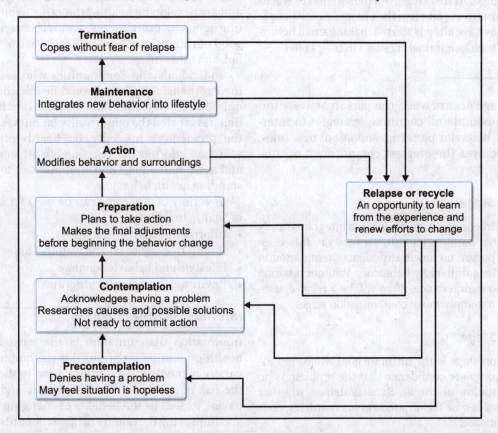

Figure 4.2: The stages of change are rarely linear. It is more common for people to recycle several times through stages. The person who takes action and has a relapse (recycles through some or all of the stages again) is more apt to be successful the next time than the individual who never takes action.

The person may have tried changing previously, but was unsuccessful and now sees the behavior as their 'fate' or that change is hopeless.

Contemplation Stage

During the contemplation stage, the person acknowledges having a problem, seriously considers changing a specific behavior, actively gathers information and verbalizes plans to change the behavior in the near future. The person, however, may not be ready to commit the action. Some people may stay in the contemplative stage for months or years before taking action. When contemplators begin the transition to the preparation stage, their thinking is clearly marked by two changes—focusing on the solution rather than the problem and thinking more about the future than the past.

Preparation Stage

The preparation stage occurs when the person undertakes cognitive and behavioral activities that prepare the person for change. At this stage, the person makes the final specific plans to accomplish the change. Some people in this stage may have already started making small behavioral changes, such as eliminating sugar in their coffee.

Action Stage

The action stage occurs when the person actively implements behavioral and cognitive strategies to interrupt previous behavior patterns, and adopt new ones. This stage requires the greatest commitment of time and energy.

Maintenance Stage

During the maintenance stage, the person integrates newly adopted behavior patterns into his/her lifestyle. This stage lasts until the person no longer experiences temptation to return to previous unhealthy behaviors. Without a strong commitment to maintenance, there will be a relapse, usually to the precontemplation or contemplation stage.

Termination Stage

The termination stage is the ultimate goal where the individual has complete confidence that the problem is no longer a temptation or threat. Experts debate whether some behaviors can be terminated versus requiring continual maintenance.

These six stages are cyclic; people generally move through one stage before progressing to the next. However, at any point a person may relapse or recycle to any previous stage. In fact, the average successful self-changer recycles through the stages several times before they make it to the top and exit the cycle. The majority of individuals who relapse return to the contemplation stage. During this time, they can think about what they learned and plan for the next action to be attempted. The strategies for the promotion of health should be adopted according to the needs of the people depending upon their social, cultural, economic and environmental background. The strategy is to strengthen the individual to achieve optimal health, which includes—proper health system, information and education, health research, welfare programs and healthy lifestyle.

NURSE'S ROLE IN HEALTH PROMOTION

Health promotion is an important component of nursing practice. It is a way to thinking that revolves around a philosophy of wholeness, wellness and well-being. In the past two decades, the public has become increasingly aware of and interested in health promotion. Many people are aware of the relationship between lifestyle and illness, and are developing health-promoting habits, such as getting adequate exercise, rest and relaxation; maintaining good nutritional and controlling the use of tobacco, alcohol, and other drugs.

Individuals and communities who seek to increase their responsibility for personal health and self-care require health education. The trend toward health promotion has created the opportunity for nurses to strengthen the profession's influence on health promotion, disseminate information that promotes an educated public, and assist individuals and communities to change long-standing health behaviors.

A variety of programs can be used for the promotion of health, including:
- Information dissemination
- Health risk appraisal and wellness assessment
- Lifestyle and behavior change
- Environmental control programs.

Information Dissemination

Information dissemination is the most basic type of health promotion program. This method makes use of a variety of media to offer information to the public about the risk of particular lifestyle choices and personal behavior, as well as the benefits of changing that behavior and improving the quality of life. Billboards, posters, brochures, newspaper features, books and health fairs all offer opportunities for the dissemination of health promotion information. Alcohol and drug abuse, driving under

CHAPTER 4   Promotion of Health

the influence of alcohol, hypertension and the need for immunizations are some of the topics that are frequently discussed. Information dissemination is a useful strategy for raising the level of knowledge and awareness of individuals and groups about health habits.

When planning information dissemination, it is important to consider factors such as cultural factors and different age groups. Knowing the best place and method to distribute information will increase the effectiveness. For example, older African Americans usually have strong ties to their churches for social support as well as religious practices. Knowing this, the church can often be the appropriate place to hold health fairs or even small group discussions on various health topics. It provides a stepping stone for providing information and suggesting resources for special needs; all done in a comfortable non-threatening environment for persons in that age group and culture.

It is just critical to know where people get 'misinformation'. Sending multiple mailings has become a marketing ploy for advertising 'miracle' vitamins, herbs and food supplements. These are heavily directed towards elders who may choose this route of purchasing items due to transportation problems that they may have.

Health Risk Appraisal and Wellness

Health risk appraisal and wellness assessment programs are used to appraise individuals of the risk factors that are inherent in their lives, in order to motivate them to reduce specific risks and develop positive health habits. Wellness assessment programs are focused on more positive methods of enhancement, in contrast to the risk factor approach used in the health appraisal. A variety of tools are available to facilitate these assessments. Some of these tools are computer based, and can therefore be offered to educational institutions and industries at a reasonable cost.

Lifestyle and Behavior Change

Lifestyle and behavior change programs require the participation of the individual, and are geared toward enhancing the quality of life and extending the life span. Individuals generally consider lifestyle changes after they are informed of the need to change their health behavior and have become aware of the potential benefits of the process. Many programs are available to the public, both on a group and individuals basis, some of which address stress management, nutrition awareness, weight control, smoking cessation and exercise.

Environmental Control Programs

Environmental control programs have been developed in response to the continuing increase of contaminants of human origin that have been introduced into environment. The amounts of contaminant that are already present in the air, food and water will affect the health of our descendants for several generations. The most common concerns of community groups are toxic and nuclear wastes, nuclear power plants, air and water pollution, and herbicide and pesticide use.

Health-promotion activities, such as the variety of programs previously discussed, involve collaborative relationships with both clients and physicians. The role of the nurse is to work with people, not for them, i.e. to act as a facilitator of the process of assessing, evaluating and understanding health. The nurse may act as advocate, consultant, teacher or coordinator of services. For example, the nurse's role in health promotion includes:

- Model healthy lifestyle behaviors and attitudes
- Facilitate client involvement in the assessment, implementation and evaluation of health goals
- Teach clients self-care strategies to enhance the fitness, improve nutrition, manage stress and enhance relationships
- Assist individuals, families and communities to increase their levels of health
- Educate clients to be effective healthcare consumers
- Assist clients, families and communities to develop and choose health-promoting options
- Guide client's development in effective problem solving and decision-making
- Reinforce client's personal and family health-promoting behaviors
- Advocate in the community for changes that promotes a healthy environment.

In these roles, the nurse may work with individuals of all age groups and diverse family units or concentrate on a specific population, such as new parents, school-age children or older adults. In any case, the nursing process is a basic tool for the nurse in a health-promotion role. Although, the process is the same, the nurse emphasizes teaching the client (who can be either an individual or a family unit) self-care responsibility. Adult clients decide the goals, determine the health-promoting plans and take the responsibility for the success of the plans.

A thorough assessment of the individual's health status is basic to health promotion. As nurses move toward greater autonomy in providing client care, expanded assessment skills are essential to provide the meaningful data needed for health planning. The guide to clinical preventive services provide direction for age-specific periodic health examination, assessment and counseling interventions. In addition, the nurse selects an appropriate health risk appraisal tool for use with clinical observation and assessment. The high-risk family is taught nutritional principles and helped to incorporate healthy food into their diets to prevent nutrition-related problems. Using an aggregate approach, the nurses assesses the community for aggregates at risk for malnutrition (e.g. school children, poor persons, older adults and the homeless), analyze health-risk data and work with others to institute programs to reduce their risk, thereby preventing malnutrition. Community multimedia education for malnutrition risk reduction and lobbying for legislation to promote resources for adequate nutrition within the community are examples of a community approach.

INDIVIDUAL HEALTH PROMOTION

At the individual level, the nurse helps the individual adopt a healthy lifestyle as appropriate to age, culture and resources. For the young child, this includes educating and supporting the parent to provide health-enhancing care. Using the perspective of the family as client, the approach includes the entire family and planning with the family on how to adopt healthy lifestyle activities. These activities range from balanced nutrition to planning for relaxation activities for the family. A wellness inventory helps the nurse design an intervention targeted to the family's awareness of personal self-care. At the aggregate level, the nurse educates school personnel about healthy lunches for the aggregate of students or teachers. Regardless the level of health need or the client system at which care begins, the ultimate goal of the nurse is health promotion of the total community and its constitutes. Participating with community leaders and citizens to establish nutrition education, and making nutritious foods available to all community members are examples of a community-level approach.

Although, an important starting point is the care of the failure of thrive child, the nurse must recognize that solving the immediate problem is not sufficient. The child's health problem is viewed within a broader context of an optimally healthy child, family, aggregate of children and community. This approach necessitates not that the nursing interventions be limited to solving the immediate problem of weight gain, but rather that care be oriented toward interventions that promote optimal health for the child, family, aggregate of high-risk children and the total community.

A second example concerns a referral of a middle-aged man with coronary heart disease (CHD) (Table 4.1). The immediate goal of the nurse is to provide care that will help the individual client to resolve his/her illness. Therefore, teaching him/her about the effects and side effects of the medications and how to monitor the condition at home are important interventions. Within the context of predisposing genetic, lifestyle and environmental factors relative of CHD, the family members are also given information about illness, including early recognition of signs and symptoms for themselves. Assessing the prevalence of CHD among high-risk aggregates is also an important aspect of illness care. An example is providing certificate in Panchayat Raj classes in Karnataka to monolingual Kannada speaking persons in the community. At their community level, it is important to assess whether there are adequate providers and resources for identifying and treating heart disease in the community.

Prevention care is also addressed at the individual level by teaching measures, such as stress reduction, low-fat nutrition and progressive exercise, to prevent recurrence of the disease. For high-risk family members, low-fat nutrition, smoking cessation and regular moderate exercise are important preventive measures. Providing exercise programs to workers in high stress and sedentary occupations is an example of an aggregate level preventive intervention, and multimedia campaigns to provide intensive education to the community about prevention of heart disease during the particular month of each year are an example of a community intervention.

Health promotion care similarly includes encouraging individuals to adopt a health-promoting lifestyle and helping them to become aware of their own power to do so. The nurse can also encourage families to incorporate health-promoting activities into their daily lives. This might include taking walks, swimming together or joining an intergenerational baseball or bowling team in which families compete with other families. Aggregates can also benefit from heart-healthy classes or activities that are cultural specific to particular aggregates, such as Indian women or Indian teenage girls. These activities can include stress management, well-balanced nutrition, exercise or any other topic that can promote heart health. When looking at the total community, an example of a health promotion intervention is participating in a coalition to plan for parks and recreation areas within the community that are safe and accessible to the population.

Table 4.1: Community health levels of care: Coronary heart disease (CHD)

Focus of care	Client system			
	Individual	Family	Aggregate	Community
Illness care	• Administer medications • Monitor heart rate of individual client in the home setting	• Teach signs/symptoms of CHD to high-risk family members	• Assess prevalence of CHD in the community • Teach classes for specific high-risk groups about what to do in an emergency	• Assess the community for accessibility and adequacy of care providers for client with heart disease
Illness/Disease	• Teach low-fat nutrition, progressive exercise and relaxation to client, to prevent recurrence of heart disease	• Teach low-fat nutrition and importance of regular exercise, and relaxation to high-risk family members to prevent heart disease	• Develop classes for specific high-risk groups about cardiovascular risk reduction	• Community-wide multimedia education for cardiovascular risk reduction
Health	• Empower individual to adopt health promotion lifestyle	• Plan with family to incorporate health-promoting activities into lifestyle	• Provide group education (classes) regarding benefits of regular exercise	• Work with community leaders and citizens to establish safe parks for community activities

In summary, the concepts of health, health promotion and community are inextricably linked. It is difficult to discuss one without including the others. It is also important that nurses examine their definitions and beliefs about each concept as the basis for their practice. The essence of the community-oriented nursing perspective is the ability to see the totality of community, while addressing its component parts and at the same time, to see the total needs for health protection, illness and disease prevention, and illness care and management. It is the integrative relationship among all these levels that distinguishes community oriented from nursing in more circumscribed settings, such as hospitals and clinics.

A rural health outreach program serves migrant workers, their families and other vulnerable populations in the local community. The program's goals include increased knowledge about risk factors, services and self-care, improved community health, increased access and affordability of individual, and community level health promotion services and reduced barriers to health services. The program offers health promotion and disease prevention educational materials, and classes in English and Spanish throughout the regions in church, schools, community centers, fire departments and migrant camps. In addition, clinics have been established in eight local sites across the country. Lay health promoters from the migrant community have been trained to deliver basic health education and resource information. Clinic services include health risk appraisal, disease screening, immunizations, health education, counseling and referral. Funding from a variety of public and private sources supports the program. It is essential that the program show effective outcomes, if it is to sustain funding.

CONCLUSION

Health promotion is the process of enabling people to increase control over and to improve health in respect of physical, mental, social and spiritual well-being. The prior condition required for health education includes education, enabling act and mediation. Here the education will help people to adopt healthy lifestyles, once they are aware about advantages of healthy practices and hazards of unhealthy practices. The education is improving people to adapt healthy practices and enable the people to develop the ability or means to do accordingly, i.e. an individual need to have control over unhealthy practices, which are injurious to health. Control over unhealthy practices and adoption of healthy practices help to achieve the given health. There are different interests related to health practices prevailing in a community or within society. So, there is need to mediate those different health practices to the people by Health Personnel including Nursing Personnel and social groups come to compromise for the promotion of health. For the promotion enabling act are needed, which means a status empowering a person or body to take certain action, especially to make regulation for enabling laws relative to prevention of accidents, food adulterations, etc. The promotion of health can be achieved through taking adequate nutrition, daily exercises, getting good sleep and rest, maintaining proper environmental sanitation, proper personal hygiene, leading good and healthy lifestyle, undergoing periodical health check-up getting timely immunizations and solving proper education, etc.

Maintenance of Health

CHAPTER 5

INTRODUCTION

The chapter 'Maintenance of Health' will be a continuation of previous chapter on 'Promotion of Health'. It deals with the concept of health protection, preventive health services, disability, limitation and rehabilitation. Level and Clark (1965) define three levels of prevention—primary, secondary and tertiary. There are five steps that describe these levels:

1. Health promotion.
2. Specific protection are primary preventions.
3. Early diagnosis.
4. Prompt treatment to limit disability are secondary preventions.
5. Restoration and rehabilitation are tertiary preventions.

In the model used by Leavell and Clark, primary prevention precedes any disease symptoms. The purpose of primary prevention is to encourage optimal health and to increase the person's resistance to illness (Edelman and Mandle, 1986). Examples of primary prevention include health education concerning the hazards of smoking and specific protection against a particular disease such as the vaccine against poliomyelitis.

The second level, secondary prevention, presumes the presence of a disease or illness. Screening procedures such as a blood sugar test for a client with diabetes mellitus and the Denver developmental screening tests to assess developmental delays, are the facets of secondary prevention. Screening procedures facilitate early discovery and allow treatment to begin before the illness progresses. Disability limitation, another step in secondary prevention is also more effective in the early stages of a disease.

Tertiary prevention relates to situations where a disability is already present. The goal of tertiary prevention is to restore individuals to their optimal level of functioning within the limitations imposed by their condition. The interventions related to these levels of prevention are discussed as follows with preview of health promotion.

HEALTH PROMOTION

Health promotion is a behavior directed toward achieving a greater level of health. Illness prevention is a behavior directed toward reducing the threat of illness or disease and health maintenance is directed toward keeping a current state of health. Health promotion is a behavior motivated by the desire to increase well-being and actualize human health potential. Health protection or illness prevention is the behavior motivated by a desire to actively avoid illness, detect it early or maintain functioning within the constraint of illness.

To achieve health and continuously remain healthy, the individuals are required to adopt some preventive, promotive and protective measures. These measures help to maintain the health. The main health maintenance strategies include nutrition, exercise, hygiene, reduce stress, healthcare services, safe environment, etc.

Health promotion activities take place before disease occurs and can be considered as a part of geared toward raising the level of the health and well-being of the individual, family or community. These activities can be carried out on a government level (e.g. a national program to improve knowledge of nutrition) or on a personal level (e.g. an individual exercise program).

Health promotion programs on an individual level can be active or passive. With passive strategies, the client is recipient of the health promotion effort. Many health professionals participate in national programs to define and institute these passive strategies. Examples of passive government strategies are maintaining the cleanliness of water and promoting a healthy environment by enforcing sewage regulations to decrease the spread of disease. Active strategies depend on individuals' commitment and involvement in adopting a program directed toward their health promotion. Active strategies are more important; in that they encourage individuals to take control of their lives and assume the responsibility for their health. Examples of active strategies that involve changes in lifestyle are:

1. A diet management program to improve nutrition.
2. A self-help program to reduce stress related to parenting.
3. An exercise program to improve muscle strength and endurance.
4. A combination diet and exercise regime for weight reduction or control. For optimal health and well-being, a combination of both active and passive strategies is suggested (Edelman and Mandle, 1986).

Nutrition Education and Interventions

Nutrition is the sum of all the interactions between organism and the food it consumes. In other words, nutrition is 'what a person eats and how the body uses it'. Nutrition has an impact on health. Nutrition is organic and inorganic substances found in foods and are required for body functioning. People require essential nutrients in food for the growth and maintenance of all body tissues and the normal functioning of all body processes. The food or food component, if not consumed in proportion to requirement, leads to some health problems. For example, eating too less or more nutrients will determine health. Eating too many calories leads to obesity, causing hypertension and diabetic mellitus. Less intake of calories and proteins in children leads to malnutrition, which results in marasmus and kwashiorkor. So, both inadequate and excessive intake of nutrients results in malnutrition. These nutritional interventions comprise food distribution and nutrition improvement of vulnerable groups; child feeding programs; food fortification; nutrition education, etc.

Good eating habits means holding down the amount of fat (saturated), cholesterol, sugar, salt and include a wide variety of plant foods such as whole grain foods, beans, nuts, fresh fruits and vegetables in the diet, and some long range effects of certain excess nutrients are among many factors involved in certain diseases such as coronary artery disease and cancer, etc.

Some foods are used for decreasing the risk of diseases such as roughage diet that decreases the chances of constipation, thereby reducing chances of cancer. So, individuals have to take well-balanced diet to stay healthy. So, there is a need to take properly balanced diet throughout life to prevent illness and maintenance of health to keep people/person healthy.

Health Education

Health education is one of the most cost-effective interventions. A large number of diseases could be prevented with little or no medical intervention, if people were adequately informed about them and if they were encouraged to take necessary precautions in time. Recognizing this truth, the WHO constitution states that "the extension to all people of the benefits of medical, psychological and related knowledge is essential to the fullest attainment of health." The targets for educational efforts may include the general public, patients, priority groups, health providers, community leaders and decision-makers.

Lifestyle and Behavioral Changes

The conventional public health measures or interventions have not been successful in making inroads into lifestyle reforms. The action of prevention in this case, both individual and community responsibility for health, the physician and in fact, each health worker acting as an educator than a therapist. Health education is a basic element of all health activity. It is of paramount importance in changing the views, behavior and habits of people.

Since the health promotion comprises a broad spectrum of activities, a well-conceived health promotion program would first attempt to identify the 'target groups' or at-risk individuals in a population and then direct more appropriate message to them. Goals must be defined. Means and alternative methods of accomplishing them must be explored. It involves 'organizational, political, social and economic interventions, which is designed to facilitate environmental and behavioral adaptations that will improve or protect health'.

Exercise

Exercise is the physical activity performed to maintain muscle tone and joint mobility, to enhance physical functioning of the body systems and to improve physical fitness. Activity and tolerance is the type and amount of exercise or daily living activity an individual is able to perform without experiencing adverse effects.

Immobility affects almost every body organ and systems adversely. Complications also include psychological problems. The problems of immobility include diseases such as osteoporosis and atrophy, contractions, diminished cardiac reserve, orthostatic hypertension, venous stasis, edema, thrombus formation, decreased metabolic rates, negative nitrous oxide (N_2O) balance, decreased respiratory movements and pooling of secretions,

CHAPTER 5 — Maintenance of Health

urinary stasis, retention and infection, constipation are varying emotional problems.

Exercise, by contrast, provides many benefits to the same body organs and systems. It is directed toward physical fitness. Physical exercises strengthen body muscles, bones and immune system. Exercise in case of heart disease, strengthen the heart muscles, thereby reducing risk of heart attack. Exercise such as stretching, aerobic and anaerobic helps in keeping the body physically fit. Stretching increases the ranging motions, walking and running improve cardiovascular system.

Hygiene

Hygiene is the science of health and its maintenance. Personal hygiene is the self-care by which people attend some functions such as bathing, toileting, general body hygiene and grooming. Hygiene is the highly personal matter determined by individual values and practices. It involves care of the skin, hair, nails, teeth, oral and nasal cavities, eyes, ears, perineal and genital areas. These hygiene conditions prevent the entry of pathogens and prevent infection.

Hygiene for maintenance of health includes food hygiene. Food hygiene is important to prevent the occurrence of diseases. Food hygiene includes hygiene practices in food production, food handling, food distribution and serving all types of food such as fruits, vegetables, meat, milk, fish, etc. Improper hygiene in food leads to diseases such as typhoid, diarrhea, etc. Proper washing of hands, and washing of fruits and vegetable before eating should be practiced in daily life for the maintenance of health.

Stress-free Life

Stress is a state of physiological and psychological tension that affects the whole person physically, emotionally, intellectually, socially and spiritually. Usually the effects are mixed, because stress affects the whole person. Physical stress can threaten a person's physiological homeostasis. Emotionally, stress can provide negative or non-constructive feelings about the self. Intellectually, stress can influence a person's perceptual and problem-solving abilities. Socially, stress can alter a person's relationship with others and spiritually stress can challenge ones belief and values.

Many illness have been linked to stress. Such as metabolic disorders (e.g. diabetes), skin disorders (e.g. eczema, pruritus, urticaria), respiratory disorders [e.g. asthma, fever, tuberculosis (TB)], cardiovascular disorders [coronary artery disease (CAD), essential hypotension] gastrointestinal disorder (e.g. constipation, diarrhea, duodenal ulcers, anorexia nervosa and obesity), menstrual irregularities, musculoskeletal disorders (rheumatoid arthritis, low back pain, etc.).

The cognitive indicators or thinking responses to stress include problem solving, structuring, self-control, suppression and fantasy. The interventions for clients who are stressed, are aimed at encouraging health promotion strategies (i.e. exercise, healthy diet, adequate rest and time management), minimizing anxiety, mediating anger, teaching about specific relaxation techniques and implementing crisis intervention are needed. So, for maintenance of health, people need to take or implement stress-reduction measures.

Stress can be the result of uncertainty, workload, low income and dissatisfaction of job. When stress remains for long period, there will be a negative impact on health. Simple stresses can be easily reduced and homeostasis is maintained. In order to cope up with stress, relaxation techniques are used such as biofeedback, meditation, deep breathing, walking, gardening, yoga, massage, listening to music, watching television, etc. These techniques increases the persons capability to cope up with stress.

Healthcare Services

Healthcare system is the totality of services offered by all health disciplines. Previously, the primary purpose of a healthcare system was to provide care to the ill and injured. However, with increasing awareness of health promotion, illness prevention and level of wellness, healthcare systems are changing. The services provided by a healthcare system are commonly categorized according to type and level. The three types of healthcare services are often described in a way correlated with levels of disease prevention as given below:

1. Health promotion and illness prevention (primary prevention).
2. Specific protection.
3. Early diagnosis and treatment (secondary prevention).
4. Rehabilitation and health restriction (tertiary prevention).

Primary Prevention

Primary care is providing of integrated, accessible healthcare services by medical doctors/clinicians, who are accountable for addressing large majority of personal healthcare needs, developing a sustained partnership with patients and practicing in the context of family and community. Primary health care is the essential care made universally accessible to individuals and families in a community. Health care is made available to them through their full participation and is provided at a cost that community and country can afford. Primary care is a part of primary health care. Although, primary care practitioners are encouraged to consider the clients' biopsychosocial needs, interventions are directed primarily at the pathophysiologic process. The public health refers to organized community efforts designed to prevent disease and promote health. In India, we have subcenters, primary health centers, community health centers, major hospitals at district level, medical college hospitals, cater the healthcare needs of the people. In addition, private clinics, private hospitals and corporate hospitals are there to cater the healthcare needs of community in which people consult clinicians/doctors to keep their health maintained, and minor problems treated by clinics and health centers. The minor problems that are not treated properly, may lead to major health problem. Therefore people consult proper doctor/clinician for the adverse effects; they can approach hospitals for further treatment and other services. In this way, available healthcare services help to maintain health of the people.

SPECIFIC PROTECTION

To avoid disease altogether is the ideal protection, but this is possible only in a limited number of cases. The following are some of the currently available interventions aimed at specific protection:
1. Immunization.
2. Use of specific nutrients.
3. Chemoprophylaxis.
4. Protection against occupational hazards.
5. Protection against accidents.
6. Protection from carcinogens.
7. Avoidance of allergens.
8. Control of specific hazards in the general environment, e.g. air pollution and noise control.
9. Control of consumer product quality and safety of foods, drugs, cosmetics, etc.

Health Protection

The term 'health protection', which is quite often used, is not synonymous with specific protection. Health protection is defined as the provision of conditions for normal mental and physical functioning of the human being individually and in the group; it includes the promotion of health, the prevention of sickness and curative and restorative medicine in all its aspects. In fact, health/community development program, associated with activities such as literacy campaigns, education and food production. Thus, health protection covers a much wider field of health activities than specific protection.

Early Diagnosis and Treatment

A World Health Organization (WHO) Expert Committee defined early detection of health impairment as "the detection of disturbances of homeostatic and compensatory mechanism, while biochemical, morphological and functional changes are still reversible." Thus, in order to prevent overt disease or disablement, if possible, the criteria of diagnosis should be based on early biochemical, morphological and functional changes that precede the occurrence of manifested signs and symptoms. This is of particular importance in chronic diseases.

Early detection and treatment are the main interventions of disease control. The earlier a disease is diagnosed and treated, the better it is from the point of view of prognosis and preventing the occurrence of further cases (secondary cases) or any long-term disability. It is same as stamping out the 'spark' rather than calling the fire brigade to put out the fire.

Strictly speaking, early diagnosis and treatment cannot be called 'prevention', because the disease has already commenced in the host. However, since early diagnosis and treatment intercepts the disease process, as much as the goal of prevention 'to oppose or intercept a cause to prevent, or dissipate its effect'.

Early diagnosis and treatment, though not as effective and economical as 'primary prevention', may be critically important in reducing the high morbidity and mortality in certain diseases such as essential hypertension, cervical and breast cancer. For many others such as tuberculosis, leprosy and sexually transmitted disease (STD), early diagnosis and treatment are the only effective mode of intervention. Early effective therapy has made it possible to shorten considerably the period of communicability and reduce the mortality from acute communicable diseases.

Mass Treatment

A mass treatment approach is used in the control of certain diseases such as yaws, pinta, bejel, trachoma and filaria. The rationale for a mass treatment program is the existence of at least four to five cases of latent infection for each clinical case of active disease in the community. Patients with a latent (incubating) infection may develop disease at any time. In such cases, mass treatment is a critical factor in the interruption of disease transmission. There are many variants of mass treatment—total mass treatment, juvenile mass treatment, selective mass treatment, depending upon the nature and prevalence of disease in the community.

Disability Limitation

When a patient reports late in the pathogenesis phase, the mode of intervention is disability limitation. The objective of this intervention is to prevent or halt the transition of the disease process from impairment to handicap.

Concept of Disability

The sequence of events leading to disability and handicap have been stated as follows:

    Disease → Impairment → Disability → Handicap

The WHO has defined these terms as detailed below.

Impairment: It is defined as "any loss or abnormality of psychological, physiological or anatomical structure or function." For example, loss of foot, defective vision or mental retardation. An impairment may be visible or invisible, temporary or permanent, progressive or regressive. Further, one impairment may lead to the development of 'secondary' impairment as in the case of leprosy, where damage to nerves (primary impairment) may lead to plantar ulcers (secondary impairment).

Disability: Because of an impairment, the affected person may be unable to carry out certain activities considered normal for his/her age, sex, etc. This inability to carry out certain activities is termed 'disability'. A disability has been defined as "any restriction or lack of ability to perform an activity in the manner or within the range considered normal for a human being."

Handicap: As a result of disability, the person experiences certain disadvantages in life and is not able to discharge the obligations required of him/her and play the role expected of him/her in the society. This is termed 'handicap' and is defined as "a disadvantage for a given individual, resulting from an impairment or a disability that limits or prevents the fulfillment of a role that is normal (depending on age, sex, and social and cultural factors) for that individual."

The intervention in disability will often be social or environmental as well as medical; while impairment, which is the earliest stage, has a large medical component, disability and handicap, which are later stages, have large social and environmental components in terms of dependence and social cost.

Disability Prevention

Another concept is 'disability prevention'. It relates to all the levels of prevention:
1. Reducing the occurrence of impairment such as immunization against polio (primary prevention).
2. Disability limitation by appropriate treatment (secondary prevention).
3. Preventing the transition of disability into handicap (tertiary prevention).

The major causes of disabling impairments in the developing countries are communicable diseases, malnutrition, low quality of perinatal care and accidents. These are responsible for about 70% of cases of disability in developing countries. Primary prevention is the most effective way of dealing with the disability problem in developing countries.

Rehabilitation

Rehabilitation has been defined as "the combined and coordinated use of medical, social, educational and vocational measures for training and retraining the individual to the highest possible level of functional ability." It includes all measures aimed at reducing the impact of disabling and handicapping conditions, and at enabling the disabled and handicapped to achieve social integration. Social integration has been defined as the active participation of disabled and handicapped people in the mainstream of community life.

Rehabilitation medicine has emerged in recent years as a medical specialty. It involves disciplines such as physical medicine or physiotherapy, occupational therapy, speech therapy, audiology, psychology, education, social work, vocational guidance and placement services. The following areas of concern in rehabilitation have been identified:
1. Medical rehabilitation: Restoration of function.
2. Vocational rehabilitation: Restoration of the capacity to earn a livelihood.
3. Social rehabilitation: Restoration of family and social relationships.
4. Psychological rehabilitation: Restoration of personal dignity and confidence.

Rehabilitation is no longer looked upon as an extracurricular activity of the physician. The current view is that the responsibility of the doctor does not end when the temperature touches normal and retrained to live and work within the limits of his/her disability, but to the hilt of his/her capacity. As such medical rehabilitation should start very early in the process of medical treatment.

Example of rehabilitation are—establishing schools for the blind, provision of aids for the crippled, reconstructive surgery in leprosy, muscle re-education and graded exercises in neurological disorders such as polio, change of profession for a more suitable one and modification of life in general in the case of tuberculosis, cardiac patients and others. The purpose of rehabilitation is to make productive people out of non-productive people.

It is now recognized that rehabilitation is a difficult and demanding task that seldom gives totally satisfactory results, but needs enthusiastic cooperation from different segments of society as well as expertise, equipment and funds, which are not readily available for this purpose even in affluent societies. It is further recognized that interventions at earlier stages are more feasible, will yield results, and are less demanding of scarce resources.

Environment

A comprehensive approach to health promotion requires environmental modifications such as provision of safe water, installation of sanitary latrines, control of insects and rodents, improvement of housing, etc. The history of medicine has shown that many infectious diseases have been successfully controlled in western countries through environmental modifications, even prior to the development of specific vaccines or chemotherapeutic drugs. Environmental interventions are nonclinical and do not involve the physician.

Living in safe environment help to maintain the health of the individual. A safe home requires well-maintained flooring and carpets, a non-skid bathtub/shower face/bathroom, functioning smoke alarms that are strategically placed and knowledge of fire escape routes. Outdoor areas such as swimming pool need to be safely secured and maintained. Adequate lighting, both inside and outside, will minimize the potential for accidents.

In the workplace, machinery, industrial belts and pulleys and chemicals may create danger. Worker fatigue, noise and air pollution or working at greater heights/in subterranean areas may also create occupational hazards. Healthcare workers need to maintain an awareness of potential risks and adequate street lighting, safe water and sewage treatment, and regulation of sanitation in food buying and handling, all contribute to a healthy and hazard-free community. A safe and secure community strives to be free of excess noise, crime, traffic congestion, dilapidated housing or unprotected creeks and landfills, and environment should be free from rodents and insects.

There should be a good social interaction and people should be satisfied at their workplace, home, etc. So, health is maintained by providing safe surroundings to man in which he/she lives. In other words, safe environment help in the maintenance of health of people, who are living in the community.

TYPES OF HEALTH PROMOTION PROGRAMS

A variety of programs can be used for the promotion of health, including:
1. Information dissemination.
2. Health appraisal and wellness assessment.
3. Lifestyle and behavior change.
4. Worksite wellness programs.
5. Environmental control programs.

Information Dissemination

Information dissemination is the most basic type of health promotion program. This method makes use of a variety of media to offer information to the public about the risk of particular lifestyle choices and personal behavior as well as the benefits of changing that behavior and improving the quality of life. Billboards, posters, brochures, newspaper features, books and health fairs all offer opportunities for the dissemination of health promotion information. Alcohol and drug abuse, driving under the influence of alcohol, good nutrition and hypertension are some of the topics frequently discussed. Recently, information about acquired immunodeficiency syndrome (AIDS), including how it is transmitted, techniques for prevention and the issue of sexual responsibility has been distributed. The intent is to reduce unjustified fear, correct the misinformation, and educate the public about this disease. Information dissemination is a useful strategy for raising the level of knowledge and awareness of individuals and groups about health habits.

Health Appraisal and Wellness Assessment Programs

Health appraisal and wellness assessment programs are used to apprise individuals for the risk factors that are inherent in their lives in order to motivate them to reduce specific risks and develop positive health habits. Wellness assessment programs are focused on more positive methods of enhancement, in contrast to the risk factor approach used in the health appraisal. A variety of tools are available to facilitate these assessments. Some of these tools are computer based and can therefore be offered to educational institutions and industries at a reasonable cost.

Lifestyle and Behavior Change Programs

Lifestyle and behavior change programs require the participation of the individual and are geared toward enhancing the quality of life and extending the life span. Individuals generally consider lifestyle changes after they have been informed of the need to change their health behavior and become aware of the potential benefits of the process. Many programs are available to the public, both on a group and individual basis, some of which address stress management, nutrition awareness, weight control, smoking cessation and exercise.

Worksite Wellness Programs

Worksite wellness programs are found in a variety of settings and are generally developed to serve the needs of individual spending a great deal of time in the work environment. These include programs that address air quality standards for the office, classroom or plant; programs aimed at specific population such as accident prevention for the machine worker or back-saver programs for the individual involved in heavy lifting; programs to screen for high blood pressure or health enhancement programs such as fitness information and relaxation techniques.

Environmental Control Programs

Environmental control programs have been developed in response to the recent growth in the number of contaminants of human origin that have been introduced into our environment (Logan and Dawkins 1986). The amount of contaminants that are already present in the air, food, and water, will affect the health of our descendants for several generations. The most common concerns of community groups are toxic and nuclear wastes, nuclear power plants, air and water pollution, and herbicide and pesticide spraying.

SITES FOR HEALTH PROMOTION ACTIVITIES

Health promotion programs are found in many settings. Programs and activities may be offered to individuals and families in the home or in the community setting, at schools, hospitals or worksites. Some individuals may feel more comfortable having the nurse, diet counselor or fitness expert come to their home for teaching and following up individual needs. This type of program, however, is not cost-effective for most individuals. Many people prefer the group approach, find it more motivating, and enjoy the socializing and group support. Most programs offered in the community are group oriented.

Community Health Programs

Community health programs are frequently offered by cities and towns. This type of program depends on the current concerns and the expertise of the sponsoring department or group. Program offerings may include health promotion, specific protection, and screening for early detection of disease. The local health department may offer a townwide immunization program or blood pressure screening. The fire department may disseminate fire prevention information; the police may offer a bicycle safety program for children or a safe-driving campaign for young adults.

Hospitals began the emphasis on health promotion and prevention by focusing on the health of their employees. Because of the stress involved in caring for the sick and the various shifts that nurses and other healthcare workers must work, the lifestyle and health habits of healthcare employees was seen as a priority.

Programs offered by healthcare organizations initially began with the specific focus of prevention, i.e. infection control, fire prevention and fire drills, limiting exposure to X-rays and the prevention of back injuries. Gradually, issues related to the health and lifestyle of the employee were addressed with programs such as smoking cessation, exercise and fitness, stress reduction, and time management. Increasingly, hospitals have offered a variety of these programs and others (e.g. women's health) to the community as well as to their employees. This community activity of the healthcare institution enhances the public image of the hospital, increases the health of the surrounding population and generates some additional income.

School Health Promotion Programs

School health promotion programs may serve as a foundation for children of all ages to learn basic knowledge about personal hygiene and issues in the health sciences. Because school is the focus of a child's life for so many years, the school provides a cost-effective and convenient setting for health-focused programs. The school nurse may teach programs about basic nutrition, dental care, activity and play, drug and alcohol abuse, domestic violence, child abuse, and issues related to sexuality and pregnancy. Classroom teachers may include health-related topics in their lesson plans, e.g. the way that the normal heart functions or the need for clean air and water in the environment.

Worksite Health Promotion Programs

Worksite programs for health promotion have developed the need for business to control the rising cost of health care and employee absenteeism (Greiner 1987). Many industries feel that both employers and employees can get benefit from healthy lifestyle behavior. The convenience of the worksite setting makes these programs particularly attractive to many adults who would otherwise not be aware of them or motivated to attend them. Health promotion programs may be held in the company cafeteria so that employees can watch a film or have a group discussion during their lunch break. Program offerings include diet, relaxation techniques or physical fitness. Benefits to the worker may include an increased feeling of well-being, fitness, weight control and decreased stress. Benefits to the employer may include an increase in employee motivation and productivity, an increase in employee morale, a decrease in absenteeism, and a lower rate of employee turnover, all of which may decrease business and healthcare costs.

NURSE'S ROLE IN HEALTH PROMOTION AND ITS MAINTENANCE

Changes in the healthcare system, the demands of society, environmental and social issues, and the increased use of modern technology have all affected the role of the nurse. Clients are spending less time in acute care facilities. The focus is shifting to community and preventive nursing services. Nurses, as the largest group of healthcare workers, must prepare for the shift in emphasis and anticipate the nursing services that consumers will require. The nurse may act as advocate, consultant, teacher or coordinator of service. For example, the nurse's role in health promotion accompanying is detailed in Box 5.1. In this role, the nurse may work with all age groups or be limited to a specific population, e.g. new parents, school-age children or senior citizens. In any case, the nursing process is a basic tool for then nurse in a health promotion role. Although the process is the same, the emphasis is on teaching the client self-care responsibility. The clients decide the goals, determine the health promotion plans and take the responsibility for the success of the plans. The steps of the nursing process in health promotion are health assessment, formulation of a nursing diagnosis, development of a health promotion/protection plan, implementation of the plan and evaluation.

Box 5.1: Nurse's role in health promotion

- Model healthy lifestyle behaviors and attitudes
- Facilitate client involvement in the assessment, implementation and evaluation of health goals
- Teach clients self-care strategies to enhance fitness, improve nutrition, manage stress and enhance relationships
- Assist individuals, families and communities to increase their levels of health
- Educate clients to be effective healthcare consumers
- Assist clients, families and communities to develop and choose health-promoting options
- Guide clients' development in effective problem solving and decision-making
- Reinforce clients' personal and family health-promoting behaviors
- Advocate in the community for changes that promote a healthy environment

CONCLUSION

Maintenance of health is an important health promotional activity, need to be carried for target groups to achieve the health and continued to be healthy to lead their preventive life and its maintenance. The three levels of prevention help in the promotion of health and its maintenance. Health promotion programs are found in many settings. Health promotion activities carried out in worksite includes health assessment, stress management, prevention of accidents, prohibit smoking, nutritional education, exercise and stress. Health promotional activity of adolescents are carried out to reduce behavioral and lifestyle problems and for prevention of risk-taking behavior such as reckless driving, indulging in several activities and antisocial behaviors, etc.

Health promotion activity requires involvement of parents, education and non-educational actions in school. Health promotion activity very well need workers, children and elderly person according to small changes in the developmental process. Health status are conditions related to disease, nutritional condition and pregnancy (women) and others.

SECTION 2

Determinants of Health

Part I : **Eugenics as Determinant of Health**
  Eugenics

Part II : **Environment as Determinant of Health**
  A. *Physical Environment*
  - Water as a Determinant of Health
  - Air as a Determinant of Health
  - Light as a Determinant of Health
  - Ventilation as a Determinant of Health
  - Noise as a Determinant of Health
  - Radiation Exposure as a Determinant of Health
  - Climate as a Determinant of Health
  - Housing as a Determinant of Health
  - Sanitation: Disposal of Waste
  - Communication, Infrastructure Facilities and Linkages

  B. *Biological Environment*
  - Forestation
  - Bacterial and Viral Agents: Host and Immunity
  - Arthropods
  - Rodents
  - Food Hygiene

  C. *Sociocultural Environment*
  - Sociocultural Determinants
  - Introduction to Lifestyle
  - Lifestyle: Hygiene
  - Lifestyle: Physical Activity
  - Financial Management

Part I

Eugenics as Determinant of Health

- Eugenics

Part 1

Eugenics as Determinant of Health

Eugenics

CHAPTER 6

INTRODUCTION

The determinant refers to a cause, which occur in a particular way; to be the decision factor in or, which firmly decides. The 'determinants' is a factor, which determines the nature or outcome of something. For example, the gene determining the character and development of particular cells in an organism.

Health is multifactorial. Multiple variables influence a person's health status. Some of these are internal factors such as the person's culture and physical environment. In other words, the factors, which influence health can be both internally (within the individual) and externally in the society in which the person lives. There are number of factors affecting both individual and gray's (community) health, which includes eugenics, environment, food hygiene, sociocultural system, lifestyles, hygiene, physical activity and financial.

Eugenics is the science of using controlled breeding to increase the occurrence of desirable, i.e. human biology, which includes genetic inheritance and the process of maturation and aging as well as the complex network of structures and systems that compose the human body (internal environment). Environment, i.e. external environment consists of those things to which individual are exposed after conception and birth such as physical, biological and psychosocial:

1. Physical environment includes housing, water, air, light, noise and excrete disposal with which man is in constant interaction.
2. Biological environment includes all living things and surroundings including the man. For example, animals, rodents, microorganisms and plants. Some of them are useful to human life and some others are harmful to human health, e.g. pathogenic, bacteria, virus, etc.
3. Psychosocial environment or personal environment, which includes the individual ways of lining sociocultural aspects, lifestyles, home, school, workplace and at neighbor, etc.

GENETICS

Genetics is the branch of biological science, which deals with the transmission of characteristics from parents to offspring. Human genetics has emerged as a basic biological science for understanding the endogenous factors in health and disease, and the complete interaction between natures and nurture. The discovery of biological role of nucleic acids, the uncovering structure of genetic information and its role in regulating life process and their importance are still under process in certain studies. Prior to study of eugenics, we should know the related concepts of genetics such as chromosomes, genes, etc.

Nucleic Acid

Nucleic acid contains the genetics instructions for the development and function of living things. All known cellular life and some viruses contain deoxyribonucleic acid (DNA). The main role of DNA in the cell is the long-term storage of information. It is often compared to a blueprint, since, it contains the instructions to construct other components of the cell such as proteins and ribonucleic acid (RNA) molecules. The DNA segments that carry genetic information are called genes, but other DNA sequences have structural purposes or are involved in regulating the expression of genetic information (Figs 6.1A to D).

Any of the group of complex compounds found in all living cells and viruses are composed of purines, pyrimidines, carbohydrates and phosphoric acid. Nucleic acid in the form of DNA and RNA control cellular function and heredity.

Chromosome

In the nucleus of each cell, the DNA molecules is packed into thread-like structures called chromosomes. Each chromosome is made up of DNA and proteins that are found in cells. A chromosome is a singular piece of DNA,

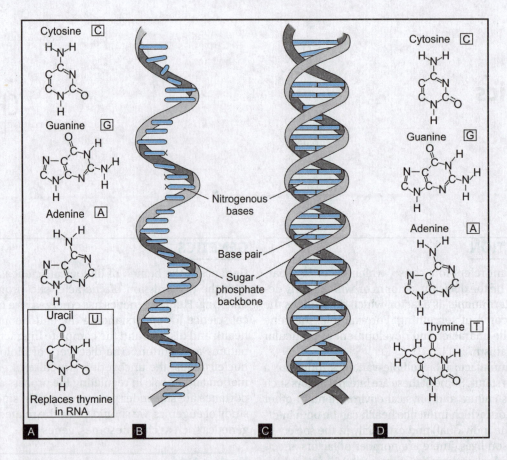

Figures 6.1A to D: Nucleic acids. **A.** Nitrogenous bases of ribonucleic acid (RNA); **B.** Structure of RNA; **C.** Deoxyribonucleic acid (DNA) structure; **D.** Nitrogenous bases of DNA.

which contains many genes, regulatory elements and other nucleotide sequences. Chromosomes also contain DNA-bound proteins, which serve to package the DNA and control its functions. The word chromosome comes from the Greek (chroma means 'color') and (soma means 'body') due to their property of being stained very strongly by some dyes. Chromosomes vary extensively between different organisms. Chromosomes are packaged by proteins into a condensed structure called chromatin.

Chromosomes are not visible in the cell's nucleus not even under a microscope, when the cell is not dividing. However, the DNA that makes up chromosomes, becomes more tightly packed during cell division and then visible under a microscope. Most of the researchers who know today about chromosomes was learned by observing chromosomes during cell division. Each chromosome has a constriction point called centromere, which divides the chromosome into two sections or 'arms'. The short arm of the chromosome is labeled as 'p arm'. The long arm of the chromosome is labeled as 'q arm'. The location of the centromere on each chromosome gives the chromosome its characteristic shape and is also used to describe the location of specific genes (Fig. 6.2).

In humans, each cell normally contains 23 pairs of chromosomes, for a total of 46. In which, 22 pairs are called autosomes, which look alike in both males and females. The 23rd pair is the sex chromosomes, which differs between males and females. Females have two copies of the X chromosome, while males have one X and one Y chromosome (Fig. 6.3).

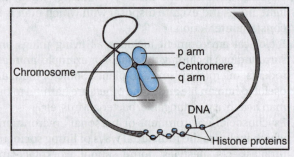

Figure 6.2: Structure of chromosome

CHAPTER 6 — Eugenics

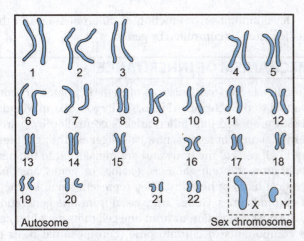

Figure 6.3: Structure of 23 pairs of human chromosomes

Functions of Chromosome

- Chromosomes contain genes; all the hereditary informations are located in the genes
- Chromosomes control the synthesis of structural proteins and thus helps in cell division and cell growth
- They control cellular differentiation
- By directing the synthesis of particular enzymes, chromosome control cell metabolism
- Chromosomes can replicate themselves or produce their carbon copies for passage to daughter cells and next generation
- Chromosomes produce nucleoli for synthesis of ribosomes
- Their haploid or diploid number respectively brings about gametophytic and sporophytic characteristics to the individual
- Chromosomes form a link between the offspring and the parents
- Some chromosomes called sex chromosomes (e.g. 'X' and 'Y') determine the sex of the individual
- Through the process of crossing over, chromosomes introduce variations
- Mutations are produced due to change in gene chemistry.

All the hereditary information is located in genes. They control the synthesis of structural proteins and then helps in cell division and cell growth, and also control cellular differentiation. Chromosomes can replicate themselves and produce their carbon copies for passage to daughter cells and next generation. Their haploid or diploid number respectively brings about gametophytic and sporophytic characteristics to the individual and they form a link between the offspring and the parents.

Chromosomal aberrations are disruptions in the normal chromosomal content of a cell and are a major cause of genetic conditions in human beings such as Cri-du-chat syndrome, Down syndrome, Klinefelter's syndrome, Turner's syndrome, triple X syndrome, etc. Previously, genetics has focused on the inheritance of hereditary disorders affecting only a small proportion of the population. Recently, genetic and technological advances are helping to better understanding the genetic changes impact on human variation as well as the development of cancer, Alzheimer's disease, essential hypertension, heart diseases, mental illness, diabetes and other multifactorial diseases that are prevalent in adults. Recently, number of studies related to new applications of genetic information resulted in providing a new and better understanding of the genetic contribution to diseases, the development of pharmacogenetics and the development of genetic tests to identify the risk of developing genetic disorders. This genetic revolution and shift to new genetics has created a demand for health professionals in a number of clinical specialties, who understand the genetic contribution to disease risk, the impact on disease management, and the genetic educational needs of patient and families.

Characteristics and Structure of Genes

The term 'gene' was introduced by Johannsen in 1909. Prior to him, Mendel had used the word 'factor' for a specific, distinct and particular unit of inheritance that takes part in expression of a trait. Johanssen has defined gene, as an elementary unit of inheritance, which can be assigned to a particular trait. Morgan's work suggested gene to be the shortest segment of chromosome, which can be separated through crossing over, can undergo mutation and influence expression of one or more traits (Fig. 6.4).

Presently, a gene is defined as a unit of inheritance composed of a segment of DNA or chromosome situated at a specific locus (gene locus), which carries coded information associated with a specific function and can undergo crossing over as well as mutation. Some of the specific features of genes are:

1. Specific portion of the DNA code is called gene, which has genetic information.
2. The term gene is often used to refer genetic material on a chromosome that code for a trait. For example, one person has a gene for hair color.
3. A unit of genetic material, which is able to replicate.
4. It is a unit of recombination or capable of undergoing crossover.
5. It is a unit of genetic material, which can undergo mutation.

6. A unit of heredity connected with somatic structure or function that leads to a phenotype expression.
7. A gene is the basic physical and functional unit of heredity.
8. Genes, which are made up of DNA, act as RNA instructor to make molecules, called proteins.
9. In humans, genes vary in size from a few hundred DNA bases to more than 2 million bases. The Human Genome Project has estimated that humans have between 20,000–25,000 genes.
10. Every person has two copies of each gene, one inherited from each parent. Most genes are the same in all people, but a small number of genes (less than 1% of the total) are slightly different between people. Alleles are forms of the same gene with small differences in their sequence of DNA bases. These small differences contribute to each person's unique physical features.

Functions of Genes

- Genes are components of genetic material and are thus unit of inheritance
- They control the morphology or phenotype of individual
- Replication of genes is essential for cell division
- Genes carry the hereditary information from one generation to next
- They control the structure and metabolism of the body
- Reshuffling of genes at the time of sexual reproduction produce variation
- Different linkages are produced due to crossing over
- Genes undergo mutation and change their expression
- New genes and consequently new traits develop due to reshuffling of different parts of genes
- Genes change their expression due to position effect
- Differentiation or formation of different type of cells, tissues and organs in various parts of the body is controlled by the expression of certain genes and nonexpression of others

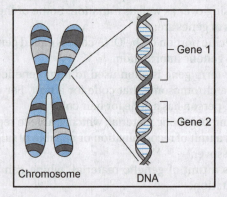

Figure 6.4: Structure of gene [genes are made up of deoxyribonucleic acid (DNA), each chromosome contains many genes]

- Development or production of different stages in the life history is controlled by genes.

MECHANISM OF INHERITANCE

Heredity is the transmission of genetic character from parents to the offspring (Fig. 6.5). Gregor Johann Mendel (1866) proposed that inheritance is controlled by paired germinal units or factors, now called genes. They are present in all cells of the body and are transferred to the next generation through gametes. Factors or genes are thus physical basis of heredity. They represent small segment of chromosomes. Genes are passed from one generation to the next generation or from one cell to its daughter cell as components of chromosome (chromosomal basis of heredity). The genetic material present in chromosomes is DNA. Genes are the segment of DNA called citrons. Therefore, DNA is the chemical basis of heredity.

Inheritance refers to how genetic information is passed down from one generation to next generation. The basic features and mechanism of inheritance are as follows:

1. Genes or chromosomes are physical basis of inheritance.
2. Person inherits half of the genetic information from each parent.
3. Every gene has two copies of genes, and each parent contributes for one copy of gene to their offspring.
4. Genes for different traits are inherited separately from one another. For example, the gene for hair color is not linked with the gene for height. A child may have his mothers' hair color, but may not her height. For the most part, each trait is inherited separately.

Laws of Inheritance

Mendel has given following laws of inheritance.

Law of unit inheritance (paired factors/genes): A character is represented in an organism or person by at least two factors. The two factors lie on the two homologous chromosomes at the same locus. They may represent the same (homozygous, e.g. 'TT' in case of pure tall and 'tt' in case of dwarf) or alternate expression (heterozygous, e.g. 'Tt' in case of heterozygous tall) of the same character. Factors representing the alternate or same form of a character are called alleles.

Law of dominance: In heterozygous individual, a character is represented by two contrasting factor called alleles. Out of the two alleles, only one is able to express its effect in the individual. It is called dominant allele. The other allele, which does not show its effect in the heterozygous individual called recessive allele.

Law of independent assortment: According to this principle or law, the two factors of each character assort or separate independent of the factors of other characters at the time of gamete formation and get randomly rearranged in the offspring.

CHAPTER 6 — Eugenics

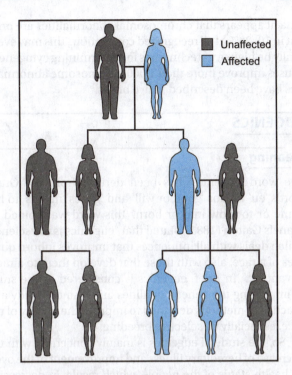

Figure 6.5: Mechanism of inheritance

Chromosomal Aberrations (Chromosomal Mutation)

1. Chromosomal aberrations are disruptions in the normal chromosomal content of a cell and are a major cause of genetic conditions in human such as Down syndrome.
2. In other words, they are changes in the number and/or arrangement of genes in the chromosomes.
3. Change in number of chromosomes is known as aneuploidy or numerical aberration.
4. Change in arrangement of genes in the chromosomes is known as numerical aberration.
5. Chromosomal aberrations may involve change in single chromosome, known as intrachromosomal aberrations.
6. Chromosomal aberrations may involve changes in two chromosomes, known as interchromosomal aberrations.
7. They are also termed as chromosomal abnormalities. Some chromosome abnormalities do not cause disease in carriers, such as translocations or chromosomal inversions, although they may lead to a higher chance of having a child with a chromosome disorder. Abnormal numbers of chromosomes or chromosome sets, aneuploidy, may be lethal or give rise to genetic disorder.
8. Chromosomal abnormalities result in a proportion of congenital anomalies, developmental and intellectual disabilities and behavioral difficulties. The majority of spontaneous abortions (about 50–60%) are the result of chromosomal abnormalities, particularly, if they occurs early, numerical changes happens in chromosomes.

Chromosomal aberrations can lead to a variety of genetic disorders. Human examples include some of the genetic disorders or genetic diseases as detailed below.

Cri-du-chat: It is caused by the deletion of part of the short arm of chromosome 5. 'Cri-du-chat' means 'cry of the cat' in French, and the condition was so-named because affected babies make high-pitched cries that sound as a cat. Affected individuals have wide-set eyes, a small head and jaw, and are moderate-to-severe mentally retarded and very short.

Wolf-Hirschhorn syndrome: It is caused by partial deletion of the short arm of chromosome 4. It is characterized by severe growth retardation and severe to profound mental retardation.

Down syndrome: Usually it is caused by an extra copy of chromosome 21 (trisomy 21). Characteristics include decreased muscle tone, stockier build, asymmetrical skull, slanting eyes and mild-to-moderate mental retardation.

Edwards syndrome: It is the second most common trisomy after Down syndrome. It is a trisomy of chromosome 18. Symptoms include mental and motor retardation and numerous congenital anomalies causing serious health problems. About 90% die in infancy; however, those who live past their first birthday usually are quite healthy thereafter. They have a characteristic hand appearance with clenched hands and overlapping fingers.

Patau syndrome: Also called D-syndrome or trisomy 13. Symptoms are somewhat similar to those of trisomy 18, but they do not have the characteristic hand shape.

Aberration idic(15): Abbreviation for isodicentric 15 on chromosome 15; also called by the following names due to various researches, but they all mean the same; idic(15), inverted duplication 15, extra marker and partial tetrasomy 15.

Jacobsen syndrome: Also called terminal 11q deletion disorder. This is a very rare disorder. Those affected have normal intelligence or mild mental retardation, with poor expressive language skills. Most have a bleeding disorder called Paris-Trousseau syndrome.

Klinefelter's syndrome (XXX): Men with Klinefelter's syndrome are usually sterile and tends to have longer arms and legs, and to be taller than their peers. Boys with the syndrome are often shy and quiet, and have a higher incidence of speech delay and dyslexia. During puberty, without testosterone treatment, some of them may develop gynecomastia.

Turner syndrome (X instead of XX or XY): In Turner's syndrome, female sexual characteristics are present, but underdeveloped. People with Turner's syndrome often have a short stature, low hairline, abnormal eye feature and bone development, and a 'caved-in' appearance to the chest.

XYY syndrome: XYY boys are usually taller than their siblings. Similar to XXY boys and XXX girls, they are somewhat more likely to have learning difficulties.

Triple X syndrome (XXX): XXX girls tend to be tall and thin. They have a higher incidence of dyslexia.

Small supernumerary marker chromosome: This means there is an extra abnormal chromosome. Features depend on the origin of the extra genetic material. Cat-eye syndrome and idic(15) are both caused by a supernumerary marker chromosome, as is Pallister-Killian syndrome.

Incidence of Chromosomal Aberration

The incidence of the specific chromosomal abnormalities found is summarized in Table 6.1. Autosomal trisomies account for about 25%, sex chromosome abnormalities for about 35% and structural rearrangement for about 40%. These figures represent only a small fraction of chromosomal abnormal conception. Naturally exercises considerable selection, as only small percentage of these abnormal conceptions survives to term. Between 10 and 20% of all recognized conception ends in spontaneous abortions.

Table 6.1: Incidence of selected chromosomal abnormalities in live born children

Abnormality	Incidence
Autosomal trisomies	
Trisomy 21 (Down syndrome)	1:650–1:1,000*
Trisomy 13 (Patau syndrome)	1:4,000–1:10,000*
Trisomy 18 (Edward's syndrome)	1:3,500–1:7,500*
Sex-chromosome disorders	
45 X (Turner's syndrome)	1:2,500–1:8,000†
47 XXX (triple X)	1:850–1:1,250†
47 XXY (Klinefelter's syndrome)	1:500–1:1,000‡
Other sex-chromosome abnormalities	
Male	~1:1,300‡
Female	~1:1,300†
Structural abnormalities	
Rearrangement (e.g. translocation, duplications)	~1: 440*

*Live births; †live female birth; ‡live male birth.

Studies of the products of spontaneous abortion have detectable chromosomal abnormalities. Approximately 95–99% of all Turner's syndrome embryos are spontaneously aborted, as are about 95% of those with available data, it appears that chromosomal abnormalities are present in 10–20% of all recognized conception. This may eventually be higher, as techniques for determining cytogenetic causes improve more than 1,000 chromosome abnormalities have been described in live births.

EUGENICS

Meaning

The word 'eugenics' has been derived from the Greek words 'eu' means 'good or will' and 'genes' means 'to become or to grow into or born'. This word was coined by Francis Galton (1883), stated that "eugenics is the science, which deals with all influences that improves inborn qualities of a race, also with those that develop them to almost advantage." In brief, eugenics is considered as the study of improving the genetic qualities and also the study and practice of methods designed to improve the quality of the race, especially by selective breeding.

So, the study of eugenics is mainly concerned with the decrease of hereditary illness and improvement of the overall health status of the people, which results in decreasing genetic morbidity. The main goal of eugenics is to improve the genetic composition of population; and main objectives of the study of eugenics are to reduce the economic burden of the country due to hereditary diseases, to decrease the human suffering and to produce healthy and intelligent people in the community. Nurses have the responsibility to reduce human suffering through providing proper education among community in which one way of promoting health of the community is by using eugenic measures.

Definitions

Eugenics is a social philosophy, which advocates the improvement of human hereditary traits through various forms of intervention. Throughout history, eugenics has been regarded by its various advocates as social responsibility, to create healthier and more intellectual people, to save resources and lessen human suffering.

The term eugenics is often used to refer the movements and social policies that were influential during the early 20th century. In the historical and broader sense, eugenics can also be a study of improving human genetic qualities. It is sometimes broadly applied to describe any human action, whose goal is to improve the gene pool. Some forms of infanticide in ancient societies, present-day prenatal testing, preimplantation genetic testing are referred as eugenics.

Eugenics was an international scientific, political and moral ideology and movement, which was at its height in first half of the 20th century and was largely abandoned after the Nazi holocaust and its future associations with racisms. Its advocates regarded it as a social philosophy for the improvement of human hereditary traits through various forms of intervention. Today, it is widely regarded as a brutal movement, which inflicted massive human rights violations on millions of people.

In India, since ancient period, there are some of the social eugenic movements are practiced. For example, among many social groups marriages are avoided within close-related subcastes and marriage is allowed outside the certain close-related paternal and maternal subcastes. The eugenics movement arose in the 20th century as two wings of a common philosophy of human worth. Francis Galton, who coined the term eugenics in 1883, perceived it as a moral philosophy to improve humanity by encouraging the ablest and healthiest people to have more children. The Galtonian idea of eugenics is usually termed positive eugenics. Negative eugenics, on the other hand, advocated culling the least able from the breeding population to preserve humanity's fitness. The eugenics movements in the United States (US), Germany and Scandinavia favored the negative approach.

Purpose of Eugenic Movements

- To develop a genetically strong human population, which is free from diseases and suffering
- To improve the human hereditary through various interventions
- To improve human race, which is healthier, intelligent and more productive.

Gregor Mendel, who was the first person to describe the elements of hereditary genes. His observations and analysis of observable features of pea plant led him to conclude that specific traits and particular factors were passed on unchanged, from a parent plant to the next generation. Some last several decades, several scientific discoveries have provided more and more information about how genes function and how they contribute to human health and disease. Now, the genetics is the branch of biological sciences, which deals with the transmission of characteristics from parents to offspring. In other words, genetics is the study of inheritance of disease in families, mapping of diseased genes to specific location on chromosomes, analysis of molecular mechanism through which it gives cause of disease and the diagnosis, and treatment of genetic diseases. Genes are genetic material on chromosomes that code for trait, e.g. one person has a gene for eye color.

Significance of Eugenics in Health Promotion

Eugenics is a social philosophy, which advocates the improvements of human hereditary traits through various forms of intervention. It has been regarded by its various advocates as social responsibility to create healthier and more intellectual people, to save resources and lesser human suffering. It means to say that eugenic helps to develop a genetically strong human population, free from diseases and sufferings to improve the human hereditary through various interventions and to improve human race, which is healthier, intelligent and more productive.

Classification of Eugenics

Eugenic movements are broadly classified into two categories, i.e. positive and negative eugenics.

Positive Eugenics

1. Positive eugenics is aimed to encourage reproduction among the genetically advantage people.
2. Possible approach includes financial and political stimuli, targeted demographic analysis, in vitro fertilization (IVF), egg transplantation and cloning to improve the genetic composition of the population by encouraging the carriers of desirable genotypes to assume the burden of parenthood.
3. Current positive eugenic movements are preimplantation genetic testing, prenatal testing and screening, premarital and preconception genetic counseling, genetic engineering, discouraging consanguineous marriages.

Negative Eugenics

1. Negative eugenics is aimed at lowering fertility among the genetically disadvantaged people.
2. This includes abortions, sterilization and other methods of family planning. Hitler sought to improve the German race by killing the weak and defective. This was negative eugenics, but nobody in civilized world would improve the human race by these means. The people, who were suffering from serious hereditary disease are sterilized or otherwise debarred from producing children.
3. Other historical examples of negative eugenics movement are state-sponsored discrimination-forced sterilization of person deemed genetically affected and disabled people.

Ethical and Moral Status of Eugenics

However, developments in genetic, genomic and reproductive technologies at the end of the 20th century have raised many new questions and concerns about, what exactly constitutes the meaning of eugenics? What its ethical and moral status is in the modern era? There are various ways of eugenics are helpful in reducing morbidity due to hereditary diseases among society/community. These include positive eugenics and negative eugenics.

Positive eugenics seeks to improve the genetic composition of the population by encouraging the carriers of desirable genotypes to assume the burden of parenthood.

Negative eugenics is aimed at lowering the fertility among the genetically disadvantaged people by various ways such as abortions, sterilization and other method of family planning. But, these eugenics measures are considered as immoral and leads to controversies in the society that there are chances of occurrence of new hereditary illness due to fresh mutations and hidden carriers of recessive type. However, it may be hoped that if eugenic measures be applied, hereditary illnesses would become less frequent.

Other Eugenic Measures

Marriage Counseling

Marriages among heterozygous parents of any defects can give rise to affected children. That is to say that marriages among the persons who are suffering with congenital abnormalities, mental retardation, gout, sickle cell anemia (SCA) may increase the risk of the defective children. Marriages among close blood relations (consanguineous marriage) or when blood relatives marry each other, the offspring of the traits are controlled by recessive genes and those are determined by polygenes, e.g. phenylketonuria (PKU), albinism, alkaptonuria, etc. In consanguineous marriages, there may be premature deaths and late marriage may increase the risks of genetic disorders such as Down syndrome and trisomy 21. So, marriage restrictions among genetically disadvantaged individuals are considered and helps in achieving the genetic health among population. When nurses come across with such family or persons, they will be advised about genetic risks and convince them to have a restriction followed about marriage and it is important to have healthy family/get healthy children.

Birth Control Measures

When marriage occurs between two individuals who are either carrier or diseased, they can adapt birth control measures, so no child is born with defective genotype. One of the aim of birth control measure as eugenics is to reduce the frequency of genetic disorder and disability in the community. Nurse who comes across such people can be advised to undergo or adapt suitable birth control measures such as contraception, sterilization or medical termination of pregnancy (MTP) to reduce the occurrence of hereditary/genetic disorders among people who lived in community.

EARLY DIAGNOSIS AND TREATMENT

Early diagnosis of some of the genetic disorders can help to correct the deformity or disorder, which includes genetic testing. The genetic test is 'the analysis of human DNA, RNA, chromosomes, protein and certain metabolites in order to detect heritable disease-related genotypes, mutations, phenotypes or karyotypes for clinical purposes'. The genetic testing identifies changes in chromosomes, genes or proteins. Most of the time, testing is used to find changes that are associated with inherited disorder. The results of genetic test can confirm or rule out a suspected genetic condition or help determine a individual's chance of developing or passing on a genetic disorder. Several genetic tests are currently used and more are being developed, which includes:

1. Preimplantation genetic diagnosis: Detection of disease-causing gene alteration in human embryo just after IVF.
2. Prenatal testing: Detect changes in fetus' genes or before birth.
3. Newborn screening: Identify infants who have an increased risk for developing genetic disorder, e.g. PKU, SCA and hypothyroidism.
4. Predictive genetic testing: Detect gene mutations associated with disorder.
5. Carrier testing: Asymptomatic persons, who may be carrier of one copy of gene alterations that can be transmitted to future children. For example, X-linked inheritance.
6. Diagnostic testing: Rule out a specific genetic disorder.
7. Forensic testing: Use DNA sequences to identify person for legal purpose and others.
8. These genetic tests help to early screening and preventive measures; future planning and life preparation; lifestyle adoptions, decreased confusion, uncertainty and anxiety; relieves psychological stress; reproductive choice; informed extended family and reduce the medial follow-up cost, if any negative results found.

EUTHENICS

Euthenics is the manipulation of environment in order to improve genotype, since there is a relationship between human genetics and environments. For example, environmental factors are involved such as smoking, diet, lack of exercise, obesity are leading to cancer, hypertension, diabetes mellitus and heart diseases, which can cause abnormalities in genetic constitution. Hence, it is required to provide stable environment to achieve normal genetic constitution. Since the existence of the world, the man has been adapting environment to genes more than adapting his genes to environment. It is considered that improving the genotype has no significance, if access to suitable environment is not provided. For example, specific protective measures can also be used to reduce the risk for diseases due to exposure of mutagens such as ultraviolet (UV) rays, radiations such as wearing lead aprons, when exposed to X-rays or radiations. These protective measures reduce the risk of mutation, thereby reducing morbidity and improving the health leading to chances of getting healthy population.

GENETIC COUNSELING

In response to increasing knowledge of the role of genetics in health and diseases, Reed proposed the term 'genetic counseling' in 1947. Although giving genetic advice and transmission of certain traits were not new ideas.

'Genetic counseling is a communication process, which deals with the human problems associated with the occurrence or the risk of occurrence of a genetic disorder in a family'.

In other words, 'genetic counseling is the process by which patients or relatives at risk of an inherited disorder, are advised of the consequences and nature of the disorder, the probability of developing or transmitting it, and options open to them in management and family planning in order to prevent, avoid or ameliorate it. This complex process can be seen from diagnostic (the actual estimation of risk) and supportive aspects'.

Genetic counseling is offered to people with genetic or inherited diseases and their families and to individuals (often children with birth defects or development delays), who are suspected of having a genetic condition. These services help families and their healthcare providers make informed decisions about their health care. In some cases, families use the information they get in a genetic evaluation to help them make reproductive decisions.

Purpose

Genetic counselors provide supportive counseling to families, service as patient advocates and refer individuals and families to community or state support services. Counseling process involves an attempt by one or more appropriately trained person to help the individual or family:

- To comprehend the medical facts including diagnosis, the probable course of the disorder and the available management
- To appreciate the way hereditary contributes to the disorders and the risk of recurrence in specific relatives
- To understand the options for dealing with the risk of occurrence
- To choose the course of action, which seems appropriate to them in view of their risk and family goals, and in accordance with that decision
- To make the best possible adjustment to the disorder in an affected family member and/or the risk of recurrence of that disorder.

Beneficiaries

- People who have a birth defect or genetic condition
- Parents, who have had a child with a birth defect or genetic condition
- Parents, who have a child with development delay, mental retardation or other problems with growth and development
- Women who had three or more miscarriages, or infertility from an unknown cause
- Pregnant women or couples considering having children in which:
  - The mother will be 35 years or older at the time of delivery
  - The couples are blood relatives (second cousins or closer)
  - Testing during the pregnancy indicated that baby may have a birth defect or genetic condition
  - There is a family history of birth defects, mental retardation or genetic diseases.
- People concerned that they may have inherited a tendency to develop cancer
- People concerned that they may have inherited a tendency to develop a neurologic condition such as Huntington's disease (Huntington's chorea)
- A person whose doctor or healthcare provider has recommended a genetic evaluation or genetic testing.

Genetic counseling can be seen from diagnostic and supporting aspects. For example, information provided by nurses during antenatal period to detect fetal abnormalities such as spina bifida or neurological disorder by amniocentesis.

Another example, if any person earlier born in family was having problem, then after making a pedigree, nurses will know the chances of occurrence of diseases in offspring. This information provided by nurse regarding cost of correction of disease, prognosis and burden on the family, will help family members to take decision regarding continuation of pregnancy or its termination. In the same way other diseases such as hydrocephalus, SCA, congenital abnormality, etc. can be brought under control.

So, genetic counseling involves information of various ways of eugenics to people to reduce the further occurrence of genetic disorder. Genetic counseling is offered to people with genetic or inherited diseases and their families, and to individuals (often children with birth defects or development delays), who are suspected having a genetic condition. These services help families and their healthcare providers make decision about their health care.

Nurses work as a member of healthcare team and act as a patient advocate as well as genetic resources to physicians. Nurses are present at high risk or specialty prenatal clinic that offers prenatal diagnosis, child care centers and adult genetic centers. Genetic counseling can occur before conception to adulthood. Genetic counseling may be perspective or retrospective:

1. Prospective genetic counseling: Allows for the true prevention of disease. This approach requires identifying heterozygous individual for any particular defect by screening procedures and explaining them the risk of having affected children, if they marry another heterozygous person of the same gene. If marriage can be prevented, it reduces the prospects of giving birth to affected children will diminish, e.g. thalassemia.
2. Retrospective genetic counseling: Allows the hereditary disorder that has already occurred within the family. Here, genetic advice is mainly sought in connection with congenital abnormalities, mental retardation, mental illness and inborn error of metabolism and premarital advice.

For this, the World Health Organization (WHO) recommends the establishment of genetic counseling centers in sufficient numbers in regions where infection and nutritional disorders have brought under control and in areas, where genetic disorders have estimated a serious health problem, e.g. SCA and thalassemia. The methods of retrospective counseling are contraception, MTP and sterilization depending upon the attitudes and cultural environment of the couple involved.

Phases

Assessment Phase

Assessment phase is the primary beginning phase of counseling in which following tasks are accomplished:
- Initial interview with counselee and family for preparation of counselee for genetic counseling
- Collect family history and other relevant histories, prepare and analyze pedigree
- Carry out primary assessment of counselee, physical examination, etc.
- Considering potential diagnosis based on collected information.

Diagnostic Phase

In some cases, the goal of a genetic evaluation is to make a diagnosis of a particular genetic condition or syndrome. This is commonly the case, when a child is born with multiple birth defects or problems with growth and development. In other cases, the diagnosis already is known and the genetic counselor or geneticist probably will confirm the established diagnosis to proceed for next phases of the following steps:

1. Confirmatory or supplementing tests or procedures such as:
   - Chromosomal analysis
   - Biochemical tests
   - Molecular DNA testing
   - X-rays, biopsy
   - Linkage analysis
   - Developing testing
   - Dermatography
   - Prenatal diagnosis
   - Immunological tests, etc.
2. Establishment of an accurate diagnosis.

Analysis Phase

Analysis phase includes following tasks:
- Literature search and review of information
- Consultation with other experts
- Compiling of information and determination of recurrence risk.

Communication Phase

Communication phase includes:
- Communication of the results and risk to the counselee and to the family, if appropriate
- Discussion of options and review of questions
- Assess the counselee's understanding about facts and relevant hereditary pattern, diagnostic and management options for disorders
- All explanation should be culturally appropriate for counselee and appropriate for their education.

Referral and Support Phase

In referral and support phase, counselor offers following services:
- Refer the individual to genetic specialist for further interventions, e.g. referral for prenatal diagnosis or treatment modalities for different disorders
- Support of decision made by counselee
- Psychological support should be provided throughout the process
- Follow-up and evaluation.

ROLE OF NURSES IN GENETIC COUNSELING

Nurses work as members of a healthcare team and act as a patient advocate as well as genetic resource person to physicians. Genetic nurses are present at high risk or specialty prenatal clinics that offer prenatal diagnosis, pediatric care centers and adult genetic centers. Genetic counseling can occur before conception (i.e. when one or two of the parents are carriers of certain trait) to adulthood (for adult onset genetic conditions such as Huntington's disease or hereditary cancer syndromes). Following are the main roles of general genetic nurses have to accomplish during genetic counseling:

1. Receive the client and family and make them comfortable in assessment room for genetic counseling.
2. Obtain prenatal, family and other health histories from individual and family.
3. Conduct a primary physical examination and collect other relevant information.
4. Identify families at risk, investigate the problems present in the family, interpret information about the disorders, analyze inheritance patterns and risks of recurrence and review available testing options with the family.
5. Prepare and analyze pedigree to establish information about hereditary pattern.
6. Provide psychological support to individual and family throughout the counseling.
7. Collect other related information from individual and family, e.g. any prior test report or documents.
8. Obtain an informed written consent for any planned genetic test or intervention.
9. Encourage the individual and family to ask question as much as they can, to understand about all aspects of disorders and to families, who may be at risk for a variety of inherited conditions.
10. Establish a plan of care with the family and coordinate with other healthcare professionals.
11. Maintain privacy and confidentiality of all information related to individual and family, only disclose the information as per individual's wish and permission.
12. Provide the referral guidance to individual for genetic specialist for further interventions.
13. Coordinate for available community resources to help individual and family to provide available help.
14. Be available for the individual and family for any genetic services through the course of disorders.
15. Ensure follow-up and supportive services to individual and family during entire course of need.

CONCLUSION

In human beings, there are 23 pairs of chromosomes. The chromosome consists of a continuous DNA structure. Structural chromosomes as aberrations occur due to either deletion are translocation of chromosomes. Genetic disorders are chromosome abnormalities (structural) either sex chromosome or autosomes. As stated earlier, each individual has 23 pairs of chromosomes (23 from mother, 23 from father). These chromosomes are condensed chromatins. On chromosomes, genes are located. These genes occur in pairs. Depending upon the genes, whether alike or different, the genes are homologous and heterozygous. These normal genes due to exposure of mutagens, can be converted into abnormal genes. These abnormal genes lead to diseases. Sometimes the chromosomes content of cell is disrupted either due to gain or loss of chromosome, or duplication of gene on chromosomes or problems with division. These all lead to genetic diseases of either autosomes or sex chromosomes. These can be reduced if assessed, planned and treated as early as possible. Eugenic is the science, which deals with improvement in the inborn qualities of a race, so considered as health promotional measure. The positive eugenic measures include euthenics, genetic counseling, marriage restriction, birth control, early diagnosis and treatment; and the negative eugenic measures include abortion, sterilization, etc. These eugenic measures can be used by community health nurse in cooperation with health department and other departments to reduce morbidity associated with genetic problems. The community health nurses can inform the risks and benefits associated with appropriate measures to reduce hereditary diseases.

Part II

Environment as Determinant of Health

A. *Physical Environment*
- Water as a Determinant of Health
- Air as a Determinant of Health
- Light as a Determinant of Health
- Ventilation as a Determinant of Health
- Noise as a Determinant of Health
- Radiation Exposure as a Determinant of Health
- Climate as a Determinant of Health
- Housing as a Determinant of Health
- Sanitation: Disposal of Waste
- Communication, Infrastructure Facilities and Linkages

Part II

Environment as Determinant of Health

9. Physical Environment
10. Water as a Determinant of Health
11. Air as a Determinant of Health
12. Light as a Determinant of Health
13. Ventilation as a Determinant of Health
14. Noise as a Determinant of Health
15. Radiation Exposure as a Determinant of Health
16. Climate as a Determinant of Health
17. Housing as a Determinant of Health
18. Sanitation: Disposal of Wastes
19. Communication, Infrastructure Facilities and Linkages

Water as a Determinant of Health

CHAPTER 7

INTRODUCTION

The term 'environment' is defined to include all that is external to the human body. Here, the environment refers to the internal and external factors that affect the health of the people. A clean, beautiful and hazard-free environment is a great asset to health. The health status of an individual, a community or a nation is determined by the interactions of internal environment of the man himself/herself and the external environment, which surrounds him/her. So, an environment is one of the major determinants of health status of the human beings.

Environment is the external factor(s) present around man and has got an influence on the health of the human being. According to ecologists, health is a state of dynamic equilibrium between man and his environment and when this equilibrium is disturbed, ill-health (disease) occurs.

Such an environment has been divided into four components:
1. Physical environment.
2. Biological environment.
3. Social environment.
4. Cultural environment.

The term 'environmental health' previously familiarized an 'environmental sanitation'. The word 'sanitation' means 'the science of safeguarding health'. Sanitation is defined as 'a way of life'. It is the quality of the living that is expressed in the clean home, the clean form, the clean business, the clean neighborhood and the clean community. Being a way of life, it must come from within people; it is nourished by knowledge and grows as an ideal in human relations. The World Health Organization (WHO) defines environmental sanitation as "the control of all those factors in man's physical environment, which exercise or may exercise a deleterious effect on his/her physical development, health and survival." The factors that influence the health of the people will include food, water, housing, clothing and sanitation.

Environmental is all the external conditions surrounding human beings such as air, water, light, etc. Environment, if gets polluted, affects the living as well as non-living components. Air is part of external environment, which a man needs to live. If air gets polluted, then it affects the health and requires measures to control air pollution. In the same way light, housing, impure water, improper sanitation also affects human beings. The community health nurses, while visiting homes, doing survey or working at health centers, can teach public regarding the prevention and control of pollution. She/He can identify the cases suffering due to pollution of water, poor housing, pollution of air and can refer for appropriate treatment for the control of disease, and can prevent the complications.

Environmental sanitation now being replaced by environmental health has been defined as "the aspect of public health concerned with all the factors, circumstances and conditions in the environment or surroundings of humans that can exert an influence on human health and well-being." The health of the environment is a long-standing public health problem for which every gains seem to be met with new problems.

India is still lagging far behind many countries in the field of environmental health. Only 31% of the rural population has access to potable water supply and only 0.5% enjoys basic sanitation. The basic problems of safe water supply and sanitary disposal of human excreta are yet to be solved. Most of the ill-health in the country is due to defective environment. High incidence of diarrheal diseases and other preventive and infectious diseases, especially amongst infants and children are due to lack of safe drinking water and poor environmental sanitation.

The need of environmental health is to create and maintain ecological conditions that will promote health and thus prevent disease. One of the important public healthcare elements is safe drinking water sanitation. More than a billion people in developing countries lacked access to safe drinking water and laced an adequate system for disposing off their excreta. Feces deposited near homes, contaminated drinking water, fish from polluted rivers and coastal waters and agricultural produce fertilized with human waste are all health hazards. Water quantity is as important as water quality. Without sufficient water in or near home, hygiene becomes difficult or impossible. The lack of water supply and sanitation is the primary reason why disease transmitted via feces are so common. The most important symptom of these diseases is diarrhea and intestinal worm infestations. Inadequate water supply increases the risk of schistosomiasis, skin and eye infections and guinea worm disease.

Achievements of health for all are concerned with a healthy environment, healthy lifestyle and require initiatives by the individual, the family and the community. A new initiative is aimed at providing universal coverage of water supply and sanitation services. Much of the ill-health in India is due to poor environmental sanitation, i.e. unsafe water, polluted soil, unhygienic disposal of human excreta and refuse, poor housing, insects and rodents. Air pollution is also a growing concern in many cities. The high death rate, infant mortality rate, sickness rate and poor standards of health are in fact largely due to defective environmental sanitation. Improvement of environmental sanitation is therefore crucial for the prevention of disease and promotion of health of individuals and communities.

PHYSICAL ENVIRONMENT

This consists of non-living things and certain physical forces/energy present around man. These are water, air, soil, housing, radiation, light, ventilation, noise, refuse, wastes, etc.

WATER

Water is a primary necessity of life, without water, terrestrial animals and vegetable life must cease to exist. Water helps the man in many ways, i.e. it replaces loss of fluids from tissues; maintains fluidity of blood and lymph, helps in excretion of waste products, acts as a vehicle of dissolving food, helps in digestion, and regulates body temperature.

Purpose of Water

As already mentioned, water is the necessity of life, which is required for many purposes as described below:
1. Domestic purposes: Water is required for drinking, cooking, etc. Washing, personal cleanliness, cleaning of car sheds and flushing latrine.
2. Public purposes: Water is required for public cleansing, fire fighting, maintenance of public gardens, swimming pools and numerous other civic purposes.
3. Industrial purposes: Some industries such as the iron, pharmaceutical, steel and paper industries need lot of water.
4. Agricultural purpose: For cultivation of food, fruit, vegetables and raw materials water is essential. So, it is a very essential factor in socioeconomic and cultural development of the community as a whole.

Requirement of Water

It is difficult for a man to survive without water. It is an essential constituent of men, animals, plants and all storable matters. There is an increase utility of water by human beings such as cooking, drinking, bathing, washing, etc. Advanced civilization and technology has increased the utility of water more enormously. It is used for the following purpose. Its requirement depends upon the purposes.

Domestic Purposes

Water is required for drinking, cooking, bathing, washing of clothes, utensils, cleaning of places, flushing. In India, daily requirement of water per capita is 135 liters according to IS 1172 (1971):
- Cooking (5 L)
- Drinking (5 L)
- Bathing (50 L)
- Washing clothes (25 L)
- Washing utensils (15 L)
- Cleaning places (10 L)
- Flushing (25 L).

Industrial Purposes

Water requirement differs depending upon the type of industry, hotel, power station and the city in which it is existing. As in case of sugar industry, the water requirement is 10 L/kg and in case of steel industry, it is 50 L/kg.

Public Utility

Water is used for public buildings other than residential purposes such as for hostels, schools, road washings, public gardens, nursing homes, hospitals, etc. Water requirement for hospitals with beds not exceeding 100 is 340 L/day/capita and for beds exceeding 100 is 455 L/capita/day. Water consumption for nursing homes and medical quarters is 135 L/day/capita.

Chapter 7: Water as a Determinant of Health

Extinguishing Fires

Water is used by municipal body for adequate protection against fire. During fire, large quantity of water is required to be supplied to fire spot, but in comparison to total consumption, it is small.

Agriculture Use

Water is utilized for irrigation purposes, which is the required need of plants and crops for growing. Water is considered as an essential factor in the socioeconomic development of country. Unclean and inadequate water supply undoubtedly contribute substantially to the risks of diarrheal diseases thereby increasing morbidity and mortality. But clean water can reduce the health problems thereby reducing the economic burden on the nation. The consumption of water depends upon climatic conditions, standard of living and habits of the people. A daily supply of 150–200 liters (35–40 gallon) per head is considered as adequate allowance. In general, we need 30 gallon of water per head per day. In hospitals, people need 40–50 gallon per head per day. In Kolkata, due to climatic conditions people need 70 gallon per head per day. Drinking water should be safe and agreeable to use or wholesome; such supply of water may be termed as 'acceptable' or 'potable'. Potable water may be defined as:
- Free from pathogenic agents
- Free from harmful chemical substances
- Pleasant to the taste
- Usable for domestic purposes.

In brief, potable water means that water, which is physically, chemically and bacteriologically suitable for drinking. A safe water supply is more important to the health of the people than any drug or thing.

Sources of Water (Fig. 7.1)

Rain Water

Rain is the main source of all water. A part of the rain water sinks into the ground to form groundwater; part of it evaporates back into the atmosphere and some runs off to form streams and rivers, which flow ultimately into the sea. Some of the water in the soil is taken up by the plants and is evaporated in turn by the leaves:

1. Rain water is the purest water in nature. Physically, it is clear, bright and sparkling. Chemically, it is very soft water containing only traces of dissolved solids.
2. Rain water becomes impure when it passes through the atmosphere. It picks up suspended impurities from the atmosphere such as dust, soot, microorganisms and gases such as carbon dioxide, nitrogen, oxygen, and ammonia. Gaseous sulfur and nitrogen oxides are emitted from power plants that use fossil fuels. These gases react with atmospheric water forming dilute solution of sulfuric and nitric acid. These acids have serious impacts on surface water quality and on plants, etc.

Surface Water

Surface water originates from rain water, which includes rivers, tanks, lakes, wadis (water source, which are dry, except in rainy season), man-made reservoirs and seawater. Surface water is prone to contamination from human and animal sources. It is never safe for human consumption unless subjected to sanitary protection and purification.

Impounding reservoirs

These are artificial lakes constructed usually of earthwork or masonry in which large quantities of surface water is stored. Dams built across rivers and mountain streams also provide large reserves of surface water. Water draining into the

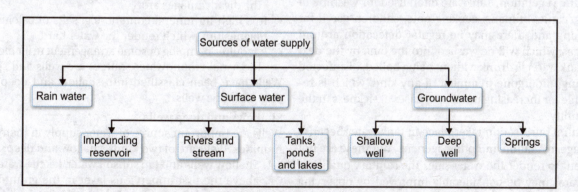

Figure 7.1: Sources of water

reservoir is called 'catchment area'. Storing water for long periods in reservoirs is the growth of algae and other microscopic organisms, which impart bad tastes, and odors to water:

1. Impounding reservoirs water is usually clear, palatable and ranks next to rain water in purity. The water is usually soft and considered to be free of pathogenic organisms.
2. The upland surface water derives its impurities from the catchment area, the sources being human habitations and animal keeping or grazing.

Rivers and stream

Almost all rivers furnish a dependable supply of water. The river water is always polluted and is quite unfit for drinking without treatment:

1. River water is turbid during rainy season; it may clear in other seasons. River water contains dissolved and suspended impurities of all kinds including bacteria and other organisms.
2. The impurities of river water are derived from surface washings, sewage, sullage water, industrial and trade wastes, and drainage from agricultural areas. The customs and habits of the people such as bathing, animal washing and disposal of the dead, all this add to the pollution of water.
3. Self-purification in river water occurs by natural forces of purification such as dilution, sedimentation, aeration, oxidation, sunlight, plant and animal life. However, river water needs purification before it can be used for drinking purposes.

Tanks

Tanks are the important source of water supply in some Indian villages. Tanks are recipient of contamination of all sorts. They are full of silt and colloidal matter, especially immediately after rain. The older tanks may be full of aquatic vegetation. Tanks are often used for washing of clothes, cattle, humans, cooking pots; children use it for swimming and there may be regular defecation around the edges, which will be washed into the tank by the next rain. Tank water is drunk without being boiled, disinfected or having undergone treatment of any kind, which is responsible for increasing number of cases of sickness in the community.

Natural purification takes place in tank water because of storage, oxidation and other agencies, but these are not sufficient to render the water safe. The sanitary quality of tank water may be considerably improved by observing the following:

- The edges of the tank should be elevated in order to prevent the entry of surface washings
- There should be a fence around the tank to prevent access to animals
- No one should be permitted to get into the tank directly
- There should be an elevated platform from where people can draw water
- The weeds should be periodically removed
- The tank should be cleaned at the end of the dry season.

From a practical point of view, it is not possible to prevent pollution of tanks as the people who consume the tank water are often among the poorest in the country and do not have sanitary concepts. It is believed that the simplest solution consists of subjecting the tank water to some sort of sand filtration. The addition of chlorine would undoubtedly add to the value of sand filtration (Fig. 7.2).

Seawater

Seawater is plenty, but it has some disadvantages. It contains 3.5% of salt in solution. Offshore waters of the oceans and seas have a salt concentration of 30,000–36,000 mg/L (30–36 L) of dissolved solids including 19,000 mg/L of chloride, 10,600 mg/L of sodium and 1,270 mg/L of magnesium. Desalting and demineralization process involves heavy expenditure. Seawater is used with treatment, where there is no other source of water.

Groundwater

Rainwater percolating into ground constitutes groundwater. Since, there is a limit to groundwater people should withdraw only quantities of water that can be renewed.

Groundwater is the cheapest, most practical and superior to surface water, because the ground itself provides an effective filtering medium.

The advantages of ground water are:
- It is likely to be free from pathogenic agents
- It usually requires no treatment
- The supply is likely to be certain even during dry season
- It is less subject to contamination than surface water.

The disadvantages are:
- It is high in mineral content, e.g. salts of calcium and magnesium, which render the water hard
- It requires pumping or some arrangement to lift the water.

The usual groundwater sources are wells and springs. Wells have been classified into shallow and deep wells, dug, and tube wells.

Shallows and deep wells

Wells are important source of water supply in many communities. Wells are of two kinds, shallow and deep:

1. Shallow wells and tap subsoil water, i.e. the water from above the first impervious layer in the ground. They yield limited quantities of water and the water is notoriously liable to pollution unless care is taken in well-construction.

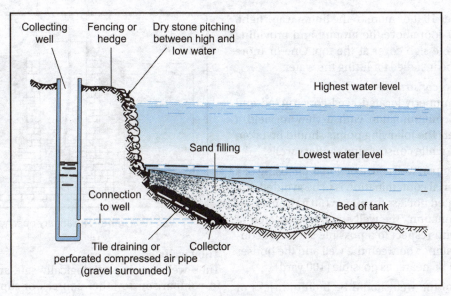

Figure 7.2: Slow sand filtration of tank water

2. A deep well is one, which taps water from the water-bearing stratum below the first impervious layer in the ground. Deep wells are usually machine dug and may be several hundred meters deep. Deep wells furnish the safest water and are often the most satisfactory sources of water supply. Shallow wells are liable to pollution from neighboring sources of contamination such as latrines, urinals, drains, cesspools, soakage pits and collections of manure. Shallow wells are not safe to community, if they are not made sanitary. A deep well is not safe if it is open, poorly constructed and not protected against contamination. Near the sea, there is danger of infiltration of seawater in deep wells and may make the water not fit for domestic use (Fig. 7.3).

Wells may also be classified according to the method of construction into dug wells and tube wells. Two types of dug wells exist in rural areas; the unlined katcha well and the masonry or pucca well. The katcha well is a hole dug into the water-bearing stratum. The pucca well is an open well-built by stone bricks. Steps are constructed into these wells to enable people to descend into the well to fetch water or quench their thirst. In these wells, there is considerable personal contact between the user and the water.

Some people may even wash their faces, hands and feets, which is a common Indian custom. The open dug wells and stepwells are not safe to the community. The points of difference between a shallow well and deep well are set out in Table 7.1.

Table 7.1: Differences between a shallow well and deep well

Features	Shallow well	Deep well
Definition	Taps the water from above, the first impervious layer	Taps the water from below, the first impervious layer
Chemical quality	Moderately hard	Much hard
Bacteriological quality	Often grossly contaminated	Taps pure water
Yield	Usually goes dry in summer	Provides a source of constant supply

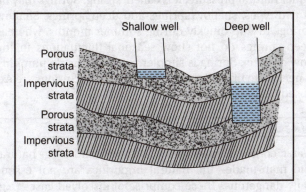

Figure 7.3: Shallow and deep wells

The unlined katcha wells may be made sanitary by deepening the bottom, installing a hand pump with screen and filling the well with coarse sand up to the water level and with clay above that level. When the material used for filing is completely consolidated a platform and drainage may be constructed. Masonry well, improvement consists of making the upper 10 ft or more of the lining watertight, raising the lining 1 foot above the ground and providing a reinforced concrete slab cover at the top. One or more hand pumps may be installed for lifting the water.

Sanitary well and its construction
A sanitary well is properly located, well-constructed and protected against contamination with a view to yield a supply of safe water. The following points should be taken into consideration, while constructing sanitary wells.

Location: The first step in well construction is choosing of a proper site. If bacterial contamination is to be avoided, the well should be located not less than 15 m (50 ft) from likely sources of contamination. The well should be located at higher elevation with respect to a possible source of contamination. The distance between the well and the houses of the users should be nearer as possible (100 yard).

Lining: The lining of the well should be built of bricks or stones set in cement up to a depth of at least 6 m (20 ft) so that water enters from the bottom and not from the sides of the well. The lining should be carried 60–90 cm (2–3 ft) above the ground level.

Parapet: There should be parapet wall up to a height of at least 70–75 cm (28 inch) above the ground.

Platform: There should be a cement concrete platform round the well extending at least 1 m (3 ft) in all directions. The platform should have gentle slope outwards toward a drain built along its edges.

Drain: There should be a pucca drain to carry off spilled water to a public drain or a soakage pit constructed well beyond the 'cone of filtration' (area of drainage) of the well.

Covering: The top of the well should be closed by a cement concrete cover, because the bulk of the pollution is introduced into the well directly through the open top.

Hand pump: The well should be equipped with a hand pump for lifting the water in a sanitary manner. When a pump is fitted, there is marked improvement in the bacteriological quality of the water. The hand pump construction should withstand rough handling by the people and there should be an efficient maintenance service of hand pump.

The consumers observe certain basic precautions at the individual and family level. For example, strict cleanliness should be enforced in the vicinity of the well; personal ablutions, washing of clothes and animals and the dumping of the wastes should be prohibited. Ropes and buckets from individual homes should not be used for drawing water supply from the well. Water from the well should be carried in clean sanitary vessels to individual houses (Fig. 7.4).

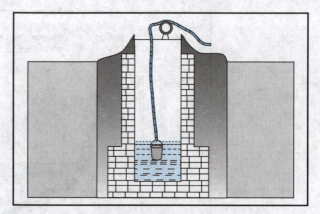

Figure 7.4: Sanitary open well

Tube wells
Tube wells are bacteriologically safe and are also cheap in comparison to other sources of supply. Shallow tube wells or 'driven wells' have become the largest individual source of water supply to the rural community. The tube well consists of a pipe (usually galvanized iron) sunk into the water-bearing stratum and fitted with a strainer at the bottom, and a hand pump at the top. A water-tight concrete platform with a drain should be provided. The area within 15 m of the tube well should be kept free from pollution with liquid and solid wastes. The hand pump should be kept in good repair. The life of the tube well varies from place to place depending upon the type of strainer, quality of underground water and the nature of soil. An average well may last for a period of 5–10 years; in some cases, tube wells have given satisfactory service even after 30 years. Deep tube wells or bored wells are sunk by drilling through successive substrata of gravel or rock until a suitable supply of groundwater is located; may be costly to construct and to operate are in many ways the ideal supply, and yield is normally very high.

Springs
When groundwater comes to the surface and flows freely under natural pressure, it is called 'spring'. Springs may be of two types, shallow springs and deep springs. Shallow springs dry up quickly during summer months, whereas deep springs do not show seasonal fluctuations in the flow of water. Spring is simpler to exploit, as no pumping is needed to bring the water to the surface. Springs are exposed to contamination.

WATER POLLUTION AND ITS HAZARDS

Water contains impurities of various kinds, e.g. natural and man-made. The natural impurities are not essentially dangerous. These comprise of dissolved gases (e.g. nitrogen, carbon dioxide, hydrogen sulfide, etc. that may

CHAPTER 7 — Water as a Determinant of Health

be picked up during rainfall) and dissolved minerals (e.g. salts of calcium, magnesium, sodium, etc.), which are natural constituents of water following its contact with soil; suspended impurities (e.g. clay, slit, sand and mud) and microscopic organisms. These impurities are derived from the atmosphere, catchment area and the soil.

The indicators of pollution include the amount of total suspended solids, biochemical oxygen demand (BOD) at 20°C, concentration of chlorides, nitrogen and phosphorus, and absence of dissolved oxygen. Even if the source of water supply and its treatment are of a high standard, water pollution may still occur as often happens, due to corrosion of pipelines, leaky points and cross-connections between water supply pipes and sewage drainage pipes. Surveillance has to be exercised at every point in the distribution system to ensure supply of safe water to the consumer.

Some of the new pollutants are not easily removed by conventional water treatment or purification processes and also water is associated with the following:

1. Dental health: The presence of fluoride at about 1 mg/L in drinking water is known to protect against dental carries, but high level of fluoride cause mottling of the dental enamel.
2. Cyanosis in infant: High nitrate content of water is associated with methemoglobinemia. This is a rare occurrence, but may occur when surface water from farmland is treated with a fertilizer and gain access to the water supply.
3. Cardiovascular diseases: Hardness of water appears to have a beneficial effect against cardiovascular disease.
4. Some diseases are transmitted because of inadequate use of water such as shigellosis, trachoma and conjunctivitis, ascariasis, scabies.
5. Some diseases are related to the disease carrying insects breeding in or near water, e.g. malaria, filarial, arboviruses, onchocerciasis and African trypanosomiasis. Water pollution seems to be an inevitable consequence of modern industrial technology, the problem now is to determine the level of pollutant that permits economic and social development without presenting hazards to health. In India, water pollution is becoming a serious problem. To protect water from being contaminated, in 1974, Parliament passed The Water (prevention and control of pollution) Act. The Act seeks to provide legal deterrent against the spread of legislation.

Sources of Water Pollution

Water pollution is broadly defined as the addition of substance that changes the natural qualities of water. Substances, which can pollute water and pose health hazards include waterborne viruses and bacteria, waste, heat, radioactivity, industrial pollutants, oil spills, and undergoing pollution from dumping. The more serious aspect of water pollution is that it is caused by human activity urbanization and industrialization.

The sources of pollution resulting from these human activities are as follows:

1. Sewage, which contains decomposable organic matter and pathogenic agents, e.g. infective organisms.
2. Industrial trade and wastes, which contain toxic agents ranging from metal salts to complex synthetic organic chemicals, e.g. effluents from pulp and paper industry, textile, sugar, steel industries, jute mills, distillers and coal washeries, metal salts, wastes, etc.
3. Agricultural pollutants, which comprise fertilizers and pesticides, e.g. irrigation water carrier's fertilizers and pesticides to rivers, well and ponds.
4. Physical pollutants include heat (thermal pollution), radioactive substances and carcinogenic agents, etc. Heat by deoxygenation of water also causes thermal pollution.

As already stated, the drinking water comes either from surface sources or underground sources. Drinking water can be contaminated in one of the following four ways:

1. When water has never been treated with protective chemicals.
2. When deficiencies exist in the distribution system (e.g. sewage and drinking water lines are crossed).
3. When deficiencies exist in treatment system.
4. When a proper functioning system is unable to remove contaminating agents or chemicals.

Hazards of Water Pollution

The hazards of water pollution are classified into two groups:

1. Biological hazards.
2. Chemical hazards.

Biological Hazards

Biological hazards include diseases caused by the presence of an infective agent or an aquatic host in water. The infectious diseases resulting from water pollution can be classified into four groups depending upon the ways in which their incidence can be lessened by improvement in water supply:

1. Waterborne diseases are those in which infectious agent remains alive in drinking water, e.g. cholera, typhoid, paratyphoid, gastroenteritis, bacteria and viruses, viral hepatitis, poliomyelitis, etc. The incidence of these diseases can be reduced by the purification of water.

2. Water-washed diseases include infection of the outer body surfaces, e.g. bacillary and amoebic dysentery, trachoma, skin ulcers, scabies, typhus and gastroenteritis. The incidence can be reduced by augmenting water quantity.
3. Water-based infections are due to the presence of an aquatic host. Thus, guinea worm, fish tapeworm are caused by *Cyclops*, schistosomiasis is caused by snails. Some infections can occur when the skin comes in contact with water or through drinking water, e.g. roundworm, whipworm, threadworm, hydatids disease (helminthic infections), Weil's disease (leptospiral infection).
4. Water breeding or water proximity diseases are caused by mosquitoes or flies living near aquatic conditions.

The features of waterborne epidemics include outbreaks expensive in nature; marked geographical and seasonal distribution; affects all ages except infants who do not drink water and both sexes are equally affected.

Chemical Hazards

Chemical hazards are an increasing incidence in chemical pollutants in the public water supplies. These pollutants include detergents, solvents, cyanides, heavy metals, minerals and organic acids, nitrogenous substances, bleaching agents, dyes, pigments, sulfides, ammonia, toxic and biocidal organic compounds, etc. These may affect man's health in aquatic life, e.g. fish used as human food.

Presence of toxic and inert substances lead, arsenic, mercury, cyanide, insecticides lead to concern poisoning (e.g. lead poisoning) and the substances, which may affect health, are fluoride, iodine and nitrates, etc.

For example, deficiency of iodine causes goiter, deficiency of fluoride leads to caries, excess of fluoride leads to dental and skeletal fluorosis, excess of nitrate (NO_3) (over 45 mg/L) may lead to methemoglobinemia.

PURIFICATION OF WATER

The objective of purification of water is to remove the dissolved and suspended impurities of water as shown in Figure 7.5.

Purification of Water on a Large Scale

The purification of water by treatment is to produce water that is safe and wholesome. The method of treatment to be employed depends upon the nature of raw water and the desired standards of water quality. For example, groundwater (e.g. wells and springs) may need no treatment other than disinfection. Surface water (e.g. river water), which tends to be turbid and polluted requires extensive treatment. Water purification systems comprise of storage, filtration and disinfection.

Storage

Storage provides a reserve of water from which further pollution is prevented. This is natural purification and the process takes place as follows:

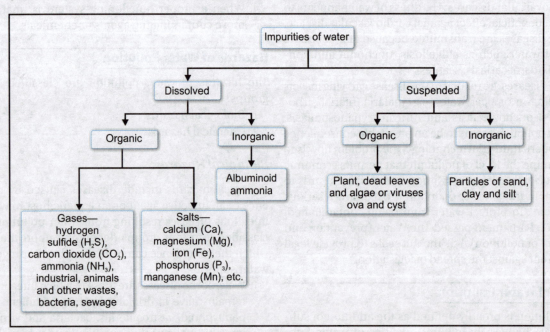

Figure 7.5: Impurities of water

1. **Physical:** By mere storage, the quantity of water improves. About 90% of the suspended impurities settle down in 24 hours by gravity. The water becomes clearer. This allows penetration of light and reduces the work of the filters.
2. **Chemical:** Certain chemical change also takes place during storage. The aerobic bacteria oxidize the organic matter present in the water with the aid of dissolved oxygen. As a result, the content of free ammonia is reduced and a rise in nitrates occurs.
3. **Biological:** A tremendous drop to take place in bacterial count during storage. The pathogenic organisms gradually die out. It is found that when river water is stored, the total bacterial count drops by as much as 90% in the first 5–7 days. This is one of the greatest benefits of storage. The optimum period of storage of river water is considered to be about 10–14 days. If the water stored for long periods, there is likelihood of development of vegetable growths such as algae, which impart a bad smell and color to water.

Filtration

Filtration is the second stage in purification of water and quite an important stage, because 98–99% of the bacteria are removed by filtration, apart from other impurities. Two types of filters are in use, the 'biological' or 'slow sand' filters and the 'rapid sand' or 'mechanical' filters. A brief description of these filters is given below.

Biological filter

Biological filters were first used for water treatment in 1804 in Scotland and subsequently in London. They are generally accepted as the standard method of water purification. The various elements of a slow sand filter are shown in Figure 7.6. Essentially these consist of the following:
- Supernatant (raw) water
- A bed of graded sand
- An underdrainage system
- A system of filter control valves.

Supernatant water

The supernatant water above the sand bed, the depth varies from 1 to 1.5 m. It provides a constant head of water so as to overcome the resistance of the filter bed and thereby promote the download flow of water through the sand bed, and also it provides waiting period of some hours (3–12 hour, depending upon the filtration velocity) for the raw water to undergo partial purification by sedimentation, oxidation and particle agglomeration. The level of supernatant water is always kept constant.

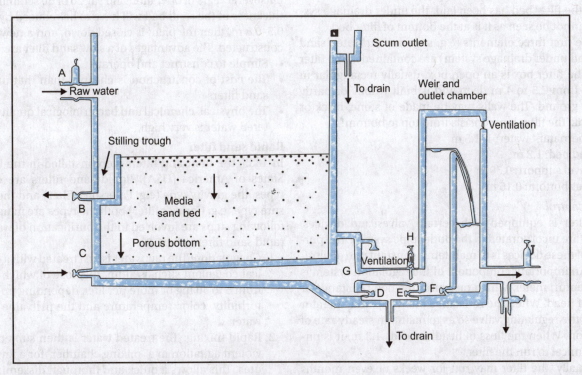

Figure 7.6: Slow sand filter (biological filter). **A.** Raw water inlet; **B.** Supernatant water to waste; **C.** Filtered water for backfilling; **D to F.** Drain valves; **G.** Venturi meter; **H.** Rate of flow control valve; **I.** Filtered water to waste; **J.** Filtered water to clear well.

Sand bed

The thickness of the sand bed is about 1 meter. The sand grains are carefully chosen preferably rounded an 'effective diameter' between 0.2 and 0.3 mm. The sand should be clean and free from clay and organic matter. The sand bed is supported by a layer of graded gravel.

The sand bed presents a vast surface area and it is subjected to a number of purification processes, mechanical straining, sedimentation, absorption, oxidation and bacterial action, all playing their part. The designed rate of filtration of water normally lies between 0.1 and 0.4 m^3/h of bed surface. When the filter is newly laid, it acts merely as a mechanical strainer, but very soon, the surface of the sand bed gets covered with a slimy growth known as 'schmutzdecke,' vital layer, zoogleal layer or biological layer. The layer is slimy and gelatinous and consists of thread-like algae and numerous forms of life including plankton, diatoms and bacteria. It may take several days for the vital layer to form fully. The vital layer is the 'heart' of the slow sand filter. It removes organic matter, holds back bacteria and oxidizes ammoniacal nitrogen into nitrates, and helps in yielding bacteria-free water (Fig. 7.7).

Under drainage system

Under drainage system consist of porous or perforated pipes, which serve the dual purpose of providing an outlet for filtered water and supporting the filter medium above. Once the filter bed has been laid, the under drainage system cannot be seen as it is at the bottom of filter bed.

The first three elements (e.g. supernatant water, sand bed and under drainage system) are contained in the filter box. The filter box is an open box, usually rectangular in shape from 2.5 to 4 m deep and is built wholly or partly below ground. The walls may be made of stone, brick or cement. The filter box consists from top to bottom:
- Supernatant water: 1–1.5 m
- Sand bed: 1.2 m
- Gravel support: 0.30 m
- Filter bottom: 0.16 m.

Filter control

The filter is equipped with certain valves and devices, which are incorporated in the outlet pipe system. The purpose of these devices is to maintain a constant rate of filtration. An important component of the regulation system is the 'Venturi meter,' which measures the bed resistance or 'loss of head'. When the resistance builds up, the operator opens the regulating valve so as to maintain steady rate of filtration. When the 'loss of head' exceeds 1.3 m, it is uneconomical to run the filter.

Usually, the filter may run for weeks or even months without cleaning. When the bed resistance increases to such an extent that the regulating valve has to be kept fully open,

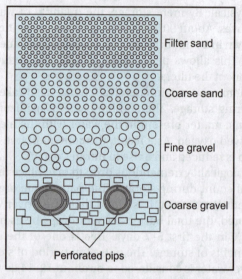

Figure 7.7: Layers of graded gravel

it is time to clean the filter bed, since any further increase in resistance is bound to reduce the filtration rate. At this stage, the supernatant water is drained off and the sand bed is cleaned by 'scrapping' off the top portion of sand layer to a depth of 1 or 2 cm. This operation may carry out by unskilled laborers using hand tools or by mechanical equipment. After several years of operation and say 20 or 30 scrapings, the thickness of the sand bed will have to be reduced by about 0.5–0.8 m, then the plant is closed down, and a new bed is constructed. The advantages of a slow sand filter are:
- Simple to construct and operate
- The cost of construction is cheaper than that of rapid sand filters
- The physical, chemical and bacteriological quality of filtered water is very high.

Rapid sand filter

In 1885, the first sand filters were installed in the United States of America (USA). Rapid sand filters are of two types, the gravity type (e.g. Paterson's filter) and the pressure type (e.g. Candy's filter) both the types are in use. The following steps are involved in the purification of water by rapid sand filters (Fig. 7.8):

1. Coagulation: The raw water is first treated with a chemical coagulant such as alum, the dose of which varies from 5 to 40 mg or more per liter, depending upon the turbidity, color, temperature and the pH value of the water.
2. Rapid mixing: The treated water is then subjected to violent agitation in a 'mixing chamber' for a few minutes. This allows a quick and thorough dissemination of alum throughout the bulk of the water, which is very necessary.

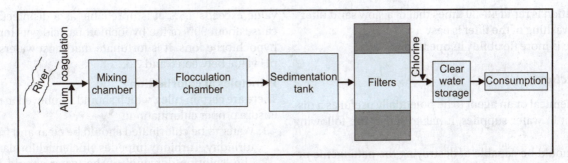

Figure 7.8: Rapid sand filtration plant

3. **Flocculation:** The next phase involves a slow and gentle stirring of the treated water in a 'flocculation chamber' for about 30 minutes. The mechanical type of flocculator is the mostly widely used. It consists of a number of paddles, which rotate at 2–4 rpm. The paddles rotate with the help of motors. These slow and gently stirring results in the formation of a thick, copious, white flocculent precipitate of aluminum hydroxide. The thicker the precipitate or flock diameter, the greater the settling velocity.
4. **Sedimentation:** The coagulated water is now led into sedimentation tanks where it is detained for periods varying from 2 to 6 hours when the flocculent precipitate together with impurities and bacteria settle down in the tank. At least 95% of the flocculent precipitate needs to be removed before the water are admitted into the rapid sand filters. The precipitate or sludge, which settles at the bottom is removed from time to time, without disturbing the operation of the tank. For proper maintenance, the tanks should be cleaned regularly from time to time; otherwise they may become a breeding ground for mollusks and sponges.
5. **Filtration:** The partly clarified water is now subjected to rapid sand filtration.
6. Each unit of filter bed has a surface of about 80–90 m² (about 900 ft²). Sand is the filtering medium. The 'effective size' of the sand particles is between 0.4 and 0.7 mm. The depth of the sand bed is a layer of graded gravel which is about 30–40 cm deep (1½ ft). The gravel supports the sand bed and permits the filtered water to move freely towards the underdrains. The depth of the water on the top of the sand bed is 1.0–1.5 m (5–6 ft). The underdrains at the bottom of the filter bed collect the filtered water. The rate of filtration is 5–15 m²/h. A view of the rapid sand filter is given in Figure 7.9.

As filtration proceeds, the 'alum floc' not removed by sedimentation is held back on the sand bed. It forms a slimy layer comparable to the zoogleal layer in the slow sand filters. It absorbs bacteria from the water and effects purification. Oxidation of ammonia also takes place during the passage of water through the filters. As filtration proceeds, the suspended impurities and bacteria clog the filters. The filters soon become dirty and begin to lose their efficiency. When the 'loss of head' approaches 7–8 ft, filtration is stopped and the filters are subjected to a washing process known as 'backwashing'.

Rapid sand filters need frequent washing daily or weekly depending upon the loss of head. Washing is accomplished by revering the flow of water through the sand bed, which is called 'backwashing'. Backwashing dislodges the impurities and cleans up the sand bed. The washing is stopped when clear sand is visible and washed water is sufficiently clear. The whole process of washing takes about 15 minutes. In some rapid sand filters, compressed air is used as part of the backwashing processes.

The advantages of rapid sand filter over the slow sand filters are:
- Rapid sand filter can deal with raw water directly, no preliminary storage is needed
- The filter beds occupy less space

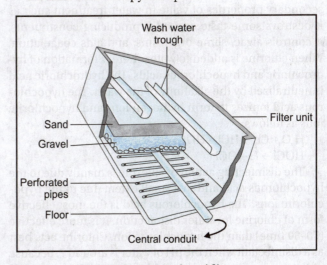

Figure 7.9: Rapid sand filter

- Filtration is rapid 40–50 times that of a slow sand filter
- The washing of the filter is easy
- There is more flexibility in operation.

Disinfection

For a chemical or an agent to be potentially useful as a disinfectant in water supplies, it has to satisfy the following criteria:

1. It should be capable of destroying the pathogenic organisms present within the contact time available and not unduly influenced by the range of physical, and chemical properties of water encountered particular temperature, pH and mineral constituents.
2. It should not leave products of reaction, which render the water toxic or impart color or otherwise make it nonpotable.
3. It should have ready and dependable availability at reasonable cost permitting convenient, safe and accurate application of water.
4. It should possess the property of leaving residual concentration to deal with small possible recontamination.
5. It should be amenable to detection by practical, rapid and simple analytical techniques in the small concentration range to permit the control of; efficiency of the disinfection process.
6. The term disinfection is synonyms with chlorination in practice.

Chlorination

Chlorine kills pathogenic bacteria, but it has no effect on spores and certain viruses (e.g. polio, viral hepatitis) except in high doses. Chlorine also has several important secondary properties of value in water treatment such as it destroys some taste and odor producing constituents, it controls algae, slime organisms, and aids coagulation. When chlorine is added to water, there is formation of hydrochloric and hypochlorous acids. The hydrochloric acid is neutralized by the alkalinity of the water. The hypochlorous acid ionizes to form hydrogen ions and hypochlorite ions as follows:

$$H_2O + Cl_2 \rightarrow HCl + HOCl$$
$$HOCl \rightarrow H + OCl$$

The disinfecting action of chlorine is mainly due to the hypochlorous acid and to a small extent due to the hypochlorite ions. The hypochlorous acid is the most effective form of chlorine for water disinfection. It is more effective (70–80 time) than the hypochlorite ion. Chlorine acts best as a disinfectant when the pH of water is around 7, because of the predominance of hypochlorous acid. When the pH value exceeds 8.5%, it is unreliable as a disinfectant, because about 90% of the hypochlorous acid gets ionized to hypochlorite ions. It is fortunate that most waters have a pH value between 6 and 7.5.

Principles of chlorination

There are certain rules, which should be obeyed in order to ensure proper chlorination:

1. Water to be chlorinated should be clear and free from turbidity. Turbidity impedes efficient chlorination.
2. The 'chlorine demand' of the water should be estimated. The chlorine demand of water is the difference between the amount of chlorine added to the water and the amount of residual chlorine remaining at the end of a specific period of contact (usually 60 minute) at a given temperature and pH of the water. In other words, it is the amount of chlorine that is needed to destroy bacteria and oxidize all the organic matter and ammoniac substance present in the water. The point at which the chlorine demand of the water is met then it is called 'breakpoint'. If further chlorine is added beyond the breakpoint, free chlorine (HOCL and OCL) begin to appear in the water.
3. Contact period: The presence of free residual chlorine for a contact period of at least 1 hour is essential to kill bacteria and viruses. It is noted that however, chlorine has no effect on spore protozoan cyst and helminthic ova except in high doses.
4. The minimum recommended concentration of free chlorine is 0.5 mg/L for 1 hour. The free residual chlorine provides a margin of safety against subsequent microbial contamination such as may occur during storage and distribution.
5. The sum of the chlorine demand of the specific water and the free residual chlorine of 0.5 mg/L constitutes the correct dose of chlorine to be applied.

Method of chlorination

For disinfecting large scale of water, chlorine is applied either as chlorine gas on chloramine or perchloric acid.

Chlorine gas

Chlorine gas is the first choice because it is cheap, quick in action, efficient and easy to apply. Since, chlorine gas is an irritant to the eyes and poisonous, specific equipment known as 'chlorinating equipment' is required to apply chlorine gas to water supplied. Paterson's chloronome is one such device for measurer regulating and administering gaseous chlorine to water supplies.

Chloramine

Chloramines are loose compounds of chlorine and ammonia. They have a less tendency to produce chlorine tastes and give a more persistent type of residual chlorine.

The greatest drawback of chloramines is that they have a slower action than chlorine and therefore they are not being used to any great extent in water treatment.

Perchloron or high-test hypochlorite
Perchloron or high-test hypochlorite (HTH) is a calcium compound, which carries 60–70% of available chlorine. Solutions prepared from HTH are also used for water disinfections.

Breakpoint chlorination
When chlorine dose in the water is increased, a reduction in the residual chlorine occurs, due to destruction of chlorine by the added chlorine. The end products do not represents any residual chlorine. This fall in residual chlorine will continue with further increase in chlorine dose and after a stage, the residual chlorine begins increase in proportion to the added dose of chlorine. This point at which the residual chlorine appears and when all combined chlorine have been completely destroyed is the breakpoint dosage. Breakpoint chlorination achieves the same results as super chlorination in a rational manner.

Superchlorination
Superchlorination is followed by dechlorination comprises the addition of large doses of chlorine to the water and removal of excess of chlorine after disinfection. This method is applicable to heavily polluted waters, whose quality fluctuates greatly.

Orthotolidine test
Orthotolidine (OT) test enables both free and combined chlorine in water to be determined with speed and accuracy. The test was developed in 1918. The reagent consists of analytical grade OT dissolved in 10% solution of hydrochloric acid. When this reagent is added to water containing chlorine, it turns yellow and the intensity of the color varies with the concentration of the gas. Then yellow color is produced by both free and combined chlorine residuals. OT reacts with free chlorine instantaneously, but reacts more slowly with combined chlorine.

The test is carried out by adding 0.1 mL of the reagent to 11 mL of water. The yellow color produced is matched against suitable standards or color disks. Commercial equipment is available for this purpose. It is essential to take the reading within 10 seconds after the addition of the reagent to estimate free chlorine in water. The color that is produced after a lapse of 15–20 minutes, is due to the action of both free and combined chlorine.

Orthotolidine-arsenite test
Orthotolidine-arsenite (OTA) test is a modification of the OT test to determine the free and combined chlorine residuals separately. Further, the errors caused by the presence of interfering substances such as nitrites, iron and manganese all of which produce a yellow color with OT are overcome by the OTA test.

Chlorine alternatives
Now, many chlorine alternatives are receiving renewed interest. Ozone is showing the greatest promise and ultraviolet (UV) irradiations limited usefulness as complimentary agents for chlorine in water disinfection.

Ozonation
Ozone is a relatively unstable gas. It is a powerful oxidizing agent. It eliminates undesirable odor, taste and color and removes all chlorine from the water. Most importantly, ozone has a strong virucidal effect. It inactivates viruses in a matter of seconds, whereas few minutes are required to inactivate them with either chlorine or iodine. This has prompted many municipalities to consider ozone for potable water treatment.

Ozone decomposes and disappears, but there is no residual germicidal effect. So, ozone should be used as a pretreatment of water to destroy not only viruses and bacteria but also organic compounds that are precursors for undesirable chloro-organic compounds that form when chlorine is added. A carefully controlled minimum dose of chlorine is added to the water before is pumped into the distribution system. Thus, ozonation is usually employed in combination with chlorination. The two methods complement each other taking advantage of the best features each. The ozone dosage required for potable water treatment varies from 0.2 to 1.5 mg/L.

Ultraviolet irradiation
Ultraviolet irradiation is effective against most microorganisms known to contaminate water supplies including viruses. This method of disinfection involves the exposure of a film of water up to about 120 mm thick to one or several quartz mercury vapor are lamps emitting UV radiation at a wavelength in the range of 200–295 mm. The water should be free from turbidity and suspended or colloidal constituents for efficient disinfection.

The exposure is for short period, no foreign matter is introduced and no taste, and odor produced. Overexposure does not result in any harmful effects. Therefore, no residual effect is available. The apparatus needed is expensive.

Multi-stage Reverse Osmosis Purification of Water

Multi-stage reverse osmosis purification process is used to make water both chemically and microbiologically potable by reducing the total dissolved solids, hardness, heavy metals, and disease causing bacteria, virus, protozoa and cysts.

The various elements of a typical multistage reverse osmosis process is shown in Figure 7.10.

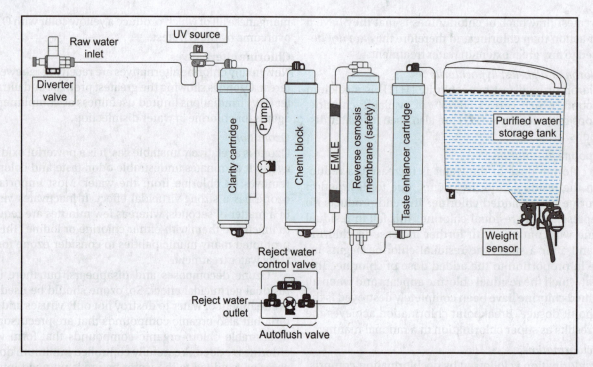

Figure 7.10: Multi-stage reverses osmosis purification of water (EMLE, electric membrane life enhancer; UV, ultraviolet)

The clarity cartridge removes the suspended particles such as dust, mud and sand from the water. The reverse osmosis cartridge reduces the total dissolved solids, hardness and heavy metals such as arsenic, lead, mercury and eliminates microorganisms.

Purification of Water on Small Scale

Purification of Water on Domestic Level

There are three methods available for purifying water on an individual or domestic scale, boiling, chemical disinfection and filtration. These methods can be used singly or in combination.

Boiling

Boiling is a satisfactory method of purifying water for household purpose. To be effective, the water must be brought to a 'rolling boil' for 5–10 minutes. It kills all bacteria, spores, cysts, ova and yields sterilized water. Boiling also removes temporary hardness by driving off carbon dioxide and precipitating the calcium carbonate. The taste of water is altered, but is harmless. While boiling is an excellent method of purifying water, it offers no 'residual protection' against subsequent microbial contamination. Water should be boiled preferably in the same container in which it is to be stored to avoid contamination during storage.

Chemical Disinfection

Bleaching powder/Chlorinated lime

Bleaching powder or chlorinated lime ($CaOCl_2$) is a white amorphous powder with a pungent smell of chlorine. When freshly made, it contains about 33% of 'available chlorine'. It is, however, an unstable compound. On exposure to air, light and moisture, it rapidly loses its chlorine content. But when mixed with excess of lime, it retains its strength, this is called 'stabilized bleach'. Bleaching powder should be stored in a dark, cool, dry place in a closed container that is resistant to corrosion.

Chlorine solution

Chlorine solution may be prepared from bleaching powder. If 4 kg of bleaching powder with 25% available chlorine is mixed with 20 liters of water, it will give a 5% solution of chlorine. Ready-made chlorine solutions in different strengths are also available in the market. Like bleaching powder, the chlorine solutions are subject to losses on exposure to light or on prolonged storage. The solution should be kept in a dark, cool and dry place in a closed container.

High-test hypochlorite (perchloron)

High-test hypochlorite (HTH) is a calcium compound, which contains 60–70% available chlorine. It is more stable than bleaching powder and deteriorates much less on storage. Solutions prepared from HTH are also used for water disinfections.

Chlorine tablets

Under various trade names, halazone tablets are available in the market. They are quite good for disinfecting small quantities of water, but they are costly. The National Environmental Engineering Research Institute, Nagpur has formulated a new type of chlorine tablet, which is 15 times better than ordinary halogen tablets. These tablets are manufactured in various strength and are now available in plenty in the Indian market at a cheaper rate. A single tablet of 0.5 g is sufficient to disinfect 20 liters of water.

Iodine

Iodine may be used for emergency disinfections of water. Two drops of 2% ethanol solution of iodine will suffice for 1 liter of clear water. A contact time of 20–30 minutes is needed for effective disinfection. Iodine does not react with ammonia or organic compounds to any great extent; hence it remains in its active molecular form, over a wide range of pH values and water conditions, and persists longer than either chlorine or bromine. Iodine is unlikely to become a municipal water supply disinfectant in broad sense. High costs and the fact that the element is physiologically active (thyroid activity) are its major disadvantages.

Potassium permanganate

Once widely used, it is no longer recommended for water disinfection. Although a powerful oxidizing agent, it is not a satisfactory agent for disinfecting water. It may kill *Vibrio cholerae*, but is of little use against other disease organisms. It has other drawbacks too such as altering the colors, smell and taste of water.

Filtration in Small Scale

Water can be purified on a small scale by filtering through ceramic filters such as Pasteur-Chamberland filter, Berkefeld filter and Katadyn filter. The essential part of a filter is the 'candle', which is made of porcelain in the Chamberland type and of kieselguhr or infusorial earth in the Berkefeld filter. In the Katadyn filter, the surface of the filter is coated with a silver catalyst so that bacteria coming in contact with the surface are killed by the 'oligodynamic' action of the silver ions, which are liberated into the water. Filter candles of the fine type usually remove bacteria found in drinking water, but not the filter passing viruses. Filter candles are liable to be logged with impurities and bacteria. They should be cleaned by scrubbing with a hard brush under running water and boiled at least once a week. Only clean water should be used with ceramic filters. Although ceramic filters are effective in purifying water, they are not quite suitable for widespread use under Indian conditions (Fig. 7.11).

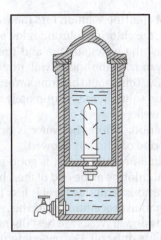

Figure 7.11: Berkefeld filter

Disinfecting Wells on Mass Scale

Wells are the main source of water supply in the rural areas. The need often arises to disinfect them, sometimes on a mass scale during epidemics of cholera and gastroenteritis. The most effective and cheapest method of disinfecting wells is by bleaching powder by using the following procedure:

1. Find the volume of water in a well:
   - Measure the depth of water column 'h' meter
   - Measure the diameter of well 'd' meter
   - Take the average of several readings of the above measurements
   - Substitute 'h' and 'd' in:

   $$\text{Volume (liters)} = \frac{3.14 \times d^2 \times h}{4} \times 1{,}000$$

   - One cubic meter = 1,000 liters of water.

2. Find the amount of bleaching powder required for disinfection: Estimate the chlorine demand of the well water by 'Horrocks' apparatus and calculate the amount of bleaching powder required to disinfect the well.

   Roughly, 2.5 g of good quality bleaching powder would be required to disinfect 1,000 liter of water. This will give an approximate dose of 0.7 mg of applied chlorine per liter of water.

3. Dissolve bleaching powder in water: The bleaching powder required for disinfecting the well is placed in a bucket (not more than 100 g in one bucket of water) and made into a thin paste. More water is added till the bucket is nearly three fourths full. The contents are stirred well and allowed to sediment for 5–10 minutes when lime settles down. The supernatant solution, which is chlorine solution is transferred to another bucket and the chalk or lime is discarded (the line sediment should not be poured into the well as it increases the hardness of well water).

4. Delivery of chlorine solution into the well: The bucket containing the chlorine solution is lowered, some distance below the water surface and the well water is agitated by moving the bucket violently both vertically and laterally. This should be done several times so that the chlorine solution mixes intimately with the water inside the well.
5. Contact period: Before the water is drawn for use a contact period of 1 hour is allowed.
6. Orthotolidine-arsenite test: It is good practice to test for residual chlorine at the end of the 1 hour contact. If the 'free' residual chlorine level is less than 0.5 mg/L, the chlorination procedure should be repeated before any water is drawn. Wells are best disinfected at night after the day's draw off. During epidemics of cholera, wells should be disinfected every day.

Double Pot Method

The double pot method is an improvement devised by the National Environmental Engineering Research Institute, Nagpur, India. This method uses two cylindrical pots, one placed inside the other. The inside height and diameter are 30 cm and 25 cm respectively for the outer pot. A hole of 1 cm in diameter is made in each pot in the inner pot the hole is in the upper portion, near the rim and in the outer pot; it is 4 cm above the bottom (Fig. 7.12).

A mixture of 1 kg of bleaching powder and 2 kg of course sand (approximately 2 mm in diameter) is prepared and slightly moistened with water. The inner pot is filled with this mixture up to 3 cm below the level of the hole. The inner pot is introduced into the outer one and the mouth of the pot is closed with polyethylene foil. The use of two pots makes it possible to have larger holes without the risk of over chlorination.

The double pot is lowered into the well by means of a rope attached to the well kerb. The pot should be immersed at least 1 meter below the water level to prevent damage by the buckets used for drawing water. It has been found that this device works satisfactory for 2–3 weeks in small household wells containing about 4,500 liters of water and having a draw off rate of 360–450 L/day.

GUIDELINES FOR POTABLE WATER BY WHO

The WHO has published guideline for drinking water quality intended for use by countries as a basis for the development of standards, which, if properly implemented will ensure the safety of drinking water supplies. In order to define standards, it is necessary to consider these recommendations in the context of prevailing environmental, social, economical and cultural conditions. The guideline

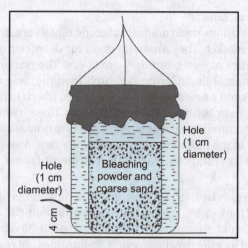

Figure 7.12: Double pot

for drinking water quality recommended by WHO (1993 and 1996) relate to the following variables:
- Acceptability parameters
- Microbiological parameters
- Chemical parameters
- Radiological parameters
- Biological aspects.

Acceptability Parameters

Physical Parameters

The ordinary consumer judges the water quality by its physical characteristics. The provision of drinking water which is not only safe but also pleasing in appearance, taste and odor is a matter of high priority. The supply of water, i.e. unsatisfactory in this respect will undermine the confidence of consumers. Leading to use of water from less safe source. The acceptability of drinking water can be influenced by many different constituents. These are as given below.

Turbidity

On esthetic grounds, drinking water should be free from turbidity. Turbidity in drinking water is caused by particulate matter that may be present as a consequence of inadequate treatment or from resuspension of sediment in the distribution system. It may also be due to the presence of inorganic particulate matter in some groundwater. Turbidity interferes with disinfection and microbiological determination. Water with turbidity of less than 5 nephelometric turbidity units (5 NTU) is usually acceptable to consumer.

Color

Drinking water should be free from color, which may be due to the presence of colored organic matter (primarily humic substances), metals such as iron and manganese or highly colored industrial waters. Consumers may turn to alternative, perhaps unsafe, sources when their water is colored to an esthetically displeasing degree. The guideline value is up to 15 TCU can be detected in a glass of water.

Taste and odor
Taste and odor originate from natural and biological sources or processes, from contamination by chemicals, or as a by-product of water treatment (e.g. chlorination). Taste and odor may develop during storage and distribution. It is indicative of some form of pollution or malfunction during water treatment or distribution. The cause should be investigated particularly if there is substantial change. An unusual taste or odor might be an indication of the presence of potentially harmful substances—health-based guideline value is proposed for taste and odor.

Temperature
Cool water is generally more palatable. Lower water temperature tends to decrease the efficiency of treatment process including disinfection and may thus have a deleterious effect on drinking water quality. However, high water temperature enhances the growth of microorganisms and taste, odor, color and corrosion problem may increase. No guideline value is recommended since its control is usually impracticable.

To sum up, we cannot judge the quality of drinking water by physical characteristics alone. A detailed chemical and microbiological examination is also needed for complete assessment.

Inorganic Constituents

Chlorides
All waters including rain water contain chlorides. In the neighborhood of the sea, the salinity of water varies from place to place. First to all it is necessary to determine the normal range of chlorides of the unpolluted surface and groundwater in the given locality. Any excess over the normal range should arouse suspicion of water contamination. The standard prescribed for chloride is 200 mg/L. The maximum permissible level is 600 mg/L.

Hardness
Public acceptability of the degree of hardness may vary considerably from one community to another depending on local conditions. The taste threshold for the calcium ion is in the range of 100–300 mg/L depending on the associated anion and the taste threshold of magnesium is probably less than that for calcium. In some instances, water hardness in excess of 500 mg/L is tolerated by consumers.

Depending on the interaction of other factors such as pH and alkalinity, water with a hardness of approximately 200 mg/L may cause scale deposition in the distribution system and will result in excessive soap consumption and subsequent scum formation. On heating, hard water forms deposits of calcium carbonate scale. Soft water with a hardness of less than 100 mg/L on other hand have a lower buffer capacity and so be more corrosive for water pipes.

Ammonia
The term ammonia (NH_3) includes the non-ionized and ionized. Ammonia in the environment originates from metabolic, agricultural and industrial processes and from disinfection with chloramine. Natural levels in ground and surface water are usually below 0.2 mg/L. Anaerobic groundwater may contain up to 3 mg/L. Intensive rearing of farm animals can give rise to much higher levels of surface water. Ammonia contamination can also rise from cement mortar pipe linings. Ammonia in water is an indicator of possible bacterial sewage and animal waste pollution. Ammonia can comprise disinfection efficiency result in nitrite formation in distribution systems, can cause the failure of filters for the removal of odor problems.

pH
One of the main objectives in controlling the pH is to minimize corrosion and incrustation in the distribution system. pH levels of less than 7 may cause severe corrosion of metals in the distribution pipes and elevated levels of certain chemical substances such as lead may result. At pH levels above 8, there is a progressive decrease in the efficiency of the chlorine disinfection process. An acceptable pH drinking water is between 6.5 and 8.5. In the absence of a distribution system, the acceptable range of pH may be broader.

Hydrogen sulfide
The taste and odor threshold of hydrogen sulfide in water are estimated to be between 0.05 and 0.1 mg/L. The 'rotten eggs' odor of hydrogen is particularly noticeable in some groundwaters and in stagnant drinking water; the distribution system as a result of oxygen depletion and the subsequent reduction of sulfate by bacterial activity. Sulfide is oxidized rapidly to sulfate in well-aerated water and hydrogen sulfide levels in oxygenated water supplies are normally very low. The presence of hydrogen sulfide in drinking water can be easily detected by the consumer and requires immediate corrective action.

Iron
Anaerobic groundwater may contain ferrous iron at concentrations of up to several milligrams per liter without discoloration or turbidity in water when directly pumped from the well. On exposure to the atmosphere, however, the ferrous iron oxidizes to ferric iron giving an objectionable reddish brown color to the water. Iron also promotes the growth of 'iron bacteria', which derive their energy

from the oxidation of ferrous iron to ferric iron and in the process deposit a slimy coating on the pipe. At level above 3 mg/L, iron stains laundry and plumbing fixtures.

Sodium

The taste threshold concentration of sodium in water depends on the associated anion and the temperature of the solution. At room temperature, the average taste threshold for sodium is about 200 mg/L.

Sulfate

The presence of sulfate in drinking water can cause noticeable taste. Taste impairment varies with the nature of the associated action. It is generally considered that taste impairment is minimal at levels below 250 mg/L. It has been found that addition of calcium and magnesium sulfate (but not sodium sulfate) to distilled water improves the taste; optimal taste was recorded between 270 and 90 mg/L for the two compounds respectively.

Total dissolved solids

Total dissolved solids (TDSs) can have an important effect on the taste of drinking water. The palatability of water with a TDS level of less than 600 mg/L is generally considered to be good. Drinking water becomes increasingly unpalatable at TDS level greater than 1,200 mg/L. Water with extremely low concentrations of TDS may be unacceptable because of its flat, insipid taste. The presence of high level of TDS may also be objectionable to consumers owing to excessive scaling in water pipes, heaters, boilers and household appliances. Water with concentrations of TDS below 1,000 mg/L is usually acceptable to the consumers.

Zinc

Zinc imparts an undesirable astringent taste to water. Tests indicate a taste threshold concentration of 4 mg/L (as zinc sulfate). Water containing zinc at concentrations in excess of 5 mg/L may appear opalescent and develop a greasy film on boiling, although these effects may also be noticeable at concentrations as low as 3 mg/L. Drinking water seldom contains zinc at concentrations above 0.1 mg/L, levels in tap water can be considerably higher, because of the zinc used in plumbing material.

Manganese

Manganese concentrations below 0.1 mg/L are usually acceptable to consumers; this may vary with local circumstances. At levels above 0.1 mg/L manganese in water supplies stains sanitary ware and laundry, and causes an undesirable taste in beverages. It may lead to accumulation of deposits in the distribution system. Even at concentration of 0.02 mg/L, manganese will often form a coating on pipes, which may slough off as a black precipitate.

Dissolved oxygen

Water with dissolved oxygen content is influenced by the raw water temperature, comparison, treatment and any chemical or biological processes taking place in the distribution system. Depletion of dissolved oxygen in water supplies can encourage microbial reduction of nitrate to nitrite and sulfate to sulfide giving rise to odor problem. It can also cause an increase in the concentration of ferrous iron in solution. No health-based guideline value has been recommended.

Copper

The presence of copper in a water supply may interfere with the intended domestic use of water. It increases the corrosion of galvanized iron and steel fittings. Staining of laundry and sanitary ware occurs at copper concentrations above 1 mg/L.

Aluminum

The presence of aluminum at concentrations in excess of 0.2 g/L often leads to deposition of aluminum hydroxide floc in distribution system and the exacerbation of discoloration of water by iron.

Microbiological Aspects

Bacterial Indicators

Natural and treated waters vary in microbiological quality. Ideally, drinking water should not contain any microorganisms known to be pathogenic. It should be free from bacteria indicative of pollution with excreta. Failure to provide adequate protection, effective treatment and disinfection of drinking water will expose the community to the risk of outbreaks of intestinal and other infectious diseases. Those at greatest risk of waterborne diseases are infants and young children, people who are debilitated or living under insanitary conditions, the sick and elderly. For them, the infective dose is significantly lower than the healthy population. The potential consequences of microbial contamination are such that its control must always be of paramount importance and must never be compromised. The primary bacterial indicator recommended for this purpose is the coliform group of organisms as a whole. Supplementary indicator organisms, such as fecal streptococci and sulfite-reducing clostridia may sometimes be useful in determining the origin of fecal pollution as well as in assessing the efficiency of water treatment processes.

Coliform organisms

The 'coliform' organisms include all aerobic and facultative anaerobic, gram negative, nonsporing, motile and non-motile rods capable of fermenting lactose at 35–37°C in less than 48 hours. The coliform group includes both fecal and non-fecal organisms. Typical example of the fecal group is *Escherichia coli (E. coli)* and of the non-fecal group *Klebsiella aerogenes*. From a practical point of view, it is assumed that all coliforms are of fecal origin unless a non-fecal origin can be proved.

There are several reasons why coliform organisms are chosen as indicators of fecal pollution rather than the waterborne pathogens directly:

1. The coliform organisms are constantly present in great abundance in the human intestine. It is estimated that an average person excretes 200–400 billion of these organisms per day. These organisms are foreign to potable waters and hence their presence in water is looked upon as evidence of fecal contamination.
2. They are easily detected by culture methods—as small as one bacteria in 100 mL of water, whereas the methods for detecting the pathogenic organisms are complicated and time consuming.
3. They survive longer than the pathogens, which tend to die out more rapidly than coliform bacilli.
4. The coliform bacilli have greater assistance to the forces of natural purification than the waterborne pathogens. If the coliform organisms are present in water sample, the assumptions is the probable presence of intestinal pathogens.

Fecal streptococci

Fecal streptococci regularly occurs in feces, but in much smaller numbers than *E. coli*, in doubtful cases, the finding of fecal streptococci in water is regarded as important confirmatory evidence of recent fecal pollution of water. Streptococci are highly resistant to drying and may be valuable for routine control testing after laying new mains or repairs in distribution systems or for detecting pollution by surface run off to ground or surface waters.

Clostridium Perfringens

Clostridium perfringens also occur regularly in feces, through generally in much smaller numbers than *E. coli*. The spores are capable of surviving in water for a longer time than organisms of the coliforms group and usually resist chlorination in the doses normally used in waterworks practice. The presence of spores of *C. perfringens* in natural water suggests that fecal contamination has occurred and their presence in the absence of the coliform group suggests that fecal contamination has occurred, and their presence in the absence of the coliform group suggests that fecal contamination occurred at some remote time. Its presence in filtered supplies may indicate deficiency in filtration practice.

Virological Parameter

Virological parameter is recommended that to be acceptable, drinking water should be free from any viruses infections for man. Disinfection with 0.5 mg/L of free chlorine residual after contact period of at least 30 minutes at a pH of 8.0 is sufficient to inactive virus. This free chlorine residual is to be insisted in all disinfected supplies in areas suspected of endemicity of hepatitis A to take care of the safety of supply from the virus point of view. This incidentally takes care of safety from the bacteriological point of view as well. For other areas, 0.2 mg/L of free residual chlorine for half-an-hour should be insisted. The turbidity condition of 1 BNUT or less must be fulfilled prior to disinfection of water, if adequate treatment is to be achieved. Ozone has been shown to be effective viral. Disinfectant, preferably for clean water, if residuals of 0.2–0.4 mg/L are maintained for 4 minutes, but it is not possible to maintain a ozone residual in distribution system.

Biological Aspects

Protozoa

Species of protozoa known to have been transmitted by the ingestion of contaminated drinking water include *Entamoeba histolytica*, *Giardia* species and rarely *Balantidium coli*. These organisms can be introduced into water supply by human or in some instances, animal fecal contamination. Drinking water should not contain any pathogenic intestinal protozoa. Rapid or slow sand filtration has been shown to be effective in removing a high proportion of pathogenic protozoa. Standard methods are not currently available for the detection of pathogenic protozoa in water supplies in the context of a routine monitoring program.

Helminths

The ineffective stage of many parasitic roundworms and flatworms can be transmitted to man through drinking water. A single mature larva or fertilized egg can cause infection and such infective stages should be absent from drinking water. However, the water route is relatively unimportant except in the case of *Dracunculus medinensis* (guinea worm) and the human *Schistosoma*, which are primarily hazards of unpiped water supplies. Source protection is the best approach to prevention. The methods for detection of these parasites are unsuited for routine monitoring.

Free-living Organisms

Free-living organisms that may occur in water supplies include fungi, algae, etc. The most common problem with these is their interference in the operation of water treatment process, color, turbidity, taste and odor of finished water.

Chemical Aspects

The health risk due to toxic chemicals in drinking water differs from that caused by microbiological contaminants. These are few chemical constituents of water that can lead to acute health problems except through massive accidental contamination of a supply. Moreover, experience shows that in such incidents, the water supply becomes undrinkable owing to unacceptable taste, odor and appearance.

The chemicals selected for the development of guideline value include those considered potentially hazardous to human health; those detected relatively frequent in drinking water and those detected in relatively high concentrations. The problem associated with chemical constituents of drinking water arise primarily from their ability to cause adverse health effects after prolonged periods of exposure; particular concern are contaminants that have cumulative toxic properties such as heavy metals and substances that are carcinogenic.

The presence of certain chemicals in excess of prescribed limits may constitute ground for rejection of the water as a source of public wider supply. These substances may be inorganic or organic.

Inorganic Constituents

Inorganic constituents include arsenic, cadmium, chromium, cyanide, fluoride, lead, mercury, nickel, nitrate, selenium, etc.

Arsenic

Arsenic is introduced into water through the dissolution of mineral and ones from industrial effluents and from atmospheric deposition, concentrations of ground water in some areas are sometimes elevated as a result of erosion from natural sources. The average daily intake of inorganic arsenic in water is estimated to be similar to that from food. Intake from air is negligible. A provisional guideline value for arsenic in drinking water is 0.01 mg/L is established.

Cadmium

Cadmium metal is used in the steel industry and in plastics. Cadmium compounds are widely used in batteries. It is released to the environment in waste water and diffuse pollution is caused by contamination from fertilizers and local air pollution. Contamination in drinking water may also be caused by impurities in the zinc of galvanized pipes and some metal fittings, although levels in drinking water are usually less than 1 mg/L. Absorption of cadmium compound is dependent on the solubility of the compound. Cadmium accumulates primarily in the kidneys and has a long biological half-life in humans of 10–35 years. A guideline value for cadmium is established at 0.003 mg/L.

Chromium

Chromium is widely distributed in the earth's crust. In general, food appears to be the major source of intake. The absorption of chromium after oral exposure is relatively low and depends on the oxidation state. The guideline value for chromium is 0.05 mg/L, which is considered to be unlikely to give rise to significant health risks.

Cyanide

The acute toxicity of cyanide is high cyanides can be found in some foods, particularly in some developing countries and they are usually found in drinking water, primarily as a consequence of industrial contamination. Effects on thyroid and particularly the nervous system were observed in some populations as a consequence of the long-term consumption of inadequately processed cassava containing high levels of cyanide. The guideline value of 0.007 mg/L is considered to be safe.

Fluoride

Fluoride accounts for about 0.3 g/kg of the earth's crust. Inorganic fluorine compounds are used in the production of aluminum and fluoride is released during the manufacture, and use of phosphate fertilizers, which contain up to 4% fluorine. Levels of daily exposure of fluoride depend on the geographical area. If diets contain fish and tea, exposure via food may be particularly high. In specific areas, other foods and indoor air pollution may contribute considerably to total exposure. Additional intake may result from the use of fluoride toothpastes.

Exposure to fluoride from drinking water depends greatly on natural circumstances. Levels in raw water are normally below 1.5 mg/L, but groundwater may contain about 10 mg/L in areas rich in fluoride containing minerals. High fluoride levels, above 5 mg/L have been found in several countries (e.g. China, India and Thailand). Such high levels have at times led to dental or skeletal fluorosis. Fluoride is sometimes added to drinking water to prevent dental caries. Soluble fluorides are readily absorbed in the gastrointestinal tract after intake in drinking water. The guideline value suggested is 1.5 mg/L in setting national standards for fluoride. It is particularly important to consider climatic conditions, volume of water intake and intake of fluoride from other sources (e.g. food, air).

Lead

Lead is present in tap water to some extent as a result of its dissolution from natural sources, but primarily from household plumbing systems containing lead in pipes, solder, fittings or the service connections to homes. The amount of lead dissolved form the plumbing system depends on several factors including pH, temperature, water hardness and standing time of the water with soft, acidic water being the most plumbosolvent.

Placental transfer of lead occurs in humans as early as 12 weeks of gestation and continues throughout development. Young children absorb four to five times as much lead as adults and the biological half-life may be considerably longer in children than in adults. Lead is a general toxicant that accumulates in the skeleton. Infants, children up to 6 years of age and pregnant women are most susceptible to its adverse health effects. Lead also interferes with calcium metabolism both directly and by interfering with vitamin D metabolism. Lead is toxic to both central and peripheral nervous system inducing subencephalopathic, neurological and behavioral effects. Renal tumors have been induced in experimental animal exposed to high concentrations of lead compounds in the diet and it is grouped in group B (possible human carcinogen). The health-based guideline value of lead is 0.01 mg/L.

Lead is exceptional in that most lead in drinking water arises from plumbing in buildings and the remedy consists principally of removing plumbing and fittings, which contain lead. This requires much time and money, and it is recognized that not all water will meet the guideline immediately. Measures to control corrosion should be implemented.

Mercury

Mercury is present in inorganic form in surface and groundwater at concentrations usually less than 0.5 mg/L. The kidney is the main target organ for inorganics mercury, whereas methylmercury affects mainly the central nervous system. The guideline value for total mercury is 0.001 mg/L.

Nitrate and nitrite

Nitrate and nitrite are naturally occurring ions that are part of the nitrogen cycle. Naturally occurring nitrate level in surface and groundwater are generally a few milligrams per liter. In many groundwaters, an increase of nitrate level has been observed owing to the intensification of farming practice. In some countries, up to 10% of the population may be exposed to nitrate levels in drinking water of above 50 mg/L.

In general, vegetables are the main source of nitrate intake when levels in drinking water are below 10 mg/L. When nitrate level in drinking water exceeds 50 mg/L, drinking water will become the main source of total nitrate intake. The guideline value for nitrate in drinking water is solely to prevent methemoglobinemia, which depends upon the conversion of nitrate into nitrite. Bottle-fed infants of less than 3 months of age are most susceptible.

The guideline value should not be expressed on the basis of nitrate nitrogen, but on the basis of nitrate itself, which is the chemical entity of concern of health and the guideline value for nitrate is 50 mg/L.

As a result of recent evidence of the presence of nitrite in some water supplies, it was concluded that a guideline value of 3 mg/L for nitrite should be proposed. Because of the possibility of simultaneous occurrence of nitrate and nitrite in drinking water, the sum of the ratios of the concentration of each to its guideline value should not exceed 1, that is given in the following equation:

$$\frac{\text{Concentration of nitrate}}{\text{Guideline value of nitrate}} + \frac{\text{Concentration of nitrite}}{\text{Guideline value of nitrate}} = < 1$$

Selenium

Selenium level in drinking water vary greatly in different geographical areas and are usually much lesser than the guideline value of 0.01 mg/L. Foodstuffs are the principal source and the level depends according to geographical area of production. Selenium is an essential element for humans and forms an integral part of the enzyme glutathione peroxidase. Most selenium compounds are water soluble. In humans, the toxicity of long-term exposure are manifested in nails, hair and liver.

Polynuclear aromatic hydrocarbons

A large number of polynuclear aromatic hydrocarbons (PAHs) from a variety of combustion and pyrolysis sources have been identified in the environment. The main source of human exposure to PAHs is food with drinking water contributing only minor amounts. Little information is available on the oral toxicity of PAHs, especially after long-term exposure. Benzo(a)pyrene, which constitutes a minor fraction of total PAHs have been found to be carcinogenic in mice by the oral route of administration. Some PAH compounds have been found to be carcinogenic by non-oral routes. Benzo(a)pyrene has been found to be carcinogenic in a mutagenic of in vitro and in vivo assays. The following recommendations are made for the PAH group:

1. Because of the close association of PAH with suspended solids, the application of treatment, when necessary to achieve the recommended level of turbidity will ensure that PAH levels are reduced to a minimum.
2. Contamination of water with PAH should not occur during water treatment or distribution. Therefore, the use

of coal-tar-based and similar materials for pipe lining and coatings on storage tanks should be discontinued.
3. In situation where contamination of drinking water by PAH has occurred, the specific compounds present and the source of contamination should be identified as the carcinogenic potential of PAH compound varies.
4. Pesticides: These are important in connection with water quality include chlorinated hydrocarbons and their derivatives, persistent herbicides, soil insecticides, pesticides that are easily leached out from the soil and pesticides that are systemically added to water supplies for disease vector control. The recommended guideline value is set at a level to protect human health as follows (Table 7.2).

Table 7.2: Pesticides and their concentration

Pesticides	Upper limit of concentration (mg/L)
Aldrin/Dieldrin	0.03
Chlordane	0.2
2,4-D	30
Heptachlor and heptachlor epoxide	0.03
Heptachlorobenzene	1
Lindane	2
Methoxydhlor	20
Pentachlorophenol	9 (P*)

*P, provisional value

Drinking water consumption and body weight
The average daily per capita consumption of drinking water is usually found to be around 2 liter, but there are considerable variations between individuals as water intake is likely to vary with climate, physical activity and culture, e.g. at temperature above 25°C, there is a sharp rise in fluid intake, largely to meet the demands of an increased sweat rate. In developing the guideline values for potentially hazardous chemicals, a daily per capita consumption of 2 liter by a person weighing 60 kg was generally assumed. However, such an assumption may underestimate the consumption of water per unit weight and this exposure are for those living in hot climates as well for infants and children, who consume more fluid per unit weight than adults. Where it was judged that this segment of the population was at a particularly high risk from exposure to certain chemicals, the guideline value was derived on the basis of a 10 kg child consuming 1 liter of water per day or a 5 kg infant consuming 0.75 liter of water per day.

Health-risk assessment
For most kinds of toxicity, it is generally believed that there is a dose below which no adverse effect will occur. For chemicals that give rise to such toxic effects, a tolerable daily intake (TDI) can be derived.

Tolerable daily intake
The TDI is an estimate of the amount of a substance in food or in drinking water, expressed on a body weight basis (mg/kg of body weight) that can be ingested daily over a lifetime without appreciable health risk.

The ADI are established for food additives and pesticide residues that occur in food for necessary technological purpose or plant protection reasons. For chemical contaminants, which usual have no intended function in drinking water the term TDI is seen as more appropriate than ADI, as it signifies permissibility rather than acceptability.

No-observed-adverse-effect level
The no-observed-adverse-effect level (NOAEL) is defined as the highest dose or concentration of a chemical in a single study found by experiment or observations that cause no detectable adverse health effect. Whenever possible, the NOAEL is based on long-term studies, preferably of ingestion in drinking water.

Lowest-observed-adverse-effect level
Lowest-observed-adverse-effect level (LOAEL) is the lowest observed dose or concentration of a substance at which there is a detectable adverse health effect. When LOAEL is used instead of NOAEL, an additional uncertainty factor (UF) is normally used.

Uncertainty factors
The applications of UF have been widely used in the derivation of ADI for food additives, pesticides and environmental contaminants. The derivation of these factors requires expert judgment and a careful sifting of the available scientific evidence.

In the derivation of the WHO drinking water quality guidelines values, UF were applied to the lowest NOAEL or LOAEL for the response considered to be most biologically significant and were determined by consensus among a group of experts using the approach outlined below (Table 7.3).

Table 7.3: Source of uncertainty and their factors

Source of uncertainty	Factors
Interspecies variation (animal to humans)	1–10
Interspecies variation (individual variation)	1–10
Adequacy of studies or database	1–10
Nature and severity of effect	1–10

The total UF should not exceed 10,000. If the risk assessment would lead to a higher uncertainty factor then the resulting TDI would be so imprecise as to lack meaning. For substances, which UF were greater than 1,000 guideline values are designated as provisional in order to emphasize the high level of uncertainty inherent in these values.

Derivation of guideline value using a TDI approach
TDI can be calculated by following formula:

$$TDI = \frac{NOAEL/LOAEL}{UF}$$

where,
  TDI: Tolerable daily intake
  NOAEL: No-observed-adverse effect level
  LOAEL: Lowest-observed-advise-effect level
  UF: Uncertainty factors.

The guideline value (GV) is then derived from the TDI as follows:

$$GV = \frac{TDI \times bw \times p}{C}$$

where,
  bw: Body weight (60 kg for adult, 10 kg for children, 5 kg for infants)
  p: Fraction of the TDI allocated to drinking water
  C: Daily drinking water consumption (2 liter for adults, 1 liter for children and 0.75 liter for infants).

Radiological Parameters

The effects of radiation exposure are called 'somatic', if they become manifest in the exposed individual and 'hereditary' if they affect the descendants. Malignant disease is the most important delayed somatic effect. For some somatic effects such as carcinogenesis, the probability of an effect occurs, rather than its severity is regarded as a function of dose without a threshold (stochastic effect). Whereas for other somatic effects, the severity of the effect varies with dose without threshold may therefore exist for such effects. The aim of radiation protection is to prevent harmful non-stochastic effects and to reduce the probability of stochastic effects to a level deemed acceptable.

Radioactivity in drinking water should not be kept within safe limits; it should be also within those limits and kept as low as reasonably possible. The guideline values recommended take account of both naturally occurring radioactivity and any radioactivity that may reach the water source as a result of man's activities. From a radiological point of view, they represent a value below which water can be considered potable without any further radiological examination.

The activity of a radioactive material is the number of nuclear disintegration per unit of time. The unit activity is becquerel (Bq); 1 Bq = 1 disintegration per second. Formerly, the unit of activity was Curie (Ci). The proposed guideline values are:
- Gross alpha activity 0.1 Bq/L
- Gross beta activity 1.0 Bq/L.

SURVEILLANCE OF DRINKING WATER QUALITY

The activities that ideally should be included in the surveillance function are:
1. Approval of new sources (including private owned supplies).
2. Watershed protection.
3. Approval of the construction and operating procedures of waterworks, including:
   a. Disinfection of the plant and of the distribution system after repair of interruption of supply.
   b. Periodic flushing programs and cleaning of water storage facilities.
   c. Certification of operators.
   d. Regulation of chemical substances used in water treatment.
   e. Cross-connection control, backflow prevention and leak detection control.
4. Sanitary surveys.
5. Monitoring programs including provision for central and regional analytical laboratory services.
6. Development of codes of practice for well construction, pump installation and plumbing.
7. Inspection quality control in bottled water and ice manufacturing operations.

Surveillance of drinking water is essentially a health pleasure. It is intended to protect the public from waterborne disease. The elements of a surveillance program are explained below.

Sanitary Survey

Sanitary survey is an on-the-spot inspection and evaluation by a qualified person of the entire water supply system. The purpose of the survey is detection and correction of faults and deficiencies. A sanitary survey is essential for adequate interpretation of laboratory results.

Sampling

Sampling of water should be done with the thoroughness of a surgical operation with the observation of similar aseptic precautions for upon it depends the results of analysis. It should be carried out by competent and trained personnel in strict accordance with the methods, and frequency of sampling prescribed in the WHO guidelines for drinking water quality or the Indian Council of Medical Research (ICMR), 'Manual of Standards of Quality for Drinking Water Supplies'.

Samples for Physical and Chemical

Sample should be collected in clean glass stoppered bottles made of neutral glass of capacity not less than 2 liters. Stoppered glass bottles technically known as 'Winchester quart bottles' are suitable. Before collecting the sample, rinse the bottle well three times with the water, filling it each time about one third full. Then fill it with the water, tie the stopper tightly down with a piece of cloth over it and seal the string.

Samples for Bacteriological Examination

Bacteriological sample should be collected in clean sterilized bottles made of neutral glass of capacity 200–500 mL and provided with a ground glass stopper having an overlapping rim. The stopper must be relaxed by an intervening strip of paper to prevent breakage of the bottle during sterilization or jamming of the stopper. The stopper and the neck of the bottle should be protected by a paper or parchment cover. If the water to be sampled to contain or is likely to contain chlorine, a small quantity of sodium thiosulfate (0.1 mL of 3.0% solution or a small crystal of the salt) should be added to the bottle before sterilization. Sterile sampling bottles should be obtained from the laboratory, which is to carry out the analysis. The sampling bottle should not be opened until the moment at which it is required for filling.

Collection of the sample from a tap

When the sample is to be taken from a tap in regular use, the tap should be opened fully and the water run to waste at least for 2 minutes in order to flush the interior of the nozzle and to discharge the stagnant water in the service pipe. In case of samples to be collected from taps, which is not in regular use, the tap should be sterilized by heating it either with a blow lamp or with an ignited piece of cotton soaked in methylated spirit, until it is unbearably hot to the touch. Then the tap should be cooled by allowing the water to run to waste before the sample is collected.

The bottle should be held near the base with one hand and the other on stopper, and paper cover over it to be removed together and held in the fingers. The sample bottle should be filled from a gentle stream of water from the tap, avoiding splashing. The collection of samples from taps, which are leaky should be avoided, because the water might run down outside of the tap and enter the bottle causing contamination; if this cannot be avoided special precautions should be taken to clean the outside of the tap and to flame it sufficiently to ensure sterility.

Collecting sample from rivers, lakes, reservoir, wells, etc.

Samples from rivers and streams should not be taken near the tank or too far away from the point of draw off. For collecting samples directly from river, lake, tank, well, etc. A bottle with a string attached to the neck, which is fully wrapped in paper and sterilized should be used. Before taking the sample, the paper cover should be removed, taking care not to allow the sides of the bottle to come in contact with anything, another long clean string should be tied to the end of the sterilized string and the bottle lowered into the water and allowed to fill up. The bottle should be then raised and the stopper with cover must be replaced.

Another method of collecting samples from rivers or reservoirs is to hold the bottle by the bottom and plunge its neck downward below the surface of the water. The bottle is then turned until the neck points slightly upwards, the mouth being directed toward the current. If no current exists, as in a reservoir, a current should be artificially created by pushing the bottle horizontally forward a direction away from the hand. When full, the bottle is raised rapidly above the surface and the stopper replaced.

If a sample is to be taken from a well fitted with a pump, the water should be pumped to a waste for about 2 minutes and the sample collected from the pump delivery or from a tap on the discharge.

Transport and storage of samples

The bacterial examination of the sample should be commenced as soon as possible after collection. Where, this is not feasible, the sample should be kept in ice until it is taken for analysis. All such iced samples should be taken for analysis within 48 hours after collection. Samples not preserved in this manner should not be accepted for bacteriological examination. Certain particulars reading the date and time of collection and dispatch, source for water, particulars recent rainfall, and findings of the sanitary survey should also be supplied with the sample.

Bacteriological Surveillance

The tests usually employed in water bacteriology are presumptive coliform test for the detection of fecal streptococci and *Clostridium perfringens,* and colony count. A complete bacteriological examination consists of all these tests.

Presumptive Coliform Test

Multiple tube method: This test is based on estimating the most probable number (MPN) of coliform in 100 mL of water. The test is carried out by inoculating measured quantities of the sample water (0.1, 1.0, 10, 50 mL) into tubes of McConkey's lactose bile salt broth with bromocresol purple as an indicator. The tubes are incubated for 48 hours. From the number of tubes showing acid and gas, an estimate of the MPN of coliform organisms in 100 mL of the sample water can be obtained from statistical tables. This result is known as 'presumptive coliform count', the presumption being each tube showing fermentation contains coliform organisms. The reaction may occasionally be due to the presence of some other organisms or combination of organisms.

Confirmatory Tests

The next step is to confirm the presence of coliform organisms in each tube showing a presumptive positive reaction. Such confirmation is not generally required in case of unchlorinated water, but is required in case of chlorinated water. Confirmation is done by subculturing each presumptive positive tube in two tubes of brilliant green bile broth, one of which is incubated at 37°C for up to 48 hours for confirmation of the presence of coliform organisms; and the other incubated at 44°C inspected after 6–24 hours to decide whether or not *E. coli* is present. *E. coli* is almost the only coliform organisms, which is capable of producing gas from lactose at 44°C. Further confirmation of the presence of *E. coli*, if desired can be obtained by testing for indole production at 44°C.

Membrane filtration technique: In some countries, membrane filter technique is used as a standard procedure to test for the presence of coliform organisms. A measure volume of the sample is filtered through a membrane specially made of cellulose ester. All the bacteria present in water are retained on the surface of the membrane and by inoculating the membrane face upwards on suitable media and at appropriate temperature. It is possible to count the colonies and obtain results within 20 hours as compared to 72–96 hours required for the usual multiple tube technique.

Detection of Fecal Streptococci and Clostridium perfringens

The presence of fecal streptococci and *C. perfringens* provide useful confirmatory evidence of the fecal pollution of water in doubtful cases.

Colony count: The colony counts on nutrient agar at 370°C and 220°C are frequently used in the bacteriological examination of water. Colony counts provide an estimation of the general bacterial purity of water. A single count is of a little value, but counts from the same source at frequent intervals may be of considerable value. A sudden increase in the colony count may be given at earliest as a indication of contamination. The recommended plate count on yeasts extract agar after incubation at 220°C for 7 days might serve as the best general purpose indicator of microbiological quality, because of bacteria growing at 220°C after 7 days incubation can increase enormously.

Biological examination: Water may contain microscopic organisms such as algae, fungi, yeast, protozoa, rotifers, crustaceans, minute worms, etc. These organisms are collectively called 'plankton'. The plankton organisms produce objectionable tastes and odors in water. They are an index of pollution. The degree of pollution is assessed qualitatively and quantitatively by noting the type and number of organisms prevailing in water.

Chemical surveillance: Chemical surveillance of drinking water is assuming greater importance in view of industrial and agricultural pollutants finding their way into raw water sources. Tests for pH, color, turbidity, chlorides, ammonia, chlorine demand and residual chlorine are the basic tests. Regular measurement of chlorine residuals supply may in part replace bacteriological surveillance. Tests for iron and manganese are required when these substances are present in the raw water with sufficient amount to influence water treatment. Complete chemical analysis would include analysis for toxic metals, pesticides, persistent organic chemicals and radioactivity.

HARDNESS OF WATER

Hardness refers to the soap-destroying power of water. The consumer considers hard water, if large amount of soap is required to produce lather. The hardness in water is caused mainly by four dissolve compounds. These are:
- Calcium bicarbonate
- Magnesium bicarbonate
- Calcium sulfate
- Magnesium sulfate.

The presences of anyone of these compounds produce hardness. Chlorides and nitrates of calcium and magnesium, iron, manganese and aluminum compounds also cause hardness, but as they generally are present in such small amounts.

Hardness is classified as carbonate and noncarbonate. The carbonate hardness, which was formerly, designated as 'temporary' hardness; due to the presence of calcium and magnesium bicarbonates. The non-carbonate hardness formerly designated as 'permanent' hardness is due to calcium, magnesium sulfate, chlorides and nitrates.

Hardness in water is expressed in term of 'milliequivalents per liter (mEq/L). 1 mEq/L of hardness producing ion is equal to 50 mg $CaCO_3$ (50 ppm) is 1 liter of water. The soft and hard water are used when the levels of hardness are detailed in Table 7.4.

Table 7.4: Hardness of water

Classification	Level of hardness (mEq/L)
Soft water	Less than 1 (< 50 mg/L)
Moderately hard	1–3 (50–150 mg/L)
Hard water	3–6 (150–300 mg/L)
Very hard water	Over 6 (> 300 mg/L)

Drinking water should be moderately hard. Softening of water is recommended when the hardness exceeds 3 mEq/L (300 mg/L). Hardness in water presents several disadvantages both to the domestic and industrial consumer. These may be stated as follows:

1. Hardness in water consumes more soap and detergents.
2. When hard water is heated, the carbonates are precipitated and bring about furring or scaling of boilers, this leads to great fuel consumption, loss of efficiency and may sometimes cause boiler explosions.
3. Hard water adversely affects cooking; food cooked in soft water retains its natural color and appearance.
4. Fabrics washed with soap in hard water do not have a long life.
5. There are many industrial processes in which hard water is unsuited and gives rise to economic losses.
6. Hardness shortens the life of pipes and fixtures.

Removal of Hardness

The methods of removal of hardness are briefly stated as below.

Temporary Hardness

Boiling: It removes the temporary hardness by expelling carbon dioxide and precipitating the insoluble calcium carbonate. It is an expensive method to soften water on a large scale:

$$Ca(HCO_3) \rightarrow CaC_3 + H_2O + CO_2$$

Addition of lime: Lime softening not only reduces total hardness but also accomplishes magnesium reduction. Lime absorbs the carbon dioxide and precipitates the insoluble calcium carbonate. In the Clark's method of softening water, one ounce of quick lime is added to every 700 gallons of water for each degree (14.25 ppm) of hardness:

$$Ca(OH)_2 + Ca(HCO_3) \rightarrow 2CaCO_3 + 2H_2O$$

Permanent Hardness

- Addition of sodium carbonate
- Base exchange process.

Addition of sodium carbonate: Sodium carbonate (soda ash) removes both temporary and permanent hardness as given below:

$$Na_2CO_3 + Ca(HCO_3) \rightarrow 2NaHCO_3 + CaCO_3$$
$$CaSO_3 + Na_2CO_3 \rightarrow CaCO_3 + Na_2SO_4$$

Base exchange process: In the treatment of large water supplies, the permutit process is used. Sodium permutit is a complex compound of sodium, aluminum and silica ($Na_2Al_2Si_2O\,H_2O$). It has the property of exchanging the sodium cation for the calcium and magnesium ions are entirely removed by base exchange and the sodium permutit is finally converted into calcium and magnesium permutit. By this process, water can be softened to zero hardness. Since, water of zero hardness is corrosive and a part of the raw water is mixed with the softened water to secure the desired hardness. After permutit has been used for sometime, it loses its effectiveness, but it may be regenerated by treating with concentrated solution of sodium chloride or brine, and washing away the soluble calcium and magnesium chloride formed. Permutit process removes both temporary and permanent hardness.

Fluoridation of Water

Fluorine is one of the constituents naturally present in water supplies. In fact, the main source of fluorine is drinking water. Deficiency of fluorine in drinking water is associated with dental caries and excess with dental and skeletal fluorosis. Leading worker in India regard fluorine in concentration of 0.5–0.8 ppm in drinking water as optimum (a concentration of 1 ppm is regarded as optimum in temperature climates, because the consumption of water is low). The term 'fluoridation' has been given to the process of supplementing the natural fluoride content of potable water to the point of optimum concentration. The WHO in 1969, recommended fluoridation of community water supplies in areas, where the total intake of fluorides by the population is below the optimal levels for protection against dental caries.

In some areas, water may contain a high level of fluorides. In such communities, water is defluoridated by phosphate to reduce fluorides to optimum levels.

Selection and Distribution of Water

While selecting a source, attention must be given to possible future developments that may influence the continued suitability of the source and the following:
1. Quantity (source capacity): The quantity of water should be sufficient to meet continuing water demands, taking into account daily and seasonal variations, and projected growth in the size of the community being served.
2. Quality: The quality of raw water should be such that with appropriate treatment, it meets the drinking water standards.
3. Protection: The watershed must be protected from pollution with human excreta, industrial discharge and agricultural runoff.
4. Feasibility: The source should be available to reasonable cost.
5. Treatability: The raw water should be treated adequately under locally prevailing conditions.

Potential new source should be examined in the field by qualified and experienced sanitary surveyors and physical, bacteriological and chemical analysis should be carried out for a period covering seasonal variations prior to final selection of the source. Such information is essential in order to define appropriate water treatment requirements and necessary pollution control measures to protect raw water resources. It is referable to choose the source that requires the least treatment. The source should be protected from contaminants emanating from septic tanks, sewers, cesspools, sullage water and flooding from contamination by users. Maintaining adequate residual chlorine levels in the distribution system is the most reliable indicator of protection against contamination resulting from cross-connection, back siphon age, leaks, etc.

There are two main systems of water distribution, the intermittent supply and the continuous supply. In the intermittent system, water is delivered only during fixed hours. The disadvantages of the intermittent system are:
1. The pipes may be empty during times of emergency.
2. People need to store water in containers, which may not be clean always. The safe water is likely to be rendered unsafe through improper storage.
3. When the pipes are empty, there is negative pressure and by what is known as back siphoning, bacteria and foul gases may been sucked in through leaky joints. A number of recorded outbreaks of typhoid and of relapsing fever, among other diseases have be traced back to the contamination of water in the intermittent, piped water supplies. Flowing water available for 24 hours, therefore, desirable, although it may entail some wastage of water through misuse. The supply of water in most cities in India is intermittent.

Sanitation of Swimming Pool

Swimming pool water is exposed to contamination and organisms from skin and nasopharynx. The health hazards associated with swimming pools are:
1. Fungal and viral infections of the skin. This includes *Epidermophyton* and *Trichophyton* species, which produce 'athlete's foot'. The papilloma virus is the inciting agent of 'plantar warts'.
2. Infections of the eye, ear, nose and throat.
3. Infections of the upper respiratory tract.
4. Intestinal infections.
5. Accidents.

The recommended area is 2.2 m^2 (24 ft^2) per swimmer. Rules and regulations governing the use of the pool should be posted in conspicuous place for the information of the users. These are:
1. Persons suffering from skin diseases, sore eyes, cold, nasal or ear discharge or any other communicable disease should not be allowed into the swimming pool.
2. Bathers are strictly instructed to empty the bladder and if necessary use the toilet.
3. A cleansing shower bath in the nude with soap and water is required before entering the pool.
4. Spitting, spouting of water, blowing nose, etc. are prohibited.
5. The environment of the swimming pool including the shower rooms, walk ways and pool decks should receive proper disinfection to destroy bacterial, viral and fungal agent's swimming pools are equipped with rapid sand filters.

The filtering is continuous such that all water is refiltered in less than 6 hours. Part of the water up to 15% should be replaced by fresh water every day. The function of water replacement is to remove solutes nitrogen derived from the bathers. These solutes have the capacity to reduce the bactericidal activity of chlorine. Chlorination is the most widely used method of pool disinfection. Various workers have stated that a continuous maintenance of 1.0 mg/L (1 ppm) of free chlorine residual provides adequate protection against bacterial and viral agents. The pH of water is kept between 7.4 and 7.8. The bacteriological quality of water should reach nearly as possible, the standards prescribed for drinking water.

The National Water Supply and Sanitation Program was launched in 1954 by the Government of India as part of the health plan to assist states to provide adequate water supply and sanitation facilities in the entire country. Provisions have been made in the successive Five-year plan to improve the water supply. To secure freedom from waterborne diseases, people must recognize safe water as a 'felt' health need and give up their old unhygienic habits of polluting water supplies. In these circumstances, health education emerges as an important weapon in creating among people for desire of higher standards of life.

Water Conservation

Trend and rainfall decline and rapid urbanization with industrialization has created increasing demand for water. Growing water shortage is already causing problems in several areas and available resources such as river, ponds and lakes are shrinking causing more and more pressure on subsoil water resources. The rate of water extraction is exceeding the replenishment that takes place by natural processes—mainly recharge due to rainfall. This is causing alarming fall in subsoil water levels, which is going down in and around several cities. Development of agriculture dependent on tube wells has further worsened the situation. The underground water resources, therefore, urgently need conservation. The term conservation implies both protection of water resources and further building up the precious water reserves. Conservation of water resources requires the following.

Prevention of Wastage

Widespread awareness need to be developed among people about economical use of water. It has to be propagated that people should make an effort not to waste water and help in reducing consumption of the invaluable water reserves. Efficient water management can substantially reduce total water requirement of communities. Domestic consumption of water can be reduced by individuals and by cultivating better habits in kitchen and bathroom use to avoid free running of water.

Water Harvesting

Simple innovative ideas such as water harvesting are extremely important to preserve and buildup underground water reserves in urban and semi-urban areas, where considerable water is drawn out by tube wells for domestic consumption. Vast quantity of rainwater is normally discharged into drains. The rainwater can be easily added to the underground reserves by diversion of rainwater from rooftops and courtyards into soaking pits or trenches, instead of drains. It is also viable to clean and tilter this water and divert into existing tube wells or wells. Various economic designs are suggested by agencies such as Central Ground Water Board (CGWB), United Nations Children's Fund (UNICEF), etc. suitably large pit is filled in layers with big stones followed by gravel and sand. Collected rainwater from rooftops is brought into the pit by PVC pipes. The rainwater filtered through these layers, then travels by a polyvinyl chloride (PVC) pipe connecting bottom of the pit into the nearby well or tube well (Fig. 7.13).

Role of Community Health Nurses in Connection with Water

Since, the responsibility of environmental health in connection with water is fixed to some extent to the other health workers in the community, the community health nurse also plays an important role to ensure proper water supply and its advantages are dealing with hazards of water pollution. Here, they have to play a role of advocates for safer environmental health.

Nurses must help people to learn both how to conserve water and how to avoid polluted water. As nurses make visits in the community, they can continuously assess for water pollution. Look at the household or city drinking water to determine, if it is discolored or has any obvious particles in it.

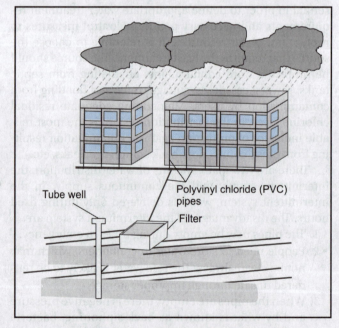

Figure 7.13: Water harvesting in a tube well

CHAPTER 7 — Water as a Determinant of Health

Nurses should encourage clients to report signs of impure water and to test their own water resources, especially if it comes from a source not regulated by city or state guidelines for water safety. Nurses should be vigilant for any illness that might be associated with water used for drinking, swimming or bathing.

The provisions of water supply are the responsibility of the engineers, but it is the duty of health workers including nurses to ensure that the water is safe to drink. In collaboration with male health assistants, the community health nurses should also prepare to shoulder certain responsibilities as listed below:

- Survey the water sources in the community
- Chlorinating the public water supply sources
- Ensuring the pumps fitted to the community wells is intact, if not report to the persons concerned
- Educating the public about the importance of safe drinking water
- Advising methods for water disinfection
- Taking certain steps during epidemic to safeguard the health of the people.

The educational activities of nurses in connection with the water in a community should include the teaching of the following:

- The health hazards attached to drinking water from surface sources
- The importance of drinking chlorinated water
- The importance of boiling water
- The safe ways of storing water and of drawing water from storage tank and containers
- The waterborne diseases and their prevention
- The importance of keeping the areas clean around open water supplies
- Community responsibilities for cleanliness of water resources
- The need for the community to seek advice whenever problems relating to supply and utilization of water arise.

WATER ACT (PREVENTION AND CONTROL OF POLLUTION), 1974

Water Act was enacted on 23rd March, 1974 to implement the decision reached at Stockholm conference under Article 252 section I of Indian Constitution. It is a social welfare legislation enacted for the purpose of:

- Prevention and control of water pollution
- Maintaining or restoring of wholesomeness of water
- Establishing pollution control boards
- Assigning powers and functions relating water pollution to boards.

The Act has been adopted by states of Assam, Bihar, Gujarat, Haryana, Himachal Pradesh, Jammu and Kashmir, Karnataka, Kerala, Madhya Pradesh, Rajasthan, Tripura and West Bengal and all Union Territories of 23rd March, 1974. The state of Uttar Pradesh adopted it on February 3, 1975.

Definitions

Water Pollution

1. Contamination of water or alteration of physical, chemical and biological properties of water.
2. Discharge of sewage or trade effluent.
3. Discharge of gaseous substance, which may or is likely to:
   a. Create nuisance.
   b. Render the water harmful or injurious to public health, safety, domestic, commercial, industrial, agricultural uses, the life and health of animals, plants or aquatic life.

Also, a members of board, sewer, sewage, effluent outlet, etc. has been defined in detail. Board means Central Board or State Board.

Central and State Pollution Control Boards

Central/State Board shall consist of the following members:

1. A full time chairman, being a person having special knowledge or practical experience in respect of matters relating to environmental protection, to be nominated by central/state government, as the case may be.
2. Officials, not exceeding five to be nominated by respective government
3. Persons, not exceeding five, to be nominated by central government from amongst the members of state board, and in the case of state boards, to be nominated by state government from amongst the members of local authorities.
4. Nonofficials, not exceeding three to be nominated by respective government to represent the interest of agriculture, fishery, industry, trade or any other interest which in the interest of government ought to be represented.
5. Two persons to represent the companies or corporations owned, controlled or managed by the central government, state government, as the case may be, to be nominated by that government.
6. A full time member—secretary, possessing qualifications, knowledge and experience of scientific, engineering or management aspects as pollution control, to be appointed by respective government.

Maximum number of members of the board is 17 including Chairman and Member—Secretary. A member can hold office for a term of 3 years. A member can be removed, if they fail to attend three consecutive meetings without sufficient reason. A member can be disqualified by the following conditions:
- Solvency
- Unsound mind
- Conviction court
- Abuses position
- If he/she is a partner in the firm dealing with supply of machinery or other related material:
    - A Board shall meet at least once in every 3 months.
    - Two or more states or state and union territory can have a joint board.

Functions of Central Board

The main functions of Central Pollution Control Board (CPCB) are:
1. Cleanliness of rivers, fresh waters and wells in different areas of the states.
2. Advice the central government on water pollution issues.
3. Coordinate the activities of state boards and resolve disputes among them.
4. Carry out and sponsor investigation and research relating to water pollution and provide technical assistance and guidance to state boards.
5. Training of persons engaged in programs for control of water pollution.
6. Organize comprehensive programs for pollution control, e.g. through mass media.
7. Lay down or modify the standards for streams and wells in consultation with concerned state government.
8. Plan nationwide programs for analyzing the samples of water, sewage of trade effluent.
9. Establish or recognize laboratories for analyzing the samples of water, sewage or trade effluent.
10. Perform the functions of state boards/union territories.

Powers of Central Board

1. Central board is more powerful than a state board. In case of conflicts between a central board and state board, the central board prevails.
2. When the central government is of the opinion that any state Board has failed to comply with the directions given by central board, the central board may then be directed by the central government to take over the state board function.
3. Central board can demand state of purity and wholesomeness of water from state boards if some complaints arise.

Functions of State Board

Functions of state board are:
1. To plan a comprehensive program to prevent water pollution in streams and wells.
2. To advice the state government on water pollution issues and location of industries.
3. To encourage, conduct and participate in the investigations and research relating to problems of water pollution.
4. To inspect sewage or trade effluents, works and plats for the treatment of sewage and trade effluents.
5. To develop economical and reliable methods of treatment of sewage and trade effluents.
6. To evolve method of utilization of sewage and suitable trade effluents in agriculture.
7. To evolve efficient methods of disposal of sewage and trade effluents.
8. To establish or recognize laboratories for analyzing samples of water from sewage or trade effluents.
9. To lay down standards of treatment of sewage and trade effluents.

Powers of State Board

1. State board has powers to make survey of any area of industry.
2. It has the power to take samples of water of any sewage or trade effluent for the purpose of analysis.
3. The official has the power to enter any building to examine any plant or record.
4. It has the power to order closure of any industry or stoppage of supply of electricity and water.

Punishment or penalty
1. Failure to comply with the directions of the board to give information will lead to imprisonment for up to 3 months or a fine up to ₹10,000 or both.
2. If anybody destroys property of board will lead to imprisonment for up to 3 months or a fine up to ₹10,000 or both.
3. Anybody, who pollutes water will, lead to imprisonment from 1½ to 6 years and a fine up to ₹5,000.
4. Any person, who interferes with monitoring device (meter or gauge), will lead to imprisonment for up to 3 months or a fine up to ₹10,000.
5. If any offence is committed by company, the director or manager of the company will be punished.

CHAPTER 7 — Water as a Determinant of Health

6. Court shall take cognizance of any offence under this act, if the complaint is made by:
   a. Board or any authorized officer.
   b. Any person who has given notice of not less than 60 days.
7. Parliament amended the Water Act in 1988 to make it more effective and also to deal with air pollution.

CONCLUSION

Man can survive for 5 weeks without food, but not more than five days without water, so it is difficult for a man to survive without water. Water is essential as it is the predominant constituent of cell for both plants and animals. In that way 70% of body weight is due to water only. Water has got an influence on the health/life of an individual both directly and indirectly. It is related directly because water is essential for digestion, regulation of body temperature, removal of wastes from the body through fears, perspiration, urination and feces and for lubricating joint or also act on a buffer by actualizing the acids produced by the body. It is a vehicle for all metabolize process in the body. Deficiency of water on the body causes dehydration, acidosis, shock, urinary tract infections, indigestion and constipation. The daily requirement of water for drinking purpose is above 2.5 liters per head. Water also has an influence upon the health of the human being directly or indirectly portable water is a safe and wholesome, which is free from pathogens and harmful chemical substances, pleasant to taste and usable for domestic purposes.

Water is said to be contaminated when it contains pathogens or harmful chemical substances and it is said to by polluted when it contains substances or impurities affecting physical quality of water such as color, odor, taste and morbidity. The sources of water are rain, surface water and subsurface water. Water if polluted needs to be treated before use, so as to reduce the morbidity and mortality associated with water. Water can be purified by self-purification of natural water system purification of water at large scale and small scale purification of water requires either one or combination of two or more methods, i.e. storage, filtration and disinfection.

Air as a Determinant of Health

CHAPTER 8

INTRODUCTION

Air is essential for maintenance of life. It supplies oxygen to human body, which is essential for life. Clean air is necessary for our health and longevity. An average person breaths 16 kg of air each day, which is about six times of food and water intake. The oxygen in the air is the life force in each cell of the body. Certain functions of the body carried out by the air transmitted stimuli are hearing and smelling. In the same way, certain deviations of the body are conveyed by the air, e.g. various disease and allergens are transmitted by the air. Appreciation of the value of fresh air is among the factors, which have lessened disease and mortality. Pure air acts as natural tonic and it increases the power of resistance.

Man needs oxygen to live and gets oxygen from air. No one can think of a life without air. It is most precious resource. Air is present in atmosphere. Troposphere is the lowest layer of atmosphere in which the organisms operate. It is the region of strong air movements and cloud formations. A mixture of gases; water vapor and dust occurred in troposphere in extremely variable concentrations. The air in troposphere, which we breath consists of about 78.1% nitrogen, 20.73% oxygen, 0.93% argon and 0.03% carbon dioxide (CO_2) and the rest is made up of neon, krypton, methane, helium, nitric oxide, etc. In addition of gases, water vapor and suspended matter such as dust, bacteria, spores and vegetable debris.

The layer of greatest interest in pollution control is troposphere. Pollution problems result from confluence of atmospheric contaminants.

Air has two important functions, i.e. interchange of gases during respiration and regulation of body temperature. Air is a mechanical mixture of gases. The composition of air in inspiration and expiration is detailed in Table 8.1.

Table 8.1: Composition of air in respiration

Gases	Inspired air (%)	Expired air (%)
Oxygen	20.94	16.40
Nitrogen	79	79.00
Carbon dioxide	0.40	4.40

Apart from supplying the life-giving oxygen, air and atmospheric conditions serve several functions. The human body is cooled by the air contact, the special senses of hearing and smell function through air transmitted stimuli and disease agents may be conveyed by air. Pollution of air by dust, smoke, toxic gases and chemical vapors are resulted in sickness and death. Human beings need a continuous supply of air to exist. The requirement for air is relatively constant (about 10–20 m^3/day).

Air is a mechanical mixture of gases. The normal composition of external air by volume is approximately—nitrogen 78.1%, oxygen 20.93% and CO_2 0.03%. The balance is made up of other gases, which occur in traces, e.g. argon, neon, krypton, xenon and helium. In addition to these gases, air also contains water vapor, traces of ammonia and suspended matter such as dust, bacteria, spores and vegetable debris.

Impure air: It means the presence of impurities in air. These impurities occur due to respiration, combustion of coal, gas or petrol, decomposition of organic matter, etc. These impurities in air can be corrected by natural self-cleaning mechanism such as wind, sunlight, rain and plant life.

Air becomes impure by respiration of human beings and animals; combustion of coal, gas, oil; decomposition of organic matter and trade, traffic and manufacturing processes, which gives off dust, fumes, vapors, and gases. Under ordinary conditions, the composition of outdoor air is remarkably constant. Because it is brought about by certain self-cleansing mechanisms that operate in nature, which includes:

1. Wind: It dilutes and sweeps away the impurities by its movement. Because of wind movement, impurities do not accumulate in anyone place.
2. Sunlight: The atmospheric temperature and sunlight play their own part by oxidizing impurities and killing bacteria.
3. Rain: It cleans the atmosphere by removing the suspended and gaseous impurities.
4. Plant life: The green plants utilize the CO_2 and generate oxygen. This process is reversed during the nighttime. When the rate of pollution becomes too high or when the cleansing process becomes ineffective, it constitutes a health hazard.

CHANGES IN AIR DURING OCCUPANCY

Room occupied by human beings impair the quality of air. The changes in air take place in confined places are both chemical and physical.

Chemical Changes

The air becomes progressively contaminated by CO_2 and the oxygen content decreases due to metabolic processes. An average person at rest gives off 0.7 ft^3 of CO_2 per hour. This may increase up to 2 ft^3 during physical activity. In a mixed gathering comprising all age groups, the per capita output of CO_2 is taken as 0.6 ft^3 per hours.

Physical Changes

The physical changes that occur due to human occupancy are as detailed below.

Rise in temperature: The indoor temperature tends to rise as a result of the emanating of body heat. A man at times gives off approximately 400 British thermal unit (BTU) per hour. One BTU is the quantity of heat required to raise the temperature of 1 pound of water by 1°F under conditions of physical exertion, the heat output may go up to 40,000 BTU.

Increase of humidity: There is an increase in the relative humidity due to moisture evaporated from the skin and lungs. The expired air contains about 6% of water vapor. An adult person at rest releases an average 700 g of water vapor per 24 hours in the form of perspiration. It has been calculated that human being releases 18.4 g of water vapor per hour when sleeping and up to 175 g of water vapor, when engaged in really vigorous exercise.

Decrease in air movement: In crowded places, the natural movement of air is impeded.

Body odors: Unpleasant odors arise from foul breath, perspiration, bad oral hygiene, dirty clothes and other sources. The production of body odors depends upon the social status, age and personal hygiene of the people.

Bacterial pollution: The exhaled air contains microorganisms in suspension. These are principally saprophytic bacteria and may include pathogenic bacteria. These organisms are discharged into the air during conversation, coughing, sneezing and loud talking.

Vitiated air: In confined places, the chemical and physical changes occur in air and vitiate the air. In chemical changes, the CO_2 level in the confined placed or closed room without any ventilation is increased. These depend upon the number of persons releasing CO_2 in air. Not only chemical but also physical changes such as rise in temperature, increase in humidity, unpleasant odors and increase in microbial contents also occur. These changes occur due to decreased air movement. If this vitiated air is not replaced, then adverse effects on health such as discomfort and decreased efficiency, headache, drowsiness and inability to concentrate are seen. So, proper ventilation is required in overcrowded and closed areas to decrease the impact of adverse effects. Studies have shown that chemical and physical changes within the air produce adverse health effects.

Knowledge of the ways of air to be vitiated helps in understanding the impact on the health. Creating an awareness of the relative methods of getting pure form of air such as proper ventilation will help in reducing the morbidity associated with pollution.

Unless the vitiated air is replaced by fresh air, it may adversely affect the comfort, health and efficiency of the occupants. It is known that a feeling of suffocation or discomfort is experienced by the occupants in insufficiently ventilated rooms and also complaints of headache, drowsiness and inability to concentrate. There is also the risk of droplet infection and lowered resistance to disease (on prolonged exposure). Discomfort is a subjective sensation, which people experience in ill ventilated and crowded rooms. It was believed to be increased CO_2 rooms and decreased oxygen, resulting from respiration. Recent studies shown that, the causes of discomfort are not due to chemical changes, but physical changes such as temperature, humidity, air movement and heat radiation. These factors determine the 'cooling power' of the air with respect to the human body.

THERMAL COMFORT

Thermal comfort is a complex entity. To express thermal comfort and heat stress following indices used from time to time.

Air temperature: It is used as an index of thermal comfort, but it was realized that air temperature alone was not an adequate index of thermal comfort.

Air temperature and humidity: It is considered together to express thermal comfort; even this was found be unsatisfactory.

Cooling power: Air temperature, humidity and air movement were considered together and expressed as 'cooling power' of the air. An instrument was devised by Hill called 'kata thermometer' to measure the cooling power. Researchers have shown that the kata cooling powers are also not reliable indices of comfort conditions.

Effective temperature: It is an arbitrary index, which combines into a single value, the effect of temperature, humidity and movement of the internal air on the sensation of warmth or cold fell by the human body. The numerical value of effective temperature is that of the temperature of still and saturated air, which would induce the same sensation of warmth or cold as that experienced in the given conditions.

Corrected effective temperature (CET): It is an improvement over the effective temperature index. Instead of the dry bulb temperature, the reading of the globe thermometer is used to allow for radiant heat, i.e. the CET. Scales deal with all the four factors namely, air, temperature, velocity, humidity and mean radiant heat. Whenever a source of radiant is present, it is preferable to take CET. The CET may be readily obtained from prepared nomograms by reference of the globe thermometer temperature, the wet bulb temperature and air speed. At present, effective temperature and CET scales are widely used as indices of thermal comfort (Fig. 8.1).

McArdle's maximum allowable sweat rate: McArdle and associates took 4.5 L of sweat excreted in 4 hours as the maximum allowable seat rare compatible with physiological normal reaction of acclimatized, healthy young men for repeated exposures of heat. They prepared a chart from which the 'predicted 4-hour sweat rate' (P4SR) can be obtained from any combination of dry and wet bulb temperature of the air, mean radiant air temperature and air velocity under different work intensity. McArdle has put P4SR value of 3 as upper limit of comfort zone.

Comfort zones may be defined as the range of effective temperatures (ETs) over which the majority of adults feel comfortable. There is no unanimous decision on a single zone of comfort for all people because comfort is quite a

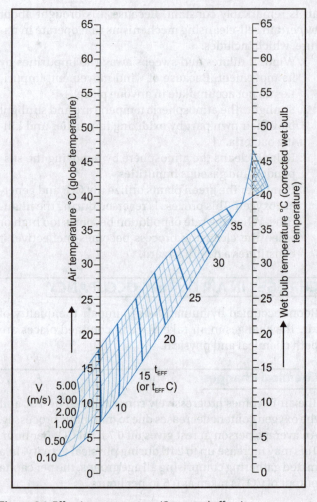

Figure 8.1: Effective temperature/Corrected effective temperature nomogram for lightly clothed men (V, velocity of air in meter per second; $T_{EFF}C$, corrected effective temperature).

complex subjective experience, which depends not only on physical, physiological factors but also on psychological factors that are difficult to determine. Considering only the environmental factors, 'comfortable thermal conditions are those under which a person can maintain normal balance between production and loss of heat at normal body temperature and without sweating. Comfort zones evaluated in India are given in Table 8.2.

Comfort zones is the range of corrected effective temperature in which the individual or the worker in an industry, feels comfortable. The criteria of comfort zone are:
- Corrected effective temperature: 25–27°C (77–80°F)
- Relative humidity: 30–65%
- Dry kata: 6 and above
- Wet kata: 20 and above
- Predicted 4-hour sweat rate: 1–3 L.

Table 8.2: Comfort zone evaluation

Corrected effective temperature	
Description	Temperature (°C)
Pleasant and cool	20
Comfortable and cool	20–25
Comfortable	25–27
Hot and uncomfortable	27–28
Extremely hot	28+
Intolerably hot	30+
Predicted 4-hour sweat rate (P4SR)	
Description	Sweat rate (L)
Comfort zone	1–3
Just tolerable	3–4.5
Intolerable	4.5+

The P4SR is applicable only in that situation where sweating occurs.

AIR POLLUTION

Air pollution problem started due to industrialization, population explosion and automobile revolution. All those conditions are making earth's environment inhospitable for future generations. The release of poisonous gases and smoke of vehicles and combustion disturb the balance and effect the health of living. Non-living components of biosphere are also affected. But, sometimes natural resources of pollution are volcanic, eruptions, dust storms and forest fires, etc.

Definition

Air pollution occurs due to presence of undesirable substances entering the atmosphere. So, air pollution is the presence of the substances, which are either present, where it does not belong or at levels greater than the particular level in the environment. In other words, air pollution is defined as the presence of poisonous gases in the atmosphere to such concentration that they produce undesirable effects on environment and are detrimental to health.

According to American Medical Association "Air pollution is the excessive concentration of foreign matter in the air, which adversely effect the well-being of an individual or causes damage to property."

According to Engineer's Joint Council, USA, "Air pollution means the presence in the outdoor atmosphere of one or more contaminants such as dust, fumes, gas, mist, odor, smoke or vapor in quantities of characteristics and of duration as to be injurious to human, plant or animal life or to property, which reasonably interferes with the comfortable enjoyment of life and property."

Air pollution is also defined as pollution of air with unwanted gases emitted from factories, power stations, exhaust and vehicles.

Pollute means contaminate with harmful or poisonous substance. The phenomenon called 'pollution' is an inescapable consequence of the presence of man and his activities. The term 'air pollution' signifies the presence in the ambient atmosphere of substances (e.g. gases, mixture of gases and particular matter) generated by the activities of man in concentrations that interfere with human health, safety or comfort or injurious to vegetation, animals and other environmental media resulting in chemicals entering the food chain or being present in drinking water, and thereby constituting additional source of human exposure. The direct effect of air pollutants on plants, animals and soil can influence the structure and function of ecosystems including self-regulation ability, thereby affecting the quality of life.

Sources of Air Pollution

- Domestic sources: Burning of fire wood, kerosene oil, coal, etc.
- Industrial sources: Factories of iron and steel, paper, cement, fertilizers, thermal power plant, petroleum refineries, etc.
- Vehicular sources: Motor vehicles, railways, ships, aeroplanes, etc.
- Miscellaneous: Tobacco smoking, nuclear explosions, forest fires, volcanoes, burning of refuse, dust storm, ocean spray, etc.

Causes of Air Pollution

Natural Causes

1. Volcanic eruptions: It release many gases and volcanic ash, which cause air pollution.
2. Forest fires: It release smoke and harmful trace gases in the atmosphere.
3. Electronic storms and solar flares cause the air to be polluted by the release of harmful chemical substances in air.
4. Dust storms: It carry harmful pathogenic spores or bacteria in air, which affect the health of people.
5. Breakdown of methane: When methane (CH_4) or marsh gas, which is produced from decaying of vegetable matter is broken down, it releases carbon monoxide (CO) air, which affects the lungs.

6. Pollen, fungal spores, cyst or bacteria: These are natural contaminant, which are usually present in the air.
7. Decayed vegetable matter: In marshy places, i.e. anaerobic decomposition of organic matter results in the release of marsh gas, which pollute the air.
8. Miscellaneous: Salt spraying from oceans is one of the natural cause of air pollution.

Man-made Causes

Man-made causes are a number of anthropogenic sources, which poses several problems endangering the life and property.

The main sources of air pollution are:

1. Automobiles: Motor vehicles are a major source of air pollution throughout areas, mainly in urban areas. Automobiles emit hydrocarbons, CO, lead, nitrogen oxides and particulate matter in air as the byproduct of the combustion of fossil fuels.

    Exhaust of automobiles and industries release hydrocarbon and nitrous oxides, an interaction occurs in these in presence of sunlight and air stagnation resulting in the production of photochemical smogs. The adverse effects include degradation of rubber, cellulose, respiratory and cardiac problems. The formation of photochemical smog is given below.

$$\text{Hydrocarbons} + N_2O \xrightarrow[\text{Air stagnation}]{\text{Sunlight}} \text{Photochemical smog}$$

    In strong sunlight, certain of these hydrocarbons and oxides of nitrogen may be converted in the atmosphere into 'photochemical' pollutants of oxidizing nature. In addition, diesel engines, when misused or badly adjusted are capable of emitting black smoke and malodorous fumes.

2. Industrialization: Industries are the source of a wide variety of air pollution through gases, dust, fumes, tars, etc. The gases, which are produced by industries are SO_2 gas, ammonia (NH_3), nitrous dioxide (NO_2), hydrogen chloride (HCl), hydrogen fluoride (HF), hydrogen sulfide (H_2S), etc.

3. Industries: These emit large amounts of pollutants into the atmosphere. Combustion of fuel to generate heat and power produces smoke, SO_2, nitrogen oxides and fly ash. Petrochemical industries generate hydrogen fluoride, hydrochloric acid and organic halides. Many industries discharge CO, CO_2, ozone, hydrogen sulfide and SO_2. Industries discharge their wastes from high chimneys at high temperature and high speed.

4. Deforestation: It means cutting of trees. If less of plan life and more of human beings then it means more of CO_2 in air. This result in high concentration of CO_2 in air resulting ill health effects on people.

5. Domestic sources: Domestic combustion of coal, wood or oil result smoke, dust, SO_2 and nitrogen oxide. In 1952, in London, disaster occurred due to coal burning in which 1,000s of people died.

6. Smoke: The most direct and important source of air pollution affecting the health of many people is tobacco smoke. Even those who do not smoke may inhale the smoke produced by others (passive smoking).

7. Overpopulation: It has resulted in air pollution due to deforestation, industrialization. Even more release of CO_2 by increased number of people and reduced number of plants in the air causing air pollution.

8. Advanced agriculture technology: Techniques such as spraying of crops for pests and weed control releases many pollutants in air such as chlorinated hydrocarbons, organic phosphates, arsenic, lead, etc.

9. Nuclear energy: To have power, man is involved in many nuclear energy activities, which involve the use of radioactive materials. Nuclear explosions used in war result in radioactive fallout of strontium-90, cesium-137 and iodine-131, which result in a wide variety of defects in human population.

10. Miscellaneous: These comprise burning refuse, incinerators, pesticide spraying, natural sources (e.g. windborne dust, fungi, molds, bacteria) and nuclear energy programs. All these contribute to air pollution.

Classification of man-made pollution sources
- Stationary sources, e.g. industries
- Mobile sources, e.g. automobiles
- Area sources, e.g. towns and cities.

The level of atmospheric pollution at any one time depends upon meteorological factors, e.g. topography, air movement and climate. Winds help in the dispersal and dilution of pollutants. If the topography is dominated by mountains (or tall buildings), the winds become weak and calm, and pollutants tend to concentrate in the breathing zone.

The vertical diffusion of pollutants depends upon the temperature gradient. When there is a rapid cooling of lower layers of air (temperature inversion), there is little vertical motion and the pollutants, and water vapors remain trapped at the lower level, the result is 'smog'. The temperature inversion, which is more frequent in winter months than in spring or summer, is a threat to human health.

Air Pollutants

Classification of Air Pollutants

Air pollutants have been classified according to the origin and according to state of matter.

According to origin
1. **Primary pollutants:** The pollutants, which are directly emitted from the source and are found in atmosphere are primary pollutants, e.g. smoke, dust, ash, nitrogen oxides, fumes, mist, sprays, etc.
2. **Secondary pollutants:** These are formed by the chemical interaction between primary pollutants and atmospheric constituents in the atmosphere. These secondary pollutants result from:
   - Photochemical reactions
   - Hydrolysis or oxidation reaction, e.g. ozone, sulfur, trioxide, aldehydes, etc.

According to state of matter (Box 8.1)
1. **Gaseous air pollutants:** These pollutants are present in gaseous state at normal temperature and pressure such as SO_2, CO_2, etc.
2. **Particular air pollution:** These are suspended droplets, solid particles or mixture of two. The particulate matter differ in terms of density and size. Particulate air pollutants are aerosols, dust, smoke, fumes, mist, fog, protozoa, fungal spores and volcanic dust.

Box 8.1: Air pollutants

Gaseous air pollutants
• Carbon monoxide
• Carbon dioxide
• Oxides of nitrogen and sulfur
• Hydrocarbons
• Oxidants such as ozone
• Chlorofluoromethane
Metallic air pollutants
• Cadmium
• Lead
• Zinc
• Iron
Particulate air pollutants
• Aerosols
• Dust
• Smoke
• Fumes
• Mist
• Fog
• Fly ash
• Soot
• Bacteria, fungi, spores, volcanic dust

The important substances, which pollute air are CO, CO_2, hydrogen sulfide, SO_2, sulfur trioxide (SO_3), nitrogen oxides, fluorine compounds, organic compounds (e.g. hydrocarbons, aldehydes, ketones, organic acid, etc.), metallic contaminants (e.g. arsenic, zinc, iron resulting from smelting operation), radioactive compounds, photochemical oxidants (e.g. ozone). Others include asbestos, beryllium, mercury, benzene, fluorides, vinyl chloride, lead and radiation.

Pollutants may be in the form of solids, liquids (vapors) or gases. The combination of smoke and fog is called 'smog'. These may be particulate matters, gasses or metals:
- **Particulate matters:** Dust, smoke, soot and grit, etc.
- **Gases:** CO, CO_2, hydrogen sulfide (H_2S), methane (CH_4), NO_2, sulfur dioxide (SO_2), methyl isocyanate (MIC), fluorohydrocarbons, etc.
- **Metals:** Arsenic, beryllium, copper, zinc, lead carcinogens, etc.

Air Pollutants and their Effect on Health

Carbon monoxides

Sources of carbon: Transportation sources, forest fires, charcoal stoves and gas heaters and solid waste disposal and CO effect on health includes on health includes:
- Affects human metabolism
- Affects central nervous system—giddiness, exhaustion, etc. the mechanism is as follows:

$$CO + Hemoglobin\ (Hb) \longrightarrow Carboxyhemoglobin\ (COHb)$$

Thereby, this reduces oxygen carrying capacity:
- Affects cardiovascular system
- Decreases vision
- Acts as asphyxiant.

Carbon monoxide is a product of incomplete combustion of carbon containing materials such as in automobiles, industrial process, heating facilities and incinerators. Estimates of man-made CO emission vary from 350 to 600 million tons per annum. Concentrations in urban areas depend on weather and traffic density. It varies with the density of petrol-powered vehicles and most cities have CO peak levels that coincide with the morning and evening rush hours. The fluctuation in ambient concentrations is slowly reflected in the carboxyhemoglobin levels in humans, as it takes 4–12 hours for approximate equilibrium between air levels and blood levels to occur. Thus, environmental concentrations tend to be expressed in terms of 8 hours average concentrations.

Sulfur dioxide

Sulfur dioxide results from the combustion of sulfur-containing fossil fuel, the smelting of sulfur-containing

ores and other industrial processes. Domestic fires can also produce emissions containing SO_2. Acid aerosol sulfuric acid (H_2SO_4) is a strong acid that is formed from the reaction of (SO_3) gas with water. Sulfuric acid is strongly hygroscopic –80 mg/m³ is considered safe limit in atmosphere. Oxides of sulfur are SO_2 and SO_3. Sources are burning of solids and fossil fuels as well as vehicles. Their effect on the health includes:
- Irritation of respiratory tract
- Bronchitis.

Lead
The combustion of alkyl-lead additives in motor fuels accounts for all lead emission into the atmosphere. An estimated 80–90% lead in ambient air derives from the combustion of leaded petrol. The mining and smelting of lead ores create pollution problems in some areas. Children up to 6 years of age are at increased risk for lead exposure as well as for adverse health effect, as children have behavior characteristic (outdoor activity), which increases the risk of lead exposure. The sources of lead are motor fuels and mining and smelting of lead ores and its effects on health includes:
- Hematological problems
- Neurological problems resulting change in behavior characteristics.

Carbon dioxide
Carbon dioxide is a natural constituent of the air. It does not take part in any significant chemical reactions with other substances in the air. However, its global concentrations are rising above the natural level by an amount that could increase global temperature enough to affect climate markedly. CO_2 is less dangerous than CO and it has major effect on earth causing increase in temperature. Sources of CO_2 are deforestation, fossil fuel combustion and its effects on health includes nausea and headache.

Hydrocarbons
Man-made sources of hydrocarbons include incineration, combustion of coal, wood, processing and use of petroleum. Hydrocarbons exert their pollutant action by taking part in the chemical reactions that cause photochemical smog. The sources of hydrocarbons are natural fires, incomplete combustion from incinerations, processing of petroleum, car engines, forest fires and agricultural burning and its effect on health are hydrocarbons take part in chemical reaction to produce photochemical smog, thereby resulting in irritation of respiratory tract, bronchitis, laryngitis, etc.

Cadmium
The steel industry, waste incineration, volcanic action and zinc production seem to account for the largest emission. Incineration is increasingly chosen as a method of refuse disposal. This source of atmospheric cadmium pollution is of growing concern. Tobacco contains cadmium and smoking may contribute significantly to the uptake of cadmium. Cigarettes may contain from 0.5 to 3 mg cadmium per gram of tobacco.

Sources of cadmium are:
- Steel industry
- Waste incinerations
- Volcanic action
- Tobacco.

It effect on health are long-term exposure to cadmium can cause damage to kidneys.

Hydrogen sulfide
Human activities can release naturally occurring hydrogen sulfide into ambient air. Hydrogen sulfide can be formed whenever element sulfur or sulfur-containing compounds come in contact with organic material at high temperatures. Hydrogen sulfide is formed during coke production, in viscose rayon production, using the sulfate method, sulfur extraction process, oil refining and in tanning industry. Hydrogen sulfide is the main toxic substance involved in livestock rearing systems with liquid manure storage. The first noticeable effect of hydrogen sulfide at low concentration is its unpleasant odor. Conjunctival irritation is the next subjective symptom. Workers exposed to hydrogen sulfide concentrations of less than 30 mg/m³ are reported to have rather diffuse neurological and mental symptoms.

Ozone
Ozone is one of the strongest oxidizing agents. In the troposphere, the ozone producing and ozone scavenging processes, involve absorption of solar radiation by nitrogen dioxide. The maximum ozone concentrations of volatile are not only organic compounds and nitrogen oxides but also their ratio. At intermediate ratio (4:1–10:1) conditions are favorable for the formation of appreciable concentration of ozone. Ozone is the secondary type of air pollutant, which is produced by chemical interaction between primary pollutants and atmospheric constituents. Its effect on health includes:
- Irritation to eyes
- Irritation of nose and throat
- Cough
- Headache
- Laryngitis, pharyngitis
- Irritation to respiratory tract.

Polynuclear aromatic hydrocarbons
Polynuclear aromatic hydrocarbons (PAHs) are large group of organic compounds with two or more benzene rings.

They are formed mainly as a result of pyrolytic processes, especially the incomplete combustion of organic materials as well as in natural PAH in the air; the best known is benzo[a]pyrene (BaP). The relation between the amount of BaP and some other PAH is termed the 'PAH profile'. Under special conditions, PAH can increase to very high concentrations indoors. In India, the BaP exposure averaged about 4 mg/m^3 during cooking with biomass fuels.

The concentrations of BaP in a room extremely polluted with cigarette smoke can be 22 mg/m^3. Chimney sweeps and tar workers were dermally exposed to substantial amounts of PAH and there is sufficient evidence of skin cancer. Studies in coke, oven workers, coal gas workers and employees in aluminum production plants provide sufficient evidence of the role of PAH in the induction of lung cancer.

Particulate matter

Airborne particulate matter represents a complex mixture of organic and inorganic substances. Mass and composition tend to divide into two principal groups, i.e. coarse particles larger than 2.5 mm in aerodynamic diameter, and fine particles smaller than 2.5 mm in aerodynamic diameter. The smaller particles contain the secondarily formed aerosols (gas to particle conversion), combustion particles and recondensed organic, and metal vapors. Aerosols are released as the emissions from aeroplane and deplete the ozone layer, and allowing the ultraviolet (UV) rays to reach the earth.

Dust particles remain suspended in air and can cause respiratory problems. Fly ash and soot, which are added in air by burning of coal can cause respiratory problems.

Arsenic: Sources of arsenic are coal and oil furnaces, glass manufacturing, etc. and its effect on health includes:
- Jaundice
- Damage to kidneys
- Cancer of skin and lung.

The large particles usually contain earth's crustal material and fugitive dust from roads and industries. Particulate matter of respirable size may be emitted from a number of sources, some of them natural (e.g. dust storms) and many others that are more widespread and more important (e.g. power plants and industrial processes, vehicular traffic, domestic coal burning, industrial incinerators). The majority of these non-natural sources are concentrated in limited portions of the territory, i.e. the urbanized areas, where populations are also concentrated. About 100 mg/m^3 is considered maximum safe limit of particulate matter in air.

Indoor air pollution (Table 8.3) contributes to acute respiratory infections in young children, chronic lung disease and cancer in adults, and diverse pregnancy outcomes (such as stillbirths) for women exposed during pregnancy. Studies have shown that up to half of adult women (few of whom smoke) suffer from chronic lung and heart diseases.

Table 8.3: Sources of indoor air pollutants

Pollutants	Sources
Respirable particles	Tobacco smoke: Stove, aerosol sprays
Carbon monoxide (CO)	Combustion equipment: Stove, gas heaters
Nitrogen dioxide	Gas cookers, cigarettes
Sulfur dioxide	Coal combustion
Carbon dioxide (CO_2)	Combustion, respiration
Formaldehyde	Particle board, carpet adhesives, insulation
Other organic vapors (benzene, toluene, etc.)	Solvents, adhesives and resin products aerosol sprays
Ozone	Electric arcing, ultraviolet (UV) light sources
Radon daughters	Building material
Asbestos	Insulation, fireproofing
Mineral fibers	Appliances

The best indicators of air pollution are SO_2, smoke and suspended particles. These are monitored on a daily over several sites are given below:

1. *Sulfur dioxide:* This gas is a major contaminant in many urban and industrial areas. Its concentration is estimated in all air pollution surveys.
2. *Smoke or soiling index:* A known volume of air is filtered through a white filter paper under specified conditions and the stain is measured by photoelectric meter. Smoke concentration is estimated and expressed as micrograms/cubic meters or air as an average level over a period of time.
3. *Grit and dust measurement:* Deposit gauges collect grit, dust and other solids. There are analyzed monthly.
4. *Coefficient of haze:* A factor used particularly in the United States of America (USA) in assessing the amount of smoke or other aerosol in air.
5. *Air pollution index:* It is an arbitrary index, which takes into account one or more pollutants as a measure of the severity of pollution.

On the basis of the evidence concerning adverse effects, judgments about the protection factors needed to minimize health risks are made. Averaging times were included, since the time of exposure is critical in determining the toxicity.

Biological Pollutants

1. Pathogens (microbes), spores, etc.
2. Although the earth's atmosphere extends to several kilometer above the surface, it is only the first 30 km that hold the major portion of the atmospheric gasses. Man is concerned only with the first 8–10 km of the atmosphere.
3. Degree of air pollution is influenced by topography, i.e. atmospheric temperature, humidity, atmospheric pressure and air movement.
4. Pollutants are affected by sunlight and temperature inversion.

Sunlight

The UV rays of the sun act on the oxides of nitrogen and other hydrocarbons, and form photo-oxidants, which are irritant to conjunctiva, nose, throat and respiratory mucous membrane.

Temperature Inversion

Normally, the air near the surface of the earth is warmer than the air higher up. So warmer air, being lighter, moves up, expands and becomes cool. Thus, the pollution is diluted and dispersed, while the air of the upper layer being cool and heavy, and comes down (turbulent flow).

Under exceptional conditions, as in deep valleys, the temperature gradient is reversed, i.e. the air near the surface of the upper layer becomes warm. The temperature rises with increase in altitude. So, the normal upward movement of air is impeded. Pollutants become locked up and their concentration rises steeply.

If fog is present under such conditions of temperature inversion, water vapor condenses around the smoke particles and forms 'smog' (water vapor + smoke = smog). Intense smog is lethal. Such temperature inversion often persists for several days resulting in acute episodes of respiratory illness, suffocation and death. Highly susceptible population groups are young children, elderly people and those suffering from lung diseases and heart diseases.

The famous episodes of acute illness and deaths due to general atmospheric pollution by temperature inversion are Meuse Valley disaster (Belgium) in December 1930, lasted for 5 days, killing 63 people and many cattle. Donora (Pennsylvania) disaster in 1948 took the life of 20 people and hundreds became ill. London disaster in 1952 (England) was the deadliest smog history, due to domestic coal burning, when more than 4,000 people died. Bhopal gas tragedy in India in 1984 killed thousands of people and it was due to leakage of MIC gas in Union Carbide industry. This was an example of toxic pollution of air and not due to photo-oxidants.

Effects of Air Pollution

Air pollution can affect by two ways, i.e. health aspects and socioeconomic aspects.

The effect of air pollution (Fig. 8.2) on an individual depends upon the extent to which an individual was exposed to damaging chemicals. The main two factors are considered to check the harm to be cause to an individual. They are:

1. Duration of exposure.
2. Concentration of chemicals.

On the basis of these factors the health effects can be seen as short-term and long-term effects.

Health Aspects

The health effects of air pollution are both immediate and delayed. The immediate effects are borne by respiratory system, the resulting state is acute bronchitis. If the air pollution is intense, it may result even in immediate death by suffocation. The delayed effects most commonly linked with air pollution are chronic bronchitis, lung cancer, bronchial asthma, emphysema and respiratory allergies. The major air pollutants, their source and adverse effects on health are given in Table 8.4.

Air pollution damages the human respiratory and cardiorespiratory system in various ways. The elderly people,

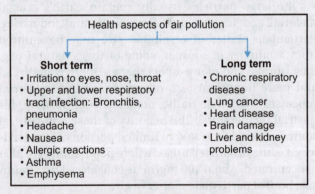

Figure 8.2: Effect of air pollution

Table 8.4: Major air pollutants, their sources and adverse effects

Noxious agents	Source	Adverse effects
Oxides of nitrogen	Automobile exhaust gas stoves and heaters, wood-burning stoves, kerosene space heaters	Respiratory tract irritation, bronchial hyperactivity, impaired lung defenses, bronchiolitis obliterans
Hydrocarbons	Automobile exhaust, cigarette smoke	Lung cancer
Ozone	Automobile exhaust, high-altitude aircraft cabins	Cough, substernal discomfort, bronchoconstriction, decreased exercise performance, respiratory tract irritation
Sulfur dioxide	Power plants, smelters, oil refineries, kerosene space healers	Exacerbation of asthma and chronic obstructive pulmonary disease (COPD), respiratory tract irritation, hospitalization may be necessary and death may occur in severe exposure
Lead	Automobile exhaust using lead gasoline	Impaired neuropsychological development in children

children, smokers and those with chronic respiratory difficulties are most vulnerable. Studies have shown that a sudden increase in the air pollution has often been associated with immediate increase in morbidity and mortality.

Social and Economic Aspects

Social and economic aspects comprise destruction of plant and animal life; corrosion of metals; damage to buildings; cost of cleaning and maintenance, and repairs and esthetic nuisance. Air pollution also reduces visibility in towns. It can soil and damage clothing.

Delayed and Chronic Effects

Delayed and chronic effects of air pollution are chronic bronchitis, bronchiectasis, emphysema, chronic obstructive pulmonary disease (COPD), bronchial asthma and even lung cancer.

Global Effects of Air Pollution

Acid Rain

Acid rain is the end result of several processes occurring in the atmosphere. Sulfur dioxide emitted from combustion of coal produces sulfuric acid by getting dissolved in water vapor of the atmosphere. Similarly, CO_2 produces carbonic acid and nitrogen dioxide produces nitric acid. Thus, the rainfall containing sulfuric acid, carbonic acid and nitric acid produces devastating ecological effect by causing acidification of soil and water. Trees killed by acid rain results in deforestation, desertification and erosion of soil, thus disturbing the ecosystem. Acidification of water bodies destroys aquatic life including fish. Destruction of food crops effects food production also.

Global Warming

Global warming is a phenomenon occurring in the troposphere. Normally, the atmospheric gases have a 'greenhouse effect', i.e. the glass of a greenhouse, allow light and warmth to reach the earth, but they do not allow warmth to be lost, thus maintaining life on earth.

With air pollution, the gases such as CO_2, methane and chlorofluorocarbons, and accumulation of ozone. All the troposphere elevates the global temperature beyond the desirable level resulting in global warming and affecting the ecosystem.

In the past 10 years, a rise of 0.3–0.6°C has been noticed. This results in the following effects:
- Increase in the dryness of the climate
- Reduction in the world food production
- Melting of polar ice caps
- Increase in sea level resulting in floods
- Smog formation
- Increased incidence of skin cancer and cataract
- Spread of tropical diseases to temperate regions.

Effects of Depleted Ozone Shield

Normally, ozone layer of the earth filters the harmful UV rays of the sun and prevents them from reaching the surface of the earth. Because of air pollution, ozone layer begins to thin out and results in the following effects:
- Inhibitions of photosynthesis (due to burning of leaves, retardation of growth of plants, fall in the crop yield, aging of plants, etc. all due to air pollution)
- Disruption of marine food chain
- Impairment of human immune mechanism, predisposing for infections
- Ocular damage (cataract)
- Skin cancers (melanotic and nonmelanotic)
- The UV rays also cause damage of small forms of life such as plankton, pollen grains and nitrifying soil bacteria.

On Animals

Cattle become weak and cachexia. Yield of animal products become less.

Miscellaneous Hazards

Socioeconomic hazards are as follows:
- Damage to buildings such as old monuments
- Damage to metals, alloys, textiles, rubber and works on wood, bronze and stone (such as painting, carvings)
- Repairs of these cost millions of rupees (thus time, money and energy are wasted).

Indicators of Air Pollution

Following indicators are employed for monitoring of air pollution:
1. Sulfur dioxide index: This is estimated by lead peroxide device.
2. Smoke index (soiling index): A known volume of air is filtered through a disk of filter paper. The discoloration produced is measured against the standards in photoelectric meter. Result is expressed as Coh units per 1,000 linear feet in air.
3. Suspended particles (measurement of dust and grit concentration): The amount of dust particle present in the given volume of air is measured by using an instrument, 'midget impingers' and is expressed in milligram per cubic meter of air.
4. Air pollution index: It is an arbitrary index, considering one or more pollutants as a measure of severity of pollution. For example, employed in USA—10 times SO_2 concentration plus twice CO concentration plus twice the coefficient of haze. It is considered as an alarm, when this value becomes more than 50.
5. Coefficient of haze: It is the amount of smoke or other aerosol per cubic meter of air.
6. Other parameters are lead, CO, NO_2 and oxidants.

Prevention of Air Pollution

The World Health Organization (WHO) has recommended the following procedures for the prevention and control of air pollution:
1. Containment: It is prevention of escape of toxic substances into the ambient air. Containment can be achieved by a variety of engineering methods such as enclosure, ventilation and air cleaning. A major contribution in this field is the development of 'arresters' for the removal of contaminants.
2. Replacement: Replacing a technological process causing air pollution by a new process that does not increased use of electricity, natural gas and central heating in place of coal has greatly helped in smoke reduction. Now there is a move to reduce lead in petrol, which is a cumulative poison.
3. Dilution: It is valid so long as it is within the self-cleaning capacity of the environment. For example, some air pollutants are readily removed by vegetation. The establishment of 'green belts' between industrial and residential areas in the attempt at dilution. The capacity for dilution is however, limited and trouble occurs, when the atmosphere is overburdened with pollutants.
4. Legislation: Air pollution is controlled in many countries by suitable legislation, e.g. clean air acts. To decrease the nuisance of air pollution, the Government of India has enacted Air (Prevention and Control of Pollution) Act in 1981.
5. International action: The WHO established an international network of laboratories for the monitoring and study of air pollution. The network consists of two international centers at London and Washington, three centers at Moscow, Nagpur and Tokyo, and 20 laboratories in various parts of world. These centers will issue warning of air pollution, where and when necessary.
6. Disinfection of air has received much attention. The methods employed are:
   a. Mechanical ventilation: This reduces vitiated air and bacterial density.
   b. The UV radiation: This has been found to be effective and infectious disease wards. Since direct exposure to UV rays is a danger to the eyes and skin, the UV lamps are shaded and located in the upper portion of the rooms near the inlet of air.
   c. Chemicals mists: Triethylene glycol vapors have been found to be effective air bactericides, particularly against droplet nuclei and dust.
   d. Dust control: Application of oil to floors of hospital wards reduces the bacterial content of the air. Air disinfection is still in the experimental stage.

Control of Air Pollution

Air pollution can be control by three measures:
1. Engineering technology.
2. Legislations.
3. General measures.

Engineering Technology

1. Location of the industries: Industries must be located far away from the human habitations and where topography of the soil is favorable.

CHAPTER 8 — Air as a Determinant of Health

2. **Replacement measures:** Within the industries, the processes causing air pollution should be replaced by the processes preventing air pollution. For example, using electricity instead of fuels, using liquefied petroleum gas (LPG), smokeless fuel, i.e. in the place of coal, etc.
3. **Containment measures such as:**
   - Controlling the production of dust by wet method
   - Prevention of the escape of dust into the atmosphere by using enclosures hood, exhaust pipes for removal
   - Increasing the height of smoke vent, etc.

Legislation Measures

To control air pollution, Government of India has enacted some acts such as Indian Factories Act, Prevention and Control of Air Pollution Act, Smoke Nuisance Act, etc.

General Measures

- Control of traffic by construction of bypass roads
- Maintenance of vehicles by periodical servicing, mixing of petrol and oil in proper proportions, use of unleaded petrol to the vehicles, fitting the catalytic converter to the exhausts pipes of four wheelers, which convert the harmful gas into harmless gas
- Establishment of 'green belts', i.e. growing plants and trees between the industries and the residential areas, so that the leaves absorb CO_2 and give out oxygen
- Health education of the people about hazards of air pollution and their role in the prevention and control of air pollution
- Population control.

ROLE OF NURSES IN PREVENTION AND CONTROL OF AIR POLLUTION

Keeping in view of above discussion, community health nurse has to educate the public regarding the following.

There are a number of methods, which are effective in prevention and control of air pollution, which are as follows:

1. **Prevention and correction of air pollution at source:** As industries are the main source of air pollution so the formation of pollutants and emission of pollutants can be reduced at the source. This can be achieved by substituting the raw material with another material, which reduces the formation of pollution. This can be done by modifications in the existing process such as washing of coal before pulverization can reduce the emission of fly ash. Even modification in the existing equipment can reduce the air pollution.

   Methods of prevention and control of air pollution at source:
   - Substitution
   - Modifications in process or technique
   - Modifications of the equipments.

2. **Installation of pollution control equipments:** Sometimes pollutants are present in high concentration at the sources because of not possibility of controlling the escape of pollutants, then pollutant control equipments removes the gaseous pollutants by increasing their distance from the main source thereby diluting and diffusing the pollutants with air. There are a number of pollution control devices such as cyclone separator, gravitational setting chamber, etc.

3. **Diffusion of pollutants:** Diffusion is another way to control the air pollution. This can be achieved by the use of tall stacks, which can penetrate and disperse the contaminants in the upper atmospheric layers. But this depends on the temperature, speed and direction of wind.

4. **Plant the trees:** Plants help in controlling the air pollution by making use of CO_2 released during respiration by man and release the oxygen, which is utilized by human beings. This way the air is being purified. So plenty of trees should be planted near high-risk areas of pollution, i.e. establishment of green belts.

5. **Zoning:** It means separate areas for industries and industries should be far from the residential area. This method is adopted at the time of planning the cities. The industrial estate of Bengaluru is divided into heavy, medium and light zones.

6. **Disinfecting the air:** Vitiated air can be reduced by mechanical ventilation UV lamps after shading can be place at the inlet of air to disinfect the air. Even vapors such as triethylene glycol act as bactericides. If oil applied to floors, then there will be reduced chances of having bacteria content in air.

These methods of disinfection of air need to be experimented. Air pollution is a constant and menacing problem throughout the world, due to man's own activities such as industrialization and urbanization. It is increasing progressively during the past few decades. Air pollution is not only a public health problem but also an economic problem. For presence and control of air pollution the act is prevailing in India are as follows.

Air Act or Air (Prevention and Control of Pollution) Act, 1981

Air Act was framed in the year 1981, but enacted on March 29, 1982 for the effective prevention, control and abatement of air pollution in the country.

The Air Act extends to whole of India and is a welfare legislation dealing with the special civil of pollution. Therefore, it is considered a modern act of special act.

Central and State Pollution Control Boards (constituted under water act, 1974) shall exercise the power and perform functions for the prevention and control of air pollution to improve the quality of air.

Measures to Control Air Pollution

The Air Act was amended in 1987 to remove the difficulties encountered during implementation, to confer more powers on the implementing agencies and to impose more stringent penalties for violation of the provisions of the act. Definition of air pollutant was amended to include noise also. Section 19 was added [air pollution control area (APCA) can be declared].

The state government, after consultation with state board can:
1. Declare any area within the state as 'APCA'. This power provides measures, which are preventive in nature, particularly use of only approved appliances in the premises.
2. Prohibit the use of any fuel other than an approved fuel in any APCA.
3. Prohibit the burning of any material (other than fuel) in any APCA:
   a. The state government has to notify this declaration in the official gazette.
   b. No person without the previous consent of the state board in writing can operate any industrial plant in APCA.
   c. No person, operating an industrial plant in any APC area shall discharge the emission of any air pollutant in excess of the standards laid down by the state board.
   d. Emission of air pollutants in excess of the standards laid down by state board is an offence and punishable under Section 37 of Air Act. Therefore, in such cases, board can lodge and application to the court.
   e. On receipt of application, the court can order the person to check the emission of air pollutants or can authorize the board to implement the directions. All expenses incurred by the board shall be recoverable form the person concerned.

Any Person, Authorized by the Board, has the Right to Enter any Place

1. For the purpose of performing his/her duty.
2. For the purpose of determining whether the provisions and directions given under this act are being complied with.
3. For the purpose of examining or testing any control equipment, industrial plant, record, register or any other document:
   a. Any obstruction or wilful delay is offence, which is punishable.
   b. State board has the power to obtain any information from a person carrying on any industry.
   c. State board has the power to take samples of air or emission. The board has set a procedure to be followed in this connection.

Penalties

1. Violation of act under any circumstances—imprisonment from 1½ to 6 years and fine (no limit).
2. Whosoever damages the property of board—imprisonment up to 3 months or fine up to ₹10,000 or both.
3. Offence by a company or government department—punishment to the director of company or head of government department according to offence:
   - Court shall take cognizance of any offence if the complaint is made by:
     - Board or its authorized officer
     - Any person who has given notice of not less than 60 days.
5. State government has the powers to supersede state board if the board persistently makes default in the performance of its functions.
6. Central government has the powers to make rules.

CONCLUSION

The term environmental sanitation is replaced by environmental health. Environment get polluted due to industrialization, deforestation, open defecation, fire smoke, improper disposal of waste, etc. The environmental pollution affects living as well as non-living components. Air pollution is the presence of excessive concentration of foreign matter in air. This can occur due to natural or man-made causes. Air pollution has an impact on health of people such as headache, laryngitis, pharyngitis, asthma, nausea, lung cancer, etc. The pollution of air can be minimized by preventing and correcting the pollution at source, diffusing pollutants, zoning and disinfection the air. According to WHO, containment, replacement and dilution are the methods or controlling air pollution. Air constitute the immediate physical environment. It is such as important environment factor, i.e. without air life would not have excessed on earth the public health importance of air is that not only it is not breathing purpose, cooling of body, hearing and smelling but also it act as a vehicle of transmission of diseases results is even epidemics and pandemics air is said to have become polluted, when it contain these foreign substance such as dust, bacterial, spore, gases, etc. in excessive concentration, so as to affect the health of human beings and animals and causes damage to plants and properties. Prevention and control of air pollution can be achieved by three measures—engineering technology, legislation and general measures—control of traffics greenbelt health education and population stabilization.

Light as a Determinant of Health

CHAPTER 9

INTRODUCTION

Good light is essential for efficient vision. Imperfect light is one of the causes of ill health and accidents. It can damage the eyesight and produce physical and mental discomfort. Visible light has a varying wavelength of electromagnetic waves from 380 nm (violet) to 760 nm (red).

LIGHT

Measurement of Light

Measurement of lighting includes the foot-candle and lumen type. The four measurements of lights are as follows:
1. The luminous intensity or power of artificial light is measured by the standard 'candle'.
2. The amount of light given off by burning of a sperm wax candle burning 120 grains per hour is called one candlepower.
3. The illumination received from one candle at a distance of 30.48 cm is known as 10.76 lux.
4. The illumination is measured by an instrument called photometer. A minimum of at least 64.58 lux illumination is required for clear visibility for performance of work.

The light is also measured by other parameters such as:
- Luminous flux (flow of light), expressed in lumens
- Illumination (amount of light reaching a surface) expressed as lux per unit area
- Luminance (brightness, i.e. amount of light reflected from a surface) expressed as lamberts.

Foot candle: It is the intensity of light desired at a point placed at a distance of 38.5 cm^2 from a light source of standard candlepower. It is an old unit of measurement.

Lumen: Amount of light, which falls as on 929 cm^2 of surface from a distance of 38.5 cm from one lighted by standard candle source.

Essentials of Good Lighting

Essentials of good lighting are:
1. Sufficiency and uniformity in distribution: Light should be adequate and uniform in distribution without causing eye strain (193.75–215.28 lux).
2. Absence of glare: The glare causes confusion and strain. It should not fall directly on the eye of the worker.
3. Sharp shadow is disturbing and also it should not be patchy, as it can lead to accident. Fluorescent strip lighting is practically shadowless.
4. Overbright light: If light is overbright, it dazzles and causes eye strain. In industry, the dazzle of light from a bright surface is a constant source of trouble. It can be overcome by painting the machine.

Source of Light

In environment, sources of light vary widely in the intensity of their emission of light. Common high-intensity sources are sun (natural source) and lasers, electric weldings, lamps and artificial sources. Broadly, sources of light (Fig. 9.1) can be divided into two groups:
- Natural sources
- Artificial sources.

Natural Light

Natural light is obtained not only from the sky but also from reflection. Natural lighting depends upon the time of the day, season, weather and atmospheric pollution. It is better and cheaper than artificial light. It depends upon designs, orientation, location, type and size of the house. North and south facing gives uniform illumination and whitewashing gives a good light. For proper natural light, minimum area for windows or doors available in the household should be:
- Living and bedrooms: 1/10 of the total room area
- School room: 1/5 of the total room area

CHAPTER 9 — Light as a Determinant of Health

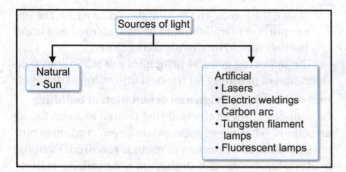

Figure 9.1: Sources of light

- Factory: 1/5 of the total room area
- Cow shed: 1/5 of the total room area.

Windows should be located high. Modern factories cannot depend upon natural light always.

Artificial Light

The best form of artificial lighting is the electric tube light (filament lamp and fluorescent lamp). It does not vitiate the air and gives of minimum heat. Gas lighting either coal gas or acetylene, or petrol gas is liable to pollute air with carbon monoxide and a considerable amount of heat. Lighting standard for some places include the following:
- Living room: 75.35 lux
- Stairs: 21.55–43.05 lux
- Class and library room: 107.64 lux
- Hotel: 64.58 lux
- Office general: 107.64 lux
- Hospital ward: 32.29 lux
- Industrial processes: 59.20 lux
- Operation theater: 1,076.39 lux.

Factors Essential for Good Lighting

Good lighting is essential for efficient vision. If the lighting conditions are not ideal, the visual apparatus is put to strain, which may lead to general fatigue and loss of efficiency. For efficient vision, the following light factors are essential.

Sufficiency

The lighting should be sufficient to enable the eye to discern the details of the object as well as the surroundings without eye strain. An illumination of 161.45–215.27 lux is accepted as a basic minimum for satisfactory vision.

Distribution

For efficient vision, the distribution of light should be uniform, having the same intensity over the whole field of work. If there are contrast differences in light, it will strain eyes and affect adversely the visual acuity.

Absence of Glare

Glare is excessive contrast. Glare may be a direct glare from the light source or reflected glare from sources such as table tops and polished furniture. It causes annoyance. The eye cannot tolerate glare, because it causes acute discomfort and effective vision.

Absence of Sharp Shadows

Slight shadows are inevitable, but sharp and contrasting shadows are disturbing. Similar to glare, shadows cause confusion to the eye and therefore should be present in the field of vision.

Steadiness

The source of light should be constant. It should not flicker because flickering causes eye strain and may lead to accidents.

Color of Light

Natural light has a soothing effect on the eye. The artificial light should, as far as possible, approximate the daylight color.

Surroundings

For efficient vision, color schemes in rooms are important. Ceilings and roofs should have a reflection factor of 80%. There should not be much reflection from the floor, not more than 15–20%. Contrasting colors are often used to prevent accidents, e.g. culverts, bridges, etc.

Units of Light

Light containing all visible waves is perceived as white. There are considerable confusion about units of light measurement (Fig. 9.2). There are four measures of importance:

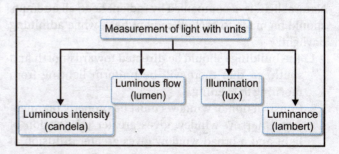

Figure 9.2: Units of light

- Luminous intensity: Point of source brightness or dullness
- Luminous flux: Flow of light
- Illuminance: Light reaching the surface
- Luminance: Light reflected by the surface.

For each of these four measures, again there are a number of terms and also a great variety of names. The four measures are:
1. Luminous intensity, which is the 'power' of a light source considered as a point radiating in all directions; this is measured as candelas or candlepower.
2. Luminous flux, which is the flow of light related to unit of solid angle measured in lumens.
3. Illumination or illuminance, which is the amount of light reaching a surface measure in lux per unit area.
4. Brightness or luminance, which is the amount of light reflected from a surface measured in lamberts.

METHODS TO IMPROVE LIGHTING

Now, we shall discuss briefly about natural illumination and artificial illumination, i.e. natural light and artificial light and methods to improve them.

Natural Illumination

Natural Lighting

Sun is the natural source of light and it is accompanied by heat. There are a number of factors, which affect the natural light illumination. These are:
- Weather
- Time of the day
- Season
- Design, location and orientation of building
- Atmospheric pollution.

Natural lighting is derived from the visible sky reflection. More light comes to the rooms by reflection from light-colored objects. Efficient utilization of natural light calls for careful design, location and orientation of buildings and relationship between buildings (town planning). Natural light is accompanied by radiant heat; all attempts should be made to exclude radiant heat, while admitting daylight:
1. The buildings should be directed towards north and south, so that there will be uniform lighting from morning to evening.
2. Construction of windows must be properly planned. A tall narrow window gives greater penetration of light and a broad window gives greater diffusion of light.
3. Inside the rooms, the ceiling should be white, the upper portion of walls should be light colored and lower portion should be slightly dark colored.

The following general principles are taken into consideration in planning for the best utilization of daylight.

Proper location, design and orientation of building

Careful designing of the building related to room facing directions, windows of appropriate size according to purpose of room and interiors of room is required. Even the relationship between buildings is required. To achieve uniform lighting, wherever possible, schools, factories, buildings and laboratories should be north or south oriented as in east and west facing building/room, window shades are used to protect direct entry of sunlight. Illumination is subject to variation in east and west facing buildings.

To achieve illumination of light in rooms, window's size, shape and location of window opening are most important. While talking about interiors of rooms, proper illumination is achieved, if the ceiling is white and walls of upper portion is light color and lower portions of dark tint. In east facing rooms, morning sun cast yellow glow in rooms, so with too much orange or yellow color may be stifling in this light. On the other hand, in western facing windows, orange, red, yellow glow of sun will overwhelm any room with orange or red color scheme. Natural light is best achieved through placement of windows, skylight reflections and penetration and doorways.

Orientation

The brightness of the sky is not constant on the east and west, and therefore the illumination is subject to variation in buildings facing east or west. Further, the direct penetration of sunlight from the east or west may heat up rooms unduly in the tropics, especially during summer. Buildings are therefore oriented, whenever possible, toward north or south for uniform illumination. When a building faces east and west, window shades are provided to protect against the direct penetration of sunlight.

Removal of obstructions

Removal of obstruction items either wholly or partially is likely to give the most effective single improvement in lighting. One of the important ways to achieve natural light illumination is removal of obstruction in the path of flow of light to rooms.

Windows

Windows should be properly planned, as the natural lighting within any room is influenced by the amount of visible sky, size, shape and arrangement of the window openings.

A tall window gives greater diffusion of light. Window area is correlated to the purpose the room is intended to serve. North facing rooms receive less direct sunlight and are cooler, while the south facing rooms receive more intense light and are warmer. Tall windows penetrate more light in rooms, but broader windows diffuse more light. Windows size appropriate to room will provide appropriate illumination.

Interior of the rooms
For full benefit of the natural illumination, the ceiling should be white; the upper portion of the walls should be lightly tinted and lower portion should be somewhat dark, so as to give comfortable contrast to the eyes.

Daylight illumination is liable to change from moment to moment; it is not measured in terms of foot-candles. Reliance is placed on a factor called daylight factor (DF). It is the ratio of illumination at a given point to illumination at a point exposed simultaneously to the whole hemisphere of the sky (taken as 5381.95 lux) excluding direct sunlight. The daylight factor may be summarized as follows:

$$DF = \frac{\text{Instantaneous illumination indoors}}{\text{Simultaneously occurring illumination outdoors}} \times 100$$

The DF in a building may be rapidly determined by a modified photoelectric meter known as a DF meter. It is recommended that in living rooms, the DF should be at least 8% and in kitchens about 10%.

Advantages of having natural light: It has the biological effects as described below:
- Reduces bilirubin level in case of premature infants having hyperbilirubinemia
- Maintains the biological rhythm of body
- Stimulates melanin synthesis
- Activate the precursors of vitamin D
- Maintain the adrenocortical secretion.

Artificial Illumination

Artificial Lighting
Artificial light is required, when there is less or no natural light because of weather or time of day. With the advanced technology, artificial light can be produced by using tungsten filaments, lamps or fluorescent lamps. Even lasers and electric weldings or carbon can produce artificial light.

Daylight should be implemented by artificial illumination in adequate illumination. Artificial lighting should be as close as possible to daylight in composition.

Depending on the type of projection of light towards working area, or upwards or downward and of reflection basis, it is divided into five types:
1. Direct lighting: In this, 99-100% of the light is projected directly toward the working area. Direct lighting is efficient, economical, but tends to cut sharp shadows. It should be directed not into the eyes.
2. Semidirect lighting: Here, 10-40% of the light is projected upwards, so that it is reflected back on the object by the ceiling.
3. Indirect lighting: Light does not strike a surface directly because of 90-100% of the light is projected toward the ceiling and walls. This gives a general illumination of the whole room, but not of any object.
4. Semi-indirect lighting: Here, 60-90% of the light is directed upwards and the rest downwards.
5. Direct and indirect lighting: Here, light is distributed equally. No one system can be recommended to the exclusion of others.

Electric light is the best method of providing artificial illumination. There is no combustion nor there is any reduction in the oxygen content of atmosphere. It gives good, steady and bright light. The different types of electric lights (Table 9.1) are:
1. Filament lamps (incandescent lamps): In this type, the tungsten filament is heated and light is emitted. Only 5% of the current is available for lighting and remaining 95% is expended as heat. The hotter filaments produce the bluer light. Accumulation of dust on the bulb reduces illumination by 30-40%. The bulbs and shades therefore should be cleaned frequently.
2. Fluorescent lamps: These are economical in the use of electric current; they are cool and efficient; the light emitted, stimulates natural light. The lamps consist of a glass tube filled with mercury vapor and an electrode fitted at each end. The inside of the tube is coated with fluorescent chemicals, which absorb practically all the ultraviolet (UV) radiation and remit the radiation in the visible range.

Table 9.1: Emission of energy by lamps

Lamps	Light (%)	Heat (%)
Filament	5	95
Fluorescent	21	79

Different types of fluorescent lamps are:
1. Neon-filled sodium discharge lamp: This gives yellow light.
2. Mercury vapor lamp: It consists of a glass tube, filled with mercury vapor and an electrode fitted at each

end. The inside of the tube is coated with fluorescent chemicals, which absorbs UV radiation and remits the radiation in the visible range.
3. Cold cathode neon lamps: They are used for decorative purpose.
4. Shadowless lights: They are specially necessary in operation theaters.

In addition, other sources of artificial light are:
1. Gas light: In this type, there is burning of the coal gas in an incandescent burner having a mantle. The light is steady and bright, but it produces too much heat and emits disagreeable smell.
2. Gas burner: Oil lamps, candle and acetylene gas.

Standards of Lighting

The eye responds to a range of illumination ranging from 0.1 (full moonlight night) to 100,000 lux (bright sunshine). There is considerable confusion about standards because of the adaptability of the eye. The visual efficiency increases with the increase of illumination, but the curve flattens out at higher levels. The law of diminishing return applies a useful 'rule of thumb', i.e. the illumination level should be 30 times higher than the level at which the task can just be done. There are no exact lighting standards. For practical situations and various activities, the following values (in lux) have been suggested by the illuminating engineering society:
- Visual task: Illumination
- Casual reading: 100
- General office work: 400
- Fine assembly: 900
- Very severe tasks: 1,300–2,000
- Watchmaking: 2,000–3,000.

The observation that daylight could cause the in vitro degradation of bilirubin is now being used as a therapeutic measure in premature infants with hyperbilirubinemia. Other effects of light include effect on physical activity, the stimulation of melanin synthesis, the activation of precursors of vitamin D, adrenocortical secretion and food consumption.

Criteria for Good Lighting

For proper visualization of an object, good light is required; otherwise there will be strain on eyes. Following is the criteria for good light:
- Proper illumination
- Uniform distribution
- Not too bright light
- Absence of flickering
- No sharp shadows or contrasting shadows
- Too bright light
- Too light illumination
- Thermal effect of light.

Proper illumination: The light will enable to know the details of an object without putting too much strain on eyes. The illumination requirement differs depending upon the area, but 161.45–215.27 lux is the basic minimum requirement for satisfactory vision.

Illumination requirements are as follows:
- Satisfactory vision: 161.45–215.27 lux, without eye strain
- Stairs: 53.81 lux
- Corridors: 1,076.39 lux.

Uniform distribution: The light should fall over the whole or the area of work with same intensity, so that there can be proper uniform distribution of light and a person is able to perform the work without any eyes strain.

Not too bright light: As bright light causes constriction of pupils, thereby putting more strain to eye to see an object in detail, because of less area of visualization created by constricted pupils. Sometimes glare light, unable a person to visualize the objects. Many times in nights, glare light of vehicles causes confusion among the riders, leading to accidents. Bright light reduces the critical vision ability, so the light should not be too bright.

Absence of flickering: There should not be any flickering in light; it should come from a constant source. Flickering light unable a person to focus on the object and even more strain in put on the eye, because of presence and absence of light alternatively on the object.

No sharp or contrast shadows: Sharp shadows of objects produced by light can cause confusion and these should not be present in field of vision, but slight shadows do not create problems.

Too bright light: This injures the eye through photochemical reaction in retina. If an individual has sustained exposure exceeding 0.1 mW/cm^2, then the chances of having blue light injury and an exposure of more than 10 W/cm^2 for even a small period of time can cause retinal burn depending upon the image size.

Too light illumination: If illumination is not adequate, then the individuals can have eye strain and seasonal affective disorders.

Thermal effect of light: Too much heat caused by light can cause injury to iris, lens, cornea and skin due to exposure to laser radiations produced by an artificial laser light.

Poor Lighting

Poor lighting has bad effects on health, which includes:
- Eye strain
- Annoyance
- Discomfort
- Accidents
- Injury to eye
- Retinal burn.

Prevention of Effects of Poor Lighting

- Proper illumination
- Appropriate training
- Proper design of buildings
- Proper design of equipments
- Protective eye shields
- Not to look directly to the sources of light, which are large and bright enough to cause retinal damage such as solar eclipse
- Avoid looking directly to high-intensity sources such as lasers or carbon arc
- Proper planning of town or city, i.e. distance between the building and windows, and door facing directions of light.

Proper light in homes, schools, offices and work places reduce the chances of occurrence of eye strain problems, discomfort, annoyance, etc. by which, the productivity and efficiency will be increased. Use of protective eye devices at the time of exposure of high-intensity light will reduce the diseases as well as economic burden on the individual/family and nation. It is the nurse, who can make community aware of the ill effects of light and how these can be easily prevented by taking simple measures.

CONCLUSION

Light constitutes an important physical environment of human beings. It is also a form and a source of energy. Without light, living will not be comfortable. It is essential for vision. Light may be from natural source or artificial source. Excessive bright light or glare results in glaring, blurring of vision, discomfort and accidents, and poor lighting results in nystagmus, headache, accidents, visual strain, etc.

The observation that daylight causes degradation of bilirubin is now employed as a therapeutic measure among premature newborns with physiological jaundice. Other biological effects of light are stimulation of melanin synthesis and synthesis of vitamin D in the skin.

Natural source of light is the sun. The visible rays of the sunlight constitute the solar spectrum 'VIBGYOR', which can be seen in the rainbow. The sun rays beyond the spectrum are invisible. The rays beyond the violet end are UV rays and the rays beyond the red end are infrared rays. Both have got therapeutic uses. For carrying out the work efficiently with efficient vision, following 'daylight factors' are essential:

- Sufficient illumination of 161.45–215.27 lux
- Uniform distribution in the working place
- Absence of glare (i.e. glare is excessive contrast, e.g. headlight of a vehicle at night, the same light during day time does not cause glare because of absence of contrast)
- Absence of sharp shadows
- Steadiness of source of light
- White color of the light
- Contrast surroundings.

Light, i.e. visible light should have proper illumination, uniform distribution, not too bright light, no sharp shadow and absence of flickering. Poor lighting has an impact on health such as eye strain, annoyance, discomfort, injury to eye and retinal burn. This can be prevented by proper illumination, appropriate training, proper designing of building equipments, protective eye shields and health education, etc.

Ventilation as a Determinant of Health

10 CHAPTER

INTRODUCTION

Most of the ill effects attributive to bad air is due to overcrowding. The supply of fresh air and removal of inside stale air from the rooms of building is called ventilation of building. Ventilation is the process of removal of vitiated air and supply of fresh quality air, i.e. in regard to the temperature, humidity and purity. A well-ventilated building is a sign of health and comfort for inmates. Proper ventilation is important to control humidity and to prevent condensation. The objectives of ventilation includes:
- To provide constant fresh air
- To remove unpleasant odor, which has resulted from humidity and warmth
- To check the breeding of bacteria.

Now, ventilation implies not only the replacement of vitiated air by a supply of fresh outdoor air but also control of the quality of incoming air with regard to its temperature, humidity and purity with a view provide a thermal environment that is comfortable and free from risk of infection.

STANDARDS OF VENTILATION

The standards of ventilation have been based on the efficiency of ventilation in removing body odor. According to Gupta BR and Arora NL, for good ventilation by natural methods, the aggregate area of door and window openings should not be less than one seventh of floor area of rooms and in addition to every 10–15 m³ capacity of a room, a ventilation having 0.15 m² of an area should be provided just below the roof slab, but not above 3.5 m from the floor level.

Cubic Space

Standards for the minimal fresh air supply ranging from 300 to 3,000 ft³/h/person. The widely quoted standard a fresh air supply of 3,000 ft³/h/person on the following grounds. It was observed that so long as the amount of carbon dioxide (CO_2) due to respiration was not more than two parts in 10,000 parts of air, the air of the rooms seemed fresh and did not sensibly differ from outdoor air. Assuming that an average person expires 0.6 ft³ of CO_2 per hour, and that 0.0002 ft³ of CO_2 in 1 ft³ of air as the 'permissible impurity', it was calculated that 0.6/0.0002 or 3,000 ft³ of air would require by a man at rest per hour.

Air Change

Air change is more important that the cubic space requirement. It is recommended that in the living rooms, there should be two or three air changes in 1 hour; in work rooms and assemblies four to six air changes. If the air is changed more frequently, i.e. more than six times in 1 hour, it is likely to produce a drought, which should be avoided. Based on this concept, it is now considered that a space of 1,000–1,200 ft³ per person is quite sufficient. The number of air changes per hour is calculated by dividing the total hourly air supply to the room by the cubic capacity of the room. In addition to this, air change is also important in living room, two to three air changes per hour and in assembly hall four to six air changes are required.

Air space of a room can be determined by multiplying the length, breadth and height of a room up to 304.8 cm only. Height above 304.8 cm should not be considered. The space occupied by furniture and other contents of the room should be deducted from it. An oil lamp burning in the room will pollute the air as much as five to six persons taken together indoors. Minimum air spaces required per head are as follows:
- Residence: 1,000 ft³ per adult, 500 ft³ per child and 50 ft³ minimum per worker
- General hospital: 1,200 ft³ per patient
- Infectious disease: 1,400 ft³ per person
- Lodging house: 400 ft³ per person
- Shop: 300 ft³ per person
- Soldier: 600 ft³ per soldier.

Floor Space

Floor space per person is even more important than cubic space. Heights in excess of 304.8–365.76 cm are ineffective from the point of view of ventilation, as the product of respiration tends to accumulate in the lower levels. Therefore, in circulating cubic space requirements, heights over 304.8–365.76 cm is not taken into account. The optimum floor space requirements per person vary from 50 to 100 ft^2.

TYPES OF VENTILATION

Ventilation is of two types:
1. Natural ventilation.
2. Artificial ventilation.

Natural Ventilation

Natural ventilation is thought of a low-energy cooling strategy, which provides comfort at a low capital and maintenance cost. The main consideration of adopting natural ventilation is climate. Building shape is crucial in creating the wind pressure that will drive the air through the opening in rooms such as windows, doors, etc. There are many benefits such as it is easily available and economical. But the disadvantages is that quality of air can be impure due to nearness of industrial area main two reasons for natural ventilation. These are:
1. To control the indoor quality air.
2. To control the temperature during summer.

Natural ventilation is of two types:
1. Wind-driven ventilation.
2. Stack-driven ventilation.

Wind-driven Ventilation

Wind plays an important role in ventilating the building with fresh air. Cross ventilation is one of the example of wind-driven ventilation. In this, wind will hit one side of building, the air will speed up in order to flow around the building to opposite side. This will happen when both the windows of opposite direction open. This depends upon three factors:
1. Perflation and aspiration of the wind.
2. Difference of temperature.
3. Diffusion of gases.

Natural ventilation helps considerably, if the buildings are constructed with sufficient open space around and by having large number of windows, preferably opening direct into the outside air. Cross ventilation (Fig. 10.1) means perflation between windows and other opening placed opposite to each other. Naturally, cross ventilation becomes impossible in 'back-to-back' houses.

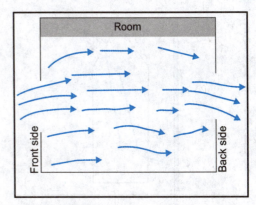

Figure 10.1: Cross ventilation

Perflation and aspiration of the wind: Perflation means blowing of the air through a room, when the doors and windows are open, which is a natural result of air movement. When air is moving, it drives the air before it, lessens the pressure around it and causes the surrounding air to move towards it by aspiration.

Effects of difference of temperature: Air always flows from high density to low density. Outer cooler air is of high density, rushes in through every opening of the room (or through the inlets placed at lower level). Inside air of the room being of lower density moves up.

Greater the difference of temperature between the outer cooler air and the inner warmer air, greater will be the velocity of the incoming air, until the temperature of both outside and inside air becomes equal. Since the incoming air gets warmed up, a constant current is maintained. This is the basis of natural ventilation. The reverse process takes place in the tropics, where the outside air is better than the inside air. But in cold countries, fires are used inside the room to keep the inside air warm.

Diffusion of gases: This means passing of the air through the smallest openings or spaces such as cracks and crevices. This is a very slow process and is very small. As a ventilation agent, it is of little value.

During ventilation, perflation occurs when the wind blows through a room. If any obstruction is in room, then a pressure of suction as is created at its tail end and air passes resulting aspiration. Air when enters through the openings of the room into, then it is known as diffusion. It means wind is drawn into the room by diffusion and perflation. Cross ventilation and aspiration result into exist of stale air from the room.

Stack-driven Ventilation

Stack-driven ventilation occurs (Fig. 10.2) when there is difference in adjoining volumes of air, i.e. between the

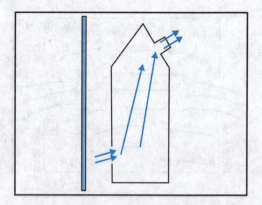

Figure 10.2: Stack-driven ventilation

density of air as air flows from high density to low density. Low density occurs in women air, will rise above the cold air by creating an upward air stream. For achieving the stack effect, the room should have higher aperture for the escape of warm air and a lower aperture for entry of cool dense air.

Artificial Ventilation

Artificial ventilation may be of the following types:
- Exhaust ventilation
- Plenum ventilation
- Balanced ventilation
- Air conditioning.

Exhaust Ventilation

In vacuum system (exhaust system or extraction system) foul, vitiated air is extracted or exhausted to the outside by using exhaust fans, operated electrically.

As air is exhausted, a vacuum is created, which induces fresh air to enter the room through windows, doors and other inlets. Exhaust ventilation is generally provided in large halls and auditorium, cinema halls and are fixed near the roof for removal of vitiated air. The exhaust fans are housed in apertures in the external walls, high up near the roof, which facilitates removal of the upper layers of the heated light air. The ventilation may be regulated by adjusting the speed of the fans. Local exhaust ventilation is widely used in industries to remove dusts, fumes and other contaminants at their source.

Plenum Ventilation

Plenum ventilation type, fresh air is pushed or propelled or blown into the room by centrifugal fans or high-pressure fans. This creates a positive pressure and displaces the vitiated air (Fig. 10.3). Plenum or propulsion system is used for supplying air to air-conditioned buildings and factories. Air is delivered through ducts at desired points. It is limited in use.

Balanced Ventilation

In balanced ventilation both types of fan are used such as exhaust and blowing. Exhaust fans remove the dirty air, while blowing fans blow the fresh air in the room.

Balanced system: In this type, there is a combination of both exhaust system and plenum systems of ventilation. This is used in large halls with extensive sitting capacity. This is also used in air conditioning (AC) system.

Air Conditioning

In this system, the outer air is 'conditioned or controlled' with reference to physical and chemical conditions, such as cleaning (free from pathogens, dirt and dust), adjustment of humidity, which will be most comfortable and then letting into the room at a measured rate and volume of flow without producing draught and exhausted through ducts.

These are being increasingly used in an operation theaters of the hospitals, in hotels, restaurants, offices commercial firms, cinemas, aeroplanes, railways, etc. Where the temperature difference between the outside air and air-conditioned room is very large, 'transition rooms' are provided, so as to prevent sudden exposure to high or low temperature.

The advantages of artificial methods of ventilation are the constancy and the facility with which fresh air is supplied under all conditions, whereas natural ones though less costly are not under human control being subjects to atmospheric conditions.

Air condition supplies fresh air with control of physical temperature, humidity, air movement and bacterial

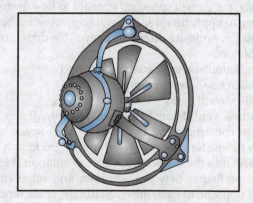

Figure 10.3: Propeller fan with motor

pollution) and chemical (CO_2 concentration) conditions of atmosphere. It is widely used in homes, institutions, industries and hospitals. So as to avoid the health problems related to sudden change in temperature (outside and inside) due to AC inside the room, there is need to have transitional rooms.

Health Hazards and its Prevention

Poorly ventilated houses will have change in physical and chemical conditions of atmosphere inside the house. Increase humidity can cause the growth and reproduction of molds, house dust mites or fungal growth resulting from dampness. These airborne pollutant can give rise to symptoms of rhinitis, conductivities, eczema, cough and wheeze. In confined space with no ventilation, for prolonged periods can cause discomfort, headache, confusion and respiratory diseases.

Prevention
1. In physical locations and orientations of building, a designer must consider fluctuating temperature, humidity, speed of wind and direction of wind, while preparing layouts of buildings. Outdoor pollution also need to be considered, while designing the building.
2. Windows should be designed to allow natural ventilation. As the amount of air that flows through a window depends upon the area and vertical distribution of opening.
3. Artificial ventilation can be used, if natural ventilation is not achieved such as exhaust fans, AC, etc.
4. Clothes should not be dried in homes unless in a dryer ventilation to external air.

Good Ventilation

Disadvantage of natural ventilation includes velocity of air cannot be regulated and temperature and humidity cannot be adjusted. Moreover, natural ventilation acts better in winter and in cold countries. Good ventilation requires a sufficient number of doors and windows with cross ventilation and should be provided in a room as given below.

Inlets and Outlets

Inlet is an entrance through which fresh air enters the room. The foul air escapes through the outlet. It is very essential to have inlets and outlets in every room for the purpose of ventilation. They should be placed 152.4–182.88 cm above the level of floor. This prevents drought during cold weather and dust, and dirt during the summer season. It is always desirable to have several small inlets than one or two large ones.

External Ventilation

Proper ventilation requires some open space or part in front of the house or round it. Lower floors of tall buildings in cities facing narrow streets are devoid of sunshine and pure air.

Artificial Ventilation

Artificial ventilation is the replacement of foul air by fresh air through some artificial means. There are four methods:
1. Propelling fresh air or plenum system.
2. Extraction of foul air or exhaust system.
3. Combination of both or balance system.
4. Air conditioning.

Propelling fresh air or plenum system
In this method, fresh air is mechanically driven into the room by centrifugal fans to create a positive pressure and displace the foul air. Air is also introduced into the room through air diffusion, which consists of baffles or circular plates, which separate the air in the form of cone rather than direct gap.

Extraction of foul air or exhaust system
In this method, foul air of the room is extracted by means of exhaust fans. Exhaust fans are fitted in the aperture of external wall high up near the roof. The ventilation is regularized by adjusting the speed of the fan.

Combination of both or balanced system
In this, both the methods exhaust and plenum are combined. This is meant for big halls and factories. The velocity of fresh air is about 15,240–18,288 cm per minute. If it goes through a washers, velocity is reduced.

Extractions are usually 15,240–21,336 cm per minute. In industrial and lofty buildings, the plenum system is toward ceiling.

Air conditioning
Air conditioning is a process by which the air is simultaneously purified, cooled or heated according to need with control of moisture content. In other words, temperature, humidity and air movements are regulated with elimination of dust, bacteria, odor and toxic gases affecting human health and comforts. It is necessary required in large institutions, hospitals or operation theaters, industrial buildings, dwelling houses in the tropical countries, etc.

Generally, the difference in temperature of the outside air and that of the air-conditioned room should not be more than 20°F. The difference of 10–15°F is desirable. The main advantage of artificial ventilation is that it is under human control. However, it loses much of its freshness and may cause discomfort.

Estimation of Amount of Fresh Air Required

de Chaumont has recommended 3,000 ft³ of fresh air per hour per person based on a point that a person entering a room from outside should not perceive any smell or stuffiness. The stuffiness occurs in a room when the CO_2 concentration exceeds 0.02%.

The amount of fresh air to be delivered per hour to an occupied room, can be calculated by the formula:

$$D = E/P$$

where,

D: Amount of fresh air to be delivered to a room
E: CO_2 exhaled per hour per person (a person at rest gives off 0.6 ft³ of CO_2 per hour)
P: Limit of respiratory CO_2 per ft³ of air (i.e. 0.02 ft³ of CO_2 per 100 ft³ of air, e.g. 0.002 in one ft³).

$$D = \frac{0.6}{0.0002}$$

So, 3,000 ft³ of air required per person per hour, CO_2 being taken as an indicator. A child requires about 200 ft³ of air per hour. However, this standard of ventilation is no longer followed.

Air change: For a person to get 3,000 ft³ of air per hour and occupying a room of 100 ft³, the air should be changed 30 times per hour or if person occupies a room of 1,000 ft³, air requires to be changed only three times. This causes a disagreeable draught specially in cold weather. Otherwise, it does not cause any perceptible draught.

Floor area: This is an important standard of ventilation. The optimum floor area per person in a house recommended is 50–100 ft² results in overcrowding favoring spread of droplet infections. In general hospital, it should be 150 ft² and infectious diseases hospital, it should be 200 ft²/person.

CONCLUSION

Ventilation means not only the replacement of vitiated air (stagnant, warm and moist air) by the drier, cooler and moving air but also control of the quality of incoming air with reference to temperature, humidity and purity in order to provide a comfortable environment without the risk of infection. Internal ventilation is with reference to the ventilation of the rooms and external ventilation is with reference to outside air. External ventilation is done by making the streets broad, building houses with sufficient gap in between and to sufficient height, watering the streets to lay the dust, by keeping plenty of open spaces and parks, etc. Mainly there are two systems of ventilation, namely natural and artificial, depending upon the motive power, which originates them.

Natural ventilation depends on three forces, i.e. perflation and aspiration of wind, differences of temperature and diffusion of gases. Artificial or mechanical ventilation of four types, i.e. vacuum system, plenum system, balanced system and air conditioning.

Noise as a Determinant of Health

CHAPTER 11

INTRODUCTION

Noise is unwanted sound or a sound without agreeable musical quality. Noise as 'unwanted sound' is subjective because of the fact that one man's sound may be another man's noise. So, noise is, 'wrong sound, in the wrong place, at the wrong time'. Man is living in an increasingly noisy environment. Noise has become a very important 'stress factor' in the environment of man. The term 'noise pollution' has been recently coined to signify the vast cacophony of sounds that are being produced in the modern life leading to health hazards.

NOISE

Source

The sources of noise are many and varied. These are automobiles, factories, industries, air crafts, etc. noise levels are particularly acute near railway junctions, traffic round about, bus terminuses and airports. Use of pressure horns, recreational noise of loudspeakers with full volume during festivities particularly at night are other sources of noise production. The domestic noises from the radios, transistors, television (TV) sets all add to the quantum of noise in daily life.

Properties

Noise has two important properties such as loudness or intensity and frequency.

Loudness

Loudness depends upon the amplitude of the vibrations, which initiated the noise. The loudness of noise is measured in decibels (dB). When we say that sound is 60 dB, it means that it is 60 dB more intense than the smallest distinguishable noise or the 'reference' sound pressure, which is understood to be 0.0002 microbar or dynes cm^2. A dyne is 1/1,000,000th of atmospheric pressure. Normal conversation produces a noise of 60–65 dB; whispering, 20–30 dB; heavy street traffic, 60–80 dB; and boiler factories about 120 dB. A daily exposure up to 85 dB is about the limit people can tolerate without substantial damage of hearing.

The human ear responds in a non-uniform way to different sound pressure levels, i.e. it responds not to the real loudness of sound, but to perceived intensity. A weighting curve, called curve A has been constructed, which takes into account the subjective effects of that sound. Acceptable dB noise levels are given in Table 11.1.

The permissible noise levels differences are given in Table 11.2.

Table 11.1: Acceptable noise levels

Locality	Place	Sound pressure level (dB)
Residential	Bedroom	25
	Living room	40
Commercial	Office	35–45
	Conference	40–45
	Restaurants	40–60
Industrial	Workshop	40–60
	Laboratory	40–50
Educational	Classroom	30–40
	Library	35–40
Hospitals	Wards	20–35

Table 11.2: Permissible noise levels in different areas

Areas	Noise level	
	Day time (6 AM to 9 PM)	Nighttime (9 PM to 6 AM)
Industrial	75	65
Commercial	65	55
Residential	55	45
Silence	50	45

Frequency

Frequency is denoted as Hertz (Hz). 1 Hz is equal to 1 wave per second. The human ear can hear frequencies from about 20 to 20,000 Hz, but this range is reduced with age and other subjective factors. The range of vibrations below 20 Hz are infra-audible; and those above 20,000 Hz ultrasonic. Many animals (e.g. dogs) can hear sounds inaudible to the human ear. Sometimes noise is expressed in psychoacoustic terms, the phone. The phone is psychoacoustic index of loudness. It takes into consideration intensity and frequency. The sound level of some of the noises are given below (Table 11.3). The basic instruments used in studies on noise are:

1. The 'sound level meter', which measures the intensity of sound in dB or dB(A).
2. The 'octave band frequency analyzer,' which measures the noise in octave bands. The resulting plot shows the 'sound spectrum' and indicates the characteristics of the noise, whether it is main high pitched, low pitched or of variable pitch.
3. The 'audiometer', which measures the hearing ability. The zero line at the top in the audiogram represents normal hearing. Noise-induced hearing loss shows the characteristic dip in the curve at the 4,000 Hz frequency.

Effect of Noise Exposure

The effects of noise exposure are of two types, they are auditory and nonauditory.

Auditory Effects

1. Auditory fatigue: It appears in the 90 dB region and greatest at 4,000 Hz. It may be associated with side effects such as whistling and buzzing in the ears.

Table 11.3: Sound level of some of the noises

Source of noise	Sound level (dB)
Whisper	10
Speech, 2–3 people	73
Speech on radio	80
Music on radio	85
Children shouting	79
Children crying	80
Vacuum cleaner	76
Piano	86
Jet take off	150

2. Deafness: It is a serious pathological effect. Deafness may be temporary or permanent. Temporary deafness results from a specific exposure to noise; the disability disappears after a period of time up to 24 hours following the noise exposure. Mostly, it occurs in frequency range between 4,000 and 6,000 Hz. Repeated or continuous exposure to noise around 100 dB may result in a permanent deafness; in this inner ear damage may vary from minor changes in the hair cell endings to complete destruction of the organ of Corti. When this occurs as a result of occupation in industries, it is called occupational deafness. Exposure to noise above 160 dB may rupture the tympanic membrane and cause permanent loss of hearing.

Non-auditory Effects

1. Interference with speech: The frequencies causing most disturbances to speech communication lie in the 300–500 Hz range. Such frequencies are commonly present in noise produced by road and air traffic. For good speech intelligibility, it is considered that the speech sound level must exceed the speech interference level (SIL) by approximately 12 dB.
2. Psychological response: Neurotic people are more sensitive to noise than balanced people. Workers exposed to higher intensity of noise in occupational capacities, were often irritated, short tempered and impatient and more likely to resort to agitation and disrupt production.
3. Efficiency: Where mental concentration is to be undertaken, a low level of noise is always desired. Reduction in noise has been found to increase work output.

4. Physiological changes: Temporary physiological changes occur in the human body as a direct result of noise exposure includes a rise in blood pressure (BP), a rise in intracranial pressure, an increase in heart rate and breathing, and an increase in sweating. General symptoms such as giddiness, nausea and fatigue may also occur. Noise interferes with sleep. Noise is also said to cause visual disturbance.

Measures to Control Noise

The following measures may control noise.

Careful Planning of Cities

In planning cities, measures should be taken to reduce noise include division of the city into zones with separation of areas concerned with industry and transport; the separation of residential areas from the main streets by means of wide green belts. House fronts should be lie not less than 15 m from the road and the intervening, space should be thickly planted with trees and bushes, and widening of main streets to reduce the level of noise penetrating into dwellings.

Control of Vehicles

Heavy vehicles should not be routed into narrow streets. Vehicular traffic on residential streets should be reduced. Indiscriminate blowing of the horn and use of pressure horn should be prohibited.

To Improve Acoustic Insulating of Building

From the acoustic standpoint, the best arrangement is construction of detached building rather than a single large building or one that is continuous. Installations that produce noise or disturb the occupants within dwellings should be prohibited. Buildings should be soundproof, where necessary.

Industries and Railways

Definite areas must be earmarked, outside residential areas, for industries, for railways, marshaling yards and similar installations. If it is not possible, protective green belts must be laid down between the installations and residential areas.

Protection of Exposed Persons

Hearing protection is recommended for all workers who consistently exposed to noise louder than 85 dB in the frequency bands above 150 Hz. Periodical audiogram checkups and use of earplugs, ear muffs are also essential as the situation demands.

Legislation

Legislation providing for controls, which are applicable to a wide variety of sources. Workers have the right to claim compensation, if they have suffered a loss of ability to understand speech.

Noise Pollution and Legislative Measures

Noise is defined as a loud, unpleasant or unwanted sound that disturbs unwilling eras. It adversely affects the physiological and mental health.

Noise is measured in units called dB. Noise above 115 dB is regarded as highly disturbing. The World Health Organization (WHO) recommends an industry noise limit of 75 dB. Vehicles create noise of about 90 dB, jets of about 150 dB and rockets of 180 dB. A sound above 80 dB causes noise pollution.

Legislative measures

Various legislative measures are as follows:
1. Excessive noise has been recognized as a crime under Section 268 of Indian Penal Code (IPC) (Nuisance Act, 1860).
2. Noise has been recognized as a pollutant under Section 6-2.6 of Environment Protection Act, 1986. This act has been amended in 1989 to prescribe day and night limits of noise level.
    An area with 100 m radius around a hospital, institution or court can be declared a 'silence zone'. The use of vehicular horns, loud speakers and bursting crackers is banned in a silence zone under this act.
3. Under Section 133 of IPC, the use of loudspeaker is a public nuisance.
4. The provisions under Motor Vehicles Act, the Factories Act, the Railways Act and Aircraft Act are not sufficient.

To control this means, there is need of a separate Noise Pollution Act.

What to do for Seek Redressal?

Before proceeding to seek redressal from others, we should be aware of the following facts:
1. It shall be the duty of every citizen of India to protect and improve the natural environment [Article 51-A Clause (g) of constitution].
2. We must have the knowledge about our environment. For this, environmental education is necessary for

every citizen to know that we all share common environment and it is the property of all on this earth, and not only one segment.

3. We must develop a habitual love for pollution free environment. In the words of Dewan (1987) "We are traditionally pollution loving nation." We pollute air by bursting crackers on Diwali and on many other occasions. We pollute rivers by disposing dead bodies and other waste. We take so much wood from our trees that trees have become scarce in many areas. We are primarily a vegetarian nation, yet our wildlife is on the edge of extinction. We believe in open latrines. Municipalities allow the city waste and industrial effluents to flow in open drains. Our Jagratas, Akhand paths, Azans, etc. remain incomplete without the use of loudspeakers and amplifiers. Most people of our country are ignorant about deteriorating environment, but even awakened persons are not well-versed with the rights in the constitution and how to seek help of court.

We must have knowledge about the laws made for compensation of loss of lives by pollution and control the person who are polluting are polluting by creating noise, discharging effluents in air and water, ruthlessly exploiting the natural resources and doing loss to the wild life.

How can we Seek Redressal?

Article 21 of the Constitution guarantees, the right to life and it includes right to clean unpolluted air, water and environment. Under this article, one can seek help of court or State Pollution Control Board to take action against a polluter.

Redressal through court

Law of tort and the pollution

A common law of tort is the action against the polluter and is one of the major and the oldest law to abate pollution. Most pollution cases in tort law fall under the categories of nuisance negligence and strict liability:

1. Section 268 of IPC deals with the person found guilty of public nuisance, which causes injury, damage or annoyance to public and its property is a punishable offence.
2. A plaintiff (one who sues in law court) in a tort (private or civil wrong) action may sue for damage or an injunction (judicial order to restrain). While damages are the monetary compensation payable for the commission of a tort, an injunction is a judicial process in which a wrongdoer is restrained from pursuing such acts.

Law of crime and pollution

Crime and pollution is actually a mixture of law of tort and IPC procedures as it has made provisions for the Code of Criminal Procedure and provide speedier remedy against public nuisance. The public duty of the Magistrate to come to the rescue of citizen in such cases has been emphasized.

A public nuisance is an unreasonable interference with a general right of the public. It is to be noted that a private dispute, e.g. dispute between two neighbors only, is actionable in tort, persons who pollute the environment by domestic, urban or industrial wastes, or cause loud and continuous noises affecting the health and comfort of these dwelling the neighborhood (e.g. an instrument, noise producing installation in a factory or a shop) are liable to prosecution for causing a public nuisance.

Indian Penal Code and pollution

The IPC has made direct provision under Section 133 of IPC and gave powers to the District Magistrate or Subdivisional Magistrate or other Executive Magistrate to pass an order (for the person who creates public nuisance) on receiving the report of a police officer or other information (including complaint made by a citizen) and on taking such evidence as thinks fit.

The order is conditional as it is only a preliminary order. When a person fails to appear and show cause (against the order), or when the court is satisfied on the evidence adduced that the initial order was proper, the order is made final otherwise it is vacated.

If the final order is defined or ignored, Section 188 of IPC comes into play. According to it, if such disobedience causes or tends to cause danger to human life, health, safety, causes or tends to cause a riot or affray shall be punished for 6 months imprisonment or fine up to ₹1,000 or both.

Direct action

The Environment Act, 1986 (Section 7) prohibits every person carrying on any industry from discharging or emitting any industry any environmental pollutant in excess of prescribed standard. In such cases, we can serve a direct notice to the polluter. If the polluter fails to comply with the provisions of Section 7, we can lodge a complaint against the polluter in the court after 60 days of serving the notice.

Limitations of Laws

All acts have drawbacks, short comings or lacunae, which can be summarized as follows:
- The laws are not comprehensive in nature
- The laws are fragmented and haphazard
- Many of the laws are outdated
- Powers given to implementing machinery are inadequate
- Litigation process is very slow.

Education

People's participation can be taken by education, then through all available media is needed to highlight the importance of noise as a community hazard in noise control programs.

CONCLUSION

Noise is a wrong sounds, in the wrong place at the wrong time noise has become a very important factor in the environment of man. The term noise pollution has been recently coined to signify the vast cacophony of sounds that are being produced in the modern life leading to health hazards. Noise has two properties, i.e. loudness or intensity and frequency. The effective of noise exposure are two types such as auditory effect and non-auditory effect. Auditory effects are auditory fatigue and deafness. Non-auditory effects are interference with speech, annoyance, efficiency, physiological charges and diseases affecting health. The control of noise can be made is careful planning of cities, control of vehicle to improve acoustic insulation of building, protection of noise exposing persons, health education and legislation.

Radiation Exposure as a Determinant of Health

CHAPTER 12

RADIATION

Radiation is the action of process of radiating, i.e. energy emitted as electromagnetic waves are subatomic particles, radiation sickness or illness caused by X-rays or other radiation. Radiation is defined as a form of energy, emitted from a matter in all directions, in the form of waves carrying a quantum of energy or emitted in the form of fast-moving subatomic particles or nucleotides. Such energy is emitted from a matter as a result of electrical excitement or internal changes. The energy that is emitted, depends upon the wavelengths. Shorter the wavelength, greater is its energy value and vice versa. Wavelengths are expressed as alpha (α).

Sources of Radiation

The sources of radiation to which man is exposed are divided into two groups, i.e. natural and man-made source.

Natural Sources

Man is exposed to natural radiation from time immemorial. Natural background radiation arises from three sources.

Cosmic rays

The cosmic rays, which originate in outer space are weakened as they pass through the atmosphere. At ordinary living altitudes, their impact is about 35 mrad a year. At altitudes above 20 km, cosmic radiation becomes important. It has been calculated that a commercial jet pilot receives about 300 mrad per year from cosmic radiation.

Environmental sources

The source are of two types, terrestrial radiation and atmospheric radiation.

Terrestrial radiation: Radioactive elements such as thorium, uranium, radium and an isotope of potassium (^{40}K) are present in man's environment, e.g. soil, rocks and buildings. It is estimated that man derives about 50 mrad per year from terrestrial radiation. Some areas exist (e.g. Kerala in India), where there are rock formations containing uranium; it can be high as 2,000 mrad a year.

Atmospheric radiation: The external radiation dose from the radioactive gases radon and thoron in the atmosphere is rather small, about 2 mrad per year.

Internal radiation

Man is also subjected to internal radiation, i.e. from radioactive materials include minute quantities of uranium, thorium and related substances, and isotopes of potassium (^{40}K), strontium (^{90}Sr) and carbon (^{14}C). Internal radiation is thought to inflict about 25 mrad a year on the body as a whole, but may be as high as 70–80 mrad. All in all, it is estimated that the total natural radiation to which the average person is subjected, comes to approximately 0.1 mrad a year.

Man-made Sources

Man is exposed to artificial or man-made sources.

X-rays: The greatest man-made sources of radiation exposure to the general population at the present time are medical and dental X-rays. Two distinct groups are involved:
1. Patients.
2. Radiologists and medical technicians.

When optimum radiographic techniques are employed, the skin dose to the patient from a single X-ray film varies roughly from 0.02 to 3.0 mrad.

Radioactive fallout: Nuclear explosions release a tremendous amount of energy in the form of heat, light, ionizing radiation and many radioactive substances. The important being the isotopes of carbon (^{14}C), iodine (^{131}I), cesium (^{137}Cs) and strontium (^{90}Sr) are considered most important because they are liberated in large amounts and remain radioactive for many years. The half-life of ^{90}Sr is about 28 years and that of ^{137}Cs is 30 years. These radioactive particles released into atmosphere, float down to earth for some years afterwards. Because of air currents, the particles are distributed fairly evenly over the whole human race. Measurements made in 1963 in Germany Federal Republic (FR), a country where there had been no explosions, showed that a dose of 33 mrem per person was received from this source.

Miscellaneous: Some everyday appliances (e.g. TV sets, luminous wrist watches) are radioactive. But, radiation from these sources at present is too small to be important.

Hazards of Radiation

Radiation Hazards and Nuclear Medicine

Nowadays, ionizing radiation has been used in many walks of life such as medicine, industry, chemical, agriculture, etc. Manipulation of radioactive materials may involve health hazards as ionizing radiation is silent, unseen and unfelt. Its presence can be made known only by means of special instruments; some of the damaging effects on human system may not develop until many years of exposure.

Many elements have radioactive isotopes. Nuclei of these atoms are unstable and because of instability, they emit radiation till they become stable. Duration of radioactivity lasts from the fraction of second to million years. They emit three types of radiation such as α and β particles, γ rays besides X-rays, which are electromagnetic radiations artificially produced by electric machines and cosmic rays.

Cosmic rays: These originate in outer space. As they pass through atmosphere, they get weakened.

Terrestrial: Radioactive elements such as thorium, uranium and radium present in soil rocks in; more in United States (US). In Kerala, rock formation containing uranium has been found.

Atmospheric: Radioactive fallout is rather small.

Man-made sources: Medical and dental X-rays. Two groups of man-made sources are involved. Here patients, radiologists and technicians are affected.

Radioactive fallout: Nuclear explosion releases tremendous amount of energy in the form of heat, light, ionizing radiation and many radioactive substances.

Medical uses: In medical diagnosis and treatment, and in preventive medicine.

Mode of entry: Medical, dental X-rays, radioisotopes, occupational exposure and nuclear radiation fallout, and exposure through cut surfaces.

The generally accepted limits for maximum permissible exposure of entire body are 5 roentgens per year in the instance of occupational exposure and 0.5 roentgens per year for those not occupationally exposed. Lethal dose is 600 roentgens. Routine radiation exposure from chest X-ray is 1.0 roentgen, if applied to the chest only. The use of X-ray machines should be carefully evaluated by the physician in each case to assure that the benefit of the X-ray outweighs its contribution to cumulative exposure.

The radiation status of an individual is the sum of all his/her exposure to radiation from diagnostic and therapeutic procedures, from cosmic rays and other environmental exposure including occupational exposure. Human race has always been exposed to ionizing radiation of cosmic origin and from natural sources in the environment and within body. A 70-year-old person has been exposed on an average to a total of about 9 roentgens of radiation, but is increased due to great increase in use of artificial sources of radiation.

Effects of Radiation on Health

Epidemiological points of radiation on health include the following:

- During pregnancy, both mother and fetus are at risk
- Children are 10 times more susceptible than adults to radiation hazards
- Malnourished and debilitated individuals are at a greater risk than the healthy counterpart
- Drugs such as metronidazole and bromouridine increases the susceptibility to radiations
- People living at high altitudes are at a greater risk than those at sea level
- Keralites living in coastal areas are at a greater risk because of monazite sand
- Persons working in the following occupations are at a higher risk—uranium mines, atomic power generation, radiology department, watch and television factories, jet navigation, nuclear submarines, laboratories of radioactive isotopes, sterilization of drugs, bandages and sutures, etc.

The biologic effects of ionizing radiation may be divided into two separate groups as detailed below.

Somatic Effects

A dose of 400–500 roentgens on the whole body is fatal in about 50% of cases and that of 600–700 roentgens in practically every case. A dose of 25–50 roentgens to the whole body was found to affect the white blood corpuscles and to produce mild lassitude and softening of the muscles. The delayed effects take time to develop; the latent period may vary from a few weeks to years. It is now fairly well established that delayed effects are mainly of three kinds such as leukemia, malignant tumors and shortening of life.

Genetic Effects

While somatic effects are recognizable within the life span of the irradiated person, genetic effects would be manifested in the more or less remote offspring. Genetic effects result from injury to chromosomes, chromosomal mutations and point mutations. Chromosomal mutation is associated with sterility. Point mutation affects the genes.

TYPES OF RADIATION

Radiation are classified into two groups namely ionizing and non-ionizing radiations (Table 12.1) depending upon the ability to penetrate the tissue, energy and cause destruction of the tissue or not respectively.

Table 12.1: Ionizing and non-ionizing radiation

Rays	Wavelengths [in millimicrons (mµ) or nanometers (nm) 1 nm = 1/1,000 µ]
Ultraviolet rays	20–400 nm
Visible light	400–700 nm
Infrared rays	700–1,000 nm (1 mm)
Microwaves	1 mm–1 m
Radiofrequency waves	1 m–1 km
Laser radiation	

NON-IONIZING RADIATION

Non-ionizing radiation do not penetrate the body tissues, but they are absorbed by the superficial tissues such as skin and eyes. Depending upon their increasing wavelength (or decreasing frequency), they are classified under the following headings.

Ultraviolet Rays

Sources
Natural source is sun. As they are coming from sun, maximum rays are more absorbed by ozone of the atmosphere, but still the effects are more at higher altitudes than at sea level and in summer than in rainy days.

Artificial sources are many, such as mercury vapor tubes, carbon-arc, electric welding, etc.

The high-risk persons for natural source are farmers, shepherds, sailors, road builders, fisherman and those skating on snow. The artificial sources are arising from electric welders and cinema projector workers.

Since the UV rays do not penetrate the tissues, but are absorbed, the effects are primarily on the skin and eyes. From the natural sources, the effects are more on the skin and from artificial sources, the effects are more on the eyes. This effects depend upon the duration of exposure, intensity of exposure and the individual susceptibility. Health hazards of UV rays have two types of effects on the skin, which includes:
- Short-term effects
- Long-term effects.

Short-term effects
Short-term effects are immediate effects, as follows:
1. Melanin pigment, which is normally present in malpighian layer, migrates upwards into the corneum causing darkening of the skin (suntan).
2. Histamine is released resulting in erythema, edema, blisters and even ulcers depending upon the quantity released.
3. Thickening of all layers of epidermis—a protective mechanism.
4. Synthesis of vitamin D takes place and rickets is prevented (the last two are useful to the body).

Long-term effects
Long-term effects are delayed effects, as follows:
- Degeneration of skin
- Decrease in elasticity
- Cancer of the skin (squamous cell carcinoma, rodent ulcer).

For all these effects, black individuals are less susceptible than white persons. The effects on the eyes includes the following:
1. From the natural source, the effects are:
   - Snow blindness: Common among those skating on the snow, because UV rays reflect from the snow causing keratitis
   - Burns: Inside the nose, common among skaters, because of the reflection from the snow
   - Eclipse blindness: Due to direct gazing at the sun, specially on the solar eclipse.
2. From the artificial sources, the effects are:
   - Conjunctivitis, keratitis and photophobia
   - Flash burns (welder's flash) from arc welding
   - Corneal ulcer (in later stages).

The effects can be prevented by:
- Education of workers about hazards and prevention
- Personal protection by clothing, goggles, visors, etc.
- Regulation of exposers.

CHAPTER 12: Radiation Exposure as a Determinant of Health

Visible Light

The natural source is sun and artificial sources are bulbs, candles, neon-tube lights, oil lamps, etc. The hazards of visible lights are:
- Poor lighting: Result in eye strain, visual fatigue, accidents, nystagmus (in the mines)
- Bright lighting: Direct light result in glaring, blurring of vision and accidents.

Direct light from the sun on the eyes result in scotoma (a blind spot), conjunctivitis, keratitis and photophobia.

Infrared Rays

The natural source is sun and artificial sources are fire, molten metal, red-hot objects, etc.

High-risk groups blast furnace workers, blacksmith, kiln and oven workers, stokers, etc.

The information of infrared rays are on the skin, it causes flushing, burns and even ulcers. On the eyes, it may cause cataract.

Microwaves

Microwaves are used in radar communication in ships and airplanes.

Prolonged exposure may result in cataract and microwave sickness characterized by headache, giddiness, loss of memory, fatigue, etc.

Radiofrequency Waves

Radiofrequency waves are used for wireless transmission. They are also employed in radios, television stations and from satellites. They are not absorbed and therefore they are harmless to the body.

Laser Radiations

Laser stands for light amplification by stimulated emission of radiation. It is an instrument, which generates extremely intense, monochromatic, coherent light, passing in unidirectional beam, carrying intense heat. Skin and eyes are susceptible. It causes thermal burns on the skin and corneal damage, opacification of the lens and burning of the retina, thus resulting in cataract and/or blindness.

Electromagnetic Radiations

In electromagnetic radiations, the energy is emitted in the form of very short frequency waves, each wave length measuring one fourth of a mm, carrying intense energy. These are not liberated in continuous waves, but in discrete units called quanta. For example, X-rays and gamma rays (γ).

The X-rays are artificially produced and emitted from intact atoms; they are of lower intensity, capable of penetrating about 25 cm into the tissues, used for diagnostic purposes.

The γ rays are naturally produced, emitted spontaneously during disintegration by the atom, which are more intense than X-rays and are capable of penetrating about 50 cm into the tissues, used for sterilization of plastic materials, intrauterine devices (IUDs), catgut, sutures, bandages, etc. However, electromagnetic radiations are thousand times weaker than corpuscular radiations.

Particulate Radiations

Particulate radiations are made up of subatomic particles or nucleotides. Depending upon whether they are positively charged or negatively charged or not charged at all, they are called α particles, β particles and neutrons respectively.

Alpha Particles

Alpha particles are made up of helium nuclei, consisting of two protons and two neutrons. They are positively charged. They are the most intense form of ionizing radiation. They do not have the penetrating capacity (hardly 0.05 mm) unlike that of electromagnetic radiations, but they are hazardous when inhaled, ingested or implanted subcutaneously. They are emitted spontaneously from unstable radioactive elements such as uranium, thorium, radium and plutonium. The α particles are nearly 10 times more harmful than X-rays.

Beta Particles

Beta particles are negatively charged, consisting of electrons. They have more penetrating capacity than alpha particles, i.e. 0.06–4 mm, but the intensity of ionization is 1/100th of α particles. They are also emitted spontaneously from the radioactive elements.

Neutrons

Neutrons are neutrally charged, i.e. uncharged. They do not act directly. They import energy to other atoms, which then become unstable and release β particles causing ionization.

The period after which the emitting power of an atom is reduced to half, is called 'half-life'. Longer the half-life of an atom, greater is its health hazard.

Some of the other ionizing radiations are photon rays, meson rays, proton-antiproton collisions, neutron-antineutron collisions, etc.

IONIZING RADIATION

The term ionizing radiation is applied to radiation, which has the ability to penetrate tissues and deposit its energy within them. Ionizing radiation may be divided into two main groups:
1. Electromagnetic radiations: X-rays and γ rays.
2. Corpuscular radiations: α particles, β particles (electrons) and protons. Some common types of environmental radiations are as given in Table 12.2.

These are capable of penetrating the body tissues, deposit the energy and cause destruction of the tissues. Such ionizing radiations are emitted from the atomic particles.

An atom is the smallest unit of an element, which cannot be split further. Such an atom has definite proportion of electrons and protons become dissimilar and is said to have become unstable. Such an unstable atom tries to attain stability. In such an attempt, it emits energy in the form of rays and particles, carrying intense energy, which have got ability to penetrate the body tissues, deposit the energy resulting in destruction of the tissues. This is called 'ionization' or 'ionizing radiation'.

Table 12.2: Environmental radiations

Types of radiation	Approximate penetrating ability		
	Air	Tissue	Lead
α particles	4 cm	0.05 mm	0
β particles	6–300 cm	0.06–4.0 mm	0.005–0.3 mm
γ rays	400 m	50 cm	40 mm
X-rays	120–240 m	15–30 cm (some components are very high)	0.3 mm

'At-risk' group are persons working in radiotherapy, radiology, nuclear medicine and soldiers exposed to nuclear explosions in the war.

Depending upon the type of the energy emitted from an unstable atom, whether it is in the form of waves or subatomic particles, the ionizing radiations are of two types:
- Electromagnetic radiations (or photon radiations)
- Corpuscular radiation (or particulate radiations).

Sources of Ionizing Radiation

The sources of ionizing radiation are of two types—natural and artificial.

Natural Sources

Natural sources are external and internal.

External sources: These include are sun, atmosphere and earth.

Sun: The radiations coming from the sun are called 'cosmic radiations' (cosmos = sun). They originate from the sun. They are positively charged protons. Their penetrating capacity is minimal. As they pass through the atmosphere, they are weakened. Their effect is 35 mrad per year.

Atmosphere: Sources are originate from the atmospheric gasses such as radon and thoron. They have an impact of 2 mrad per year. Their effect is minimal. Environmental pollution with these gasses occur through the processes such as processing of uranium and thorium ores, operation of nuclear reactors, testing of nuclear weapons, etc.

Earth: The earth is called 'terrestrial radiations'. They originate from the radioactive substances such as ores of radium, actinium, uranium and thorium present in the earth's crust (soil) or rocks and buildings. Their effect is 50 mrad per year. But in Kerala, it is about 2,000 mrad per year because of the monazite sand.

Internal sources: These sources originate from the radioactive elements stored in the body tissues, such as radioactive isotopes K^{40}, I^{131}, C^{14}, Sr^{90}, Cs^{137}, etc. These internal radiations inflict about 25 mrad per year. The last two Sr^{90} and Cs^{137} remain active for many years.

Artificial Sources

Artificial sources are man-made sources. These radiations are used for medical purposes such as X-rays, radioactive isotopes and also for non-medical purposes such as television and watch industries agriculture, atomic power generation, nuclear explosions (ware fare), etc. The radiations from the sources of non-medical purposes are too small.

Health Hazards of Ionizing Radiations

Health hazards are acute and chronic effects.

Acute Effects

Acute effects occur when the body is exposed to heavy (1 Gy) or very heavy (1–9 Gy) doses of radiation for short period of time. This is usually accidental. The condition is called 'acute' radiation syndrome,' which occurs in the following four stages:

1. **Prodromal stage:** Characterized by anorexia, nausea, vomiting, prostration, fatigue and sweating. Diarrhea and oliguria may occur in fulminating cases, lasts for 8–48 hours.
2. **Latent stage:** This is an asymptomatic stage, lasts for 1–2 weeks.
3. **Stage of overt illness:** Symptoms reappear characterized by fever, anemia, leukopenia, paralytic ileus, paresthesia, motor disturbances, ataxia, disorientation, autonomic collapse indicating involvement or injury to central nervous system (CNS), lasts for 3 weeks.
4. **Recovery stage:** Lasts for about 15 weeks.

Exposer to massive doses of more than 10 Gy may cause death, in a day or two from cerebral edema or cardiac failure.

Treatment

- Strong supportive care by prophylactic antibiotics
- Bone marrow transplantation
- Ion exchange carriers or chelating agents to be applied to facilitate the excretion of inhaled or ingested radioactive nucleotides.

Chronic Effects

Chronic effects are the delayed effects. Grouped into two groups—somatic and genetic.

Somatic effects: Earliest effect is on the eyes, resulting in cataract. Skin lesions appear late. They include erythema, edema, blisters and ulcers. Still later hyperkeratosis and atrophy of the sebaceous glands occur. Skin lesions are common with b particles and cataract with neutrons.

The other delayed somatic effects are cancer of the lung, skin, blood, aplastic anemia and tumor induction. These delayed somatic effects are seen among those exposed to less than 1 Gy over a long period of time. Fetal somatic effects are malformation and microcephaly.

Genetic effect: These occur when gonads are exposed and chromosomes are injured:

1. Chromosomal mutations result in still-births, congenital defects, neonatal deaths and even sterility.
2. Point mutations are due to injury to genes resulting in Down syndrome, Huntington's chorea, polycystic kidney and hemophilia.

Thus, somatic effects are seen within the life span of the affected individual, whereas genetic effects are seen in the next generation. Factors influencing radiation hazard are detailed as follows.

Type of tissue involved: Tissues such as gonads, lymph nodes, bone marrow and thyroid glands are highly susceptible.

Type of ionizing radiation: Electromagnetic radiations are less harmful compared to corpuscular radiations, but they are more frequently used than latter. Among the electromagnetic radiations, X-rays are more commonly used than γ rays.

Area of the body exposed: Larger the surface area of the body exposed, more will be the bone marrow depression and therefore severe will be the hazard.

Protective clothing: Reduces the effect.

Other factors: These are intensity of the radiation, duration of exposure and individual susceptibility are other influencing factors.

The α particles are 10 times as harmful as X-rays, β particles or rays; γ, α particles luckily have little penetrating force. On the other hand, they are quite dangerous, if radioactive substance has entered the body (by inhalation or through a wound). Gamma rays and X-rays have short wavelengths; they are deep penetrating radiations. X-rays are man-made, while γ rays are emitted spontaneously by radioactive elements during their disintegration. Otherwise, there is no material difference between γ rays and X-rays. Cosmic rays also contain ionizing radiations.

The term 'non-ionizing radiation' refers to several forms of electromagnetic radiation of wavelength longer than those of ionizing radiation. As wavelength elongates, the energy value of electromagnetic radiation decreases. So, all non-ionizing forms of radiation have less energy than cosmic; γ and X-radiation includes UV radiation, visible light, infrared radiation, microwave radiation and radiofrequency radiation.

RADIATION MEASUREMENTS

The activity of a radioactive material is the number of nuclear disintegration per unit of time. The unit of activity is a becquerel (Bq); 1 Bq is equal is to one disintegration per second. Formerly, the unit of activity was curie (Ci) and 1 Bq corresponds approximately to 27 Pci. The potency of radiation is measured in three ways:

1. **Roentgen:** It is the unit of exposure. It is the amount of radiation absorbed in air at a given point, i.e. number of ions produced in 1 mL of air.
2. **Rad:** It is the unit of absorbed dose. It is the amount of radioactive energy absorbed per gram of tissue or any material 1 mrad—0.001 rad.
3. **Rem:** It is the product of the absorbed dose and the modifying factors. The rem indicates the degree of potential danger to health.

The radiation to which the average citizen is exposed is made up almost of the fast moving, highly penetrating

X-rays and γ rays, where rem and rad are equal. The radiation units (viz. roentgen, rod, rem) are being replaced by new International System of units (SI units), which are:
1. Coulomb per kilogram (C/kg) replacing the roentgen; 1 roentgen is equal to 2.58×10^4 C kg^{-1}. It is the unit for exposure. There is no special name for this.
2. Gray (Gy) replacing the rad, it is the unit of absorbed dose defined as the two dose of ionizing radiation that impart 1 J of energy to 1 kg of absorbing material; 1 rad is equal to 0.01 Gy.
3. Sievert (SV) replacing the rem and it is the SI unit of dose equivalent. The dose equivalent to 1 SV is equal to 100 rem.

Dose Equivalent

As all types of radiations do not produce the same biological effect unit of energy absorbed, the concept of dose equivalent (H) has been introduced. The dose equivalent, M (Sievert) is equal to the absorbed dose D (rays), multiplied by a quality factor Q, which depends upon the density of ionization produced in the tissue by the radiation:
$$H = DQ$$
The factor Q for X-rays, any rays and electrons are equal to 1, whereas for particles, it is 20.

PROTECTIVE MEASURES AND RADIATION

As stated earlier, the amount of radiation received from outer space and background radiation has been estimated to be 0.1 rad a year. The additional permissible dose from man-made sources should not exceed 5 rad a year. The X-rays constitute the greatest hazards. In routine fluoroscopy, a dose of 4 rad is delivered to a part of the body for 1 minute. This implies that unnecessary X-ray examinations should be avoided, especially in the case of children and pregnant women. It also implies adequate control and surveillance of X-ray installations, protection of workers, improvement in techniques and improvements leading to dose reduction. Effective protection measure includes proper use of lead shields and lead rubber aprons. Lead aprons (0.5 mm of lead) will reduce the intensity of scattered X-rays over 90% and should be worn by all workers regularly associated with X-ray procedures. Workers must wear a film badge or dosimeter, which shows accumulated exposure to radiation since last time the instrument was changed. Besides, periodic medical examinations, regular working hours, recreation and holidays must be ensured to workers that maintain their state of health. Radiation protection is called radiation hygiene. The International Commission on Radiological Protection (ICRP), the International Atomic Energy Agency (IAEA) and the World Health Organization (WHO) have been active in maintaining radiation-hygiene. The ICRP recommended that the genetic dose to the whole population from all sources additional to the natural background radiation should not exceed 5 rem over a period of 30 years. The WHO has published permissible radiation levels in drinking water. The IAEA's main concern has been to promote peaceful uses of atomic energy and to assure that these uses do not imperil peace or health.

PREVENTION AND CONTROL OF RADIATION HAZARDS

Radiation hazards are easily prevented by primary and secondary prevention.

Primary Prevention

Primary prevention is by the following measures—safety of the machine, man environment and other measures.

Safety of the Machine

1. Machine should be of approved quality and installed properly.
2. Periodical servicing and proper maintenance.
3. Use of efficient filters so that unwanted radiations are excluded.
4. Operated on high kilo voltage (KV) with fast films and image intensifier, so that exposer is reduced to minimal dose.
5. The machine is connected to the door in such a way that it should stop functioning automatically, the moment the door is opened accidentally.

Safety of the Worker

1. Preplacement examination of the worker to exclude contraindications, if any, for fitting the job to the worker (ergonomics).
2. Health education about radiation hazards and avoiding unnecessary exposer.
3. Regulation of exposure, so that exposure is limited by provision of holidays and recreation, and also by rotation of the worker.
4. Personal protection by wearing:
   a. Filter respirators/masks.
   b. Spectacles with reflecting mirrors; visors while doing arc welding.
   c. Lead aprons, lead gloves, (lead reduces the intensity over 90%).
   d. Pocket dosimeter (this is a monitoring device, worn on the collar by the worker, same dosimeter

CHAPTER 12 — Radiation Exposure as a Determinant of Health

to be worn by the same individual, which records the cumulative dose of the radiation received by that individual). It is sent to atomic research center, where it is analyzed and report is given about the dose or radiation received more than the permissible limit of 5 rad per year, clinical examination and differential count is done.

- e. Use of lead boxes to keep radium needless and radioactive isotopes.
- f. Use of long forceps to handle radium needles.
- g. Use of shield between the source and the recipient.
- h. By avoiding eating or drinking in the working room.

Safety of the Environment

Air, soil and water should be clean and pure. They should be free from pollution.

Other Measures

Measures such as specification of the room of cobalt unit or X-ray machine and disposal of radioactive wastes:

1. Specification of the room of cobalt unit and X-ray machine include:
   a. Walls must be thick and made of concrete.
   b. Roof must be high.
   c. Wet mopping of floor to be done (good housekeeping).
   d. Vacuum cleaning of the room.
   e. Lead protected doors.
   f. Lead glasses to be used for windows.
   g. Exhaust system of ventilation.
   h. Controlling machine should be as far away as possible from the worker.
   i. Enclosure of the machine, ventilated hoods, splash-trays control the release of dust in the environment.
2. Disposal of radioactive wastes include:
   a. By putting in a steel case and embedding deep in the sea bed at 1,800 m deep.
   b. By putting it in an underground concrete seal.
   c. By burning in a special incinerator provided with filters and very tall stacks.

Secondary Prevention

1. Early diagnosis/detection: It is done by periodical analysis of dosimeter.
2. Treatment:
   a. For leukemia: By prednisolone, vincristine, daunorubicin and arabinosylcytosine.
   b. For bone marrow aplasia: By antibiotics and blood transfusion.
   c. For bone sarcoma: By amputation followed by chemotherapy.

If the individual is accidentally exposed and the radioactive material has entered the system, the person is immediately decontaminated as follows:

1. If implanted, the skin is excised, the radioactive material is removed, the area is washed with hot water and soap followed by application of citric acid.
2. If swallowed, the adsorbent such as Prussian blue or ion exchange agents are given followed by emetics and salt purgatives. Diethylene triamine pentaacetic acid (DTPA) is effective.

Control of Health Hazards of Radiation

Personal protection and general guidelines:

1. Protective clothing and other devices.
2. Workers for general medical examination including examination of skin, nail, blood, urine feces and sputum.
3. Special medical check-up in cases of overexposure.
4. Suspension of jobs or given job free from radiation hazard.
5. Protective clothing put on in laboratories should not be worn in non-active rooms.
6. Operators of X-rays should never stand in the beam of X-ray. Fluoroscopic examination should be conducted quickly and with minimum dose over 100 kV in rooms with protective walls.
7. Health education.
8. Unsealed radioactive isotopes should be used in special laboratory. Floor should be covered with linoleum, work place with non-absorbing covers.
9. Radioactive liquid wastes should not be disposed into river and sewers. Solid waste should be kept separate.
10. Responsibility of health physician, engineer, doctor and physicist.
11. Workers under continuous observation with the help of film badge or pocket dosimeter.
12. Maximum permissible dose should not be exceeded.

Climate as a Determinant of Health

CHAPTER 13

INTRODUCTION

Climate change is a complex phenomenon of many factors such as heat, cold, air movement, rainfall, moisture, dryness, sky, altitude and solar radiation, electricity, ionization, and cosmic factors, and on the geological and radioactive conditions of soil. This is influenced by various factors such as sea, hill, desert, vegetation and forest, etc. All the above factors affect the health of people, but the principal factors of climate, which affects the health, are:
- Amount of sunlight (sunshine)
- Variations of external temperature
- Humidity
- Atmospheric pressure
- Air movement
- Altitude.

Sunlight is good for health and well-being. It has infrared rays and ultraviolet rays. They are not only important for good health but also for curative effects. It prevents rickets. The vitamin D produced by the exposure to sunlight in the skin of human beings and animal passes into the milk of the mother. The elements, which comprise the meteorological environment, are:
- Atmospheric pressure
- Air temperature
- Humidity
- Rainfall
- Direction and speed of wind
- Movement of clouds and character of weather.

The term 'climate' is a geographical concept representing a summation of the whole range of meteorological phenomena.

ATMOSPHERIC PRESSURE

The atmosphere (envelope of the air) is about 200 miles thick (320 km). The air of the lower level is much denser and heavier than the upper layer.

The atmospheric pressure at sea level is 790 mm Hg. This is called 'one atmosphere of pressure'. The atmospheric pressure falls as the altitude increases as in high mountains and rises as altitude decreases as in deep mines. Thus, at an altitude of 100,000 feet above the sea level, the atmospheric pressure is less than 10 mm Hg and for every 33 feet below the sea level, the atmospheric pressure increases as the rate of '1 atmosphere', i.e. when a person descends 33 feet (as in mines), he/she is exposed to an atmospheric pressure of 2 atmospheres, i.e. 760 × 2 = 1,520 mm Hg.

The instruments used for measuring atmospheric pressure are known as barometers. There are three well-known kinds of barometer such as Fortin's barometer, aneroid barometer and barograph. The 'Kew pattern' station barometer is widely used.

Aneroid Barometer

The aneroid barometer is a barometer, which is derived from the name 'aneroid' means 'devoid of fluid'. It does not contain mercury or any other fluid. It consists of a cylindrical metal box with partial vacuum. It has an elastic metal top, which is sensitive to changes in the atmospheric pressure (Fig. 13.1). The pressure changes are transmitted from the metal top to a pointer through a series of springs. The pointer moves on a dial and indicates atmospheric pressure. It is not pressure instrument. Since it is a handy apparatus, it is used while climbing the mountains or in aeroplanes.

Barograph

Barograph is a modified aneroid barometer in which the pointer records the pressure changes on a graph continuously.

CHAPTER 13   Climate as a Determinant of Health

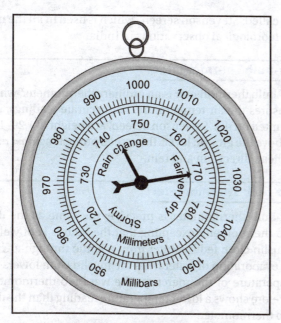

Figure 13.1: Aneroid barometer

Influence of Atmospheric Pressure on Health

The influence of atmospheric pressure on health is considered under two headings:
1. Effects of diminished atmospheric pressure.
2. Effects of increased atmospheric pressure.

Effects of Diminished Atmospheric Pressure

The effects occur in high altitudes, because air becomes rarefied (less dense), temperature of air also becomes less and the partial pressure of oxygen also becomes less. Man cannot survive at an altitude of 25,000 feet without breathing equipment. However, human body has a remarkable power of adjusting itself to low oxygen pressure provided the change is made slowly and persons can live for long period at heights of 15,000–20,000 feet without ill effects. This adjustment of the body is called 'acclimatization'. The physiological changes are:
- Increase in rate and depth of respiration (to minimize the difference between the oxygen of the air and oxygen of the blood)
- Increase in the hemoglobin content of the blood
- Increase in the cardiac output.

But sudden exposure to high altitude above 10,000 feet results in 'acute mountain sickness' (or aviator sickness) due to rarity of atmosphere and deficiency in oxygen. This is characterized by headache, mental fatigue, irritability, irrational behavior, loss of muscular coordination, insomnia, nausea, vomiting, breathlessness, and in severe cases, there may be bleeding from the nose, ringing in the ears, palpitation and even collapse. Excessive secretion of lymph results in hemoconcentration. Later, there will be chronic anoxemia due to low oxygen tension in the blood.

Later as the pulmonary edema develops, the respiration becomes deep and irregular (Cheyne-Stokes breathing). The person also develops oliguria, mental confusion, hallucinations, later develops stupor, convulsions, coma and death supervenes. The only treatment is to carry that person to lower altitude as soon as possible.

Effects of Increased Atmospheric Pressure

The effects occur in low altitudes, as in mines and under the water in sea. The increased pressure of air produces effects of opposite nature. The effects are best observed in persons working in diving bells, compressed air chambers (Caisson's), etc. and the symptoms produced in known as 'Caisson's disease', wherein the person exposed to high pressure, the gases in the air such as oxygen, carbon dioxide and nitrogen are dissolved in the blood and tissues, depending upon their partial pressures and the whole body is thus saturated with air. Nitrogen exerts narcotic action leading to loss of mental function and consciousness. The excess of CO_2 enhances the narcotic action of nitrogen. Excess of oxygen leads to convulsions and death.

When the person comes up to the surface (i.e. during decompression), the process is reversed. The absorbed gases are released from blood and tissues. Oxygen is retained and the nitrogen is liberated causing bubbles in the tissues, and gas emboli in blood vessels (air embolism) resulting in fatality.

As a rule, the workers do not suffer when they are in the caisson, but grave symptoms occur after they return to the outside air. It is called 'decompression sickness', characterized by euphoria, sensation of increased strength, respiration becomes deeper and quicker, and the heart becomes stronger and slower. These may be followed by nasal voice, disturbance in hearing, changed sense of smell or taste and rarely hemorrhages from the mouth, tympanic cavity, and even from the lungs. There may be perspiration with a feeling of fatigue and weakness.

Sudden decompression results in severe pain in the muscles and joints of the extremities, called 'bends' or 'screws'. This is often referred to as 'compressed air sickness'. There may be vertigo, chokes, unconsciousness or collapse. Pulmonary air embolism may result in sudden death, due to cardiac tamponade.

The effects of atmospheric pressure on health are as detailed below.

Acute mountain sickness: This is a relatively common, harmless and transient condition characterized by headache, insomnia, breathlessness, nausea, vomiting and impaired vision.

High altitude pulmonary edema: The symptoms generally appear on about the 3rd day at high altitude and are indistinguishable from those of ordinary mountain sickness. But as pulmonary edema develops, the patient develops a cough and may experience irregular or Cheyne-Stokes breathing, oliguria, mental confusion, and hallucinations, stupor, seizures and coma. The condition is rare below 12,000 ft (3,600 m). The patient should be carried to lower altitudes as soon as possible.

Low altitudes: The atmospheric pressure increases by one atmosphere for every 33 ft depth below sea level. The greatest depths so far reached are the equivalent of 10 atmospheres. When man is exposed to high pressure, the gases in the air namely oxygen, carbon dioxide (CO_2) and nitrogen are dissolved in the blood, and tissues proportionately to the partial pressure of these gases. Excess concentration of nitrogen exerts a narcotic action leading to loss of mental functions and consciousness; excess of CO_2 increases the narcotic action of nitrogen; excess of oxygen can lead to convulsions and death. When the person comes up to the surface, the gases, which are dissolved in the blood under pressure are released and cause air embolism, the effects of which are fatal.

AIR, TEMPERATURE AND ITS TOOL FOR MEASUREMENT

The temperature of air varies in different parts of the day and also in different seasons. The factors, which influence the temperature, are latitude of the place, altitude, direction of wind, and proximity of sea. The temperature of the ground surface is always higher than that of the air.

Thermometers are the instruments used for measuring temperature. Mercury thermometers are widely used, as mercury boils at a high temperature, has a regular expansion and its level can be easily been. Alcohol thermometers are also used. Alcohol has the advantage of not solidifying even at the lowest known temperature. The essential conditions for the use of the thermometers are:
1. The air should have free access to the bulbs of thermometers.
2. The thermometer should be protected against radiant heat. These conditions are fulfilled by mounting the thermometers on a special approved screen called 'Stevenson screen', which is used in all the meteorological observations in India.

Dry-bulb Thermometer

Dry-bulb thermometer is an ordinary thermometer, which measures the air temperature. For accurate readings, it is mounted on the 'Stevenson Screen', at a height of 1.20–1.80 m above the ground level. The screen protects against radiant heat, direct sun and rain.

Wet-bulb Thermometer

Wet-bulb thermometer is precisely the same as the dry-bulb thermometer excepting that the bulb is kept wet by a muslin cloth fed by water from a bottle through a wick. The evaporation of water from the muslin cloth lowers the temperature of the mercury. The wet-bulb thermometer therefore shows a lower temperature reading than the dry-bulb thermometer.

Maximum Thermometer

Maximum thermometer is a mercury thermometer so designed that there is a very fine constriction near the neck of the bulb. When the temperature rises, mercury expands, when the temperature falls, mercury cannot get back the bulb. The end of the mercury thread at the distal end gives the maximum temperature reached. The thermometer is set each time by swinging briskly, when the mercury retreats into the bulb.

Minimum Thermometer

Minimum thermometer is an alcohol thermometer. The liquid inside the minimum thermometer is spirit in which a dumb-bell shaped index is immersed. When the temperature of air falls, the spirit drags the index toward the bulb end; when the temperature rises, the spirit expands and runs past the index, not displacing the index, thus recording the lowest temperature.

Globe Thermometer

The globe thermometer is used for the direct measurement of the mean radiant temperature of the surroundings. The instrument consists of hollow copper bulb 6 inches (15 cm) in diameter and is coated on the outside with matte black paint, which absorbs the radiant heat from the surrounding objects. A specially calibrated mercury thermometer is inserted, with its bulb at the center of globe. The globe thermometer registers a higher temperature than the ordinary air temperature thermometer, because it is affected both by the air temperature and radiant heat. The globe thermometer is also influenced by the velocity of air movement. The standard globe instrument reaches equilibrium with its environment in 15–20 minutes.

Wet-globe Thermometer

Wet-globe thermometer is designed for environmental heat measurement. It consists of a dial thermometer with the heat-sensing portion enclosed by a blackened copper sphere that is completely covered with wet black cloth. The wet-globe exchanges heat with the surroundings by conduction, convection, evaporation and radiation similar to the way a perspiring man does, so the equilibrium temperature of the globe provides a comprehensive measure of the cooling capacity of the work environment (Figs 13.2A and B).

Silvered Thermometer

The bright metallic surface reflects as much of the incident radiant heat as is given, a more accurate reading of the air temperature.

Kata Thermometer

The kata thermometer is quite sensitive to slight air movements. It can record air velocities as low as 10 ft/min. Kata means 'down'. The kata thermometer is an alcohol thermometer with a glass bulb 4 cm long and 1.8 cm in diameter (refer Figs 13.2A and B).

The readings on the stem are marked from 100 to 95°F. Two instruments are used, the bulb of one is covered with a wet muslin cloth, the wet kata and the other dry kata. Before taking the readings, the bulbs are immersed in hot water, then warm them slightly above 130°F, when the alcohol rises into a small reservoir at the top of the instrument. The bulb of the dry kata is wiped dry. Then both the instruments are suspended in air at the point of observation. The temperature in seconds required for the spirit to fall from 100 to 95°F is noted with a stop watch. This is repeated at least four times. The first reading is discarded and the average of the last three is taken. The length of time depends upon the 'cooling power' or the air. Each kata has a 'factor' called kata factor marked on the stem. This factor is determined for each instrument by the manufactures. This factor, divided by the average cooling time gives the rate of cooling in millicalories per square centimeter per second. The kata thermometer was originally devised for measuring the 'cooling power'

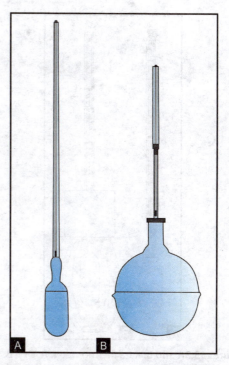

Figures 13.2A and B: Thermometer. **A.** Kata thermometer; **B.** Globe thermometer.

of the air. A dry kata reading of 6 and above, and a wet kata reading of 20 and above were regarded as indices of thermal comfort. The kata thermometer is now largely used as an anemometer for recording low air velocities rather than the cooling power of the air (Figs 13.3A and B).

Six's Maximum and Minimum Thermometer

A combination of maximum and minimum thermometers and gives a double reading. It is an 'U-shaped' glass tube with a bulb at each end, containing mercury in the middle portion. Both the tubes are above the mercury and one bulb contain alcohol, and the part of the other bulb contains alcohol vapor and air. In each stem, there is an iron index, which may be moved by a magnet. With the rise of air temperature, the alcohol expands and pushes the mercury along with the index recording the maximum temperature of the place in 24-hour cycle. With the fall of temperature, the alcohol contracts and the mercury falls, pushing the index in the other column recording the minimum temperature of the place in a 24-hour cycle. Thus, highest and lowest temperatures can be recorded by the indices in the right and left limb respectively. Both the indices are set again before the thermometer is placed for the next day's recordings (Fig. 13.4).

Since, it is not an accurate measurement, this instrument is not used in the Indian meteorological department.

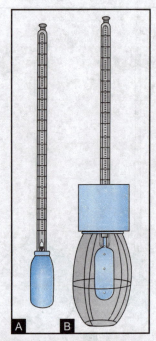

Figures 13.3A and B: Kata thermometer. A. Dry; B. Wet.

Vacuum or Solar Radiation Thermometer

A mercurial thermometer having the bulb coated with black color to absorb the sun's rays. The bulb is placed in a vacuum glass case in order to prevent the black paint from being washed off by the rain. The glass case also protects the bulb from loss of heat, which would otherwise take place. The instrument is placed horizontally 4 ft above the ground level and exposed to the direct rays of the sun (Fig. 13.5).

The difference between the maximum reading in the sun and minimum in the shade is the amount of solar radiation.

Terrestrial Thermometer

A minimum shade thermometer, placed 4 inch above the ground on the grass or on a black board, if grass plot is not existing and temperature in recorded. Similarly, it is recorded in the shade.

Effects of High Temperature

Heat stress, result of higher temperature is the burden of heat that must be dissipated, if the body is to remain in thermal equilibrium. The factors, which influence heat stress are metabolic rate, air temperature humidity, air movement and radiant temperature. The amount of heat gained by the body must be equaled by the amount of heat lost from it.

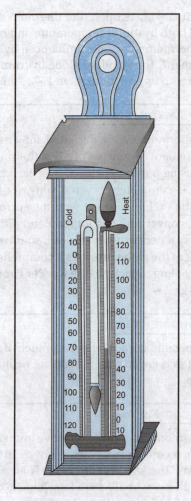

Figure 13.4: Six's thermometer

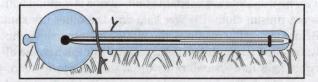

Figure 13.5: Vacuum or solar radiation thermometer

Many heat stress indices have been devised, but none is adequate to be valid in all possible complexities of work rate, air temperature, air movement, etc. These include equatorial comfort index, heat stress index and predicted 4 hours sweat rate (P4-SR). The important ones are detailed below.

Heat Stroke

Heat stroke is attributed to failure of the heat-regulating mechanism. It is characterized by very high body temperature, which may rise to 110°F (43.3°C) and profound disturbances including delirium, convulsions, and partial and complete loss of consciousness. The skin is dry and hot. Classically, sweating is absent or diminished, but many victims clear-cut heat stroke perspire profusely. The outcome is often fatal, even when patients are brought quickly to medical attention; death/case ratios of 40% or more have been reported. The treatment consists of rapidly cooling the body in ice water bath till the rectal temperature falls below 102°F (38.9°C). The rectal temperature should be monitored continuously, both to monitor the efficacy of hypothermia treatment and to guard against the development of clinically significant hypothermia, which can occur if cooling is continued too long. Further treatment is supportive and directed toward the many potential complications of hyperthermia. Hypovolemia, hyperkalemia, rhabdomyolysis, hypocalcemia and bleeding diathesis may require intensive supportive treatment. The patient should be kept in bed for several days until the temperature control becomes stable.

Heat Hyperpyrexia

Heat hyperpyrexia is attributed to impair functioning of the heat-regulating mechanism, but without characteristic features of heat stroke. It is arbitrarily defined as a temperature above 106°F. It may proceed to heat stroke.

Heat Exhaustion

Unlike heat stroke, heat exhaustion is not because of failure of thermoregulation. It is milder illness than heat stroke and is caused primarily by the imbalance or inadequate replacement of water and salts lost in perspiration due to thermal stress. Heat exhaustion typically occurs after several days of high temperature. Body temperature may be normal or moderately elevated, but it is uncommon to exceed 102°F (38.90°C). The symptoms, primarily dizziness, weakness and failure, are those of circulatory distress. It may be severe enough to require hospitalization, especially in elderly patients. Treatment is directed toward normalizing fluid and electrolyte balance.

Heat Cramps

Cramps occur in persons who are doing heavy muscular work in high temperature and humidity. There are painful and spasmodic contractions of the skeletal muscles. The cause of heat cramps is loss of sodium and chlorides in the blood.

Heat Syncope

Heat syncope is a common ill effect of heat. In its milder form, the person standing in the sun becomes pale, his/her blood pressure falls and collapses suddenly. There is practically no rise in body temperature. The condition results from pooling of blood in lower limbs due to dilation of blood vessels, with the result that the amount of blood returning to the heart is reduced, which in turn is responsible for lowering of blood pressure and lack of blood supply to the brain. This condition is common among soldiers when they are standing for parades in the sun. Treatment is quite simple. The patient should be made to lie in the shade with head slightly down; recovery usually comes within 5–10 minutes.

Prevention of Ill Effects of High Temperature

The ill effects of high temperature may be prevented by observing the following precautions.

Replacement of water: Persons working under conditions of high temperature have to drink cool water. It has been found in India that a man doing hard work in the sun requires about 1 L of water per hour. For a sedentary worker, the requirement is nearly half of this quantity. There is a widespread belief that extra salt intake during the summer helps prevent the ill effects of heat. The normal intake of salt in the Indian diet is far more than is actually needed. Further, salt losses through sweat in small amount since the concentration of salt in sweat are considerably low. Therefore, there is no need to add salt to water.

Regulation of work: The duration of exposure to a hot environment should be cut down. There should be periods of rest in between intense work. If signs, such as headache and dizziness appear, the person should be moved to a cooler environment, and the necessary treatment is given.

Clothing: The clothing worn should be light, loose and of light colors.

Protective devices: Protective goggles, shields and helmets are helpful.

Work environment: The temperature and humidity in the work environment may be controlled by proper ventilation and air conditioning.

Effects of Low Temperature

Injury due to cold may be general or local. In general cold injury (hypothermia), the individual is said to be suffering from exposure to cold. This is characterized by numbness, loss of sensation, muscular weakness, desire for sleep, coma and death. Local cold injury may occur at temperature above freezing (wet-cold conditions) as in immersion or trench foot. At temperatures below freezing (dry-cold condition), frostbite occurs; the tissue freeze and ice crystals form in between the cells. Frostbite is common in high altitudes. It is extremely important to dress up according to temperature with which the part of body will be in contact. The affected part should be warmed using water at 44°C. Warming should last about 20 minutes at a time. Intake of hot fluids promotes general rewarming.

HUMIDITY

Humidity or moisture is always present in the atmosphere. The amount of moisture, which air can hold, depends upon its temperature. If the air is cooled, the excessive moisture precipitates for the particular temperature. This is called 'dew point'. Humidity may be expressed as absolute humidity or relative humidity.

Absolute Humidity

Absolute humidity is the weight of water vapor in a unit volume of air. It is expressed as gram per kilogram or gram per cubic meter of air.

Relative Humidity

Relative humidity (RH) is the percentage of moisture present in the air, complete saturation being taken as 100. The greater the relative humidity, the nearer the air to saturation. Relative humidity expresses the moisture content of air. There is no evidence that humidity has an effect on physical health, although it definitely has an effect on comfort. If the RH exceeds 65%, the air inside the room feels sticky and uncomfortable. Better ventilation serves to lower such humidity. The RH below 30% is also unpleasant. Permanent exposure to such low humidities can cause drying of nasal mucosa, which may predispose to infection (e.g. sore throat, cough). There are several instruments, which may be used for measuring humidity. The ones commonly used are described below.

Dry- and Wet-bulb Hygrometer

Dry- and wet-bulb hygrometer is the most widely used instrument for measuring humidity. The instrument consists of two similar thermometers—a dry-bulb thermometer and a wet-bulb thermometer, which are mounted side by side on a stand. The dry bulb measures the air temperature (DBT). The bulb of the second one is covered with a gauze or wick and is kept moist. The wet-bulb temperature (WBT) is usually lower than the DBT. If both the readings are same, it indicates that the atmosphere is 100% saturated with moisture, which never occurs in reality. After obtaining the readings of the dry-and wet-bulb thermometers, the corresponding RH can be found from specially constructed psychrometric charts or slide rule. Humidity values are high in early morning and near the minimum value in the afternoon at about 15:00 hours. For accurate readings of the wet-bulb thermometer, the air should pass over the bulb with a speed of about 800 ft/min; the sling psychrometer (described below) achieves this when rotated rapidly (Fig. 13.6).

Sling psychrometer

The sling or whirling psychrometer consists of two mercury thermometers (wet and dry) mounted side by side, on a suitable wooden frame and provided with a handle for rotating the instrument. The underlying principle is that by rotating, the bulbs are exposed to air at a definite velocity. The wet bulb is first moistened with distilled water and the instrument is whirled or rotated standing with the back to the sun, for about 15 seconds at the rate of four revolutions per second, so as to obtain the desirable air speed of about 5 m/s. The reading of the wet bulb is then noted. The instrument is again whirled for about 10 seconds and the wet bulb reading is noted. This is repeated several times till two successive readings of the wet bulb are identical. The reading of the dry bulb is then noted.

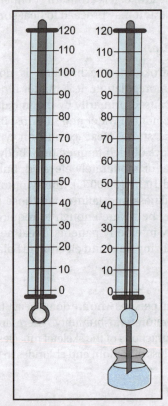

Figure 13.6: Dry- and wet-bulb thermometers

By use of suitable tables or charts, the relative humidity of the air may be obtained from the readings of the psychrometer (Fig. 13.7).

Assmann psychrometer

Assmann psychrometer is a portable, specially designed to give accurate measurement of the wet- and dry-bulb temperature of the air. In this instrument, air is drawn at a speed higher than 5 m/s by a clock-work fan. The bulbs of the thermometer are protected from the effects of solar radiation, so that the instrument can be used even in strong sunshine.

RAIN

The term precipitation is the collective term used for rain, snow, hail, dew and frost, i.e. all forms of water precipitated from the atmosphere. It is measured by rain gauges. The rain gauge prescribed by the Government of India for use at rainfall measuring stations in India is known as the 'Symon's rain gauge'. The funnel for receiving the rainfall has a diameter of 5 inch.

Great care is exercised in selecting a suitable site for the erection of rain gauge. The rain gauge should be set on a level ground, away from trees, buildings or other obstructions. The rule, which must be strictly adhered to in the erection of a rain gauge is that its rim should be exactly horizontal and 1 foot above the ground level, the instrument have been fixed in a masonry or concrete foundation. The rainfall is measured in millimeters per a time unit (mm/day; mm/month).

WIND

Wind plays an important role in the climate. The air velocity is measured by an instrument called anemometer.

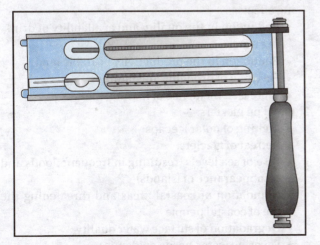

Figure 13.7: Sling psychrometer

It consists of four hemispherical cups, attached to the ends of two crossed metal arms. There is vertical spindle, which is attached to the 'anemometer box.' The velocity of the wind is indicated on a counter called cyclometer, placed in the anemometer box.

Wind velocities are normally recorded in open flat at a height of 10 m. Velocities are measured in meters per second (m/s). When the wind speed is 0.5 m/s, it is described as complete calm with smoke rising vertically; when it is 3.3 m/s, it is described as slight breeze with leaves rustling; when it is 10 m/s, it is described as strong wind with larger branches of trees moving; when it is 15–20 m/s, it is called storm; when it is 25–30 m/s, it is called gale and over 30–35 m/s, it is called hurricane.

Wind Direction

The wind direction is observed by an instrument called 'wind vane'. There is an arrow, which turns freely about a vertical axis. The wind vane is erected at a height of 10 meter above the ground level. If the arrow is motionless for 3 minutes, the wind is described as 'calm'. The wind direction may also be noted by letting off bits of paper in the air, which gives the approximate direction. Directions are grouped into 4 main categories, i.e. [north (N), east (E), south (S) and west (W)] and 8-16 subcategories.

CLOUDS AND WEATHER

In all meteorological stations, clouds are observed for their form, amount, direction and height. Such observations give an insight into the sequence of weather in the particular locality. From the state of the sky and evolution of clouds, weather is described as fine weather, fair weather, unsettled weather, bad weather and thunderous sky. Meteorological satellites are now being used for automatic picture taking to give an idea of the clouds. The satellites can also measure temperature and humidity in the atmosphere.

CLIMATE CHANGE AND ITS IMPACT ON HEALTH

The climate change has been a constant and menacing problem and it is on the increase due to increased population growth.

During 2007, we consumed more than 30 billion barrels of oil per day. In addition, we used 3 billion tons of coal. Burning of these fuels has resulted in causing air pollution by increasing the concentrations of carbon dioxide, nitrous oxide, methane, chlorofluorocarbons and depletion of ozone layer in the earth's atmosphere.

Normally, these gases (CO_2, CH_4, N_2O chlorofluorocarbons, etc.) trap sufficient heat, coming from the Sun, to sustain life on earth. These prevent the heat from being radiated out. Thus, they act as the glass of a greenhouse. Therefore, they are called 'greenhouse gases' (GHGs). Without greenhouse effect, life would not have been existed on earth. The earth's over all surface temperature is about 15°C and it is being maintained by the carbon cycle and the ecological system (i.e. excess temperature is cooled by ice caps). Accumulation of these GHGs in the atmosphere result in trapping more heat and rise of the surface temperature of the earth. This effect is called 'global warming', by which our life/health is put into danger.

GLOBAL WARMING

From the last 8,000 years, earth's surface temperature is raised by 1°C only. As on today, it is 15°C. From the last 100 years, the surface temperature has raised by ½°C and at this rate of global warming, it is estimated that within another 50 years (by 2050), the temperature would rise by 2.5°C and by the end of this century, by another 2.5°C. A rise in temperature of 2°C could trigger irreversible and catastrophic state of global warming. The earth, which was similar to an icebox has started burning. All because of human activities only.

Developed countries are the worst polluters (US, Russia and Japan in that order). About 55% carbon emission is produced by 15% of the population. This is likely to double in another 150 years. This leads to an effect called, 'runaway greenhouse' effect. This is found in the planet Venus, where the surface temperature is 860°F (480°C) and CO_2 concentration is 97%, nitrogen is hardly 3% and clouds are of sulfuric acid, making the planet hottest, next to sun in the solar family.

Thus, the effects of climate change originate mainly from the industrialized countries, but the health risks are concentrated in the poorest developing nations that have contributed least to the problem, including India. The health impacts will be disproportionately greater in the vulnerable groups of population in the developing and under developed countries. The population that are hit hardest are the very young, the malnourished, the elderly, medically infirm and socially disadvantaged group. The countries with high levels of poverty, malnutritions, weak health infrastructures and poor political unrest will be least able to cope up.

Without effective action to mitigate and adopt to climate change, the burden of climate sensitive diseases such as malnutrition, diarrheal disease, malaria and dengue fever will be greater and that will be more difficult and costly to control.

Thus, keeping in view the overwhelming evidence that climate change presents growing threat to public health/global health, WHO's selection of the theme for World Health Day 2008, 'Protecting Health from Climate Change', is both timely and relevant.

There is sound evidence that global warming is now unequivocal. The effects on global climate system could be abrupt or irreversible, sparing no country, causing more frequent and more intense heat waves, rain storms, tropical cyclones and tidal surges in sea level this very century. Food and water shortage will put the health security of millions of people at stake. These will threaten human health security and cost lives.

Hazards of global warming are:
- Acid rain
- Shift in hydrological cycle
- Effect on glaciers
- Air pollution
- Disturbances of ecological system
- Ozone depletion.

1. **Acid rain:** The SO_2 and NO_2 coming from the industries combine with oxygen and moisture of the air and form dilute mixture of sulfuric acid, nitric acid (and carbonic acid) in the clouds. When the acid rain falls on earth, it results in the following effects:
   - Destruction of food crops
   - Deforestation (dense forests become scrub jungles)
   - Desertification
   - Erosion of soil
   - Acidification of water bodies
   - Destruction of aquatic life.
2. **Shift in hydrological cycle:** This results in the following effects:
   - Reduction in the quality and availability of drinking water
   - Reduction in the productivity of arable land
   - Favoring of droughts and famines
   - Increased incidence of malnutrition.
3. **Effect on glaciers:**
   - Melting of polar icecaps
   - Retreat of glaciers
   - Rise of sea levels (resulting in frequent floods and disappearance of islands)
   - Inundation of coastal areas and threatening the life of coastal people
   - Degradation of surface water quality
   - Favoring water-borne epidemics.

4. Hazards of air pollution:
   - Respiratory diseases (allergic, infectious and carcinogenic)
   - Decreased vital capacity of lungs
   - Animals (cattle) become weak (animal yield becomes less)
   - Destruction of historical monuments
   - Heat waves, heat stress
   - Smog formation in valleys
5. Effects of ecological disturbance:
   - Increased frequency of natural disasters (e.g. rainstorms, hurricanes, floods, cyclones, etc.)
   - Alteration of vector ecology favoring their propagation and transmission of vector-borne diseases [e.g. malaria, filariasis, dengue fever, Japanese encephalitis (JE), etc.]
   - Destruction of coral reefs (the great barrier reef of Australia, which took lakhs of years for its construction will be lost in another 50–100 years affecting the life of more than 1,500 species of aquatic life, which depend on these coral reefs).
   - Economic loss.
6. **Ozone depletion:** Normally ozone layer acts as a barrier to the harmful effects of UV rays. Depletion of zone allows harmful rays from the sun resulting in increased incidence of skin cancer and cataracts.

Global health is thus affected mainly by global warming supplemented by natural disasters, terrorism, increased population growth, displacement and migration of people. It is difficult to reverse over human time scales. This has jeopardized the hopes of achieving Millennium Development Goals. The possible health impacts are shown in Figure 13.8.

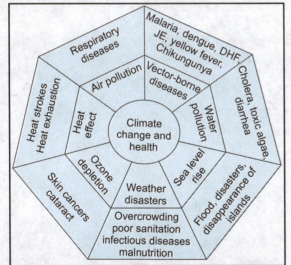

Figure 13.8: Possible health impacts due to climate change (DHF, dengue hemorrhagic fever; JE, Japanese encephalitis)

It is a challenge to achieve the goal of net zero carbon emission. It is a challenge for each one of us. The challenge is daunting, perplexing, intense and wide. It calls for a preventive, public health approach. It is a shared international responsibility. There is a need to strengthen the existing public health system rather than inventing the new system. People must tackle the issue on all fronts and they have to 'Thing Globally, Act Locally' (World Health Day Theme, 1990). 'One Planet One Family', we have to save our beautiful planet Earth by adopting following containment measures.

CONTAINMENT MEASURES

- Encourage greeneries, they act as most effect carbon sinks
- Opt for electric cars, which are emission free and eco friendly; saves fuel
- Tap the sun and use solar power plants
- Encourage community biogas plants, which prevent the use of firewood
- Beat the wind by wind mill to obtain power supply
- Improve water harvesting system
- Save the wet lands to recharge ground water, they help to preserve flora and fauna
- Use solar lantern for rural home lighting
- Mitigate disasters
- Ban the plastic bags, which are not eco friendly; not only carbon emissions occur while they are manufactured but also noxious fumes are released while they are burnt or disposed off
- Avoid leisurely car drives and walk as much as possible
- Save the rivers from sewage and industrial waste
- Save Himalayas
- Avoid using papers and use E-mail so that trees can be saved
- Use bicycle, which is a zero pollution vehicle (being a good exercise prevents obesity and improves health).

Today, global health is being affected very prime cause is human activities only such as urbanization, deforestation, vehicular of fossil fuel (coal and petroleum product ground), nuclear explosions, use of chemical supplemented by natural disasters. All these climate change, which in turn has affected to mental determinants of health—air, food and water.

Emission of greenhouse gases into the atmosphere have been increasing ever since the beginning of the industrial revolution. A major component of emission of CO_2 is from the combustion of fossil fuels. It is generally conceded that the main effects of this include an increase of about 3°C in the average global surface temperature by the year 2030, a rise in the sea level by 0.1–0.3 m by 2050 and an increase in the occurrence of extreme climatic events such as cyclones, heat waves and draughts. The temperature rise overwhelms the capacity of man species to adapt. A change of the magnitude would affect global ecosystems, sea levels and ocean currents, prevailing winds, fresh water supplies, agriculture, forests, fisheries, industry, transport, urban planning, demographics and human health. Some effects are mutually reinforcing, so a small additional change in the existing trend could have massive consequences, in accordance with the mathematics of catastrophe theory.

Changes in the configuration of jet stream, prevailing winds and ocean currents could alter the distribution of rainfall in many regions, making some wetter, other drier. The summers are becoming hotter. Temperature zone warming induces a decline in soil moisture that impairs grain production. This will also change the distribution of vegetation. The distribution of insect vectors of disease will change. The 'heat island' phenomenon that makes cities warmer than surrounding; rural areas will lead to longer and more severe heat waves, than we are accustomed to now.

CONCLUSION

Meteorology is the study of the process and phenomena of the atmosphere, especially as a means of weather forecasting or the climate and weather of a region. Climate change is a complex of many factors such as heat, cold, etc. The components of meteorological environment include atmosphere pressure, air temperature, humidity, air movement (air velocity, the direction and speed of the wind) and rainfall. The net effects of all these elements on the health and well-being of human life, animal life and vegetable life for the period of month or year is called climate and with reference to a particular stated period or time is called weather.

Housing as a Determinant of Health

CHAPTER 14

INTRODUCTION

Residential environment (housing) is a part of total environment affecting the health of an individual and the community to great extent. Housing is defined as a physical structure, which provides safety, security and shelter to the members living in and the environment including services and facilities necessary for maintaining optimum health by those members. It is the place where the members spend most of their lifetime and are reared, thus determining the culture (social and civil life) of the family, good house protection from bad weather and accidents. Houses help us to meet physiological and psychological need by providing the following.

PHYSICAL NEEDS OF HOUSE

1. House should have living room according to number of people, drawing room, guest room, sickroom, and study room for children and place for recreation with sunlight and cross ventilation.
2. It should be free from objectionable odor and air movement with a noise level below 50–70 dB.
3. It should have adequate light with tap water supply or tube well.
4. It should have good drainage for water and rooms should be damp proof.
5. It should have proper place for collection of refuse and its disposal.
6. It should have bathroom and sanitary latrine within the reach of the people in the house.
7. It should have pucca floor.
8. It must be protected from rain, sun, wild animals, rodents and snakes.

Aesthetic satisfaction in the house, good location and open space to some extent meets psychological need. 'Housing' in the modern concept includes not only the 'physical structure' providing shelter, but also the immediate surroundings and the related community services and facilities. It has become part of the concept of 'human settlement', which is defined as "all places in which a group of people reside and pursue their life goals; the size of the settlement may vary from a single family to millions of people."

The World Health Organization (WHO) expert group (1961) on public health aspects of housing prefers to use the term 'residential environment', which is defined as the physical structure that man uses and the environs of the structure including all necessary services, facilities, equipment and devices needed for desired.

HOUSING

Goals of Housing

Goals are statements about desirable or projected conditions; the generally accepted goals of housing.

Shelter: The house should provide a sanitary shelter, which is a basic need.

Family life: The house should provide adequate space for family and related activities, viz. preparation and storage of food, meeting, sleeping, individual activities and other basic activities. The adequacy of housing at this level has been found to have a direct impact on such things as worker productivity and family stability.

Access to community facilities: A third element of housing is accessibility to community services and facilities such as health services, school, shopping area, places of worship, etc.

Family participation in community life: Family is part of the wider community. Community is important to family in many ways, it can offer help in times of need; it is an important source of friends. Communities are able to pool their efforts and improve their living conditions.

Economic stability: Housing is a form of investment of personal savings. It provides for economic stability and well-being of the family.

The implementation of social goals in housing requires that government should:
- Introduce social housing schemes
- Establish both minimum and maximum standards
- Create financial and fiscal institutions geared to helping low-income people obtain credit for building or improving their houses.

Housing Requirements

Location: The house should be located on dry, non-caving ground having an independent unit and should be nearer to shopping place, recreational facilities, educational centers, emergency services and transport system.

Construction: The house should be so strongly constructed as to withstand the vagaries of nature such as landslide, floods or earthquake, etc. and also it should be safe and secured.

Sanitation: From the point of view of health, there should not be overcrowding and there must be sufficient light and ventilation, sufficient water supply and proper arrangements for drainage of liquid waste in the house. Provision should be made for insect proofing and rodent proofing also, cleanliness to be maintained in and around the house.

Comfortable house lives: For this there must be ideally separate kitchen, store room, bedrooms, a common living room for the entire family and a corridor.

Criteria for Healthful Housing

An expert committee of the WHO recommended the following criteria for healthful housing:
1. Healthful housing provides physical protection and shelter.
2. Provides adequacy for cooking, eating, washing and excretory functions.
3. House is designed, constructed, maintained and used in a manner such as to prevent the spread of communicable diseases.
4. Provides for protection from hazards of exposure to noise and pollution.
5. House is free from unsafe physical arrangements due to construction or maintenance and from toxic or harmful materials.
6. Encourages personal and community development, promotes social relationships reflects a regard for ecological principles and by these means promote mental health.

Housing Standards

Housing standards vary from country to country depending upon the socioeconomic status, family size and composition, cultural practices and climate conditions.

The standards are no longer confined to narrow health criteria such as per capita space and floor space. Social and economic characteristics such as family income, family size and composition, standard of living, lifestyle, stage in life cycle, education and cultural factors must be taken into consideration in determining housing standards. Because of cultural diversity and other factors such as climate and social traditions, standards of housing must vary from region to region.

Urban Housing

Minimum standards are still maintained by building regulations, the aim being improvement of housing and environmental condition for the majority of families within the limits set by available sources and objectives. The standards recommended in India for urban housing are as follows.

Site selection
1. The site or the ground selected should be high and only to drain the water. The soil should be of gravel nature. Made soil (i.e. ground leveled by dumping refuse) is very unsatisfactory for building purposes for at least 20–25 years and damp sites should be avoided. It should have proper approach roads and away from traffic and industries. The subsoil water should be below 304.8 cm.
2. The site should be elevated from its surroundings, so that is not subject to flooding during rains.
3. The site should have an independent access to a street of adequate width.
4. It should be away from the breeding places of mosquitoes and flies.
5. It should be away from nuisances such as dust, smoke, smell, excessive noise and traffic.
6. It should be in pleasing surroundings.

Foundation

Foundation must always be solid and substantial. The foundation is laid with a bed of cement concrete over the stones to cover the trench. The object is to prevent subsidence of the building. The width of the foundation should never be less than 25 inch. In addition to this bed of concrete, a layer of impervious material known as 'damp proof course' should be laid horizontally along the entire thickness of each wall at plinth level. This prevents the upward progress of the moisture.

Walls
The walls are constructed with cement and bricks or stones, with a minimum thickness of 9 inch obtained by laying the bricks lengthwise and crosswise in alternate layers. The walls are then plastered so that it should neither absorb heat nor it should conduct the heat. Painting of the walls renders the surface impervious and enables easy wash. The walls should be:
- Reasonably strong
- Should have a low-heat capacity, i.e. should not absorb heat and conduct the same
- Weather resistant
- Unsuitable for harborage of rats and vermin.
- Not easily damaged
- Smooth: These standards can be attained by 9 inch brick wall, plastered smooth and colored cream or white.

Floor area
Floor area should be air and water tight; surface should be smooth, facilitate easy wash and should be damp proof. The concrete floor should be covered with patent stone slabs or in better class houses, with marble slabs or tiles.

The floor area of a living room should be at least 120 ft^2 for occupancy by a single person. The floor area available in living rooms per person should not be less than 50 ft^2; the optimum is 100 ft^2. The optimum floor area per person in the living room should be 50–100 ft^3, but it should never be less than 50 ft^3.

Roof
Flat roofs should have sufficient slope to drain rainwater. Height of the roof should not be less than 10 ft as the heat radiated from the roof is in inverse ratio to the square of its distance.

Sloping roofs may be either of tiles, slates, thatch, corrugated iron, asbestos, etc. A double roof with a space between will make a very cool covering to a dwelling. The roof should have a low-heat transmittance coefficient.

Rooms
The number of living rooms depends upon the size of the family to prevent overcrowding. The number of living rooms should not be less than two, at least one of which can be closed for security. The other may be open on one side if that side is a private courtyard. The number and area of rooms should be increased according to size of family, so that the recommended floor space per person may be made available.

Doors and windows
Every living room should be provided with at least two windows and one of them should open directly to the open space. Doors and windows should open directly to the open space; and should be so placed as to allow cross ventilation (i.e. air should pass through one end and come out at the other).

The windows should be placed at 30 inch (2½ ft) above the floor level (not above 3 ft) and the window area should be one fifth of the floor area of the room. Doors and windows combined should have two fifth of the floor area. Ventilation grills should occupy 2% of the floor area placed near the ceiling and facing open space outside. Doors and windows can be made mosquito proof with wire gauze.

Lighting
The daylight factor should exceed 1% over half the floor area. The room is said to be adequately lighted, when one can read or write in the center of the hall without the help of artificial light during daytime.

Kitchen
Every house should have separate kitchen room, should neither be near a privy (toilet) nor so placed as to allow the smoke and smell of cooking getting into the rest of the house. It should not be exposed to dust and impurities getting into it. It should have adequate light and ventilation. Provision must be made for storing food grain, fuel [liquid petroleum gas (LPG) cylinders] and utensils. There should be sufficient water supply and drainage facility. The floor of the kitchen must be impervious.

Water closets or privies
Minimum one sanitary privy is a must for every house, preferably on the leeward side. It should have good ventilation. It should always be clean and dry.

Bathroom
Bathroom should also be on the leeward side of the house with drainage facility for the sullage water.

Utility
Provision should be made for washing utensils and clothes.

Water supply
There must be sufficient supply of safe and wholesome water. There may be individual water source for the house with a tube well, during the time of scarcity of water supply.

Setback
For proper lighting and ventilation, there should be an open space all-round the house, this is called 'setback'. This also prevents 'back-to-back' houses. Balcony should

be provided in the multistoried buildings. The question of open space becomes more a luxury than necessity in cities, where the value of land is very high.

In rural areas it is recommended that the built-up areas should not exceed one third of the total area; in urban areas, where land is costly, the built-up area may be up to two thirds. The setback should be such that there is no obstruction of lighting and ventilation. The floor should be pucca and satisfy the following criteria:

1. Setback should be impermeable, so that it can be easily washed and kept clean and dry. Mud floors tend to break up and cause dust; they are not recommended.
2. The floor must be smooth and free from cracks and crevices to prevent the breeding of insects and harborage of dust.
3. The floors should be damp proof.
4. The height of the plinth should be 2–3 ft.

Refuse and garbage

Refuse such as ash, dust, waste paper, rags and garbage, vegetable and animal matter, collected in metal receptacles at least twice daily and emptied into the public dustbin at regular hours.

The liquid refuse such as wash water from the kitchen, bathroom and other washing places such as utility and also the human excreta must be drained by underground drainage system.

Privy

A sanitary privy is must in every house, belonging exclusively to it and readily accessible. In the more developed areas of the world, the majority of dwelling units are equipped with water carriage systems.

Cubic space

Unless means are provided for mechanical replacement of air the height of rooms should be such as to give all air space of at least 500 ft^3 per capita, preferably 1,000 ft^3.

Other provisions

In the construction of houses, efficient space utilization, storage for household goods and personal belongings and home safety measures should be incorporated. Provision must also be made for draining their vehicles, if any. Provision must also be made for draining the rainwater. Domestic animals if any must be away from the living rooms. Electrification must be proper and safe.

Rural Housing

The following minimum standards have been suggested in rural areas:

1. There should be at least two living rooms.
2. Ample veranda space may be provided.
3. The built area should not exceed one third of the total area.
4. There should be a separate kitchen with a paved sink or platform for washing the utensils.
5. The house should be provided with a sanitary latrine.
6. The window areas should be at least 10% of the floor area.
7. There should be a sanitary well or a tube well within a quarter of a mile from the house.
8. It is insanitary to keep cattle and livestock in dwelling houses. Cattle sheds should be at least 25 ft away from dwelling houses. A cattle shed should be open on all sides; an area 8 × 4 ft is sufficient for each head of cattle.
9. There should be adequate arrangement for the disposal of waste water, refuse and garbage.

Standards of rural housing

- Built-up area should be about 60% of the total site
- There must be sufficient space around the house for adequate lighting and ventilation
- The area of doors and windows should be about 25% of the floor area
- Preferably two living rooms at least
- Separate kitchen with a provision for washing utensils
- Provision for washing the clothes
- Soakage pit for disposal of sullage water coming from bathroom and kitchen
- House should be provided with a RCA latrine (RCA stands for Research-cum-Action project)
- The source of water should be within the reach of about 400 m
- Livestocks such as cattle, pigs, sheep, etc. should be away from the human dwellings
- There must be manure pit arrangements for the disposal of kitchen waste and domestic refuse.

Effect of Housing on Health

Housing is part of the total environment of man and being a part, it is to some extent responsible for the status of man's health and well-being. It is difficult, however to demonstrate the specific cause and effect relationships because housing embraces so many facets of environment. Poor standard of housing associated with defective ventilation and overcrowding affects the health of the residents physically, mentally and socially, resulting in increased morbidity and mortality.

Overcrowding is said to have occurred based on the following three criteria:

1. Floor area (person ratio): On the basis of floor area, the accepted standards are:
   - 110 ft^2 or more—2 persons
   - 90–110 ft^2—1½ person (a child between 1 and 10 years is considered as half person or half unit)

- 70–90 ft²—1 person
- 50–70 ft²—½ person (a child below 1 year is not counted).

2. Room (person ratio): On the basis of room-person ratio, the accepted standards are:
   - 1 room—2 persons
   - 2 rooms—3 persons
   - 3 rooms—5 persons
   - 4 rooms—7 persons
   - 5 rooms or more—10 persons (additional two for each further room).
3. Sex separation: On the basis of sex separation, overcrowding is considered, if two persons over 10 years of age of opposite sex unless husband and wife are obliged to sleep in the same room.

If the definition of health given by WHO is applied, we have also to take into consideration the broader aspects of mental and social well-being of individuals and families, i.e. factors related to satisfaction of physiological, psychological and social needs.

Physiological Effects

The ill-ventilated, dirty and overcrowded houses are responsible for various diseases listed below:
- Respiratory: Common cold, tuberculosis (TB), influenza, diphtheria, bronchitis and measles
- Skin infections: Scabies, ringworm, leprosy and other skin disorders
- House flies: Mosquitoes, rats and flies spread disease
- Threadworm due to sleeping together, especially among children
- Accident due to some defects in the home
- High morbidity and mortality rates are observed in substandard housing conditions
- Children have defective vision and hearing. They have higher mortality from TB, chronic bronchitis and rheumatic heart disease.

Psychosocial Effects

Psychosocial effects must not be overlooked. The sense of isolation felt by persons living in the upper floors of high buildings is now well known to have harmful effects. Often, also, people living in densely populated urban areas feel a similar sense of isolation, which may lead to neurosis and behavioral disorders.

TOWN PLANNING

Towns are growing with industrialization as industrial centers. These towns have grown up haphazardly, creating congestion, ill health and slums mostly due to lack of proper planning. Growth of industries encouraged migration from rural to urban areas. Moreover, due to abolition of Zamindari and land ceilings laws, people are shifting from villages to towns. There has been rapid process of urbanization creating congestion, ill health and increased mortality.

The above facts have made it necessary for careful town planning with proper housing, provision of adequate protection, water supply and sanitary latrines are responsible for waterborne and respiratory diseases. The busters are being created in the cities and industrial areas. Such an area is usually located in the peripheral part of the city. In order to avoid new slum and improve the existing slums necessary actions under the law and housing schemes are necessary. Both the central as well as state government has been interested in improving the slums.

OVERCROWDING IN THE HOUSE AND HEALTH

Overcrowding refers to the situation in which more people are living within a single dwelling than there is space for, so that movement is restricted, privacy secluded, hygiene impossible, rest and sleep difficult. In general, the risks as regards physical health are clear enough. Infectious diseases spread rapidly under conditions of overcrowding. The effects on psychosocial health are not so clear-cut, viz. irritability, frustration, lack of sleep, anxiety, violence and mental disorders. Children are said to be more affected. In short, it is a psychosocial stress leading to unhappiness and very probably to psychosomatic and mental disorders.

Overcrowding associated with poor ventilation (and poor housing) causes rise of temperature, excessive humidity and air stagnation of the room, which lowers the vitality of the inmates and makes them more susceptible to diseases. Respiratory diseases spread by droplet infection very fast such as TB, measles, influenza, streptococcal throat infections, acute rheumatic fever, common cold, diphtheria, whooping cough, bronchitis, etc. contagious diseases such as scabies, impetigo, ringworm, leprosy, trachoma, conjunctivitis also spread. Overcrowding has a bad social effect especially when persons of opposite sexes occupy the same sleeping room.

On the other hand, isolation or loneliness felt by the person, living alone in the house may result in neurosis, psychosis, behavioral disorders and also habits such as alcoholism and drug addiction.

Sex Separation

Overcrowding is considered to exist if two persons over 9 years of age, not husband and wife, of opposite sexes are obliged to sleep in the same room.

INDICATORS OF HOUSING

In recent years, the use of indicators has become widespread for the measurement of quality of life. The indicators for housing may be classified as:

Physical: These are based on construction, floor space, cubic space, room height, persons per room, rooms per dwelling, environmental quality and sanitation. For example, air, light, water, noise, ventilation, drainage facilities, sewage disposal, etc.

Economic indicators: These are cost of the building, rental levels, taxes, expenditure on housing, etc.

Social indicators: The following were proposed at an interregional seminar on the social aspects of housing organized by the United Nations (UN) in 1975.

Indicators related to prevention of illness due to:
- Inadequate sewage and garbage collection
- Associated with contaminated water source
- Frequency of insect-borne diseases
- Overcrowding
- Accidents
- Proximity to animals
- Access to medical facility.

Indicators related to comfort:
- Thermal
- Acoustic
- Visual
- Spatial.

Indicators related to mental health and social well-being:
- Frequency of suicides in the neighborhood
- Neglected and abandoned youth in the neighborhood
- Freshness of psychoses and neuroses
- Drug abuse (including alcohol) in the neighborhood.

HOUSING PROBLEM

In India, housing problem has assumed serious proportions in recent times due to population explosion, migration of population due to industrialization and urbanization, eruptions of slums, faulty methods of construction of houses, lack of provision of protected water supply, disposal of refuse and excreta, etc. have given rise to following problems:

1. Nonavailability of houses: So, the homeless are forced to live on pavements, in railway and bus stations or among the discarded truck bodies, rail carriages, etc.
2. Substandard houses and slums: These are poorly constructed houses with lack of lighting, ventilation and drainage facilities. New slums are constantly growing up and old ones are getting expanded.
   The situation is still made worse by overcrowding, by keeping the raw materials of the domestic industry and even domestic animals.
3. Dilapidated and crumbling houses: Frequently, these are due to use of poor construction materials by the contractor.
4. A reasonably good house in bad surroundings: In the vicinity of cesspools, open drains, offensive trades, noisy industries, liquor shops and red-light areas.
5. A house with a bad social environment such as uncooperative attitude and quarreling after consuming alcohol and also prostitution, gambling, etc.

Measures to Solve Housing Problem

1. Provision of good quality houses or tenements to the poorest of poor.
2. Provision of sites with loan on easy terms to the landless poor.
3. Improvement of existing slums by providing basic amenities such as street lights, protected water supply, drainage facilities, community latrines, etc.
4. Encouragement of owners of large establishments to built quarters for their employees.
5. Construction of shelters for the street children.

The programs related to above activities are Indira Awaas Yojana, Ashraya Program and Nirman Kendra. In every country, where housing conditions in general are unsatisfactory the need for government intervention has been recognized. The approach to public policy on housing in India is indicated in the Five-Year Plans. In 1952, a separate ministry of works and housing was created at the center. The Government Housing Programs consist of two categories—public sector housing and social housing schemes. The former provides mainly for government employees, while the latter attempts to provide assistance particularly to low and middle income groups through various housing schemes. For promoting housing activities, statutory housing boards have been established at the state level. The four organizations, viz. National Buildings Organization (NBO), National Buildings Construction Corporation Limited, Housing and Urban Development

Corporation (HUDCO) and the Hindustan Housing Factory are functioning under the aegis of the Union Ministry of Works and housing to deal with various aspects of housing.

CONCLUSION

Housing is the physical structures, which provide protection against storm, lighting, snowfall, rain, etc. Houses not only protect and provide physical protection, but it is the immediate surrounding and the related community. It provides shelter to the intimate and sufficient space persons to live in. It protects against harmful effects of naturally occurring changes in the environments. Housing also prevents from the pollution exposure, which are hazardous to health and prevents the spread of community disease through proper designing and construction of houses. Housing should be constructed in proper selection of site for property amenities, orientation for which proper design needed. In relation to drop proof, doors, windows, stairs, roadside margin, rooms, floor, walls, open space, basic amenities and other facilities. Poor housing leads to many health-related respiratory problems such as asthma, arthritis it due to damp and moldy conditions. Allergic conditions such as rhinitis, conjunctivitis, eczema, cough (due to airborne pollutants), accidents (due to slippery floor, poisoning) due to combustion of appliances and stoves (carbon monoxide) unhygienic conditions can exacerbate the disease caused by mosquitoes, house flies, fleas, etc. and also scabies, ringworm impetigo, and psychosocial stress occurs among inmates due to overcrowding. So, good housing needed for healthy living.

Sanitation: Disposal of Waste

CHAPTER 15

INTRODUCTION

In earlier days sanitation was centered on the sanitary disposal of human excreta. Even now, for many people, sanitation still means the construction of latrine. Actually, the term sanitation covers the whole field of controlling the environment with a view to prevent disease and promote health. The increased demand for utility of services for both domestic and industrial use leads to an accumulation of waste products in water, air and on the ground. Inadequate supply and distribution of poor quality of water for drinking and domestic uses increase the likelihood of exposure to gastrointestinal infections. Storage of water for domestic use in uncovered storage tanks, and accumulation of surface water and sewage due to inadequate drainage will (where climatic conditions are favorable) provide conditions suitable for the dissemination of filariasis, malaria, and other vector-borne diseases. Lack of sanitary facilities leading to fouling of the ground and accumulation of garbage causes pollution of the soil and spread infestations. The concentration of industries in and around the community not only creates greater demand in water supplies and drainage, housing and transport sources but also creates its own problems of waste disposal, air, water and soil pollution.

WASTE AND REFUSE

The waste products of the community living are refuse, human excreta and sewage.

The term 'waste' is applied to unwanted or discarded waste matter, while 'refuse' means the solid discarded material produced by human habitation except human excreta. The accumulation of solid wastes in many environments constitutes a positive health hazard because of the following reasons:
- The organic portion of solid wastes ferments and favors fly breeding
- The garbage and refuse attract rats
- The pathogens may be conveyed to man through flies and dust
- There is a possibility of water pollution by rain water passing through deposits of fermenting refuse
- There is a risk of air pollution, if there is accidental or spontaneous combustion of refuse
- Piles of refuse are a nuisance from an esthetic point of view, i.e. bad smell and bad sight.

Disposal of wastes is now largely the domain of sanitarians and public health engineers. However, health professionals need to have a basic knowledge of the subject since improper disposal of wastes constitute a health hazard. Further the health professional may be called upon to give advice in some special situations, such as camp sanitation or coping with waste disposal problems, when there is a disruption or breakdown of community health services in natural disasters. These aspects are considered in this section.

Solid Wastes

'Solid wastes' include garbage (food wastes), rubbish (paper, plastics, wood, metal, throw-away containers, glass), demolition products (bricks, masonry, pipes), sewage treatment residue (sludge and solids from the coarse screening of domestic sewage), dead animals, manure and other discarded material. Strictly speaking it should not contain night soil. The output of daily waste depends upon the dietary habits, lifestyles, living standards and the degree of urbanization and industrialization. The per capita daily solid waste produced ranges between 0.25 and 2.5 kg in different countries.

Solid waste, if allowed to accumulate is a health hazard because:
- It decomposes and favors fly breeding
- It attracts rodents and vermin

CHAPTER 15

Sanitation: Disposal of Waste

- The pathogens, which may be present in the solid waste, may be conveyed back to man's food through flies and dust
- There is a possibility of water and soil pollution
- Heaps of refuse present an unsightly appearance and nuisance from bad odors.

Improper disposal of solid wastes increases incidence of vector-borne diseases. There should be efficient systems for its periodic collection, removal and final disposal without risk of health. The sources of refuse include the following:

1. Street refuse: It is the refuse that is collected by the street cleansing service or scavenging. It consists of leaves, straw, paper, animal droppings and litter of all kinds.
2. Market refuse: It is refuse that is collected from markets refuse. It contains a large proportion of putrid vegetable and animal matter.
3. Refuse that is collected from stables. It contains mainly minimal droppings and left over animal feeds.
4. Industrial refuse comprises a wide variety of wastes ranging from completely inert materials such as calcium carbonate to highly toxic and explosive compounds.
5. Domestic refuse consists of ash, rubbish and garbage. Ash is the residue from fire used for cooking and heating. Rubbish comprises paper, clothing, bits of wood, metal, glass, dust and dirt. Garbage is waste mailer arising from the preparation, cooking and consumption of food. It consists of waste food, vegetable peelings and other organic mailer. Garbage needs quick removal and disposal because its ferments on storage.

Storage of Refuse

Dustbins made of galvanized iron sheets are suitable receptacles, placed at a fair distance from the house. If it is covered with a lid, people will not open it, but throw the refuse around it. If not covered, the dogs, pigs and other animals scatter the contents, thus creating nuisance.

In the developed countries, the dustbins will have 'paper sack'. When the paper sack is filled, it is removed from the bin and a new sack is placed inside. The municipal workers remove the refuse periodically.

The galvanized steel dustbin with close fitting cover is a suitable receptacle for storing refuse. The capacity of a bin will depend upon the numbers of users and frequency of collection. The output of refuse per capita per day in India is estimated to vary from 1/10 to 1/20 ft^2 for a family of five members, a bin having a capacity of 5/10 or 1/2 ft^2 would be needed. If collection is done once in 3 days a bin having a capacity of 1½ or 2 ft^2 would be adequate. Recent refuse is stored in the paper sack and the sack itself is removed with the contents for disposal, and new sack is substituted. Public bins cater for a larger number of people. They are usually without cover in India because people do not like to touch them. In corporations the bins are handled and emptied mechanically by lorries fitted with cranes.

Collection of Refuse

House collection is by a far the best method of collecting refuse and people are expected to dump the refuse in the nearest public bin, which is usually not done. Refuse is dispersed all along the street and some is thrown out in front and around the house. As a result, an army of sweepers is required for sweeping the streets in addition to the gang for collecting the refuse from public bins. The open refuse cart should be abandoned and replaced by enclosed vans. Mechanical transport should be used wherever possible, as it is more practical and economical.

House-to-house collection of refuse is the best method, but that is not done. Dumping the refuse in the public dustbin is also not done properly. As a result, refuse is dispersed all along the street. The Environmental Hygiene Committee (1948) recommends:

- House-to-house collection of refuse
- Open refuse carts should be replaced by enclosed vans
- Mechanical transportation is more practical and economical.

The collection and transportation of refuse should be carried out during the early hours of the morning to minimize the nuisance. Wheel barrows are small hand pushed carts used to collect refuse from narrow lanes where big carts cannot go. The refuse collected by wheel burrows is deposited in dustbins.

Collection and removal of domestic and town refuse, apart from human excreta, by means of manual labor is called 'scavenging'.

Methods of Refuse Disposal

There are number of methods of refuse disposal, which are equally suitable in all circumstances. The choice of a particular method is governed by local factors such as cost and availability of land and labor. The common methods of refuse disposal are:

- Dumping
- Controlled tipping or sanitary landfill
- Incineration
- Composting
- Manure pits
- Burial.

Dumping

In this method, the refuse is dumped in the low-lying areas and later reclamation is done and used for cultivation purpose. Since it results in all the health hazards mentioned above, the land selected for dumping should be as far away from human habitation as possible or outside the limits of the town.

The WHO Expert Committee (1997) condemned dumping as 'a most insanitary method of disposal of refuse because of the health hazards', to be replaced by sound procedures.

Refuse is dumped in low-lying areas partly as a method of reclamation of land, but mainly as an easy method of disposal or dry refuse. As a result of bacterial action, refuse decreases considerably in volume and is converted gradually into humus. The disadvantages of open dumping are:
- The refuse is exposed to flies and rodents
- It is a source of nuisance from the smell and unsightly appearance
- The loose refuse is dispersed by the action of the wind
- Drainage from dumps contributes to the pollution of surface and ground water.

Dumping is a most insanitary method that creates public health hazards 'a nuisance and severe pollution of the environment'.

Controlled Tipping

Controlled tipping is nothing, but dumping or burial of the refuse in a sanitary way as to prevent the health hazards. The dumping site should be away from the human habitation or outside the city limits and sources of water, so that water pollution due to leaching from refuse dumps is avoided. After dumping the refuse, it is covered with a layer of earth on the top daily, so that nuisance by sight and smell, and also breeding of flies is prevented. 'Modified sanitary landfill' term is applied to those operations, where compaction and covering with earth is done once or twice a week.

Controlled tipping or sanitary landfill is differs from ordinary dumping in that the material is placed in a trench or other prepared area, adequately compacted and covered with earth at the end of the working day. Three methods are used in this operation are the trench method, the ramp method and the area method:
1. Trench method: Where level ground is available, the trench method is usually chosen. A long trench is dugout, i.e. 2–3 m (6–10 ft) deep and 4–12 m (12–36 ft) wide, depending upon local conditions. The refuse is compacted and covered with excavated earth.
2. Ramp method: This method is well-suited where the terrain is moderately sloping. Some excavation is done to secure the covering material.
3. Area method: This method is used for filling land depressions, disused quarries and clay pits. The refuse is deposited, packed and consolidated in uniform layers up to 2–2.5 m (6–8 ft) deep. Each layer is sealed on its exposed surface with a mud cover at least 30 cm (12 inch) thick. Such sealing prevents infestations by flies and rodents, and suppresses the nuisance of smell and dust.

Chemical, bacteriological and physical changes occur in buried refuse. The temperature rises to over 60°C within 7 days and kills all the pathogens, and hastens the decomposition process. Then it takes 2–3 weeks to cool down. Normally it takes 4–6 months for complete decomposition of organic matter into an innocuous mass.

Incineration

Incineration is the method of choice where suitable land is not available. Hospital refuse, which is particularly dangerous is best disposed of by incineration. Incineration is practiced in several of the industrialized countries, particularly in large cities due to lack of suitable land. Incineration is not a popular method in India because the refuse contains a fair proportion of fine ash, which makes it burning difficult. It is more expensive to separate ash and dust. Disposal of refuse by burning is a loss to the community in terms of the much needed manure.

This is process of burning the solid waste and is the most sanitary method of disposal of refuse, especially the hospital refuse because of its dangers. The incinerator consists of the following features:
- A furnace or combustion chamber lined with firebricks, where the fire is built with firewood or electricity
- A platform for tipping the refuse
- Stokers (through the openings) to bring the refuse together for burning completely
- A baffle plate to drive of all the fumes (Fig. 15.1).

By this process of burning, the refuse is reduced to about one fourth of its original weight and the organic matter is transformed into innocuous vapors—carbon dioxide and nitrogen. The residuum left after the combustion is a mass of hard material called 'clinkers', which are utilized for making the roads. It is also used as cement by powdering the clinkers and mixing with lime.

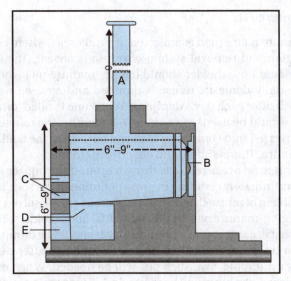

Figure 15.1: Incinerator—longitudinal section. A. Chimney; B. Charging door; C. Openings for stoking; D. Iron grating; E. Opening for removing ashes.

This method is feasible in those city areas where considerable quantity of refuse is produced daily, but sanitary land-fill sites are not available.

The incinerators built of mud or irons without bricks do not give satisfactory results. However, they are suitable for fairs and melas of short duration. The beehive incinerators have been found useful under such conditions (Fig. 15.2).

The drawback in many incinerators is that the draught is not sufficient. Therefore, they give off offensive smoke creating nuisance. To overcome this, the temperature in the furnace should be more than 1,250°F for which the chimney should be tall and draught of air adequate.

Composting

In composting method, the refuse is disposed of along with the night-soil or sewage. There are two methods—biological and mechanical.

Biological method

Biological is also called Bangalore method or anaerobic method or hot fermentation process. In this method, trenches are dug measuring 5–10 m length, 2 m breadth and 1 m depth, away from the city limits. Alternate layers of refuse and human excreta (night-soil) are put into the trench, in the thickness of 15 cm and 5 cm respectively, the first and last layer being that of refuse. The trench is then covered with excavated earth.

Within about a week intense heat is generated to about 60°C, persisting for about 2–3 weeks killing all the pathogens and the parasites. The lignins and cellulose are broken down. The end products of decomposition are acted upon by fungi and anaerobic bacteria, resulting in harmless, odorless, innocuous humans' mass, called 'compost', which has high manurial value. It is sold as organic manure, without causing any nuisance. It is ready for application to the land.

Composting is a method of combined disposal of refuse and night soil or sludge. It is a process of nature whereby organic matter reaks down under bacterial action resulting in the formation of relatively stable humus-like material, called compost, which has considerable manorial value for the soil. The principal by products are carbon dioxide, water and heat. The heat produced during composting, 60°C or higher, over a period of several days destroys eggs and larvae of flies, weed seeds and pathogenic agents. The end-product compost contains few or no disease-reducing organisms and is a good soil builder containing small amounts of the major plant nutrients such as nitrates and phosphates. The following methods of composting are now used:

1. Bangalore method (anaerobic method).
2. Mechanical composting (aerobic method).

Bangalore method (hot fermentation process)

Indian Council of Agriculture Research (ICAR) carried out investigation at Indian Institute of Science (IISc) Bangalore, a system of anaerobic composting, known as Bangalore method (hot fermentation process) has been developed. It has been recommended as a satisfactory method of disposal of town wastes and night soil.

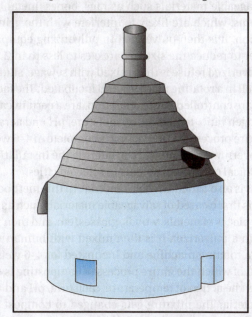

Figure 15.2: Beehive incinerator

Trenches are dug, i.e. 90 cm (3 ft) deep, 1.5–2.5 m (5–8 ft) broad and 4.5–10 m (15–30 ft) long, depending upon the amount of refuse and night soil to be disposed of. The pits should be located not less than 800 m (1/2 mile) from city limits. The composting procedure is as follows:
1. First layer of refuse about 15 cm (6 inch) thick is spread at bottom of the trench.
2. Over this, night soil is added corresponding to a thickness of 5 cm (2 inch).
3. Then alternate layers of refuse and night soil are added in the proportion of 15 cm (6 inch) and 5 cm (2 inch) respectively, till the heap rises to 30 cm (1 ft) above the ground level.
4. The top layer should be refuse, at least 25 cm (9 inch) thickness. Then the heap is covered with excavated earth; if properly laid, a man's legs will not sink when walking over the compost mass.

Within 7 days as a result of bacterial action considerable heat (over 60°C) is generated in the compost mass. This intense heat, which persists over 2 or 3 weeks, serves to decompose the refuse and night soil, and to destroy all pathogenic and parasitic organisms. At the end of 4–6 months, decomposition is complete and the resulting manure is a well-decomposed, odorless, innocuous material of high manorial value ready for application to the land.

Mechanical composting

In 'mechanical composting' compost is literally manufactured on a large scale by processing raw materials and turning out a finished product. The refuse is first cleared of salvageable materials such as rags, bones, metal, glass and items, which are likely to interfere with the grinding operation. It is then pulverized in pulverizing equipment in order to reduce the size of particles to less than 2 inch. The pulverized refuse is then mixed with sewage, sludge or night soil in a rotating machine and incubated. The factors, which are controlled in the operation, are a certain carbon to nitrogen ratio, temperature, moisture, pH and aeration. The entire process of composting is complete in 4–6 weeks. The Government of India is considering the installation of mechanical composting plants in selected cities.

This is also called 'aerobic method'. In this method, the refuse is first cleared of salvageable materials such as rags, bones, pieces of metals, woods, glasses, etc. and then powdered in a pulverizer. It is then mixed with human night soil in a rotating machine and incubated for 4–6 weeks at the end of which the entire process of composting is complete by the action of temperature, moisture, pH and aerobic bacteria. The mixture gets changed to compost. This method is in vogue in developed countries.

Manure Pits

Manure pit method is preferred in rural areas, where collection and removal system of refuse is absent. The individual householder should have a 'manure pit', where the daily domestic refuse is dumped and covered with earth after each day's dumping. When one is filled, other pit should be used. After about 4–6 months, the refuse is converted into compost, which can be used to the field as manure. This is simple and effective method.

In rural areas refuse is thrown around the houses indiscriminately resulting in gross pollution of the soil. The problem of refuse disposal in rural areas can be solved by digging 'manure pits' by the individual householders. The garbage, cattle dung, straw and leaves should be dumped into the manure pits and covered with earth after each day's dumping. Two such pits will be needed. When one is closed, the other will be in use. In 5–6 months' time, the refuse is converted into manure, which can be returned to the field. This method of refuse disposal is effective and relatively simple in rural communities.

Burial

Burial is suitable for small camps. A trench 1.5 m wide and 2 m deep is excavated, and at end of each day the refuse is covered with 20–30 cm of earth. When the level in the trench is 40 cm from ground level, the trench is filled with earth and compacted, and a new trench is dug out. The contents may be taken out after 4–6 months and used on the fields. If the trench is 1 m in length for every 200 persons, it will be filled in about 1 week.

This is also the same as trench method, but in the trenches, only the refuse is dumped and not the human excreta. At the end of each day refuse is covered with earth. When the trench is filled, new trench is dug out. After 4–6 months, the compost is removed and used as manure.

PUBLIC EDUCATION AND EXPENDITURE IN DISPOSAL

People have very little interest in cleanliness outside their homes. Many municipalities and corporations usually look for the cheapest solution, especially in regard to refuse disposal. What is needed is public education on these matters, by all known methods of health education, i.e. pamphlets, newspapers, broadcasting and films, etc. Police enforcement of the laws may also be needed at times.

If refuse disposal is to be carried out efficiently, hygienically and economically, heavy capital outlay will be

CHAPTER 15 Sanitation: Disposal of Waste

needed whatever system of disposal is adopted. In the highly industrialized countries up to 20% of municipal budgets are spent on the collection and disposal of solid wastes, and even more will be required if the job is to be done adequately.

HUMAN EXCRETA DISPOSAL

Human excreta are a source of infection. It is an important cause of environmental pollution. The health hazards of improper excreta disposal are soil pollution, water pollution, contamination of foods and propagation of flies. The resulting diseases are typhoid and paratyphoid, fever, dysentery, diarrhea, cholera, hookworm disease, ascariasis, viral hepatitis, and similar other intestinal infections and parasitic infestations, which are burden to the community in terms of sickness, mortality and a low expectation of life, leads to a basic deterrent to social and economic progress. Proper disposal of human excreta is a fundamental environmental health service to improve the state of community health.

In rural areas the majorities of them 'go to the fields' for defecation and thereby pollute the environment with human excrement. The situation is no way better in urban areas. The Health Survey and Planning Committee (1962) reported that not more than 15% of the urban population in India had the amenity of a sewerage system. Statistics indicate that the intestinal groups of diseases claim about 5 million lives every year, while another 50 million people suffer from these infections. The solution to the problem is only through hygienic disposal of human excreta, which is the cornerstone of all public health services.

The human excreta of a sick person or a carrier of disease is the main focus of infection. It contains the disease agent, which is transmitted to a new host through various channels such as water, fingers, flies, soil and food. The fecal-borne disease cycle may be broken at various levels such as segregation of feces, protection of water supplies and protection of foods, personal hygiene and control of flies. Of these, the most effective step would be to segregate the feces and arrange for its proper disposal so that the diseases agent cannot reach the new host, directly or indirectly. The segregation of the excreta by imposing a barrier called the 'sanitation barrier'. In simple terms, this barrier can be provided by a 'sanitary latrine' and a disposal pit. The more elaborate schemes envisage installation of a sewage system and sewage treatment plants.

Methods of Excreta Disposal

There are number of methods of excreta disposal. Some are applicable to unsewered areas. A classification and description of the various methods of excreta disposal is given below:

1. Unsewered areas:
   a. Service type (conservancy system) night soil is collected from pail or bucket type of latrines by human agency and later disposed of by burying or composting.
   b. Non-service type (sanitary latrines):
      i. Borehole latrine.
      ii. Dug well or pit latrine.
      iii. Water-seal type of latrines:
         - Planning, Research-cum Action Institute (PRAI)
         - Research-cum Action (RCA)
         - Sulabh shauchalaya.
      iv. Septic tank.
      v. Aqua privy.
   c. Latrines suitable for camps and temporary use:
      i. Shallow trench latrine.
      ii. Deep trench latrine.
      iii. Pit latrine.
      iv. Borehole latrine.
2. Sewered areas: Water-carriage system and sewage treatment:
   a. Primary treatment:
      i. Screening.
      ii. Removal of grit.
      iii. Primary sedimentation.
   b. Secondary treatment:
      i. Trickling filters.
      ii. Activated sludge process.
   c. Other methods:
      i. Sea outfall.
      ii. River outfall.
      iii. Sewage farming.
      iv. Oxidation ponds.
      v. Oxidation ditches.

Excreta Disposal in Unsewered Areas

Service type (conservancy system)

The collection and removal of night soil from bucket or pail latrines by human agency is called the service type or conservancy system, and their latrines are called service latrines. The night soil is transported in 'night soil carts' to the place of final disposal, where it is disposed by composting or burial in shallow trenches. Service latrines are a source of filth and insanitation. They have all the drawbacks and faults that tend to perpetuate the disease cycle, which tend to perpetuate the disease cycle of fecal-borne diseases in the community. The night soil is exposed to flies; there is always the possibility of water and soil pollution. The employment of human labor for the collecting of night soil is not consistent with human dignity and is no longer pardonable. The Environmental Hygiene Committee (1949), therefore, recommended that in unsewered areas the services latrines should be replaced by sanitary latrines, which require no service and in which excreta can be disposed of at the site of the latrine in a hygienic manner.

Non-service type of latrines (sanitary latrines)
A sanitary latrine is one, which fulfills the criteria as detailed below:
- Excreta should not contaminate the ground or surface water
- Excreta should not pollute the soil
- Excreta should not be accessible to flies, rodents, animals (pigs, dogs, cattle, etc.) and other vehicles of transmission
- Excreta should not create a nuisance due to odor or unsightly appearance.

A brief description of some of the well-known types of sanitary latrines is given below.

Borehole latrine
The borehole latrine was first introduced by the Rockefeller foundation during 1930s in campaigns of hookworm control. The latrine consists of a circular hole 30–40 cm (12–16 inch) in diameter, dug vertically into the ground to a depth of 4–8 m (13–26 ft) most commonly 6 m (20 ft). Special equipment is known as auger is required to dig a borehole. In loose and sandy soils, the hole is lined with bamboo matting or earthen ware rings to prevent caving in of the soil. A concrete squatting plate with a central opening and foot rests is placed over the hole. A suitable enclosure is put up to provide privacy. For a family of five or six people, a borehole of the above description servers well for over a year. Borehole is essentially a family type of installation and is not recommended as a public convenience because of its small capacity. When the contents of the borehole reach within 50 cm (20 inch) of the ground level, the squatting plate is removed and the hole is closed with earth. A new hole is dug and similarly used. The night soil undergoes purification by anaerobic digestion and is eventually converted into a harmless mass. The amount of sludge that accumulates has been estimated to amount of sludge that accumulates has been estimated to amount to 2.1–7.3 ft^2 per 1,000 user's days. The merits of a borehole latrine are:
1. There is no need for the services of a sweeper for daily removal of night soil.
2. The pit is dark and unsuitable for fly breeding.
3. If located 15 m (50 ft) away from a source of water supply, there should be no danger of water pollution. In spite of these merits, borehole latrines are not considered a very suitable type of latrine today. The reasons are:
   - The borehole fills up rapidly because of its small capacity
   - Special equipment, the auger, is required for its construction, which may not be readily available
   - In many places, the subsoil water is high and the soil loose; with the result it may be difficult to dig a hole deeper than 3 m (10 ft).

The borehole latrine is therefore, not very much in use today. It has been superseded by better innovations (Fig. 15.3).

Dug well latrine
Dug well latrine or pit latrine was first introduced in Singur, West Bengal in 1949–1950. It is an improvement over the borehole latrine. A circular pit about 75 cm (30 inch) in diameter and 3–3.5 m (10–12 ft) deep in dug into the ground for the reception of the night soil. In sandy soil, the depth of the pit may be reduced to 1.5–2 m (6–7 ft). The pit may be lined with pottery rings and as many rings as necessary to prevent caving in of the soil may be used. A concrete squatting plate is placed on latrine are:
1. It is easy to construct and no special equipment such as an auger is needed to dig the pit.
2. The pit has a longer life than the borehole because of greater cubic capacity. A pit 75 cm (30 inch) diameter and 3–3.5 m (10–12 ft) deep will last for about 5 years for a family of four to five persons. When the pit is filled up, a new pit is constructed. The action of the dug well latrine is the same as in the borehole latrine, i.e. anaerobic digestion (Fig. 15.4).

Water-seal latrine
Sanitary latrines for rural families are the hand flushed 'water seal' type of latrine in which the squatting plate is fitted with a water seal. The water seal performs two important functions:
1. It prevents access by flies, i.e. the night soil is sealed off from flies by a small depth of water contained in a bent pipe called trap.
2. It prevents escape of odors and foul gases, and thereby eliminates the nuisance from smell. Once the latrine is flushed, night soil is no longer visible.

CHAPTER 15 — Sanitation: Disposal of Waste

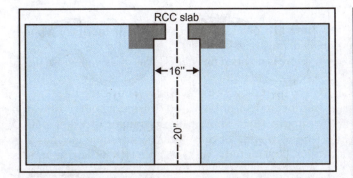

Figure 15.3: Borehole latrine (RCC, reinforced cement concrete)

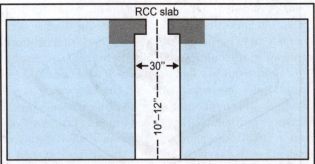

Figure 15.4: Dug well latrine

Several designs of water-seal latrine have been tested in the field and two types have gained recognition for wide use, these are:
1. The PRAI type, evolved by the Planning Research-cum Action Institute, Lucknow (Uttar Pradesh).
2. The RCA type, designed by the Research-cum Action Projects in Environmental Sanitation of the Ministry of Health, Government of India.

Of these two types, the RCA latrine has been accepted as a suitable designed for wide adoption in different parts of the country (Fig. 15.5).

The parts of a water-seal latrine, whether RCA type or PRAI type, are essentially the same (refer Fig. 15.5) the difference are in matters of minor engineering detail. The essential features of a RCA latrine and its installation are described below:

1. **Location:** The safe distance between the latrine and a source of water supply will depend upon the porosity of the soil, level of ground water, its slope and direction of flow. In general it may be stated that latrine of any kind should not be located within 15 m (50 ft) from source of water supply; and should be at a lower elevation to prevent the possibility of bacterial contamination of the water supply. Where possible, latrines should not be located in are usually subject to flooding.
2. **Squatting plate:** The squatting plate or slab is an important part of a latrine. It should be made of an impervious material so that it can be washed, kept clean and dry. If kept dry, it will not facilitate the survival of hookworm larvae. In recommending squatting plates, due consideration should be paid to the habits of Indian people who defecate in the squatting position and use water for anal washing. The slab of the RCA latrine has been designed to meet the above needs. It is made of cement concrete with minimum dimensions of 90 cm² (3 ft) and 5 cm (2 inch) thickness at the outer edge. There is a slope 112 inch

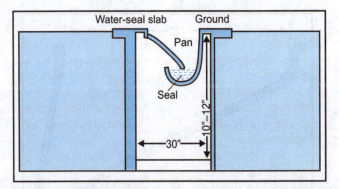

Figure 15.5: Water-seal latrine [Planning Research-cum Action Institute (PRAI) or Research-cum Action (RCA)]

towards the pan. This allows drainage into the latrine of the water used for ablution or cleansing purpose. A circular squatting plate of 90 cm (3 ft) diameter and 5 cm (2 inch) for the convenience of the users, raised footrests are included in the squatting plate (Fig. 15.6).

3. **Pan:** The pan receives the night soil, urine and wastewater. The length of the pan is 42.5 cm (17 inch). The width of the front portion of the pan has a minimum of 12.5 cm (5 inch) and the width at its widest portion is 20 cm (8 inch), there is a uniform slope from front to back of the pan is given a smooth finish (Fig. 15.7).
4. **Trap:** The trap is a bent pipe, about 7.5 cm (3 inch) in diameter and is connected with the pan. It holds the trap and the lowest point in the concave upper surface of the trap. The depth of the water seal in the RCA latrine is 2 cm (3/4 inch). The water seal prevent the access by flies and suppresses the nuisance from smell (Fig. 15.8).
5. **Connecting pipe:** When the pit is dug, away from the squatting plate, the trap is connected to the pit by a short length of connecting pipe 7.5 cm (3 inch) in diameter and at least 1 m (3 ft) in length with a bend at the end.

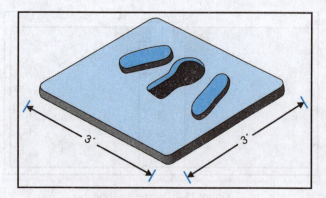

Figure 15.6: Squatting plate

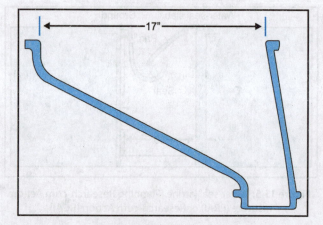

Figure 15.7: Latrine pan

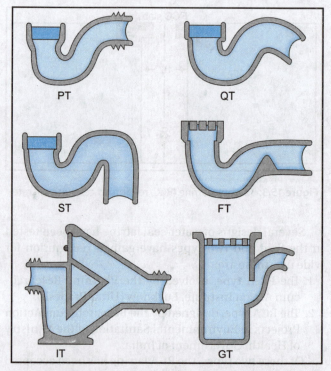

Figure 15.8: Sanitary traps (FT, floor trap; GT, gully trap; IT, intercepting trap; PT, P trap; QT, Q trap; ST, S trap).

A latrine of this type is called the indirect type because the pit sited away from the squatting plate. In the direct type there is no need for a connecting pipe. The direct type is best suited for areas where the ground is hard and does not easily cave in. The direct type is cheaper and easier to construct and occupies less space. An advantage with the indirect type is that when the pit fills up, a second pit can be put into operation by merely changing the direction of the connecting pipe. Therefore, the indirect type is usually preferred (refer Fig. 15.8)

Dug well
The dug well or pit is usually 75 cm (3 inch) in diameter, and 3–3.5 m (10–12 ft) deep and is covered. In loose soil and where the water label is high a lining of earthenware rings or bamboo matting can be used to prevent caving in of the pit. When the pit fills up, a second pit is dug nearby and the direction of the connecting pipe is changed into the second pit. When the second pit fills up, the first one may be emptied and reused.

Superstructure
The desired type of superstructure may be provided for privacy and shelter. An attractive superstructure with a neat finish is desirable as this will be generally well-maintained.

Maintenance
The life of a latrine will depend upon several factors such as care in usage and maintenance. The latrine should be used for only for the purpose intended and not for disposal of refuse or other debris. The squatting plate should be washed frequently, and kept clean and dry. People should learn to flush the pan after use with adequate quantity of water. About 1–2 liters of water are sufficient to flush the RCA latrine (Fig. 15.9). Thus, proper maintenance involves health education of the people, which is very necessary for the success of any latrine program.

Sulabh shauchalaya
The 'sulabh shauchalaya' model, the invention of a Patna-based firm, is a low-cost pour flush, water-seal type of latrine, which is now being used in many parts of India. Basically, it is an improved version of the standard hand flush latrine (e.g. RCA type). It consists of a specially designed pan and a water-seal trap. It is connected to pit 3 ft^2 and is deep. Excreta undergo bacterial decomposition, it is converted to manure (compost). The method requires

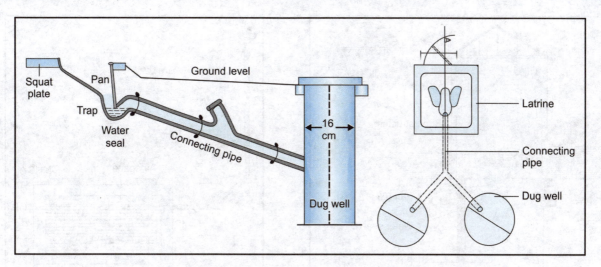

Figure 15.9: Research-cum Action latrine (indirect type)

very little water. Sulabh International, the investors not only build, but also maintain the system of sulabh community latrines. Their usual structure is a lavatory block of several dozen seats, with a bathing block adjoining. The system is to charge ₹1 per user (who is given soap powder by the sulabh attendant after use). Recently, Delhi has opted for this system in all its slums. This system has drawn praise from ecologist and planners (Fig. 15.10).

Septic tank

The septic tank is watertight masonry tank, is a satisfactory means of disposing excreta and liquid wastes from individual dwellings, small groups of houses and institutions, which have adequate water supplies, but do not have access to a public sewerage system. The main design features of a septic tank are as follows:

1. **Capacity:** The capacity of 20–30 gallons or 2½–5 ft² per person is recommended for household septic tanks. The minimum capacity of a septic tank should be at least 500 gallons. Septic tanks are not recommended for large communities.
2. **Length:** The length of a septic tank is usually twice the breadth.
3. **Depth:** The depth of a septic tank is from 1.5 to 2 m (5 to 7 ft).
4. **Liquid depth:** The recommended liquid depth is only 1.2 m (4 ft).
5. **Air space:** There should be a minimum air space of 30 cm (12 inch) between the level of liquid in the tank and the undersurface of the cover.
6. **Bottom:** In some septic tanks, the bottom is sloping towards the inlet end, this facilities retention of solids.
7. **Inlet and outlet:** There is an inlet and outlet pipe, which are submerged.
8. **Cover:** The septic tank is covered by a concrete slab of suitable thickness and provided with a manhole.
9. **Retention period:** Septic tanks are designed in this country to allow retention in undue septicity of the effluent whereas too short, period gives insufficient treatment (Fig. 15.11).

Sewage purification in septic tank

The solids settle down in the tank to form 'sludge', while the lighter solids including grease and fat rise to the surface to form 'scum'. The solids are attacked by the anaerobic bacteria and fungi, and are broken down into simpler chemical compounds. This is the first stage of purification called anaerobic digestion. The sludge is much reduced in volume as a result of anaerobic digestion and is rendered stable, and in offensive. A portion of the solids is transferred into liquids and gases (principally methane), which rises to the surface in the form of bubbles.

The liquid, which passes out of the outlet pipe from time to time, is called the 'effluent'. It contains numerous bacteria, cysts, helminthic ova and organic matter in solution or fine suspension. The effluent is allowed to percolate into the subsoil. It is dispersed by means of perforated or open-jointed pipes laid in trenches 90 cm (3 ft) deep and the trenches are then covered with soil. The effluent percolates into the surrounding soil. There are millions of aerobic bacteria in the upper layers of the soil, which attack the organic matter present in the effluent. As a result, the organic matter present in the effluent. As a result, the organic matter is oxidized into stable end products, i.e. nitrates, carbon dioxide and water. This stage of purification is called aerobic oxidation. To sum up, two stages are involved in the purification of sewage.

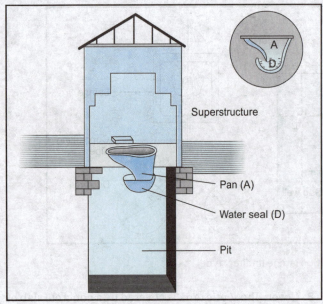

Figure 15.10: Hand flush water-seal latrine PRAI type [Planning Research-cum Action Institute (PRAI)].

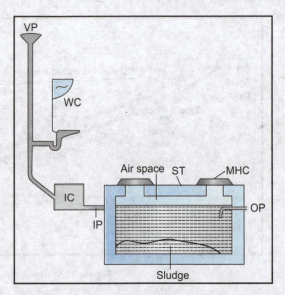

Figure 15.12: Septic tank latrine (IC, inspections chamber; IP, inlet pipe; MHC, manhole cover; OP, outlet pipe; ST, septic tank; VP, vent pipe; WC, water closet).

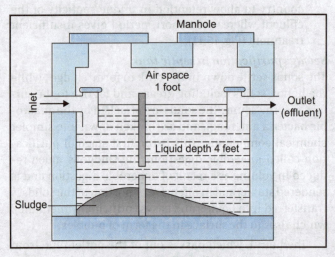

Figure 15.11: Septic tank

The first stage, anaerobic digestion takes place in the septic tank proper and the second stage, aerobic oxidation takes place outside the septic tank in the subsoil. Together, these two stages complete the purification of sewage (Fig. 15.12).

Maintenance of septic tank
1. The use of soap water and disinfectants such as phenol should be avoided, as they are injurious to the bacterial flora in the septic tank.
2. Undue accumulation of sludge reduces the capacity of the septic tank and interferes with proper working. Therefore, the contents of the septic tank should be bailed out at least once a year. This operation is called 'desludging'. The bailed out sludge is disposed of by trenching.
3. Newly built septic tanks are first filled with water up to the outlet level and then seeded with ripe sludge drawn from another septic tank, to provide the right type of bacteria to carry out the decomposition process.

Aqua privy
The aqua privy functions such as a septic tank and has been used in different regions in the country. The privy consists of a watertight chamber filled with water. A short length of a drop pipe from the latrine floor dips into the water. The shape of the tank may be circular or rectangular. The size of the tank depends upon the number of users. A capacity of 1 m^2 (35 ft^2) is recommended for a small family, allowing 6 years or more for cleansing purpose. Aqua privies are designed for public use also.

Night soil undergoes purification by anaerobic digestion. Since there is evolution of gases, vent should be provided for the escape of the gases into the atmosphere, the vent should be open above the roof dwellings. The effluent is far from innocuous. It contains finely divided fecal matter in suspension and may carry parasitic and infective agents. It should be treated in the same manner as the effluent from a septic tank by subsoil irrigation or absorption. The digested sludge, which accumulates in the tank, should be removed at intervals (Fig. 15.13).

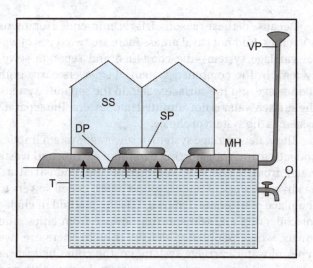

Figure 15.13: Aqua privy T tank (water tight) (DP, drop; MH, manhole; O, outlet; SP, squatting plate; SS, superstructure; VP, vent pipe).

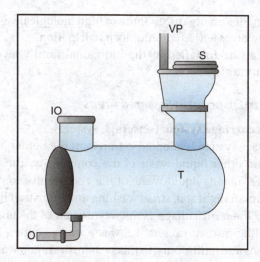

Figure 15.14: Chemical closet (T, tank; S, seat; VP, ventilation pipe; O, outlet; IO, inspection opening).

Chemical closet
The closet consists of a metal tank containing a disinfectant fluid. The active ingredients of the fluid are formaldehyde and ammonium compounds. In addition, a harmless water dye and a deodorizing substance are usually incorporated. A seat with a cover is placed directly over the tank. Nothing except the toilet paper should be thrown into the chemical closet (Fig. 15.14).

Latrines for camps or temporary use
Shallow trench latrine
Shallow trench latrine is simply a trench dug with ordinary tools. The trench is 30 cm (1 ft) wide and 90–150 cm (3–5 ft) deep. Its length depends on the number of users 3–3.5 m (10–12 ft) are necessary for 100 people. Separate trenches should be provided for men and women. The earth from the trench should be piled up at the side. People should be instructed to cover feces with earth each time they use the latrine. However, these instructions may not be carried out and it will be necessary to post sweepers in attendance to do this work. Ablution water should be provided. The shallow trench is a rudimentary arrangement for a short period (up to 1 week). When the trench is filled to 30 cm (12 inch) below ground level, it must be covered with earth, heaped above ground level and compacted; if necessary, a new trench must be dug.

Biogas plant
Deep trench latrine
Deep trench type of latrine is intended for camps of longer duration from a few weeks to a few months. The trench is 1.8–2.5 m (6–8 ft) deep and 75–90 cm (30–35 inch) wide. Depending upon the local customs, a seat or a squatting plate is provided. A superstructure is built for privacy and protection. Other requirements are the same as for shallow trench latrine.

Biogas plant
Biogas plants are also popularly known as gobargas plant. In this method not only the human night soil is disposed off, but also animal dung and left over animal feeds are also disposed.

A suitable place in the courtyard near the cattle-shed is selected. A well of about 3 meters is dug with variable diameter depending upon the size of the livestock. A small chamber called 'mixing chamber' is constructed at one end of the cattle shed near the well, where animal dung after collection from allowed in this chamber. The human night soil urine and wash water of the sanitary latrine is also drained into the same digester. An inverted dome-shaped metallic gas holder is put in the well, which holds gases produced in the digester, chiefly the methane. As the gas collects, dome rises. The gas is utilized for lighting and cooking purposes (Figs 15.15A and B).

The scum and sludge are periodically removed and disposed in trenches, which later becomes an excellent organic manure.

Benefits of biogas plant
- Human and animal excreta can be disposed simultaneously
- It is an excellent source of energy at a low cost
- Refuse can also be disposed

- Provides an organic manure of high biological value
- It involves active community participation
- It can be installed at the individual family level or community.

Excreta Disposal in Sewered Areas

Water carriage system (sewerage system)

Sewerage system is adopted to transport the human night soil and other liquid waste of the community. The term 'sewage' means liquid waste of the community containing human night soil, street washing and industrial liquid waste. The term 'sullage' is the waste water of the houses, excluding human excreta, i.e. waste water coming from kitchens and bathrooms. In this system, the liquid waste is carried away through a system of drains and underground pipes (sewers) from the houses, industries and commercial areas, through the agency of water to the place of ultimate disposal. Therefore it requires an abundant water supply. Even though the initial investment is heavy, it is cheaper in the long run and is the cleanest quickest and most sanitary method of removing night soil. For successful operations the following conditions are essential:

- An abundant supply of water
- Good drains and sewers with proper ventilation
- Sufficient slope to give the required velocity to the sewage
- Proper means for disposal and utilization of the sewage.

Because of these reasons, it is recommended for towns and cities, and not rural areas. There are two types of water carriage system—the combined and separate sewer system. In the combined system, the sewers carry both the sewage and the surface water. In the separate system, the surface water is not admitted into sewers. The separate system is the system of choice.

The water carriage system or sewerage system implies collecting and transporting of human excreta and waste water from residential, commercial and industrial areas by a network of underground pipes, called sewers to the place of ultimate disposal. It is the method of choice for collecting and transporting sewage from cities, and towns, where population density is high. There are two types of water carriage system, i.e. the combined sewer system and the separate sewer system. In the combined system, the sewers carry both the sewage and surface water. In the separate system, surface water is not admitted into sewers. The separate system is considered the system of choice today. The problem is one of the economics; a heavy outlay of capital is needed to install a water carriage system. Since water is needed for flushing the toilets and for conveying the human wastes, there can be no sewerage system without a piped water supply.

A water carriage system consists of the following elements:

- Household sanitary fittings (plumbing system of buildings)
- House sewers

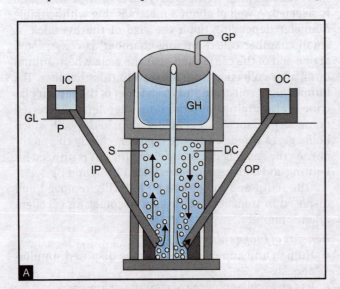
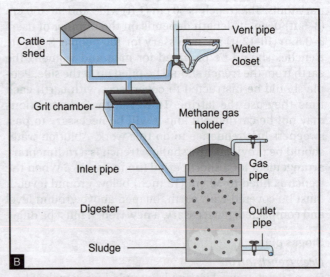

Figures 15.15A and B: Biogas plant. **A.** Plan of chamber (DC, digesting chamber; GH, gas holder; GL, ground level; GP, gas pipe; IC, inlet chamber; IP, inlet pipe; OC, outlet chamber; OP, outlet pipe; P, pipe); **B.** Plan of biogas plant implementation.

- Street sewers or trunk sewers
- Sewer appurtenances, e.g. manholes, traps, etc.

Household sanitary fittings

Where sewers exist, every house is expected to be connected to the nearest sewer. The usual household sanitary fittings are water closet, urinal and wash basin.

Water closets may be broadly divided into two types, i.e. Indian squatting type and the Western commode type. An ideal water closet bowl (western type) is shown in Figure 15.16. It is recommended that for efficient performance:

- The water seal are should not be more than 7.5 cm
- There should not be any sharp corners in the trap design
- The volume of water in trap should be as little as possible, preferably not exceeding 1.75 liters to maintain a minimum of 50 mm deep water seal
- The interior of the bowl should be vertical at least 50–75 mm just above the surface of water sea.

The water closets are provided with a 'flushing rim'. Human excreta are directly received into the water in the closet without soiling the sides. The flushing removes all traces of excreta from the sides and keeps the closet clean. The closet is connected to a small cistern by a pipe 2.5–3.75 cm (1–1.5 inch) in diameter. The flushing cistern normally holds 15 liters (3 gallons) of water and works by symphonic action. The flushing cisterns can be classified as high level, low level and integrated depending upon the height of location above the water closet bowl or pan. The Indian squatting type water closet pans are used with high-level flushing cisterns.

House sewer (drain)

The house drain is usually 10 cm (4 inch) in diameter and is laid in the courtyard about 15 cm (6 inch) below the ground level on a bed of cement concrete with sufficient gradient towards the main drain. The house drain empties the sewage into the main sewer or public drain.

Through soil pipe and house drain, removes the excreta through the agency of water immediately, thus preventing the nuisance by sight, smell and flies.

A water closet consists of two parts—closet proper and the flushing apparatus:

1. Closet proper: This is of two types—Indian and Western types. The Indian type consists of a squatting plate below, which is a pan (or basin) with a trap, opening into the connecting pipe. The squatting plate has got footrest on either side of the pan proper. All these apparatus are placed flush with the floor of the closet apartment. The western type consists of a bowl with a flushing rim near the surface and a trap below. It is called commode (Fig. 15.17).

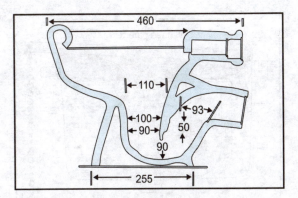

Figure 15.16: An ideal water closet (western type)

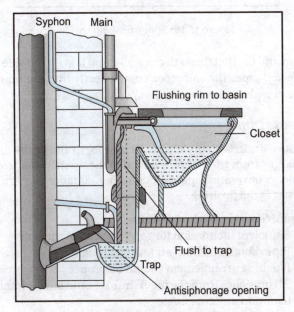

Figure 15.17: Siphonic closet

2. Flushing apparatus: This consists of a small cistern or tank placed about 1 m above the basin, holding about 15 liters of water and works by siphonic action either by pulling a chain or pedal action, or a hand button and delivers the water by pipe to flush out the excreta into the connecting pipe, keeping the closet or pan clean (Fig. 15.18).

Soil pipes

Soil pipes are the pipes laid vertically outside the wall, meant to carry the excreta from the closet to the house drain on one side and for the escape of foul gas on the other side covered with wire-gauze dome.

When several closets on different floors discharge into a common soil pipe, the transmission of excreta from the upper closets down the soil pipe may cause unsealing of the traps of the lower closets by siphon action is ensured by means of an another pipe, fixed on the crown of the

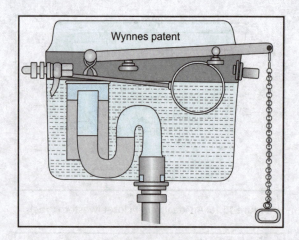

Figure 15.18: Siphon flushing cistern

trap and carried through the walls, and laid on the side of the soil pipe. The soil pipes open directly into the house drain without any intervention of a trap.

House Drain

House drain is an underground pipe for draining the discharges from the soil pipe and also the waste water from able to have an inspection chamber. Smaller the drain better is the flushing.

Requirements of a house drain
- Sufficient inclination for good velocity to the flow
- Pipes should be both air and water tight
- Flushing arrangement should be proper
- All branches from the main drain should have Y joints, to obtain an acute angle
- It should be laid on a bed of concrete.

Gully trap
Gully trap is placed in courtyards, especially where rain water and waste water pipes open. It is placed about 30 cm away from the wall and the surface opening is protected by a grating. Since there is a possibility of sweeping of the mud, debris and other particles into the gully, a provision is made for such particles to settle at the bottom of the gully trap, which can be removed periodically.

Trunk sewer
The trunk sewers are not less than 22.5 cm (9 inch) in diameter; bigger ones may be 2–3 m (8–10 ft) in diameter. They are laid on a bed of cement concrete, about gradient to ensure what is known as 'self-cleansing'. Velocity varies from 2 to 3 ft/second. The trunk sewers collect sewage from several houses and transport to the main outfall or place of final disposal.

Public sewer
Public sewer are big underground pipes, laid in concrete bed, meant for draining the sewage (liquid waste) from several houses and also other liquid waste of the community. It should have sufficient gradient to ensure 'self-cleansing' velocity. It is carried to the ultimate place of disposal.

Sewer appurtenances
Sewer appurtenances consist of inspection chambers and intercepting trap:

1. **Inspection chamber:** These are also called 'manholes'. These are masonry underground chamber, lined with cement as to make water tight and covered with air tight iron lid (Fig. 15.19). These are placed or constructed at the following sites:
   - Where the direction of the sewer is changed
   - Where two or more sewers meet
   - At distance of 100 m in long straight runs.

   The chamber permits a person to enter inside to carry out inspection, repairs and cleaning activities. Since they are at risk of gas poisoning and asphyxiation, due precautions are taken for their safety.

2. **Intercepting trap:** This is interposed between the house drain and the sewer. It is also called 'disconnecting trap' (Fig. 15.20). These are designed to remove sand, grit and grease from sewage.

Sewer accessories
Sewer accessories are manholes and traps, which are installed in the sewage system.

Manholes are openings built into the sewerage system. They are placed, whenever there is a change in the direction of sewers; at the meeting point of two or more sewers; and at distance of 100 m in long straight runs.

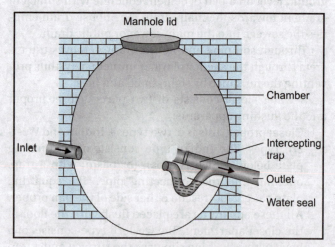

Figure 15.19: Manhole chamber

These openings permit a man to enter the sewer for inspection, repairs and cleaning. Workers entering the manholes are liable to gas poisoning and asphyxiation. Due precautions should be taken to ensure their safety. Traps are of various kinds, these are devices designed to prevent foul gases entering the houses and to remove sand, grit and grease from sewage. Traps are placed in three situations:

- Under the basin of water closets
- Where the house drain joins the public drain (intercepting trap)
- Where surface waste water enters the drains.

Sewerage system installation involves considerable planning, designing, construction, operation, maintenance and administration, each calling for specialized skills one generation.

Sewage and its treatment
Sewage is a mixture of human excreta, urine, wash water, liquid waste coming from bathrooms and kitchen, surface water and industrial liquid waste. It is dirty water with unpleasant sight and smell, which if not drained and disposed of, can contaminate sources of water and also food and vegetables resulting in diseases and deaths.

Objectives of sewage treatment
- Protection of water sources from contamination
- Protection of soil against pollution
- Protection of fish and aquatic lives
- Protection of human food, which are eaten raw
- Prevention of hazards to live-stocks
- Prevention of nuisance by sight and smell

Therefore, from hygienic and esthetic considerations, sewage treatment is also far and wide. Valuable recoveries are possible from a completely treated sewage such as nitrates, phosphates, vitamin B_{12} methane gas for lighting and cooking purposes, grease, etc.

The aim of the sewage treatment is to stabilize the organic matter by bacterial action, to utilize the innocuous products without risk to human health and to produce an effluent, which can be disposed off into land, river or sea without causing danger. Stabilization means breaking the organic matter into simpler substances, which cannot be decomposed further.

The quality or strength of the sewage is expressed in terms of biochemical oxygen demand, chemical oxygen demand and suspended solids. These indicators are required to know the amount of water needed to dilute the sewage during its final disposal.

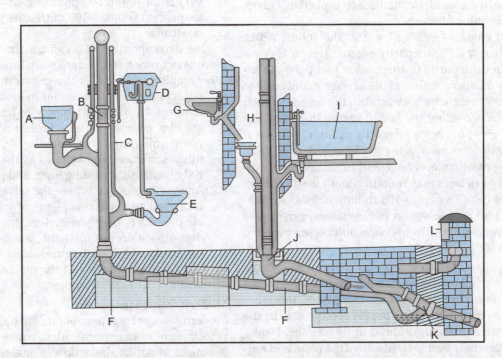

Figure 15.20: Complete system of house drainage. A and E. Two closets, which open into the soil pipe; B and C. Antisiphonage pipe; D. Flushing cistern opening into the closet; E and F. House drain laid on a bed of concrete; G. Wash basin; H. Rain water pipe; I. Bath tub—these empty into the gully trap; J and K. Intercepting trap placed in the manhole chamber intercepting the house drain from the sewer; L. Inlet opening for ventilation—the soil pipe and the ventilating pipes are carried above the roof and are protected by wire gauze; they act as outlets.

Sewage is waste water from community-containing solid and liquid excreta, derived from houses, street and yard washing, factories and industries. It resembles dirty water with an unpleasant smell. The term 'sullage' is applied to waste water from kitchens and bathrooms. The amount of sewage that flows in the sewage depends upon:

1. Habits of people: If people use more water, there will be more sewage.
2. Time of day: Sewage is subject to variations depending upon the time of day and during different seasons. In the morning, when people tend to use more water there is greater quantity and flow, in mid-day the flow is less, and again there is a slight increase in the evening. The average amount of sewage, which flows through the sewage system in 24 hours, is called 'dry weather flow'.

Prompt measure has to be taken to provide proper mean of sewage disposal, if not, the following problems will emerge:
- Creation of nuisance, unsightliness and unpleasant odors
- Breeding of flies and mosquitoes
- Pollution of soil and water supplies
- Contamination of food
- Increase in the incidence of disease, especially enteric and helminthic diseases.

Sewage contains 99.9% of water. The solids, which comprise barely 0.1%, are partly organic and partly non-organic; they are partly in suspension and partly in solution. The offensive nature of the sewage mainly due to the organic matter, which it contains, the organic matter decomposes according the law of nature during which process it gives offensive odors. In addition, sewage is charged with numerous living organisms derived from feces, some of which may be agents to disease. It is estimated that 1 g of feces may contain about 1,000 million of *Escherichia coli (E. coli)*, 10–100 million of fecal streptococci and 1–10 million spores of *Clostridium perfringens* besides several others. The average adult person excreted daily some 100 g of feces.

Goal of sewage treatment
Inadequately treated sewage should not be discharged into rivers, sea or other sources of water supply. This is because, the oxygen in the water supply is used up to by the numerous aerobic bacteria found in the sewage. Depletion of oxygen may lead to the death of the plant and animal life in water. That water may yield an offensive smell due to the release of hydrogen sulfide.

The goal of sewage treatment is to 'stabilize' the organic matter so that it can be disposed off safely; and to convert sewage water into an effluent of an acceptable standard of purity, which can be disposed off till land, rivers or sea. A standard test, which is an indicator of the organic content of the sewage, is biochemical oxygen demand. The 'strength' of the sewage is expressed in terms of:

1. Biochemical oxygen demand (BOD): It is defined as the amount of oxygen absorbed by a sample of sewage during a specified period, generally 5 days at a specified temperature, generally 20°C for the aerobic destruction or use of organic matter in living organisms. BOD values range from about 1 mg/L for natural waters, about 300 mg/L for untreated domestic sewage. If the BOD is 300 mg/L and above sewage is said to be 'strong'; if it is 100 mg/L, it is said to be 'weak'.
2. Chemical oxygen demand (COD): The COD test measures the oxygen equivalent of that portion of the organic matter in a sample, which is susceptible to oxidation matter in a sample that is susceptible to oxidation of strong chemical oxidizer. If wastes contain toxic substances, this test may be the only practical method for determining the organic load.
3. Suspended solids: The suspended solids are yet another indicator of the 'strength' of sewage. The amount of suspended solids in domestic sewage may vary from 100 to 500 ppm (mg/L). If the amount of suspended solids is 100 mg/L, the sewage is said to be strong.

The decomposition of organic matter in sewage takes place by two processes, i.e. aerobic and anaerobic processes:

1. Aerobic process: It is the most efficient method of reducing the organic matter in sewage. The process requires a continuous supply of free dissolved oxygen. The organic matter is broken down into simpler compounds namely carbon dioxide, water ammonia, nitrites, nitrates and sulfates by the action of bacterial organisms including fungi and protozoa.
2. Anaerobic process: Where the sewage is highly concentrated and contains plenty of solids, the anaerobic process is highly effective. The end products of decomposition are methane, ammonia, carbon dioxide and hydrogen. In anaerobic decomposition the reactions are slower and the mechanism of decomposition extremely complex.

Modern sewage treatment
Modern sewage treatment plants are based on biological principles of sewage purification, where the purification is bought about by the action of anaerobic and aerobic bacteria. The treatment of sewage may be divided into two stages, primary treatment and secondary treatment. Figures 15.21 and 15.22 shows the flow diagram of modern sewage treatment plant.

CHAPTER 15 Sanitation: Disposal of Waste 167

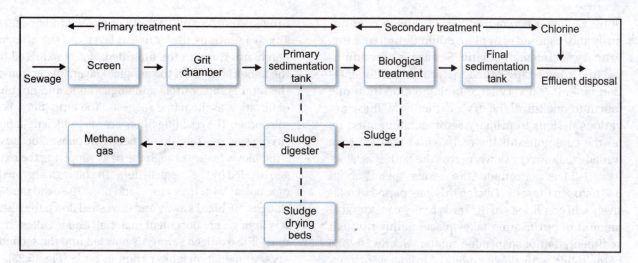

Figure 15.21: Modern sewage treatment plant

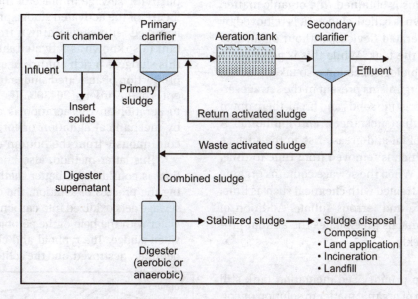

Figure 15.22: Plan of sewage treatment

Primary treatment

In primary treatment, solids are separated from the sewage party by screening and partly by sedimentation, and subjected to anaerobic digestion, which is the first stage in purification. Primary treatment constitutes:

1. Screening: Sewage arriving at a disposal work is first passed through a metal screen, which intercepts large floating objects such as pieces of wood, rags, masses of garbage and dead animals. Their removal is necessary to prevent clogging of the treatment plant. The screen consists of vertical or inclined steel bars usually set 5 cm (2 inch) apart. In some plants, the screens are of the fixed type, while in others the screens are of the moving type. The screenings are removed from time-to-time either manually or mechanically and disposed of by trenching or burial.

2. Grit chamber: Sewage is then passed through a long narrow chamber is approximately 10–20 m in length. It is so designed as to maintain a constant velocity of about 1 foot per second, with a detention period of 30 seconds to 1 minute. The function of the grit chamber is to allow the settlement of heavier solids such as sand and gravel, while permitting the organic matter to pass through. The grit, which collects at the bottom

of the chamber is removed periodically or continuously and disposed of by plain dumping or trenching.

3. **Primary sedimentation tank:** Sewage is now admitted into a huge tank called the primary sedimentation tank. It is a very large tank, holding from one fourth to one third, the dry weather flow. These are various designs in primary sedimentation tank. By far the commonest is the rectangular tank. Sewage is made to flow very slowly across the tank at a velocity of 1–2 feet per minute. The sewage spends about 6–8 hours in the tank. During this long period of relatively still conditions in the tank, a very considerable amount of purification takes place mainly through sedimentation of suspended matter. Nearly 50–70% of the solids settle down under the influence of gravity. A reduction between 30 and 40% in the number of coliform organisms is obtained. The organic matter, which settles down is called 'sludge', it is removed by mechanically operated devices, without disturbing the operation in the tank. While this is going on, a small amount of biological action also takes place in which the microorganisms present in the sewage, attack on complex organic solids and break them down into simpler soluble substances, and ammonia. A certain amount of fat and grease rise to the surface to form scum, which is removed from time to time, and disposed off. When the sewage contains organic trade wastes, it is treated with chemical such as lime, aluminum sulfate and ferrous sulfate. Addition of one of these chemicals precipitates the animal protein material quickly.

Secondary treatment

The effluent from the primary sedimentation tank still contains a proportion of organic matter in solution or colloidal state and numerous living organisms. It has a high demand for oxygen and cause pollution of soil or water. It is subjected to further treatment, aerobic oxidation by one of the following methods:

1. **Trickling filter:** The trickling filter or, percolating filter is a bed of crushed stones or clinker, 1–2 m (4–8 ft) deep and 2–30 m (6–100 ft) in diameter, depending upon the size of the population. The effluent from the primary sedimentation tank is sprinkled uniformly on the surface of the bed by a revolving device. The device consists of hollow pipes each of which have a row of holes. The pipes keep rotating, sprinkled uniformly on the surface and down through the filter, a very complex biological growth consisting of algae, fungi, protozoa and bacteria of many kinds occurs. This is known as the 'zoogleal layer'. As the effluent percolates through the filter bed, it gets oxidized by the bacterial flora in the zoogleal layer. The action of the filter is thus purely a biological one and not one of filtration as the name suggests. The term 'filter' is a misnomer. The trickling filters are very efficient in purifying sewage. They do not need rest-pauses, because wind blows freely through the beds supplying the oxygen needed by the zoogleal flora. The biological growth of zoogleal layer liver grows and dies. The dead matter sloughs off, breaks away and is washed down the filter. It is light green, flocculent material, and is called 'humus'. The oxidized sewage is now led into the secondary sedimentation tanks or humus tanks (Fig. 15.23).

2. **Activated sludge process:** It is the modern method of purifying sewage in place of the trickling filter. The 'heart' of the activated sludge process is the aeration is mixed with sludge drawn from the final settling tank (also known as activated sludge or return sludge; this sludge is a rich culture of aerobic bacteria). The proportion of activated sludge to the incoming effluent is of the order of 20–30%. The mixture is subjected to aeration in the aeration is accomplished either by mechanical agitation or forcing compressed air continuously from the bottom of the aeration tank.

This latter method, also known as 'diffuse aeration' is considered a better method of aeration. During the process of aeration, the organic matter of the sewage gets oxidized into carbon dioxide, nitrates and water with the help of the aerobic bacteria in the activated sludge. The typhoid and cholera organisms are definitely destroyed, and the coliforms greatly reduced.

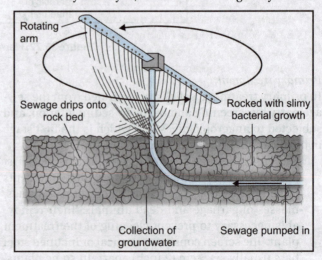

Figure 15.23: Trickling filter

Activated sludge plants occupy less space, require skilled operations. Activated sludge process is therefore, best suited for larger cities and the percolating filter for smaller towns because they are cheaper to install and easier to operate (Fig. 15.24).

Secondary sedimentation

The oxidized sewage from the trickling filter or aeration chamber is led into the secondary sedimentation tank, where it is led into the secondary sedimentation tank, where it is detained for 2–3 hours. The sludge that collects in the secondary sedimentation tank is called 'aerated sludge' or activated sludge, because it is fully aerated. It differs from the sludge in the primary sedimentation tank in that it is practically inoffensive and is rich in bacteria, nitrogen and phosphates. It is a valuable manure, if into the 'aeration tanks'. In the activated sludge process and the rest pumped into the sludge digestion tanks for treatment, and disposal.

Sludge disposal

One of the greatest problems associated with sewage treatment is the treatment and disposal of the resulting sludge. One million gallons of sewage produces 15–20 tons of sludge. The sludge is a thick, black mass containing 95% of water and it has a revolting odor. There are a number of methods of sludge disposal:

1. Digestion: Modern sewage treatment plants employ digestion of sludge as the method of treatment. If sludge is incubated under favorable conditions of temperature and pH, it undergoes anaerobic auto-digestion in which complex solids are broken down into water, carbon dioxide, methane and ammonia. The volume of sludge is also considerably reduced. It takes 3–4 weeks or longer for complete sludge digestion. The residue is in offensive, sticky and tarry mud, which will dry readily, and form excellent manure. Sludge digestion is carried out in special tanks known as 'sludge digestion tanks'. Methane gas, which is a byproduct of sludge digestion, can be used for heating and lighting purposes.
2. Sea disposal: Sea coast towns and cities can dispose of sludge by pumping it into the sea.
3. Land: Sludge can be disposed of by composting with town refuse.
4. Disposal effluent by dilution: Disposal of water courses such as rivers and streams is called 'disposal by dilution'. The effluent is diluted in the body of water and the impurities are oxidized by the dissolved oxygen in water. The diluting capacity of river or the receiving body of water and is dissolved oxygen contents are important considerations before discharging the effluent into a river or any body of water. Since people use river water for drinking purpose, the effluent must be rendered free from pathogenic organisms by adequate chlorination.
5. Disposal on land: If suitable land is available the effluent can be used for irrigation purposes (e.g. the Okhla Sewage Treatment Plant in Delhi).

Other methods

Methods of sewage disposal other than sewage treatment are as follows:

1. Sea outfall: Seacoast towns and cities may dispose of their sewage by discharging it into the sea. Purification takes places by dilution in the large body of sea water and the solids get slowly oxidized. The drawback of this method is that the offensive solid matter may be washed back to the shore and create public nuisance. In order to prevent this, the sewage outfall is designed to discharge the sewage into deep water at many points.
2. River outfall: Raw sewage should never be discharged into rivers. The present day practice is to purify the sewage before it is discharged into rivers. How far the sewage should be purified depends upon the dilution the river provides to carryon aeration and self-purification.
3. Land treatment (sewage farming): If sufficient and suitable land (porous soil) is available sewage may be applied to the land after grift removal; type of treatment is practiced in some Indian towns and cities and is known as sewage farming or broad irrigation.

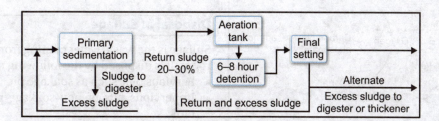

Figure 15.24: Activated sludge process

An acre of land would be required to treat the sewage of 100–300 persons. The land is first laid into the ridges and furrows. Sewage is fed into the furrows intermittently and crops are grown on the ridges. The crops that are found suitable to grow are those which do not come in contact with sewage and likely to be eaten raw. Fodder grass and potatoes seem to be the most paying crops. Fruit trees whose fruits are high above the ground (e.g. plantain) can be grown. But sugar cane, coriander, cucumber, tomato, onion, etc. should not be grown. The farm should be under the direction of a competent not be possible to operate the sewage farms. Badly managed farms stink, a condition described as 'sewage sickness' because of lack of sufficient aeration and rest pauses to the land. Alternate methods of disposal may have to be provided during the rainy season.

4. **Oxidation pond:** A cheap method of sewage treatment is the oxidation pond (Fig. 15.25), which has been referred to by many different names such as waste stabilization pond, redox pond, sewage lagoons, etc. The term 'waste' includes both sewage and industrial wastes; although, an old method of purifying sewage, oxidation pond has attracted the attention of public health engineers only recently. Over 50 ponds are working at present in India. The first large-scale installation was at Bhilai, where it serves as population of 100,000.

   The oxidation pond is an open, shallow pool 1–1.5 m (3–5 ft) deep with an inlet and outlet. To qualify as an oxidation pond, there must be the presence of algae certain types of bacteria, which feed on decaying organic matter and sunlight. The organic matter contained in the sewage is oxidized by bacteria (hence, oxidation pond) to simple chemical compounds such as carbon dioxide, ammonia and water. The algae, with the help of sunlight, utilize the carbon dioxide, ammonia and water, and inorganic minerals for their growth. Thus, there is a mutually beneficial biological balance between the algae and bacteria in oxidation ponds. Oxygen that is needed for oxidation is derived in a small extent from the atmosphere, but mostly from the algae, which liberates oxygen under the influence of sunlight. Consequently, sunlight is an important factor in the proper functioning of oxidation ponds. Cloudy weather definitely lowers the efficiency of the process.

   The oxidation ponds are predominantly aerobic during sunshine hours as well as some hours of the night. In the remaining hours of night, the bottom layers are generally anaerobic. Thus, sewage purification in oxidation ponds is brought about by a combination of aerobic and anaerobic types of bacteria. The effluent may be used for growing vegetable crops (land irrigation) or may be discharged into river or other water courses after appropriate treatment. Mosquito nuisance is avoided by keeping weed growth in the neighborhood of oxidation ponds to a minimum and the water line free from marginal vegetation. There is no odor nuisance associated with these ponds when they are properly maintained. Oxidation ponds have become an established method of purifying sewage for small communities.

5. **Oxidation ditches:** Other methods recommended are oxidation ditches and aerated lagoons. These methods make use of mechanical rotors for extended aeration. For treatment of the wastes of a population between 5,000 and 20,000 an oxidation ditch requires an area of 1 acre as compared to 22 acres for an oxidation pond, and 2.5 acres for an aerated lagoon. These are low-cost treatment methods for the purification of sewage.

Disposal of Sullage

Sullage is the waste water coming from kitchen and bathroom. It is disposed by the following methods:
- Pervious pits, such as soakage pit
- Impervious pits or non-soakage pits, such as septic tank
- Surface irrigation, such as kitchen garden
- Underground drainage or sewerage system.

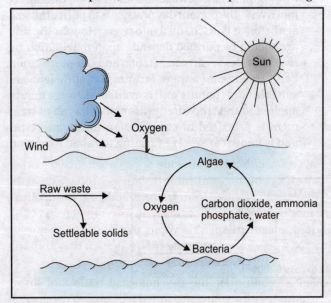

Figure 15.25: Oxidation pond

Soakage Pit

Soakage pit is also called soak pit or seepage pit. It is the simplest and cheapest method of disposal of sullage water in villages, on a small scale.

For individual houses a pit of about 1½ m³ of rectangular shape is dogged, filled from bottom to top with large stones, brick bats and gravel, lined with bricks, keeping open the joints for absorption. The topmost layer is of gravel or sand. It is covered with a gunny cloth, tarred on both sides to prevent the loose soil slipping into the trench and block it (Fig. 15.26). Bottom of the pit should be sloping away from the house. The pit is dug at a strategic point in courtyard of the house wherein sullage can be admitted.

Since the sullage contains grease, oil, detergents and solid waste, these are removed by allowing the sullage to pass through an earthen pot (matka or kerstin tin) with perforated bottom, filled with straw and grass. If not removed these will interfere with proper functioning of soakage pit. The perforated pot with grass is also therefore known as 'grease trap'. Grass has to be changed periodically, once in 10–15 days, depending upon the waste water. Use of grease trap is not essential in hot climates because fats do not solidify. It would be still better if a small grit chamber is constructed between the outlet of the house and the soakage pit. This small chamber functions like that of gully trap to remove solid waste from the sullage. T-shaped pipe connection is made between the outlet of the house and the matka.

The sullage from the house is drained to the grease trap and then to the soakage pit through submerged pipes. As the sullage passes through the grease trap, the grease, oil, garbage, food waste, grit or dust, etc. are all mechanically trapped. The sullage passes through the bottom of the trap into the soakage pit, where it gets large area for biological degradation by the aerobic bacteria in the pit, ultimately converting it into harmless inorganic substance. The water percolates into the ground.

After sometime, the pit become sullage sick, because pores become clogged. So, another pit must be constructed by the side and two pits are made to work alternatively. When one becomes sullage sick, it is drugged up and exposed to air and sun, and filled again with fresh stones and gravel.

DISPOSAL OF DEAD BODIES

Death is universal experience and every culture has some rituals associated with death. When there are many fatalities, then the collection and disposal of dead bodies is must in an appropriate way. As animals die, their body starts to decompose, emits foul smell and provides a place for breeding of various bacteria. Similarly human's body after death, if not disposed off properly, starts decomposing, resulting in bad smell (causing air pollution) and breeding place for microorganisms. It is important not only from health risk point, but also because of social and political impact. Dead bodies need to be disposed of properly considering the mental health of community in taking care of dead bodies.

As all the dead bodies are potentially infectious, so there is need to implement the standard precautions. Most of the organisms in dead bodies are unlikely to cause infection in healthy individuals, but some infections microorganisms can be transmitted to the persons handling the body with body fluids and tissue as they are in close contact with dead body. So it becomes inevitable to reduce the risk of transmission through proper handling thereby reducing the exposure to blood and body fluids. An appropriate approach should be used to minimize the risk of infection such as:

- Staff training
- Education
- Safe working environment
- Use of safety devices
- Vaccination against hepatitis B.

Health Risks (According to WHO)

Physical health risks: The wide spread belief that corpse pose a risk of communicable disease is wrong. Especially if the death resulted from trauma, bodies are unlikely to cause out breaks of diseases such as typhoid fever, cholera or plague, though they may transmit gastroenteritis or food poisoning syndrome to survivors, if they contaminate streams, wells or other water resources.

Mental health risks: The psychological trauma of losing loved ones and witnessing the death on a large scale is the greatest cause for concern. It is therefore important

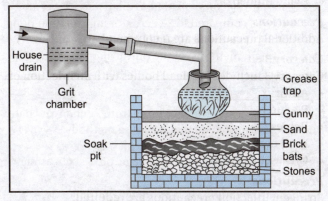

Figure 15.26: Soakage pit

to collect corpses as quickly as possible to minimize this distress. It is however, not necessary to rush their burials or cremation. This does not allow correct identifications and record taking of the details of the dead. Nor does it give the time for the bereaved to carry out the ceremonial and cultural practices, which would normally occur after a death.

Cultural and religious practices: Relief workers should respect the wishes of the families and communities of the dead to observe whatever cultural, and religious events are usually practiced on death. This is important in helping people deal with psychological impact of such disasters. Encouraging stricken communities to carry out traditional ceremonies and grieving processes sets in motion the process of disaster recovery.

Methods of disposal of bodies

The two methods of disposal of dead bodies are:
1. Burial.
2. Cremation.

Burial: It is the most common method of disposal. According to WHO the location of graveyards should be agreed with the community and attention should be given to ground conditions, proximity to ground water drinking sources (which should be at least 50 m) and to the nearest habitat (500 m). An area of at least 1,500 m² per 10,000 populations is required.

The burial site should be divided to accommodate different religious groups if necessary. Burial depth should be at least 1.5 m above the ground water label, with at least 1 m covering of soil. Burial in individual graves is preferred and can be dug manually. If coffins are not available, corpses should be wrapped in plastic sheeting to keep the remains separate from the soil. Burial procedures should be consistent with the usual practices of the community concern.

Cremation: It is the second most common method of disposal of dead bodies. Cremation method is preferred by some communities because of religious or cultural reasons. Cremation requires approximate 300 kg of wood for a single cremation. This method also causes smoke pollution. According to WHO, for this reason, cremation site should be located at least 500 m downwind of dwelling. The resultant ashes should be disposed of according to the cultural and religious practices of community.

Other Methods

Mummification: This method was practiced by the ancient Egyptians.

Burial at sea: It is a form of burial in which the dead body was drift on a boat. It is often associated with the funeral, which also involves off the corpse.

Alkaline hydrolysis: In this method, strong solution of lye is used to dissolve corpses so that the remains can be flushed down the drain.

Legal Regulation for Disposal of Dead Bodies

Regulations have been enacted for disposal of human bodies in many areas/places. It may be entirely legal to bury a dead body, but the law restricts the locations in which this is allowed, in some cases it is carried out in licensed institutions. It is considered a crime, if the dead body is not disposed properly.

Precautions for Handling and Disposal of Dead Bodies

On the basis of transmission of infection, the dead bodies are categorized under three categories and depending upon the type of category precautions are used for handling and disposal of dead bodies.

Categorization

Category 1
Category 1 includes all dead bodies other than those listed in category 2 and 3.

Precautions
Standard precautions are recommended.

Category 2
Category 2 includes the dead bodies with known:
- Human immunodeficiency virus (HIV)
- Hepatitis C
- Creutzfeldt-Jakob disease (CJD) without necropsy
- Severe acute respiratory syndrome (SARS)
- Avian influenza.

Precautions
Additional precautions are recommended.

Category 3
Category 3 includes the dead bodies with an infection of:
- Anthrax
- Plague
- Rabies
- Viral hemorrhagic fevers
- CJD with necropsy.

Precautions
Stringent infection precautions are required.

CHAPTER 15 — Sanitation: Disposal of Waste

Standard precautions for all dead bodies under category 1

1. Hepatitis B vaccination is recommended for all staff, which is likely to come in contact with dead bodies.
2. Nursing and other personnel, who handle dead body, must wear protective clothing consisting of gown/apron and gloves.
3. They should cover all cuts and abrasions with waterproof bandages.
4. Wound drainage and needle puncture holes should be disinfected with 1% household bleach and dressed with impermeable material.
5. The body should be cleaned and dried.
6. After removing protective clothing, hands should be washed thoroughly.

Additional precautions required for category 2 and 3

Additional precautions include all the precautions carried out in category 1 and additional precautions as given below:

1. Disposal linen should be discarded into red plastic waste bag, which should be accurately tied and sent for disposal.
2. Linen and protective clothing should be autoclaved or enclosed in 0.1% household bleach (1.50 dilution) for 30 minutes. All surface, which is contaminated should be disinfected with 0.1% household bleach.
3. Equipments should be autoclaved or decontaminated appropriately.
4. After removing protective clothing and gloves, hands should be washed thoroughly.

Make sure that while handling dead bodies under any category, do not smoke, eat or drink and avoid touching their own mouth, eyes, nose with their hands.

In epidemics

According to WHO, disposal of dead bodies when there is epidemic, is discussed below. Where possible, in the case of mass deaths due to infectious disease, body handling should be left to specialist medical staff. Rather than using lime for disinfection purposes, which has a limited effect on infectious pathogens, it is better to use chlorine solution or other medical disinfection for after use. It is important to make communities aware of the risks of being contagious from practices such as traditional washing of the dead. Also, any large gathering, including a funeral, can be away of spreading an epidemic. Consequently burial or cremation should take place soon after death at a site near the place of death with limits placed on the size of any gathering.

Contact with the body leads to exposure to *Vibrio cholerae* and requires careful washing of hands using soap and water.

Ebola is spread through bodily secretions such as blood, saliva, vomit, urine and stools, but can be easily killed with soap and water. Those dealing with disposal of bodies require high level of protection.

To avoid infestation with the fleas and lice that spread diseases such as typhus and plague, protective clothing should be worn. Body bags should be used to store the bodies prior to burial or cremation.

Important principles

According to WHO:
- Give priority to the living over the dead
- Dispel fears about health risks posed by corpses
- Identify and tag corpses
- Provide appropriate mortuary services
- Reject unceremonious and mass disposal of unidentified corpses
- Respond to the wishes of the family
- Respect cultural and religious observances
- Proper use of protective equipment in handling dead bodies
- Educate the public with proper sanitation and provide basic public health services to prevent outbreak of communicable diseases.

PROBLEM OF SANITATION IN INDIA

The problem of sanitation in India is that 'rural sanitation'. Studies have shown that 90% of the population 'go to the open fields' for defecation. This habit of indiscriminate fouling the surroundings with human excrement is generation old and rooted firmly in the cultural behavior of the Indian village people. In urban areas, the latrine is considered a necessary part of a house. In rural area, by and large, people have not accepted latrines with any enthusiasm, and even when installed only a few used them regularly. The problem in rural sanitation is how to overcome the resistance of the village people and induce them to use sanitary latrines. Some of the reasons found in the studies are:

- Latrines are associated with bad smell
- They are the breeding places of flies
- They are something foul and dirty so that one should not have them close to houses
- Latrines are costly and beyond their means to install
- They do not know how fecal-borne diseases are spread.

The solution of the problem lies in teaching the people first the reasons why latrines are important. The teaching should be undertaken by all known methods of health education-direct discussion, group discussion, latrine demonstrations and use of visual aids, and above all service facilities. The ultimate goal of health education will be to motivate the rural people towards acceptance and use of sanitary latrines.

SANITATION PROBLEMS AFFECTS THE PUBLIC HEALTH

First in public health importance are the many 'fecal-oral' infections acquired by consumption of contaminated food and drink. Children are particularly exposed to infection when playing or bathing in surface water. Surface water becomes contaminated with pathogens from blocked sewers and overflowing septic tanks. This contaminated surface water can infect people in many ways. Another important group of diseases related to poor drainage is transmitted by mosquitoes and malaria is the best example. Transmission can be particularly intense in urban areas, where there are relatively few animals to divert the vector species of mosquito from human blood meals. Drainage construction is an effective mosquito control measure. Urban poor may often build on land with drainage problems, but good urban planning can help to avoid making these problems worse.

FAIRS, FESTIVALS AND TRAFFIC SANITATION, AND MEASURES

1. Fairs and festival sanitation: Large number of cattle and religious fairs are being held every year in India. In addition to various festivals, these fairs and festivals vary in character and duration; because of the variable nature of fairs and festivals sanitary arrangement also vary to some extent. These fairs are the sources of spread of infections in the country. Besides fair, same type of arrangement are done for refugees, or during flood or emergency.
2. General and sanitary measures:
   a. Site selection.
   b. Formation of Mela Committees for:
      i. Funds.
      ii. Rules and control of staff.
      iii. Cooperation of different departments.
3. Water supply:
   a. Provision of safe water supply for fairs annually held and lasting for 2–3 weeks with a daily attendance of 50,000 or more people, permanent water supply at the rate of 6 gallons per day.
   b. One tap for 200 persons.
   c. Tube wells can be sunk for small fairs.
   d. Supply of water should be chlorinated and continuous.
   e. Wells in fairs and surrounding areas should be regularly disinfected with bleaching powder.
4. Disposal of refuse and human excreta:
   a. Whole area should be swept once a day, but more frequently in the areas of eating establishments.
   b. One sweeper per 100 persons.
   c. Equipment's such as wheel barrows, dustbins, carts and lorries to be provided disposal by the incineration or sanitary dumping.
   d. For disposal of excreta there should be borehole latrine or for temporary fair, shallow trench latrine.
   e. One seat for 50 persons properly fenced.
   f. Gammexane powder to be sprinkled on excreta deposited here and there on the earth.
   g. Soakage pit and urinal one for 500 persons to be provided.
5. Antifly measures:
   a. Use of gammexane on human excreta to prevent fly breeding.
   b. Proper disposal of refuse and excreta.
   c. Good general sanitation.
6. Food arrangements:
   a. Licensing of all food vendors and shops before mela begins.
   b. All rotten and exposed food should be destroyed.
   c. Sale of substandard food by taking food sample for analysis, under prevention of Food Adulteration Act, 1954, to be stopped.
7. Compulsory anticholera inoculation: It should be done in fairs. Inoculation should be arranged in rail and other transports.
8. Proper disposal of dead bodies: For both human and cattle.
9. Control of importation of infection:
   a. Arrangement for indoor and outdoor patient's saline infusion unit, ambulance, and first aid service and small laboratory.
   b. Service of voluntary organization such as National Cadet Corps (NCC), Scouts, Red Cross, etc. should be utilized. They should be given specific duty to perform.
10. Health education:
    a. A good opportunity for health education.
    b. Health exhibitions and health talks to be arranged.
    c. Arrangement of film show.
11. Accommodation:
    a. Temporary shed with water supply and electricity.
    b. Lodging house or dharamshala.
    c. No sick should be allowed to lodge.

12. Medical dispensary and hospital with necessary medicine.
13. General administration: For 53,000 persons or more, Chief Medical Officer or Civil Surgeon of the District should camp. Primary responsibility is of District Medical Officer of Health Fair should be divided in sectors and each sector should be kept under the charge of a Medical Officer assisted by the paramedical staff, such as sanitary inspectors, health inspectors, vaccinators, inoculators, disinfectors and sweepers. Duty chart should be strictly followed. Daily report should be sent to the higher authorities regularly.
14. After the fair (postmela period):
    a. Cleaning of entire area.
    b. Burning of refuse.
    c. Disinfection of wells and tanks.
15. Traffic sanitation: Sanitation of vehicle in which a man travels is important. It may be source of infection and a health hazard. An infectious passenger may be a source of danger to the healthy person.

    Sanitation in railway and steamer include supply of clean water, food, and disposal of refuse and excreta. The exhaust gases from buses are harmful. Under Indian Railways Act, a case of infectious disease cannot travel with others. A ship or aeroplane is regarded infected, if it has a case of cholera on board. Necessary actions and dichlorodiphenyltrichloroethane (DDT) spray are essential to disinfect the same.

ROLE OF NURSES IN ENVIRONMENTAL HEALTH

Community health nurses (CHN) should be advocates for transforming waste into usable products, for simply producing garbage and moving towards an integrated system of waste management. Nurses who work in the community should be aware of the types of environmental hazards present. The challenge of maintaining individual family community and worldwide environmental health and safety is tremendous. The CHN are in an ideal position to detect environmental hazards and to instruct or educate individual families, and communities on ways to avoid or alter environmental hazards.

The CHN may not always directly combat these hazards, but they do monitor, report, advise community members and serve action-oriented catalysts to initiate community activity. Water, air, soil and food hazards are only a few of the potential community hazards. To implement an ecological approach nurses must continually recognize the interaction among people and the environment in which they live. This human and environment interaction and its effects on health have been sources of concern, since early recorded events. Many problems have been solved, but new and often more difficult and resistant ones continually arise. This is what makes the role of the CHN dynamic and exciting.

CONCLUSION

Waste is a useless, unwanted material for which no use in intended. Human and animal activities generate waste. This waste can be divided into three main categories, i.e. solid, liquid or gaseous waste. Solid and liquid waste should be disposed off in a proper way, as improper disposed cause's health hazards. Improper handling and transfer of solid waste can cause the occurrence of diseases due to open sores, vectors, insects, which invade the refuse drugs. The diseases caused by solid waste pollution are plague, salmonellosis, endemic typhus, trichinosis (rodents), diarrhea, dysentery, cholera, malaria, dengue, tuberculosis (insects), poisoning death (chemicals) and cholera, GI disease, jaundice, hepatitis (due to contamination of soil and water). These are various methods for improper disposal of waste, i.e. open dumping, controlled tipping, incineration, composing, etc. The methods of sewage disposal are natural methods (land treatment and dilution) and artificial methods primary treatment and secondary treatment). The proper disposal of human excretes can be made service type latrines, non-service type latrine and latrine for semipermeable. The disposal dead bodies can be made through burial or cremation.

Communication, Infrastructure Facilities and Linkages

CHAPTER 16

INTRODUCTION

The term communication has various meanings depending on the context in which it is used. To some, communication is the interchange of information between two or more people, i.e. the exchange of ideas or thoughts. This kind of communications uses methods such as talking and listening or writing and reading. However, painting, dancing, storytelling are also methods of communication. In addition, thoughts are conveyed to others not only by spoken within words but also by gestures or body action. Communication can be transmission of feelings or more personal and social interaction between people. Thus, communication is any means of exchange information or feelings between two or more people. It is basic components of human relationship. The linkages in the physical movement of people and material from one component to the other through the traditional infrastructure system such as roads, using traditional carriages such as ambulances, jeeps, cars, trucks, motorcycles and other movable equipment. Technology also has recently caused the use of the telemedicine, telephone, fax, wireless, radio and television, computers, etc. instead of roadways for the transmittal of information and data from one component to another without necessitating the physical movement of people and materials. The information system is fast settling in as an important linkage medium, relying on the above infrastructure systems. The degree on which a community relies on either system depends upon its resources and the presence in the area of the infrastructure system.

COMMUNICATION PROCESS

The intent of any communication is to elicit a response. Thus, communication is a process. It has two main purposes to influence others and to obtain information.

The communication can be described as helpful or unhelpful. The helpful communication encourages sharing information, thoughts or feelings between more people, whereas unhelpful communication hinders or blocks the transfer of information and feelings.

Face-to-face communication involves a sender, a receiver and a response. In its simplest form, communication is a two-way process involving the sending and the receiving of a message. Because, the intent of communication is to elicit a response the process is ongoing, the receiver of the message then becomes the sender of a response and the original sender then becomes the receiver.

TYPES OF COMMUNICATION

Communication may be classified on the basis of relationship as formal and informal communication on the basis of direction or flow as downward, lateral, diagonal, external communications and on the basis of expression on verbal and non-verbal communications.

Formal Communication

Formal communication, which occurs through the official organizational channels, it follows the chain of command and determined by hierarchy or seal, or main of organization.

Informal Communication

Informal communication occurs outside the official communication networks such as talking in the lunch hour or hallways between employees. It is neither preplanned nor deliberately motivated by the management. It is neither written nor documented or recorded. It is not set with the lines of organization hierarchy. But, it has the potential to build teams, improve working relationships and generate ideas as workers are in a relaxed environment. As it has no set rules and regulations, it is not confined to a particular direction, but it just spread-like grapevine (gossip). So, it is called grapevine communication.

Downward Communication

Here, communication that flow from a higher level to a lower level in an organization, i.e. from superiors to a subordinate in a chain of command. For example, when the communication related to various schemes or plans, or programs to achieve the health flow from national level to state level, then from state level to district level and then from district levels to community health centers (CHC), primary health centers and subcenters.

Upward Communication

Here, the communication flows from bottom to the top, i.e. from subordinates to superiors from operational level to management level then to top level authorities. In other words, when the flow of communication is from lower level as in the case of implementation of health programs, problem faced, e.g. lack of resources such as men, money, material as well as achievement of target or goals of programs/schemes. The upward communication takes the forms of report giving details of subordinates performance, suggestions and complaints enquiries. This can be oral or written. This may include problems related to work confidential reports, feedback of the orders, instructions, opinions, attitude and feelings of personnel at operational levels.

Lateral Communication

Lateral communication is horizontal communication that takes place at same levels of hierarchy in an organizations or it refers to the exchange of information among employees of same level and status. For example, between auxiliary nurse midwives (ANMs) or between lady health visitors (LHVs), between community health nurses or between nurse managers, or between any horizontally equivalent organizational members. This type of communication facilitates coordination of work and saves time.

Diagonal Communication

Diagonal communications that takes place between supervising person and employees of other workgroups. It is usually does not appears on organizational chart.

External Communication

Here, communication that takes place between supervising person and external group, e.g. communication between public health nurses and Nursing Superintendent of hospital.

Verbal Communication

Verbal communication involves the use of spoken words (oral communication) or written words and depends upon language.

Oral communication: It involves exchange of information with the help of spoken words. These may be in the form of face-to-face conversation, or through mechanical, or electronic devices. Speeches, presentations and discussion are all forms of oral communication. It helps to build a rapport and trust.

Written communication: Any form of communications, which is written and documented from the sender to the receiver. For examples, letters, memos, research paper, reports, orders, instructions, statements, posters, handbooks, bulletins, notice boards, etc. Verbal communication is effective when the criteria of pace and information, simplicity, clarity and brevity, timing, relevance, adaptability and credibility are met.

Non-verbal Communication

Non-verbal communication is the communication of feelings, emotions, attitudes and thought through body movements/gesture/eye contact, etc. Non-verbal communication often reveals more about a person's thoughts and feelings. Verbal communication includes personal appearance, posture and gait, facial expressions and gestures. Eye contact is most effective in the goal to gain someone's trust; gesture allows to interesting the person showing. Movement is the key to obtain a less dull conversation that will eventually attract people to have more interest in something. Having good postures show's confidence, trust and power.

In addition to the above classifications of communications, one more typology relates to the size of the social group or the number of people involved in the experience of communication. It is ranger from intrapersonal, interpersonal group, mass and group communications.

Intrapersonal communication: It can occur on an intrapersonal level within a single individual as well as on interpersonal and group level. Intrapersonal communication is that communication, which you have with yourself, i.e. self-talk. Both the sender and the receiver of a message usually engage in self-talk. It involves thinking about the message before it is sent, while it is being sent and after it is sent, it occurs constantly and consequently, and it can interfere with a person's ability to hear a message on the sender intended. For example, when a person engage in thinking, listening, day dreaming, studying, creating, contemplating or dreaming, etc. It is an individual reflection contemplation and/or meditation (e.g. transcendental meditation).

Interpersonal communication: In which all of the activities verbal and nonverbal, people use when interacting directly with one another. In other words, interpersonal communication denotes that interactions of two or more people. The communication is direct face-to-face between two individuals for an interview, conversation, e.g. therapeutic communication promote understanding and can helps to establish relationship between the nurse and the client. Unlike, the social relationships where there may not be a specific purpose direction, the therapeutic helping relationship in client and goal directed.

Group communication: People are born into a group, i.e. family and interact with others at all stages of life in various groups. For example, peer groups, workgroup, recreational group, religious groups and soon a group is of two or more people, who have shared needs and goals, who take each other into account in their actions and who thus held together, and set apart from others by virtue of their interactions. Group exists to help the people to achieve goals that would be unattainable by individual effort alone. The communication that takes place between members of any group is called 'group dynamics'. The manner of this communication will be determined by a number of group will have an effect on the group dynamics based on that motivation for participating their similarity to other group members, the maturity of the group members in expressing their feelings and the goal of the grays.

Much of nurse's professional life is spent in a wide variety of groups, ranging from dyads to large professional organization. As a participant in a group, the nurse may be required to fulfill different role such as member or leader, teacher or learner, advisor or advice, etc. The common types of health groups include task groups, teaching groups, therapy groups and work-related social support groups. There are similarities and differences among the characteristic of these various types of groups and the role of nurses. Communication between the group and it requires leadership, equal sharing ideas, peer pressure, roles and norms. It focuses on common goals.

Mass communication: It is usually a some form of medium/media, such as print media (e.g. newspaper, magazines, electronic media such as radio, television (TV), video and computers.

BARRIERS OF COMMUNICATION

Barrier of communication refer to the factors causing an interruption in the communication, i.e. the factors, which lead to ineffective communication that includes the following:

1. Physiological barriers: The person who is unable to perceives the message due to some physiological defects, e.g. defect in the ear either internal or external.
2. Psychological barrier: The person, who is emotionally disturbed having low intelligence, suffering from neurosis, cannot communicate properly.
3. Cultural barrier: Includes certain customs, beliefs, religion, attitude, language variation, education class difference also influence as barriers of commencing.
4. Environmental barrier: Noisy environment blocks communication.

PRESENT TREND IN COMMUNICATION

As telecom network is spreading swiftly and the government is keen to provide broadband connectivity to all parts of the country, information technology can be effectively harnessed to improve the delivery of health services. According to Elizabeth Alexander and Pradeep Varma, in a situation where there is a paucity of qualified healthcare personnel, the most optimal solution is distance health care (also including telemedicine, teleconsulting, telecounseling) where expert advice can be made available at some central point and accessed as and when required by telephone or internet.

The information system such as computers, telephone, internet, etc. allow for communication and interaction between people without moving from their places of work. Even within the health facility itself, without leaving the workstations it allow people to talk through their computer screens. In this way the network of computers minimizes the movement of people and improves efficiency. This development is changing the space programs of healthcare facilities, bringing in new systems called 'paperless and/or filmless' medical documentation. This technology has also given to mankind the gift of facsimile and electronic mail transfers of information such as teleconferences, tele-education and telemedicine, which allow team performance of people even when they are physically separated by distance.

A simple computer- and system-based diagnostic application can guide the paramedic/nurse in handling common ailments directly by administering simple remedies, and only refer to secondary care for the more complex problems. The patient can get a printed registration card as well as a record of his/her consultation and the test results. But a particularly useful mechanism would be a smart card with all data written onto it. This is a need to create network in different level.

At Primary Care Level

There is need to create a dispersed network of computerized, internet-enabled centers in rural areas, all managed by technically competent, functionally English literate young men and women, who will form a resource pool through which such health services will flow. If the villagers are reluctant to visit such a center for medical purposes, the stationing of the ANM or paramedic inside the center will lend it credibility.

At Secondary Care Level

Out patients departments (OPDs) of all government hospitals, whether at the block or district level are overcrowded and it can be reduced by online connectivity of the hospitals to the PHC. And the registration (those who need to be referred to a doctor) can be completed by giving an ID in the form of a printed card, i.e. a smart card at the village. The patients who are informed by the nurse/paramedic will need to visit the hospital and the patient can directly visit a doctor with whom an appointment has already been fixed.

At Tertiary Care Level

Those patients who require specialist consultation are referred to a tertiary care hospital.

INFRASTRUCTURE FACILITIES AND LINKAGES

Infrastructure refers to the basic physical and organizational structure (e.g. buildings, roads, power supplies, etc.) needed for the operation of society enterprise. Here, means the infrastructure of the healthcare facilities, i.e. health institution, health centers and hospitals, and other health organizations. Linkages means that the action of linking or the state of being linked or a system of links. In this text, it refers to the linkages of health infrastructure of the country, which include 'center to states' to 'district to local' and so on.

A national health information infrastructure provides a framework that stakeholders can use to communicate with each other and to transform data into useful information on multiple levels. Efforts are under way throughout the world to develop integrated national and global health information infrastructures to support health improvements. The infrastructure makes it possible for people not only to use health information designed by others but also to create resources to manage their own health and to influence the health of their communities. For example, community groups could use computers to gain access to survey information about the quality of life in their neighborhoods and apply this information to create an action plan to present to local elected and public health officials.

Health system/infrastructure consists of all organizations, institutions and resource that are developed to produce health actions. A health action is that any effort whether in personal health care, public health services or through interspectral initiative whose primary purpose is to promote, restore, maintain or improve health.

Health infrastructure consists of all those people and actions whose primary purpose is to improve and maintain health. It includes not only the government hospital and the dispensaries, the doctors, nurses and other professionals working in these organizations but also the philosophy of health care, funded management of health professionals—both formal and informal, and all the health professional activities, which people carry out to remain healthy.

Health professionals need a high level of interpersonal skills to interact with diverse populations and patients who may have different cultural, linguistic, educational and socioeconomic backgrounds. Health professionals also need more direct training in and experience with all forms of computer and telecommunication technologies. In addition to searching for information, patients and consumers want to use technology to discuss health concerns, and health professionals need to be ready to respond. To support an increase in health communication activities, research and evaluation of all forms of health communication will be necessary to build the scientific base of the field and the practice of evidence-based health communication. Collectively, these opportunities represent important areas to make significant improvements in personal and community health. The integration of communication media means electronic access to health information not only via computers but also with web-enabled televisions and telephones, handheld devices and other emerging technologies. Technical literacy or the ability to use electronic technologies and application will be essential to gain access to this ability to use electronic technologies and applications, will be essential to gain access to this information.

Since, the health is the fundamental right to each individual, the country has the responsibility for their health. In India, the states are largely independent in matter relating to the delivery of health care to the people. The control of health system is through main links center, state and local or peripheral. As in figure, the structure of healthcare systems at national, state and district community (Fig. 16.1).

National Level

As national or union level, the center makes the policy, plans, guidelines and assists, and coordinates the activities of state health ministries. It also administers, union territories. Health system at national level consists of:
- Union Ministry of Health and Family Welfare
- Directorate General of Health Sources
- Central Council of Health and Family Welfare.

Union Ministry of Health and Family Welfare

Union Ministry of Health and Family Welfare is responsible for forming the health policy and for all the programs that are related to family planning in India. It has three departments under its control such as Department of Health, Department of Family Welfare and Department of Indian System of Medicine and Homeopathy (ISM and H). They are responsible for dealing the issues related to their respective departments.

Directorate General of Health Services

Directorate General of Health Services (DGHS) is the technical wing in Department of Health. The general function of DGHS includes, survey, planning, coordination, programming and appraisal of all health matters of the country, the specific functions are:
- International health relations and quarantine
- Control of drug standards, medical store depots
- Administration of postgraduate training and medical education
- Medical Research, National Health Programs
- Central Health Education Bureau
- Health intelligence
- National Medical Library.

Central Council of Health

Central Council of Health consists of Union Health Minister (Chairman) and State Health Minister (as member). The main function of the council are:

- To consider and recommend broad outlines of policies
- To make proposals for legislation on matter related to public health
- To make recommendation to Union Government, grant in aid and to review its utilization
- To establish organizations inserted with appropriate functions for providing and maintaining cooperation between center and state health administrators.

Regional or central level institutions, hospitals: Specialized hospitals at the central level provide health services to cure the problem and also research activities are carried out related to health in order to find out the cure for illness and in other areas of health.

Private clinics and hospitals: Public health engages both private and public organizations. These also provide health-related services to promote the health, and sometimes are within the reach, but at a little higher cost or sometimes unaffordable by people.

The Nation's public health infrastructure is the resources needed to deliver the essential public health services to every community people who work in the field of public health, information and communication systems used to collect and disseminate accurate data, and public health organizations at the state and local in the front lines of public health.

State Level

The organization at state level is under the state Department of Health and Family Welfare in each state headed by Minister and with Secretariat under the charge of Secretary. It has some functions, which include prevention of extension of communicable diseases, prevention of food adulteration, labor welfare, economic and social planning, and population control and family planning.

State Health Directorate headed by Director of Health and Family Welfare and Medical Education, assisted by Joint Director, Deputy Director and Assistant Director. Functions of State Health Directorate include:
- To study the health problems, to identify the health needs of people
- To make provisions for control of milk and food sanitation
- To take all the remedial action at the time of outbreak of communicable diseases
- To establish and maintain control laboratories for preparations of vaccine
- To promote health awareness among people
- To collect, tabulate and publish vital statistics
- To promote all the health program

CHAPTER 16 Communication, Infrastructure Facilities and Linkages

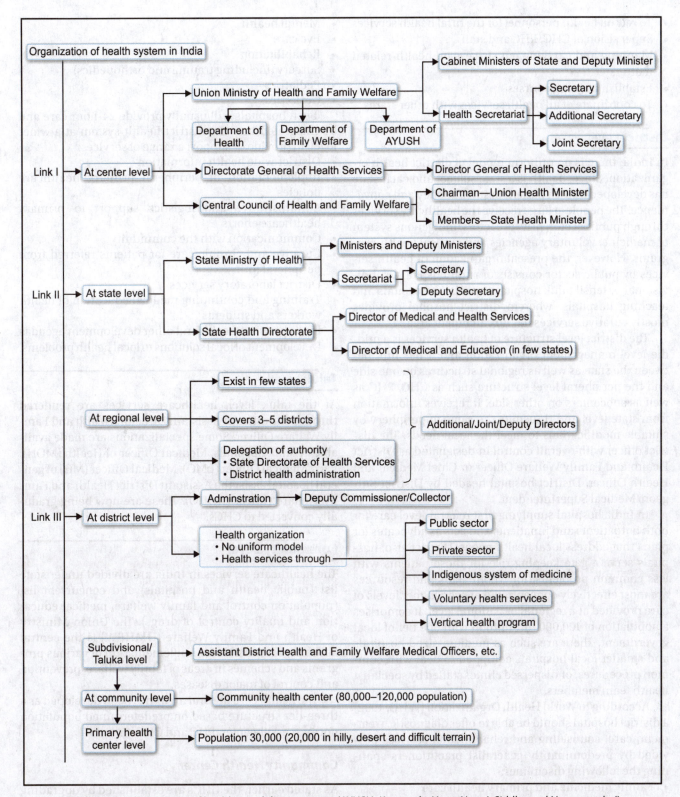

Figure 16.1: Organization of healthcare delivery system (AYUSH, 'Ayurveda, Yoga, Unani, Siddha and Homeopathy')

- To recruit health personnel for the rural health services
- Supervision of CHC, PHC and staff
- Manning and carrying out surveys on health-related matters
- Establish training courses
- To coordinate of all health services with other states.

District Level

In India, there is no uniform model of district health organization. Since, health is a state subject and each state has developed its own pattern to suit its policy and convenience. The people at large receive the healthcare services through public sector, private sectors, indigenous system of medicine, voluntary agencies and vertical health programs. However, the present organization of health services by public sector consists of rural hospitals, subdivisional or tehsil taluk hospitals, specialist hospitals and teaching hospitals, wherein district hospital provides mostly curative services has no catchment area.

The district level structure of health services is a middle level management organization and it has link between the state as well as regional structures on one side and the peripheral level structure such as CHC, PHC as well as subcenters on other side. It receives information from state level and transmits the same to periphery by suitable modifications to meet the local needs. The district officer with overall control in designated as District Health and Family Welfare Officer or Chief Medical and Health Officer. District hospital headed by District Surgeon/Medical Superintendent.

In India hospital supplying first referral-level care for both outpatients and inpatients and acts as advocates for plans that address local health needs. District also, hospitals serve a gate keeping role for those patients with less common problems, for whom skills and resources are most effectively concentrated at even higher levels of care provided at a regional or national level. It comprises a population of 100,000 to 1 million with one tier of local government. There are such as medium-sized hospitals and smaller local hospitals equipped to deal with common procedures, or dispersed clinics staffed by specialist health team members.

According to World Health Organization (WHO, 1992) a district hospital should be able to offer diagnostic, treatment, care, counseling and rehabilitation services provided by predominantly generalist practitioners spanning the following disciplines:
- Family medicine and primary health care
- Medicine
- Obstetrics
- Mental health
- Eye care
- Rehabilitation
- Surgery (including trauma and orthopedics)
- Pediatrics
- Geriatrics.

Such hospitals will usually provide 24-hour care and be integrated into the district health system at a wider level, to provide or support a range of services:
- District-wide health information
- Implementation of peripheral primary healthcare policies
- Administrative and logistics support to primary healthcare efforts
- Communication with the community
- Curative and chronic care for patients referred from peripheral units
- District laboratory services
- Training and continuing medical education of health workers and students
- Links between health and other development agendas
- Development of local solutions to local health problems.

Taluk Level

At the taluk level, healthcare services are rendered through the office of Assistant Director, Health and Family Welfare Officer. Some specializations are made available at taluk hospitals, Medical Officer of Health (MOH), Lady Medical Officer (LMO), Medical Officer (MO) of general hospital assist the Assistant District Health and Family Welfare Officer (ADHO). These are now being gradually converted to CHCs.

Community Level

The healthcare services in India are divided under state list (public health and hospitals) and concurrent list (population control and family welfare, medical education and quality control of drugs). The Union Ministry of Health and Family Welfare (UMHFW) is the central authority responsible for implementation of various programs and schemes in areas of family welfare, prevention and control of major diseases.

The health care in rural areas has been developed as a three-tier structure based on predetermined population norms, i.e. subcenter, PHC and CHC.

Community Health Center

As stated earlier, the CHCs are established by upgrading the subdistrict/taluk hospitals. Some of the block goal PHCs or by creating a new center, wherever absolutely needed. For successful primary healthcare program effect referral support is to be provided. For the purpose, one CHC has been established for every 80,000–120,000 population of rural areas and this center provides a basic specialty services in general medicine, pediatrics, surgery, obstetrics and gynecology. So, CHC forms the upper most tier in three-tier system. According to norms, a typical CHC requires to have 30 indoor beds (inpatients), with operation theater (OT), X-ray, labor room and laboratory facilities. These are established and maintained by State Government under minimum needs program/basic medical services. A CHC is the referral center for four PHCs within its jurisdiction providing facilities for obstetrics care and specialist expertise. Manpower at CHC include surgeon, physician, obstetrician and gynecologist, pediatrician and 21 paramedical, and other staffs.

Primary Health Center

Primary health centers (PHCs) comprise the second tier in rural healthcare structure envisaged to provide integrated curative and preventive health care to the rural population. It has four to six beds for inpatients and acts as a referral unit for six subcenters. These are established and maintained by State Governments under the Minimum Needs Program/Basic Minimum Services (BMS) Program.

Many rural dispensaries have been upgraded to create these PHCs and some new PHCs are designed according to needs of rural population. At present, there is one PHC covering about 30,000 (20,000 no hilly, desert and difficult terrains) or more population.

Each PHC has one Medical Officer, two health assistants (one male and one female) and health workers, and supporting staffs. Medical Officer who is incharge of the PHC supported by 14 paramedical and other staff including Nurse Midwife, ANMs, Block Extension Educator (BEE), health assistants (HA) [male (M), female (F)], Upper Division Clerk (UDC), Secondary Division Clerk (SDC), laboratory technician, drivers and group D official. The services provided here are medicare and laboratory services, maternal and child health (MCH) of family planning, safe water supply, sanitation, vital statistics and even selected surgical procedure. Training of health guides, health workers, local dais, health assistants and Accredited Social Health Activities (ASHA) workers, etc. The PHC provide curative, preventive and family welfare services. These are:
- The MCH including family planning
- Training of health guides, health workers, local dais and health assistants
- Safe water supply
- Sanitation
- Vital statistics
- National health programs
- Medical care and laboratory services
- Selected surgical procedures such as vasectomy, tubectomy and minor surgical procedures.

Subcenter

The most peripheral health institutional facility in the 'subcenter' manned by one male and one female multi-purpose health worker (HW), i.e. HW (F), ANM and HW (M). It is center, where first contact between the PHC system and community take place. The subcenter comprises the first tier in rural healthcare structure. These centers are expected to use various mediums of interpersonal communications in order to bring about behavioral changes so as to achieve health. At present, in most places there is one subcenter for about 50,000 populations, (3,000 in hilly and desert areas and in difficult terrain). The subcenters are required to providing services that are basic health services according the needs of men, women and children. In some centers, there will be one voluntary worker and usually one health assistant (F) in in-charge of six subcenters. They are provided with basic drugs for minor health problem. The services available at subcenters are MCH, family welfare, nutrition and immunization, control diarrhea and communicable diseases. A lady health worker (LHV) is incharge of six subcenters. They are provided with basic drugs for minor ailments. The services provided in the subcenter are:
- Maternal and child health
- Family welfare
- Nutrition
- Immunization
- Diarrhea control
- Control of communicable diseases.

CURRENT PROBLEMS

The main framework of the health system is based on three-tier system of health care, i.e. community-based primary health care, and hospital-based secondary and tertiary care. But, there is no infirmity as for as the development of health system is concerned in different parts of India. PHC in India is provided through government operated PHCs at village and town levels. A Medical Officer appointed at each of these PHCs and is supported to diagnose and manage all medical and surgical illness at the primary level and refer solicited patients for higher

investigations and treatment or expert opinion to centers based at the district level, the CHCs where at least one postgraduate surgeon, one physician, one obstetrician and gynecologist are posted. At present, the current problems faced by the healthcare services include are:
- Persistent gap in manpower and infrastructure in public sectors
- Suboptimal functioning of infrastructure, poor referral services
- Plethora of hospitals in government, voluntary and private sector not having appropriate manpower, diagnostic and therapeutic services, and drugs
- Availability and utilization of services that are poorest in the remote rural areas in states and districts
- Increasing dual diseases burden of communicable and non-communicable diseases because of ongoing demographic lifestyle, and environmental transitions
- Technological advances that widen the spectrum of possible interventions
- Increasing awareness and expectations of possible interventions
- Escalating costs of health care.

LINKAGES

A health system is dependent on strong and efficient linkage between and among its components/elements for it to function in its totality, allowing each component to contribute its specified role and function to the total mission. The linkages required of district health services can be broken down into four groups:
- Linkages between district hospitals and peripheral health facilities
- Linkages with the community they serve
- Linkages with tertiary referral hospitals and central government agencies
- Intersectoral linkages within the district, i.e. with education, agriculture, local government, etc.

To build strong linkages a number of factors are required such as:
- A formal organizational structure
- Informal personal relationships
- Communication systems
- Transport systems
- Integration of management and support functions, e.g. planning
- Education, training, supplies and maintenance.

Linkages are required to ensure better outcomes by the following.

Service coordination and service integration: Multiple levels of the health system are involved in dealing with the communities health problems. When services are well-coordinated and integrated then it is easier to achieve the goal. For example, in case workers in case of the prevention and treatment of diarrheal diseases in the district. The primary care workers will:
- Educate the community on hygiene practices to minimize spread
- Diagnose and manage mild and moderate cases
- Refer severe cases to the district hospital:
  - Treat severe cases
  - Perform microbiology testing
  - Monitor the case
  - Distribution of rehydration salts
  - Assist in epidemiological surveillance of the district to identify and pinpoint the source of significant outbreaks
  - Educating the patients and their families on hygiene practices as the occasion arises.

Service planning: When there will be good communication and cooperation between district and peripheral units, then it may evolve service coordination.

Logistics support: There is a range of areas where linkages and a common approach to the purchase and distribution of supplies can result in better stock management lower prices, fewer stock outages arid lower inventories, all leading to better service at lower cost.

Staff development and support: The hospital is the focal point for a range of professional and technical staff training programs.

Job satisfaction: Linkages are important to develop a sense of joint purpose and joint achievement. It enables staff to feel part of the broader strategy to improve the health of the community. Thus, linkages increase staff motivation and satisfaction, and peripheral units do not feel unsupported and district hospitals as they are convenient dumping ground for other problems.

Consequences of poor linkages: A number of problems may occur due to poor linkages.

Gaps in service: The task of finding out the source of an epidemic may be overlooked or patients may be referred to the district hospital due to lack of resources.

Service duplications: Sometime both peripheral and district services attempt to do the same task and may purchase expensive equipment for the task, when the district could have managed with only one.

Inappropriate division of tasks: Peripheral units may take on tasks, which could have been handled more efficiently at the district level and on the other hand, patients who could have been treated at peripheral units, may be treated at the district hospital at higher cost with the use of

CHAPTER 16: Communication, Infrastructure Facilities and Linkages

resources that should have been used for patients with more complex problems. Linkages must be established in multidirections horizontally and vertically.

Vertical linkage: It refers to the linkages between levels in the system of hierarchy between subcenter, PHC and CHC or between the polyclinic and the district hospital, etc.

Horizontal linkages: It means that at their own levels in the hierarchy. The facilities in horizontal linkages must be interconnected between and among themselves.

It is important that the directions of communication may be multidirectional, up and down, vertically, and to and from horizontally.

CONCLUSION

Communication is the process of sharing information in the common language. It is defined as the process of conveying information from a sender to a receiver with the use of a medium in which the information is understood in the same way by both sender and receiver. It is a process of exchanging information. There are different types of communication. Health communication means providing informations and identifying the individual, and community decisions to improve health. It encompasses the study and use and communication strategies to inform and influence individual and community decisions that enhance health. The functions of health communications are information, education, motivation, persuasion and counseling, raising morals, health developments and organization for the community. These communications can be utilized to influence the public health, advocate for policies and programs related to health, promote positive changes in the socioeconomic and physical environments, improve the deliveries of community health and healthcare service and encourage social norms. In the field of health, it takes on a wider role than mere physical infrastructure facilities, which include healthcare centers, dispensaries or hospitals need to be manned by well-trained staffs with service perspective. Health system is dependent on strong and efficient linkage between and among its components for it to function into totality or comprehensiveness to it specified role.

Part II

Environment as Determinant of Health

B. *Biological Environment*
   - Forestation
   - Bacterial and Viral Agents: Host and Immunity
   - Arthropods
   - Rodents
   - Food Hygiene

Part II

Forestation

CHAPTER 17

BIOLOGICAL ENVIRONMENT

Biological environment consists of living things around man. These are plants, animals, rodents, insects and microbes like bacteria, viruses, rickettsiae, parasites, fungi. This Chapter discuss the concepts related to plants, i.e. forestation.

The forest refers to a large area covered chiefly with trees and undergrowth. The word 'forest' has been derived from the Latin word 'foris,' which means 'outside'. Forests are national biotic type of non-renewable resources. They cover one third of total earth land and above 33% of world have been cleared, and is converted for other uses. Forest provides many benefits to human beings and plays an important role in maintaining ecosystem. According to ecologists, health as a dynamic equilibrium between man and his environment and disease, maladjustment of the human organisms to environment.

Ecology is a key word comes from the Greek 'oikos' meaning a 'house', which has its importance in the philosophy of health. Since, ecology is science of mutual relationship between living organisms and their environment, human ecology is a subset of ecology. A full understanding of health requires that humanity be seen as a part of an ecosystem. The human ecosystem includes in addition to the natural environment in all the dimensions of the man-made environment, i.e. physical, chemical, biological and psychological. Disease is embedded in the ecosystem of man. As stated earlier according to ecological concepts, health is visualized as a state of dynamic equilibrium between man and his environment. By constantly altering his environment or ecosystem by such a charities as urbanization, industrialization and deforestation land reclamation construction of irrigation canal and dams, man has creating himself new health problem. For example, man's intrusion into ecological cycle of disease has resulted in zoonotic diseases such as Kyasanur Forest disease, rabies, yellow fever, monkey fever, Lassa fever, etc. and the construction of dams, irrigation systems and artificial lake has created ecological riches favoring the breeding of mosquitoes, snails and spread of filariasis, schistosomiasis and Japanese infection.

IMPORTANCE OF FORESTS

As stated earlier, forest provide many benefits to human beings, which includes forest assist in regular recycling of water, oxygen, nitrogen and other nutrients. Since a forest is a natural, self-sustaining community, i.e. characterized by the presence of trees, which are large and generally single-stemmed plants. All the forests share the same physical characteristics, but can exist in different region under wide range of condition such as temperature, atmospheric carbon dioxide (CO_2) and type of soil available in forests. The benefits of forest will include the following.

Forests are the Source of Energy

For example, certain plants are growing in the forests are used as a source of food such as fruits, vegetables, roots and tubes of plant, which either eaten raw or cooked by human beings, and animal. And certain animals, i.e. rabbits, pig and birds are also caught by human beings for using as food.

Forest Provides Shelter

The shelter is provided for the birds, reptile, insects and mammals, wild animals, etc. that are living in the forest.

Forests Provide Products for Further Use

In forest many useful plants are growing, which helps to man for manufacture of many further products. For example, wood branches and pulp are used for manufacturing paper and rayon. Other products such as waxes, honey, musk, gums, etc. are provided by flora and fauna.

Forests Prevent Soil Erosion

Forest conserves the soil in which they bind the soil through roots and forests increase the fertility of the soil by humus, which is formed by the decay of the forest litter.

Forests Maintain the Climate

Atmosphere humidity is increased by the transpiration, which in turn causes rainfall and changes the temperature of climate to be cool.

AFFORESTATION

Forests have been influenced by human activities by influencing forest development. Often human beings manipulate forest system, so as to produce more of goods and services as desired by individual who are living in a community, since sometimes humans have controlled over the forest. When a man will start cutting the trees for his own purpose, then there will be disturbance in the ecosystem, thereby disturbing health of human beings through the effects of global warming and greenhouse effect.

Afforestation is the establishment of forest or stand of trees in an area, where there was no forest. Reforestation is the re-establishment of forest cover, either naturally (by natural seeding, coppice or root suckers) or artificially (by direct seeding or planting). Many governments and non-governmental organizations directly engage in programs of afforestation to create forests, increase carbon capture and sequestration, and help to anthropogenically improved biodiversity [in the United Kingdom (UK), afforestation may mean converting the legal status of some land to 'royal forest']. Special tools, e.g. tree planting bar are used to make planting of trees easier and faster.

DEFORESTATION

Deforestation, clearance or clearing is the removal of a forest or stand of trees where the land is thereafter converted to a non-forest use. Example of deforestation includes conversion of forestland to farms, ranches or urban use.

The term deforestation can be misused when applied to describe a tree harvesting method in which all trees in an area are removed (clear cutting). However in temperate climates, this method is in conformance with sustainable forestry practices and correctly described as regeneration harvest. In temperate mesic climates, natural regeneration of forest stands often will not occur in the absence of disturbance, whether natural or anthropogenic. Furthermore, biodiversity after regeneration harvest often mimics that found after natural disturbance including biodiversity loss after naturally occurring rainforest destruction.

Deforestation occurs for many reasons; trees are cut down to be used or sold as fuel (sometimes in the form of charcoal) or timber, while cleared land is used as pasture for liver stock, plantations of commodities and settlements. The removal of trees without sufficient reforestation has resulted in damage to habitat, biodiversity loss and aridity. It has adverse impacts on biosequestration of atmospheric CO_2. Deforestation has also been used in war to deprive the enemy of cover for its forces and also vital resources.

Disregard or ignorance of intrinsic value, lack of ascribed value, lax forest management and deficient environmental laws are some of the factors that allow deforestation to occur on a large scale. In many countries, deforestation, both naturally occurring and human induced, is an ongoing issue. Deforestation causes extinction, changes to climatic conditions, desertification and displacement of populations as observed by current conditions, and in the past through the fossil record. More than half of all plant and land animal species in the world live in tropical forests, the overwhelming direct cause of deforestation is agriculture. Subsistence farming is responsible for 48% of deforestation; commercial is responsible for 32% of deforestation; logging is responsible for 14% of deforestation and fuel wood removals make up 5% of deforestation.

Experts do not agree on whether industrial logging is an important contributor to global deforestation. Some argue that the poor people are more likely to clear forest because they have no alternatives, others that the poor lack the ability to pay for the materials and labor needed to clear forest. One study found that population increases due to high fertility rates were a primary driver of tropical deforestation in only 8% of cases.

Other causes of contemporary deforestation may include corruption of government institutions, the inequitable distribution of wealth and power, population growth and overpopulation and urbanization. Globalization is often viewed as another root cause of deforestation, though there are cases in which the impact of globalization (new flows of labor, capital, commodities and ideas) have promoted localized forest recovery.

Deforestation is defined as the unscrupulous and indiscriminate destruction of indigenous forests, and wood lands. The causes of deforestation are as follows.

Increasing population: Needs to have many facilities including shelter, food and survival facilities for which they destroy the forests step by step.

Natural calamities: Such as forest fires, pest attacks, floods, storms and lightening, etc. will spoil forests.

CHAPTER 17 — Forestation

Human activities: Such as cutting trees for agriculture, construction of roads, establishment of industries, construction of railway tracks and even carelessness. The effect of deforestation leads to reduction of stability in the ecosystem and fauna habitat will be disturbed, and also food chain will be disturbed, leading to extinction of some species.

Effects of Deforestation

In brief, the effect of deforestation leads to:
- Deprivation of shelter for birds, insects, etc.
- Deprivation of food for animals and human beings
- In atmosphere, there will be decrease of oxygen and increase of CO_2 occurs
- Scarcity of fuel woods
- Increase of draught
- Melting of ice caps and glaciers causing floods
- Loss of cultural diversity
- An occurrence of increased soil erosion and pollution
- Decreased availability of food products
- Depletion of soil nutrients
- Increased aridity
- Global warming and greenhouse effect
- Biologically, diversity reduced due to reduced genetic base.

SUSTAINING THE FOREST SYSTEM

A number of organisms exist within the forest and these organisms interact with each other playing specific role in sustaining forest system. Plants primarily produce food through the process of photosynthesis. All animals, insects and birds depend upon the plants for food and they consume food to get energy for their survival they are called consumers. The leaves and old branches from the trees fall to the ground. These along with the animal remnants are broken into smallest primary elements to be used again. Human beings are consuming as they get food from plants to get energy for their survival. Human activities such as cutting trees for residential purpose or for other benefits disturb the forest system, but man's intervention can be effective for sustaining forest system.

Changing Forest System

Forests are sensitive to climate variability such as air temperature, atmospheric CO_2, frequency and severity of wild fire and pollution. Air temperature has the likelihood of migrating tree species resulting in change in forest location, composition and productivity. Climatic changes increase the chances of diseases, which are determined to forests, thereby changing forest system. This system is a complex of interrelated living and non-living elements. Forests suggest a number of species, i.e. animals, plants, earth, air and water. The reasons for changes in composition and structure of forests include natural succession, natural disturbances and human activities.

Natural succession: This will occur naturally without the involvement of human being, i.e. due to climatic changes, one type of plant species is replaced by another. This progressive replacement of species with another is known as succession.

Natural disturbances: For example, the organisms of forest alters due to natural disturbances such as wildfire, frost, diseases of the trees, etc.

Human disturbances: Human beings also influenced the composition and structures of forests by introducing and removing species. For example, human disturbance are thinning, fires and forest logging.

MANAGEMENT OF FORESTS

Forests play an important role in maintaining aquatic and terrestrial ecosystem. As forests holds the soil, thereby preventing soil erosion and also regulate streamflow, thereby maintaining the aquatic ecosystem. Ecosystem is a natural functional unit in which there is an interaction between supporting systems. Forest management is needed to stop the ecological degradation, which can result in harmful climate conditions. Its aim is to ensure the access of forests for next generations. The measure need to be taken to conserve the forest such as avoid wastage of forest products, use alternate source of energy, i.e. cooling gas instead of woods profit deforestation. Encourage reforestation, i.e. use of pesticides (to reduce damage to forests), prevention and control of forest fire, prohibit overgrazing and afforestation.

Forests play a vital role in maintaining ecosystem. But, human activities and natural calamities have disturbed the forest system. One of the reasons for decrease forest land is population explosion. People cut the trees for the residential purpose. If this will continue then the health of the people will be disturbed due to impact of deforestation. Proper and adequate plans with implementation and evaluation need to be carried out to avoid disturbances, and to achieve the control and prevention of deforestations.

PLANS AND POLICIES FOR FORESTATION, AND PREVENTION FOR DEFORESTATION

The government should take appropriate action to prevent cutting trees to avoid disturbances in ecosystem. The certain measures already taken by the government plan and policies for forestation and prevention of deforestation are as follows.

Indian Forest Act (1927)

Indian Forest Act was passed with the following objectives:
- To conserve and protect the forests
- To ensure judicious use of forest products.

According to this act, state government may appoint three officers, but only one being Forest Officer for performing the duties of a Forest Settlement Officer under Section 4 of the act. He/She is being given the powers to declare prohibition of clearing of land, to form village forest, manage forests and protect forests, etc. If one does not follow the law, i.e. violates the law, then penalty under Section 33 of this act is an imprisonment of 6 months or more, or ₹500 penalty. This law failed to prove effective because of gross violation of rules and regulations of the act. Adequate provision for implementing and reviewing of performance of law resulted in lack of affectivity. So, further actions are required to coordinate the activities, review the legislation, study, plan and implement the rules and regulations keeping in view the extent of health hazards caused by this.

Van Mahotsav

Since 1950, Van Mahotsav is celebrated as a festival twice a year in the month of February and July. Tree plantation is carried out during the week with the purpose of land transformation. It deals with plantation of trees. It was stated by former Union Minister of Agriculture and Food, Munshi KM with the purpose that thousands of trees can be implanted by this way.

National Forest Policy (1952)

About 33% of land area of country should be covered with forest, but in India forests forms only 23% of total land area. To make up this shortfall, central and state government have started afforestation programs such as agroforestry, social forestry and urban forestry.

Chipko Movement (1973)

The Chipko Movement was started in hilly areas of Uttar Pradesh (UP) in 1970s for prevention of deforestations against relentless process of forest destruction. It spread to many districts of Himalaya in UP. The word 'Chipko' means 'embrace', i.e. villagers hug the tree and save them by caring in between the trees and contractors axe. The movement got victory in 1982 and Indira Gandhi banned the falling of trees for 15 years. Many slogans were used such as 'ecology is permanent economy' and 'embrace the trees and save them from being looted'. This was to establish the harmonious relationship between man and nature.

National Forest Policy (1988)

The policy was started with the aim to ensure environmental stability and maintenance of ecological balance including atmospheric stability, which is vital for sustenance of all forms of life of plants, animals and human beings. The integral feature of the policy was to involve women and native people. It includes the following objectives:
- Conserving the natural heritage
- Increasing forest/tree cover substantially through afforestation and social forestry programs
- Meeting the requirement for fuelwood, fodder, nonwood forest products (NWFP) and small timber of rural and tribal population
- Increasing the productivity of forests
- Encouraging efficient utilization of forest produce
- Creating a massive people's movement
- Maintaining environmental stability.

Van Sanrakshan Samiti

Government thought of involving people to manage the lands from which they get benefits. In Van Sanrakshan Samiti (VSS), the local/indigenous people were involved who were residing at the periphery of forests. Forestry Department provided technical and administrative support to VSS. The theft, fire and encroachment has reduced in the areas managed by VSS. During 1994–1998, the number of VSS increased to 5,000.

National Forestry Action Program (1999)

National Forestry Action Program is a plan of next 20 years. The purpose of the plan is to find out the issues and programs to achieve sustainable forestry development by coordinated efforts. It identifies five programs:

CHAPTER 17   Forestation

1. Protect existing forest resources: It includes forest protection, soil and water conservation and conservation of protected areas.
2. Improve forest productivity: It includes the following aspects:
   - Rehabilitation of degraded forests
   - Research and technology development
   - Development of NWFP
   - Assisting in private initiatives with community participation.
3. Reduce total demand: It can be achieved through technological interventions and alternate ways by which efficiency of forest product use can be achieved.
4. Strengthening the policy and institutional network: It aims at strengthening the central and state forestry administrations and institutions. It includes public education, research, legislation and development of information process.
5. Expand the forest area: It can be achieved by implanting trees in forest and non-forest lands with people's participation.
6. Environment Day: The United Nations organizes Environment Day on the 5th June of every year to create awareness among the people about how forestation can help in improving the environment.

ACTS REGULATING THE ENVIRONMENT NATIONAL POLLUTION CONTROL BOARD

Historical Background

History of Indian efforts for environment conservation and control of pollution is about 150 years old. Following is the brief history of Indian Laws on environment:

1. The Shore (Bombay) Nuisance Act, 1853.
2. The Indian Penal Code (IPC), 1860 gave some provisions to control nuisance (pollution). Section 268 of IPC defines public nuisances and Sections 133–144 of IPC are about abatement of public nuisance. These are only prohibitive provisions. A person guilty of public nuisance, who does not act or is guilty of illegal omission, which may cause injury, damage or annoyance to public is liable to prosecution and punishment. This section also deals with the maintenance of ecological balance of resources and their rational use without disturbing the balance of nature. But, Britishers themselves exploited the resources ruthlessly during their reign. Even in independent India, efforts to frame constituting for laws pertaining abatement of environmental pollution were made after Stockholm Conference through amendments.
3. The Indian Fisheries Act, 1897.
4. The Indian Ports Act, 1907.
5. Bengal Smoke Nuisance Act, 1905.
6. The Motor Vehicles Act, 1938.
7. Factory Act, 1948.
8. The Maharashtra Prevention of Water Pollution Act, 1953.
9. The Orissa River Pollution and Prevention Act, 1954.
10. The Prevention of Food Adulteration Act, 1954.
11. The River Boards Act, 1956.
12. Prevention of Cruelty to Animals Act, 1960.
13. The Atomic Energy Act (Radiation Protection Rules), 1962.
14. The Gujarat Smoke Nuisance Act, 1963.
15. The Insecticides Act, 1968.

In February 1971, the University Grants Commission (India) launched a symposium on the development of environmental studies in the Indian universities in collaboration with other organizations. It was a concluded that ecology and environmental issues should form part of the courses of study at all levels.

Environment Pollution and Laws in India

The real awareness about environmental protection at global level was recognized at the United Nations (UN) Conference on the Human Environment held at Stockholm (Sweden) in June, 1972. The later Prime Minister, Indira Gandhi took keen interest and initiative to take appropriate steps for the protection, and improvement of human environment. Keeping in view the need for environment protection, following Indian Laws were made to abate pollution in India:

1. Indian Forest Act, 1972.
2. Wildlife Protection Act, 1972.
3. Water Act, 1974.
4. Forest (Conservation) Act, 1980.
5. Air (Protection and Control of Pollution) Act, 1981.
6. Environment Protection Act (EPA), 1986.
7. Notification on the Coastal Regulation Zone, 1991.
8. Environment Impact Assessment of Development Project, 1994.
9. The Motor Vehicle Act, 1988.
10. Public Liability Insurance Act, 1991.
11. The National Environmental Tribunal Act, 1995.
12. National Environment Appellate Authority Act, 1997.

Indian Laws and Constitutional Amendments

Indian Constitution has specific provision for environment protection under the Chapters of 'Directive Principles of State Policy and Fundamental Duties'. The amendment, known as 42nd Amendment, of Indian Constitution added Article 48A and Article 51A(g) (Table 17.1).

Article 48A

The Article 48A deals with the Directive Principles of State Policy and states that the State shall endeavor to protect and improve the environment and to safeguard the forests and wildlife of the country.

Article 51A(g)

The Article 51A(g) deals with fundamental duties of the citizens and states that "It shall be the duty of every citizen of India to protect and improve the natural environment including forests, lakes, rivers and wildlife and to have compassion for living creatures." Thus, protection and improvement of natural environment is the duty of the state (Article 48A) and every citizen [Article 51A(g)].

Article 253

The Article 253 states that "Parliament has power to make any law for the whole or any part of the country

Table 17.1: Indian legislation and provisions

Legislation (Acts)	Provisions
Forest Act, 1972	This act stipulates that no forest land or any portion thereof may be used for non-forest purposes; it provides for the constitution of an advisory committee to advise the government on cutting the trees
Forest (Conservation) Act, 1980	This act has been passed to control deforestation, which causes ecological imbalance and results in environment degradation, it has provisions to put restrictions on the use of the forest land for non-forest purpose
Wildlife Protection Act, 1972	This act provides the constitution of a Wildlife Advisory Board, regulating the hunting of wild animals and birds, laying down procedures for declaring the areas of sanctuaries and national parks and regulation of trade in wild animals
Water (Protection and Control of Pollution) Act, 1974	Provides for the establishment of Central and State Pollution Control Boards for the prevention and control of water pollution The act seeks to control pollution primarily through standards to be laid down by the boards and the consent orders issued by them Stiff penalties are imposed for violation, the boards are given ample powers for investigation and inspection and to take samples and to establish laboratories for analysing the samples
Air (Protection and Control of Pollution) Act, 1981	Air pollution is to be controlled primarily through standards laid down (1981) by the boards and the consent orders issued by them For contravening, the standards laid down by the boards and for violating the provision relating to consent by the board, stiff penalties have been provided
Environment Protection Act, 1986	Provides for: • Covering some of the major areas of environmental hazards not covered by the existing laws • Linkages in handling matters of industrial and environmental safety and control mechanisms to guard against slow, insidious build-up of hazardous substances, especially of new chemicals in the environment • An authority not only to coordinate the activities of the various regulatory agencies, but to assume the lead role for studying, planning and implementing long-term requirements of environmental safety
The National Environmental Tribunal Act, 1995	The tribunal shall consist of judicial as well as technical members with appropriate knowledge and experience of legal administration, scientific and technical aspect of the problem related to environment and wildlife This act seeks to establish a higher powered body to decide cases related to wildlife and environment in addition to providing compensation to the people for death, injury or damage to property, or to the environment
Public Liability Insurance Act, 1991	This act provides liability insurance for persons injured by accidents with hazardous materials The measure mandates that business owner operating with hazardous waste take out insurance policies, an environmental relief fund was established and is maintained by industry operators

CHAPTER 17 — Forestation

for implementing any treaty, agreement or convention with any other country." This article enabled Parliament to enact Air Act and Environment Act to implement the decision reached at Stockholm Conference.

ACTION TAKEN BY THE GOVERNMENT OF INDIA

Formation of Ministry of Environment and Forest

On the recommendations of ND Tiwari Committee, Central Department of Environment was established in November, 1980 under the control of Ministry of Environment (renamed Ministry of Environment and Forests, April 4, 1985). This ministry handles the affair of environment, forests and wildlife. Central Pollution Control Board (CPCB) and State Pollution Control Boards (SPCB) have been formed for this purpose.

National Environment Awareness Campaign

Following important programs have been started by Government of India to create awareness amongst the people.

Environment Education

United Nations Organization (UNO) launched International Environmental Education Program (IEEP) in 1975. First World Governmental Conference of Environment Education (EE) was held in Tbilisi (Soviet Georgia) in 1977.

The Supreme Court [Writ Petition (Civil) No. 860 of 1991] has directed University Grants Commission (UGC) to prescribe a source on 'man and environment'. UGC has issued a circular to various universities to introduce the course on 'EE' (as in Punjab University). The main focus of EE is as follows:

1. Overpopulation and the ways to check its rapid growth.
2. Afforestation as a preventive to soil erosion and water pollution.
3. Afforestation to prevent air pollution, insisting on smokeless cooking.
4. Discipline in playing radio and television (TV) and a ban on use of loudspeaker.
5. Elementary knowledge of the scientific and philosophical basis of man and the environment.
6. Rules regarding disposal of household waste.
7. General principles of sanitation.

National Environmental Campaign

National Environmental Campaign was started through mass media in 1986, e.g. various TV channels such as Discovery channel, National Geographic channel, Animal Planet, etc. telecast regular programs on environment, e.g. Ham Zameen, Earth file, Wildlife, Living on Edge, etc.

Paryavaran Vahini

The Ministry of Environment and Forests has started a scheme called 'Paryavaran Vahini' or 'Environment Brigade' in 1992 to create environment awareness among common people. This people's program extends over 168 districts of India with the objective of involvement of people through active participation. Each Vahini has 20 members such as students, teacher, doctors, engineers, non-governmental organizations (NGOs), etc. belonging to different fields.

Special Drive for Rural Areas

Special awareness programs regarding environmental sanitation and use of non-conventional energy resources have been launched in rural areas.

Environment Friendly Product Scheme (1991)

Under this scheme, the environmentally unsafe (from pollution point of view) products will be tested before marketing and will bear a label 'Eco mark' (with 'earthen pot' logo). A notification regarding this was issued on February 21, 1991 covering four articles of soaps, detergents, paper and paints. In the initial stage, 16 consumable products are required to get 'Eco mark'.

Celebration of Important Days

The awareness is created by celebrating important days through media such as seminars, lectures, public meetings, TV films, audio and video cassettes, puppets shows, etc. Some important days are:

1. World Environment Day (5th June) declared at Stockholm Conference in 1972.
2. Earth Day (22nd April): 'Save Earth' from greenhouse gases (GHGs) and ozone depletion.
3. World Population Day (11th July).
4. World Health Day (7th April).
5. Antitobacco Day (31st May).
6. World Forest Day (21st March).
7. World Nature Day (3rd October).
8. National Science Day (28th February).

9. World Food Day (16th October).
10. United Nations Day (24th October).
11. United Nations International Day for Lessening Natural Disaster (13th October).
12. National Environment Awareness Month (19th November to 18th December).

The first National Environment Awareness Campaign was started in 1986 at Environment Education Center, Ahmedabad and the subject was 'Save Water'. Some important subjects under 'Environment Month' were 'flood and drought' in 1987–1988; 'Save Environment-Save Yourself' in 1990–1991; 'Peoples Participation in Global Environment Concerns' in 1991–1992; 'Biodiversity' in 1992–1993; 'Animal Welfare and Waste Management' in 1993–1994, etc.

Important National Level Awards

Ministry of Environment and Forests has instituted some national level awards for individuals and organizations with outstanding work in the field of environment protection. The main objective is to encourage the people for active participation in environment protection programs. Following is the list of such awards:

1. Pitambar Pant National Environment Fellowship Award, 1978.
2. Indira Priyadarshini Vriksha Mitra Award, 1986.
3. Indira Gandhi Paryavaran Puraskar, 1987.
4. Incentive on Hindi Books on Environment, 1987.
5. National Award for Prevention and Control of Pollution, 1991.
6. The 'Sultan Qaboos' Prize for Environment Preservation. The prize has been instituted by United Nations Educational, Scientific and Cultural Organization (UNESCO).
7. Paryavaran Evam Van Mantralaya Vishisht Vaigyanik Puraskar, 1992.
8. Maha Vriksha Puraskar, 1993.
9. Rajiv Gandhi Wildlife Conservation Award (1998).

Major Areas of Activities for Pollution Control

The main areas being looked after through law are as follows.

Air Quality Monitoring

A national network of ambient air quantity monitoring stations was initiated in 1984. Several such stations have been established in cities and towns of India. The parameters to be measured are sulfur dioxide (SO_2), Carbon monoxide (CO), nitrogen oxide (NO), suspended particulate matter (SPM), temperature, humidity, wind speed and directions.

Assessment of Water Quality

Under the National Water Quality Monitoring Program, the water quality of rivers is being monitored. The stations covering all major rivers of country monitor in respect of 19 parameters such as total dissolved solids (TDS), biological oxygen demand (BOD), metals and nitrates.

Assessment of Coastal Water Quality

The CPCB in collaboration with the Department Of Ocean Development has identified 173 monitoring stations all over the Indian Coast to assess the water quality. Four SPCB have also been involved. Data of 25 parameters are being processed to formulate schemes to control and monitor pollution of the coastal waters.

Preparation of Environmental Standards

Based on the standard prepared by CPCB and the Bureau of Indian Standard (BIS), effluent and emission standards for different kinds of industries including thermal power plants have been notified under EPA, 1986.

Enforcement of Standards

Enforcement of standards are very helpful to control pollution at source. Minimal National Standards (MINAS) have been evolved by CPCB for major categories of water and air pollution industries respectively. Those standards refer to the maximum limit of effluents and emissions that an industry may discharge into any water body or the atmosphere. The SPCBs can stipulate the same or more stringent standards for effluent and emission discharges.

Ganga Action Plan

There are 27 stations along the river at Rishikesh, Kanpur, Allahabad, Varanasi, Patna and Rajmahal. The BOD values and other parameters have been recorded to assess the pollution (refer Chapter 3 'Concepts of Nursing').

ENVIRONMENT PROTECTION ACT

The Environment Protection Act, 1986 was enacted to provide for the protection and improvement of environment, and matters connected therewith. The act consists of 26 Sections distributed among 4 Chapters and extends to the whole of India and came into force on 19th November, 1986.

Objectives of Section 1

1. The environment quality has been declining since 1960s. This has resulted in increasing pollution, loss of vegetal cover, excessive concentrations of harmful chemicals in atmosphere and threats of life support system. The concern over the state of environment has grown.
2. There are many laws existing, which concern directly or indirectly for protection of environment, but it is necessary to have general legislation for environmental protection and some hazardous areas.
3. There is urgent need for enforcement and making general legislation on environmental protection, speedy response in the event of accidents threatening environment and deterrent punishment to those who endanger human environment, safety and health.

Definitions (Section 2)

1. Environment includes water, air, land and the interrelationship, which exists among and between water, air and land, human beings, other living creatures, plants, microorganisms and property.
2. Environmental pollutant means any solid, liquid or gaseous substance present in such concentration as may be injurious to environment.
3. Environmental pollution means the presence of any environmental pollutant in the environment.
4. Hazardous substance means any substance or preparation, which by reason of its chemical or physico-chemical properties is liable to cause harm to human life, plant life, animal life or property.

Powers and Measures of the Law

Central government has the power to take all necessary measures for the purpose of protecting and improving the quality of environment, preventing, controlling and abating environmental pollution. Power of central government to take measures are:

1. It must coordinate with state government.
2. To execute nationwide programs.
3. To lay down standards of the quality of environment.
4. To lay standards for emission or discharge of environmental pollutions.
5. Restriction on location of industry in certain areas.
6. To lay down procedures and safeguards for the handling of hazardous substances.
7. To examine manufacturing processes as are likely to cause environmental pollution.
8. To prepare manuals, codes or guidelines relating to prevention or control of environmental pollution.
9. To establish environmental laboratories.
10. Collection and dissemination of information on environmental pollution.
11. Central government appoints officers for performing various functions.
12. Central government issues directions and it can order:
    a. Closures of an industry.
    b. Stoppage of the supply of water, electricity or any other service:
    - The central government can make rules for the protection of environmental quality. The rules may provide:
        - Standards of quality of air, water or soil
        - Maximum allowable limit of concentration of various environmental pollutants (including noise and dust)
        - The procedure and safeguards for handing hazardous substances
        - Restriction on the location of industry
        - Procedures and safeguards for preventing accidents.

Measure to Control Environmental Pollution

1. The act prohibits every person carrying on any industry from discharging or emitting any environmental pollutant in excess of prescribed standards.
2. Hazardous substances shall be handled only in accordance with prescribed safeguards.
3. The person in-charge of premises (industry) from where excess emission occurs is bound to inform the board. He/She is also bound to render all assistance, if called upon.
4. Any authorized officer of the board has the right to enter any place for performing his/her duty or to examine and test any equipment, and industrial plant or to determine where rules are being followed.
5. Any authorized officer of the board can take samples.
6. For the analysis of samples, government has set up environmental laboratories and appointed analysis.

Punishment or Penalties

1. Any authorized officer of the board can lodge a complaint in the court.
2. Any person can lodge a complaint in the court after a notice of at least 60 days.

3. The central government has powers to make rules regarding various matters.
4. If a person found guilty, does offense again and again then additional fine up to ₹5,000 and an imprisonment of 7 years should be extended in this case.

AIR PREVENTION AND CONTROL OF POLLUTION ACT (1981)

The Air Act was framed in the year 1981, but enacted on 29th March, 1982 for the effective prevention, control and abatement of air pollution in the country. The Air Act extends to whole of India and its welfare legislation dealing with the special evil of pollution. Therefore, it is considered a Modern Act or Special Act.

The CPCB and SPCB (constituted under Water Act, 1974) shall exercise the power and perform functions for the prevention and control of air pollutions to improve the quality of air.

Measures to Control Air Pollution

The Air Act was amended in 1987 to remove the difficulties encountered during implementation, to confer more power on the implementing agencies and to impose more stringent penalties for violation of the provisions of the act. Definition of air pollutants was amended to included noise also. Section 19 was added [Air Pollution Control Area (APCA) can be declared]. The state government, after consultation with state board can:

1. Declare any area within the state as 'air pollution control area'. This power provides measures, which are preventive in nature, particularly use of only approved appliances in the premises.
2. Prohibit the use of any other than an approved fuel in any APCA.
3. Prohibit the burning of any material (other than fuel) in any APCA:
   a. The state government has to notify this declaration in the official gazette.
   b. No person without the previous consent of the state board in writing can operate any industrial plant in APCA.
   c. No person, operating an industrial plant in any APC area, shall discharge the emission of any air pollutant in excess of the standard laid down by the state board.
   d. Emissions of air pollutants in excess of the standards laid down by state board is an offence and punishable under Section 37 of Air Act. Therefore, in such cases, board can lodge an application to the court.
   e. On receipt of application, the court can order the person to check the emission of air pollutants or can authorize the board to implement the directions. All expenses incurred by the board shall be recoverable from the person concerned.

Any person, authorized by the board, has the right to enter any place:
1. For the purpose of performing the duty.
2. For the purpose of determining whether the provisions and directions given under this act are being complied with.
3. For the purpose of examining or testing any control equipment, industrial plant, record, register or any other document:
   a. Any obstruction or willful delay is offence, which is punishable.
   b. State board has the power to obtain any information from a person carrying on any industry.
   c. State board has the power to take samples of air or emission. The board has set a procedure to be followed in this connection.

Punishments and Penalties

1. Violation of act under any circumstances: Imprisonment from ½ year to 6 years and fine (no limit).
2. Whosoever damages the property of board: Imprisonment up to 3 months or fine up to ₹10,000.
3. Offence by a company or government department: Punishment to the Director of Company or Head of Government Department according to offence:
   a. Court shall take cognizance of any offence, if the complaint is made by:
      - Board or its authorized officer
      - Any person who has given notice of not less than 6 days.
   b. State government has the powers to supersede state board, if the board persistently makes default in the performance of its function.
   c. Central government has the powers to make rules.

WATER ACT OR THE WATER (PREVENTION AND CONTROL OF POLLUTION) ACT (1974)

Water Act was enacted on 23rd March, 1974 to implement the decision reached at Stockholm Conference under Article 252, Section 1 of Indian Constitution. It is a social welfare legislation enacted for the purpose of:
- Prevention and control of water pollution
- Maintaining or restoring of wholesomeness of water
- Establishing pollution control boards

- Assigning powers and functions relating water pollution to boards.

The act has been adopted by states of Assam, Bihar, Gujarat, Haryana, Himachal Pradesh, Jammu and Kashmir, Karnataka, Kerala, Madhya Pradesh, Rajasthan, Tripura and West Bengal and all union territories with effect from 23rd March, 1974 and the State UP adopted it on February 3, 1975.

Definitions

Water pollution means:
1. Contamination of water or alternation of physical, chemical and biological properties of water.
2. Discharge of sewage or trade effluent.
3. Discharge of gaseous substance, which may or is likely to:
   a. Create nuisance.
   b. Render the water, harmful or injurious to public health, safety, domestic or commercial, industrial or agricultural uses, or the life and health of animals or of plants or of aquatic life.

Also, board and member of board, sewer, sewage, effluent outlet, etc. Have been defined in detail. Board may refer to central board or state board.

CENTRAL AND STATE POLLUTION CONTROL BOARDS

Central or State Pollution Control Board shall consist of the following members:
1. A full-time Chairman, being a person having special knowledge or practical experience in respect of matters relating to environmental protection, to be nominated by central or state government, as the case may be.
2. Officials, not exceeding five, to be nominated by respective government.
3. Persons, not exceeding five, to be nominated by central government from amongst the members of state board and in the case of state boards, to be nominated by state government from amongst the members of local authorities.
4. Nonofficials, not exceeding three, to be nominated by respective government, to represent the interest of agriculture, fishery or industry or trade, or any other interest, which in the interest of government ought to be represented.
5. Two persons to represent the companies or corporation owned, controlled or managed by the central government or state government, as the case may be, to be nominated by that government.
6. A full-time Member Secretary, possessing qualifications, knowledge and experience of scientific, engineering or management aspects as pollution control, to be appointment by respective government.

Maximum number of members of the board is 17 including Chairman and Member Secretary. A member can hold office for a term of 3 years. A member can be removed, if he/she fails to attend three consecutive meeting without sufficient reason. A member can be disqualified under the following conditions:
1. Solvency.
2. Unsound mind.
3. Conviction by court.
4. Abuses position.
5. If he/she is a partner in the firm dealing with supply of machinery or other related material:
   - A board shall meet at least once in every 3 months
   - Two or more states, or state and union territory can have a joint board.

Function of Central Board

The main function of CPCB shall:
1. Cleanliness of rivers, fresh waters and wells in different areas of states.
2. Advise the central government on water pollution issues.
3. Coordinate the activities of state boards and resolve dispute among them.
4. Carry out and sponsor investigation and research relating to water pollution and provide technical assistance and guidance to state boards.
5. Training of persons engaged in programs for control of water pollution.
6. Organize comprehensive programs for pollution control, e.g. through mass media.
7. Lay down or modify the standards for streams and wells in consultation with concerned state government.
8. Plan nationwide programs for pollution control.
9. Establish or recognize laboratories for analyzing the samples of water, sewage or trade effluent.
10. Perform for the functions of state boards or union territories.

Powers of Central Board

1. Central board is more powerful than a state board. In the case of conflicts between a central board and state board, the central broad prevails.
2. When the central government is of the opinion that any state board has failed to comply with the directions given by central board, the central board may

then be directed by the central government to take over the state board function.
3. Central board can demand state of purity and wholesomeness of water from state boards if some complaints arise.

Functions of State Board

Functions of state board are:
1. To plan a comprehensive program to prevent water pollution in streams and wells.
2. To advise the state government on water pollution issues and location of industries.
3. To encourage, conduct and participate in investigations and research relating to problems of water pollution.
4. To inspect sewage or trade effluents, works and plants for the treatment of sewage and trade effluents.
5. To develop economical and reliable methods of treatment of sewage and trade effluents.
6. To evolve methods of utilization of sewage and suitable trade effluents in agriculture.
7. To evolve efficient methods of disposal of sewage and trade effluents.
8. To establish or recognize laboratories for analyzing samples of water from sewage or trade effluents.
9. To lay down standards of treatment of sewage and trade effluents.

Powers of State Board

1. State board has powers to make survey of any area of industry.
2. It has the power to take samples of water of any sewage or trade effluent for the purpose of analysis.
3. The official has the power to enter any building to examine any plant or record.
4. It has the power to order closure of any industry or stoppage of supply of electricity and water.

Punishment or Penalty

1. Failure to comply with the directions of the board to give information imprisonment up to 3 months or fine up to ₹10,000 or both.
2. If anybody destroys property of board, imprisonment up to 3 months or fine up to ₹10,000 or both.
3. Anybody who pollutes water, imprisonment from 1½ to 6 years and fine up to ₹5,000.
4. Any person who interferes with monitoring device (meter or gauge), imprisonment up to 3 months or fine up to ₹10,000.

5. If any offence is committed by company, the Director or Manager of the company will be punished:
   a. Court shall take cognizance of any offence under this act, if the complaint is made by:
      - Board or any authorized officer
      - Any person who has given notice of not less than 60 days.
   b. Parliament amended the Water Act in 1988 to make it more effective and also to deal with air pollution.

NOISE POLLUTION AND LEGISLATIVE MEASURES

Noise is defined as a loud, unpleasant or unwanted sound that disturbs unwilling ears. It adversely affects our physiological and mental health. Noise is measured in units called decibel (dB). Noise above 115 dB is regarded as highly disturbing. The World Health Organization (WHO) recommends an industry noise limit of 75 dB. Vehicles create noise of about 90 dB, jets of about 150 dB and rockets of 180 dB. A sound above 80 dB causes noise pollution (Table 17.2).

Table 17.2: Permissible noise levels in different areas

Areas	Noise level (dB)	
	Daytime (6 AM to 9 PM)	Nighttime (9 PM to 6 AM)
Industrial area	75	65
Commercial area	65	55
Residential area	55	45
Silence zone	50	45

Legislative Measures

Various legislative measures are as follows:
1. Excessive noise has been recognized as a crime under Section 268 of IPC (Nuisance Act, 1860).
2. Noise has been recognized as a pollutant under Section 6-2.6 of EPA, 1986. This act has been amended in 1989 to prescribe day and night limits of noise level. An area with 100 m radius around a hospital or institution, or court can be declared a 'silence zone'. The use of vehicular horns, loudspeakers and bursting of crackers is banned in a silence zone under this act.
3. Under IPC Section 133, the use of loudspeaker is a public nuisance.

CHAPTER 17 — Forestation

4. The provisions under Motor Vehicles Act, the Factories Act, the Railway Act and Aircraft Act are not sufficient.
5. To control this menace, there is need of a separate Noise Pollution Act.

WHAT TO DO TO SEEK REDRESSAL?

Before proceeding to seek redressal from others, we should be aware of the following facts:

1. It shall be the duty of every citizen of India to protect and improve the natural environment [Article 51A (g) of constitution].
2. We must have the knowledge about the environment. For this, environmental education is necessary for every citizen to know that we all share common environment and it is the property of all on this earth and not of only one segment.
3. We must develop a habitual love for pollution free environment. In words of Dewan (1987) "We are traditionally pollution loving Nation. We pollute air by bursting crackers on Diwali and on many other occasions. We pollute our rivers by disposing dead bodies and other waste. We take so much wood from our trees that trees have become scarce in many areas. We are primarily vegetarian nation, yet our wildlife is on the edge of extinction. We believe in open latrines. Municipalities allow the city waste and industrial effluents to flow in open drains. Our Jagraths, Akhand paths, Azans, etc. remain incomplete without the use of loudspeakers and amplifiers. The voice must reach Gods."
4. Most people of the country are ignorant about deteriorating environment, but even awakened persons are not well-versed with the rights in our constitution and how to seek help of the court.
5. We must have knowledge about the laws made for compensation of loss of lives by pollution and control the persons who are polluting by creating noises, discharging effluents in air and water, ruthlessly exploiting our natural resources and doing loss to the wildlife.

HOW CAN WE SEEK REDRESSAL?

Article 21 of our constitution guarantees the right to life and it includes right to clean unpolluted air, water and environment. Under this article, one can seek help of Court or SPCB to take action against a polluter.

Redressal Through Court

Law of Tort and the Pollution

A common law of tort is the action against the polluter and is one of the major and the oldest law to abate pollution. Most pollution cases in tort law fall under the categories of nuisance, negligence and strict liability:

1. Section 268 of IPC deals with the persons found guilty of public nuisance, which causes injury, damage or annoyance to public and its property is a punishable offence.
2. A plaintiff (one who sues in law court) in a tort (private or civil wrong) action may sue for damage or an injunction (judicial order to restrain). While damages are the monetary compensation payable for the commission of a tort, an injunction is a judicial process in which a wrongdoer is restrained from pursuing such acts.

Law of Crime and Pollution

Law of crime and pollution is actually a mixture of Law of Tort and IPC procedures, and provides speedier remedy against public nuisance. The public duty of the Magistrate to come to the rescue of citizen in such cases has been emphasized. A public nuisance is an unreasonable interference with a general right of the public. It is to be noted that a private dispute, e.g. dispute between two neighbors only, is actionable in tort, persons who pollute the environment by domestic, urban or industrial wastes, or cause loud and continuous noises affecting the health and comfort of those dwelling the neighborhood (e.g. an instrument, noises producing installation in a factory or a shop) are liable to prosecution for causing a public nuisance.

Indian Penal Code and Pollution

Indian Penal Code has made direct provision under Section 133 and gave powers to the District Magistrate or Subdivisional Magistrate, other Executive Magistrate to pass an order (for person who creates public nuisance) on receiving the report of a police officer or other information (including complaint made by a citizen) and on taking such evidence as he/she thinks it.

The order is conditional as it is only a preliminary order. When a person fails to appear and show cause (against the order) or when the court is satisfied on the evidence adduced that the initial order was proper, the order is made final otherwise it is vacated. If the final order is defied or ignored, Section 188 of IPC comes into play. According to it, if such disobedience causes or tends to cause danger to human life, health or safety, causes or tends to cause a riot or affray shall be punished for 6 months imprisonment or fine up to ₹1,000 or both.

Direct Action

The Environment Act, 1986 (Section 7) prohibits every person carrying on any industry from discharging or emitting any environmental pollutant in excess of prescribed standard. In such cases, they can serve a direct notice to the polluter. If the polluter fails to comply with the provisions of Section 7, they can lodge a complaint against the polluter in the court after 60 days of serving the notice.

Limitations of Laws

All acts have drawbacks, short comings or lacunae, which can be summarized as follows:
1. The laws are not comprehensive in nature.
2. The laws are fragmented and haphazard.
3. Many of the laws are outdated.
4. The powers given to implementing machinery are inadequate.
5. Litigation process is very slow.

Bacterial and Viral Agents: Host and Immunity

CHAPTER 18

INTRODUCTION

Agent, host, environment model of health and illness also called ecological modes originate in the community health (Leavell and Clark, 1965) and has been expanded into a general theory of the multiple causes of disease. The model is used primarily in producing illness rather than in promoting wellness (health), although identification of risk factors than results from the interactions of agent, host and environment are helpful in promoting and maintaining health. The mode has three dynamic interaction elements, which are examined as follows:

1. Agent: It refers to any environmental factor or stressor (biological, chemical, mechanics, physical or psychological) that by its presence or absence (e.g. lack of essential nutrients) can be lead to illness or disease.
2. Host: It refers to a person(s) who may or may not be at risk of acquiring disease. Family history, age and lifestyle habits influence the host reaction.
3. Environment: All factors external to the host that may or may not predispose the person for the development of disease, physical environment includes climate, living conditions and sound (noise levels and economic levels). Several environment include interactions with others and life events such as death of a spouse.

Each of these factors are constantly interacting with others, health is an ever-changing state; when the variable are in balance, health is maintained and when they are not in balance, disease occurs.

AGENT

Diseases are produced by noxious, inimical or harmful organisms (micro or macro), substances [organic or inorganic, or force (energy)] are called agents. Some disease agent is defined as a substance, living or nonliving or a force, tangible or intangible, the excessive presence or relatively lack of which may initiate or perpetuate a disease process. When agent enters in the body of susceptible human host and multiplies, which induces change, i.e. tissue and physiological changes resulting in the disease in human beings. A disease may have single agent, number of independent alternative agent or a complex of two or more factors whose combined presence is essential for the development of the disease. The disease agents have been classified broadly into following groups.

Biological Agents

Biological agents are living agents of disease such as bacteria, virus, fungi, rickettsia, protozoa and metazoan. These agents exhibit certain host-related biological properties such as infectivity, pathogenicity, toxigenicity, antigenicity and virulence. Infectivity is the ability to invade and multiply in a host producing infection. Pathogenicity is the ability to induce clinically apparent illness and virulence is the proportion of clinical cases resulting in severe clinical manifestations including sequelae. The case fatality rate is one way of measuring illness.

Physical Agents

Physical agents include exposure to excessive heat, cold, humidity, pressure, radiation, electricity, noise, etc. may result in illness.

Chemical Agents

Chemical agents present in human body, but due to derangement of functions inside and outside the human host are of two types:
1. Endogenous.
2. Exogenous.

Endogenous are some of chemical, which are produced in the body as a result of derangement of function, e.g. urea, serum bilirubin, ketones, uric acid and calcium carbonate leads to uremia, jaundice, ketosis, gout and kidney stone respectively.

Exogenous are those arising outside the human host, e.g. allergens, metals, fumes, dust, gases, insecticides, etc.

Social Agents

The poverty, smoking, abuse of drugs and alcohol, unhealthy lifestyle, social isolation, maternal deprivation, etc. are considered as social agent.

Excess or Deficit of Certain Factors

The disease is sometimes initiated when the body encounters the agent in excessive quantity, deficit, absence or insufficiency of a factor necessary to health. These may be:
1. Chemical factors, e.g. hormones such as insulin, estrogen and enzymes [e.g. insulin deficit leads to diabetes mellitus (DM)].
2. Nutrient factors: These can be protein, carbohydrate, vitamin, minerals and water. Any excess deficiency of intake of nutrients lead to nutritional disorders, e.g. protein-energy malnutrition (PEM), anemia, goiter, obesity, vitamin deficiencies, etc.
3. Lack of structure, e.g. thymus.
4. Lack of part of structure, e.g. cardiac defects.
5. Chromosomal factor, e.g. mongolism, Turner's syndrome.
6. Immunological factor, e.g. gamma globulin, anemia.

For medical purpose, the biological agents particularly bacterial and viral agents are detailed here.

BACTERIA

Bacteria are prokaryotic microorganisms that do not contain chlorophyll. They are unicellular and do not show true branching, except in the so-called 'higher bacteria (actinomycetales)'. They measure about 0.2–1.5 millimicrons (mμ) in diameter and about 3–5 mμ in length, which is smaller than the limit of resolution of the unaided eye, hence bacteria can only be seen when magnified. Bacteria diffuse from eukaryotes in not having a nuclear membrane, nucleolus, deoxyribonucleoproteins (DNP), mitochondria, lysosomes, Golgi apparatus, an endoplasmic reticulum or sterol, they undergo mitotic division. Bacteria possess a single circular chromosome (eukaryotes have multiple linear chromosomes).

Classification

Bacteria are classified according to their shape:
1. Cocci are spherical or oval cells, e.g. pneumococci, gonococci, streptococci, staphylococci, etc.
2. Bacilli are rod-shaped cells, e.g. *Clostridium, Bacillus anthracis, Salmonella, Shigella, Mycobacterium*, etc.
3. *Vibrio* is comma shaped, curved rods and derive their name from that characteristic vibratory motility, e.g. *Vibrio cholerae*, etc.
4. Spirilla are rigid, spiral forms.
5. Spirochetes (speira means coil and chaite means hair) are flexuous spiral forms, e.g. *Treponema pallidum, Leptospira*.
6. *Actinomyces* (actis means ray and mykes means fungus) are branching of filamentous bacteria so-called because of a resemblance to the radiating rays of the sun when seen in tissue lesions.
7. *Mycoplasmas* are bacteria that do not have a cell wall and hence do not possess a fixed shape. They occur as round or oval bodies and as interlacing filaments.

Structure of Bacteria

Bacterial cell structure includes the outer layer or cell envelope consists of two components such as rigid cell wall and beneath it cytoplasmic or plasma membrane. The cell envelope encloses the protoplasm, comprising the cytoplasm (viscous watery solution), cytoplasmic inclusions such as thousands of ribosomes, granules, vacuoles and nuclear body, and various organic and inorganic solutes. The bacterial nucleus does not possess nuclear membrane. Nucleolus and nucleus does not divide by mitosis. The cell may be enclosed in a sticky layer, which may be a loose slime layer or organized as a capsule. Some bacteria carry filamentous appendages protruding from the cell surface, the flagella, which are organs of locomotion and the fimbriae that appear to be organ for attachment.

Growth of Bacteria

There are certain factors, which affect the growth of bacteria.

Nutrition

For growth and multiplication of bacteria, the minimum nutritional requirements are water, source of carbon and nitrogen, and some inorganic salts particularly phosphate, sulfate, sodium, potassium, magnesium, iron, manganese and calcium. These are normally present in the natural environment, where bacteria live, but have to be supplied in culture media. Water is the route of entry for all nutrients into the cell as well as the elimination of all waste products. It participates on metabolic reactions and also forms an essential part of the protoplasm. Some bacteria require certain organic compounds in minute quantity, e.g. vitamins.

Oxygen

Bacteria may be aerobic or anaerobic. Aerobic bacteria require oxygen for growth, e.g. *Vibrio cholerae*. Anaerobic bacteria grow in the absence of oxygen and obligate anaerobes may even die on exposure to oxygen, e.g. clostridia. Microaerophilic bacteria are those that grow best in the presence of low oxygen concentration.

Carbon Dioxide

All bacteria require small amounts of carbon dioxide (CO_2) for growth. The CO_2 are present in the atmosphere produced within the cell by cellular metabolism. Bacteria such as *Brucella abortus*, which require much higher level of CO_2 are called capnophilic.

Temperature

Most pathogenic bacteria grow at optimum temperature at 37°C. But, some cases of bacteria grow at different temperature, i.e. mesophilic bacteria (25–40°C), psychrophilic bacteria (below 200°C) and thermophilic bacteria (55–80°C).

Moisture and Drying

Water is an essential ingredient of bacterial protoplasm and hence, drying (desiccation) is lethal to cells. Spores, which are resistant to drying may survive in the dry state for several decades.

pH

The majority of pathogenic bacteria grow best at neutral or slightly alkaline pH (7.2–7.6). Some of *Lactobacilli* grow best under acidic conditions. Other examples are *Vibrio cholerae* very sensitive to acid, but tolerate high degree of alkalinity.

Light

Most bacteria grow well in the dark except photogenic. They are sensitive to ultraviolet (UV) light and other radiation, cultures die if exposed to sunlight. Exposure to lights may influence pigment production. For example, some mycobacteria form pigment only on exposure to light.

Diseases Caused by Bacteria

Bacteria are the most common infection causing microorganism. Several hundreds of species can cause disease in human beings and can live, and be transported through air, water, food, soil, body tissues and fluids, and inanimate objects. Some of the examples are given below:

1. *Staphylococcus* causes cutaneous lesions such as furuncles, styes, boils, abscess and impetigo, and number of infections, which include tonsillitis, pharyngitis, pneumonia, meningitis, endocarditis, acute osteomyelitis, food poisoning, etc.
2. *Streptococcus* causes pharyngitis, tonsillitis, influenza, bronchopneumonia, scarlet fever, skin infections in burns, wounds, cellulitis, impetigo and also rheumatic fever, acute glomerulonephritis, abscess, septicemia, etc.
3. *Pneumococcus* responsible for causing lobar pneumonia, bronchopneumonia, pneumococcal meningitis, emphysema, pericarditis, otitis media, sinusitis, peritonitis, etc.
4. *Neisseria gonorrhoeae* causes urethritis, prostatitis, salpingitis, pharyngitis, arthritis, endocarditis, neonatal ophthalmia, gonorrhea.
5. *Neisseria meningitidis* causes meningitis, meningococcal septicemia, cerebral meningitis.
6. *Corynebacterium* causes cervical lymphadenitis.
7. *Clostridium tetani* causes puerperal tetanus, tetanus neonatorum, postabortal tetanus and cephalic tetanus.
8. *Clostridium welchii* causes gangrene, food poisoning, etc.
9. *Escherichia coli* causes cystitis, pyelitis, pyelonephritis, gastroenteritis, pyogenic infection, peritonitis meningitis, septicemia, etc.
10. *Shigella* causes bacillary dysentery.
11. *Salmonella* causes food poisoning, enteric fever and septicemia.
12. *Vibrio cholerae causes* dehydration, acute gastroenteritis, hypochloremia and cholera.
13. *Mycobacterium tuberculosis* causes leprosy.

VIRUSES

Viruses are much smaller than bacteria. Due to small size and filterability, they are known as 'filterable viruses'. Most of them were too small to be seen under the light monoscopic, so they were called ultramicroscopic. Viruses do not strictly fall into the category of unicellular microorganisms, as they do not possess cellular organisms and contain only one type of nucleic acid either deoxyribonucleic acid (DNA) or ribonucleic acid (RNA), but never both. They are obligate intracellular parasites, because they lack the enzymes necessary for synthesis of proteins and nucleic acid and are dependent for replication on synthesis machinery of the host cell. They multiply by a complex process (not binary fission) and are not affected by antibacterial antibiotics.

Structure

Viruses are considered to be the smallest living units. The extracellular infectious virus particle is called 'virions'. The virion consists of nucleic acid surrounded by a protein coat (capsid). The capsid together with enclosed nucleic acid is known as 'nucleocapsid'. Capsid protects the nucleic acid from agents in the environment and sticking or absorbing to host cells. The capsid is composed of individual unit called 'capsomeres'. Virions may be enveloped or nonenveloped. The envelope is derived from the host cell membrane when the virus is released after multiplication within the host cell.

Property

Viruses contain only one type of nucleic acid either single or double-stranded DNA or RNA. Their capsid are made of proteins. Most viruses are killed easily by heat. They are generally inactivated within seconds at 56°C, within minutes at 37°C and in days at 4°C. They are stable at low temperature. They are inactivated by sunlight, UV rays and ionizing radiation. They are more resistant than bacteria to chemical disinfectant probably because they lack enzymes.

Chemical such as hydrogen peroxide, potassium permanganate, iodine and hypochlorites, formaldehyde and beta-propiolactone are all able to kill viruses and therefore used in killed vaccine preparation. Also chlorination of drinking water kills most viruses except hepatitis virus and polioviruses. The presence of organic matter in water delays the destroying of viruses.

So, viruses are ultramicroscopic and reproduce inside the living cells. They are 20–200 nm in size with different shapes, i.e. bullet and brick, round. They have central core of nucleic acid with the protein coat around it known as capsid. The subunit of capsid is capsomere and within envelope having subunits as protein on the surface known as peptomeres.

Classification and Diseases Caused by Virus

Viruses are classified into two major groups:
1. DNA viruses are poxvirus, herpes virus, adenovirus and papovaviruses, etc.
2. RNA viruses are picornavirus, paramyxovirus, orthomyxovirus, rhabdovirus, yoga virus, retrovirus, flavivirus, etc. These viruses cause many diseases. The common diseases caused by the viruses are as follows:
   a. Poxvirus: Variola major causes smallpox and cowpox virus causes cowpox.
   b. Herpes virus: Herpes simplex causes eczema genital herpes and neonatal herpes:
      - Varicella zoster causes chickenpox
      - Cytomegalovirus causes infection of salivary glands and kidneys.
   c. Adenovirus: Human adenovirus causes respiratory infections, ocular infections and genitourinary infections.
   d. Papovavirus: Papillomavirus causes cutaneous warts, genital warts and oral papillomatosis.
   e. Picornavirus: Poliovirus causes poliomyelitis and rhinovirus causes common cold (coryza).
   f. Rhabdovirus: Rabies virus causes rabies.
   g. Orthomyxovirus: Influenza virus causes influenza.
   h. Paramyxovirus: Mumps virus causes mumps and measle virus cause measles.
   i. Yoga virus: Rubella virus causes rubella, i.e. German measles.
   j. Flavivirus: Dengue virus causes dengue, i.e. breakbone fever.
   k. Retrovirus: Human immunodeficiency virus (HIV) causes acquired immune deficiency syndrome (AIDS).
   l. Hepatitis virus: Hepatitis A virus (HAV) causes hepatitis B such as HBV, HCV, HDV, HEV, HGV causes hepatitis C, D, E and G respectively.

HOST

Host refers to a person or an animal including birds and arthropods that afford lodgment to an infectious agent or a parasite. Agents even when they are potentially pathogenic and in sufficient quantity may not produce disease in individual called 'host', if the individual has the capability to ward off their onslaught. Human host is referred as the soil. The host can be diseased after the entry of pathogenic organisms or agent. The response of human host to infection depends upon many factors, which includes the following.

Human Host

Demographic Factors

The demographic factors such as age and ethnicity for example:
1. Age: Childhood is protective against coronary artery disease (CAD) and cancer, whereas old age is against infectious diseases.
2. Sex: Females do not suffer from the diseases of male reproductive organs and vice versa.
3. Ethnicity or race: The dark skin Negroes protect them against the harmful effects of UV radiation.

Biological Factors

Biological factors include genetic factors, cellular constituent of the blood, immunological factors and physiological function of the organs of the body. For example, persons with blood group 'O' are less likely to suffer from tumors of salivary gland as compared to those with blood group 'A'.

Socioeconomic Factors

Socioeconomic factors are education, occupation, stress, marital status, etc. For example, poverty may cause less intake of nutrients that leads to undernutrition, which in turn may have low resistance to infection. And continued stress causes headache, migraine, nervousness, insomnia, cavities, caries, musculoskeletal problems, fatigue, hyperacidity, amenorrhea, menstrual disorders and psychosomatic diseases.

Lifestyles

An individual lifestyle depends upon personal traits, nutrition, living habits, physical exercise and smoking, etc. For example, smoking and tobacco chewing predisposing to lung cancer, CAD, stroke, peripheral arterial obstructive disease, cancer of larynx and esophagus, chronic obstructive pulmonary disease (COPD), etc. and food habits such as eating polished rice resulting disease to beriberi, maize and jowar resulting in pellagra, etc. Eating animal fats result in CAD, etc. lack of exercise and sedentariness leads to obesity, hypertension and heart disease. Host may be of the following types:

1. Definitive host: It is a primary or final host in which the parasite undergoes sexual phase of its development in its life cycle and attains maturity, e.g. dog in hydatid disease; female *Anopheles* mosquito in malaria.
2. Intermediate host: It is secondary or alternate host in which the parasite undergoes a sexual phase of its development in its life cycle (i.e. larval stage), e.g. man in malaria and hydatid diseases, female *Culex* mosquito in filariasis.
3. Obligate host: It is compulsory host, means that only host status available for a particular disease, e.g. human being is the only host status available in measles, poliomyelitis, typhoid fever, etc.
4. Transport host: It is mechanical carrier in which the organisms remain alive, but does not undergo multiplication or development, e.g. house fly.

Human Host as Reservoir

Human host is also considered as a source or reservoir of infection for human beings. The term 'source' and reservoir are not synonymous always. Source of infection is a person, animal, arthropod, soil or the substance from which the organisms directly enter the host. The reservoir is one in which the causative organism lives, multiplies and depends primarily for its survival, i.e. the natural habitat of the organisms, such reservoir may be human, animal or soil. There are two states of reservoir:

1. Homologous reservoir state is one in which both the reservoir and the susceptible person belong to the same species, e.g. chickenpox, measles and poliomyelitis (human beings).
2. Heterologous reservoir state is one in which both the reservoir and the susceptible belong to the different species, e.g. salmonellosis (cattle-human being), rabies (dog-human being), etc.

Human reservoir: It may be case or carrier.

Case

A case is an infected person having clinical features of the disease. Such a case may be mild, moderate or severe case. Mild cases are more dangerous than the severe cases, because they are ambulatory and go on spreading the disease wherever they go. Severe cases are usually bedridden. In epidemiology, the terms used are:

1. Primary case refers to the first person developing the disease in an outbreak in the defined population.
2. Index case is the first case, which comes to the attention of the investigator.
3. Secondary cases are those who get the disease by contact from the primary case.

Carrier

A carrier is an infected person, but not having the clinical features of the disease then harboring the organisms and serve as a source of infection to others in the community.

Such carries are seen in typhoid, diphtheria, gonorrhea, AIDS, hepatitis B, meningitis, salmonellosis and amebiasis.

So, case and carriers, which harbors the agent are the potential source of infection to human population.

Classification of carrier
According to the stage in the disease cycle, there are three types of carriers namely, incubating, convalescent and contact or healthy carrier.

Incubatory carrier
In this type, carriers shed the infectious agent during incubatory period of disease. Incubatory carrier is one who spread the disease during the incubation period itself, i.e. before the onset of disease itself. This state occurs in diseases such as measles, mumps, diphtheria, poliomyelitis, pertussis, influenza and hepatitis A and B. After the incubation period, individual develops signs and symptoms and become a case.

Convalescent carrier
In this type, carriers shed the infectious agent during convalescence period, i.e. here one who is acting as a carrier during the period of convalescence (recovery time) from illness. That means such a person is getting cured clinically, but not bacteriologically may be incomplete course of treatment, e.g. diphtheria, typhoid, amebiasis, cholera, dysentery, etc.

Healthy or contact carrier
It is one in which person is subclinically infected and act as a source of infection to others, i.e. healthy carriers are those who have developed carrier state without suffering from overt disease, but nevertheless, shedding the disease agent. The nursing personnel, the patient's attendants or the family members who are in close association with the cases often become healthy carriers. They never suffer from a disease. Depending upon the duration of carrier state, they are grouped into temporary and chronic carriers.

Temporary carrier
Temporary carriers are those, who shed the infectious agent for a short period of time or for several days. All incubating, convalescent and all contact carriers are temporary carriers. Temporary carriers are the carriers who shed the infectious agents for short period of time.

Chronic carriers
Chronic carriers are those, who are transmitting the disease for a long period of time; several weeks to several months. This occurs due to persistence of the organisms in the organ such as gallbladder in typhoid, tonsils in diphtheria, liver in hepatitis B, etc.

Depending upon the route of exit and portal of exit, the carrier is also grouped into the following:
- Urinary carriers, where the focus of organisms is the kidney as in typhoid
- Intestinal carrier, where the focus of organism is the intestine as in typhoid, amebiasis
- Biliary carriers, where the focus of organisms is the gallbladder as in typhoid
- Cutaneous carriers as in staphylococci
- Nasal carriers as in nasal diphtheria
- Genital carriers as in gonorrhea and AIDS.

IMMUNITY

Immunity is the protection against infectious disease based on the immune systems. The structure of this system comprises of bone marrow, thymus, lymph glands, spleen, Peyer's patches, tonsils and adenoids. The system consists of different cells, which includes:

1. The B cells or B lymphocytes: These are so named, because although derived from bone marrow, they undergo maturation in B lymphocytes in the bursa equivalent.
2. The T cells or T lymphocytes: These are so named, because although derived from bone marrow, they undergo maturation in thymus.
3. Miscellaneous cells such as plasma cells, epithelial cells, macrophages, follicular dendritic cells, polymorphs and mast cells.

Immunity is the host defines against infection. It is the body's ability to recognize, destroy and eliminate antigenic material foreign at its own. So, 'immunity' refers to the resistance exhibited by the host towards injury caused by microorganisms and their products.

Classification
Immunity can be classified as innate (native) or acquired. Acquired immunity can be further divided into active and passive and both of these can be natural or artificial.

Innate or Native Immunity
Innate immunity is the resistance to infection that an individual possess by virtue of his/her genetic and constitutional makeup. Because of this, humans do not become infected by plant viruses and they are not susceptible to these infections. Within the species, different races may show differences no susceptibility to infections, this is known as 'racial community'. Several factors influence the innate immunity in an individual include age, hormones and nutrition.

CHAPTER 18 Bacterial and Viral Agents: Host and Immunity

Age: The very young and the very old are more susceptible to infectious disease than the rest, e.g. fetus in utero is normally protected from maternal infections by the placental barrier.

Hormones: Hormonal disorders such as DM, hypothyroidism and adrenal dysfunction are associated with enhanced susceptibility to infection, e.g. high incidence staphylococcal sepsis in diabetes.

Nutrition: The relationship between malnutrition and immunity is complex, but in general both humoral and cell-mediated immune processes are reduced, thereby causing immunodeficiency which leads to malnutrition.

Acquired Immunity

The resistance that an individual acquires during life is known as 'acquired immunity'. Acquired immunity is of two types.

Active immunity

Active immunity is the resistance developed by an individual as a result of stimulation by an antigen. An antigen is any substance, which when introduced into the body will stimulate an immune response. This response is also known as adaptive immunity, as it represents the adaptive response of the host to a specific pathogens or other antigen:

1. Active immunity involves an active response by the host and results in the production of various substances and immune cells.
2. Active immunity occurs only after a lag period, which is required for the immune system to react.
3. Active immunity is long-lasting. If an individual who has actively immunized against an antigen experiences the same antigen again. The immune response occurs more quickly and is stronger than during the first encounter. This is known as secondary response.
4. Active immunity is associated with immunological memory. This means that the immune system 'remembers' antigen to which it has been exposed and responds more quickly when it is exposed again.
5. Active immunity is more effective and gives better protection than passive immunization.

Active immunity in which immunity develops is a result of infection or due to immunization. It is associated with the presence of antibodies. It is also associated with the cells having specific action against foreign or particular infectious agent. It depends upon:
- Cellular response
- Humoral response
- Combination of both the response. On the basis of these responses immunity is cellular, humoral or combination of both. Active immunity is acquired by the following ways:
    - Clinical infections such as chickenpox
    - Subclinical infection such as polio
    - Immunization with an antigen.

Whenever an antigen enters by any of the above ways, then the body shows two types of responses:
1. Primary response.
2. Secondary response.

Primary response
Antigen enters for the first time in human body, who has never been exposed to it. The antibody in response to antigen appears as immunoglobulin M (IgM) type. Its level rises for 2–3 days, then falls and in the meanwhile if sufficient antigen stimulus is present, then IgM antibody appears and reaches its peak level within 7–10 days and then it declines over a period of weeks or months. There are number of factors in which nature and extent of primary response depends. These factors include dose of antigen, nature of antigen, the route of administration and the nutritional status of host. The outcome of the primary response is the production of both memory cells by ('B' and 'T' lymphocytes). The memory cells provide immunological memory that can be achieved after immunization, which is the main purpose of immunization.

Secondary response
Secondary response is the booster response, which involves the brief production of IgM and more prolonged production of IgG antibody.

Humoral immunity

In this, on the entry of antigen, specific antibodies are produced, which comes from B cells. B cells are bone marrow-derived lymphocytes. These specific antibodies circulate in the body and neutralize the antigen or microbe. These antibodies are specific, because they react against the same antigen, which have provoked their production.

Cellular immunity

Cellular immunity is responsible for immunity against many diseases such as tuberculosis, etc. It is effective against most of infectious disease. T lymphocytes secrete lymphokines, which stimulate macrophages and perform phagocyte function. For example, the baby born with defect in humoral antibody production can live up to 6 years of life without any replacement therapy. 'B' and 'T' lymphoid cells, accessory cells and human killer cells' joint function constitute complex events of immunity. It is most important that vaccines should be effective against both humoral and cellular responses. The immunity is the combination of both.

Types of active immunity

Active immunity may be of two types:
1. Natural active immunity results from either a clinical or an in apparent infection by microbes. A person, who has recovered from an attack of measles develop natural active immunity. For many viral diseases, immunity is usually lifelong, whereas for bacterial diseases immunity is of shorter duration.
2. Artificial active immunity is the resistance induced by vaccines. Vaccines are preparation of live or killed microorganism, or their products used for immunization.

Passive immunity

The resistance that is transmitted passively to a recipient in a readymade form is known as 'passive immunity'. Here, the recipient is immune system plays no active role:
- In passive immunity, there is no antigenic stimulus, instead, performed antibodies are administered
- In passive immunity, there is immediate protection with no lag period
- In this immunity, there is no secondary response
- In this, the response is less effective than that by active immunity.

Types of passive immunity

Passive immunity may be of two types:
1. Natural passive immunity: It is the resistance passively transferred from mother to baby. In human infants, maternal antibodies are transmitted predominantly through the placenta. The human colostrum, which is also rich in IgA antibodies is resistant to intestinal digestion and gives protection to the neonate. It is only at the age of 3 months that the infant begins to be able to make an immune response until then maternal antibodies give passive protection against infectious diseases to the infant.
2. Artificial passive immunity: It is the resistance passively transferred to a recipient by the administration of antibodies, these are used for prophylaxis and therapy.

So, passive immunity is the production of antibodies in one body and then transfer to another person body in order to protect against diseases. It means, readymade antibodies are transferred to human body to achieve protection against diseases. The passive immunity is induced by administrative of antiserum or immunoglobulin, or transfer of maternal antibodies to fetus across placenta or transfer of lymphocytes.

Herd Immunity

Herd immunity refers to the overall level of immunity in a community and is relevant in the control of epidemic diseases. Large proportion of individual in a community (herd) is immune to a pathogen. The herd community is low, epidemic diseases are likely to occur when a suitable pathogen is introduced due to the presence of large number of susceptible individuals in the community. Eradication of communicable diseases depend on the development of high level of immunity in individuals. Herd community can be increased by vaccination of large number of people in the community. So, herd community is the immunity developed in a large proportion (i.e. 80%) of individuals in a population, reduces the likelihood of epidemics arising in that community caused by the pathogen against which the immunity has been raised.

Herd community or community immunity describes a type of immunity that occurs where the vaccination of a portion of the population (herd) provides protection to unprotected individuals. Vaccination acts as a sort of immunological barrier in the spread of the disease, slowing or preventing further transmission of the disease to others. The herd structure is never constant due to new births, deaths and population mobility. An on giving immunization programs will keep the herd immunity at a very high level.

Contact Immunity

Contact immunity is the property of some vaccines, wherein contact of unimmunized individuals with a vaccinated individual can confer immunity, e.g. oral polio vaccine (OPV), i.e. children immunized with OPV shed the live virus in their feces for few days after immunization. Immunized family member, who is exposed to this shed virus usually develops immunity as well.

IMMUNIZATION AND IMMUNIZING AGENTS

Immunization is a procedure in which immunobiological substance are administered to strengthen the defense (immune) mechanisms as to protect the individual against the disease. There are two types of immunizations, i.e. active and passive.

Active Immunizations

Active immunizations consist of administration of antigen such as Bacille Calmette-Guèrin (BCG), diphtheria, pertussis-tetanus (DPT), measles vaccine (MV), OPV, etc.

It is an active process in which immunity is produced after sometime (i.e. 10–15 day). In this, immunity lasts longer. Here, reticuloendothelial cells are encountered. It is usually given before exposure to disease and usually not associated with reactions. So, it is very useful, but never used for treatment purposes.

Passive Immunizations

Passive immunization consists of administration of antibodies such as antidiphtheria serum (ADS), antitetanus serum (ATS), etc. Here, reticuloendothelial cells are not encountered, so it is a passive process in which immunity is produced instantaneously. Immunity last for stated period and is often associated with reactions. Usually, it is given after exposure to the disease and often used as part of treatment, e.g. tetanus, diphtheria, it is less useful.

Immunizing Agents

Immunity against specific disease is developed through the administration of immunizing agents. They have been classified into three groups:

1. Vaccines.
2. Immunoglobulin.
3. Antisera.

Vaccines

Vaccines are the antigenic substances, which when administered in an individual, stimulate the production of specific antibodies and protect the individual against that particular disease. Therefore, they are used for active immunization.

Types
Vaccines are grouped into four groups:
1. Vaccines included in the National Immunization Schedule BCG, OPV, DPT, MV, diphtheria toxoid (DT) and TT.
2. Vaccines are commercially available, but not included in the schedule, which includes hepatitis B vaccines, hepatitis A vaccines, measles, mumps, rubella (MMR) vaccine, rubella vaccine, typhoid vaccine (both oral and parenteral), *Haemophilus influenzae* b vaccine (Hib vaccine), ARY, meningococcal vaccine, Kyasanur forest disease (KFD) vaccine, chickenpox vaccine (Varilrix).
3. Vaccine under experimental phase: Rotavirus (RV) vaccine, HIV vaccine, dengue fever vaccine, cytomegalovirus vaccine, antimalaria vaccine, anti-leprosy vaccine (candidate vaccines), birth control vaccines, split virus and recombinant vaccines.
4. Prospective vaccines: Synthetic peptides, anti-idiotype vaccines, naked DNA vaccines, split virus vaccines and recombinant vaccines.

The vaccines are of following types:
- Live vaccines
- Killed vaccines
- Toxoids
- Cellular fractions
- Subunit vaccines
- Recombinant vaccines
- Combined vaccines
- Tissue culture vaccines and related vaccines (or terms).

Live vaccines
Live vaccines are so-called because, the organisms (antigen) in the preparation are living, but attenuated, i.e. they are made to retain the antigenicity and to loose pathogenicity. Since, the organisms are living, they multiply in the body after administration and so the antigenic stimulus becomes more than what is administered and the production of the antibody is also quick and more, thereby the immunity is also long-lasting. Usually, they are given in single dose, except OPV. Thus, live vaccines are safe, effective and more potent with long-lasting immunity and require single dose compared to killed vaccines. There are no untoward reactions. The only limitation is to maintain the 'cold chain' to retain the potency of the vaccines. Live vaccines should not be given to persons with immune deficiency states such as AIDS, steroid therapy, radiotherapy, chemotherapy for malignancy and acute febrile conditions. These are absolute contraindications.

However, pregnancy is not an absolute contraindication, but a relative contraindication, i.e. if the merits are more than the demerits, vaccine can be given during pregnancy also. For vaccines such as OPV, tissue culture antirabies vaccine, there are no contraindications at all. For example, for live vaccine BCG, OPV, MV, MMR, RV, oral typhoid vaccine, influenza live vaccine and yellow fever (17D) vaccine.

Killed vaccines
In this type, the organisms are inactivated or killed by heat, or chemicals such as phenol, β-propiolactone (BPL). Usually, they are given in multiple doses in the primary course (two booster doses) followed by booster dose subsequently. Immunity lasts shorter than live vaccines and reactions are also frequent. Thus, compared to live vaccines, killed vaccines are less safe, less effective and less potent with short-lasting immunity requiring multiple doses.

For example, cholera vaccine, plague vaccine, BPL, anti-rabies vaccine (ARV), influenza-killed vaccine, Salk polio vaccine, Japanese encephalitis (JE) vaccine, KFD vaccine, yellow fever vaccine, etc.

Toxoids
Toxoids are modified toxins. The toxins of the organisms are modified (detoxified) so as to maintain only antigenicity and not pathogenicity (toxicity). Thus, they are used as vaccines. They also require multiple doses in the primary course followed by booster doses. They are quite safe and effective, e.g. DT, TT.

Cellular fractions
Cellular fraction vaccines are prepared from the extract of the bacterial cell wall or capsule. They are also safe, effective and some require booster doses, e.g. meningococcal vaccine, pneumococcal vaccine, parenteral vaccine and typhoid vaccine.

Subunit vaccine
Subunit vaccine is prepared from a component of the virus, e.g. influenza vaccine.

Recombinant vaccines
Recombinant vaccines are genetically engineered recombinant DNA vaccines, i.e. the subunit of the virus (antigen) is inserted into the genome of another avirulent virus and vaccines are prepared, e.g. hepatitis B vaccine.

Combined vaccines
Combined vaccines are so-called because the preparation contains more than one antigen. Therefore, they are also called 'mixed vaccines', e.g. DPT, DT, measles, mumps, rubella and varicella (MMRV). The merits are:
- The individual is simultaneously protected against two to three diseases
- One antigen enhances the effect of other antigen
- It reduces the number of visits to the clinic and becomes economical.

Tissue culture vaccines
Tissue culture vaccines are prepared by culturing the viruses in special cells such as chick embryo cells, Vero cells of kidney of monkeys, human embryonic lung fibroblasts, etc. They are highly safe, antigenic, effective, stable, potent, protective and purified. They are costly and are given in multiple doses. For example:
- Purified chick embryo cell vaccine (PCECV)
- Purified Vero cell rabies vaccine (PVRC)
- Human diploid cell vaccines (HDCV), all used against rabies.

Related vaccines (terms)
1. Polyvalent vaccines: Vaccine containing more than one strain of the same species, e.g. OPV (trivalent vaccine), influenza vaccine.
2. Adjuvant vaccines: Adjuvants such as aluminum phosphate are used to enhance the antigenic property. But, they are painful and often result in fever. For example, purified toxoid adsorbed on aluminum phosphate (PTAP) tetanus toxoid.
3. Freeze-dried vaccines: These are the vaccines, which are frozen and died. Therefore, they are in the form of powder. Hence, they are always supplied along with diluents. Such vaccines are highly stable and retain the potency for a long time than liquid vaccines. Diluents have to be added only at the time of use along the side wall of the vial. After adding the diluents, the vial should not be shaken, but rolled between the fingers to prevent the formation of forth. It should be used as early as possible, but not beyond 30 minutes. Freeze-dried vaccines could be live or killed vaccines, e.g. BCG, PVRV (diluent sterile normal saline) MV, MMRV, yellow fever (17D) vaccine, purified chick embryo cell vaccine (PCECV) and JEV; diluent is sterile distilled water.

Immunoglobulins

Immunoglobulins are readymade antibody preparations obtained from human beings. They produce immunity instantaneously. Therefore, they are used for passive immunizations, i.e. for those who are at risk such as young close contacts and not immunized before. Since, their human preparation reactions are nil. They are of two types:
1. Human normal immunoglobulins.
2. Human specific immunoglobulins.

The advantage of immunoglobulin are that it is free from hepatitis B, used as immunoglobulin M (IgM) because of small volume and if properly stored, the antibody content can be kept stable.

Human normal immunoglobulins
Human normal immunoglobulin is prepared from the pooled plasma of at least 1,000 (multiple) donors. It is a general antibody preparation. It consists of IgGs. It produce instantaneous, but temporary immunity, e.g. against viral hepatitis A. It is given to those, who are traveling to endemic areas. This should be given simultaneously along with live vaccines, because this IgG will interfere with the development of immunity. If this is given first, live vaccine should not be given for 12 weeks and if live vaccines are given first, this should not be given for 2 weeks.

Human specific immunoglobulins
Human specific immunoglobulin is prepared from the plasma of those persons, who have been recently immunized or recovered from the disease. Therefore, this contains specific antibodies, which is highly safe, effective and

costly. Passive immunity lasts longer than that of human normal immunoglobulin. Not only it is used for passive immunization (i.e. for postexposure prophylaxis) but also it is used as a part of treatment to neutralize the circulating toxins in the patient (i.e. for both prophylaxis and therapeutic measures) as in rabies and tetanus. For example:

- Human rabies immunoglobulin (HRIg)
- Human tetanus immunoglobulin (HTIg)
- Hepatitis B immunoglobulin (HBIg)
- Varicella zoster immunoglobulin (VZIg).

These can be used simultaneously along with active immunization, unlike human normal immunoglobulin. Human immunoglobulin preparations are viscous in nature. So, they require big bore needles to inject. They are given deep intramuscularly.

Adverse reactions of immunoglobulins
1. Local such as pain, abscess.
2. Systemic reaction: It occurs within minutes or hours. Depending upon this, systemic reactions are of two types as detailed below.

Rapid systemic reaction: It occurs within minutes of administration, such as flushing, rigor, flank pain, dyspnea, shock, etc.

Late systemic reactions: It includes urticaria, arthralgia, pyrexia or diarrhea, which can occur within hours or days. These are usually severe.

Antisera

Antiserum is the term applied to materials in animals such as horse and passive immunization is achieved by administration of antisera and it exists for small number of diseases given below:

- Diphtheria
- Tetanus
- Gas gangrene
- Rabies
- Botulism.

Antisera are the specific immunoglobulins prepared from the plasma of immunized animals such as horses. They are cheap and less effective. Immunity lasts for about 2–3 weeks only. Reactions are frequents because of animal proteins. So test dose is a must. For example:

- Anti-tetanus serum
- Anti-diphtheria serum
- Equine rabies immunoglobulin (ERIg)
- Anti-snake venom (ASV)
- Anti-gas gangrene serum.

Related immunoglobulin preparation is Rh antibody prevent erythroblastosis fetalis.

Chemoprophylaxis

Chemoprophylaxis is another type of specific measure to protect the susceptible, i.e. it is a prophylactic (preventive) chemotherapy. If given to uninfected person to prevent the occurrence of the infection, it is called 'primary chemoprophylaxis' and if given to an infected person to prevent the development of the disease, it is called 'secondary chemoprophylaxis'.

Secondary chemoprophylaxis is given for those who are at risk of getting the disease. For example, diaminodiphenylsulfone (DDS) given to the family members (contacts) of lepromatous leprosy case, isoniazid (INH) to the young children of the open case of pulmonary tuberculosis, penicillin eyedrops to the newborn of a mother suffering from gonorrhea and tetracycline for a contact of pneumonic plague. General measures for the protection of susceptible are:

1. Improvement in the quality of life such as good living condition, with clean sanitation in and around the house, with adequate lighting and ventilation along and with good nutrition, etc. will protect the individuals against many communicable diseases. This is how all developed countries are free from common infectious diseases.
2. Legislative measures: Government of India has implemented certain acts for the protection of the health of the people, e.g. Indian Factories Act, Prevention of Food Adulteration Act, etc.
3. Health education: People are educated about the protection of their health by adopting certain healthy lifestyle such as personal hygiene, avoiding habits such as smoking and drinking alcohol, getting immunization, using sanitary latrine, etc.

Hazards of Immunization

Hazards of immunization are grouped into the following groups:

1. Reactions inherent to inoculation: These may be local or general. Local reactions are pain, swelling, nodule, sterile abscess, redness and tenderness at the site of inoculation. General reactions are fever, malaise and headache.
2. Reactions due to faulty techniques: Faulty technique may be in the production of vaccine (such as inadequate attenuation or detoxification), inadequate dosage (such as under dosage or overdose age), improper route of administration (such as giving subcutaneously instead of intradermally), improper

constitution instead of intradermally), improper constitution with wrong diluent, improper sterilization of syringes or needles, ignoring the contraindications, etc.

3. Reactions due to hypersensitivity: This can be immediate or delayed. Immediate reaction is anaphylactic shock, which is dangerous characterized by hypotension, rapid thread feeble pulse, perspiration, cyanosis, cold extremities and collapse. Delayed reaction (or serum sickness) is characterized by pyrexia, arthralgia, myalgia, urticaria and edema.
4. Neurological complications such as postvaccinal encephalitis, postvaccinal neuroparalysis follows administration of BPL, ARV, Guillain-Barré syndrome following administration of swine influenza vaccine. Another example is subacute sclerosing panencephalitis (SSPE) following measles vaccine, etc. these are often fatal.
5. Provocative reactions: This means occurrence of a disease, which is totally unconnected with the immunizing agent, e.g. development of poliomyelitis following the administration of triple antigen (DPT). The mechanism is that the pain of the vaccine triggers the latent infection of poliomyelitis into a clinical attack or the pain reduces the incubation period.
6. Other reactions: The following are the reactions:
    a. Damage to the fetus following rubella vaccination to the pregnant mother.
    b. Toxic shock syndrome due to contamination of measles vaccine with *Staphylococcus aureus*.

CONCLUSION

An agent may be living or nonliving, tangible or intangible or substances that perpetuate the disease process. The disease agents have been classified into biological (e.g. bacteria, virus, fungi, etc.), physical agent (e.g. heat, cold, pressure, humanity, sound, electricity, etc.), chemical agents [endogenous (e.g. urea, calcium carbonates, ketone bodies, etc.) and exogenous (e.g. metals, fumes, dust, gases, etc.)] and mechanical agents (mechanical forces), and nutrient agents (e.g. protein, fats, carbohydrates, vitamin, mineral). Bacteria and virus are free living organisms causing variety of health problems. Human host is referred as the soil and considered as a source of reservoir of infection in human beings. Community is the body's ability to recognize, destroy and eliminate antigenic material foreign to his own. It is of two types, i.e. active immunity and passive immunity. Natural immunity is required and artificial immunity is created by giving vaccines and immunoglobulins. The immunity protects the individual against infections.

Arthropods

CHAPTER 19

INTRODUCTION

The term 'arthropoda' is derived from Greek words 'arthron' means jointed and 'poda' means foot. Accordingly, arthropods are creatures having jointed legs. Other characteristic of arthropods are absence of vertebrae, bilateral symmetrical body consisting of segments, chitinous exoskeleton and power of ecdysis, i.e. molding. Internally, the body is filled with colorless fluid, i.e. hemocele in which the internal organs are bathed, the heart dorsally; the central nervous system (CNS) ventrally and in between there is alimentary canal. Their respiratory system consists of air tubes, which open by a series of pores called spiracles. Sexes are separate.

CLASSIFICATION OF ARTHROPODS

Arthropods have distinctive features such as body, legs, antennae and wings. Body is divided into head, thorax and abdomen and having three pairs, four pairs or five pairs of legs. Depending upon these distinct features, they are classified into three classes, i.e. insecta, arachnida and crustacea.

Insecta

Insecta has a cylindrical shape of body, i.e. divided into head, thorax and abdomen, and one pair antennae in head. Some are winged and some are wingless. It has three pairs of legs and it is living on land. For example, mosquitoes and flies (winged), fleas, bugs and lice (wingless). This class is comprised of following categories with examples are given in Table 19.1.

Arachnida

Arachnida has a circular or oval-shaped body is divided into cephalothorax and abdomen, and has no antennae and wings, and it is living on land, e.g. ticks, spiders and scorpions. The arthropods of this class have four pairs of legs. It has main two categories, i.e. ticks and mites.
1. Ticks: Hard ticks, soft ticks.
2. Mites: Chikungunya, itch mite, trombiculid.

Table 19.1: Classification of insecta with examples

Insecta	Examples
Mosquitoes	*Anopheles,* culicines
Flies	Housefly, sandfly, tsetse fly, black fly
Human lice	Human head lice, human body lice, crab lice
Fleas	Rat fleas, sand fleas

Crustacea

Crustacea has a pear-shaped body that is divided into cephalothorax and abdomen. It has two pairs of antennae in head and has no wings, but it has five pairs of legs and found in water. For example, cyclops, crabs, lobsters and prawns.

All arthropods are not harmful. In fact most of them are faithful friends and servants of human beings. For example, the World Health Organization (WHO) process of food production depends on the pollination carried on the bees and butterflies. Only a few arthropods are responsible for causing or more commonly transmitting disease and also causing minor lesions (due to bite of some arthropods such as hemorrhage, puncture, blisterations, erythema, etc.) allergic reactions (e.g. urticaria from bite of human flea, sandfly and bed bugs), dermatitis by coconut mites, asthma, eczema; secondary infections (due to bite wounds of sand flea and eye mites); entomophobia (unusual fear of bite or strong fear of contact of arthropod); envenomation (toxic reactions following bite or sting, or contact of arthropod), scabies and myiasis.

DISEASES CAUSED BY ARTHROPODS

Insecta as Vectors

Diseases caused by insecta class or arthropods insecta have been discussed below.

Mosquito

- *Anopheles:* Malaria
- *Culex:* Filaria
- *Aedes aegypti:* Yellow fever, dengue, dengue hemorrhagic fever
- Mansonoides: Chikungunya fever.

Flies

- Housefly: Diarrhea, dysentery, typhoid, paratyphoid gastroenteritis, cholera, poliomyelitis, conjunctivitis, trachoma, jaws, anthrax, amebiasis, etc.
- Sandflies: Oriental sore, oraya fever, sandfly fever, kala-azar
- Tsetse flies: Sleeping sickness
- Black flies: Onchocerciasis.

Human Lice

The threat associated with body lice is not the louse itself, but is associated with bacterial diseases:
- *Borrelia recurrentis (B. recurrentis):* Relapsing fever
- *Bartonella quintana:* Trench fever
- In head of lice causes: Pediculosis.

Fleas

- Rat fleas: Bubonic plague *Hymenolepis diminuta (H. diminuta),* endemic typhus
- Sand fleas: Tetanus and gas gangrene frequently occur due to secondary infection.

Reduviid Bugs

Chagas disease is caused by reduviid bugs.

Arachnida as Vector

Following are the types of diseases caused by this class of arthropods arachnida:
- Ticks:
  - Hand ticks: Viral encephalitis, tick typhus, viral fever, viral hemorrhagic fever, tick paralysis, etc.
  - Soft ticks: Q fever, relapsing fever, etc.

Mites

- Itch mite: Scabies
- Trombiculid mite: Scrub typhus, rickettsialpox.

Crustacean as Vector

- Diseases caused by cyclops, are guinea worm disease, fish tape worm disease.

MECHANISM OF TRANSMISSION OF DISEASE

A vector is an invertebrate (arthropod) that capable of transmitting disease from the source or reservoir of infection, or spreading of the disease. Vectors transmit disease by two broad mechanisms, i.e. mechanical and biological.

Transmission

In spread of arthropod borne diseases following types of transmission is involved:
- Direct contact
- Mechanical transmission
- Biological transmission.

Direct Contact

The disease such as scabies and pediculosis are transmitted by arthropods that are directly transferred from man-to-man through close contact.

Mechanical Transmission

In mechanical mechanisms, the arthropod carries the infection material passively transmits the pathogens without biting, e.g. housefly mechanically lifts up the pathogen from the filthy substances and deposit over eatable and contaminate foods. The diseases such as diarrhea, dysentery, trachoma, typhoid and paratyphoid caused by housefly are transmitted mechanically. In this, the transmission occurs by the mechanical transportation of infectious agents through soiled feet of flying arthropods and passage of organisms through its gastrointestinal tract (GIT). There is no development of infectious agent on or within vector.

Biological Transmission

In biological mechanism, the disease agent forges parasitic relationship with arthropod. Here, it is an arthropod, which transmits the pathogen indirectly by biting the reservoir and sucking the blood-containing pathogens. Subsequently, the pathogens undergo biological development inside the body of the vector for a specific period, only after which the vector can spread the disease, e.g. mosquitoes, rat flea, cyclops, etc.

In biological mechanisms of transmits, there are two types of transmission, i.e. noncyclic and cyclical transmission. If the organism spends its whole life cycle in either the human or arthropod hosts, then the transmission is called noncycled. But, if it spends one half of its cycle in the arthropods and the other in the human host, the transmission is called cyclical. In biological transmission, infectious agents undergo replications/multiplication/development in the vector and the vector cannot transmit infection before completion of an incubation period. Biological transmission is of three types:

1. Propagative: Plague, bacilli in rat fleas.
2. Cyclopropagative: Malaria parasite in anopheline mosquito.
3. Cyclodevelopment: Filaria in *Culex*.

Non-cyclic Transmission

In non-cyclic transmission there are three types, which includes the following.

Propagative: Here, the pathogen organism multiplies in the body of the arthropod without invading its germplasm. For example, bubonic plague by rat flea, trench fever by the louse, yellow fever virus in rat flea, yellow fever virus in *Aedes* mosquito.

Transovarial: Here, the pathogenic organism invades the germplasm and gets incorporated into it with the result that the progeny is automatically infected and hence capable of transmission, e.g. the spread of Rocky Mountain spotted fever and the hard tick.

Transovarial transstadial: In this transmission, the adult arthropod is not in picture at all, for it does not bite man or animals. Larva bites and in the process pickups the causative agent, but itself does not spread the diseases as it does not bite a second time. The organism is incorporated into the deoxyribonucleic acid (DNA) of its ovum and is passed down to progeny. For example, scrub typhus is spread by the *Trombicula* mite.

Cyclic Transmission

In cyclical transmission there are two types, which includes the following.

Cyclopropagative: Here, the organisms divide and subdivides inside the vector body, so that at the end of extrinsic incubation periods thousands of progeny are produced. So, the pathogens undergo not only multiplication, but also cyclic development inside the body of vector, e.g. spread of malaria by the female *Anopheles* mosquito.

Cyclodevelopmental: Here, the organisms does not multiply inside the body of the vector, it merely undergoes maturation. If the arthropod has picked up a pair of organisms, at the end of the extrinsic incubation period, there is still be only two. So, here the pathogen undergo only developmental changes, but multiplication only inside vector, e.g. bancrofti inside *Culex* mosquito transmitting filariasis. One guinea worm embryo grow in cyclop.

CLASSES OF ARTHROPODS

In India, diseases produced by arthropods constitute major health problem in rural and urban. Arthropods comprise varied living things in the surrounding of human being.

For public health importance, there are five classes of arthropods, which include mosquitoes, flies, fleas, lice and bugs of class insecta; ticks, mites of class arachnida and cyclops of class crustacea. Brief description and control measures of these arthropods are as given below.

Mosquitoes

Mosquitoes are the small biting insects, are found all over the world. There are 30 genera and 100 types of species. Fortunately, only four generic transmits diseases, namely *Anopheles, Culex, Aedes* and *Mansonia* (Fig. 19.1).

Morphology

The mosquito is a small (1.5–2.5 mm), long limbed, narrow winged, buzzing and flying insect. It has three pairs of legs and one pair of antennae. It has a cylindrical body, divisible into head, thorax and abdomen (Figs 19.2A to C).

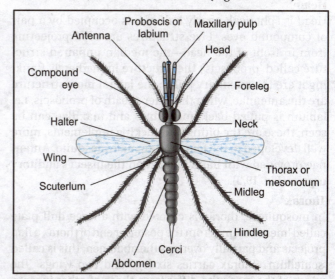

Figure 19.1: Female *Anopheles* mosquito (wings spread out and maxillary palps slightly separated)

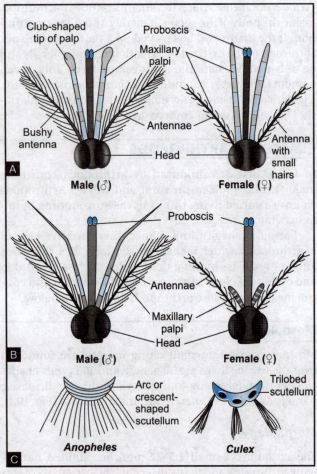

Figures 19.2A to C: Head of *Anopheles* and *Culex*

Head

Head is spherical; nearly half of it is occupied by a pair of compound eyes. Five structures are seen projecting from in front of the head—the median unpaired structure called 'proboscis'; the structure immediately flanking it are the maxillary pulps; the lateral most structure are the antennae, when the outer sheath of proboscis, i.e. labium is pulled back, mandibles and maxillae can be seen; these are the biting and sucking implements, more well developed in the female than male mosquito. Antennae provided with hairs that act on the insect's auditory organs (Fig. 19.3).

Thorax

In mosquitoes, thorax is covered with a large dull plate called 'mesonotum'. From the posterior end of thorax a flap projects and partially overlaps the abdomen, this is called 'scutellum'. Thorax carries six legs and two wings. The wings of the mosquito differ from those of other insects, than scales are present over their veins and along their lower margins. Flight wings are held out at right angle to the long axis of thorax. When the mosquito is resting they are folded one on another and overlap abdomen (Fig. 19.4).

Abdomen

The abdomen is long and cylindrical. Developmentally it consists of 10 segments in the adult mosquito, but only eight can be counted. At the posterior end of the abdomen the reproductive organs of the insect are seen. They are prominent, large and curved inward (i.e. claspers) in the male, and are small and rounded (cerci) in the female.

Life Habits

Female mosquitoes live for 5–7 weeks male for many days. Male mosquitoes feed on fruit juices, vegetables, sap, nectar, etc. Females require blood that obtain by biting man, animals or birds. The first class protein of blood is necessary for the maturation of their ova. Except *Aedes*, the other mosquitoes are night biters. Daytime they hide in shady places away from wind and sunlight (i.e. under leaves, bushes, tree holes, animal sheds, inside shoes, under cots, behind clothing, etc.). Mosquitoes breed in water.

Anopheles: Prefers clean water free of organic matter such as wells, roof reservoirs, cisterns and flooded basement.

Culex: It is like to breed in dirty water contaminated with organic matter, i.e. ditches, cesspools, septic tank, pit latrines, blocked drains, etc.

Aedes: Breeds in small amount of water held in artificial containers such as coconut shells, broken pots, tree holes, discarded tires, urns, jars, animal boroughs, roof gutters, etc.

Mansonia: Breeds in water on whose surface aquatic plants growing such as *Pistia*, *Eichhornia*, Slovenia type, etc.

Life Cycle

The life cycle of the mosquito is characterized by complete metamorphosis. The stages of egg, larva, pupa and adult have no resemblance to each other.

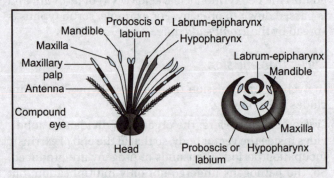

Figure 19.3: Mouthparts of mosquito (female *Anopheles* and cross section through proboscis)

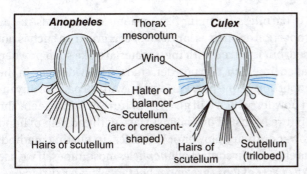

Figure 19.4: Thorax of *Anopheles* and *Culex* showing scutellum and halter (dorsal view)

Egg
The egg is ovoid or shaped-like a spindle, cigar or flask. Immediately after emerging from the pupa stage, the male and female soon thereafter lay eggs in batches of 100–300 at intervals of 2–3 days, a total of about 10 batches. Eggs are deposited singly in the case of *Anopheles* and *Mansonia* and cemented together to a form a raft in the case of *Culex* and *Aedes*. The anopheles eggs are provided with lateral floats too. *Mansonia* pastes the eggs the under surface of the leaves and aquatic plants.

Larva
After 1–2 days the egg hatches into a larva (wiggler). The larva is a 0.5–1 mm long non-winged, legless and cylindrical creature. It has a dorsoventrally flattened head adorned with two prominent and two non-prominent eyes, a globular thorax with a number of hairs, and spines along its margins, and a segmented abdomen. At the junction of the final two abdominal segments either a tube, i.e. the air tube or the siphon tube exists, or two openings flush with the body, i.e. air aperture is present (Fig. 19.5).

The larva feeds voraciously on algae, bacteria, diatom, jute fibers, etc. It is a restless and active creatures. When the water surface is distributed, it dives to the bottom with the speed of light. Motility is made possible by twitching of the body. The larva rises to the surface of water and breaths through the air apertures of the siphon tube. However, the *Mansonia* larva breaths through the rootlets of the aquatic plant, in other words it takes oxygen present in the tissues of rootlets.

Pupa
After 4–10 days and many moltings, the larva is changed into a pupa or a tumbler. It is cephalothorax forming the dot and curved abdomen the tail. It builds a hard covering around itself. It breaths, but does not feed, since it has enough food stored gathered during the preceding stage. It is a sensitive creative and if water is disturbed it dives to the bottom (Fig. 19.6).

Adult
After about 2–3 days an adult mosquito complete with wings, legs and mouth parts emerges. Under the pressure of the adult, the pupal ease breaks open. The adult sits, while on the split case to dry its wings, before commencing its terrestrial life. The time required for life cycle is 7–14 days.

Transmitting of Diseases
The diseases transmitted by female mosquitoes, i.e. *Anopheles* mosquitoes transmit malaria; *Culex* mosquitoes transmit filariasis, Japanese encephalitis, Rift Valley

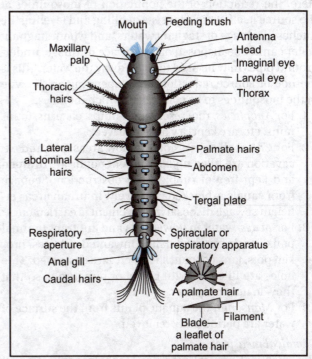

Figure 19.5: Dorsal view of *Anopheles* larva

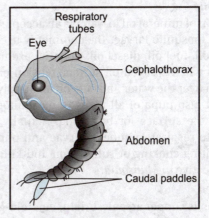

Figure 19.6: Pupa of mosquito

fever and Murray Valley fever. *Aedes* mosquitoes transmit yellow fever, chikungunya, dengue fevers, Ross river fever, etc. *Mansonia* transmits rural filariasis.

Mosquito Control Measures

Mosquito control can be achieved through antiviral measures, antiadult measures and personal prophylaxis.

Antilarval measures

Antilarval measures are grouped into physical, chemical and biological control methods.

Physical measures

Here, the reduction of the population of mosquitoes at the source itself, which consists of filling and leveling the ditches, drainage of stagnant waters, and where stagnant water cannot be disposed off by surface drainage, underground pipes may be used to drain away the water. This is method of 'source reduction'. It is depending on the type of the mosquitoes to be controlled, which includes:

1. For *Anopheles*, roof reservoirs, sumps, cisterns, fountains, etc. are kept dry once in a week.
2. For *Culex*, all depressions, hollow areas, pits and excavation are filled up. Permanent ponds are drained and kept free of rubbish and obstruction. Seepage from canals is blocked effectively. In urban areas efficient sewage disposal management is carried out.
3. For *Aedes*, water in flower pots and ant traps, animal pans, etc. is changed daily. Unwanted old tires, broken pots, jars, coconut shells, etc. are destroyed. Tree holes are filled up with gravel or punctured, so that they do not hold water.
4. For *Mansonia*, the aquatic plants from the surface of water are periodically removed.

Chemical measures

The chemical control measures include application of mineral oil, use of Paris green and larvicides.

Mineral oils

Application of mineral oil to water is an accepted method to control mosquito larvae. The commonly used oils are kerosene oil, fuel oil, diesel oil, malarial aroma oil, etc. These oils when sprayed on surface tension of water, it forms film over the water and cuts off air supply not only larvae but also pupa of all types of mosquitoes, which comes to the surface for breathing. Actually, oil penetrates into respiratory tube of larvae and pupae, clogs then resulting choking or suffocation and killing them. Oil not effective in *Mansonia*.

Paris green

Paris green is copper arsenic, bright, emerald-green colored powder insoluble in water, but soluble in dilute acid. It is harmless for man, fish or domestic animals in the proportion applied as larvicide. Paris green on such is not used, but is mixed with inert materials-like soap powder, slaked lime, ash, talc powder, charcoal powder, etc. in the proportion of one part Paris green with 99 parts of any inert powder, which will give 1% mixture of Paris green. The mixture is dusted on water surface with the help of hand blower or rotary blower or sprinkles. In dusting method, it is effective in control of *Anopheles* mosquitoes. If we use 1 kg of actual Paris green per hectare of water surface.

Larvicides

Most effective larvicides are abate, fenthion and chlorpyrifos. They are organophosphorus compounds, which are quickly dissolved in water. The requirement of abate 50–112 gram per hectare of water surface, like wise fenthion 22–112 gram per hectare and malathion 224–672 gram per hectare of water surface.

Abate: It is being low in toxicity is used as larvicide in artificial water reservoirs and domestic water containers for controlling breeding of *Aedes* mosquitoes in a concentration of 1 ppm and also control larvae or *Anopheles stephens* in wells.

Fenthion: It is a colorless oily liquid, insoluble in water, but soluble in organic solvents. It is a contact and stomach poison with good penetration power and residual action.

Organochlorine compound: Such as dichlorodiphenyltrichloroethane (DDT) are not used because of risk of water contaminants.

Biological measures

In biological measures, using of larvivorous or larvicidal fish, which feed on the larvae of the mosquitoes. There are two types of fishes, i.e. the surface feeders and bottom feeders. Surface feeders fishes are helpful in controlling mosquitoes. *Gambusia affinis*, *Aplocheilus panchax* and *Lebistes reticulatus* are very useful. For *Anopheles*, *Gambusia*, guppy or *Lebister* fish are grown and then released into wells, ornamental ponds and clean water collections. For *Aedes* and *Mansonia* biological control is not possible.

Antiadult measures

Antiadult measures used to control the mosquitoes include residual syrups, space sprays and genetic control:

Residual sprays: Includes DDT, [benzene hexachloride (BHC) lindane 0.5 g/m^2], organophosphorus compounds—malathion, parathion, fenthion, dichlorides. Now, the resistance to these insecticides becomes more and more. The average duration of effectiveness of DDT from 6 to 12 months and lindare, malathion and orthoisopropoxyphenyl methylcarbamate (OMS-33) is 3 months.

Space sprays: Include pyrethrin and pyrethroids, and residual insecticide are the insecticides. It is an extract of flowers of *Chrysanthemum cinerariaefolium*. Pyrethrum is sprayed on door and windows are kept closed for half-an-hour. At small scale, i.e. for houses hand gun with fire nozzle is used and large scale, power sprayers are used. Residual insecticides such as malathion, fenitrothion for fogging is used as insecticides.

Genetic control: Laboratory grown sexually potent, but sterile mosquitoes are released in the community for the control of malaria and filaria. The technique of genetic control includes male sterile techniques, cytoplasmic incompatibility, chromosomal translocations, sex distortion and gene replacement.

Personal protection measures
The measures for personal measures are simply disallowed the access of mosquitoes to man there by prevent the transmissions of mosquito-borne diseases. These are all defensive mechanisms, which include use of mosquito nets, screening of building and use of repellents.

Nets: Sleeping inside the mosquito net provides protection against mosquito bites and other biting insects during night times. The net cloth should be preferably white, so that other insects will be visible. Net should be tucked under the matters all round. There should not less single hole in the net. The net should not have diameter of opening more than 0.0475 inch and within one square inch there should be 150 holes.

Repellents: The repellents are applied to skin over the exposed parts of the body, drive away the mosquitoes on coming near the person for biting. The repellents keeping away the mosquitoes. There are number of repellents are available into the market. Usually, they do not produce any side effects that are very rare.

Housefly

Housefly (*Musca domestica*) a filth-inhabiting and filth-loving domesticated or synanthropic insect is a gray-colored, broad and burly creature. It has a 6–7 mm long body and 14 mm wide wingspan. Its body divided into head, thorax and abdomen (Fig. 19.7).

Morphology

Head
The head measures more in breadth than the length. A pair of large compound eyes occupies most of it. In the male, they are closely and the female widely set. In the anterior part of the head there is proboscis that projects at right angle to the long axis of the head. It is suited for

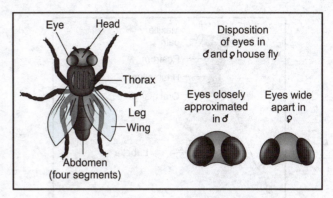

Figure 19.7: Housefly (*Musca*)

sucking and sponging projects and retracts the proboscis at its will. A disk-shaped structure called oral disk is situated at the tip of proboscis, it is covered with a film of sticky secretion. Head bears a pair of short antennae. A hairy structure called arista present at their tip. Arista is real feeling organ of fly (Figs 19.8 and 19.9).

Thorax
The thorax of housefly is decorated with 3–4 longitudinal stripes. It carriers one pair of halters and three pairs of legs, wings, when folded do not overlap, part of the abdomen is being visible in the gap between them. The legs are covered with brush-like hairs and end in claws. Between the claws there are present lobulated structures called pulvilli. In between lobes of each pulvillus there are hollow hairs, which are bathed in an oily secretion (Fig. 19.10).

Abdomen
The abdomen of housefly gray black in the male and yellow-black in the female, consists embryologically of eight segments in the male, and nine in the female, actually only four are visible in each sex (Fig. 19.11).

Life Habits

Housefly lives for 1–2 months or up to 8 months (when it hibernates). It feeds on liquids such as milk, buttermilk, sputum, water stools, body discharge, etc. by sucking them up.

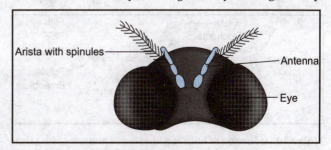

Figure 19.8: Head of housefly enlarged to show antenna

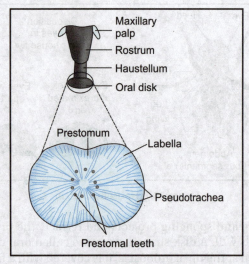

Figure 19.9: Proboscis of housefly

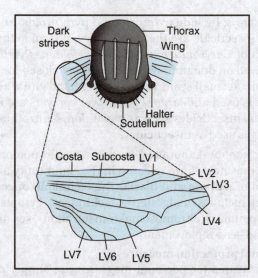

Figure 19.10: Thorax of housefly (dorsal view) with magnified view of wing venation (LV, longitudinal vein)

It also devours solid things that form man's food, but in this case it first spits on them and when its saliva liquefies them, it sponges and draws them up. Its range of flight is 1–3 km. Housefly is active during daytime. At night it rests in projections, hanging wires, edges of plants, walls of animal shelters, exterior surfaces of building, fences, shrubs, trees, etc. From time to time it cleans its proboscis with its forelegs and the hind part of the body with hind legs. Female housefly lays eggs in batch of 100–150 eggs at semiweekly intervals. The eggs are laid in putrefying organic matter, such as human excreta, animal dung, decaying food, vegetable refuse and animal remains.

Life History

The development of housefly occurs in four stages and marked by complete metamorphosis. The egg is 1 mm long, white and banana shaped. It looks like an unpolished grain of rice. In 8–12 hours, the egg hatches into a larva (maggot) a wedge-shaped, legless and hairless creature. Slightly larger than egg at first, it gradually grows to its full size of 10 mm. Their growth is the result of ingestion of enormous food that is possible on account of its ravenous appetite. Unlike adult larvae, it is nocturnal in habit, hiding in the depth of organic matter during the daytime. After 5 days and two moltings, the larva shifts to a dry, compact inorganic soils, burrows into it, and there changes itself into a dark brown, bird-shaped pupa (chrysalis). Pupa uses the old larval skin to make a protective covering for itself. After another 5 days, the pupa moves vertically upward and the adult housefly emerges (Fig. 19.12).

Housefly Transmitting Diseases

Housefly larvae cause myiasis. The disease transmitted by houseflies includes enteric fever, shigellosis, salmonellosis, cholera, amebiasis, giardiasis, balantidiasis, yaws, ascariasis, trichuriasis, poliomyelitis, hepatitis A and enteric viral diseases. Housefly is only a mechanical vector, it passively carries the infective material from the feces to food or sometimes from ocular, or cutaneous lesions directly to the eye or abraded skin of a person. The following factors of housefly help it to transmitting diseases:
- Housefly keeps traveling between feces and food
- It has oral disk, brush-like bristles on its leg and hairs, the infective material at readily sticks to these
- It has the habit of periodically cleaning hind abdomen with its legs; this results in the abdomen becoming smeared with the infected matter
- The infective organisms ingested by the housefly remain alive in its intestines and are excreted alive in its feces and vomits.

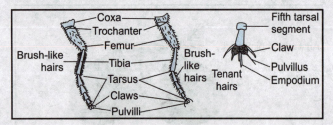

Figure 19.11: Foreleg of housefly, hind leg of housefly, fifth tarsal segment of leg to show tenant hairs

CHAPTER 19 — Arthropods

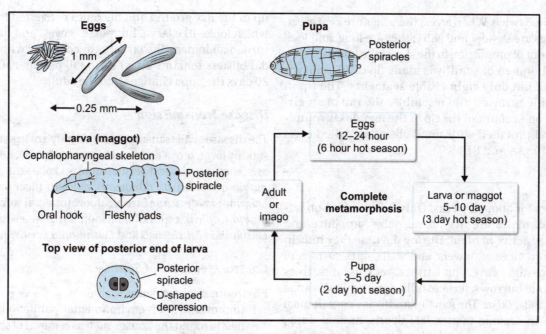

Figure 19.12: Life cycle of housefly

Control Measures of Houseflies

Corrective measures
Improvement of environmental sanitation, which consists of the following measures to eliminate their breeding places:
- People who used to open air defecation are advised to use sanitary latrines; the traps prevent flies from gaining access to the feces
- Proper disposal of human feces by underground drainage system
- Proper and speedy disposal of refuse and garbage by incineration, composing or sanitary landfill
- Refuse particularly its organic matter is disposed of by incineration, sanitary landfill or burial
- Make provision of sanitary latrines
- Sanitary disposal of animal excreta and quick removal, and burial of remains of slaughter houses
- People are encouraged and assisted to build biogas plants or convert the cattle dung into dung cakes.

Offensive measures
Offensive measures include antiadult measures and antilarval measures, which are used to destroy the houseflies:
1. Antiadult measures includes use of insecticides (pyrethrum extract of kerosene spray), use of baits (powder poisoned with organic phosphorus compounds), tangle food poison bait (mixture of milk and formalin), trapping (mixture of resin, groundnut oil and Vaseline smear over both sides of paper or ribbon, which attracts flies, are sucked and die) and use of fly swatter.
2. Antilarval measures include spraying of organic phosphorus insecticides, e.g. diazinon, dichlorvos and dimethole over the breeding places, proper composing of rubbish, and refuse also can control larvae.

Defensive measures
Defensive measures include the screening of doors and windows of the house with wire mesh, air conditioning of the houses (by those who can afford). Use of housefly repellents, food hygiene and food protection such as covering milk, meat, sweet, etc.

Sandfly

Sandfly is a small (2 mm long), light to dark brown-colored, hair, long-limbed insect. Its body divided into head, thorax and abdomen:
1. The head is filled up by twin compound eyes. It carries proboscis with well-developed blade-like biting parts in the female, but poorly developed in the male. Proboscis is flanked by four curved palpi. Lateral to them on either side are the antennae made up of articulating segments. The points of the segments are covered with a whorl of hairs.
2. The thorax of the sandfly is covered with a sentellum. It carries three pairs of legs and a pair each of wings, and halteres. The wings are lanceolate and covered thickly with hairs. The second longitudinal vein is

branched twice. When at rest the wings are kept erect. The legs are slender and hairy; they are long, and look much out of proportion to the size of the body.

3. The abdomen of sandfly is made up of 10 embryological, but only eight visible segments. The tip in the male is raised and resembles the tail of an airplane on account of the tip of the females is rounded, and provided with small elevation called cerci (Figs 19.13A and B).

Life Habits

Sandfly live for about 2 weeks. Only females feed on human blood. Males are live on vegetable sap, juice and nectar. They active at night. During daytime they hide in crack and crevices of flowers, and walls, dark corners of rooms, limestone caves, pit latrines, rock fissures, trees holes, animal burrows, termite hills, etc. The usual range of flight is 100–200 m. The female sandfly lay eggs in most earth rich in organic matter, leaf debris, animal dung, insect remain, etc. Eggs are laid in batches of 20–70. The usual breeding places are the backyard of houses, the vicinity of animal shelters and tree holes (Fig. 19.14).

Life Cycle

Sandfly undergoes complete metamorphosis, changing from egg, through larva and pupa to adult in 40–50 days. The egg is torpedo-shaped marked with white striations when first laid, it gradually turns black. After 6–9 days the egg hatches into larva. The larva is 5 mm long when fully grown. It is made up of three thoracic and nine abdominal segments. Several rows and spines occur on its body. Four stout bristles, two long and two short, are present at the tip of its body, these are called 'caudal bristles'. The larva has voracious appetite. It feeds on putrid organic matter, lit is capable of going down the soil or dust heap to the extent of 30 cm. After 20–30 days, the larva climbs up to the dry ground and becomes converted into pupa, which looks-like larva, but possess eyes, and has an upturned abdomen. The larval skin complete with the caudal blisters remains attached to tail of pupa, after about 20 days the pupa changes into the adult.

Disease Transmission

The diseases will transmitted by sandfly are leishmaniasis, sandfly fever, oroya fever and verruga peruana. Leishmaniasis such as visceral leishianmasis, kala-azar by *Leishmania donovani* (*L. donovani*), chiclero ulcer (cutaneous *Leishmania mexicana*), tropical sore (oriental sore by *Leishmania tropica*), espundia, nasopharyngeal leishmaniasis, *Leishmania braziliensis* and *Leishmania peruviana*.

Control Measures of Sandfly

Environmental measures include:

1. Improvement of environmental sanitation (cleanliness) around the houses such as removal of shrubs and vegetation within 50 yards of human residential area.
2. Engineering measures such as filling up of the cracks and crevices of the house walls, floors by cement plastering and doors by proper wick.
3. Keeping location of cattle sheds and poultry houses away from the human habitants/human living places.
4. Chemical control by spraying of human dwelling, cattle sheds and other places is done with lindane once in 3 months or with DDT.
5. Sleeping inside fly nets (300 mesh/cm^2) and smearing repellents on the lower part of the body are done for personal protection.

Tsetse Fly

Tsetse fly or *Glossina* belongs to hematophagous or blood sucking group of flies. They are voracious blood suckers of animals and skin darken gradually. Both the sexes bite. They are living in dense forest areas because of shade and moisture. They require loose soil and nearby watery source by laying eggs (Fig. 19.15).

Morphology

Tsetse flies are larger than housefly in size, brown in color measuring about half-an-inch. At rest wings overlap each other and cover the abdomen dorsally completely. Head bears a pair of large compound eyes with a median proboscis, which is rigid, nonretractable, adopted for biting, sucking the blood, and pair of maxillary palpi one on either side of the proboscis. The palpi area also

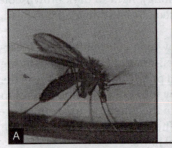
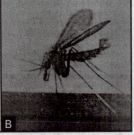

Figures 19.13A and B: Phlebotomine sandflies (*Lutzomyia longipalpis*) showing the hairy body and wings, the generally mosquito-like stance and appearance except for the characteristic position of the wings, held in a V over the back. **A.** Living female; **B.** Living male.

CHAPTER 19 — Arthropods

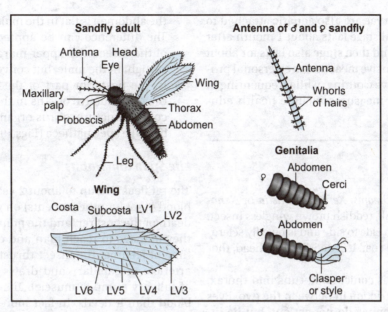

Figure 19.14: Sandfly

long as proboscis and they protect the proboscis. A pair of three segment antennae is also found. The venation in the wings are the same type as in housefly except than the fourth vein is curved twice. Abdomen reveals six segments.

Life History

Tsetse fly has peculiar history then gravid female does not lay eggs, but directly gives birth to larva, one at a time, at 10 days interval. Therefore, it is viviparous or larviparous. The larva is a fat maggot, having two black small spherical structures, the polyneustic lobes in the lost abdominal segment. The larval stage last hardly for 30–60 minutes.

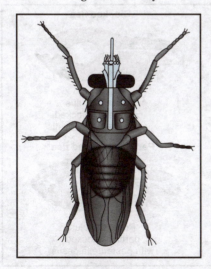

Figure 19.15: Tsetse fly

Larva goes deep into the soil and pupa develops. Pupa is barrel-shaped structure, having holopneustic lobes at the posterior end. It takes rest for 1–2 months and then comes to surface of the soil at the time of emergence of young adult. Thus, the history is that of complete metamorphosis. This tsetse causes sleeping sickness.

Control Measures

1. Offensive measures are destruction of wild animals on which the flies feeds, now it is prohibited.
2. Spraying of 20% dieldrin insecticide from the aircraft to cover the large are of forest.
3. Defensive measures in personal protection by chemo prophylaxis.
4. Corrective measures area cleaning of vegetation along the banks of rivers, supplemented by insecticides.
5. No human habitation to be allowed within 450 m of fly breeding zones.

Black Fly

Black fly is black-colored, small, robust fly found in forest areas. Only female bite, it is a vicious blood sucker of cattle and occasional bites man. It breeds on fast flowing water.

Black flies are responsible for the transmission of onchocerciasis in Africa, Mexico and South America. *Simulium indicum* is Indian species not transmit any diseases so far. The eggs are laid in the submerged stones and water weeds. The larvae are also aquatic attached to stones and weeds. Larval stage lasts about 1 month after which pupae come out and then stage also lasts for about 2–3 weeks interval. Defensive measures are personal protection by using protective clothing, while frequenting in forest areas. Corrective measures include health education (Fig. 19.16).

Rat Flea

Morphology

The rat flea, *Xenopsylla cheopis, Xenopsylla astia* or *Xenopsylla braziliensis* is a small, reddish brown wingless insect. It is body is flattened from side to side and is heavily sclerotized covered with a hard coat. It is divisible into head, thorax and abdomen:

1. The head of rat flea is conical and runs into thorax, there being no constriction in between the two. Eyes are pigmented. Antennae do not get out, but lie in-grooves. The head bears a proboscis and two pair of palpi. The proboscis is well developed in both sexes. It is suited for piercing and sucking, the blade-like mandibles and labrum epipharynx are responsible for piercing, and sucking respectively.
2. Thorax is made up of three segments. The first one, prothorax, is decorated with a row of stout spins called comb.
3. Attached to the thorax are three pairs of well-developed legs that terminate in strong claws. The hindmost legs are the most developed, they are connected to and controlled by strong thoracic muscles.
4. The abdomen of rat flea is made of 10 segments. The first nine are more or less similar in shape and size. The last is smaller than the rest. The dorsal surface of the abdomen is flat in the male, convex in the female. The difference can be appreciated in the side view of the insect; the upper margin of the body will be straight in the male, but convex in the female.
5. In the posterior part of the abdomen are situated the reproductive organs in the male, there is a long-coiled structure, cirrus organ; in the female, a short bag-like spermatheca (Figs 19.17 and 19.18).

Life Span and Habits

The rat fleas live up to about 2 years. Both sexes feed on blood of rat (or other rodents) on which they live. On the death of the host rat (and the nonavailability of a rodent) they manage to reach man and drink blood too. At the time of feeding, the insect thrusts its proboscis into an arteriole or capillary and draws in blood with the aid of salivary pump (a muscle). The rat flea sucks up more blood than it needs, in fact more than what it stomach can hold, with the result that some blood goes out of the anal opening (and is used as food by the larva). The range of exclusion of the rat flea is limited to the body of its host.

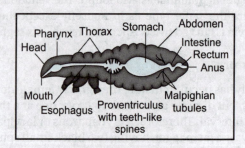

Figure 19.17: Alimentary canal of flea

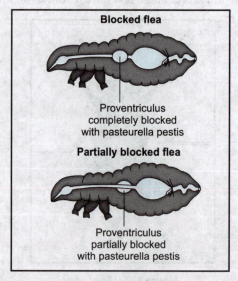

Figure 19.18: Blocked and partially blocked flea

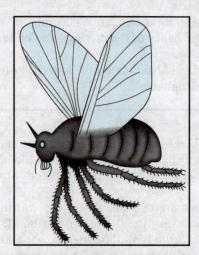

Figure 19.16: *Simulium* (black fly)

It deftly crawls in between the host's hairs. When it is forced to leave the dead rat, the flea no longer crawls, but moves about by hopping 10 cm, if it is gorged up with blood, otherwise 15 cm, an activity that is possible on account of its strong hind legs and its well-developed thoracic muscles (Fig. 19.19).

Life Cycle

The life cycle of the rat flea exhibits complete metamorphosis. The egg is small (0.5 mm), ovoid and glistening white when laid, and turning dull yellow ultimately. After 2–4 hours the egg hatches into a larva, 2–6 mm long becomes worm. Its head is covered with backwardly directed hairs. It feeds on rat feces, organic debris and bold that escapes from the alimentary tract of the adult rat flea. It propels itself by jerky movements of its body. After 7–10 days the larva becomes changed into an ovoid pupa provided with a sticky case. Dirt and debris stick to the pupae case so much so that it is difficult to locate pupae of rat fleas.

Disease Transmitted

The disease actively transmitted by the rat flea is bubonic plague and endemic (murine) typhus. The accidental ingestion of the rat flea (usually by children) results in the transmission of *Hymenolepis nana* and *H. diminuta* infestations.

Transmission of plague

When a flea bites a rat suffering from plague, it ingests *Yersinia pestis*. Over the next 3 days (the extrinsic incubation period) the bacilli multiply and form a 'plague mass' inside the proventricularis. The flea is now said to be 'blocked', totally or partially depending on the size of the mass. In the meanwhile the rat dies from plague. Its body cools down, whereupon the fleas leave it and hop about in search of a new host.

If they happen to reach a man, they bite him/her. Sucking is not easy on account of the obstruction of proventricularis. The flea therefore makes powerful sucking efforts. During this process it vomits out a bit of the plague mass, which immediately contaminates the bite wound. The swallowed blood does not quench the insect's thirst on account of the obstruction, so it goes on biting repeatedly (till it dies of starvation) with each successive bite the chances of transmission of plague increase.

Transmission of endemic typhus

The flea transmits this disease, primarily from rat to rat; secondarily, rat to man. By biting an infected rat, the insect ingests the causative agent *Rickettsia mooseri* (or *Rickettsia typi*). After multiplication in the cells lining the insects gut, the organisms are excreted in its feces.

In the meanwhile the host dies. The rat flea abandons the dead rat and goes in search of a live alternative. If it alights on a human being it bites him to satisfy its hunger. At the same time it defecates. The organisms in the feces contaminate the bite wound and produce infections.

Control Measures

1. Environmental control: Sanitary measures such as keeping the environment free from unhygienic conditions, which can lead to breeding of fleas should be adopted. It also requires engineering measures such as filing of crevices, etc.
2. Chemical control: 10% of DDT is used. The spray is applied to floors and walls up to a height of about 1 feet.
3. Protection against fleas: Repellents such as diethyltoluamide is used, which is impregnated on clothings. By this the fleas are repelled at least for a week.

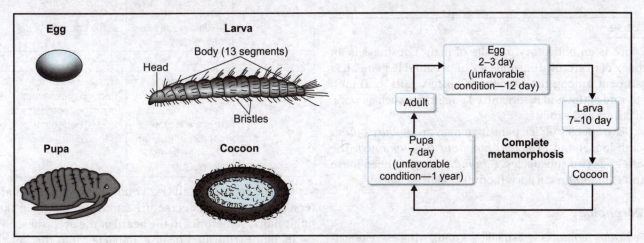

Figure 19.19: Life cycle of flea

4. Rodent control: Fleas control measures also require rodent control measures.

Species sanitations are not possible. Professional rat catchers and those who visit areas infested with rodents protect themselves by wearing gumboots and pants with its bottom impregnated with N, N-diethyl meta-toluamide (DEET) or a synthetic pyrethroid. The larva of a rat fleas are killed inside the rat burrows through blowing methoprene into them.

The most efficient method of a flea control is the destruction of adult fleas with the applications of the dust of hexachlorocyclohexane (HCH), malathion, bendiocarb, diazinon, carbaryl or fenitrothion, depending on their susceptibility. For killing fleas on domestic rats, the insecticide powder is dusted with the aid of a hand duster in patches about 0.5 cm thick and 20–25 cm long. Dusting is done along the bottom of walls, along floors up to 20–30 cm from the wall, along rafters and beams, on top of the walls, along floors up to 20–30 cm from the wall, along the rafters and beams, and on top of the wall if a gap exists between it and the roof. It is also done on piles of wood, timber, debris and rubbish. All rat burrows are identified in and around the house, and about 30 g other dust is blown into each one of them. This will also kill the immature stages of the flea.

Dichlorvos resin strips are employed to kill fleas in warehouse and containerized cargo insufflation of ships, and aircraft with cyanogen kills the rodents, and the fleas on them at one stretch. The killing of rat alone is inadvisable; in that case, the fleas leave the dead rat and go in search of alternative hosts.

For killing the fleas on wild rodents, the method of choice is to employ bait boxes containing 50–90 g of HCH dust with food bait. These boxes are kept in the fields and other areas that are infested with wild rodents. The bait attracts the rodents. As they enter the box, their fur picks up the insecticide. Fleas thereon are killed.

Louse

Louse is an obligatory parasite of man. Lousiness is an index of overcrowding and lack of personal hygiene. It is rampant among the inmates of hostels, jails, barracks, etc. and at times of disorganized conditions such as wars, disasters and exodus.

Two species of lice parasitize man are *Phthirus pubis* (crab louse) and *Pediculus humanus* (*P. humanus*). The latter has two subspecies. *P. humanus* capitis head louse and *P. humanus* corporis (body 9 or clothes louse).

Morphology

Pediculus humanus is a small (2–3 mm), wingless, elongated, flat bodied and thick skinned, grayish to reddish-brown colored insect. Its body is divided into head, thorax and abdomen:

1. The head of the louse is cone shaped with the base of the cone contiguous to the thorax. Set in the head are two inconspicuous simple eyes. A proboscis and two short antennae make up the mouth parts that lack palpi proboscis is hidden in a pouch called staber sac situated on the under surface of head. It is bought out only at the time of feeding. The antennae, unlike those of the other insects, arise from the sides of the head and project out at right angles to the long axis of head (Table 19.2).
2. The thorax of louse is squarish. It is built up of three segments. The dents between them are distinct along the side and indistinct elsewhere. Thorax carried three pairs of well-developed legs, but no wings or halters. At the tip of each leg is a large recurved claw. A projection called the tarsal thumb is present on the penultimate segment of the leg. The insect can bring it in opposition to its claw.
3. The abdomen of the louse is longer than the head and thorax combined. It is composed of seven segments. In the male the tip of abdomen is rounded and bears a spine-like penis in the female it is bifid (Fig. 19.20).

Table 19.2: Differences between head louse and body louse

Feature	Head louse	Body louse
Nomenclature	It is *Pediculus humanus* (*P. humanus*) capitis	It is *P. humanus* corporis
Habit	It is found on hairs of scalp	Found on body hairs and bugs in seams of clothes
Oviposition	Eggs are laid in occipital region About 150 eggs are laid at the rate of 5–6 daily	Eggs are laid on body, hairs and clothes About 300 eggs are laid at the rate of 8–10 daily
Longevity	4 week	6 week
Made of spread	Usually spreads from person to person when they are in close contact or through common items like combs	Usually it spreads through the medium of clothes, combs, caps, towels, bed sheets or pillow covers, etc.

Pthirus pubis is small (1–22 mm), grayish (reddish after a meal) and squash creature found commonly in the pubic hairs, sometimes in the beard or the eyelashes.

Its blunt truncated head is impacted into the upper border of its thorax. It has a pair of simple eyes and a pair

CHAPTER 19 — Arthropods

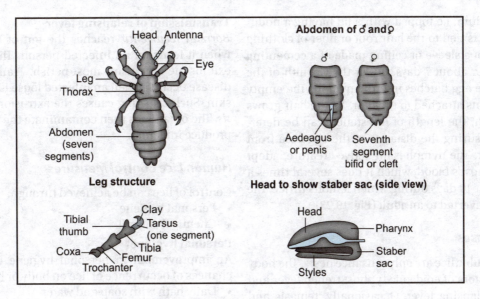

Figure 19.20: Female louse (*Pediculus humanus*)

of short antennae. The thorax and abdomen are fused to form a hexagonal structure. The thorax carries three pairs of legs. The first pair is thin. The second and third pairs are very powerful, and carry large claws. The insect uses these for gripping the coarse (but not fine) hairs. Crab louse infestation (phthiriasis or crabs) spreads from person to person through sexual intercourse (Figs 19.21 and 19.22).

Life Span and Habits

The louse has a life span 4–6 weeks. Lice, both male and female, feed on blood of the host. They feed at short and each time, swallow more than what is needed. The excess blood escapes in feces as such or after partial digestion. Mating occurs at frequent intervals. The female body louse lays about 10 eggs at a time about 30 times in all. The female head louse lays about five eggs each time, repeating the process 20 times in her life span.

The head louse inhabits the hair upon its host's head and the body louse lives in the underclothing. To clasp the hair or garment fiber the louse uses its claw and tarsal thumb. The louse deserts its host when an attack of fever makes person skin hot or a spell of hard work makes it wet with perspiration. After desertion the lice seek out a new host. The lice are capable of leaving their normal hosts and switching over to another either by themselves (as happens when the tow come close together) or by passive transference through the intermediary of combs, hats, pillow covers, etc.

Life Cycle

The development of the adult from the egg occurs through incomplete metamorphosis. There are only two immature stages, egg and nymph. The nymph resembles the adult, but it is similar and sexually immature. The egg of louse or nit is small (0.8 mm), pinkish and ovoid.

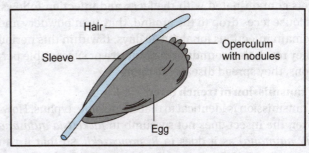

Figure 19.21: Egg or nit of louse

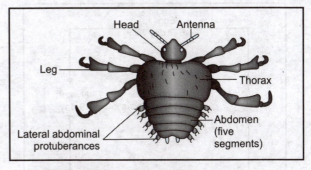

Figure 19.22: *Pthirus pubis* (pubic or crab louse)

It is operculum, i.e topped with a lid having a nodular surface. Nit is tied to the hair root or fiber of clothing with the help of a sleeve or ceiling made of a cementing substance. After about 7 days, under the warmth of the host's body, the egg hatches into the nymph. The empty egg case remains attached to the hair. As the hair grows by 1 cm/month, the length of infestation can be determined by measuring the distance of the egg case from the root of hair. The nymph is an active creature, adopt in sucking its host's blood, which it does several times a day. After about 10 days during which it molts thrice, the nymph gets converted to an adult (Fig. 19.23).

Lice and Diseases

The head and pubic lice are only nuisance pests. The body lice are the vectors of epidemic typhus, trench fever and louse-borne relapsing fever. Occasionally, teniasis and *Dipylidium caninum* infestation too are louse borne.

Transmissions of epidemic typhus

Biting an individual suffering from epidemic typhus infects the body louse. *Rickettsia prowazekii (R. prowazekii)* multiply in the cells of its midgut. About 7 days, later the organisms start appearing in the insect's feces. If the louse is transferred to another person and it bites him/her and defecates on his/her skin the bite wound gets contaminated with the feces and infection follows. If louse feces drop to the ground, they turn powdery and remain infectious for about 60 days. If within this period they reach the wounds or conjunctiva or susceptible persons, they spread diseases to them.

Transmission of trench fever

Transmission is identical to that of epidemic typhus. However, the insect does not succumb to *Rickettsia quintana (R. quintana)* as it does to *R. prowazekii*, so that it can transmit trench fever throughout its unabridged life span.

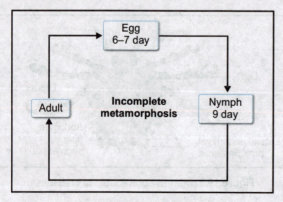

Figure 19.23: Life cycle of louse

Transmission of relapsing fever

Borrelia recurrentis reaches the gut of the body louse, when it feeds on an infected person. There is no scope exit for the organisms most perish. Transmission of the disease occurs, when an infected louse is crushed on the skin. Such crushing causes the extrusion of *B. recurrentis*. The organisms then contaminate the bite wound and produce infection.

Human Lice Control Measures

Control of lice can be achieved through:
- Personal hygiene
- Chemical control.

Personal hygiene

An improvement in personal hygiene can reduce the chances of occurrence of lice on body or hairs:
- Daily bath with soap and water
- Frequent washing of long hairs
- Change and launder clothes
- Autoclaving of clothes and bedding in case of body lice
- Improving living standards.

Head lice: Malathion solution (0.5%) is used and kept for 12–24 hours, after that the hairs are washed, malathion kills the nits and lice.

Body lice: Malathion 1% is applied in powder form to the inner surface of clothings. One application of 1% malathion is enough to eradicate infestations, but a second application is required after 7 days. The required amount is about 50 g (2 ounce) of insecticidal powder.

Species sanitation: Daily bathing (including washing of hairs) with soap followed by wearing of washed and laundered clothes will prevent the breeding of lice. Elimination of crab lice is possible through the shaving of pubic hairs.

Physical killing: The immature stages and adult of lice are picked up by combing the hairs with a fine comb, and killed by pressing them between the two thumbs.

The lice and nits living in the underclothing as well as those that have spread to the bedsheets, towels, etc. are killed by disinfection with steam under pressure.

Chemical control

Insecticides are also used to control the lice. For the control of head and pubic louse, one of the following liquid formulations is used:
1. About 0.5% deodorized malathion lotion in isopropyl alcohol.
2. 1% lindane in coconut oil or as an aqueous suspension.
3. 0.3% bioallethrin shampoo.
4. 1% carbaryl lotion.

About 10 mL is applied to the head or pubic region until thoroughly wet. Bath is taken 12 hours afterwards in the case of lindane; and 24 hours later in case of the rest of the preparations.

If necessary, treatment is repeated 3 weeks later. For the control of body louse, 1% malathion or carbaryl dust in talc is used. The whole body, the underclothing and bedding are dusted with 30–40 g of the dust. A bath is taken 24 hours later. Clothing is boiled, washed and laundered.

When school children are treated for louse infestation, they are given insecticidal packets or pouches with the advise to use them on their siblings at home. For emergency delousing, a hand or machine-operated duster with 10 dusting heads is used. With the aid of this 10% DDT dust is blown down collar, up the sleeves and down beltline of 10 persons at a time.

BUGS

Bugs are insects of varied shapes and sizes. They possess dorsoventrally flat bodies and the mouth parts are adapted for piercing and sucking. Some are winged and some wingless. They are oviparous and metamorphosis is incomplete.

The bugs of public health impotence are the bed bug and the *Triatoma* bug (reduviid bug).

Bed bugs

The species that survive on man are *Cimex lectularius* in temperate countries and *Cimex hemipterus* (or *Cimex rotundatus*) in tropical countries such as India, which are reddish brown in color (Fig. 19.24).

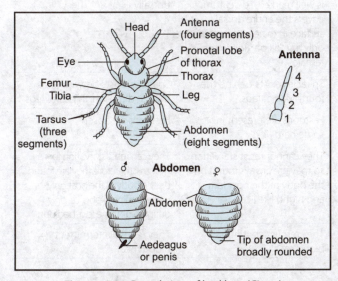

Figure 19.24: Dorsal view of bed bug (*Cimex*)

They do not act as vectors in transmission of any disease. However, they are suspected to transmit certain disease such as leprosy, plaque, kala-azar, typhus, relapsing fever and Rocky Mountain spotted fever, but not proved.

Bionomics

Both sexes bite and suck blood. They are nocturnal in habit usually. The adults and nymphs resist starvation for 6 months or even more and look like a brown leaf the moment they get blood feed, they swell and regain normal reddish brown color. On the body they possess stink glands and hence the bed bugs give out a peculiar smell described as buggish odor.

Even through the bed bug does not transmit any disease, it is mainly a source of nuisance due to the bite and consequently causes irritation, discomfort, excoriation of skin and disturbs sleep.

Control Measures

1. Offensive measures consist of exposure of bug infested articles to direct sunlight or pouring boiling water on them. Application of direct heat (or flaming) to bug infested steel cots is also effective. Spraying of the insecticide, consisting of a mixture of β-hexachlorocyclohexane (BHC) and malathion in their daytime hideouts like cracks and crevices of the walls, fissures in furnitures, etc. also help to achieve good results.
2. Defensive measures consist of using repellants.

Ticks

Morphology

Ticks or acari are spider-like creatures. They are of two types:
1. Hard or ixodid as ticks, characterized by the presence of a chitinous shield, scutum, covering the whole body in males, but only half the body in female.
2. Soft or argasid as ticks characterized by the absence of the scutum. The hard ticks are the ectoparasites of cats, dogs, rodents, etc. examples are *Dermacentor andersoni*, *Haemaphysalis spinigera* and *Ixodes pilosus*. The soft ticks are free living. They feed on cats, dogs and cattle. An example is *Ornithodoros moubata*. Both kinds of ticks bite man accidentally (Fig. 19.25).

Ticks have a sac-like body not differentiated into head, thorax and abdomen, and four pairs of legs. They do not have wings and antennae. They have no true head, but only a square structure at the anterior end of the body

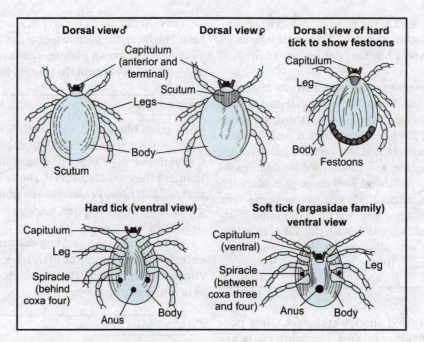

Figure 19.25: Dorsal and ventral views of hard and soft ticks

called 'basis capitulum' to which the mouth parts are attached. Basis capitulum and the mouth parts together constitute 'capitulum'. In the ticks the capitulum projects from the anterior portion of the body and looks like a head. In soft ticks capitulum lies beneath the anterior end and is not visible in the dorsal view.

The mouth parts of ticks consist of two 'chelicerae' two 'pedipalps' and a median 'hypostome'. The hypostome is finger shaped and is furnished on its underside with backwardly turned hooks. Through the hypostome the acarus attaches itself to the host and swallows the blood. The chelicerae are fitted with sharp blade-like tools used in cutting the host's skin.

Life Span and Habits

Ticks live from 2 to 5 years. They feed on the blood of their hosts. The hard ticks are found on the hosts, while the free living soft ticks are found in cracks and cervices of walls, and in wood and grassy areas. After obtaining the blood meal, the soft ticks fall back to the ground. They suck a large amount of blood so that flat on an empty stomach, they become globular at the end of the blood meal. Tick lays eggs on the ground. The female tick drops down to the ground and deposits all her around 5,000 eggs, and then dies. The female soft tick lays eggs in batches of 20–100 a day for several days (Table 19.3).

Table 19.3: Differences between hard tick and soft ticks

Hard ticks	Soft ticks
They belong to the family ixodidae	They belong to the family argasidae
Capitulum is anterior in position	Capitulum is ventral in position
Scutum is present	Scutum in absent
Dorsally sexual dimorphism is well marked, i.e. scutum covers the entire dorsal surface in male and covers only a small portion in the female	Sexual dimorphism is absent dorsally
Spiracles exists behind the fourth pair of legs	Spiracles exists between the third and the fourth pair of legs
Festoons are present in some hard ticks	Festoons are absent
They cannot resist starvation so they are always found on the body of the host (day and night) like lice	They can resist starvation for months; therefore they are found on the body of the host only, while feeding blood, i.e. only during nighttime (e.g. bed bugs)
They require continuous blood meal	They require intermittent blood meal

Contd...

Contd...

Hard ticks	Soft ticks
They are always found on the body their hosts	They are found in cracks and crevices during daytime, and on the body of the host during nighttime
Gravid female lays 100–1,000 of eggs at one sitting	Eggs are laid in batches of 20–100 over a long period of time
Nymphal stage is one	Nymphal stages are five
Important species are *Dermacentor andersoni*, *Haemaphysalis spinigera*	Important specimen is *Ornithodoros moubata* (refer Figs 19.22A and B)
Diseases transmitted are tick typhus (Africa), tick paralysis, tularemia, viral encephalitis, hemorrhagic fever (KFD*), human babesiosis. Rocky Mountain spotted fever (USA), Q fever (in United States of America and Australia)	Diseases transmitted is endemic relapsing fever, caused by *Borrelia duttoni*, a spirochete

*KFD, Kyasanur forest disease

Life Cycle

Ticks develop through four stages that exhibit incomplete metamorphosis. The larva and nymph resemble the adult; the former has only six legs; though nymph has eight legs, it differs from the adult only in being sexually infantile. The egg is small, spherical and shiny. After about 30 days it hatches into a larva or 'seed tick'. The larva patiently waits for the approach of an animal. The moment a suitable one comes by, it jumps on to it and stays there till it had satisfied its hunger. Thereafter it drops back to earth. After about 2 months the larva changes into a nymph such as the larva, on the first opportunity it attaches itself to a host, drinks its blood and then falls back to ground. After about 6 weeks the nymph changes into the adult tick (Figs 19.26A and B).

Diseases Transmitted by Ticks

A direct pathogenic effect is tick paralysis. This has been discussed earlier. Ticks transmit disease to man accidentally. When man brushes the animals infested with ticks, it later get transferred to him/her and bite him/her. There are two distinct mechanisms of transmission of diseases. One is true of Q fever, the other of all other diseases.

Transmission of Q fever

Ticks pick up *Coxiella burnetii* by biting an animal suffering from Q fever. In due course the organisms are excreted in tick feces. When feces dry up they become airborne. A person who inhales them contracts the infection.

Transmission of diseases other than Q fever

Biting animals suffering from the corresponding disease infects ticks. Contamination of bite wound with these results in the transmission of the corresponding disease.

CONTROL OF TICKS AND MITES

Control measures of ticks and mites are as follows:
1. Environment control: Environmental control require engineering measures such as filling of crevices in grounds.
2. Chemical control: Chemical control is achieved by using 1–2 pounds per acre of DDT, malathion, lindane, etc. Animals such as dogs can be treated with insecticidal spray.
3. Protection against ticks and mites: Wear protective clothing impregnated with insect repellent. Repellents used are indalone, benzyl benzoate.

Soft ticks are controlled by filling up the cracks and crevices of walls and by indoor residual spraying with malathion, lindane or fenthion. Grass, bushes and low-tree limbs around the houses are cut. For the control of hard ticks the camping sites are sprayed with malathion, lindane or fenthion. Persons who visit tick-infested sites protect themselves by smearing their body with 5% dimethyl phthalate and impregnating their clothing with it. After a person and his/her pets return from a visit to a tick

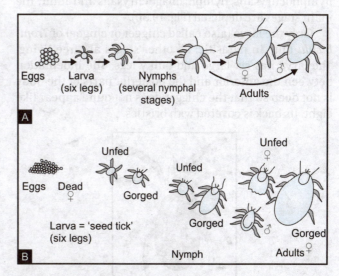

Figures 19.26A and B: Tick life cycles. **A.** Argasidae; **B.** Ixodidae.

infested area, their body is inspected for ticks. If found they are grasped close to the skin and pulled upwards with even pressure. They are disposed off by immersing them in a bottle-containing alcohol.

Trombicula

Morphology

The important species of *Trombicula* mites are *Leptotrombidium akamushi*, *Leptotrombidium deliense*, *Leptotrombidium pallidum* and *Leptotrombidium intermedia*. *Trombicula* mite is 1–2 mm long. Its single unit saccular body has a constriction at the junction of the anterior one third and the posterior two third. This constriction gives it the shape of eight. The body of *Trombicula* mite is covered densely with hairs, of its eight legs the anterior two are most well developed and the longest. It has no wings and no antennae. The mouth parts of the mite project from the anterior tip of the body. They consist of a rudimentary hypostome, a pair of chelicerae and pair of pedipalps. Each pedipalp has a curved claw at its tip and a little above the claw, and lying in position to it, a thumb-like process (Figs 19.27 to 19.29).

Life Span, Habits and Life Cycle

The life span of *Trombicula* mite is 6 months. Adult mites are free living. They are found in soil, under the shade of shrubs or in grassy lands. They do not bite, but feed on plant juice. The life cycle of the *Trombicula* mite is marked by incomplete metamorphosis. There are seven stages each lasting about a week; egg, deutovum, larva, nymphochrysalis, nymph, imagochrysalis and adult. The main stages are depicted (Fig. 19.30).

Only the larva (also called chigger or chigoe) of *Trombicula* mite in parasitic; all other stages are free living. The larva has six large and bulky legs. The indentation between the anterior and the posterior parts of the body is not deep so that the chigger does not quite appear like eight. Its back is covered with bristles.

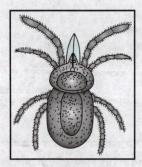

Figure 19.27: Fully grown imago of *Leptotrombidium akamushi*

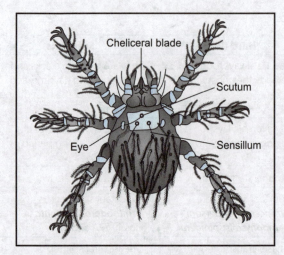

Figure 19.28: Dorsal view of *Leptotrombidium deliense*

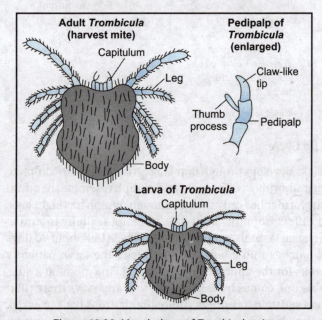

Figure 19.29: Morphology of *Trombicula* mite

Chiggers live in the ear of field rodents. They feed on the host's blood. Accidentally they bite man. The chigger feeds only once is its whole existence. After feeding it drops down to the ground there to continue its life cycle. While biting man (or rodents) the chigger secretes a substance that liquefies rickettsial pox and tularemia.

The control of this mite is possible by the following methods:
1. Outdoor spray of woodlands, bushy areas, etc. with malathion, lindane or fenthion.
2. Clearance of shrubs, bushes, grass, etc.
3. The use of repellents by persons visiting infested areas.

CHAPTER 19   Arthropods

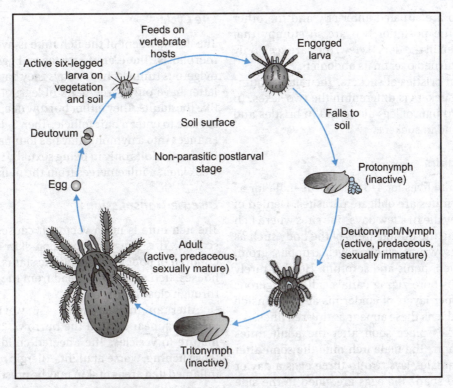

Figure 19.30: Summarized life cycle of *Trombicula* mites

Dust Mite

Dust mite (*Dermatophagoides pteronyssinus*) is commonly found in house dust (Fig. 19.31). It can cause in sensitized individuals bronchial asthma as well as extensive dermatitis. It feeds mainly on desquamated skin scales. The mites become airborne during bed making and could then be inhaled; not only the living mites but also dead one and mite feces contain potent allergens. The best method of controlling the mites would appear to be treatment of beds and settees with insecticides followed by through vacuum cleaning to remove dead mites and feces, as these could cause symptoms.

Itch Mite

Morphology

Itch mite, scab mite, *Sarcoptes scabiei, Acarus scabiei* is a strict endoparasite of man. It lives in his epidermis. It parasitize people with poor personal hygiene living under overcrowded and insanitary conditions. The itch mite is an ovoid, grayish nearly transparent and tortoise-like arthropod. The male is 0.25 mm and the female 0.4 mm long. The body of itch mite is saccular without being divided into head, thorax and abdomen, and without segmentation. A false head or capitulum projects from the anterior pole. The dorsal surface of its body is set with bristles, spines and wrinkles. The itch mite carries four pairs

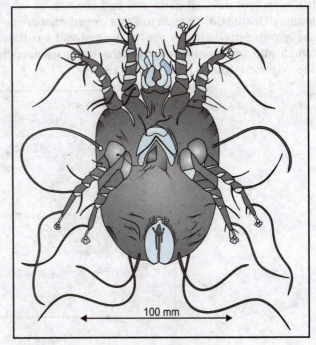

Figure 19.31: *Dermatophagoides pteronyssinus,* the house dust mite (ventral view)

of short legs. Two are situated anteriorly and the other two posteriorly. The posterior two are so stumpy that they cannot be seen in the dorsal view; they are seen only when the mite is turned over on its abdomen.

The legs end in bristles or suckers. The relative number of bristles or suckers is different in the two sexes. In the male, the third pair of legs alone end in bristles and the first, and second in suckers.

Life Span and Habits

The female itch mite lives for 4–5 weeks; the male for as many hours. Itch mites are obligate parasites. Denied of human blood, they die in a few days. The sites where itch mites are found are the humid areas of the body such as the webs of fingers, wrists, elbow, navel, arm pits, groin, beltline of abdomen, penis and scrotum. Head is rarely affected. The mites bore zigzag canals called ovigerous tunnels in the upper layers of epidermis and live inside them. With a hand lens these appear as tiny red lines.

Copulation takes place soon after the adult mites emerge from nymph. The male itch mite die soon after copulation. The females lays two to three eggs a day or throughout its life span. The eggs are glued to the side walls of the ovigerous tunnels. When the person is infected with itch mites comes into close contact with others, some of the acarids manage to reach the latter and parasitize them. Also, the itch mite reaches others through the agency of infested garments, bed sheets and other fomites. During the direct or indirect spread what are actually transferred are the newly emerged and fertilized female mites, not the older females that lie buried deep in the ovigerous tunnels (Figs 19.32 to 19.34).

Life Cycle

The development of the itch mite is by incomplete metamorphosis. There are four stages. Eggs are found in the ovigerous tunnels. In 3–4 days they hatch into larvae. The latter have only three pairs of legs; otherwise they look like the adults. They either burrow deep or come up to the surface to enter a hair follicle. Then 3 days later, the larva changes into a nymph. They has four pairs of legs and differs from adults only in being sexually immature. About 1 week later, adult emerges from the nymph.

Disease Transmission

The itch mite is not a vector. It causes a disease called scabies. This is a very common skin condition seen in children of poor socioeconomic status living in crowded houses. Itch mites are spread from the patients to others through close bodily contact.

After an incubation of 4–6 weeks, erythematous patches appear around the burrows. In a few days they mature to vesicles. The affected child complains of intense itching, worse at night. Allergic reactions by way of inflamed itch areas of skin may be present. The associated scratching leads to secondary infection with streptococci and staphylococci that produce pustules and sepsis.

Control Measures

Scabies is treated with 25% benzyl benzoate emulsion. The patient takes a hot bath with soap, scrubbing the infected parts well with brush. The heat of the bath water softens the crusts. Then 40 mL of the emulsion is applied with a brush not merely to the areas where the lesions are

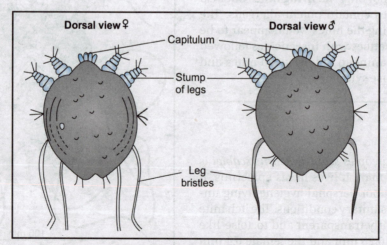

Figure 19.32: *Sarcoptes scabiei*

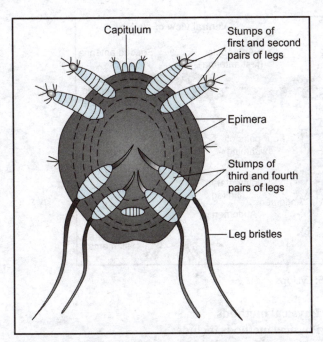

Figure 19.33: *Sarcoptes scabiei* female (ventral view)

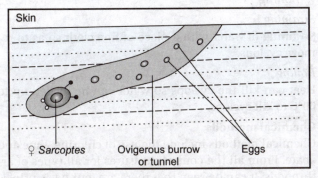

Figure 19.34: *Sarcoptes scabiei* ♀ depositing eggs in tunnel inside human skin

present, but to the entire body except the head. A second application is made 24 hours later. A bath is taken after another 24 hours. A second course of treatment after 7 days may be necessary in some cases. Used bedding, towels, clothing, etc. are boiled, dried and laundered. All other children in the patient's family, all child neighbors and all children in the patient's school are simultaneously treated. The other scabies are 5% sulfur ointment, 5% permethrin and 0.5% lindane in coconut oil.

Cyclops

Morphology

Cyclops are water fleas, crustacean belonging to the order cyclopoida. Some cyclops of medical importance are *Mesocyclops leuckarti*, *Mesocyclops hyalinus*, *Mesocyclops varicans* and *Microcyclops karvei*. Cyclops is a 1 mm tiny, white and pear-shaped crustacean. Its body is divided into three parts, cephalothorax, rest of thorax and abdomen.

The cephalothorax is the most anterior and the broadest part of the body. It is formed by the fusion of head and the first thoracic segment. Near its apex, the cephalothorax carries a single median eye. Cyclops get their name from the number and position of the eye (in Greek mythology cyclops was the one-eyed giants of Sicily). The mouth of the cyclops is situated on the ventral surface of the cephalothorax. One pair is visible from the dorsal view; only the proximal portion of the other pair is seen, as the rest is hidden under the ventral surface. The mouth of the cyclops is situated on the ventral of the cephalothorax, two pairs of maxillae and one pair of mandibles surround it (Fig. 19.35).

The rest of thorax consists of second to sixth thoracic segments. From the dorsum thorax looks to be legless. On turning cyclops over and exposing the ventral aspect five pairs of legs can be seen; the first four pairs only are functional and have enlarged tips so that they look as oars or paddles; the last pair is rudimentary.

The abdomen of cyclops is the posterior narrow part. It is made up of five segments. The last segment is forked and each branch bears a feather. The female cyclops carries two large egg-filled bag-like structures, ovisacs on the outside a fact that helps differentiate it from the male. The ovisacs arise from the point where the last thoracic segment and abdomen meet.

Life Span and Habits

The maximum life span of cyclops is 3 months. Cyclops is an aquatic arthropod and is found in step wells, ponds, tanks and other small collections of water. They feed on minute aquatic organisms. They swim about with jerky movement in their legs and antennae help them. When not swimming or feeding they rest in shady areas of the well, pond, tank, etc.

During copulation the male seizes the female with the help of the first pair of antennae. The female then sheds the eggs sacs; the fertilized eggs issue forth from the sac and remain afloat on the surface of water.

Life Cycle

The development takes place by incomplete metamorphosis. There are three stages—egg, larva and adult with the larval stage having two substages, first 'nauplius', and the second, 'metanauplius'. The eggs are very minute

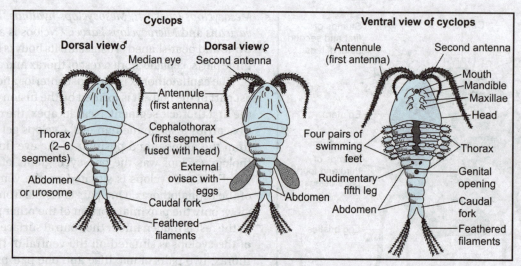

Figure 19.35: Cyclops

and are scattered in all directions by the waves. After 2–3 days they hatch into minute boat-shaped nauplius with a median eye and three pair of appendages. After about 5 days, the nauplius gets changed into metanauplius. The latter has five pairs of appendages; but for this it resembles nauplius. After 7 days the adult cyclops emerges from the metanauplius.

Cyclops and Diseases

Cyclops does not bite man. As such it is not a vector, but it is necessary for the completion of the life cycle of two long helminths *Dracunculus medinensis* (1 m long nematode also known as guinea worm) and *Diphyllobothrium latum* (*D. latum*) (3–4 m long flat helminth also called fish tapeworm). The guinea worm disease is acquired by drinking water containing cyclops that have previously ingested the larvae of the nematode. Diphyllobothrium infection is not contracted by drinking water, but by eating fish. The second of the two intermediate hosts containing the worm-like immature stage (proceroid) of *D. latum*. The fish gets infected in the first place when they feed on the cyclops that contain the embryos (coracidium) of the tapeworm. Cyclops is the first immediate host and picks up the infection by feeding on the eggs of *D. latum*.

Control Measures

Cyclops are water fleas and are present in collected fresh water areas. So the control measures should be aimed at water purification by physical, chemical and biological methods.

Physical methods

Physical methods include:
- Straining
- Boiling.

Straining

Straining of water with a piece of fine cloth so as to remove cyclops.

Boiling

Heat can kill the cyclops so water can be heated up to 60°C to kill cyclops.

Chemical methods

Chemical methods include the use of chlorine, lime and abate. From all the control measures for all types of arthropods, it can be seen that there are four basic principles for the control of arthropod borne diseases, which are as follows:
- Environmental control
- Chemical control
- Biological control
- Genetic control.

Environment control: Includes taking measures to reduce the breeding places. These are filling and drainage operations, proper disposal of refuse and waste, water management. Above all cleanliness of surroundings in and around.

Chemical control: Includes the use of various type of insecticides, which are less toxic to human beings. Biological control emphasize the use of various type of insecticides, which are less toxic to human beings.

Biological control: It emphasize the use of larvivorous and *Gambusia* fish, which eats the arthropods to minimize the occurrence of diseases caused by them. Under genetic control, certain techniques such as sterile male technique, chromosomal translocation have been found effective. One more important factor in controlling the disease is health education.

Temephos is added to the water-containing cyclops in a dose of 1 mg/L. Alternatively, superchlorination (dose 5 mg of chlorine per liter) is done followed by dechlorination. Biological control is possible by growing glass fish or barbel fish in wells, tanks and ponds.

The guinea worm disease can be controlled by boiling water or straining it through multiple layers of kerchief or by converting step wells into draw wells.

CONCLUSION

Arthropods comprise varied living things in the surroundings of man. Depending upon other destructive features, arthropods are classified into three classes; insecta, arachnida and crustacea, which include mosquitoes, flies, human lice, fleas, ticks, mites, etc. Arthropods-borne disease are major health problems. There are transmitted by direct contact, mechanically and biologically. There is a need to control arthropod-borne diseases by adopting appropriate strategies such as using antilarval measures, antiadult control measures and protecting against their bites.

Rodents

CHAPTER 20

INTRODUCTION

Rodents live in close proximity to man and form a part of man's environment. The rodents act as reservoirs of certain diseases such as plague and typhus. They are also responsible for causing health hazards in human beings. So, there is a need to control over rodents. These not only cause health hazards but also cause substantial economic loss by damaging buildings.

CLASSIFICATION

Rodents are classified into two groups:
1. Domestic rodents.
2. Wild rodents.

Domestic rodents: Rodents such as black rat and house mouse are of chief public concern as these rodents live in close association with man.

Wild rodents: Tatera indica (T. indica) and *Bandicota indica (B. indica)* are common wild rodents found in India. *T. indica* is the natural reservoir of plague.

Diseases transmitted rodents are:
1. Bacterial: Salmonellosis, tularemia, plague.
2. Viral: Hemorrhagic fever, encephalitis.
3. Rickettsial: Murine typhus, rickettsialpox and scrub typhus.
4. Parasitic: Leishmaniasis, amebiasis, Chagas disease, trichinosis and *Hymenolepis diminuta (H. diminuta)*.
5. Others: Histoplasmosis, ringworm and leptospirosis.

Rodent-borne diseases are:
1. Direct contact: By rat bite such as rat bite fever.
2. Mechanical transmission:
   a. Through contaminated water and food such as salmonellosis and leptospirosis.
   b. Through rat fleas such as plague and typhus.

RATS

Rats belong to the order rodentia, class mammalia. Like all mammals, the female rodents possess mammary glands. Rodents are characterized by having two sharp incisors in each jaw and by not having any canines. The incisors enable the rodents to gnaw and burrow. The incisors keep growing throughout life, so that if their tip is broken, new one takes place. Besides rat and mice (*Mus musculus*), some other rodents are squirrel, gerbil, rabbit, bandicoot, chinchilla, guinea pig and porcupine.

Types

Rats are of two types:
1. The roof rat (house rat, black rat or ship rat), *Rattus rattus (R. rattus)*, measures 18 cm and has a 22 cm long tail. Its body is light and slender. Its muzzle (nose) is pointed and eyes are prominent. Its ears are large and can be pulled down to a point below the level of eyes. The tip of its tail is decorated with a prominent tuft of hairs. The number of mammary glands in the female is 10. Roof rats are common in the rural than urban areas.
2. Norway rat (sewer rat, brown rat, gray rat, barn rat, wharf rat), *Rattus norvegicus (R. norvegicus)*, has a heavy, thick set and large body measuring 22 cm and short tail 18 cm. Its muzzle is blunt, eyes are small, so that it does not look as intelligent as the roof rat and ears are short and on being pulled down, barely reach the eyes. The tuft hairs at the tip of its tail is insignificant. The female possesses 12 mammary glands (Fig. 20.1).

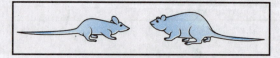

Figure 20.1: Roof rat and Norway rat

CHAPTER 20 — Rodents

Life Span and Habits

The life span of rats in nature is 9 months, but in protected laboratory conditions is 3–5 years. The roof rat lives in the space between the roofs and the wall, holes in walls, lofts, foundations, rafters, undisturbed firewood, discussed articles, drawers of discarded tables and attics. The Norway rat lives in sewer, drains and underground burrows.

At birth, the rat is blind and helpless. Its eyes become functional after 2 weeks. It depends on the mother's milk for the first 1 month of its life. Rats reach sexual maturity in 3–4 months; mating then occurs. The period of gestation is 3 weeks, about 7–8 young ones are born at parturition. A female rat may produce three litters in a year.

Rats are omnivorous, their food is the food of the people among whom they live. Rats relish fresh coconut, moist dough and fruits. Starved rats can eat anything such as paper, soap, pipe, plastic, etc. they eat 10% of their weight daily. Rats require a regular supply of water. Mice are satisfied with infrequent supply of water. The range of rats excursion is about 30 m around the place of nesting. They are nocturnal in habits and go for hunting for food at night. They run on level ground, as well as climb walls in either vase they use their whiskers to feel the way about. In exploring food, rats follow the same pathway night after night. These are called 'rat runs'. They are situated along the junction of floor with walls, overhead beams and pipes. They are distinguished by the presence of black greasy marks and rat droppings.

Rats are suspicious by nature and exhibit 'object shyness'. They avoid new objects and unfamiliar foods. If rat happens to ingest a sublethal dose of poison and recover, they avoid it for the rest of their life; this is known as 'poison shyness'.

Following are the telltale signs of rat infestation:
1. Teeth marks on wall, wood, soap, etc. These are small in the case of mice and large, if made by rats.
2. Nibbling of grains: Mice generally leave the core of grain behind; rat leaves behind grain fragments.
3. Holes in doors, screen, walls, etc. in the case of mice, the diameter is 20 mm and in rats 80 mm.
4. Rat runs.
5. Footprints: Four toes front feet, five toes back feet.
6. Droppings: Rat feces are spindle or banana shaped. Fresh ones are soft and glazed; dried ones are hard and black.

Rats and Diseases

Rats are source of nuisance and cause for insomnia. They bite the fingers, toes, ears, etc. of people sleeping on the floor; bleeding occurs and secondary infection may follow. The specific diseases connected with rats are the following:

- Diseases spread by the obligatory or incidental parasites of rats namely, fleas and mites
- Diseases contracted by eating the flesh of rat predator, pig
- Disease from consuming the food contaminated with rat dropping
- Disease resulting from wading through shallow body of water defiled by rat urine
- Diseases caused by the bite of rat.

Diseases Caused by Rats

Flea-borne diseases: These are bubonic plague, endemic typhus, *Hymenolepis nana* (*H. nana*) and *H. diminuta* infestations. These have been discussed under Rat Flea in Chapter 19 'Arthropods'.

Mite-borne diseases: The chigger of *Trombicula* mite feeds on rodent and spreads scrub typhus caused by *Rickettsia tsutsugamushi*.

Pig-borne diseases: Rats suffer from trichinosis. The adult *Trichinella spiralis* lives in their small intestine. If a pig happens to eat a rat that had died from trichinios, it too becomes infected. While the adult lives in the pig's gut, the larvae get encysted in its muscles. A susceptible person, who eats the (uncooked or improperly cooked) meat of such a pig picks up the disease.

Foodborne diseases: Salmonella typhimurium (*S. typhimurium*) and *Salmonella enteritidis* (*S. enteritidis*) live in the gut of rats. These are excreted in the feces. If foods contaminated with such feces are eaten, *Salmonella* food poisoning results.

Disease from contact with water: Leptospira icterohaemorrhagiae affects the kidney of rats and passes out in its urine. If a person wades through shallow bodies of water into which the infected rats have urinated, he/she contracts leptospirosis as the spirochetes are capable of piercing the unbroken skin.

Rat bite fevers: Are as follows:
1. Sodoku: The wound caused by the bite of the infected rat breaks down. Regional lymph glands are enlarged. The sodoku patient is febrile. The causative agent is a spirochete called *Spirillum minus*.
2. Haverhill fever: This is due to *Streptobacillus moniliformis* is characterized by fever, adenitis, exanthema and inflammation of joints.

Mouse-borne diseases: An ectoparasite of mice, *Liponyssoides sanguineus* (previously known as *Allodermanyssus sanguineus*), transmits rickettsialpox to man accidently. Foods contaminated with the droppings of infected mice can spread benign lymphocytic choriomeningitis.

Economic Impact of Rats

1. Rats devour crops and stored grains. Foods defiled by their droppings are generally discarded. It is estimated that they are responsible for the loss of one fifth of food grains in India.
2. Rats destroy eggs, chicken and grain too.
3. Rats damage soap, furniture, paper, felt, carpet, silks, laces, lead pipes, light fixtures, etc.

Control of Rats

Species sanitation, biological control, poison baiting, rodenticide application, fumigation, trapping and genetic control are the different methods of control. Species sanitation is the most effective and biological control and the least effective method. Poison baiting brings about remarkable reduction, but in the absence of other methods of control, soon the rat population expands and attains the original size. Species sanitation is done after first concluding poisoning operations. If it is done first, the rats migrate to other areas, so that very few are left behind to be killed by the subsequent poison baiting.

Species Sanitation

Following are the methods of species sanitation:
1. All food, grains, garbage, etc. are kept covered or stored in rat-proof containers.
2. Solid wastes are collected and disposed of sanitarily.
3. The living spaces under the roof and all hotels in the walls, foundations, etc. are filled up with a mixture of glass pieces and concrete.
4. All unwanted articles, old furniture, tyres, boxes, papers, rags, sacks, debris, etc. are removed to the street dustbin.
5. The space between the almirah and the wall is periodically cleaned.
6. The go downs are made rat proof thus:
   a. The floor is made of hard impervious material.
   b. All around the outer wall, a horizontal ledge (25 cm) is provided. Rats cannot negotiate such a ledge. Alternatively, a smooth paint is applied to a width of 15 cm. Windows are fitted with wire mesh and the lower part of doors are reinforced with a metal sheet.
   c. Permanent steps to the go down are not provided. Entry is with the aid of portable steps, which are kept away when not in use.
   d. All pipes, drains, cables, wires on the outside of walls are provided metal guards to prevent rodents from climbing them.
   e. The branches of the nearby trees are cut.

Biological Control

Cats, the natural predator of rats, are kept as pets. Alternatively, the rats are hunted with the aid of dogs and ferrets.

Poison Baiting

Poison baiting is the killing of rats by offering them foods mixed with rodenticides (rat poison), the chemicals capable of killing them. Rodenticides are of two types:
1. The more efficient, but slower acting anticoagulant poisons.
2. The less effective, but rapidly acting, acute poisons.

The anticoagulant, cumulative or multidose rodenticides cause the death of rats by preventing the clotting of blood and by giving rise to internal hemorrhages. Rats have to consume them daily over a couple of days. The dead rat shows blood round its mouth and anus, e.g. warfarin, coumafuryl, pindone, bromadiolone chlorophacinone and diphacinone.

Acute rodents are also called single dose of rat poisons. The best known is zinc phosphide and the next best aluminum phosphide. They release the highly toxic phosphine, when they come into contact with water. Following are some of the other acute rodenticides:
1. Scilliroside (red squill): This has emetic action and as such is safe to the domestic pets that can vomit.
2. Barium carbonate: This is a safe and simple to use as rodenticide.
3. Norbormide: This is effective against *R. norvegicus*.
4. Alpha-naphthylthiourea (ANTU): This is effective against *R. rattus*, but is not quite safe for domestic pets.

Principles of baiting

1. The bait consists of dough made from rice or wheat flour, mashed roots, vegetables or coconut. The addition of oil or sugar increases the attraction to the bait. For use in sewers, dough is mixed with wax. For killing mice, the bait is kept inside a tube. When mice come to explore the tube they pick up the poison and die.
2. The anticoagulant poisons are mixed with the bait that is then made into small moist pellets. These are kept along rat runs, near rat holes and burrows, and in dark secluded places; they are kept covered. All other

foods are excluded. The poisoned baits are kept daily for at least 2 weeks or until no more fresh carcasses of rats are noticed.

3. The acute rodenticides are not mixed with bait straight away. For the first few nights only plain bait is kept. When the rats become familiar with them, then the poison is mixed and the poisoned version is kept.
4. All dead rats are disposed of by incineration. All unconsumed baits are collected and destroyed.
5. In community, poison baiting is done in all the houses simultaneously.

Fumigation

Calcium cyanide, sulfur dioxide and methyl bromide are used as anti-rat fumigants. Cyanogas is used to fumigate burrows by special foot pump, i.e. cyanogas pump. This cyanogas when comes in contact with moisture, it leaves hydrogen cyanide, which is lethal to rats and fleas.

A spoonful of calcium cyanide powder is placed into rat holes or burrows. Alternatively with the help of a foot pump, the powder blown into rat holes and burrows, whose mouth are then sealed.

When a room to be treated with calcium cyanide, all doors and windows except one are closed. All food and drinks are removed. At first dichlorodiphenyltrichloroethane (DDT) emulsion is sprayed. Then calcium cyanide is blown into the room through the open window that is then closed. When it comes into contact with moisture left behind the DDT emulsion, it liberates hydrocyanic acid, the fumigant proper. Before re-entry the room, it is aired for at least 1 hour. Fumigation can be carried out also with carbon disulfide, sulfur dioxide, methyl bromide and chloropicrin.

Trapping

Trapping is considered as supplementary methods. Baits with indigenous foods of the area are kept in traps and because of suspicious nature of the rats, they are trapped easily. Later on they are destroyed by drowning in water.

Either the break-back trap activated by a treadle mechanisms or the Haffkine's wonder trap is used. To entice rats a bait is placed on it such as poison baiting, trapping is done in all the houses of the locality simultaneously. For the first few nights, the traps are not set, so that the rats become familiar. Gassing, drowning or incineration destroys all the trapped rats.

Genetic Control

Genetic control can be achieved by use of chemosterilants (a chemical) as they can cause temporary or permanent sterility. But, this is still in experimental stage. Male rats are sterilized by feeding them with baits mixed with chemosterilants. They are released in large numbers in the community. The mature females on mating with them to do not conceive.

Rodent Control Measures

Environmental control: In environmental control measure, sanitary measures are the most important weapon in controlling the rodents. There are three things, which are basically required such as food, shelter and water. With the decrease in these things to rodents, reduction will naturally occur among rodent-borne diseases. These environmental measures comprise:
- Proper storage of food and foodstuff
- Disposing left over foodstuff appropriately
- Collection and storage of garbage in a proper way
- Utilizing good engineering measures such as constructing rat proof buildings and blocking of rat burrow with concrete.

Chemical control: Rodenticides are used to kill the rodents. The two types of chemical control measures are listed below.

Single-dose rodenticides

These rodenticides have been grouped as 'acute' rodenticides and have lethal effect in one single dose.

According to World Health Organization (WHO), these are:
1. Requiring ordinary care:
   - Red squill
   - Norbormide
   - Zinc phosphate.
2. Requiring maximal precautions:
   - Sodium fluoroacetate
   - Strychnine
   - Fluoroacetamide.
3. Dangerous to use:
   - Arsenic trioxide
   - Alpha-naphthylthiourea
   - Gophacide
   - Phosphorus.

Most commonly used rodenticides in India are:
- Barium carbonate
- Zinc phosphide.

Barium carbonate: Baits are prepared by mixing one part of barium carbonate and four parts of flour. These baits are placed near burrows and on eating these baits, rats are killed in 2–24 hours.

Zinc phosphide: Baits are prepared by mixing one part of zinc phosphide with 10 parts of wheat or rice and a few drops of edible oil. The handling of zinc phosphide require the use of gloves as it is highly poisonous. The rats are killed in about 3 hours.

Multiple-dose rodenticides

These type of rodenticides are cumulative type and include warfarin, pindone and diphacinone. These are anticoagulants and cause internal bleeding and show death occur in 4–10 days.

CONCLUSION

Rodents live in close proximity to man and form a part of man's environment. The rodents act as a reservoir for certain diseases such as plague and typhus. Thus they are responsible for causing health hazards in human beings, so there is need to achieve control over rodents. These are not only causing health hazards but also cause substantial economic loss by damaging buildings. Rodents are controlled by careful use of rodenticides (i.e. barium carbonate, zinc phosphide, trapping, fumigation and genetic control).

Food Hygiene

CHAPTER 21

INTRODUCTION

Human beings need food for their sustenance, food has been basic to human existence. In other words, food is the prime necessity of life. Life cannot be sustained without an adequate food. People need adequate food for their growth and development. Food helps to maintain growth, repair and give energy, thereby enabling human beings to work, remain healthy and to live long. Procuring enough food for survival is the main aim of struggle in all the higher organisms.

The food we eat in our daily life has many symbolic meanings. Factors such as age, sex, genetic makeup, occupation, lifestyle, family and cultural background affects our daily food choices. Food preferences begin early in life and then change as we interact with parents, friends and our exposure to different peoples, place and situations. Many factors influence the decision about what to eat and when to eat. Amongst several factors taste, texture, cost and convenience are important things that influence the food choices. Ultimately, the reason for eating is to obtain nourishment.

Nutrition is the science of foods, the nutrients and other substances there in, there action, interaction and balance in relationships to health and disease; the process by which the organism ingests, digests, absorbs, transports and utilizes nutrients, and disposes of their end products. In addition, nutrition is concerned with social, economic, cultural and psychological implications of food and eating. In short, nutrition is the area of knowledge regarding the role of food in the maintaining of health.

Health is related to the food consumed. To maintain good health, ingesting a diet containing the nutrients in correct amount is essential. A balanced diet is one, which contain different types of food in such quantities and proportions, so that the need for calories, proteins, fats, minerals and vitamins is adequately met, and small provisions is made for extra nutrients to withstand short duration of leanness. Deficiency of any nutrients affects health of an individual. Food has not only nutrients but also has nutraceuticals, which prevent degenerative diseases where in overnutrition affects health. For example, obesity is a nutritional problem. The incidence of heart disease, hypertension, diabetes and cancer is high among obese individuals.

Good nutrition means maintaining a nutritional states that enables us to grow well and enjoy good health. Since, all foods are not the same quality from nutritional point of view, it is the capacity of an individual to include required food stuffs in such a quantity and quality, which may fulfill his/her nutritional needs. Traditionally, health care has been concern primarily with healing the sick and helping them to maintain health, but the present days, more emphasis is being given on illness prevention and community health. So, adequate nutrition is the foundation of good health and good nutrition is considered as a basic component of health, since nutrition affects human health from conception to old age. For which, people should eat hygienic food for maintaining good health.

Nurses constitute an important force in the healthcare delivery system and are supposed to provide comprehensive services to the community including nutrition, since nursing is meeting the health needs of people. Nurses are concerned about the nutritional status of people. The role of the nurse has been changed with current preventive healthcare focus and emphasis on wellness, and with the expanding responsibilities nurses are assuring in their care of clients in hospital as well as primary healthcare facilities. The knowledge of food, nutrition and food hygiene are very important.

MEANING AND DEFINITIONS OF FOOD HYGIENE

Food hygiene refers to maintaining hygienic conditions in the production, preparation, preservation, distributing and serving all types of food to people at consumption level. Food safety or food hygiene includes all conditions and measures that are necessary during production, processing, storage and distribution, and preparation of food to ensure that it is safe, sound and wholesome, and fit for human consumption according to World Health Organization (WHO).

As stated earlier, adequately hygienic food is necessary for maintaining health, vitality and well-being of an individual. Food also act as an important vehicle of transmission of disease, because its liabilities for contamination at any point during its journey from producer to consumer. So, precautions must be taken while procuring, storing, processing, cooking and serving of foods. According to Food and Agriculture Organization (FAO), food hygienic is:
1. Maintaining safe conditions for the food from the time of purchasing till the time it is served to customer.
2. Developing hygienic behavior in the employees that come in direct contact in any way with customer's meal.
3. Maintaining clean and sanitary practices and applications of an adequate pest control management.

As stated above, food also act as vehicle of transmission of foodborne diseases due to its contamination at any point that illness affect the earning capability of people. In order to avoid adverse human health effects and economic consequences due to foodborne illness, foodborne injury as well as wastage due to spoilage, everyone has to take responsibility for safe and suitable food for except, e.g. producer (farmer), processor (manufacturing), food handler and consumers. The aims of food hygiene will include to prevent foodborne diseases, preventing food poisoning and to adopt hygienic measures at all levels till consumption.

Food hygiene will be discussed on following headings:
- Food additives
- Food processing
- Safe food handling
- Personnel hygiene
- Sanitation of food establishments
- Conservation of nutrients
- Food adulteration
- Milk hygiene
- Meat hygiene
- Fish hygiene
- Food allergy.

FOOD ADDITIVES (Table 21.1)

Food additive is any substance not only naturally present in food but also added during its preparation and remaining in the finished product. Food additives are all substances added intentionally to basic food products. They include handling of substances added during the production, processing, treatment, packaging, transport and storage of a food. In general, food additives are used to decrease or improve nutritional quality, enhance appearance, increase shelf-life, reduce waste or contribute to convenience.

Food additives are legally permitted as 'non-food' substances are added to improve appearance, flavor, texture or storage properties, which include those substances that get incorporated into foods in the course of their packing, storage, transportation and handling. Additive described as generally recognized as safe (GRAS) mean that they have been used for many years without any known adverse effects, e.g. salt, sugar and vinegar. There are two categories of food additive, i.e. primary and secondary categories or direct/indirect categories.

Direct Additives

The direct additives, which are deliberately added and are safe will include:
- Coloring agents, e.g. saffron, turmeric, tartrazine and caramel
- Flavoring agents, e.g. vanilla essence, cloves and ginger
- Sweetening agents, e.g. saccharin and aspartame
- Preservatives, e.g. sorbic acid and sodium benzoate
- Palatability agents, e.g. citric acid, benzoic acid, etc.
- Stabilizing agents, e.g. gum, starch, dextrin, etc.

Indirect Additives

Indirect additives are those contaminants incidental through packing, processing steps or while transporting and they are not safe. For example, pesticides, rodenticide, arsenic, etc.

The harmful effects of food additive are allergy, food poisoning, carcinogenicity, etc. Majority of processed food, e.g. bread, biscuits, cake, jam, jellies, soft drinks, ketchup, etc. all contain additive. The prohibited additives are lead chromate, metanil yellow ferric sulfate and copper carbonate. Since, harmful effects occurring as public health problem in India, we have two regulations namely, Food Adulteration Act and Fruit Products Order to control harmful effects from additives.

Food Hygiene

Table 21.1: Food additives

Additive class	Functions	Chemical substances	Foods in which used
Anticaking, free-flowing agents	Prevent lumping and caking by absorbing moisture	Carbonates and phosphates of Ca* and Mg†, silicates of Ca, Mg, Al‡ and Na§, SiO$_2^{\|}$ and Al, Ca, K¶, Na or NH$_4^{**}$ salts of myristic acid, palmitic acid and stearic acid	Table salt, instant mix; 2% is permitted
Antimicrobial agents	Prevent the growth of bacteria, molds, fungi and yeast	Benzoic acid, esters of hydroxybenzoic acid, o-chlorobenzoic acid or salicylic acid, sulfites, sodium benzoate and sorbic acid	Squashes, crushes
Antioxidants	Prevent flavor and color changes, and retard rancidity and deterioration from exposure to oxygen	Lecithin, vitamin C and tocopherols, citric acid, tartaric acid and gallic acid, ethyl, propyl, octyl and decyl gallates (0.01%), and butylated hydroxyanisole (BHA) 0.02%	Dry mix, rosogollas, vadas, ghee and butter, edible oils and fats
Colors and adjuncts	Provide, preserve or enhance the color of food	Annatto, carotene, cochineal, chlorophyll and nitrates Red: Ponceau 4R, carmoisine erythrosine Yellow: Tartrazine, sunset yellow FCF†† Blue: Indigo carmine, brilliant blue FCF Green: Fast green FCF	Ice cream, biscuits, cakes, confectionery sweets, savories, fruit syrup, fruit squash, fruit drink and beverage, soft drink, jam (200 mg/kg permitted)
Curing and picking agents	Impart unique flavor or color to food, often increase shelf life and stability	Sodium nitrate gets converted to nitric oxide, which combines with myoglobin to form nitric oxide myoglobin; inhibits growth of *Clostridium* and *Streptococcus*	Meat
Emulsifiers	Prevent the separation of oil and water provide surface wetting, lubrication and viscosity change in combination with thickeners and fats, they give a smooth pleasing sensation in the mouth	Ammonium phosphatides, lecithin, sorbitan and polyoxyethylene in combination with fatty acids	Chocolate making, cheese making
Firming agents	To retain texture of canned fruits and vegetables	CaCO$_3^{\ddagger\ddagger}$, sodium aluminum sulfate, calcium citrate	Canned tomatoes
Flavor enhancers	Supplement enhance or modify the original flavor, or aroma of a food without contributing flavors of their own	Monosodium glutamate (up to 1%) and yeast	Masala/Spices used in noodles/Chinese cookery
Enzymes	Digestion and clarification	Pepsin, rennet, papain, amylase and pectinase	Cheese making, tenderizing meat, beverage clarifying
Neutralizing agents	To remove excess acidity	Alkaline salts of Na, K, Mg and Ca	Wine and ice cream
Stabilizing agents	Helps in ensuring a stable emulsion emulsifier/thickener	Carrageenan gums, gum Arabic	Chocolate in milk, ice cream, foam stabilizer in beer
Humectant	Prevents undesirable drying of foods and to maintain the moisture level	Glycerin, sorbitol, mannitol, dextrose and corn syrup	Shredded coconut

*Ca, calcium; †Mg, magnesium; ‡Al, aluminum; §Na, sodium; $^{\|}$SiO$_2$, silicon dioxide; ¶K, potassium; **NH$_4$, ammonium; ††FCF, four color food; ‡‡CaCO$_3$, calcium carbonate.

Contd...

Contd...

Additive class	Functions	Chemical substances	Foods in which used
Sequestrant (chelating agents)	Prevent the deterioration of food due to free metallic ions in it discoloration, flavor alteration, oxidation or turbidity formation	Calcium ethylenediaminetetraacetic acid (Ca-EDTA), phosphates such as potassium dihydrogen phosphate (KH_2PO_4) and organic acids, e.g. tartaric acid, citric acid and glycerin	Soft drinks industries, malted beverages
Flour improvers	For bleaching purpose and for dough toughening purpose by converting protein sulfhydryl (SH) group into disulfide bonds	Benzoyl peroxide, chlorine gas, ClO_2,[§§] NO_2,[∥∥] N_2O_4[¶¶] have both the properties, $KBrO_3$,[***] KIO_3,[†††] CaO_2[‡‡‡] and $Ca(IO_3)$[§§§] (oxidizing agents)	Flour
Flavoring agents and adjuvants	Impart or help impart a taste, or an aroma in food	Natural extracts and synthetic flavor chemicals are used basically they are aldehydes, ketones, hydroxy and ester or etheric in nature	Soft drinks, confectionery, chewing gum
Leaving agents and adjuvants	To increase in volume of dough or batter resulting in light fluffy and spongy, and produce or stimulate CO_2 production in baked goods	Baking powder sodium bicarbonate with another acid chemical are used basically they are aldehydes, ketones, hydroxyl and ester or etheric in nature	Bread, biscuits, cakes component such as tartaric acid or calcium hydrogen phosphate
Non-nutritive sweeteners	Provide less than 2% of the calorific value of sucrose per equivalent unit of sweeting capacity when used to sweeten foods	Aspartame (fruit flavor) acesulfame-K	Soft drinks, chewing gum, instant coffee and tea
Nutritive sweeteners	Provide greater than 2% of the calorific value of sucrose equivalent unit of sweetening capacity when used to sweeten food	Sorbitol, mannitol and other polyols	Chocolates, ice cream, pastries, jams and drinks
Propellants, aerating agents and gases	Supply force to expel a product	CO_2[∥∥∥∥] gas and Na_2CO_3[¶¶¶] or $CaCO_3$ with an acid to generate gas	Soft drinks, alcoholic beverages
Solvents and vehicles	Extract or dissolve another substance	Ethyl alcohol, propylene glycol, glycerin oils and fatty acids	Vanilla extract
Clouding agents	To produce haze in liquid foods	Calcium phosphate, cellulose derivatives, gums and starches	Liquid foods
Clarifying agents	To remove cloudiness	Bentonite, tannic acid and gelatin	Fruit juices, beer and wines
Nutritive additives	To make up for the storage or processing losses, or to fortify the product	Thiamine iron, calcium iodine lysine, vitamin A and D	Milk, salt, wheat flour, bread and vanaspati
Maintain appearance, palatability and wholesomeness	To prevent spoilage by molds, bacteria, yeast, etc.	Propionic acid, calcium and sodium salts of propionic acid, ascorbic acid, BHA, butylated hydroxytoluene (BHT), propylene glycol	Bread, pie filling, cakes, mixed potato chips, crackers, cheese, syrup, fruit juices, frozen and dried fruits, margarine, shortening, etc.

[§§]ClO_2, chlorine dioxide; [∥∥]NO_2, nitrogen dioxide; [¶¶]N_2O_4, nitrogen tetroxide; [***]$KBrO_3$, potassium bromate; [†††]KIO_3, potassium iodate; [‡‡‡]CaO_2, calcium dioxide; [§§§]$Ca(IO_3)$, calcium iodate; [∥∥∥∥]CO_2, carbon dioxide; [¶¶¶]Na_2CO_3, sodium carbonate.

CHAPTER 21 — Food Hygiene

FOOD PRESERVATION

Preservation may be defined as the state in which any food may be retained over a period of time without:
- Being contaminated by pathogenic organisms or chemicals
- Losing optimum qualities of color, texture, flavor and nutritive value.

The aims of food preservation includes:
- To decrease the process of spoilage
- To prevent the occurrence of foodborne illnesses
- To prevent the growth of bacteria and microorganisms
- To inhibit natural aging of food
- To maintain natural aging of food, texture and flavor thereby inhibiting discoloration.

Food preservation methods are vary from culture to culture. The food preservation involves the retardation of oxidation of fats, which causes rancidity.

Importance of Food Preservation

1. Food preservation adds variety to the food. For example, in the absence of fresh peas during the hot summer months, canned or dehydrated peas may be made use of.
2. Food preservation increases the shelf-life of life. Pineapples, cherries and other fruits and vegetables may be preserved by different methods for long periods of time.
3. Food preservation increases the food supply.
4. Food preservation decreases the wastage of food. Excess foods, which would have otherwise been wasted when processed and preserved, add to the existing supplies, thus, also decreasing wastage of food.
5. Food preservation decreases dietary inadequacies. Variety in diet is brought about with the help of preserved foods. For example, some Middle East countries do not grow any vegetables due to arid soil conditions. This shortcoming is overcome through the import of fresh and preserved fruits, and vegetables. However, the Middle East countries are the chief exporters of dates and dry fruits. Likewise, certain regions of a country may be lacking in particular food item, can make good, the deficiency by procuring them from various regions, where it is plentiful. In the snow-bound areas of the Himalayas most often, food is brought in from other parts of the country.

When food is available more than the present utility, it is preserved for further consumption. For example, seasonal fruit and vegetables, and food grown in plentiful are cheaper, and good quality can be preserved for further use. The objective of food preservation will include:
a. To preserve the nutritional value.
b. To protect the life of foods to add variety to food preparations, to make the food available even in off season.
c. To avoid the wasteful of food and to save time in procurement.

The preservation of food is very essential because food is liable to spoilage due to action of microorganism (i.e. mold, yeast, bacteria, etc.), insects and enzymes. The principle of food preservation will include:
- To maintain asepsis and to prevent entry of microorganisms by airtight packages
- To make free bacterial liquid by filtration through porcelain fibers
- To destroy enzymes by blanching, e.g. pasteurization of milk
- To destroy pathogens by irradiations of fruits and vegetables.

Process of Food Preservation

Prevention or Delay of Microbial Decomposition

By keeping out microorganisms (asepsis)

Nature provides protective coverings around the food in the form of shells of nuts, the skin of fruits and vegetables, the shells of eggs and the skin or fat on meat and fish. These protective coverings act as a preservative factor, thereby preventing or delaying microbial decomposition.

Even in the food industry, several aseptic methods are adopted to prevent the contamination of foods during its processing. In the canning industry, the load of microorganisms determines the heat process necessary for the preservation of food. This is better known as aseptic canning. In the dairy industry, the quality of milk is judged by its bacterial content.

Packaging of foods is also an application of asepsis. The coverings may range from simple wrappers to hermetically sealed containers of canned foods. Polythene bags and moisture proof wrapping including heavy foil, heavily mixed papers and cellophane are used.

By removal of microorganisms

Filtration is a method used for the complete removal of microorganisms and is successfully applied only to clear liquids such as water, fruit juices, beer, soft drinks and wine. The filter used in this method is made of asbestos pads, unglazed porcelain and similar materials. This filter sterilized and made 'bacteria proof' before been used as a filtration device. The liquid is filtered by forcing it under pressure through the filter.

By hindering the growth and activity of microorganisms

Growth and activity of microorganisms may be done by low temperature or drying, or providing anaerobic conditions.

When anaerobic (absence of oxygen) conditions are created, some aerobic organisms die, while the spores of others may survive, but are unable to multiply in the absence of oxygen. This principle is used as a preservative factor in canned and packaged foods.

Low temperature at which foods are preserved in cold storage slows down and sometimes prevents bacterial activity.

Drying of foods is very effective method of avoiding spoilage of food, since microorganisms cannot flourish in the absence of moisture.

Certain chemicals such as sodium benzoate and potassium metabisulfite may be used for preservation, but they should be used with great care as an excess of any of them may result in poisoning.

By killing the microorganisms using heat or radiation

Gamma rays or high speed electrons are used to destroy the microorganisms. Both types of radiations are termed as ionized radiations.

Prevention or Delay of Self-decomposition of Food

Delay of self-decomposition is done by destruction or inactivation of food enzymes by blanching. The inactivation affects many plant enzymes, which otherwise might toughness and change in color. All plant and animal tissues contain enzymes, which are highly active at room temperature and above. For each 10°C (19°F) rise in temperature, the rate of the chemical change doubles. Rancidity of fats is an excellent example of undesirable oxidation and leads to the deterioration in flavor of foods that may contain only small quantities of fat. Oxidation also leads to a loss of ascorbic acid. Plant and animal tissue fiber is softened and the surfaces of cut non-acid fruits are oxidized and become darkened as a result of enzyme action, thereby changing the color, texture and nutritive value.

Before freezing (to prevent the growth of bacteria) fruits and vegetables are blanched to inactive the oxidative enzymes. Blanching is done with hot water or steam and the extent of treatment applied varies with kind of food being treated. The brief heat treatment is supposed to accomplish reduction of the number of microorganisms on the food, enhancement of the green color of vegetables such as peas and spinach, and prevention of damage because of mechanical causes for insects and animals.

Items of food can be damaged either by insects and animals or by mishandling. Therefore, meticulous care should be exercised to minimize any damage to the foods. The entire operation of preserving foods is divided into three stages of careful handling:

1. Proper packaging.
2. Quick and effective transportation.
3. Providing good storage facilities, such as silos for grains and cold storages for fruits and vegetables.

Methods of Food Preservation

Preserving food is based upon the principles of preventing or retarding the causes of spoilage to microbial decomposition, enzymatic and non-enzymatic chemical reactions and damage from mechanical causes for insects and rodents. Food preservation can be achieved through low temperature (freezing), high temperature (pasteurizing), preservatives, osmosis and dehydration. For our convenience, there are two methods of food preservation, which includes bacteriostatic and bactericidal. Bacteriostatic methods are dehydration, coating, chilling, salting, chemicals, refrigerates and bactericidal methods are heating, smoking, canning and irradiation.

Drying

Drying is a means of preservation, which can be observed in cereal grains, legumes and nuts, which dry on the plants. Drying includes keeping the food in air or sunlight for drying, which resulting in the reduction of water activity, which is sufficient to prevent or delay the growth of organism. Removal of water from a product can be done by freezing, sun drying, by osmosis or drying by mechanical driers to retain quality during storage, dried foods have to be store in moisture proof containers. So drying includes keeping the food in air or sunlight for drying, resulting in the reduction of water activity, which is sufficient to prevent or delay the growth of microorganisms. The food, which can be dried are apples, peas, banana, mangoes, papaya, apricots raisins, etc. Dried foods are preserved because the available moisture level is so low that microorganisms cannot grow and enzyme activity is controlled. Moisture removal also results in concentration of food and thereby osmotic pressure is increased.

Freezing

Cold temperature inhibits growth of microorganism although freezing may result in the destruction of some microorganism. In slow-freezing process, the foods are placed in refrigerated rooms at temperatures ranging from −4 to −2°C may require from 3 to 72 hours under such conditions. Home freezing is done by this process (sharp freezing). Fruits and vegetables require −15 to −21°C. In quick freezing, and the low temperature used between −32 and −41°C freezes foods so rapidly that fine crystals are formed. In this process, large quantity of food can be frozen in a short period of time. The very low temperature for both freezing and holding frozen products adds to the cost, but desirable for many products in term of retention of palatability and nutritive value. Chilling helps to storing fruits, vegetables, milk, meat, egg, drinks, etc. in refrigerator. Chill refrigeration prevents the growth of organisms. Digestibility and food values are not affected. Dehydrofreezing of fruits and vegetables consist of drying the food about 50% of its weight of its original weight and volume, and then food to preserve it. The storage temperature of −18°C is usually recommended for frozen foods. So freezing is one of the commonest methods used in which the low temperature is used for preserving the food. This method involves the reduction of water activity there by inhibiting the microbial growth, e.g. potato waffles. In cold stores, freezing method is used to store large volume of food for long term.

Heating

The temperature and time used in heat processing of food depends upon the effect of heat on food and other preservation methods employed, e.g. pasteurization and canning.

Pasteurizing

Pasteurizing is a heat treatment that kills part, but not all the microorganisms present (spores are resistant to heat) and usually involves the application of temperature below 100°C. This treatment has two advantages to kill pathogenic microorganism and inactivated enzymes. The heating may be by means of steam, hot water, dry heat or electric currents and the products are cooled promptly after the heat treatment, e.g. pasteurization of milk. Since, it extends product shelf-life from a microbial and enzymatic, in some point of view when beer, wine and fruit juices are pasteurized. Preservative methods used to supplement pasteurization includes refrigeration, e.g. milk, keeping out microorganisms by usually by packing the product in a sealed container and maintenance of anaerobic conditions as in vacuum created, sealed container.

Canning

Canning is a way in which fruits and vegetables are cooked, and sealed in sterile cans and as a form of pasteurization, the cans are boiled to kill any remaining microorganisms. There are certain foods, which required only boiling for short timings, while other foods require boiling for longer time period, even some foods required pressure canning. For example, strawberries require only short boiling cycle and tomatoes require long boiling cycle and use of additives.

Canning involves the applications of temperature to food that are high enough to destroy essentially all microorganisms plus airtight sealing in sterilized container to prevent recontamination. The degree of heat and the length of time of heating vary with the type of food and the kind of microorganism that are likely to occur in it. Most canning is in 'tin cans', which are made of tin-coated steel or in glass container, but increasing use is being made of containers that are partially or wholly aluminum, are of plastics as pouches or solid containers. For example, hot food is put inside the can and again heated, then the can is sealed. This makes the can airtight.

Smoking

Smoke is an example of mixture of alcohols, acids, phenols and toxic substances, which inhibit microbial agent. Smoking is the method by which heat is used to dry the food without cooking and aromatic hydrocarbons of smoke preserve the food, e.g. smoking of meat and fish. Meat to be smoked in first, salted and then smoked. Temperature control during smoking is essential to maintain texture. So, smoking is the method in which heat is used to dry the food without cooking and aromatic hydrocarbons of smoke preserve the food, e.g. meat and fish.

Irradiation

Here, food is exposed to ionizing radiations and gamma rays. This process of irradiation is also known as cold pasteurization, so called because heat is not used for preserving food, but radiations is also known as cold pasteurizations and while using radiation safety precautions are used. Irradiation of food does not cause food become radioactive. For example, irradiation with ultraviolet rays for fruit and vegetables.

By Osmosis

High osmotic pressure may inhibit microbial growth by plasmolysis of microbial cells, but it cannot be relieved to kill organism. Yeast and molds are relatively resistant to high osmotic pressure. For instances jellies, jams and pickles are rarely affected by bacterial actions, because of their high sugar and salt content, but it is common to find mold growth on their surface, if exposed to air. Apples, guavas, grapes, bananas, sapota, mangoes and pineapples, which have pulp are suitable for making jams and jellies, there are some foods, which require addition of pectin, jellying agent to form a gel such as agar, gelatin, etc.

In jams and jellies, the concentration of sugar are done in the following process. Here water is withdrawn from microbial cells, when they are placed in solutions containing large amount of dissolved substances such as sugar or salt. As a result of this water loss, microbial metabolisms are halted. The antimicrobial effects of water loss are similar in principle to metabolic inhibitions by dehydration. Foods are also preserved by the principle of osmotic pressure in salting and pickling. Most commonly used in organic preservatives is sodium chloride. It is used in brine solution or is applied to the food. This solution is added to slowdown or prevents the growth of microorganisms.

Salting

Salting method is used to preserve the food. Salting technique draws the moisture from food by osmosis. Even nitrites and nitrates are used to preserve the food, which inhibit specific group of microorganisms, e.g. meat.

Sodium chloride or common salt is used primarily as a preservation and flavoring agent. Salt is employed to central microbial population in food such as butter, cheese, cabbages, olive, cucumber, meat, fish and bread. There are four methods of salt curing, e.g. dry salting (fish), brimming (vadu mango), low salt fermentation (chilli pickle, sauerkraut from cabbage) and pickling (lime pickle).

Pickling

Pickling method is one, which the food is preserved by using edible antimicrobial liquid. It includes two process chemical pickling and fermented pickling.

In chemical pickling the agents such as brine, vinegar, vegetable oils and many other edible oils are used. Sometimes food to be preserved is heated or boiled, so that food becomes saturated with pickling agent, e.g. pickles, corned beef, mixed vegetables, achar, herrings, etc.

When the food is fermented, it produces preserving agent by process of production of lactic acid. For example, curtido or kimchi fermented pickles, etc. The pickles may be divided into three categories:

1. Sweet pickles, e.g. tomato and mango sweet.
2. Sour pickles, e.g. mango pickles and lime pickle.
3. Fermented pickle, e.g. cucumber pickles, cabbage pickle, chilli pickles, meat and sausages.

Jellying

Jellying is the way in which the food, which is solid, is cooked to form a gel with or without adding a material such as sipunculid worms. There are some foods, which required addition of pectin (jellying agent) to form a jelly such as agar, gelatin, but in some foods pectin is naturally present.

Vacuum packing

Vacuum packing is the method of preserving the food in which air tight bags or bottles are used for storing the food. The vacuum created in the container reduces the oxygen demand of bacteria for their survival, i.e. inhibit the aerobes and delay the growth of bacteria, thereby preventing the spoilage.

Adding of Preservative

The preservatives are chemical agents, which serve to retard, hinder of mask undesirable change in food. These changes may be caused by microorganisms, by the enzymes of food or by purely chemical reaction. According to Prevention of Food Adulteration (PFA), there are two classes of preservation such as class I and II. Class I are GRAS, which includes salt, sugar, spices, vinegar and edible vegetable oils. Class II preservatives is benzoic acid and its sodium and potassium salts, sorbic acids and its sodium and potassium salts. Food preservation is often used in mixed form or in conjunction with other methods of preservations.

The important preservatives agents in pickles are salt, vinegar, sugar, oil spices and condiments.

Sugar

The food, which we need to be preserved is cooked in sugar to the point of crystallization and the outcome product is dried and stored such as apples, peaches, apricots, plums, etc. Sometimes, alcohol is combined with sugar to preserve food. The food is preserved due to high sucrose concentration, which creates too high osmotic pressure not allowing the microorganism to grow or survive.

Jugging

Jugging is used to store meat after cutting in small pieces with gravy or brine in airtight containers. Enriched atmosphere is used to preserve grain. At bottom of grain, a block of dry ice is kept and excess of gas is burped. By this method, grain can be preserved for 5 years.

Food preservation methods include all those methods in which the pathogens causing spoilage are killed or such atmosphere is provided in which either microbial growth does not occur or prevent its delay. Such methods cause:

CHAPTER 21 — Food Hygiene

- Reduction of water activity
- Low oxygen tension
- Enriched carbon dioxide atmosphere
- Reduction of intracellular pH
- Creation of high osmotic pressure
- Dehydration of the food
- Inhibition of the growth of toxins
- Inactivation of vegetative bacteria such as yeast or molds by pressure.

High pressure for preserving food

High pressure for preserving food is the method in which a vessel is used to keep and process the food exerting 70,000 pounds per square inch pressure to disable the growth of harmful microorganisms so to reduce the process of spoilage.

Food preservation is the way of treating and handling the food by vast range of methods, tools and combination of ingredients with an effect to preserve the food value. For preserving food, the food additives are used. Food additives are non-food substances, which are added to:

- Increase the shelf-life of food
- Improve the taste of food
- Change the color and texture of food.

So that food can be preserved for a particular period of time. The food additives are classified according to the particular function, they perform, such as:

1. Coloring agents: Turmeric, Deggi mirch and saffron.
2. Flavoring agent: Vanilla, strawberry, mango, essence, etc.
3. Sweetening agents: Saccharin.
4. Preserving agents: Sodium benzoate, sorbic acid.
5. Acid imparting agents: Citric acid and acetic acid.

FOOD PROCESSING (PREPARATION)

Food is prepared for eating purpose by cooking with the application of heat. There are a vast range of methods used for cooking. Various instruments such as griddle (tawa) on heat, tandoor, frying pan, etc. are used to prepare the food. Griddle is used for making chapati, paratha and tandoor for making naan, kulcha, tandoori roti and tandoori chicken. Tandoor is a cylindrical coal fire oven.

Most of the food consumed will need some form of cooking and preserving before they are fit for serving and consumption. Fruits and some vegetable used in salad or chutney are consumed uncooked. Food is prepared for eating purpose by cooking. There are many advantages of cooking will includes:

- It increase palatability of the food
- It makes mastication easier and renders the easy digestion of food
- It sterilizes the food by destroying microorganism and parasitic ova and eggs
- It lends a new flavor and thereby stimulates digestive juices
- It introduces the variety, i.e. many different types of dishes can be prepared from the same ingredients
- Proper cooking, increases the acceptability of food and improves the appearance of food.

During cooking, heat may be transferred to the food by conduction, convection, radiation or by the energy of microwaves (electronic heat transfer). Water or steam and air or fat, or combinations of these are used as cooking media. Air or fat are used in dry heat. Methods of cooking are classified according to moist heat, dry heat and combination of both:

- Moist heat, e.g. boiling, simmering, poaching, stewing, blanching, steaming and pressure cooking
- Dry heat, e.g. roasting, grilling/broiling, toasting, baking, sautéing and frying
- Combined, e.g. braising.

Various methods are used for cooking such as deep frying in oil (bhatura, puri and golgappa), boiling (pulses, for making soups), steaming (vegetables), baking (for breads), grilling (for meat). These are the most common methods used for preparing dishes in India.

Application of these methods change the flavor, texture, consistency, appearance and nutritional properties. For preparing food, the ingredients are appropriately selected, measured and combined in an order to achieve the desired taste, smell without losing the nutritive value of the food. The heat is used for preparing the food so as to kill or delay the growth of microorganisms, to prevent foodborne illnesses.

METHODS OF FOOD PREPARATION

Boiling

Boiling is cooking foods by just immersing them in water at 100°C and maintaining the water at that temperature till the food is tender. Rice, dal, pulses, roots tubers are cooked in this way. Boiling generally used in combination with simmering or other methods, e.g. cooking rice, vegetables, dal over boiling may result in loss of vitamins and minerals. To prevent this, cooked water used in soups, rasam, sambar and dal.

Simmering

In simmering, foods are cooked in a pan with a well-fitting lid at temperature just below boiling point (82–99°C) of the liquid in which they are immersed. For example, foods have to be cooked for a long time to make it tender as in the case of cheaper cuts of meat, fish, cooking custards, kheer, vegetables and carrot halwa. These methods are employed in making soups and stocks.

Stewing

In stewing method, foods are cooked in pan with a tight-fitting lid, using small quantities of liquid to cover only half the food. Here, comparatively smaller amount of liquid used and prolonged low degree of heat is applied. Food is half covered with liquid and as soon as it reaches boiling point, the heat is reduced to make it simmer for a prolonged time (2-4 hour) depends upon the nature and volume of the foods being stewed. For better results, using a pan with well-fitting lid to prevent evaporation. The nutrients, which escape while stewing are not lost, but are present in the liquid, which is served with stew. Stewing is used for cooking meat and Bengal grams. The cooking meat and vegetables together make the dish attractive and nutritious since no liquids are discarded.

Steaming

In steaming, the food are cooked in steam. The steam is generated from vigorously boiling water or liquid in a pan, so that the food is completely surrounded by steam and not in contact with the water and liquid. The water should be boiled before the food is placed in the steamer. Here, the food gets cooked at 100°C. Recipes made by steaming are idli, dhokla, rice or ragi puttu, idiyappam, appam, puttu, etc.

The principle is employed in pressure cooker, in which food is cooked by the heat of direct steam. Food is cooked in pressure cooker, it is also called steaming. Pressure cooking is better method of cooking, since it saves nutrients, fuel and time. In pressure cooker, escaping steam is trapped and kept under pressure, so that the temperature of the boiling water and steam can be raised from 100 to 120°C and reduce cooking time for which domestic pressure cookers are available.

Poaching

Poaching is a process in which foods are cook by simmering in a small amount of liquid. Cook without its shell in or over boiling water, e.g. egg.

Blanching

Blanching is a process in which foods are immersed in hot boiling water for a few minutes prior to processing (frozen dried or canned). It helps in removal of peel, inactivation of enzymes that oxidize vitamin C and removal of gas:
1. Parboiling: By this method, the nutrients lost is minimized in the rice.
2. Parching (puffing): In this method, the cereals (jowar, maize and rice) are moistened and then heated. While heating, the escaping water causes the grain to swell. For example, murmura and popcorn. Starches in the grain are broken down to singular compounds, which improves their digestibility. It leads to some loss of lysine.

Roasting

In roasting method, food is smeared with a little fat and exposed directly to heat or flame. Chicken or tender mutton may be cooked by this method. It is also called 'barbeque' when food is cooked uncovered in heated metal or frying pan. The method is known as pan broiling or roasting, e.g. groundnut and chapati.

Grilling/Broiling

Grilling/Broiling consists of placing the food below or above, or in between red hot surface. When under the heater, the food is heated by radiation only. This results in the browning of food. Then the heat is more slowly conducted the surfaces of the food downwards. As heating is most superficial, grilled foods are usually reversed and rotated. So, it is cooked by direct heat. It can be done either in a grill or a direct on flame. It is very quick method. For examples, foods cooked by grilling are cob on the corn, papad, brinjal, phulkas, sweet potato, kebab and cheese tomatoes. Barbeque or roasting is also made by this method.

Toasting

Toasting is used to describe the process by which bread slices are kept under the grill or between two heated elements to brown from both sides of the bread at the same time. This can be adjusted to give the required degree of brownness through temperature control.

Baking

In baking, food gets cooked by hot air. It is a dry heat method of cooking, but the action of dry heat is combined with that of a steam, which is generated while the food is being cooked. Baking is done in hot air oven. It is an inexpensive and slow method of cooking. Food is enclosed by hot air, so that it gets heat from all sides. The cooking temperature varies from 250 to 500°F (120–260°C). The foods prepared by baking are custards, pies, biscuits, pizzas, puffs, buns, bread, cakes, tandoori chicken, tandoori meat and fish. The oven has to be heated slightly more than the required temperature before placing food in it. The principle involved in cooking is baking as the air inside that oven is heated by a source of heat either electricity or gas, or wood in case of tandoori. The oven is insulated to prevent the outside temperature from causing fluctuations in internal temperature of the equipment. The methods of heat transfer involved are radiation from the source of heat to the metal wall at the base of the oven, by conduction through the heated air currents setup in the oven to the food.

Sautéing

In sautéing, fat as medium of cooking. This method involves cooking in just enough oil to cover the base of the pan. The food is tossed occasionally or turned over with a spatula to enable all the pieces to come in contact with oil and get cooked evenly. The heat is transferred to the food mainly by conduction. Foods cooked by this method are generally vegetables used as side dishes in a menu.

Frying

In frying method, food is cooked in fat or oil. There are two type of this method shallow fat frying and deep fat frying. In shallow frying, oil or fat will be used, but not enough to cover it. Heat is transferred to the food partially by conduction by contact with heated pan and partially by the convection currents of the food. This prevents local burning of food by keeping away the intense heat of frying pan. The shallow frying needs less quantity of oil and then suitable to cook egg, omelet, sausages, dosa, paratha, chapati, fish cutlets and tikkis.

In deep frying, food is completely immersed in hot oil and cooked vigorously in convection currents and cooking in uniform on all sides of foods. Cooking can be rapidly completed in deep frying because of high temperature used is 180–220°C. This method needs more quantity oil and it is used to cook samosa, papads, chips, chakli, pakoda, bajji and bonda, etc.

SAFE FOOD HANDLING

Food preparation and service requires handling of material, which are extremely venerable to becoming the media of contamination, thereby leading to the spread of infection and disease. In household cooking as well as in public catering, food safety that includes hygiene and sanitation (Table 21.2) plays a vital role in promoting and protecting the health.

Table 21.2: Different aspects of food safety (hygiene and sanitation)

Environmental hygiene	Hygienic food handling	Personal hygiene
Site	Receiving	Dress
Structure	Storage	Grooming
Furniture and fittings	Pre-preparation	Health
Ventilation	Holding	
Lighting	Serving	
Water supply	Cleaning	
Waste disposal	Dish washing	

Hygiene refers to general cleanliness of the environment and the people in working situation, while sanitation involves the activities, which help to bring about and maintain healthy and hygienic conditions free from the hazards of infection and diseases.

Environmental Hygiene and Sanitation

Environment refers to the total environment in which food is delivered, prepared and served:
1. The site should be free from air pollution and infestations by insects, rats, flies, fleas, etc.
2. The materials selected for construction need to be nonabsorbent and noncorrosive to facilitate easy cleaning of walls, floors, ceiling and other surfaces.
3. The surfaces of walls, partitions and floor should be made of impervious material with no toxic effect in intended use.
4. Walls and partitions should have a smooth surface up to a height appropriate to operation.
5. The floors should be constructed to allow adequate drainage and cleaning.
6. Ceilings and overhead fixtures should be constructed and finished to minimize the build-up of dirt and condensation, and shredding of particles.
7. Windows should be easy to clean, to minimize the build-up of dirt and where necessary, be fitted with removable and cleanable insect proof screens, where necessary should be fixed.
8. Doors should have smooth, non-absorbent surfaces and be easy to clean and where necessary disinfected.
9. Working surfaces that come into contact with food should be in sound condition, durable and easy to clean, maintain and disinfect. They should be made

off of smooth, non-absorbent material, inert to food, to detergents and disinfectants under operating conditions.
10. Proper maintenance of equipment, furniture and fittings help in preventing accumulation of dust and dirt. All equipment, utensils and surfaces should be cleaned after each usage.
11. Well-ventilated food service establishments keep the temperature conducive and bring down the carbon dioxide content in air.
12. Poor lighting reduces the efficiency of people at work and makes dirt, grease and infestation not easily detectable.
13. Clean and safe water used for drinking, cooking and utensil cleaning ensures prevention of food and waterborne illnesses.
14. Frequent disposal, cleaning and disinfection prevent putrefaction of garbage, which attracts insects and rodents.

Food Handlers

Proper food handling includes the prevention of contamination during the processing stages before they are served to customers.

Food should be handled in hygienic way and should be stored in a place, which is free from pests, chemicals, physical and microbiological agents.

Principles of handling of food
- Keep the hands clean
- Touch the food as little as possible
- Do not allow sick person to handle the food
- Wash the hands between handling of different foods especially after handling raw meat.

Following are the important things to remember to prevent food from contamination by food handlers:
1. Food handlers need to be medically examined at time of employment and day-to-day health appraisal of food handlers is required to find out the food handlers who are suffering from jaundice, diarrhea, vomiting, fever, sore throat, nausea with infected skin lesions or having discharge from ear, nose, throat or eye. Then he should not be allowed to handle the food in food establishments.
2. Food handlers should wear protective clothing, foot wear and the head should be covered.
3. Food handlers should not smoke, spit, chew or sneeze, or cough in food establishments, i.e. it should be refrained.
4. Education to the food handlers regarding:
   a. Personal hygiene—handwashing.
   b. Tying/Restraining hairs.
   c. White clean overall.
   d. Food handling techniques.
   e. Importance of cleanliness of utensils carrying food.
   f. Control of insects and rodents.

PERSONNEL HYGIENE OF FOOD HANDLER

1. Personnel engaged in food preparation and service need to wear clean uniforms, hair nets or caps, while on duty. Personnel need to wear protective clothing and have to wash their hands before entering food establishments.
2. Finger nails should be kept short and clean, if any, must be covered with water proof dressings.
3. People with colds, sore throats, boils or diarrhea should not handle food. Regular medical checkups to ensure good health are important.
4. Hand should be washed well with soap before handling food. Spitting or smoking in the kitchen or service areas should be prohibited. All kitchen cloths and hand towels must be washed in hot water.

Hygienic Food Handling

1. Food supplies should be purchased from reliable source and should be checked, sorted, cleaned and immediately used or stored.
2. Perishables must be stored in suitable temperature or frozen to prevent spoilage. Dry foods must be stored in closed tins and protected from insects and rodents.
3. Foods not requiring cooking must be prepared with a minimum of handling. Raw fruits and vegetables must be washed well before cooking or serving.
4. Foods should be cooked soon after pre-preparation such as washing, cutting, etc. Cooking meat should be done with extra care to see that the internal temperature is high to make it safe for consumption.
5. During the holding time between cooking and serving, hot food should be kept above 63°C, cold foods below 3°C, and frozen foods below 0°C.
6. Serving area, tableware and serving equipment, and crockeries must be cleaned and dry at all times.
7. Quick and complete clearing of the table minimizes the chance of cross contamination.
8. Dish washing is an area, where sanitary hazards can be easily created, if good care is not taken as crockeries, cutleries, pans and pots come in direct contact with food.

Food Hygiene

Storage

Food storage includes keeping/storing food at proper temperature and in a proper way to keep food clean and safe before it is consumed by the customer. It is necessary to store onions and potatoes separately. If stored together, the gases released from onions can spoil the potatoes.

Food becomes hazardous to health due to improper storage. In general, most bacteria are inactivated at freezing point, i.e. 0°C and below. Between 1.7 and 4.4°C they start becoming active, but grow slowly. As the temperature rises, the activity increases becoming optimum at 37°C, which is the normal body temperature. The temperatures at which food need to be stored to prevent their deterioration through contamination by microorganism, the escaping water causes the grain to swell. For example, murmura, popcorn, etc. Starches in the grain are broken down to simpler compounds, which improve their digestibility. It leads to some loss of lysine.

Principles of Food Storage

1. Keep hot food above 140°F.
2. Keep cold food below 41°F.
3. Store food in a clean and dry area.
4. Keep all the food covered to protect from dust, sneezes, etc.
5. Keep the storage area free from rats, mice and insects.
6. Poisonous material should be kept away from food area.
7. Do not keep the food at room temperature for longer time periods.
8. The food storage places should be easy to clean, maintain and disinfect (whenever required).
9. These food places should be properly designed to protect the food from cross contamination and preventing the food stuffs during and between operations, i.e. procedures.
10. The food storage places should be away from:
    - Environmentally polluted areas
    - Flooding areas
    - Infestations of pests
    - The areas from where it is difficult to remove waste—solid or liquid.
11. Storage place should be built of durable material.
12. Food need to be stored under adequate temperature and for adequate timing as the most common cause of foodborne illness or spoilage of food in inadequate food temperature. The temperature for the food stuff is maintained on the basis of:
    - Nature of food, i.e. its water activity and pH
    - Shelf-life of food.
13. The food storage places should be prevented from contamination by foreign bodies such as metal shards, from machine dust or fumes, etc.
14. The storage places should be washed thoroughly cleaned and disinfected after removal of raw food and whenever required. It is especially in case of meat or poultry. It is necessary to wash the utensils, equipment, which is used for cutting or storage, etc.
15. Cross contamination of food at storage places should be prevented from direct and indirect contact with pathogens, which can be transmitted from one food to another.
16. Adequate method for storing the food should be adopted such as chilling, thermal processing, etc.

Sprouting (Germination)

The pulse (green gram, Bengal gram) grains are moistened and stored in wet condition for 24–48 hours and the grain sprout. The process increases vitamin C content by about 10 times. The content of thiamine, riboflavin and niacin is almost doubled. Iron becomes free and hence available. The digestibility increases due to breakdown of cell walls. Sprouting fenugreek (methi) seeds reduce its bitter taste.

Fermenting

In fermenting method, the microorganisms multiply under the processing conditions, e.g. making curd from milk, processing of rice and urad dal for idli, etc. In curds, the lactose is converted into lactic acid. The enzyme in the starch releases carbon dioxide to cause bubbles. Fermentation doubles the thiamine, riboflavin and niacin contents. Iron availability is also increased.

Liming

Liming means introduction of lime in foods such as buttermilk, rasam, fermented mixture. It prevents destruction of thiamine and riboflavin.

SANITATION OF FOOD ESTABLISHMENTS (RESTAURANTS, EATING HOUSES)

The following minimum standards have been suggested under the Model Public Health Act (1955) for restaurants:
1. Location: It should not be near any accumulation of filth or open drain, stable, manure pit and other sources of nuisance.
2. Floor should be higher than the adjoining land, made with impervious material and easy to keep clean.

3. Rooms should be accommodative for maximum of 10 persons.
4. Walls should be impervious and easily washable.
5. Lighting and ventilation should be adequate.
6. Kitchen: The floor to be impervious, smooth, non-slippery and easy to keep clean door and windows to be rat-proof, fly-proof and of self-closing type. There must be smoke pipe and ventilators.
7. Store room: There must be provision for storing the food grains and also cooked food separately.
8. Furniture's should be strong and easy to keep clean and dry.
9. Collection of refuse: There must be provision for collection, storage and transportation of refuse.
10. Water supply should be of independent source, continuous, adequate and safe.
11. Washing utensils: There must be provisions for washing of the utensils and crockery followed by disinfection in hot water.

Sanitation of food establishments not only depends upon the physical environment of the setup but also upon the state of personal hygiene and habits of the food handlers. They may be carriers of various diseases such as typhoid, diarrheal disease, dysenteries, enteroviruses, viral hepatitis, amebiasis, ascariasis, streptococcal and staphylococcal infections. Therefore, the following measures must be taken care of the food handlers:

1. Before placement thorough medical examination to exclude the presence or suffering of the systemic diseases.
2. Day-to-day health appraisal should be made.
3. They should abstain from their duty whenever they develop septic skin lesions, respiratory and intestinal symptoms, otitis media or any other wound till they are cured bacteriologically.
4. They should undergo periodical medical checkup.
5. They should take the treatment promptly.
6. They are educated to maintain a high standard of personal hygiene on the following aspects:
   a. Hairs: Use scarfs to prevent failing of the hairs on foods.
   b. Hands: Finger nails should be kept trimmed and free from dirt, hands to be scrubbed and washed with soap and water before handling the food and after using toilet.
   c. Overalls: Clean and white overalls should be worn by them.
   d. Habits: The hazards of unguarded coughing, sneezing in the vicinity of the food, smoking in the food premises, etc. must also be told.

Food Purchase

The consumers should purchase the food, which is not spoiled and which cannot deteriorate the health of human beings. There are certain principles, which should be kept in mind, while purchasing the food:

1. Do not purchase a food from which the odor comes.
2. Look for the expiry data of food products and do not purchase outdated packages of food.
3. Purchase the labeled products to know the type of ingredients used.
4. Purchase the products labeled 'keep refrigerated' only if they are stored in the refrigerated case and are cold to touch.
5. Purchase the canned foods, which are free from dents, cracks and bulging lids, etc.
6. Before purchasing check for any hole, tear or open containers.
7. Avoid sampling raw food, if you do not know where the products are harvested or packaged.
8. Do not purchase cracked eggs.
9. Do not purchase anything with storage color or odor.
10. Purchase the food from food outlets, which are clean and the food handlers should also be clean with tidy clothes and restrained hairs. So do not purchase the food from sloppy or dirty food handlers.
11. Avoid purchasing the unwrapped or half cut items as they can be contaminated from insects, dusts, etc.
12. Do not purchase perishable food items (meat, eggs, and dairy products) that have been at room temperature for long periods of time.
13. Check for any old adulterant in food, and if found adulterated, do not purchase adulterated food.
14. Check for food additives on the label of container. Always check for nature and quantity of food.

Transportation of Food

Food should be transported after segregating the spoiled food (unfit for consumption) under adequate temperature and packed in a hygienic way. To preserve the nutritive value of food these must be kept in mind. While other things included for food safety, while preparing/cooking food include:

1. Thoroughly wash all fruits and vegetables in clean water, so as to remove all the harmful pathogens, insects, chemicals or soil.
2. Raw and ready to eat (prepared food) should be kept separately to avoid cross contamination.
3. Cutting boards should be washed and sensitized. Hot water and soap followed by a rinse should be used for washing the cutting boards.

CHAPTER 21 — Food Hygiene

4. Plastic cutting boards should be used at place of wooden, as plastic cutting boards are less porous and less likely to harbor bacteria. As cutting boards can be a place for breeding bacteria.
5. Keep the food cold at a below 5°C and hot at 60°C or hotter. Avoid keeping the food in temperature danger zone (5–57°C), i.e. 41–135°F.
6. Use separate knives, chopping boards, etc. for raw food and cooked food.
7. Use clean and dry utensils for cooking.
8. Food should be cooked to over 75°C as this temperature kills most of bacteria.
9. Thaw the frozen food on the bottom self of refrigerator and keep it in refrigerator till it is to be cooked.
10. Maintain hygiene of the area (kitchen) to maintain food hygiene, while preparing food:
    a. The cooking area including floors, walls, ceilings, counters and appliances should be clean.
    b. Wash the dishes immediately after eating so that no residue is dried in the dishes.
    c. Launder the kitchen clothes and towels especially after cleaning raw animal products.
    d. Dry the dishes appropriately as the bacteria can remain over there after cleaning with damp cloth.
    e. Bacteria grow quickly in high-risk foods, when kept in (5–60°C), i.e. this temperature zone is known as temperature danger.
11. Personal hygiene of an individual, who is cooking the food need to be maintained.
12. While cooking, keep the face away, if sneezing or coughing occurs and cover the mouth and nose with a tissue, while preparing food and then wash the hands afterwards.
13. Cover the cut or sores on the hands, while preparing or cutting the food before preparation.
14. Check the food before preparing for its spoilage, i.e. check for odor from food.
15. Use two plates and two pairs of tongs, i.e. one set for raw meat and one set for cooked meat to prevent contamination.
16. Wash hands frequently after using toilet before preparing food and after handling raw meat.
17. Do not chop or cut fresh vegetables on a cutting board, which is used for raw meat.
18. Do not cut the food into very small pieces.
19. Wash the knife and vegetables before cutting them.
20. Do not keep the cut food uncovered and cook the food in a covered container so as to prevent contamination.
21. Preserve the nutritive value of food while cooking.
22. Do not cut the food into too smaller pieces.
23. Wash the food before cutting.
24. Use appropriate temperature as excessive cooking can cause loss of nutritive value of food.
25. Do not throw the water in which pulses were soaked. Try to soak the pulse after removing any foreign matter such as dust, grit, etc. utilized the same water for cooking in which the pulses were soaked.
26. Mix the ingredients into appropriate amount, while preparing the food to preserve the taste and texture of food.
27. Add the ingredient at proper time, so as to prevent the loss of nutritive value. As in case of use of iodized salt. If added at time of frying the mixture of onions, garlic and tomato for preparing gravy, the iodine will evaporate from the iodized salt, losing the nutritive value of iodine. So it is required that it should not be added at that time.
28. Unhygienic preparation and storage also cause spoilage, thereby reducing the nutritive value of food.

CONSERVATION OF NUTRIENTS

Before Cooking

- Foods should be kept clean and dry, and stored in airtight containers
- Undermilled or hand-pounded rice to be preferably used
- Sprouting of the pulses improves the nutritive value
- Washing of the food item and to be done with minimum quantity of water
- Too small cutting and too early cutting of vegetables before cooking to be avoided to prevent the loss of vitamins and minerals
- Ghee, butter, oil, etc. should be kept sealed in a cool and dry place to prevent rancidity

During Cooking

- Vegetables are put in the boiling water instead of boiling them in water
- Vegetables should not be cooked for more than 15 minutes
- Baking soda should not be used because loss of vitamins is more in alkaline medium
- Potatoes and sweet potatoes should be cooked without peeling; it is preferable to cook them in cooker
- Milk should be rapidly brought to boiling point and then cooled quickly as in pasteurization

- Eggs are best cooked below the boiling point
- Salt should be added late, since addition of salt before boiling hastens the loss of nutrients
- Addition of little acid such as tamarind, lemon juice, vinegar, citric acid, while cooking conserves the nutrients
- Use of iron knives and cast iron pans increases the iron content
- Steam heating is preferable to use of boiling, because the loss of nutrients is almost nil
- Both shallow and deep frying of foods in oil causes loss of nutrients. Loss is less in deep frying because of the oil coating.

After Cooking

- Repeated reheating is avoided
- Food to be eaten, while it is hot.

Food Consumed

Food consumed by people should be safe and wholesome, prepared and cooked in a hygienic way and the person consuming should handle the food hygienically to prevent the occurrence of foodborne illnesses.

Important Points on Food Consumption

1. Never consume rotten or spoiled food or food with change of texture or odor.
2. Make sure that the consumer washes the hands before and after consumption of food and after using toilet.
3. Do not sneeze or cough over eating food, so if sneezing or coughing is felt by consumer while eating, keep the face away from food.
4. Do not eat or consume the food, which is half cut or cut into pieces and left uncovered or left over food.
5. Avoid eating quickly canned bread and cakes as there are more chances of botulism, which can kill or sicken the person by eating the product.
6. Do not boil the food in researchable bags before consuming as these bags have low melting point. Low boiling point used for preparing food, will not be able to kill bacteria such as *Salmonella* in food. So food prepared after boiling along with researchable bag should not be consumed.
7. The sanitation places, where the people consume food should have minimum standards as suggested for restaurants and eating houses in India under Model Public Act, 1955.
8. It should not be located near open drains or other sources such as stable or manure pits.
9. The floor of eating places should be higher than adjoining land.
10. The materials used for flooring and walls up to 3 feet should be impervious, so that floor and walls can be easily cleaned.
11. There should be adequate light and ventilation.
12. The rooms (dining rooms) of eating places for one person should not be less than 100 sq ft.
13. The kitchen of eating places should have minimum 60 sq ft area and windows of 25% of floor area and ventilation of 2% of floor area. The doors and windows of kitchen should be rat and fly proof, i.e. no rat, insect could enter kitchen, floor of kitchen should not be slippery and it should be easy to clean and made up of impervious material.
14. The storage facilities for storing the food should be in a separate room for cooked and uncooked food stuff with adequate temperature. It should be easy to clean and free from insects and rodents.
15. There should be adequate independent continuous water supply.
16. Eating places should have washing facilities for cleaning and disinfecting the utensils. Utensils should be washed in hot water and then disinfected.
17. The furniture of eating places should be clean and dry.

Food Fortification

The food is fortified with minerals and nutritive elements will help in reducing some of nutritional deficiency disorder. Such as iodine deficiency disorder, occurring due to low iodine content in soil. To prevent iodine deficiency disorders, salt (common item of food) is iodized by the process of fortification to prevent morbidity and mortality due to iodine deficiency. "Food fortification is the process whereby nutrients are added to food (in relatively small quantities) to maintain or improve the quality of diet of a group, community or a population."

Criteria for Food Fortification

1. The food must be consumed daily by larger section or whole of population.
2. The nutrient added should not cause hazardous effect, if consumed in excess.
3. The added nutrient should not cause any change in food in relation to smell, taste or appearance.
4. The cost of food, which is fortified, should not be beyond the reach of population, who are in need.

Food fortification is a process wherein nutrients are added in small quantities to the foods to maintain or to

CHAPTER 21 — Food Hygiene

improve the quality of food, aimed at prevention and control of some nutritional disorders as long-term measures are:

- Addition of vitamin A and D to vanaspati and milk (2,500 IU of vitamin A and 175 IU of vitamin D per 100 g)
- Addition of potassium or sodium iodide to common salt (iodization of salt) for the prevention and control of endemic goiter
- Addition of iron salts to common salt for the prevention of nutritional anemia
- Addition of lysine to wheat flour, while making bread
- Twin fortification of common salt with iron and iodine
- Fluoridation of water for the prevention of dental caries
- For fortification, the nutrient and the vehicle should fulfill the following criteria
- The vehicle must be consumed consistently by the community as a part of the regular diet
- The nutrient should not be hazardous
- The nutrient should not undergo any change in taste, smell, appearance or consistency
- The cost of fortification should not be beyond the reach of the people.

FOOD ADULTERATION

Food is required by man for energy, growth and maintenance of health. If the quality of food is not good and contains harmful substances, it becomes a health hazard for the consumer. Such type of food in which harmful substances are there and is not safe for consumption purposes is called adulterated food.

Adulteration means the addition of such substance in the food, which are harmful, toxic and cause deterioration of health. It consists of mixing, substitution, concealing misbranding and addition of toxicants. If food is adulterated, the consumer has to pay more for lower quality and it deteriorates his health. This practice of food adulteration varies from place to place any country to country.

Food adulteration consists of large number of practices such as mixing, substitution, removal, concealing the quality, selling decomposed products, misbranding (giving false labels), addition of toxicants, etc. Food adulteration is a social evil. This is done by the traders because of their greed for money.

The disadvantages for the consumer are:
1. Consumer is paying more money for food stuff of lower quality.
2. He/She is at a risk of ill health, e.g. epidemic dropsy, allergy, gastritis, testicular damage, etc. There are various adulterants, which are added to increase the quantity of food, its self-life flavor, texture and appearance. These adulterants are chemical, physical and biological in nature. These adulterants produce many effects on our body. They can cause:

- Kidney stones
- Gallstone
- Nausea
- Vomiting
- Dehydration
- Ulcers
- Acidity
- Gas and burning sensation in chest
- Meningitis
- Cancer.

The possible food adulterants are given in Tables 21.3 and 21.4.

Adulteration of food refers to the addition of such substances in the food, which are harmful, toxic and cause deterioration of health according to PFA and food adulteration includes:
1. Intentional addition, substitution or abstraction of substances, which adversely affect the purity and quality of foods, i.e. water to milk.
2. Incidental contaminants of foods with deleterious substances such as toxins and insecticide due to ignorance, negligence or lack of storage facility, e.g. removal of fat from milk.

Table 21.3: Food adulterant

Food materials	Common adulterant
Cereals (rice, wheat)	Stone, sand, grit
Dal (Bengal gram)	Kesari dal (lathyrism)
Milk	Addition of water, removal of cream
Ghee	Addition of starch (waterborne disease), addition of vanaspati
Butter	Starch, animal fat
Turmeric powder	Lead chromate powder (metanil yellow) (lead poisoning)
Black pepper	Dried seeds of papaya
Chilli powder	Brick powder
Tea leaves	Husk of black gram, reuse of tea leaves
Coffee seeds	Tamarind seeds
Baking powder	Citric acid
Honey	Sugar, jiggery
Sugar	Chalk
Mustard seeds	Seeds of prickly poppy (epidemic dropsy)

Contd...

Contd...

Food materials	Common adulterant
Edible oil	Mineral oil
Ice cream	Starch, cellulose, washing powder
Asafetida	Resins, gums
Jaggery solution	Honey (vice versa)
Coffee powder	Chicory
Non-alcoholic beverages	Non-permitted colors, saccharin, dulcin, lead, arsenic, dirt and filth

Table 21.4: Food articles and their adulterants

Food article	Adulterants
Milk	Water, synthetic milk from shampoos, detergents and low quality refined oil
Suji	Iron filings, grits to add weight
Tea	Used tea leaves
Red chilli	Brick powder or colored saw dust
Coffee powder	Chicory roots
Mustard oil	Argemone oil
Black pepper	Papaya seeds
Urad dal	Crushed black stones
Wheat flour	Araroot, starch or maida to make it white
Pan masala	Saccharin
Coriander powder	Horse dung powder
Cumin (jeera)	Colored grass seeds
Sweets	Artificial colors and flavors
Mushrooms	Dipped in sodium potassium-based bleach to keep white
Desi ghee	Vanaspati or vegetable oil
Jaggery	Metanil yellow
Ground sugar	Washing soda
Haldi	Starch colored with metanil yellow
Achar, chutneys	Pure acetic acid instead of vinegar
Noodles and macaroni and soups	Ajinomoto flavoring agents
Sago	Sand and talcum powder

3. Contamination of food with harmful insects, microorganism, e.g. bacteria, fungus, molds, etc. during production, storage and handling.

Adulterant refers to any material, which is employed or which could be employed for the purpose of adulterants.

Intentional adulterants

Intentional adulterants are sand, marble chips, stones, mud, chalk powder, water, mineral oil and coltra, dyes, etc. These adulterants cause harmful effects on the human beings. Now food adulteration is a social evil. It consists of large number of practices such as mixing, substitution, removal concealing the quality, selling decomposed products, misbranding (giving false label), addition of toxicants, etc. This is done by the traders because of their greedy for money. If food is adulterated, the consumer has to pay more for its low quality and it deteriorates the health of individual and individual at risk of ill health. Since, the adulterants are chemical, physical and biological in nature and produce many ill effects on the body, which includes kidney stones, gallstones, nausea, vomiting, dehydration, ulcers, acidity, gas, burning sensation of chest, meningitis, cancer, allergy, etc.

Incidental Adulterants

Contamination of Foods with Harmful Microorganisms

Raw foods such as meat, fish, milk and vegetables grown on sewage are likely to be contaminated with harmful microorganisms. These are generally destroyed during cooking or processing of food. Some of the microorganisms may survive due to inadequate heat processing. Further, some of the foods, if consumed in the raw state, may cause food poisoning. Recent studies have shown that food grains, legumes and oil seeds, when stored in humid atmosphere are infected by pathogenic fungus that can cause serious illness. The pathogenic microorganisms commonly contaminated foods and are responsible for causing serious illness are listed and briefly described in the following (Table 21.5).

Metallic Contamination

Lead is a toxic element and contamination of food with lead can cause toxic symptoms. For example, turmeric is coated by illiterate manufacturers in India with lead chromate. Lead brings about pathological changes in the kidneys, liver and arteries. The common signs of lead poisoning are nausea, abdominal pain, anemia, insomnia, muscular paralysis and brain damage. Fish caught from water contaminated with mercuric salts contain large amounts of mercury. The organic mercury compound methyl or dimethyl mercury is the most toxic. The toxic effects of methyl mercury are neurological. When the

Food Hygiene

Table 21.5: Foodborne diseases caused by some pathogenic organisms

Pathogenic organisms	Food commonly involved	Ill effects and diseases
Bacterial		
Bacillus cereus	Cereal products	Nausea, vomiting and abdominal pain
Clostridium botulinum (toxins)	Defectively processed meat and fish	Botulism (muscular) paralysis, death due to respiratory failure
Clostridium perfringens (welchii)	Defectively processed meat, fish and egg products, raw vegetables grown on sewage	Nausea, abdominal pain and diarrhea
Salmonella	Foods kept exposed or those sold in unhygienic surroundings	Salmonellosis (vomiting diarrhea and fever)
Shigella sonnei	Exposed foods are kept in unhygienic surroundings	
Staphylococcus aureus	Foods kept exposed, food items from unhygienic surrounding	Bacillary dysentery, increased salivation, vomiting, abdominal pain and diarrhea
Streptococcus pyogenes		Scarlet fever, septic, sore throat
Fungal		
Aspergillus flavus (aflatoxin)	Corn and groundnut	Liver damage and cancer
Claviceps purpurea (ergot)	Rye and pearl millet infested with ergot	Ergotism (burning sensation in extremities), peripheral gangrene
Fusarium sporotrichioides	Cereals and millets infected with *Fusarium*	Alimentary toxic aleukia
Penicillium islandicum	Rice	Liver damage
Parasitic		
Trichinella spiralis	Pork and pork products	Nausea, vomiting, diarrhea, colic and muscular pains (trichinosis)
Ascaris lumbricoides	Raw vegetables are grown in sewage farms	Ascariasis
Entamoeba histolytica	In sewage farm the raw vegetables are grown in a suitable condition	Amebic dysentery
Ancylostoma duodenale (hookworm)	The raw vegetables are grown in sewage farms	Epigastric pain, loss of blood and anemia

brain is affected, the subject becomes blind, deaf and paralysis of the various muscles make cripple. The other elements, which are toxic in small doses are cadmium, arsenic, antimony and cobalt. Toxic effects of metallic contamination are given in Table 21.6.

Tests for Adulterants

Physical tests

- *Argemone mexicana* seeds are black in color, but not uniformly smooth and round
- Kesari dal is wedge shaped
- Iron fillings in tea can be separated by using magnet
- Ergot seeds are lighter than bajra and float in water
- Sand, gravel, pebbles can be observed and removed physically.

Chemical tests

The chemical test for the following adulterants:

1. Metanil yellow: This is used in haldi (turmeric) powder. 2 g of sample is added to 5 mL of alcohol and shake. A few drops of concentrated HCl are then added. Pink color indicates presence of metanil yellow.
2. Starch: This is added to milk. Little iodine is added to the sample of milk. Development of blue color indicates the presence of starch in milk.
3. Argemone oil: This is added to mustard oil. 5 mL of nitric acid is added to 5 mL of suspected mustard oil and heated for about 5 minutes. Development of red color indicates the presence of argemone oil.
4. Artificial red color to chillies: A piece of cotton soaked in liquid paraffin is rubbed with a sample of chillies powder. Cotton becomes red with artificial color.

Table 21.6: Toxic effects of some metals and chemicals

Name	Food commonly involved	Toxic effects
Arsenic	Fruits sprayed by lead arsenate and drinking water	Dizziness, chills, cramps, paralysis leading to death
Barium	Foods contaminated by rat poison (barium carbonate)	Violet peristalsis, muscular twitching and convulsions
Cadmium	Fruits juices and soft drinks that comes in contact with cadmium and plated vessels, crabs, oysters and kidneys	Excessive salivation liver, kidney damage; prostate cancer multiple fractures (painful Itai-Itai disease reported from Japan due to cadmium poisoning)
Cobalt	Water and beer	Cardiac failure
Copper	Acid foods in contact with tarnished copperware	Vomiting, diarrhea and abdominal pain
Lead	Some processed foods, lead water pipes	Paralysis and brain damage
Mercury	Mercury fungicide treated seed grains or mercury contaminated fish particularly pike, tuna and shellfish	Paralysis, brain damage and blindness
Tin	Canned food	Colic, vomiting and photophobia
Zinc	Foods stored in galvanized iron ware	Dizziness and vomiting
Pesticides	All types of foods	Acute or chronic poisoning causing damage to liver, kidney, brain and nerves leading to death
Diethylstilbestrol	Present in meat of stilbestrol fed animals and birds	Teratogenesis and carcinogenesis
Antibiotics	Meat from animals fed antibiotics	Drug resistance, hardening of arteries and heart diseases

Prevention and Control of Food Adulteration

Prevention and control of food adulteration by food standards and legal measures.

Food Standards

Codex Alimentarius
Codex Alimentarius Commission (CAC) is a principle organ of the joint FAO/WHO food standards, program. This has formulated food standards for the international market. The standards prepared by CAC have been accepted internationally.

Prevention of food adulteration standards
The PFA standards are the standards laid down under the Prevention Food Adulteration Act (1954) by the Central Committee of the Food Standards (CCFS) to obtain minimum level of quality of food stuffs. These standards are statutory and there is a legal backing to it. Any food that does not confirm to the minimum standards is said to be adulterated.

Agmark standards
Agmark standards are prescribed by the Directorate of Marketing and inspection by the Government of India. This gives the assurance of quality of the food stuff.

Indian standards institution
Indian standards institution (ISI) are prescribed by the Bureau of Indian Standards. The Agmark and ISI standards are not mandatory, but purely voluntary. They express degrees of excellence above PFA standards. The presence of ISI mark also gives the consumer an assurance of the good quality of the product.

At international level
Food standards are setup by CAC, the principle organ of joint FAO/WHO food standards programs.

At national level
Government of India has established food standards under PFA Act, 1954 by CCFS, these mandatory so as to achieve a minimum level of quality of food stuffs under Indian conditions.

Other standards
The other standards are:
1. Established are Agmark and standards: These are set up by Directorate of Marketing and Inspection of the Government of India by introducing an Agriculture Produce Act in 1937. A sample is:
Agmark Besan
SL No. B-162002
Grade-standard

Place of packaging
Date of packaging
Net weight

Agmark seal ensures the quality and purity of product and grades are incorporated as 1, 2, 3, 4 or special, good, fair and ordinary.

2. Bureau of Indian Standards are the standards, which are used by manufacturers of the product after the production of product as per Indian standards after obtaining a license from the bureau.

Prerequisite for obtaining a license from bureau
- Manufacture has the facility as required for manufacturing and testing the product
- Follow quality assurance scheme of bureau
- Pays the fee as stipulated.

Then the license is granted for a period of 1 year, which can be renewed on the basis of satisfactory operations of scheme. This scheme is voluntary in nature.

Legal Measures

Prevention of Food Adulteration Act, 1954

The need for the Central Legislation regarding prevent of food adulteration was felt in 1937, when the committee was appointed by Central Advisory Board of Health recommended it. This adulteration of foodstuff is included in the Constitution of India under Concurrent List (III).

The bill regarding prevention of food adulteration was passed by both the Houses of Parliament. This bill received the assent of President on 29th September, 1954. On 1st June 1955, 'Prevention of Food Adulteration Act, 1954' came into force. Later on this act was amended in the year 1964, 1971, 1976 and 1986.

Objectives
- Protect the public from poisonous and harmful foods
- To prevent the sale of substandard food
- To protect the interest of the consumers by eliminating fraudulent practices.

With the objectives of ensuring pure and wholesome quality food to the consumers, to protect their health from the fraudulent practices of traders and to encourage fair trade practices, Government of India enacted an Act called, PFA Act in 1954 and amended three times respectively during 1965, 1976 and 1986 to make it more stringent. The State Government enforces the act.

The act provides protection against adulteration or contamination, the food that may have deleterious effects on consumer's health. The act also deals with the frauds that can be perpetrated by the dealers by supplying cheaper and adulterated foods. The acts regulates the use of chemicals, pesticides, flavors and other additives in food preparation. Dumping of substandard foods are also controlled under this act. However, provisions are made under this act for enrichment and fortification of foods.

It is defined that 'adulterant' is a material, which is employed for the purpose of adulteration and an article is deemed to be adulterated:

1. If it is sold by a vendor and is not of the nature demanded by the purchaser, and is not of the quality, which it purports to be.
2. If the article contains any other substance, so as to affect injuriously the nature or quality thereof.
3. If it is substituted wholly or partially by an inferior substance.
4. If the constituent of the article is abstracted partially or wholly as to affect the quality.
5. If the article has been prepared, packed or kept under insanitary conditions and become contaminated as to cause injury to the health.
6. If the article consists of filthy, rotten, putrid or decomposed substance and is unfit for consumption.
7. If the article is obtained from the diseased animal.
8. If the article contains any poisonous substance.
9. If the article contains prohibited preservative or coloring matter in excess of the prescribed limits.
10. If the quality of the article falls below the prescribed limits.

The rules are framed by an expert body called CCFS. According to the rules, any food that does not conform to the minimum standards is said to be adulterated. Powers are given to the state governments to appoint Public Analyst and Food Inspectors, who control the food supply, storage and marketing of foods. A chain of 82 states food laboratories and four central (regional) food laboratories are working in the country for the purpose of the PFA Act. It is the duty of the food inspector to draw and dispatch the sample of suspected food article to the laboratory for testing.

If the adulteration is proved, the trader is awarded a minimum imprisonment of 6 months and a fine of ₹1,000. If the adulteration results in grievous health problem or even death, the punishment will go up to life imprisonment and fine of ₹5,000.

With the amendment in 1986, the consumer and the voluntary organizations have been empowered to take the samples of food.

According to the act, a food article is considered to be adulterated if it:
- Has any other substance injurious to health
- Contains cheaper or inferior substitution wholly or partially

- Prepared or packed under insanitary conditions
- Is rotten decomposed, insect infested or filthy
- Is obtained from diseased animal
- Contains any poisonous or deleterious substance
- Contains excessive or some other coloring matter than prescribed
- Is contained in the container of poisonous or deleterious substance
- Contains any prohibited preservative
- Is of low quality, below the prescribed standard.

Prohibition of sale of certain admixture under this act. Sale of certain products by themself or by servant, or by agent is not permitted when:

- The cream contains less than 25% of milk fat or which has not been prepared from milk
- Water is added to milk
- Matter other than fat is added to ghee
- Two or more eligible oils are mixed to form edible oil
- Skimmed milk is considered and sold as whole milk
- Curd made of substances other than milk
- Any article is added beyond the prescribed limit for sweeting the food.

Definition of Term

Adulterant: Any material, which could be employed for the purpose of adulteration.

Adulterated: An article or food deemed to be adulterated.

Central food laboratory: Any laboratory or institute established under Section 4.

Committee: Means CCFS constitute under Section 3.

Food: Any article used as food or drink for human consumption other than drugs and water are includes:
1. Any article, which ordinarily enters into or is used in the consumption, or preparation of human food.
2. Any flavoring matter or condiments.
3. Any other article, which the central government may be having regard to its use, nature, substance or quality, declare by notification in the official gazette as food for the purpose of this act.

Classification of Food

Food has been classified according to origin, chemical composition, nutritive value and function (Table 21.7). Proteins are made of amino acids (the smaller unit). There are 24 amino acids, out of which few are essential. The proteins are required for body building, wear and tear of tissue, maintaining osmotic pressure and synthesis of antibodies, hemoglobin. Fats are high-energy foods. Besides providing energy, fats act as vehicle for fat-soluble vitamins. Carbohydrates are main source of energy. Cellulose of carbohydrates contributes to dietary fiber. The vitamins and minerals are protective foods. The energy produced per gram is as follows.

Table 21.7: Classification of food

Origin	Origin Chemical	Nutritive value	Function
Animal	Proteins Fats	Pulses Vegetables	Body building foods
Vegetable	Carbohydrates Minerals Vitamins	Sugar and jaggery Fats and oils Cereals and millets	Energy giving foods Protective foods

Consumer Protection Act, Initiatives 1986

The main object of the act is to promote and protect the rights of the consumer, with regard to defective goods, deficiency of services, overcharging or any unfair trade practices. In this, complains can be referred to the District Consumer Redressal Forum. The Forum can order the opposite party for removal of defect, replacement of goods, return of the prices or charges, or order of payment of the compensation for the loss, or damages suffered due to deficiency of services. Appeals can be made to state commission and then to the appellate body of National Commission.

In India, there are four food laboratories for analysis of food supplies, which includes Central Food Laboratory, Kolkata; Food Research and Standardization Laboratory, Ghaziabad; Public Health Laboratory, Pune and Central Food Technological Research Institute (CFTRI), Mysore. In addition some states have their own laboratories.

Codex Alimentarius, which means 'food law' or food code in Latin is combined set of standards, codes or practices and other model regulation available for countries to use and apply to food in international trade. The objective of this commission is to protect the health of consumers and facilitate international trade.

Hazard Analysis Critical Control Point

Hazard analysis critical control point (HACCP) is recognized throughout the world. It is a food safety management too, i.e. applied to determine significant hazards pertaining to specific products and process, and control the occurrence of such hazards. It is preventive in its approach and it aims to prevent rather than detect problems.

CHAPTER 21 — Food Hygiene

Central Committee for Food Standards

The central government constitutes a committee called CCFS to advise central as well as state government on matters arising out of administration of act and to carry out other functions assigned under this act. The Central Committee shall have the members:

1. The Director General, Health Services, ex-officio, who shall be the Chairman.
2. The Director of Central Food Laboratory or in a case where more than one central food laboratory is established and the Directors of such laboratories, and ex-officio.
3. Two experts nominated by the central government.
4. One representative:
   a. From each departments of food and agriculture in Central Ministry of Food and Agriculture.
   b. From each of Central Ministries of Defence, Commerce, Industry, Railways and Supply as nominated by central government.
5. One representative nominated by government of each state.
6. Two representative nominated by central government to represent agricultural, commercial and industrial interest.
7. Five members representative nominated by government, the consumers, interest one of whom will be from hotel industry.
8. One representative of medical profession nominated by Indian Council of Medical Research (ICMR).
9. One representative nominated by ISI.

The members of the committee entitled to hold the office for 3 years and are eligible for renomination:

1. The central government shall appoint a secretary to the committee, who will perform such duties as prescribed or delegated to him/her by committee.
2. The central government with consultation of committee will make rules regarding functions of Central Food Laboratories and local area.
3. The central or state government may appoint such persons as it thinks fit as Food Inspectors for local areas is assigned by the central or state government. The powers of Food Inspectors will be:
   a. To take sample of any item of food from a person, who is selling.
   b. Any person, who is preparing or delivering the article to purchaser.
   c. A consignee after delivery of article.

Functions of center according to act

- Proper coordination, monitoring, surveillance of program throughout the country
- Organization of training, i.e. in service training programs for food inspectors, analyst and senior officers concerned with the implementation of act.

Procedure for sampling and analysis

The Food Inspector has the authority to enter and take the samples as well as can inspect the place, where:
- Food is manufactured
- Food is stored
- The food is exhibited for sale.

For this, the Food Inspector issue notice in writing to the seller indicating his/her intention. Three samples are taken and on the samples, the signature of seller is affixed. One sample is sent to public analyst under intimation to the local health authority for further reference.

Penalties

If the food is found to be adulterated, then punishment is given:

1. If the adulteration is proved, then a minimum imprisonment of 6 months and a minimum fine of ₹1,000.
2. If the food adulteration has rendered food injuries to cause death or severe injury, then seller shall be punishable with imprisonment for a term, which will not be lessen than 3 years, but can extend up to term of life and with a fine ₹5,000.

Drug and Cosmetic Act, 1940

The Drug and Cosmetic Act, 1940 is extended throughout the India to maintain the quality of drugs and cosmetics, so as to prevent the hazardous effects on health. The main purpose of this act is to prevent the import, manufacture, distribution and sale of misbranded, adulterated, spurious drugs and cosmetics. This act was amended from time to time. The list of amending acts is as below:

- The Repealing and Amending Act, 1949
- The Adaptation of Law Orders, 1950
- The Drugs Act, 1951
- The Drugs Act, 1955
- The Drugs Act, 1960
- The Drugs Act, 1962
- The Drug and Cosmetic Act, 1964
- The Drug and Cosmetic Act, 1972
- The Drug and Cosmetic Act, 1982
- The Drug and Cosmetic Act, 1995.

Cosmetic

Cosmetic means any article intended to be rubbed, poured, sprinkled or sprayed on or introduced into, or otherwise applied to the human body or any part thereof cleaning, beautifying, promoting attractiveness or altering appearance and includes any article intended for use as a component of cosmetic.

Drug
1. All medicines for internal or external use of human beings or animals and all substances intended to be used for or in diagnosis, treatment, mitigation and prevention of any disease, or disorder in human beings, animals including preparations applied to human body for the purpose of repelling insects and mosquitoes.
2. Such substances intended to affect the structure or any function of the human body, intended to be used for the destruction of vermin or insects, which cause disease in human beings or animals, as may be specified from time to time by central government by notification in the official gazette.
3. All substances intended for use as components of a drug including empty gelatin capsules.
4. Such devices intended for internal or external use in diagnosis, treatment, mitigation prevention of disease or disorder in human beings or animals, as may be specified from time to time by central government by notification in the official gazette after consultations with board.

Drugs Technical Advisory Board

The central government constitutes a board as 'Drug Technical Advisory Board' to advise the central and state government on technical matters arising out of the functions assigned to it by this act. The board shall consist of:
1. The Director General of Health Services.
2. The Drugs Controller, India.
3. The Director of the Central Drugs Laboratory, Central Research Institute, Indian Veterinary Research Institute and Central Drug Research Institute.
4. The President of Medical Council of India and Pharmacy Council of India.
5. Two persons nominated by central government from among persons, who are in-charge of Drug Control in India.
6. One person to be elected by the Executive Committee of the Medicals Council of India from among teachers in medicine or therapeutics on the staff of an Indian University or a college affiliated there to.
7. One pharmacologist to be elected by the governing body of the Indian Council of Medical Research.
8. One person to be elected by the Council of the Indian Pharmaceutical Association.
9. Two persons holding the appointment of government analyst under this act, to be nominated by central government.

Tenure of elected and nominated members:
1. The elected and nominated members of board shall hold office for 3 years, but shall be eligible for renomination and re-election.
2. The board with the approval of government will make by laws fixing a quorum and regulating its own procedure and the conducts of all business to be transacted by it. And board may constitute the subcommittees and may appoint to such subcommittees for not exceeding 3 years, as it may decide or temporarily for consideration of particular matters, persons who are not members of the board.
3. The central government shall appoint a person to be secretary of the board and shall provide the board with such clerical and other staff as the central government considers necessary.
4. The Central Drug Laboratory: The central government shall establish a central laboratory under the control of a director appointed by the central government to carry out the functions entrusted to it by this act or any rule made under this act.
5. The Drugs Consultative Committee: The central government may constitute an advisory committee to be called 'Drug Consultative Committee' to advise the Central Government, State Government and Drugs Technical Advisory Board on any matters to secure uniformity throughout in administration of the act in India. It consists of two nominated members by central government nominated and one from each state government nominated by the concerned state government. This committee shall meet, when required to do so by the central government and shall have powers to regulate its own procedure.

According to the act, some specification for drugs and cosmetics given below.

Misbranded drugs: A drug shall deem to be misbranded:
1. If it is colored, coated, powdered or polished that damage is concealed or it is made appear of better, or greater therapeutic value than it really is.
2. If it is not labeled in the prescribed manner.
3. If it label or container, or anything accompanying the drug bears any statement, design or device, which makes any false claim for the drugs or which is false or misleading in any particular.

Misbranded cosmetic: A cosmetic shall be deemed misbranded:
1. If it contains a color, which is not prescribed.
2. If it is not labeled in a prescribed manner.
3. If the label or container, or anything accompanying the cosmetic bears may statement, which is false or misleading in any particular.

Adulterated drugs or cosmetic: A drug or cosmetic deemed to be adulterated:
1. If it consists, in whole or part of any filth, putrid or decomposed substance.

2. If it has been prepared, packed or stored under insanitary conditions, whereby it may have been rendered injurious to health.
3. If its container is composed in whole or in part of any poisonous or deleterious substances, which may render the contents injurious to health.
4. If it bears or contains for purpose of coloring other than one, which is prescribed.
5. If it contains any harmful or toxic substance, which may render, it injurious to health.
6. If any substance has been mixed therewith so as to reduce its quality or strength.

Spurious drugs and cosmetics: A drug or cosmetic to be spurious:
1. If it is imported under a name, which belongs to another drug.
2. If it is an imitation of or a substitute for another drug or resembles another drug in a manner likely to deceive or bears upon it or upon its label, or container the name of another drug/cosmetic unless it is plainly and conspicuously marked as to reveal its time character and its lack of identity with such other drugs.
3. If the label or the container bears the name of an individual or company purporting to be manufacturer of the drug or cosmetic, which individual or company is fictitious or does not exist.
4. It is purports to be the product of a manufacturer of whom it is not truly a product.
5. If it has been substituted wholly or in part by another drug/cosmetic or substances.

Powers of inspectors
An inspector may within the local limits of area of his/her appointment can inspect any premises, wherein any drug or cosmetic is being manufactured, sold, stocked or exhibited or offered for sale. Inspector may take sample of drug or cosmetic, where the drug or cosmetic is manufactured, sold, stocked, exhibited or offered for sale or distributed, and from any person, who is in course of conveying, delivering or preparing to deliver such drug or cosmetic to a purchaser or a consignee. For taking the sample, Inspector shall intimate such purpose in writing in the prescribed form to the person from whom he/she takes the sample. He/She shall divide the sample into three or four portions and effectively seal and suitably mark the same and permit such person to add his/her own seal and mark them.

One portion sent to Government Analyst for test, one portion shall produce before court, if any instituted in respect of the drug and third, were taken, he/she shall send the person, if any, whose name, address and other particulars have been disclosed under Section 18 (a). After getting the report of the test from the Government Analyst, he/she has to send the copy of the report to a person from whom the sample was taken and shall retain one copy for use in any prosecution in respect of sample. The cost of the test or analysis made by Central Drugs Laboratory under Subsection (4) shall be paid by the complainant or accused as directed by court.

Penalty
1. Any drug or deemed to be adulterate under Section 17 (a), but not being a drug referred in Clause (a) or without a valid license as required under Clause (c) of Section 18, shall be punishable with imprisonment for a term not less than 1 year, but which may extend up to 3 years with fine of ₹5,000, provided the court for any adequate and special reasons to be recoded in judgment impose a sentence of imprisonment for less than ₹500.
2. Any drug deemed to be spurious is punishable for a term of 3 years, which can extend up to 5 years and a fine of ₹5,000. Provided the court for any adequate reason, impose a sentence of imprisonment less than 3 years, but not less than 1 year:
   a. Any cosmetic deemed to be spurious under Section 17 (c) shall be punishable with imprisonment for a term, which may extend to 3 years with fine and any cosmetic other than cosmetic referred to in Clause (i) above in contravention of any provision shall be punishable with imprisonment for a term, which may extend to 1 year or with fine, which may extend up to ₹1,000 or both.
   b. To conclude about penalty, violation of law by any person, corporate manage, owner or manufacturer is liable for punishment of imprisonment for a term, which may extend from 3 to 10 years and a fine of ₹500–10,000 or both.

MILK HYGIENE

Milk is highly valued for its nourishing properties, but it is also prizes for its versatile. Served on its own hot or cold risk is a soothing and nourishing drink. Milk is used or combination with cereal and pulses in the preparation of payasam or kheer. Milkshakes prepared with fruit pulp, i.e. banana, mango and sapota. Milk is generated with lactobacilli and curd is prepared, also by diluting it buttermilk is prepared. Coffee and tea are consuming red with milk. Like this so many form of milk is used to consume by everyone in the community. So, it is very important to maintain milk hygiene, as milk is one of the efficient vehicle by which human health can be deteriorated; the milk contributes can occur due to reflected animal producing milk, the milk handlers and the environment, i.e. keeping the month in extra-minded containers or presence of dust or flies over milk, is open containers. In order to get safe and clean milk, it is necessary to have their milk from clean and healthy animal, and the milk handler should be free from communicable disease and should wash their hands before milking and also the environment in which the animal lives should be clean, the vessel used for milk storing should be clean and covered, and milk should be keeps below 1°C.

Since, milk is a good medium for the growth of microorganism and more over it is difficult to keep the milk clean, fresh and satisfactory level and it is most commonly adulterer. As stress earlier milk is liable for communication also from animal, human beings and environment such as water, dust flies, vessels, etc.

It is important to maintain milk hygiene as milk is one of the efficient vehicle by which human health can be deteriorated. The milk contamination can occur due to three reasons as follows:
- Infected animal producing milk
- Human handlers
- Environment: Keeping the milk in contaminated containers or presence of dust, or files over milk in open containers. In order to get safe and clean milk, it is necessary to have:
  – Milk from clean and healthy animal
  – The milk handlers should be free from communicable diseases and should wash their hands before milking
  – The environment in which the animal lives should be clean, the vessels used for milk storing should be clean and covered. And milk should be kept below 10°C.

Milkborne Disease

Milkborne diseases can be transmitted from consuming contaminates milk. The milkborne diseases are classified into two groups:
1. Disease of animals transmitted to man through milk, e.g. zoonoses such as salmonellosis, brucellosis, bovine tuberculosis, Q fever, anthrax and encephalitis.
2. Disease of man transmitted to other through milk may be due to adulteration and milking, adding contaminates water, e.g. amebiasis, giardiasis, ascariasis, streptococcal infection and staphylococcal, food poisoning, paratyphoid, ehlers, shigellosis and diphtheria.

The milkborne disease is prevented by procuring clean and safe milk through hygienic diary pasteurization and sterilization.

Hygienic Diary

The requirements of hygienic diary require that:
- Animals producing milk should be free from diseases
- Milking houses should have clean premises is free from dust and flies
- Milk handled should be free from communicate diseases and this should maximum a high standard of personal hygiene
- Wherever possible milking machines should be used
- Utensils of milk should be clean; water supply should be clean and safe
- Bottling storage and chilling should be done in clean surrounding
- Virus tests facilities of milk should be available for dairy laboratory.

Pasteurization

Pasteurization is a process of preservation of milk, where in the milk is heated to such a temperature and for such a period of time so as to destroy all the pathogens in at and to preserve the nutritive value of it without changing color, smell, taste, flavor and composition. Thus, in the singles safest, cheap and modern methods are used for safe milk. In this process also 95% bacteria are destroyed.

Pasteurization is of three types:
1. Holder method: The milk is heated to 65°C and maintaining the temperature for 30 minutes and then suddenly cooled to below 5°C, it prevents growth of organism. Holder method is a British method, generally used in rural area.
2. High temperature and short time process (HTST): It is a flash process in which milk is heated 72°C and maintained at least 15 seconds and then rapidly cooled to less than 5°C. It is a American process.
3. Ultra, high temperature (UHT): In this UHT process-milk heated in two stages. In first stage, heating is done under normal pressure to 88°C for few seconds and in second stage, it is heated to 125°C under pressure for few seconds only. Then it is rapidly cooled and bottled as quickly as possible. After bottling, the milk is kept cold until reaches to consumers.

Phosphate test, methylene black tests, standard plate count and coliform count are used to test pasteurization.

Sterilization

Sterilization is done in milk cookers by heating milk to 100°C (212°F) for 20-30 minutes. This process helps to destroy 100% pathogens including spores. Test for milk adulterations includes tests for specific gravity, fat content, iodine test and cane sugar.

MEAT HYGIENE

Meat include all flesh foods such as mutton, pork, beef, poultry, veal of calves, etc. Unhygienic conditions of meat results in the presence and growth of microorganisms in meat, which if consumed can cause diseases. The source of meat diseases are infected animals or unhealthy animal, human handler, slaughter houses and meat storage places.

The diseases transmitted through meat are cysticercus cellulosae of *Taenia solium* (through pork), of *Taenia saginata* (through beef), liver flukes through sheep, i.e. *Fasciola hepatica*, *Trichinella spiralis* (through pork) and also bacterial infections such as anthrax, actinomycosis, tuberculosis and food poisoning (botulism through canned food).

For having clean and safe meat or to prevent meatborne illnesses:

1. Unhealthy animals should not be used as a meat, i.e. animals before slaughtering and after slaughtering should be examined by veterinary staff, so that infected animal or infected organ should not be eaten by human beings.
2. The environment of slaughter house is of paramount importance to prevent contamination of meat. The place where animals are kept should have sanitation and the vessel or place for storing should be clean.
3. The walls, floor or ceiling should be easy to clean, otherwise it will allow the pathogenic organisms to grow or will provide the space for insects, rodents and flies, etc.
4. The waste materials of animals need to be collected and disposed of separately and appropriately to provide safe environment in the slaughter house.
5. Meat should be strong in a fly proof and rat proof rooms.
6. The temperature for string meat overnight should be below 5°C.
7. Meat should be transported at adequate temperature and in fly proof area.
8. Meat handlers should also be free from communicable diseases. Meatborne diseases are:
   - Tapeworm infestation
   - Tuberculosis
   - Anthrax
   - Actinomycosis
   - Food poisoning.

People have accustomed to eat, should eat meat to prevent meatborne diseases. For which people should eat meat from healthy animal. Before slaughtering any animal, they should be examined by the veterinary personnel, so that animal what have above meatborne animal should be avoided for eating. And maintain certain hygiene standard for slaughter houses. The slaughter houses are one, where animals are killed for the purpose of consumption of the flesh. The hygiene standard will include the following:

- Slaughter house should be minimum 100 feet away from residential area
- The floor should be above the ground level and made of imperviously material with slope and channel
- The walls should be covered with tiles or glazed bricks to a sufficient height
- All refuse, blood, manure and garbage are placed in vessels and removed as early as possible
- Dogs and other such animals should not be allowed in the premises
- Employees must be clean and wear clean outer clothes
- Butchers also maintain personal hygiene and are healthy
- The instrument used must be sterilized.

FISH HYGIENE

Fish is an intermediate host of certain parasite (tapeworm) may carry virus (type A), *Vibrio proteolyticus* (leads to food poisoning), *Salmonella* species, *Clostridium botulinum* type 'T', etc. Consumption of certain fish may give rise to food poisoning and urticaria. So, people eating fish should check the fish before purchasing and preparing that the signs of fresh fish that should be:

1. Firm, and stiff to touch, but not soft or pulpy.
2. When held flat on the hand, the tail should not drop.
3. Eyes should be clear and bright, not sunken.
4. Gills should be bright red nor muddy or pale.
5. Scales not easily detachable.
6. Fish can be a host of microorganisms such as:
   - Parasitic: Tapeworm
   - Virus: Type A
   - Other microorganisms are:
     - Vibrio parahaemolyticus
     - Clostridium botulinum type E, etc.

7. Check the fish for sings of freshness before purchasing and preparing food. These signs are:
   - Bright red gills
   - Clear prominent eyes
   - State of stiffness.

When the fish begins decomposition, body becomes flaccid, blood will run out, on cutting as a dull red liquid with offensive odor. So, it should be checked before food for its freshness and then can be prepared to eat.

In this way, other foods like egg should be examined for any cracked shell as it can be area of entry of pathogens and wash the out shell before boiling or cooking egg.

FOOD ALLERGY

In addition, fruits and vegetables also a part of food constituent and importance source of infection. These also required proper hygienic measures at production, storage, transportation, handling and consumption.

Some people will have inherent or idiosyncrasy to certain foods such as milk, meat, egg, fish, poultry, fruits, etc. and manifest an urticaria, asthma, eczema, diarrhea, and others. Sensitivity to gluten in responsible for malabsorption syndrome.

CONCLUSION

Food hygiene means all measures adopted during production, processing, storing and distributing food to make food safe and wholesome, so that is fit for consumption and does not cause foodborne illnesses. Due to environmental causes, food may lack nutritive value, such as decrease iodine content in food in hill area. Then in order to prevent deficiency disorders, food can be fortified by which people are able to get the same nutrient. Food fortification is addition of minerals and nutritive elements in food. This helps in prevention of nutritional deficiency diseases. Food should be handled and stored in a proper way. Food should not be kept above 140°F and below 41°F. It needs to be kept in a clean dry area. According to WHO, there are certain principles of food storage. Food additives are used to preserve the food for prolonged time period. There prevent spoilage, growth of bacteria and mycobacteria, thereby reducing the foodborne diseases. Milkborne diseases can be reduced by using pasteurized milk meatborne illnesses can be reduced by antemortem and postmortem examination of animals for slaughtering and cooking under hygienic conditions. Food poisoning can occur due to unhygienic food consumption. To early detect food poisoning, the community should be educated regarding signs and symptoms of treatment, so that the foodborne diseases can be controlled. Adulterated food, if consumed produces many effects on our health such as kidney stones, gall stones, dehydration, cancer, etc. The public should be educated about Food Adulteration Act, so that appropriate action against the people who do adulteration, can be taken. This will reduce the adulteration of food, thereby decreasing the chances of diseases due to adulterated food.

Part II

Environment as Determinant of Health

C. *Sociocultural Environment*
- Sociocultural Determinants
- Introduction to Lifestyle
- Lifestyle: Hygiene
- Lifestyle: Physical Activity
- Financial Management

Sociocultural Determinants

CHAPTER 22

INTRODUCTION

Sociocultural environment comprises of both social and cultural aspects. Social environment consists of occupation, literacy, income religion standard of living, lifestyle, availability of health services, etc. and cultural environment consists of knowledge, attitude, beliefs, practices, traditions, culture, customs, habits, etc. Such as environment of man is being polluted due to industrialization, urbanization and such other human activities. Man only is responsible for the pollution of his environment.

The concept of culture, race and ethnicity play a strong role in understanding human behavior. In everyday living, these three terms are often used incorrectly. Nurses are expected to understand the meaning of each, when providing culturally competent health care to clients of diverse culture.

Culture is a set of beliefs, values and assumptions of life that are widely held among a group of people and that are transmitted intergenerationally (uniform). It is a dynamic process that develops over time and is resistant to change.

Culture is complex whole, which includes knowledge, beliefs, art, morals, law, customs and any other capability acquired by man or a member of society. —*Tylor*

In sociology, the word 'culture' is used to denote acquired behavior, which is shared by and transmitted among members of society or community.

Race is primarily a social classification that relies on physical markers such as skin color to identify group membership. Individuals may be of the same race, but of different cultures.

Ethnicity is the shared feeling of peoplehood among a group of individual. —*Cigar and Davidhizar*

Ethnicity reflects cultural membership and is based on individual sharing similar cultural patterns such as beliefs, values, customs, behaviors and traditions that overtime creates a common history that is exceedingly resistant to change. Ethnicity represents the identifying characteristics of culture such as race, religion or national origin. It is influenced by education, income level, geographical location and association with individual from ethnic groups other than once own.

CUSTOMS AND TABOOS

Customs and taboos are various types of culture exist in the community within each culture. These customs start even before birth and continue till life. Even after death all rituals are performed according to customs of the culture.

Customs

Customs refer to practices that have been often repeated by a multitude of generations, practices that tend to be followed simply, because they have been followed in the past. —*Davis*

Customs are the uniform approved ways of acting, which followed are customs, transmitted from generation to generation by tradition and usually made effective by social approval. —*Anderson and Parlor*

Custom is a broad term embracing all the folkways and mores. Any routine activity in itself is a habit from the point of view of the individual person, but when it becomes general among the folk, it is known as folkways, for example, exchanging greetings, shaking hand, wearing dress, etc. The mores are folkways, which have added to them through some reflection, the judgment that group welfare in particularly depending on them. They are the strong ideas of right and wrong, which require certain acts and forbid others. So, more are beliefs in rightness and wrongness of act.

Taboos

When an activity or action violates the behavior considered appropriate by a group is considered as taboos; an action or activity prohibited and forbidden in the taboos. If anyone transgress, then it is ostracized by others or in extreme instances are killed, i.e. taboos are something, which are forbidden or avoided for religion or social reason.

Custom play an important role in the community. They are also considering as norms of action or rule, which includes that:

- Customs are so powerful that no one can escape their range, since it is an important means of controlling social behavior
- Customs is obeyed more spontaneously because that grows slowly, e.g. people follow similar behavior pattern
- Customs in fact is the repository of our social heritage
- Customs play an important role in personality building, e.g. from birth to death, individual is under the influence of customs, since it mold attitudes and ideas
- Customs create habits: Though customs is the result of habit, however there are many customs, which may give rise to habits and suggested there, e.g. custom create habits and habits create customs.

Influence of Customs on Health

As stated earlier, customs regulate and control the social behavior. These customs differ from society to society, country to country or community to community. Sometimes, simpler customary action of the culture of society can be thus interpreted as improper by another, even it is difficult to convince about the rational and irrational nature of customs because dissatisfaction, which later on can cause various problems particularly psychosocial satisfaction and approval. And sometimes if carried out certain customs can affect the health status of the individual, e.g. using ash or coffee powder on the umbilicus of newborn and not feed the colostrum to neonate such as various customs may accompany pregnancy, childbirth and weaning, the aim being successful reproduction and protects the life of mother and child. To some extent, some of these traditional customs are helpful and some are not scientific indeed may be positively harmful due to many superstitious beliefs are associated with religion, illness is often taught/thought of as a result of evil spirits, i.e. mental illness.

The cultural practices, which have influenced the health and disease are as follows:

1. Nutrition during pregnancy: During pregnancy women are advised not to take healthy food in some cultures. It is said with the aspect of childbirth, it will be easy if the child is of small size. Such unhealthy practice leads to low-birth-weight babies.
2. Breastfeeding: It has been observed that in some cultures mothers are not allowed to feed the baby for the first 3 days. This is bad and irrelevant practice affecting health of neonate.
3. Feeding of girl child: In some culture it is practiced, where the women and girl child will eat the leftover food in family and they are even not provided with adequate food, which can cause malnutrition, harmful infestation and decreases immunity.
4. Handwashing: In some culture, handwashing is common before and after meal as a good custom, which removes the germs from hands and prevents ingestion of microorganisms with food. Now it is widely practical.
5. Bathing: In most of the customs, bathing is good tradition of maintaining personal hygiene, so on to prevent occurrence of certain diseases.

Certain practices related to hygiene, food, marriage, birth are dealt in detailed as below.

Customs and Hygiene

As stated earlier some customs related to personal hygiene includes the following.

Handwashing: Romans, Hebrews and Egyptians have the tradition to wash their hand before and after meals. Guests who do not wash their hands before meal considered of having not a good manner, by the Greeks, usually servants are used to offer vessel of water, so on to carry out the custom of handwashing. Now everywhere it is used, since it is good custom to remove the germs from hand and to prevent ingestion of microorganism along with food.

Bathing: In India, there are occasions in which baths are meant for some purposes such as festivals and women after menstruations have to take bath for purifying themselves. In some religions, even priest advices ceremonial baths after the childbirth. These baths are apart from regular bath. All bathing is good tradition to prevent certain diseases.

Food Customs and Practices

Food consumption has been influenced by the customs and beliefs. In India, majority of Hindus preferred vegetarian food and majority of Muslim's and Christians prefer red non-vegetarian food. In certain religions, garlic and onion are prohibited. In certain religion, e.g. Jainism eating dinner before sunset is considered good.

Usually Muslims will not eat pork; similarly Hindus will not like to eat beef. Some foods such as meat, fish, jaggery, etc. are considered as hot food, since they generate heat, while foods such as curd, milk and some vegetables are cold foods.

Hindus observe fasts in certain occasion and Muslim observes fast in Ramzan time; to some extent it good. But fasts have influence the health and sometimes it can deteriorate the health for diabetes and pregnant women:

1. Eating of the food and diet has been influenced by the customs and beliefs. People are vegetarian and non-vegetarian because of their religion or customers. Such as in Hindus society, vegetarianism is being honored and in Muslim, Christians non-vegetarian food is preferred. Even in vegetarian diet, eating pattern is not same. In certain religions, garlic and onion is not eaten. Timings of eating dinner also different according to religion such as in Jainism eating dinner before sunset is considered good. In case of non-vegetarian diet different types of non-vegetarian items are eaten by different religions according to the customs such as Muslims like beef and Hindus, pork.
2. Hot and cold foods concept is also prevalent. Some foods such as meat, fish, jaggery are considered as hot because they are considered as they generate heat, while foods such as curd, milk, some vegetables and lemon are cold foods.
3. Adulteration of milk with water is based on the belief that if pure milk is boiled then the milk of the donor animal will be either reduced or dried up.
4. Sadhus consume charas, ganja, bhang, which is not considered good for the health and is spreading among general population especially younger.
5. Fasts have influenced the health and sometimes can deteriorate the health such as Karva Chauth fast, if kept by a pregnant women or a diabetic lady. In Muslims, Ramzan are observed by them and Hindus observe fasts on certain occasions such as Janmasthmi, Karva Chauth, Rama Navami, etc. and also in certain days such as Monday (Shiv pooja), Tuesday (Hanuman pooja), etc.
6. According to certain religions, customs related to eating are followed by women such as women eat left over food of husbands. This is still prevalent in certain village societies.
7. The custom of offering a prayer before eating was in order to distract any negative spirits that might have infested. Even before a feast of celebration, primitive peoples used to make sacrifices to their Gods that the food, which they intended would not poison them. This custom of sacrifice and prayer before a feast became a custom. In Koran, it is written "eat the good things that we have provided for you and be grateful to God."
8. Food kinship form earliest times has provided an elementary form of hospitality. In many villages, hospitality and friendship are expressed by eating together among in Muslims. Eating and drinking from common utensil is considered as a sign of brotherhood.
9. Making use of eating utensils and dining table etiquette are considered as appropriate for high social class from the primitive societies.

Marriage and Customs

In some community, marriage through purchase was quite likely to have a bride for a youth. In tribal cultures, betrothals were commonly arranged by parents between their infant daughters and their future husbands. But in modern community, marriages on the basis of mutual love of opposite sexes are able to determine marriage is acceptable.

In India, many marriages are arranged and parents select the partner for their son or daughter. Some customs early marriages are still prevalent in tribal and villages, which are not good. The consanguineous marriages can cause hereditary disease among children. In some religions polyandry type of marriage, which are present today leads to sexually transmitted diseases (STDs). The customs related to endogamy, i.e. marriage within family, relatives is still prevalent, effects on physical and mental health. Sexual intercourse during menstruation is forbidden and sexual relations between male and female in certain society not allowed according to their customs, which is a good practice. Some of the points are detailed below:

1. In some societies, marriage through purchase was quiet likely to have a bride for a young man.
2. In tribal culture, betrothals was commonly arranged by parents between their infant daughters and their future husbands.
3. In modern societies, marriages on basis of mutual love (opposite sex are able to determine their marriage) is acceptable.
4. In many societies, the man has to prove his ability to guard his wife and their family from dangers.
5. In several societies marriages are arranged and parents select the partner for their son or daughter, such type of marriages are commonly prevailing in India.
6. Customs also dictates that the bride always stands to the left of the groom during ceremony.
7. The horoscope of the prospective bride and groom to be certain are checked to make sure that they are compatible.

8. Traditional Hindus continue the ancient practice of infant betrothals.
9. The date of a Hindu marriage is set by a priest, who examines the couple's horoscope for the most favorable day.
10. Early marriage, which is still prevalent in tribal and village areas is not considered good in spite of the age fixed for male and female for marriage by law.
11. Consanguineous marriages, which can cause hereditary diseases among their children is most common among certain religions.
12. Polyandry type of marriage present in Todas of Nilgiri Hills can cause venereal diseases among them.
13. Polygamy is still continued in religious groups who justify plural marriages ordained by diet they worship.
14. Customs related to endogamy, i.e. marriage within family and relatives is still prevalent, which has an effect on physical and mental health. Even it causes, discrimination among different castes.

Customs and Other Practices

1. In order to have oral hygiene, twigs of neem, ash, charcoal and toothbrush are used. Use of charcoal is not considered as good customs, because it spoils the teeth.
2. Certain customs encourages smoking of beedis, pipe and cigarettes have been practices. It is very dangerous habits, which leads to certain health problem such as tuberculosis, oral cancer, lung cancer, bronchitis, coronary artery disease (CAD), etc.
3. Muslims women practices purdah system, which deprives them for the beneficial effects of sunrays and increases incidence of health.
4. According to certain customs people have to sleep on the ground can cause insect bites, Which may lead to ill health.

Customs and Childbirth

1. In some society, newborn children are not allowed to breastfeeding for 3 days and keeping child on water only, and sugar solution is bad practice.
2. According to certain society, prolonged feeding without weaning is not a good practice, but prolonged feeding, weaning and exposure to the baby to sun is good practice.
3. Deliveries conducted by untrained dais are not safe, since they use unsterile and unclean technique.
4. Branding of skin, which is a tradition customs among certain is considered not safe if unsterile or unclean technique are used.

5. Among Muslims circumcision of newborn babies is custom should be performed with sterile equipment and clean technique.
6. Certain community apply kajal for the newborn babies' eyes are in practice. Sometime it is harmful as it can cause eye infection and can transmit trachoma. Paste of turmeric on forehead is neither good nor bad custom.

Superstitions

1. Certain diseases are considered to occur due to wrath of Gods and Goddesses.
2. Hysteria and epilepsy is considered as the problem occurring due to intrusion of spirit, but it is a health problem and requires proper medical treatment.
3. Impure water of rivers is drunk by people, while considering it a pure/holy water.

So, culture influence health and diseases. The harmful activities of culture can cause morbidity and mortality among people. But good cultural practices maintain health of the people, who are living in the community.

Taboos are prohibition or restriction imposed on certain actions or words by social customs. Taboos set persons or objects apart as sacred, prohibited or accursed. There are universal taboos for the society to continue to evolve. Acts that were considered forbidden at one time have developed into acceptable social activity. For example, couple found to be kissing in public not appropriate in India, but some other country it is appropriate. Marriage between close blood relatives is prohibited and polygamy type marriages are not acceptable. Bathing naked in open area is forbidden.

MARRIAGE SYSTEM

Marriage is a relationship between a man and woman, who are permitted to have children. In India, marriage is performed according to traditional Hindu law. It is a sacrament and is obligatory for every Hindu. Marriage is considered as the union between two joint families rather than two young people. Marriage is defined as a 'relatively permanent bond between permissible mates' by Lowie. According to Horton and Hunt, "marriage is the approved social pattern whereby two or more persons establish a family."

Marriage system in India differ in almost all societies, because of the existence of one or other form of marriage. Each type/form of marriage has its advantages and disadvantages.

Marriage is an institution, which admits men and women to family life. It is a stable relationship in which a man and a woman are socially permitted to have children, the right to have children implying the right to sexual relations:

1. Marriage involves the social sanction generally in the form of civil or religion ceremony authorizing two persons of opposite sexes to engage in sexual and other consequent, and correlated socioeconomic relations with one another.
2. Marriage is the approved social pattern whereby two or more persons establish a family.
—Horton and Hunt
3. Marriage denotes those unequivocally sanctioned unions, which persists beyond sexual satisfaction.
—Lowie

It is relatively permanent bond between permissible mates. So, marriage is a more or less permanent association of one or more male with one or more female for the purpose of giving social sanction to progeny satisfaction of biological and social needs, and fulfilment of dharma.

Importance of Marriage

1. Marriage is the powerful instrument of regulating the sex life of humans.
2. Marriage regulates sex relations, it prohibits sex relations between the closest relatives called incest taboos; it also puts restrictions on the premarital and extramarital relations.
3. Marriages lead to the establishment of family, i.e. sexual satisfaction offered by marriage results in self-perpetuations; it is here the children are born and brought up.
4. Marriage provides way for economic cooperations in which the clear-cut division of work on the basis of sex between husband and wife helps smooth running of family.
5. Marriage contributes to emotional and intellectual interstimulation of the partners.
6. Marriage aims at social solidarity.

Types of Marriages and Their Impact on Health

The main types of marriage are polygamy, monogamy and group marriages. These are discussed in relation to their impact on health.

Polygamy

Polygamy is a type of marriage, where a person having two or more partners. There are two types, which includes polygyny and polyandry:
1. Polygyny is type of marriage in which one man marries two or more wives at a time. In India, it is still prevalent among Muslims. It was present among Hindus at the time of rule of kings. Kings used to capture the women by force and made them as his wives. Sometimes they used to purchase women as their wives.

Advantages: This type of marriage system, checks on prostitution, as man can satisfy his sexual desire with more than two wives.

Disadvantages: Are as follows:
- Polygyny form of marriage also has an impact on health of man and women and also lowers the status of women in society
- It creates jealousy among family members
- Economic burden on head of family is increased.

2. Polyandry is the marriage of one woman with several men, i.e. it is form of marriage in which one woman marries more than one man at a given time. It is of two types:
   a. Fraternal polyandry: In this type of marriage, one woman marries to all the brothers and the children are regarded as the offsprings of eldest brother.
   b. Non-fraternal polyandry: In this form of marriage, one woman marries to more than one man, who are not the brothers and one husband is chosen by special rituals as the father of the children born out of such type of families.

Advantages: Are as follows:
- Population control is achieved through the polyandry type of marriage system, i.e. it controls the growth of population
- It strengthens the economic conditions of family
- There are less chances of dispute for property, as property does not get divided.

Disadvantages: Are as follows:
- This type of marriage has an impact on the health of women such as acquired immunodeficiency syndrome (AIDS), infertility, pelvic inflammatory disease, etc.
- It is difficult for women to satisfy the sexual desire of several husbands
- It is easy for man to get divorce
- There can be reduction in population.

Monogamy

Monogamy is the form of marriage, which one man marries one woman at a time. This is the most widespread form of marriage found among the primitive as well as the civilized community. Since, there is one-to-one ratio in almost all societies, only monogamy can provide marital opportunity and satisfaction to all the individuals. It is economically better suited and promotes better understanding between husband and wife. It contributes to family peace, solidarity and happiness. It contributes to stable family and sex life. It helps for better socialization, here aged parents are not neglected. Moreover, it provides better status for women.

Advantages: Are as follows:
- Parents can give proper attention for upbringing of their children
- It creates affection and sincere devotion.

Disadvantages: It can cause extramarital relations.

Companion Marriages

Companion marriages are the type of marriage in which marriage is on the basis of understanding that marriage can be dissolved by mutual consent as long as there is no children. It is better than love or trail marriage. It can cause quick marriage and quick divorce.

Group Marriage

Group marriage means the marriage of two or more women with two or more men. Here, the husbands and wives are common wives and husbands. It is rare. The children are regarded as the children of the entire group.

Marriage Restrictions

The restrictions of marriage may be studied under three aspects, i.e. endogamy, exogamy and incest taboo.

Endogamy

The marriage is performed within the same class or caste of first partner. In India, such type of marriage system is still prevalent, as Brahmins can marry only in Brahmins. Intercaste or interclass marriage is prohibited. Following are the further subdivisions of endogamy such as:
- Tribal endogamy
- Caste/Subcaste endogamy
- Class endogamy.

As the words tribal, caste, subcaste and class, the marriages are restricted respectively.

Each type of marriage system has its advantages and disadvantages. Some forms of marriage has an impact on physical and psychological health. Polyandry, polygyny type of marriage is considered as an obstacle in the way of social progress. It creates psychological problems because of jealous, stress on the head of family member in case of polygyny. Psychological problems can also occur among companionate marriage system, because of quick divorces. Sometimes the mate choice selected by parents in case of arranged marriage or in case of chosen by one of partner can be wrong and it can doom the family to unhappiness.

Marriage is a bond, which is indissoluble in life according to Hindu shastra with the social development, awareness of right of women and availability of the Hindu Marriage Act of 1955 has made possible to women to divorce her husbands, if unable to live with them, but these divorces has increased more of psychological problems among people, because of instability of family.

Exogamy

Exogamy is almost the opposite of endogamy, it is a rule of marriage in which an individual has to marry outside his own group. It prohibits marrying within the group. Here, a man seek a wife out of his own class. Exogamy has assumed various form in India:
1. Gotra exogamy: In Hindu, practice of one marrying outside own 'gotra'.
2. Pravara exogamy: Those who belong to the same pravara cannot marry among themselves.
3. Village exogamy: It is practice of marrying outside their village.
4. Pinda exogamy: Those who belong to same pinda (common parenting) cannot marry within themselves.

Incest Taboo

Incest taboo is a social norm common to virtually all societies, prohibits sexual relationship between certain culturally specified relatives, e.g. marriages between brother and sister, between parents and children is prohibited.

Problems of Marriage

Each type of marriage has its own merits and demerits. Some forms of marriage have an impact on physical and psychological health. Polyandry, polygamy type of marriages is considered as an obstacle in the way of social progress because it creates psychological problems because of jealous, stress on the head of the family member in case of polygamy. Psychological problems can also occur among companion marriage system, because of quick divorce. Sometimes, the mate choice selected by parents in case of arranged marriages or in case of chosen by one of partner can be wrong and it can doom the family to unhappiness. The major problem related to marriage includes the following:
1. Unequal status of women: In Indian society, women do not enjoy equal status or rights with men in social, political, religious and economic field. Still women depend on one or the other after their births. Before marriage, she depends on her father, after marriage on her husband, in old age on her sons. From cradle to the grave has to bear degradation and insult:
   a. Women still do not enjoy the equal rights with men in social, political, religious and economic field.

b. In endogamy system of marriage of family, if a person falls in love with a partner outside the caste, class or tribe, then it can lead to fights, murders, etc.
2. **Dowry:** This system is considered as commercial aspects of marriage. Dowry is the property, cash, gold, etc. that women brings or given to her at the marriage. Dowry has turned to be serious problem resulting in family violence and disorganization. It leads to different types of cruelty toward bride, i.e. physical and mental torture, starving, insulting, taunting and even killing. Now, the Dowry Prohibition Act is there to eliminate evils of the system. But still it is prevalent.

Due to this dowry system, parents sometimes have to marry their daughter to a boy who is not fit for her in age, education or health, etc. Even parents commit theft just to arrange the dowry for their daughter. Dowry Prohibition Act is there to eliminate the evils of the system, but still this is prevalent.

The other problem related to marriage and family are infertility, changing gender role, divorce due to westernization, mental stress, domestic violence, social crimes, legal disputes related to property, etc. Social reformers such as Raja Ram Mohan Roy, Mahatma Gandhi started the reform movement to put an end to such inhuman practices, get an acts passed to bring an end to some evil practices, which includes the Hindu Marriage Act (1955), the Hindu Succession Act (1956), the Dowry Prohibition Act (1985), etc.

FAMILY STRUCTURE

Family has traditionally been defined using the legal notions of relationships such as biological/genetical blood ties adoption, guardianship or marriage. Now, the family has been promulgated that moved beyond the traditional blood, marriage and legal constriction:
1. Family is the biological, social unit composed of husband, wife and children. —*Elliott and Merrill*
2. Family is a group defined by a sex relationship and enduring to provide for the procreation and upbringing of children. —*Hanson*
3. Family is a group of persons united by the ties of marriages, blood or adoption, constituting single household, interacting and intercommunicating with each other in their respective social roles of husband and wife, mother and father, son and daughter, brother and sister, and creating a common culture.
—*Burgess and Locke*

Family is recognized as a focal point of health care. Family is considered as the right place for integrated preventive, promotive, curative and rehabilitative services. Family is also considered as a unit of health service, as health care is centered on the family, the first contact for providing health service as on going, care for acute or chronic problems. Community health nurse as a primary care provider provides integrated services to the people of family during home visits and at subcenters, primary health centers, community health centers to achieve optimum level of functioning of all individuals in family. So, it becomes necessary for her to understand the structure of the family. As in each family various stages of family life cycle can be seen, which have an impact on health.

Functions

Historically, families that performed the following function, which are considered healthy and good (Hanson):
- Families exist to achieve financial survival; some families are economic units of which all members contribute and from which all family members benefit
- Families exist to reproduce the species
- Families provide protection from hostile forces
- Passing along the culture including religion faith is an important function from family
- Families educate (socialize) their young
- Families confer status in society.

So, the above function performed by families are economic, survival, reproduction, protection, cultural heritage, socialization of young and conferring the status.

Definitions of Family Structure

Family structure refers to the characteristic and demographic (i.e. age, sex, number) of individual members, who make up family unit. More specifically, the structure of family defines the roles and the positions of family members.

Family structure is defined on the member composting of family, its size and type, and also articulation of the members of which the family is composed of. It also includes the relationships parameters. Family structure of each family is different because of variation in membership, size and type. As the family can have two parents, single parent, small size, larger size and depending upon kinship, it can be nuclear, extended or joint family. An individual may participate in a number of family experiences over a time. For example, a child may spend the early formation years in the family of origin (mother, father, siblings); experience some years in a single parent family, because of divorce and participate in a step family relationship when the single parent who has custody remarries, etc. Over family structures that are currently experimental will emerge as a everyday natural families, e.g. family in which the members are not related by blood or marriage, but who provide the services, caring, love, intimacy and interaction needed by all persons to experience a quality of life.

Family structure of each family is different, because of variation, membership, size and type. As a family can have two parents, single parents, small size, larger size (number of members in family) and depending upon kinship, it can be nuclear, extended or joint family.

Even cultural, socioeconomic status of family also varies among families. Within family each individual goes through a succession of developmental stages, through different rates and at slightly different stages. Age is an index positioning individuals a developmental sequence. The lifespan of an individual is divided into different periods, the names have been given to each period.

Neonate

Neonate includes the time period from birth till 28 days. It is a time of radical adjustment as from internal environment to external environment. It may be easy for some neonates to make adjustment so difficult for other. The attitude of family members toward the neonate greatly influences the kind of adjustment neonate make to postnatal life. Even the postnatal care is important in determining the kind of adjustment the neonate will make. Negative parental attitude and improper postnatal care can interrupt the life cycle of neonate through which he/she has to go in future.

Infant

As some of the infants are born prematurely and some postmaturely, then it is obvious that all infants will not go through the same level of physical and mental development. This time period of infancy is most hazardous period in the lifespan. As physical and psychological hazards during this time period can affect the present and future adjustments.

Toddler

Toddler stage is the period after infancy, when a child tries to have autonomy. The main problem during this period is the temper tantrum, which need to be dealt carefully.

Child

Children comes in the age of childhood, which is further divided into:

- Early childhood
- Late childhood.

Early childhood: It extends from 2 to 6 years. Variations occur in emotional pattern, emotions are thought to be intense at certain ages especially between the ages to 2 and 4, e.g. temper tantrum. Family size influences the frequency and intensity of emotions such as in small families, jealous is found to be much more as compared to large families. Envy is more common in large families, because of more members and less possessions the children have. Social environment also influences the development of a child. It has been seen that the child with siblings has more temper tantrum than the only child. If the social contacts with others are enjoyed by the children, then their attitude toward future social contacts will be more favorable. During this period, child develops the pattern of early socialization.

Late childhood: It is marked by conditions that affect a child's personal and social adjustments. This is marked by entering the child into first grade. Due to new demands and expectations most children are in state of disequilibrium as they are emotionally disturbed and it is difficult for them to live and work as changes take place in attitudes, values and behavior. Late childhood is regarded as quarrelsome age by many parents as it is the time when family fights are common and the emotional climate of the family is disturbed.

It is clearly not understood about the conditions, which facilitate or deviate the normal development of a child. Even some children with unfortunate disadvantage develop an emotional security and healthy personality. Mental disorders occurring during period appear to be associated with poor socioeconomic status. Some of the problems such as Juvenile delinquency, antisocial behavior can develop due to psychological and environmental conditions.

Adolescent

Adolescence is thought as the period of 'storm and stress', as emotional tensions occur due to physical and glandular changes taking place within the body. Some adolescence experience an emotional instability from time to time. They are often tense and uncontrolled, but an improvement occurs in emotions with each passing year. During this period, adolescents achieve emotional maturity, if they do not learn to get a perspective on situation, an emotional reaction can occur. They need to learn to use emotional catharsis to clear there pent-up emotional energy. They are influenced by peer group and social insight is improved. During this period, many adolescents feel that their parent do not understand them and their behavior is old fashioned.

Adult

Early adulthood is a time period, when the young adult makes adjustment to new patterns of life and is expected to play new roles, i.e. role of a spouse, parent and breadwinner. New attitude, interests and values are developed to play these roles. Parenthood is one of the most important roles in the family life cycle as this is the formation phase of family. As the problems during parenthood occur in the major areas of adjustments, so they require adequate guidance and counseling.

Old Age/Elderly

Old age is considered as a period of decline and is characterized by certain physical and psychological changes. The physical cause of decline is a change in the body cells not due to specific disease, but due to aging process. During this period, sometimes unfavorable attitude toward self, other people, work and life in general occurs due to senility, the changes are the same as occur in the changes in the brain tissue. Aging affects different people differently, so it is difficult to classify as the typical traits of old age. It is a general rule that physical changes precedes the mental changes, but sometimes the reverse is true. As people are never static, they constantly change and old age is the closing period in the life cycle.

When one envisions a family, the first image that comes to mind is a mother and father, the husband and wife and their children usually a boy and a girl. A family of parents and their offspring is known as the nuclear family. The relatives of nuclear families such as grandparents or aunts and uncles comprise the extended family. In some families, members of extended family live the nuclear family. Such multigenerational families were more common during last century, but are still seen today in many cultures as well as in many North American homes. Although members of the extended family may live in different areas, they are frequent source of support and companionship of the family.

The family is frequently defined as two or more persons, who related through marriage, blood, birth or adoption (Duvall, 1977). Although this definition characterizes a large number of families, it does not adequately describe the membership of many families today. In many family groups, there are no legal or blood relationships among members. As the structure of the family has become more diverse, it has been necessary to define the family forms seen in today's society. To provide flexibility in the study of families, Friedman (1981) defines the family as "A family is composed of people (two or more), who are emotionally involved with each other and live in close geographical proximity." Emotional involvement is demonstrated through caring and commitment to a common purpose.

The family is the basic unit of the society. Its major roles are to protect and socialize its members. Among the many functions it serves of prime importance is the role of the family plays in providing emotional support and security to its members through love, acceptance, concern, holds families together, give family members a sense of belonging and develops a sense of kinship.

In addition to providing an emotionally safe environment for members to thrive and grow, the family is also a basic unit of physical protection and safety. This is accomplished by meeting the basic needs of its members; food, clothing and shelter. Provisions of a physically safe environment require knowledge, skills and economic resources.

Type of families: Families have been described as below.

Nuclear family

Nuclear family consists of husband, wife and their children. In such type of families husband plays a dominant role, but in nuclear families presently opposite can also occur. As the family does not have any uncle, aunt or grandparent, the more of burden of rearing of children lies on nuclear family, but the advantage of having nuclear family is the more intimate husband-wife relationship.

Joint family

The joint family is one where the husband, wife, children live with their uncles, aunts and grandparents. All the men in the family are related by blood. They have the common property. The main moto of joint family system is unity.

There are advantages and disadvantages of nuclear and joint family system. In joint family system there is responsibility of sharing in all matters, which provides social security. In case of nuclear family, close intimate relationship among husband and wife exists.

Family in Modern Society

In modern society, the economic resources needed by the family are secured by adult members through employment or government programs. The family also protects the physical health of its members by providing adequate nutrition and healthcare services. Nutritional and lifestyle practices of the family not only influence the health of family members but also directly affect the developing health attitudes and lifestyle practices of children.

In addition to providing an environment conductive to physical growth and health, the family creates an atmosphere that influences the cognitive and psychosocial growth of its members. Children and adults in healthy, functional families receive support, understanding and encouragement as they progress through predictable development stages, as they move in or out of the family unit and as they establish new family units. In families, where members are physically and emotionally nurtured, individuals are challenged to achieve their potential in the family unit. As individual needs are met, family members are able to reach out to others in the family and community, and to society.

The family is a major educator of its members. Parents are often called child's first teachers. This early learning plays an influential part in the development of a child's attitudes about family, education, health, work and recreation. These attitudes persist throughout their lives. In addition, families play a major role in the transmission of religious, cultural and society values. As the family socializes its new members to the expectation of home, community and society, it provides a place of warmth, acceptance and nurturing that insulates its members from the demands of society.

STATUS OF SPECIAL GROUPS

Women

In India, the status of female or women are still not as reached the satisfactory level. Indian women do not enjoy equal rights with men in social, political, religious and economic field. An Indian girl has disadvantage right from birth, i.e. right after birth, female is dependent on one or others. As stated earlier, before marriage she depends on her father, after marriage on her husband and in old age on her son. She cannot live independently according to her own likes and dislikes. From the cradle to the grave, womb to tomb has to bear degradation and insult. Even social prejudices against her were so firmly established that she had hardly any opportunity, freedom or chances of development and self-expression.

In endogamy system of marriage of family, if a individual fall in love with a partner outside the caste, class, a tribe, then it can lead to fights, murders, etc. Another problem related to marriage is dowry system. Due to this dowry system parent sometimes have to marry their daughter to male, who is not fit for her age, education or health, etc. and may commit theft just to arrange dowry.

Women are under-represented in governance and decision-making positions. Most women do not have any autonomy in decision-making in their personal lives and women face violence inside and outside the family as well as at the working places. Many instances have seen rape and incidence of sexual harassments on women.

Human and Communities

Health throughout women's life span is closely related to their communities. Many factors such as the food they eat, the work they perform, their exposures to toxic agents, their substance use and the injuries they encounter are linked to their social and physical environment. Violence in their communities, available health services, employment opportunities, wages and transportation are also among the factors that influence, worsens health. Women suffer from hunger and poverty greater than man. The major areas, which affect women status are malnutrition, poor health, lack of education, overwork, unskilled, mistreatment and powerlessness.

Human and Customs

Certain customs in rural area that women will eat at last throughout life, which means they have to take meals after the male members have eaten their meal. Such customs of eating left meal result in malnutrition in female members including girl child. Because to these practice women suffer not only from nutritional deficiencies disorders but also they suffer from poor reproductive health. They may be due to lack of education that the girl child is disadvantage from education.

Women and Work

In addition, women have to perform the work throughout the day. They do more work as compared to men. Nowadays women have to work outside the home, because of their job, but they have to do all the household chores and have to take care of children with respect to their food, education and other care, etc. This overwork sometime leads to more stress on women. Although they work whole days hard, they are not treated properly by their family members in some families. Some husbands are abusing their wives by using abusive language. This type of mistreatment or ill treatment, females may go to depression and commit suicide. Since, females have still suffer from powerlessness that they are not able to take their own decision about their marriage, health, reproductive health, begetting children, kind of job, education and so many things.

Woman and Family

In practice, women shoulder the responsibility for well-being of their family members, but they are denied access to education, health services, job training and freedom to utilize family planning services. All of which reflect on the status of women. For which in 80s, the Department of Women and Child Development were created to formulate and implement the policies related to women and child welfare. The major programs were social legislation, education, employment and income generating and accommodation for working women. In which:

1. There are legal measures to remove social prejudices and social inequalities, which the women suffers from (e.g. Constitution, 1950).
2. The education schemes are making special effects, which are underway to improve the literacy rate among women and promoting girls education, and started adult education centers, where the education in relation to health, nutrition and child care are provided. The scheme also provides a platform for rural and poor women to share their ideas and ways to tackle the problems.
3. Employment and income generation schemes are to train women belonging to weaker sections of society and to provide employment. In 1977, scheme was launched to provide vocational training and employment and also providing residential care of the distress women. Now, number of voluntary organizations are working for the development of women, which include Indian Red Cross Society, Mahila Mandal, Indian Council for Women Welfare, All India Women Conference and so on.

The steps have taken by the government and non-government agencies for the improvement of status of women have shown that there is some improvement, but still there is a need to take suitable actions in all spheres of national life such as economic, social and also political.

Children

Children are the valuable assets of a nation. They need to be protected and well looked after, if a country in all spheres of human activity. Today's children are tomorrow's citizens. Their care should be of prime importance. A proper and comprehensive health care can develop the good citizen and it leads to good nation, which have the good standards parameter of health, and can present as a healthy nation at international level.

India has the larger child population in the world with more than one third of its population below the age of 18 years. 1 out of 16 children die before they attain age of 1 year and 1 out of 11 die before they are 5 years old. India is the home to highest number of child laborers and sexually abused children in the world. So, in countries like India the condition of child labor is alarming and dissatisfactory. A glance at child labor in India convinces that child labor is underpaid, brutally exploited; physically and mentally deprived of all opportunities. As a result, the children fail to develop their full social and economic potentialities, which would enable them to grow as a useful member of the community. This fact perpetual the cycle of social and economic backwardness among the future generation.

In India, there is 40% of child malnutrition of the developing countries. Malnutrition in children is generally caused by combination of factors such as inadequate or inappropriate food intake, gastrointestinal parasite, childhood diseases and improper care during illness. And other causes related to malnutrition, lack of public healthcare services, poor access to healthcare facilities, declining expenditure and public health in states, and lack of awareness of prevention child health care, etc. tell the factions may increase the mortality rates of children.

And children are deprived of even the scarce social benefits once available, they are displaced by forced and economic migration, increasing the children subsisting on the streets, more and more children are being trafficked within and across borders, and increased numbers of children are involved in part or full-time labor. Many children dropout in elementary education. Every year 12 million girls are born, but 3 million girls will die before attaining 15th year. Method of these deaths occur in the 1st year of life and it is estimated that every sixth female death is directly due to gender discrimination. Sex selective abortion, which is known as feticide is taking a heavy toll. In India, alone there are over 4 lakh children languishing in commercial sex exploitation. They confine themselves to the red light areas, the pimps and henchmen are the role models and this becomes a way of life for them.

Role of Family in Health and Disease

Family performs a number of functions, which are related to health behavior and health, as the family is group of biologically related individuals:

1. Care during pregnancy, birth of a child and postnatally (antenatal, intranatal and postnatal period): The care provided during these periods differ from family to family, society to society and from time to time. It depends upon:

- Level of knowledge
- Attitude of family
- Economic conditions
- Customs, beliefs and values of family
- Traditional ideas.

Whenever a health worker tries to improve the health of an antenatal or postnatal mother or child, he/she has to face the obstacles (traditional ways supported by religion). It is difficult to change the complex variations.

Adequate and proper care provided about nutrition, feeding, hygiene, sleep, clothing, etc. helps to maintain the health of mother as well as of child. The care provided during this period has an important bearing on the infant and maternal morbidity and mortality.

2. Care of the diseased or injured: The attitude of family, society toward sick or injured, who needs care and attention differs. The type of illness also determines the kind of attitude of family members. It depends upon:
   - Understanding of illness
   - Dependency on family member
   - Acute/Chronic illness
   - Economic conditions
   - Beliefs of family related to illness
   - Capability of family members in providing care
   - Attitude of family members.
3. Care of the aged or elderly: In joint family system, a number of women and men biologically related are social support for the elderly in provided physical and psychological care to elderly at home. This care depends upon:
   - An understanding of:
     - Physical needs
     - Psychological needs of elderly.
   - Attitude of family or society toward elderly.
4. Socialization and personality formation: Family plays a vital role in teaching the members especially the young ones the value of society and in transmission of culture, information, beliefs, moral values. Family head gives punishments and rewards for the bad and good conduct respectively.

Family helps its members to withstand the stress and strain. It also provides the external environment for its members where the members interact with each other and other members of society, thereby developing overall personality of an individual.

Family provides an opportunity to its members to release tension, so that mental equilibrium is attained and a stable relationship can be maintained with others. As certain disease such as peptic ulcer, colitis and high blood pressure occur due to stress. Reduction in stress factors can reduce the chances of developing the diseases.

5. Reduction of genetically hereditary diseases: There are certain diseases, which are transmitted to off springs through genes such as hemophilia, diabetes, color blindness, schizophrenia, psychoneurosis, etc. The attitude of family members can be changed through guidance and counseling toward adopting family planning methods in spite of conceiving. It is also seen that congenital malformation is more common among consanguineous marriages. The family plays a vital role in carrying out such type of marriage, because of their traditions and beliefs in developing harmonious relationship between close blood relations.
6. Reduction in antisocial behavior: As the broken families are considered as pathogenic factors in child development. The children of these families can develop psychopathic behavior, immature personality. Such type of children indulge in prostitution or crime activities.

All these can be reduced by reducing the number of broken families. Parents should establish harmonious relationship for normal growth and development of their children.

To conclude, it can be said that family has a vital role in health and disease. So, the community health nurse needs to have thorough understanding of the members, its size and type, so that health can be achieved optimally.

Children Welfare Measures

Rights of the Child

United Nations Declaration of Right of Child, United Nations proclaimed on 20th November (1959) the importance of children right and called upon the nations to observe every June 21st as the International Day of the Children's Rights. United Nation General Assembly declared 1979 as the International Year of the Child. According to the declaration of the rights of child's:

1. The right to affection, love and understanding.
2. The right to adequate nutrition and medical care.
3. The right to free education.
4. The right to full opportunity for play and recreation.
5. The right to name and nationality.
6. The right to special care, if the child is handicapped.
7. The right to be first among the first to receive relief in times of disaster.

8. The right to learn to be useful member of society and to develop individual ability.
9. The right to be brought up in a spirit of peace and brotherhood.
10. The right to enjoy these rights, regardless of race, color, sex, religion, national or social origin.

Indian Constitutional Provision for Children

There are several constitutional provisions made in India to protect children, which includes:
- Article 15: The right of the state to make special provision for women and children
- Article 24: No child below the age of 14 shall be employed to work in any hazardous employment
- Article 39(c): Children of tender age should not be abused and that they should not be forced by economic necessity to enter vocations, institute to their age and strength
- Article 39(f): Children to be given opportunities and facilities to develop in a healthy manner, and in conditions of freedom, and dignity that childhood and youth be protected against exploitation, moral and material abandonment
- Article 45: Free and compulsory education for all children until they complete the age of 14.

Accordingly in India, the number of act have been passed to protect the children:
- Child Labor Act, 1986
- Children Act, 1960
- Juvenile Justice Act, 1986
- Child Abuse Prevention and Treatment Act, 1974
- Health Maintenance Organization Act, 1973
- Education for all Handicapped Children Act, 1975.

National Policies for Children Welfare

In India, several measures have been undertaken by the government to improve health of the people and much importance for the care of children because today's children are the citizens of tomorrow's. So, to improve the health conditions of the children Government of India adapted 'National Policy on Children in August, 1974.' Keeping in view of the constitutional provisions, the United National declaration of the right of the out Government Adopted National Policy, 1974.

The programs in National Policy for Children introduced are:
- Integrated Child Development Services (ICDS) scheme
- Child Welfare Services
- Welfare of the Handicapped Children
- Child Survival and Safe Motherhood (CSSM) Program.

ICDS program

The ICDS program provides integrated package of early childhood services:
- Supplementary nutrition
- Immunization
- Health checkup and health records
- Nutrition and health education
- Non-formal preschool education.

Child welfare services

Child welfare services seek to provide supportive services to the families of the children, which include providing, preventive, promotive, development and rehabilitation services. There are many child welfare agencies in India, which are Indian Council for Child Welfare (ICCW), Central Social Welfare Board, Kasturba Gandhi Memorial Trust and Indian Red Cross Society. These agencies have got branches all over the country to provide day care services, holiday homes, recreation facilities.

Welfare of the handicapped children

Lot of Indian had taken initiative for the prevention of handicappers. They are:
1. Primary prevention includes genetic counseling, at risk approach, immunization, nutrition and others.
2. Secondary prevention includes early diagnosis of handicap, treatment and training and education (vocational guidance).

CSSM program

The CSSM program includes essential newborn care, immunization, appropriate management of diarrhea, appropriate management of acute respiratory infection (ARI) and vitamin A prophylaxis.

India has made an improvement in the states of children ensuring their basic rights. There has been overall progress as child survival rate has gone up due to decrease in infant mortality rates as well as decrease in school dropouts. But still there is need to improve the children status in all respects.

Elderly People

The population of the old or people of 60 and above age are estimated to be about 60 million in India and it account for 6.3% in the total population of the country. Once the aged commanded great respect due to traditional norms and value, but with the disintegration of the joint family system. The changes in social values, social structures and economy have undergone a change. Their children are neglecting these elderly people and they feel unwanted. The generation gap is widening and the children find it difficult to adjust with their elderly parents. Consequently, the aged peoples are suffering from problems.

The elderly people are vulnerable to mental morbidity because of biological, psychological and social factors. There is decline in mental functions such as intelligence, thinking, memory, ability to take decision, etc. This leads to poor comprehension, slow reaction and inability to learn new skills.

Majority of old people are not earning member and depend on others. This leads to decline in their status, self-respect and confidence. The death of spouse brings loneliness and old people find it difficult to adjust themselves to the new situation. They get isolated.

CONCLUSION

Each individual in the society acquires beliefs, customs and traditions in their everyday social interaction, which is known as process of socialization. Each society has its rules to maintain the relationships of authority and subordinate.

These rules, laws and enactments are social control measures. There are customs in society from which no one can escape and is divided into pathways and mores.

Culture is socially acquired learned behavior transmitted from generation to generation, when the people of different cultures come in contact and diffusion of culture occurs, then it is known as acculturation. This acculturation can result due to industrialization, trade, education, conquest, etc. Society is never static, it is dynamic within society, there exist a number of social problems, which affect a large number of people. These social problems hinders the welfare of society. Customs are norms of action. These can be rational or irrational. In case of irrational harmful type of customs, health of an individual can deteriorate. But if harmless, then does not affect the health. There is need to reform irrational harmful customs by education, information and motivation.

Marriage system has an impact on health of people such as polygyny and polyandry marriage system. These type of marriage system can increase the chances of sexually transmitted diseases, stress, jealous, etc. Within family, the individuals are biologically related. The family play a role in health and disease by caring or ignoring its member's health. Females have disadvantaged right from birth. They suffer from hunger and poverty. They are discriminated, which can be seen from the reports related to malnutrition, lack of education, powerlessness and poor health. The department of women and child development was created to implement policies and programs related to the welfare of women and children. Even other programs are there to uplift the status of women.

Children constitutes larger population. But they suffer from malnutrition, lack of elementary education and benefits. Government of India has given provisions under constitution to protect the children. Disability can be reduced by early identification, intervention, education and legislative measures.

Community health nurse should be aware about the physical and psychological changes occurring during the life cycle of each individual. As family may have member of different stages of life cycle, which can result in problems such as problems due to generation gap. Physical and psychological changes occurring within an individual of family can result change in attitude, behavior and social interactions causing stress and crisis.

Introduction to Lifestyle

CHAPTER 23

The term 'lifestyle' is rather a diffuse concept often used to denote 'the way people live', reflecting a whole range of social values, attitudes and activities. It is composed of cultural and behavioral patterns and lifelong personal habits (e.g. smoking, alcoholism) that have developed through processes of socialization. Lifestyles are learnt through social interaction with parents, peer groups, friends, siblings, and through school and mass media.

Health requires the promotion of healthy lifestyle. A considerable body of evidence has accumulated, which indicates that there is an association between health and lifestyle of individuals. Many current-day health problems especially in the developed countries (e.g. coronary heart disease, obesity, lung cancer, drug addiction) are associated with lifestyle changes. In developing countries such as India where traditional lifestyles still persist, risks of illness and death are connected with lack of sanitation, poor nutrition, personal hygiene, elementary human habits, customs and cultural patterns.

It may be noted that not all lifestyle factors are harmful. There are many that can actually promote health, e.g. adequate nutrition, enough sleep, sufficient physical activity, etc. In short, the achievement of optimum health demands adoption of healthy lifestyles. Health is both a consequence of an individual's lifestyle and a factor in determining it.

Health is a way of life. Lifestyle refers, to the way of living or the way the people live. The way of life people in a community and their individual lifestyles have a significant impact on health. Health is related deeply to lifestyle, which includes way of living, personal hygiene, habit and behavior. Lifestyle reflects social values and attitudes, and activation of the individual.

IMPORTANCE OF LIFESTYLE

Healthcare system affected by several social trends. Important trends that affect the healthcare system are the demographic, social, economic, political and technological trends, etc.:

1. Demographic trends that influence health care include growing population, i.e. size and changing age distribution of the population, etc.
2. Social trends that influence health care includes changing lifestyles, a growing appreciation of the quality of life, changing composition of families and living partners rising household incomes and revised definitions of quality health care.
3. Economic trends concerned with changes in the use of health economics is concerned with the problems of producing services and programs and distributing them to clients.
4. Technological trend that is improved technology is rapidly changing the healthcare system and having both positive and negative effects. Increasing evidence of the effects of social, biological, economic and life events on health requires broader approach to addressing health risks. Render identified six categories of risk factors; genetics, age, biological characteristics, personal health habits, lifestyle and environment.
5. Lifestyle is determined in part by circumstances and in part by the decision made, consciously or unconsciously by people about the way, they choose to live. Lifestyle depend to a large extent on the occupation of the head of the household, the income level of the family and the things that income can purchase in the way of housing, good clothing, recreation and even education and health care.
6. A healthy lifestyle helps to promote health and poor lifestyle has ill effects on health. In the developing world, many health problems are directly attributable to the lack of basic essentials of life such as adequate nutrition and housing, resulting from widespread poverty among large segment of population of many countries. For example, in India, due to persistence of

poor traditional practices, there are risks of death and illness connected with lack of sanitation, poor nutrition, self-care, habits, customs and cultural patterns. Health can be enhanced through balanced lifestyle. A balanced lifestyle means having the sight amount of rest, work, physical activity, sleep, leisure and recreation in individual daily life. The main advantage of a balanced lifestyle is that it provides the time to recuperate and restore energy. When an individual is sleeping his/her nervous system is inactive, his/her eyes are closed and postural muscles are relaxed.

LIFESTYLE RISKS AND HABITS

Personal habits continue to contribute to the major causes of morbidity and mortality. The pattern of personal habits and lifestyle risks defines the individual and family lifestyle risks. The family is the base unit within which health behaviors including health values, health habits and health risk perceptions is developed, organized and performed. Families maintain major responsibility for determining what food is purchased and prepared, setting sleep patterns, planning family activities, setting and monitoring norms about health and health risk behaviors, determining when family member is ill, determining when healthcare should be obtained and carrying out treatment regimen. More than half of all deaths were attributed to heart disease or cancer, both of which identify diet as a major causative factor. General guidelines include eating a variety of foods; maintaining health and weight; choosing a diet, low in fat and cholesterol, including plenty of vegetables, fruits, and grain products; limiting use of sugars, salts and sodium; and consuming alcohol only in moderation. Since human host is referred to as 'soil and the disease agent as seed'. In some situations, host factors play a major role in determining the outcome of an individual's exposure to infection (e.g. tuberculosis). The host factors may be classified as:

1. Demographic characteristics such as age, sex, ethnicity.
2. Biological characteristics such as genetic factors, biochemical levels of the blood (e.g. cholesterol), blood groups and enzymes, cellular constituents of the blood, immunological factors and physiological function of different organ systems of the body.
3. Social and economic characteristics such as socioeconomic status, education, occupation, stress, marital status, housing, etc.
4. Lifestyle factors such as personality traits, living habits, nutrition, physical exercise, use of alcohol, drugs and smoking, and behavioral patterns, etc. The association of a particular disease with a specific set of host factors frequently provides an insight into the cause of disease.

Substance use and abuse is a major contributor to morbidity and mortality. For example, tobacco use has been identified as the simple and most preventable cause of death. It has been associated with several types of cancer, coronary heart disease, low birth weight, premature births, sudden infant death syndrome and chronic obstructive pulmonary disease. Further, more passive smoke has been linked to disease in nonsmokers and children. Another example that drug and alcohol use associated with transmission of human immunodeficiency virus (HIV), fetal alcohol syndrome, liver disease, unwanted pregnancy, delinquency, school failure, violence and crime. Similary to this lifestyle factors such as smoking, alcohol use, diet and physical activity. Cigarette smoking is risk factors for heart disease, cerebrovascular disease and cancer. Alcohol consumption is associated with injuries and many diseases. In addition to circumstantial factors, there are also elements of personal decision-making that enters into an individual or family lifestyle regardless of income. Malnutrition is most usually associated with poverty, but it may also result from poor choice in the food eaten, e.g. the eating too many snacks foods and sweets instead of well-balanced foods.

Numerous other major problem that are causes of increasing concern in the health field today can also be attributed to lifestyle factors, these includes alcoholism and drug addiction. Sexually transmitted diseases (STDs) and mental health problems such as suicides, affecting increasing number of young people.

LIFESTYLE AND BEHAVIORAL CHANGES

The conventional public health measure or interventions have not been successful in making inroads into lifestyle reforms. The action of prevention in this case, is one of individual and community responsibility for health, the physician and in fact each health worker acting as an educator than a therapist. Health education is a basic element of all health activity. It is of paramount importance in changing the views, behavior and habits of people.

Since health promotion comprises a broad spectrum of activities, a well-conceived health promotion program would first attempt to identify the 'target groups' or at risk individuals in a population and then direct more appropriate message to them. Goals must be defined as means and alternative means of accomplishing them must be explored. It involves, 'organizational, political, social and economic interventions designed to facilitate environmental and behavioral adaptations that will improve or protect health'.

NURSES ROLE IN LIFESTYLE ISSUES

Nurses should assess lifestyle factors of vulnerable individuals, families and groups that may predispose them to further health problems. Lifestyle factors include usual dietary patterns, exercise, rest and use of drugs, alcohol and caffeine. For example, many homeless individual eat their meals, either at shelters or at fast food restaurants. Because of the unpredictability of meals and food availability, it is often difficult for them to eat a diet that is low in fat, cholesterol and sodium, and it is particularly difficult to eat the recommended five servings of fruits and vegetable per day. Cultural preferences may also influence lifestyles and health risk behaviors. And helping vulnerable persons develop lifestyle behaviors require great sensitivity by nurses. They should focus in identifying client's priorities and helping them meet these priorities. For example, discussing exercises with homeless person requires empathy and creativity. Often vulnerable individuals and families are coping with crisis intervention strategies. After the crisis has been managed, a trusting relationship is likely to exist between nurse and client. This relationship forms the basis for health promotion interventions. Nurses must be sensitive to the lifestyles of their vulnerable clients and must develop methods of health promotion that recognize these lifestyles factor.

LIFESTYLE/HEALTH RISK ASSESSMENT

Health Risk Appraisal

A health risk appraisal (HRA) or health hazard appraisal (HHA) is an assessment and educational tool that indicates a client's risk of disease or injury over the next 10 years by comparing the client's risk with the mortality risk of the corresponding age, sex and racial group. The client's health behavior and demographic data are compared to that of a large national sample. The principle behind risk appraisal is that each person, as a member of a specific group, faces certain quantifiable health hazards and that average risks are applicable to a client, if the health professional knows the client's characteristics and the mortality of a large group of cohorts with similar characteristics.

Lifestyle Assessment

Lifestyle assessment focuses on the personal lifestyle and habits of the client, as they affects the health. Categories of lifestyle generally assessed are physical activity, nutritional practices, stress management, and habits such as smoking, alcohol consumption and drug use. Other categories may be included. Several tools are available to assess lifestyle. Pender (1987) outlines a comprehensive 10 category (100 item tool) that includes the following:

1. Competence in self-care, including dental hygiene, breast self-examination, knowledge about the danger signs of cancer, blood pressure and other healthcare practices.
2. Nutritional practices.
3. Physical or recreational activity.
4. Sleep patterns.
5. Stress management.
6. Self-actualization, including outlook on life and feelings about self, work and accomplishments.
7. Sense of purpose in life and knowledge of what is important in one's life.
8. Relationships with others.
9. Environmental control to make living areas free of hazards.
10. Use of the healthcare system.

Families are the major source of factors that can promote or inhibit positive lifestyles. They regulate time and energy, and the boundaries of the system. A number of tools exist for assessing individuals lifestyle risks, but few are available for assessing family lifestyle patterns. Although assessment of individual lifestyle contributes to determining the lifestyle risk of a family, it is important to look at risks for the family as unit. In the areas of health promotion, health protection and preventive services, lifestyle can be assessed in several dimensions. From the literature on health behavior research, the critical dimensions include the following:

- Value placed on the behavior
- Knowledge of the behavior and its consequences
- Effect of the behavior on the family
- Effect of the behavior on the individual
- Barriers in performing the behavior
- Benefits of the behavior.

It is important to assess the frequency, intensity and regularity of specific behaviors and it is also important to evaluate the resources available to the family for implementing the behaviors. Thus, items for assessment of physical activity includes, the value that a family places on the hours that a family spends in exercise, the kinds of exercise, the family does and resources available for exercise.

Lifestyle refers to a person's general ways of living including living conditions and individual pattern of behavior that are influenced by sociocultural factors and personal characteristics. In brief, lifestyle is often considered as behavior and activities over which people have control. Life choices may have positive or negative effects on health practices that have potentially negative effects on health are often referred to as risk factors. For example, overeating, getting insufficient exercise and being overweight are closely related to the incidence of heart disease, arteriosclerosis, diabetes and hypertension. Excessive tobacco is clearly implicated in lung cancer, emphysema and cardiovascular disease. An example of healthy lifestyle is regular exercise, weight control, avoidance of saturated fats, alcohol and smoking avoidance, seat belt use, bike helmet use, immunization update, regular dental checkup and regular health maintenance visits in screening exams or tests.

Health is perceived as a condition in which the person engage in effective interaction with the physical and social environment. It is a purposeful, adaptive response, physically, mentally, emotionally and socially, to internal and external stimuli in order to maintain stability and comfort (Murray and Zentner 1975). Personnel lifestyle is one of the factors affecting behavior. One's lifestyle, including patterns of eating, exercise, drinking, coping with stress and use of tobacco and drugs, together with environmental hazards are the major causes of illness. Lifestyle is influenced by cultural expectations. As the understanding of health and illness increases, it has become clear that many diseases are preventable, the effects of some diseases can be minimized, or the onset of disease can be delayed through lifestyle modification. Cancer, cardiovascular disease, adult onset diabetes, and tooth decay are among the lifestyle diseases. For example, the incidence of lung cancer would be greatly reduced, if people stop smoking. Proper nutrition, good dental hygiene and fluoride in the water supply, in toothpaste, as a topical application, or as supplements have been shown to reduce dental decay or caries, one of America's most prevalent health problems. Automobile accidents, the leading cause of death among adolescents and young adults, are frequently associated with alcohol consumption and increased risk taking.

In addition to health practices and nutrition, other important lifestyle considerations are exercise, stress management and rest. Today, health professionals have the knowledge to prevent or minimize the effects of some of the main causes of disease, disability and death. Too often, there is little consideration of health until sickness occurs. The challenge is to disseminate information about prevention and to motivate families to make lifestyle changes prior to the onset of illness. Many demands are made on today's family.

An important question is "Will people take the time to be responsible for their own health?" As stated earlier, since the health can be enhanced through balanced lifestyle. A balanced lifestyle means having, maintaining proper hygiene, right amount of rest and sleep, and physical activity. The physical activity includes recreation and sleep, sexual life, spiritual life, self-reliance dietary pattern, education and occupation. These elements of balanced lifestyles dealt is detailed in Chapters 24 and 25.

Lifestyle: Hygiene

CHAPTER 24

INTRODUCTION

Hygiene refers to the practices adopted by human beings to preserve the health as well as to improve the health. This word hygiene refers to the principles of health and sanitation to be practiced by the individuals. Hygiene is of great significance to maintain the health status of people in a community it has two aspects:
- Environment hygiene
- Personal hygiene.

TYPE OF HYGIENE

Environment Hygiene

Environment is man's external surroundings. It has two categories:
- Domestic environment hygiene
- Community environment hygiene.

Domestic Environment Hygiene

Domestic environment hygiene comprises home, proper disposal of waste, hygienic storage of food and absence of pests, rats, mice, etc.

Community Environment Hygiene

Community environment hygiene comprises areas outside the home where the community lives. It also requires proper disposal of wastes, sewage, and control of air and water pollution.

Hygiene is the science of health. The self-care measure people use to maintain their health is personal hygiene. Personal hygiene deals with matters, which are personal responsibility of every person. It is concern itself with the adjustment, which the individual must make to preserve and improve the health of their body, and mind.

Personal Hygiene

Personal hygiene may be defined as 'the measures for personal, cleanliness and grooming that promote physical and psychological well-being'. Maintenance of personal hygiene is necessary for an individual comfort, safety for which a person himself is responsible. It deals with the personal care of health so that man is able to enjoy healthy life and should get satisfaction about his/her health. As for the quality of life, health enables the individual to live most and serve best.

Maintenance of personal hygiene is necessary for an individual comfort, safety as well-being. Healthy persons are capable of meeting their own hygiene needs, whereas ill or physically handicapped persons may require the nurse's assistance to carry out routine hygiene practice, illness, hospitalization and industrialization may demand modifications in hygiene practice. In addition personal and sociocultural factors, i.e. body image, social practice, socioeconomic status, knowledge, cultural variables, personal preference, physical condition influence the client's hygiene practice. The nurse determines a client's ability to perform self-care and provides hygiene care according to the client needs, and preferences. In these situations, the nurse helps the client to continue sound hygienic practice and has an opportunity to teach the client, and family members regarding hygiene.

The main objective of personal hygiene is to maintain high standard of health. Healthy living depends upon the practice of a few principles of health and hygiene. Ill health results mostly from harmful habits. Personal hygiene is not only concerned with matters pertaining to health of a person but also includes certain personal factors conductive to good health. These factors are habits, constitution, hereditary, idiosyncrasy, temperament, cleanliness, sleep, clothing, exercise, sex, etc.

OBJECTIVES

- To keep the body such as skin of body, eyes, ears or nose, etc. in a healthy condition and free from infection
- To maintain good physique and muscle strength
- To maintain health and prevent infection.

PRINCIPLES RELEVANT TO HYGIENE

- Good hygienic practices are learned
- Hygienic practices vary because of cultural norms, knowledge and personal values, and ability to keep cleanliness
- Change occur due to change in age, which causes changes in skin, mucous membrane, hair, nails and teeth
- Skin is the first line of defense against infection and injury
- Skin and its appendages change due to the effect of drugs and therapeutic treatment
- Health of an individual and its care require nourishment, fluid intake and exercise.

FACTORS AFFECTING HYGIENIC PRACTICES

There are a number of factors, which affect the person's personal hygienic practices. These are:
- Habits
- Cultural factors
- Social practices
- Personal preferences
- Knowledge
- Body image
- Illness
- Use of drugs
- Weather
- Availability of resources such as water, soap, clothes, etc. to maintain hygiene.

HABIT

Habit plays an important part in the preservation of health. Habit grows into practice and it is said to be the second nature of human being because once it is formed, it is very difficult to get rid of. To keep one fit and ready for actions, habits decent. Habit influence should necessarily be the physical, physiological and psychosocial condition of individual. Man by birth desire to be socially well-being as man reaches adulthood earning becomes the main consideration particularly when married and as families get added up. He works more and should keep good habits. Temperament should under the control of will and he should not tilt towards bad habit (e.g. smoking, alcohol, substance abuse, gambling, etc.) as they affect the health. Health of the community also depends a great deal on the habits of each member of the community.

The development of good habits, which influence in the child, is right action and right thinking. Proper healthy habits consume the only sound foundation upon which permanent physical and mental health should be built at expected level.

Eating Habits

Eating habits it is essential to create a regular habit of taking food including water. Only wholesome food should be taken for the preservation of health. Eating time is not fixed by watch Indian families, but in India the habit of taking food is more or less fixed hours and quantities compatible with one's work. In a few families and only 10% of Indian population believe in taking regular nutritious diet at the fixed hours of the day. Food should be taken slowly after desire comes for it when the appetite particularly craves for and mind should be calm, and clear. It should be bitten 32 times. Bolting of unchewed morsels should not be done. Reading should be avoided, while taking meals. Excessive eating is not a good habit.

Food should not be taken more than actual requirements of the body since gluttony or over eating results in obesity, apart from digestive and other disorders. And too much of food should not be taken at simple sitting, but the meals should be spread out over the course of the day. It is desirable that there should be sparingly taken along with meals. Water should be taken freely between principle meals. It is good to take a glass of cold water early in the morning on rise from the bed.

Alcohol should never be encouraged with food, since it is harmful to health. Adverse effects of faulty food habits results in indigestion, constipation and obesity.

Indigestion

Indigestion occurs when the food fails to get digested properly. The causes for indigestion are as follows:
- Unbalanced diet
- Eating between meals
- Rapid eating
- Too little chewing of the food
- Constipation

CHAPTER 24 Lifestyle: Hygiene

- Unpleasing surrounding, while eating
- Eating during anger, worried or fatigue
- Disease condition such as gallstone, ulcers or chronic illness.

When indigestion occurs from any of these causes, do not eat any food and if hungry take liquid foods for the next 24 hours.

Constipation

Constipation is the failure to evacuate the waste matters from the bowel in sufficient quantity. Sedentary habits and lack of regular exercise often lead to weakening of intestinal and abdominal muscle, which results in constipation. If prolonged, it may lead to piles. As a matter of fact, the residue of the meal should be expelled out within 48 hours and if this does not take place there is stagnation in the bowel. It is reasonable to eliminate waste matter from alimentary tract as soon as possible. It has been physiologically accepted that one good motion a day is sufficient, provided adequate quantity of fecal matters is expelled out. It is healthful, ideally and practically also.

Usual causes of constipation are as follows:
- Habits of using drugs to relieve constipation upset the intestinal system
- Ignoring the call to evacuate the bowel/rectum
- Lack of exercises
- Insufficient intake of fluids and roughage in the diet
- Eating too much fats
- Hurried eating habits and too little rest
- Poor posture leads to bending of the body forward and crowding of abdominal organs lead to weakening muscles.

Specifications on constipation

To prevent constipation the following measures may be helpful:
1. Adoption of correct position and regularly attending to the nature call is most essential.
2. Drinking plenty of water between principal meals, especially a glass of water early in the morning.
3. The habit of using medicine in any form to relieve constipation is harmful and should be avoided unless it is prescribed, e.g. purgatives.
4. Faulty diet must be corrected by modification in diet and habits.
5. Diet must contain simple fibrous material in order to give sufficient bulk of stool.
6. Sufficient roughage in the diet is necessary in old age.
7. Whole wheat bread, grams, vegetables, pulses and fruits in place of meat and egg should encourage in the diet.
8. Yeast is very valuable as it contains enough vitamin B complex, which tones the nerve of the intestine and improve its power of contraction and movement of the bowel.
9. Eating some course bulky foods, e.g. green vegetables, bran, whole grain cereals, fruits with their skin.
10. Taking regularly outdoor exercise.
11. Constipation is often associated with the weakness of abdomen and pelvic muscles. In order to strengthen these muscle remedial exercises should be taken.

Obesity or overweight

Obesity is an abnormal and dangerous condition in which there is stored large surplus of fat in the body. Its accumulation beyond the normal limit, may be due to endocrine dysfunction, i.e. hypothyroidism causing an abnormally low metabolic rate, but in large majority of cases, it is due to either excessive intake of food or to a deficient utilization of the food than the produce energy. Obesity may be defined as an abnormal growth of adipose tissue due to an enlargement of fat cell size hypertrophic obesity) increase in fat cell number (hyperplastic obesity) or a combination of both obesity expressed in terms of body mass index (BMI). Overweight is usually due to obesity, but can arise from other causes such as abnormal muscle development or fluid retention. However, obese individual differ not only in the amount of excess fat that they store but also in the regional distribution of this fat within the body.

Fat in food is the most common cause of overweight, which at first may causes merely discomfort and later on menace in life. It increases susceptibility to diabetes, renal diseases, cardiac failure, disease of the arteries ever and ailments. Excessive weight of 10% above the normal increase the mortality toll, about 20% and the greater the amount of surplus weight, the higher the death toll.

The ideal height and weight chart for men and women of 25 years and above. The principle underlying in that weight should not be restricted by interfering with the normal development of bones and muscles. Obesity can be prevented in those taking too rich food, by increased exercise or in those taking too little exercise, or by food restriction (Table 24.1).

To control increased weight needs a selection of food and by restriction of its amount, which may provide proteins liberally, but should restrict fats and carbohydrates:
1. Bulk, which satisfies hunger, is achieved by the use of foods rich in water, poor carbohydrates and fats, with considerable proportion of material, which cannot be absorbed, e.g. fruits and leafy vegetables.

Table 24.1: Ideal height and weight for men and women (25 year and above)

Men		Women	
Height in cm with shoes	Weight in kg	Height in cm with shoes	Weight in kg
157	56.2–60.3	152	50.8–54.5
160	57.6–61.7	155	51.7–55.3
163	59.0–63.5	157	53.1–56.1
175	62.1–66.7	160	54.5–58.1
168	64.0–68.5	163	56.2–59.9
170	65.8–70.8	165	57.6–61.2
173	67.6–72.6	168	59.0–63.5
175	71.2–76.2	170	60.8–65.3
180	71.2–76.2	173	62.1–66.7
183	73.0–78.5	175	64.0–68.5
185	75.3–80.7	178	65.8–70.3
188	77.6–83.5	180	67.1–71.7
191	79.8–85.7	183	68.5–73.9

2. Protein food should not be reduced in amount unless the individual happens to use them in excess.
3. Starchy food should not be entirely eliminated, as the stored fat is oxidized much more readily and sagely in the presence of carbohydrates.
4. It is very dangerous to reduce weight rapidly; it should not be more than 0.5 pound or 226.5 g per day. Rapid reduction leads to the production of fatty acids in excessive amounts. These acids cannot be neutralized and lead to low alkaline reserves in the body, which in turn lead to acidosis.
5. Food restrictions to become slim should never be encouraged.
6. Weight reducing drugs should not be encouraged.

Underweight

Individual should have normal weight according to their age, sex and height. Underweight also leads to many problems. The common causes of underweight are as follows:
- Insufficient intake of food
- An unbalanced diet
- Too little sleep
- Chronic infections
- Worry.

If the individual is undernourished, he/she may look pale, have poor posture, flabby muscles, dark circles under his/her eyes, decreased appetite and he/she often shows irritation.

Drinking Habit

Drinking water is very essential and good habit for all purposes. Nowadays, there are many drinks available to people for drinking purposes, e.g. soft drinks, hot drinks, which may provide some amount of stimulation, but some are not nutritious, which include coffee, tea, Coca-Cola, alcohol, etc.

Use of coffee and tea

Coffee or tea is an ideal stimulant of body tissue when properly used, but it is abuse constitutes a problem. In moderate doses, it lessens the feelings of fatigue and is of value during hard mental and physical work, and in cases of shock.

Coffee contains caffeine, which speeds up burning of food in the tissue and increases the functional activities. It whips the brain and makes the mental process keener. As a result of its intake the heart works faster and special sense become more acute, the body thus becomes highly active and vital. The habitual use of coffee repeatedly leads to the tissue response becomes dull and exhaustion results, and if the uses goes on increasing their dose to get stimulation, which is harmful to health.

The users of coffee admit that they drink coffee for the pickup and feelings of increased strength, and freshness. They get help from coffee in getting through days of stress and strain. These people with a rapid pace of life get a temporary sense of fitness and efficiency, but actually the habit increases the underlying exhaustion of their body tissues leading to breakdown. It masks the underlying fatigue and under its influences the users perform more works than their system, and by cutting down sleep and upsetting relaxation. This combination of overwork, and lack of rest gradually leads to physical and mental breakdown.

The heart has to work harder and blood pressure may be raised. So, it has been suggested the use of coffee should be prohibited among persons with impaired health. Healthy persons may use coffee in moderation during cold season as it gives feelings of comfort and mental alertness.

Tea is freely used as a stimulant due to the presence of tannin, caffeine. Average black tea contains cellulose (40%), albumin (17.9%), tannic acid (16.4%), water (8.2%), ash (8.6%), resin (4.6%), caffeine (3.2%) and others (1.1%). Among these, caffeine is most important constituent and then comes tannic acid. Preparation of tea is important. When water begins to boil, it should be poured in a separate pot, which is warm and contains the tea leaves. Tea is infused for 5 minutes after which it should be poured off and stained. Prolonged boiling should be avoided, because the longer the tea is infused, the more tannic acid is dissolved out. Tannic acid produces constipation and the taste of the tea becomes bitter. Addition of mild renders some of the tannic acid insoluble. Increase use of tea causes constipation, dyspepsia, insomnia and nervousness. Light and hard tea may be taken up to 2–4 cups a day by a healthy person.

Use of coca and chocolates

They contain an alkaloid, closely related to caffeine called theobromine, its stimulating effects are mainly exerted on the brain and central nervous system. Tea and coffee, if taken without milk and sugar have no food value, but coca and chocolate are nutritious.

Use of alcohol

Alcohol acts as a sedative. It is a food and a narcotic, but its food value is very limited. In certain occasions, if used in small doses it may help digestion or induce sleep, but it has a devitalizing action upon the tissues, the symptoms of which range from some impairment of functions to gross degenerative poisons. The feeling of exhilaration that follows after taking a mild dose of alcohol is due to paralysis of higher nerve centers that normally provide inhibition. It bottles up the disagreeable thoughts and sensations, and produces a feeling of well-being and happiness. It kills the sense of fatigue and mental unrest. But excess of alcohol or its misuse acts slow poisons.

Now, it has become alcohol or its evil, it may cause gastrointestinal disorders, fatty degeneration of heart and liver, arteriosclerosis, peripheral neuritis, etc. in its passage through different tissues alcohols has different effects:

1. On the casual nervous system, alcohol acts as a narcotic, which may begin with the production of pleasant state or euphoria, i.e. the facing out of disturbing and unpleasant facts of life, progress to stupor, then coma and even death in rare cases. The first higher centers of the brain to be affected are those which control memory, attention, thought judgment of self-control and subsequently muscular, and sensory functions are interfered with. They lose the power of concentration and memory, and may develop dullness, and may commit some breaches of the law bringing trouble on themself, and on his/her family.
2. Alcohol increases the rate of contraction causing rapid heartbeat through the nerve tissue covering the heart.
3. By dilating the blood vessel at the surface of the body alcohol interfaces with the heart regulating mechanism producing a sense of warmth in the skin and actual loss of internal body heat. The loss can be serious in cold weather, when the body is not well-wrapped.
4. By acting on the nerve tissue, which is the special sensory organs, it can produce error, and delay in observing through eye and ear. It has very dangerous effect on person driving a vehicle or an aeroplane. In view of its slow rate of elimination from the body, these effects of alcohol usually remain for some hours after alcohol has been taken.
5. As regards to respiratory process moderate amounts of alcohol produce little effect, but large amounts may cause paralysis of the respiratory centers and lead to even death.
6. In the cases of digestive process, peristaltic action may be lessened and flow of saliva increased as also of gastric juice with the difference that this lower in pepsin contents, but higher in hydrochloric acid contents than normal—a change liable to be harmful to person suffering from peptic ulcer. Persons addicted to alcohol loss their appetite. They get nausea and vomiting in the morning, which is an expression of resentment by the outranged stomach. They suffer from gastric catarrh, windy spasms and heart burns. A'cohol, which absorbed passes through the liver and damages, leads to liver disorder.
7. Usually excessive intake of alcohol is that normal restraint in conduct may be lost, involving the risk of promiscuity and of contracting such diseases in sexually transmitted diseases (STD), gonorrhea and syphilis.

Alcoholism is a social evil; its economic and social costs are heavy. It affects the personality of the man as well as his/her social status and family relationship. Family discards his/her security and happiness of home is shattered. Alcohol develops unusual cunningness to cover up one's use of alcohol and want to maintain normal behavior with friends, and family members. Alcoholism can be easily found out by relatives and friends. The following signs may serve as guidelines:

- Drinking as guidelines
- Constantly drinking and thinking
- Getting drunk without really intending to drinking frequently
- Needing drinks at odd hours
- Making excuses for drinking.

Consumption of alcohol does not remove fatigue, but makes one unconscious of it and blunts one's recollections of the difficulties and worries of the day. The real danger of its use is its the habit-forming nature; for persons having weak self-control, it very quickly ceases to be under control, but becomes their master. It is responsible for many crimes, accidents and so many physical, physiological and psychological injuries, and diseases. Therefore, use of alcohol and other such liquids should be avoided.

Use of tobacco

Tobacco is the most common form of substance abuse, which leads to social addiction. It is used mostly in smoking, chewing and sniffing.

Smoking: It is a habit, which comes from in disciplined society. The children start smoking at a very young age in case their father is chain smoker. Smoking is injurious to health and it should not be encouraged.

It is noticed that smoking in any form is injurious to health, but nobody pay least importance to it. It has been proved that cigarette smoking, has been important factor in the development of cancer of lungs and cancer of larynx. Many cases of lung carcinoma and lip cancer are due to the use of lip tobacco, and smoking cigarette or bidi/beedi. Smokers have higher death rate from coronary heart disease and it is also one of the major causes of chronic bronchitis. The smoke of tobacco consists of a mixture of gases and various vaporized chemicals including vaporized nicotine, which is a toxic substance. A smoker gets more nicotine and tar, if he smokes cigarette to the end. When smoker inhales nicotine, which increase stimulation it further intensifies the habit of smoking. Smoking is used as a means of relaxation, especially during tension in an individual smoking tends to have 20% more illness. Smoking pipe and cigar are less dangerous, while smoking bidi, which is being used extensively throughout India is more harmful. In bidi, burning of leaf in which tobacco is wrapped for making bidi irritates the throat. Hookah smoking is a better method of smoking tobacco. When the smoke of tobacco passed through water in the hookah, nicotine is dissolved in water to a great extent and hookah fumes pass through water reservoir, and most of the alkaloids of the tobacco are precipitated in this way.

Tobacco chewing: Here the tobacco leaf is powdered and little lime is mixed, and then it is kept between the lower lip and teeth, and chewed. This habit is the worst habit; on this operation, a large quantity of saliva juice and even the particles of tobacco are swallowed, causing chronic sore throat, disorders of digestion, impaired vision and nervous tremor. This is associated with high prevalence of oral cancer, i.e. lip and tongue cancer.

Snuffing: It is another form of tobacco, which is used widely. The habitual snuff users from hypertrophy and later atrophy of nasal mucosa. This is more risky than smoking and chewing of tobacco.

Once the people addicted to use of tobacco, it is very difficult, to give up the habit. To give up smoking do not use any drugs or medicine, which has no value. Success in dropping the habit of smoking depends upon desire and will power to quit it. It requires motivation, which leads to positive action in the act of stopping smoking. It may begin with gradual withdrawal, but it usually fails. But to stop it suddenly becomes uncomfortable physically and emotionally. Most smokers crave for smoking after each meal and some during office break. In order to quit smoking change in the living pattern is required.

MAINTAINING PERSONAL HYGIENE

Personal hygiene deals with the practices adopted by individuals such as bathing, cutting nails, etc. that help in the maintains and promotion of individuals health physically, emotionally, socially and spiritually. The person adopts measures to keep his/her skin and its appendages in good condition. It includes:
- Care of skin
- Care of hands and nails
- Care of hair
- Hygiene of bowel and bladder
- Care of eyes, ears, nose and mouth.

Cultivating the habit of maintaining cleanliness is very essential for the up keep of health and for the normal growth of the body. Cleanliness is next to godliness. Dirt is not only harmful but also it is antagonistic even to very existence. Therefore, special emphasis should be paid on cleanliness with regard to the food we eat, the air we breathe, and the water we drink. While taking care of the body on relation to cleanliness, emphasis should be made to take care of skin, hairs, mouth, teeth, hands, feet, nails, eyes, ears, external genitals, etc.

Care of the Skin

The skin is an active organ with the function of protection, secretion, sensation, respiration, temperature regulation and excretion. Skin has around 2 million sweat glands, which has at least three functions, i.e. to keep body temperature normal, to keep the skin permeable and to get rid of the waste material and dirt from the body. Skin is of immense value as a lot of perspiration and excretion of solids take place through its innumerable minute pores.

CHAPTER 24 — Lifestyle: Hygiene

As a matter of fact, a great deal of work, of lungs and kidneys is, performed by the skin. The amount of sweat varies from person to person. Emotional stress, worry, fear or excitement can also cause excessive sweating. Certain parts of the body, like armpits give out an unpleasant odors from the secretion of sweat.

The skin exchanges oxygen, nutrients and fluid with underlying blood vessels, synthesizes new cells, eliminated dead and non-functioning cell. The cells of the integument requires adequate nutrition and hydration to resist injury, and disease. Adequate circulation is essential to maintain cell-life. The skin often reflects a change in physical condition by alteration in color, thickness, texture, turgor, temperature and hydration. As long as the skin remains intact and healthy, its physiological function remains optional.

Skin cleanliness is desirable from the esthetic as well as hygienic standpoint. It makes bodily comfort and self-respect. Hence, it is most necessary to keep the skin clean from dirt, so that the sweat glands may function properly. The best way to maintain cleanliness is the removal of sebaceous secretions of the skin, which is best affected by taking bath regularly by using soap and water, which should be followed by liberal application of some toilet powder containing a deodorant.

Baths

Baths are not only very necessary for cleanliness but also for their beneficial action on the skin and internal organs. The purposes of bathing are as follows:

1. Cleansing the skin removes perspiration, some bacteria, sebum and dead skin cells, which minimizes skin irritation, and reduces the chance of infection.
2. Stimulation of proper circulation is promoted through the use of warm water and gentle stroking of the extremities.
3. Improved self-image bathing promotes relaxation and feeling of being refreshed, and comfortable.
4. Reduction of body odors: Excessive secretion of sweat from apocrine glands located in the axillae and public areas causes unpleasant body odors. Bathing and use of antiperspirants minimized odors.
5. Promotion of range of motion (ROM): Movement of the extremities during bathing maintains join functions.

Regular baths and proper clothing is required to preserve the cleanliness of skin and to keep healthy. Otherwise skin problems can occur due to blockage of sebaceous glands with dirt. Baths not only help in cleaning but in maintaining good circulation of blood, a sense of freshness and tone of muscles. Baths should be taken regularly, but it may vary according to climatic conditions such as warm, cold, hot bath. Oil especially mustard oil is applied and massaged into the skin. Oiling helps to keep cool and soft skin. It should be remember, while taking care of skin that:

- Baths should not be taken after a full meal
- Special care must be taken to clean skin folds such as under chin, axilla, thighs, etc.
- In case of communicable diseases such as scabies, baths in wells or swimming pools should not be taken
- Sunbathes should be taken only a few minutes in the morning or late in evening and skin burn be prevented by over exposure of skin
- A well-balanced diet including vitamin A should be taken to keep the skin healthy
- Mosquito nets should be used to prevent certain diseases such as malaria, filaria and skin should be prevented from insect bite
- Over use of cosmetics should not be done as cosmetics can cause harm to skin
- In case of clothing, material used for clothes should not harm the skin when worn
- Clothing should be selected and worn according to the climate
- Undergarments needs to be changed frequently and those should be porous to absorb moisture.

A bath should be taken early in the morning or in the middle of the day, before taking meals. It should not be taken immediately after meals or after exhaustion due to fatigue. A good quality soap should be used, while taking bath, since the function of soap to wash away the sweat and dirt, and to emulsify the sebaceous secretions of the skin or the skin oils, thus rendering the cleansing of skin easier and quicker. Cheap toilet avoided. Baths may be classified as under:

- Cold bath 33–65°F (0.50–18.3°C)
- Tepid bath 80–90°F (26.60–32.2°C)
- Warm bath 90–98°F (32.2–36.6°C)
- Hot bath 98–10°F (36.6–37.7°C).

Cold bath

Cold bath acts as a stimulant to heart and it contracts the peripheral blood vessels. Young healthy persons should use cold water for a bath as it is invigorating, more refreshing and acts very simulative to improve the texture, tone, firmness and color of the skin, and stimulates the circulation of the blood throughout the body. It stimulates the skin and increases the power of the body to react the variation in the temperature. Cold bath should be taken as quickly as possible and body covered immediately afterwards. The first effect produce by taking a cold bath is to chill the surface of the body and that of a shock followed by constriction of superficial blood vessels, but vessels dilate very soon giving feeling of warmth, and pleasure to the individual. Some people taking plunge bath by immersing their whole body in the water (e.g. river, lake or stream) such baths are beneficial and are invigorating.

Tepid bath
Bathing in cool water can relieve tension or lower body temperature. Water temperature should be tepid (37°C or 98.6°F) rather than cold to avoid chilling and to promote slow cooling; this avoids temperature fluctuations. This type of bath is especially effective in reducing the body temperature of a small child with a fever.

Warm bath
Bathing in warm water relieves muscle tension. Water temperature should be 43°C (109.4°F). In warm bath the temperature is approximately that of the body. It is of value chiefly to clean the skin, particularly when soap is used. It does not have much stimulating effect on skin or the circulation. It soothes the nervous system and may be used to induce sleep, if taken just before retiring.

Hot bath
Hot bath has a temperature above that of the body. It raises the temperature of the surface of the body and dilates the superficial blood vessels and stimulates the sweat glands. It thus causes hyperemia through the skin by withdrawing a large quantity of blood from the interior organs. There is a danger of chilling of the body due to dilated skin vessels and so it is not advisable to go out in the cold after taking a hot bath. If hot bath is continued for long time it becomes depressing. Hot bath is not desirable for persons with heart disease. It is also not desirable to take hot bath soon after meal. Frequent hot bath in a day is not desired as an undue heat is lost. It lowers the blood pressure. It relaxes the body and removes fatigue and also means of combating insomnia. Vigorous rubbing of the body with rough and dry towel, after taking a bath is very beneficial, as it act as a massage to the skin, and provides a certain amount of bodily exercise circulation of the blood in the skin. It gives splendid feeling of glow and well-being.

Therapeutic bath
A good bath influences the structure of the skin, heart, blood pressure, respiration muscle tone, fibrous tissues and joints. There are several type of therapeutic baths such as soak, sitz baths, bran bath, electric bath, mud bath and mineral bath.

Soak bath: Local applications of water or a medicated solution can remove dead tissues or soften encrusted secretions. An aseptic technique is necessary when cleansing open or abraded areas of the skin. Soaks are also useful in reducing pain and swelling of inflamed or irritated skin surfaces.

Sitz bath: It cleanses and reduces inflammation of the perineal areas, and of a client who has undergone rectal or vaginal surgery or childbirth, or who has local rectal irritation from hemorrhoids or tissues water temperature depends on the client condition, but should be 43–45°C or 90–98°C. Cold sitz bath is more effective and relieving pain in the postpartum period.

Bran bath: It is used for removing the irritation of certain types of skin disease and for soothing effects. This type of bath is prepared by adding 1 pound of fresh bran in the 5 gallons of water at 103°F and the affected parts are bathed for 40–50 minutes keeping the temperature at about 103°F by adding hot water.

Electric bath: It is suitable for parts with impaired circulation and also in chronic rheumatism, weak muscle and flat foot, etc.

Mud bath: It is useful in chronic irritation of the skin and in constipation. Mud contains mineral matters and some of the mud may contain radioactive substances useful to the systems.

Mineral bath: Hot mineral bath in the warm space, e.g. hot springs (e.g. Rajgir in Bihar) is suitable for helping in cure of certain types of ailments. Water of such springs contains usually calcium, sulfur and radioactive substances. By taking such bath regularly for a few days in these springs, patient ailments such as gout, chronic rheumatism of muscles, joints and ligaments arthritis of septic origin, and osteoarthritis, etc. are generally benefited. Regular bath is not advisable to hypertensive and weak persons.

Bathing a client
Bathing a client is a part of total hygienic care. Bath can be categorized as cleansing or therapeutic. A physician order is necessary for bath designed for therapeutic purposes (e.g. tepid sponging) the order designates bath temperature, the body part being treated (soak) and any medicated solution used (i.e. saline, sodium bicarbonate, potassium permanganate) the complete bed bath, needed for clients who are totally depended and required total hygienic care. Bathing serves a variety of purposes including the following:
- It cleanses the skin
- It act as a skin conditioner
- It helps to relax a restless person
- It promotes circulation by stimulating the skin peripheral nerve endings and underlying tissues

- It serves as a musculoskeletal exercise through activity involved with bathing and thus improves joint mobility, and muscles tone.

Patient teaching

Teach patient not to scratch the lesions to avoid further irritation and to prevent infection.

Care of Hair

Proper hair care is important to the patients' self-image. Combing, brushing and shampooing are basic hygiene measures for all patients. Illness or disability may prevent patient from performing their own daily hair care. A bedfast patient's hair remembers that most patients are aware of their appearance at all time. Therefore, good hair care must be performed routinely at least daily to meet the hygiene needs of the patient. If the patient cannot carry out this part of his/her personal hygiene, the nurse will be required to give assistance. If the patient can take a shower or tub bath, the hair can be shampooed easily. A portable chair may be used in the shower or a chair may be placed in front of a sink.

For the helpless bedfast patient, the shampoo must be done in bed. A physician's instruction may or may not be necessary. Most facilities have portable blow dryers and curling irons available, as well as shampoo boards. Hair should be kept thoroughly clean and should always be required both by men and women. The scalp needs a good blood supply and massaging for a few minutes daily is of great benefit. Fresh air is stimulating and to go without a heat except in great heat is good. If the hair is not properly looked after, disease like ring worm and dandruff may arise. Lice may appear, if hair is kept untidy. A dry scalp, seborrhea sicca, is a condition of dandruff, i.e. epithelial scales are shed in excess. Only soft soap, shampoos should be used. A good homemade shampoo consists of 50 parts of oil of lavender. An oily scalp seborrhea oleosa is a condition of overactive sebaceous glands shampoo should be readily drying and so spirit is added to them. It is necessary to wash the hair once in a week with soap and water or soap nut solution prepared by steeping powdered soap nuts for a few hours in water (preferably hot water). Oil should not be used too frequently. It may however be used once a week after washing the hair with soap to restore natural grease. One should always practice to have one self and as far as possible avoid going to barber's shop for the purpose to avoid getting danger of infection.

Hairs reflect the general condition of the body such as change of color and texture of hairs to yellowish brown and dry hairs indicate deficiency of vitamins. The points to be keep in mind, while care of hairs are:

- Hairs should be washed regularly and depending upon the dust in the atmosphere
- Massage the scalp and brush hairs daily to improve circulation
- In case of head lice, hairs should get appropriate anti-lice treatment.

Head lice: In case of head lice or pediculosis, hairs should be treated with 1:1 ratio of kerosene and pure oil. This should be applied and managed at night and covered with a towel or cap and then next morning wash the hairs. The other treatment is 10% dichlorodiphenyltrichloroethane (DDT) powder.

Care of the Mouth/Oral Care

Oral Hygiene

Oral hygiene helps to maintain a healthy state of the mouth, teeth, gums and lips. Brushing the teeth removes food particles, plaque and bacteria massages the gums, and relieves discomfort resulting from unpleasant odors and tastes. Complete oral hygiene gives a sense of well-being and thus can stimulate appetite. Certain patients are at risk for oral disorders because of:

- Lack of knowledge about oral hygiene
- An inability to perform oral care
- An alteration in the integrity of teeth and mucosa resulting from disease or treatments.

Patient who are particularly at risk are those who are paralyzed, seriously ill have upper extremity activity limitations unconscious, confused, diabetic or no food per oral (npo) status. Patient who are undergoing radiation therapy receiving chemotherapeutic drugs or undergoing oral surgery also are at risk.

The nurse will allow the patient to brush his/her own teeth whenever possible. When the patient is unable to do so, the nurse will need to perform this procedure for them.

Tongue Care

The tongue should be cleaned by a tongue cleanser every morning.

Denture care

1. Patients should be encouraged to care of their own dentures as often for natural teeth to prevent infection and irritation.
2. If the patient becomes disabled, incapacitated or confused, the nurse must assist with denture care.
3. Dentures are expensive and easily broken, and are the patient's personal property; therefore they must be handled with care.

4. Dentures should be stored in an enclosed and labeled cup during soaking or when not worn. Patients should be discouraging from wrapping them in tissue or placing them on meal trays, since the dentures may be accidentally discarded.

In mouth, there are many species of bacteria always present as a rule; a healthy mouth is capable of dealing with these. Under conditions of sepsis, however, such as caries teeth, septic tonsils, unhealthy mucous membrane or infected sinuses, the stream of bacteria are constantly pouring into the mouth find these ideal conditions of growth, helped by remnants of food. The tongue becomes coated and sordes collect around teeth, and lips. Such a mouth may give rise to parotids, otitis media, infected of respiratory passages and via general circulation, rheumatic conditions, and remote septic foci. The tongue should be cleaned every morning, by a tongue cleanser. Mouth should be well-rinsed with some pleasant antiseptic mouthwash, such as glycerin of thymol and little of it should be used for gargling in the morning and at night after taking the last meal or drink.

The oral cavity functions in mastication, secretion of mucus to moisten and lubricate the digestive system, secretion of digestive enzymes, and absorption of essential nutrients. Common problem occurring in the oral cavity include the following:
- Bad breath (halitosis)
- Dental cavities (caries)
- Plaque
- Periodontal disease
- Inflammation of the gums (gingivitis)
- Inflammation of the oral mucosa (stomatitis).

Poor oral hygiene and loss of teeth may affect a client's social interaction, and body image as well as nutritional intake. Daily oral care is essential to maintain the integrity of the mucous membranes, teeth, gums and lips. Through preventive measures, the oral cavity and teeth can be preserved. Preventive oral care consists of fluoride rinsing, flossing and brushing.

Fluoride rinsing: Fluoride can prevent dental caries. Fluoride is a common component of many mouthwashes and toothpastes; however, people with excessive dryness or irritated mucous membranes should avoid commercial mouthwashes because of the alcohol content, which causes drying of mucous membranes. Educate clients about fluoride being an excellent preventive measure against dental caries, but excessive fluoride exposure can affect the color of tooth enamel.

Flossing: Floss daily in conjunction with brushing of teeth. Flossing prevents the formation of plaque, removes plaque between the teeth and removes food debris. Dental caries and periodontal disease can be prevented by regular flossing. Many floss holders are available to facilitate flossing.

Brushing: Teeth should be brushed after each meal. Brushing should be performed using a dentifrice (toothpaste) that contains fluoride to aid in preventing dental caries. An effective homemade dentifrice is the combination of two parts of salt with one part baking soda. Brushing removes plaque and food debris, and promotes blood circulation of the gums. Dentures should be brushed using the same brushing motion as that used for brushing teeth.

Before the procedure the nurse should:
1. Assess whether the client is able to assist with oral care and to what extent—promotes independence where possible.
2. Evaluate whether the client has an understanding of proper oral hygiene—promotes self-care and teaching.
3. Check whether the client has dentures—determine how oral care will be performed.
4. Assess whether inflammation, bleeding, infection or ulceration is present—determine how oral care will be performed and the need for additional assessment and intervention.
5. Assess what cultural practices must be taken into consideration—determine how oral care will be performed.
6. Assess whether there are any appliances or device present in the client's mouth such as braces, endotracheal tube or bridgework—determine how oral care will be performed.
7. Check the proper equipment is available to perform oral care—ensures a smooth procedure.

Care of Teeth

A tooth is a hard structure composed of dentine and the enamel covering the dentine, although it resembles bone, yet it is much harder. The enamel of teeth is the hardest tissue in the body. Once the enamel of teeth is completely formed, the cells that produced it disappear. Thus, it can then no longer receive nourishment from the body, the enamel is therefore incapable of repair. It covers only the exposed surface of the tooth, as within the jaw bone and the dentine of the tooth is covered with cement-like material called cementum. Dental hygiene is maintained by:
- Brushing
- Regular dental check up
- Diet
- Habits
- Use of fluorides.

Teeth should be cleaned at least two times a day. Toothbrush is one of the best way if used with proper technique, to remove food debris and dental plague. In case of diet, refined carbohydrates such as pastries, sugar, chocolates, etc. promote dental caries. Some of the fruits and vegetables such as apple, carrot and celery reduces the chances of dental caries. The habits such as chewing betel leaves, sucking bottle throughout the day are bad habits and can cause bad oral hygiene, so proper cleaning, and good habits can reduce the risk of dental caries.

A proper wholesome diet is necessary not only for building of strong teeth but also to ward off dental diseases. Milk, eggs, tomatoes, guavas, amlas and other citrus fruits including green leafy vegetables rich in vitamin C content should be included in daily diet. If the diet happens to be lacking in minerals and vitamin C, children may suffer from structural defects of the teeth, gums and bones. Full grown teeth also require balanced nourishment for their maintenance.

A set of sound teeth is a valuable asset because it contributes to personal appearance, in addition to providing an efficient chewing apparatus. Defective teeth make difficult or impossible the proper mastication of food and when teeth are infected, health of the body may become seriously impaired. So, it is very essential that the teeth should be regularly and thoroughly cleaned to ensure good digestion. They should be scrupulously cleaned at least twice a day. The first thing in the morning and last thing at night should be with a brush of moderate stiffness. Any place between the teeth where food gets lodged habitually and hence it is not removed promptly, and regularly is quite sure to decay sooner or later. The teeth rarely decay on a fully exposed surface. If there are cavities in the teeth they should be promptly got filled up. If they are altogether decayed and carious, they should be removed at once so that nearby teeth will not be decayed. Deposit of tartar upon the teeth should receive due attention and in this case, the teeth require scaling or else the roots will become exposed, which will eventually make the teeth loose. Children often suffer from caries either on account of deficiency of vitamin D or due to acid-forming bacteria formed on account of fermentation of carbohydrates. Especially amongst children, eating of sweets, chocolates, toffees, chewing gums, etc. are the promoting causes of dental caries or decay of teeth, because starch and sugar undergo fermentation of the mouth, and are converted to acids. Acid acts on the enamel of the teeth exerting a corroding action, destroying it and exposing underlying dentine. The microorganisms, which are teeming in the mouth subsequently, attach the exposed dentine. Therefore, natural fruits in the form of dry fruits such as figs, dates, apricots, plums, etc. may be given to children, which act as nourishing substitutes for candles.

In tropics, one has to be very careful about the occurrence of pyorrhea, alveolaris adults, which is perhaps form the scurvy due to deficiency of vitamin C. Pyorrhea is essentially a disease, which is characterized by the formation of pus pockets between the surfaces and gums, where germs freely thrive, and become a source of danger to the body. Since germs from the pyorrhea may threaten the danger of poisoning even the whole body, these germs from the pyorrhea pockets can reach any part of the body and give rise to conditions such as digestive disorders, pain in joints, eye trouble, heart and kidney diseases. Moreover, apart from these ailments, pyorrhea has its social aspects too. Pockets of pus and germs giver rise to foul breath, which may lead to avoidance of social relations, and loss of friends.

The movement of the brush should not only be from side to side, but from above downwards and inside the teeth. While brushing the teeth, sufficient pressure should be exercised, so that bristles of the brush may be forced between the teeth. All the inner, outer and biting surfaces should be brushed alike at least 5 times. Upper and lower teeth should be brushed downwards and upwards, respectively. The chewing and biting surfaces, should however be particularly at night followed by a hot, and tepid water gargles will go a long way to prevent caries, and pyorrhea. The gum tissues may be benefitted by massaging them with a fingertip smeared with toothpaste.

The use of toothbrush is not very sanitary because there is always the difficulty of keeping clean and the same brush is generally used for a considerably long period. If the toothbrush is to be used, it should be kept in boiling water for some time after use. It should be frequently changed.

In India a green neem or wicker twig, datum is used for cleansing teeth, which is very good from hygienic point of view, since it requires chewing and provides massage to the gums.

Care of Hands and Feet

Hands and feet often require special attention to prevent infection, odors and injury. Problems arise from abuse or poor care of the hands and feet, for example, biting nails or wearing ill-fitting shoes.

Hands are used to eat and work. They are generally dirty and infected. Therefore hands should be washed thoroughly with soap and water before eating food, after going to toilet. Nails need to be cut as dirt under long nail can harbor harmful organisms, which can deteriorate the health conditions. The points should be kept in mind, while taking care in case of hands are:

- Wash hands before taking meal and after going to toilet
- Cut nails short
- Keep the nail clean
- Trim the toe nails.

Assessment of the feet involves a thorough examination of all skin surfaces. The area between the toes should be carefully checked. Patients with diabetes mellitus or peripheral vascular disease should be observed for adequate circulation to the feet. The elderly are also at the risk for foot disorders, because of poor vision or decreased mobility.

Care of the hands and feet can be administered during the morning bath or at another time. Hands should be kept free from the cracks and roughness due to cold wind or constant use of antiseptic solutions. Glycerin (diluted) in account of its action of drawing fluid to it or some skin cream, which will prevent evaporation should be used until cracks heal. Scrupulous cleansing of hands with soap and water is very essential to prevent spread of infectious diseases such as cholera, typhoid, dysentery, etc. they should invariably be washed before taking meals, and during handling or preparing food.

Next to hands, the feet carry the greatest load of any part of the body, so obviously they have a tremendous effect on the rest of the body. These must be kept scrupulously clean by daily washing and carefully drying between the toes.

The feet contain many sweat glands and excessive sweating or hyperhidrosis necessitates frequent washing, and change of socks. Bromidrosis is excessive sweating with offensive odors and soreness of feet. The odor is due to composition of sweat. For this condition, the feet should be washed several times a day in boric acid solution, dried, dabbed with methylated spirit mixed with starch and boric powder. Socks and shoes must be changed each time after use; used socks washing and shoes be aired. Shoes with cork heels are good and should be washed with a spirit lotion.

Corns

Corns are caused by pressure of badly fitting shoes. The epidermis thickens and becomes thorny, and grows inward to a point. If they occur between the toes, they are kept moist and are called 'soft corns'.

Callosities

Callosities are formed as a result of pointed shoes. The great toe becomes bent in producing an angle at the junction of metatarsophalangeal joint. The head of the metatarsal is thus a projecting point on the inner border of the foot and is exposed to pressure. A callosity forms on this point of pressure and the bursa underneath becomes chronically inflamed. These conditions may be avoided by wearing suitable shoes.

Arch of the Foot

The inner bony arch should be 25.4–38.1 mm from the ground. Dropped arch is very painful and is caused for want of tone in the leg muscles with stretching of the supporting tendons, and ligaments under the arch. The chief remedies are massage of leg muscles, a built up sole, raised 6.35–12.7 mm on the inner side and provision of arch supports.

Care of the Nails

Nails require to kept clean and should be cut short periodically otherwise dirt will get lodged under them and may carry infection. The cuticle surrounding the nails should be pressed back periodically, say once or twice a week with a wooden stick. If necessary, the cuticle may be softened to bed by applying the dilute glycerin or liquid paraffin at night before retiring. As a majority of Indians eat meals with their hands and do not use spoon and forks, they should be careful about regular cleansing of their nails. The fingers should never be put in the mouth of the nose. Biting of nails with the teeth is also an unclean habit and is particularly dangerous in tropics, as intestinal infections are likely to be carried in this way to the human system. The nails should be cut horizontally, because if curved, the skin around them will be pressed over the nails and the pressure of the nails on this enfolding skin will cause symptoms usually attributed to 'ingrowing toe nails'.

Care of the Eyes

Special attention is paid to the cleaning of the eyes, ears and nose during patient's bath. The nurse often has the responsibility of assisting patients in the care of eyeglasses, contact lenses or artificial eyes. For patients who wear eyeglasses, contact lenses, artificial eyes or hearing aids, the nurse will assess the patient's knowledge and methods used to care for the aids, as well as any problems caused by the aids. Patients who cannot grasp small objects, have limited mobility in the upper extremities, have reduced or are seriously fatigued will require assistance from the nurse.

The eyes, ears and nose are sensitive and therefore extra care should be taken to avoid injury to these tissues.

Cleansing of the circumorbital (circular area around the eye) area of the eyes is usually performed during the bath and involves washing with a clean wash cloth moistened with clear water. The use of soap is generally omitted because it may cause burning and irritation. The eye is cleansed from the inner to outer canthus. A separate section of the wash cloth is used each time to prevent spread of infection. If the patient had dried exudate that is not removed easily with gentle cleansing, the nurse may first place a damp cotton ball or gauze on the lid margins to loosen secretions. Never apply direct pressure over the eyeball, because this may cause serious injury. Exudates from the eyes should be removed carefully and as often as necessary to keep the eye clean. Eyes reflect the physical health and needs at most care. Care should be taken, while reading and should be prevented from dust and even from injuries. The eyes should be cleaned and each individual should use their own bath towel and face towel.

Rubbing of eyes should be prevented, while reading books should be held 12–16 inches away from the eyes. To have good eyesight vitamin A is essential as in India most common causes of blindness is trachoma, injury, eyesore or eye infections.

The eyes are well-protected with eyelashes, tearing and a split second blink reflex and usually do not require special care. Secretions may collect along the margins of the lid and inner canthus, when the blink reflex is absent or when the eyes do not completely close. Lubricating eye drops may be ordered by the physicians. Sometimes, the eyes may be medicated and covered to prevent corneal drying, and irritation.

Many patients wear eyeglasses. This represents a large financial investment for them. Therefore, the nurse should take care when cleaning glasses and should protect them from breakage or other damage when not worn.

Eyeglasses should be stored in the case and placed in the drawer of the bedside stand when not in use to avoid accidental damage. Glasses are made of hardened glass or plastic that is impact resistant to prevent shattering, but can easily scratched. Plastic lenses require special cleansing solutions and drying tissues. Warm water is adequate to clean glass lenses and the use of a cloth to dry is best to prevent the lenses.

Most patients prefer caring for their own contact lenses. A contact lens is small, round, sometimes colored disk that fits on the cornea of the eye over the pupil. If the patient's condition does not permit him/her to remove the lenses, the nurse should seek assistance from someone who is familiar with the procedure. The lenses need not be reinserted until the patient is more capable of caring for the lenses himself/herself. It is important that the nurse protect those patients who are unable to care for their lenses properly, because prolonged wearing of contact lenses may cause serious damage to the cornea. There is a very large variety of products available for lens care. Each type of lens (hard, soft or rigid gas permeable) requires different cleansing technique. Each set of lenses is stored in a case with solution according to manufacturer's directions.

It is highly specialized receptor of the optic nerve. Its mechanism enables the light waves to reach the optic nerve endings producing sight. Eyes of the school children should be periodically examined and defects corrected, and treated. Children with such defects as myopia and those whose vision is liable to deteriorate should be kept under constant supervision, and suitable work chosen for them.

Tears have considerably bacterial power and are less injurious to conjunctiva than any other lotion. They are brought about by some emotional crisis by frustration, anger, sorrow or even by the sudden lifting of some frightening crisis. For example, when a mother finds her lost child who has not been drowned or kidnapped. Frequent bathing of eyes should not be encouraged. Disinfectant lotions should be used only when prescribed.

School children should be taught the importance of looking after their eyes. They should be asked to hold the printed page about a foot and half (0.45 m) from the eyes, and at an angle of 45–70° from horizontal surface. The light in the class room should be satisfactory and the print of the books should be large enough to prevent eye strain. An inflammation or accident of the eye should receive immediate attention.

Sore Eye

Sore eye is an infective disease and fairly widespread in villages all over the country. The infection is prevented in the discharge of the eyes and transmitted to the healthy persons through handkerchiefs or towel soiled with discharge by direct contact with eyes of an infected person. Indirectly the infections are spread through flies. When the germ of sore eye infect an individual, then transparent covering the eye called conjunctiva is damaged or it may get hurt by particles of foreign bodies such as dust particles and the eyes may therefore get red, and watery. In due course of time a discharge secretes from the eyes, which is infective and is disease producing.

Prevention
The following measures should be adopted:
- One should avoid open cases of sore eye as the disease is highly infectious
- Children with eye sore should never be allowed to mix up with the others

- Mothers should not use the end of dhotis or sarees to wipe away the eye discharge of their children
- Flies should not be allowed to sit on the sore eye
- Persons infected with sore eye should be asked to use separate handkerchiefs, towels, etc.

Generally the eye needs little daily care. Normally, eyes are continually cleansed by the production of tears and movement of eyelids over the eyes. Some clients, however, do have special eye care needs.

Contact Lenses

Self-care is the best method of care for a client with contact lenses; however, accidents or illness may render a client unable to remove, or care for the lenses. Some lenses may be left on the cornea for up to a week without damage. Most must be removed daily for cleaning and to prevent hypoxia of the cornea. It is a nursing responsibility to determine whether the client is wearing contact lenses and to properly care for the lenses, and the client's eyes. In acute situations, encourage the client to wear glasses, if possible send the contact lenses home with a family member.

Prosthetic Eyes

Some clients have an artificial eye (ocular prosthesis) in place. Artificial eyes are created to look identical to the client's biological eye. They are generally made from glass or plastic. Some artificial eyes are permanently implanted in the eye socket, but others must be removed daily for cleaning. The eye socket should be gently cleansed to remove crusts and mucus, and the prosthesis replaced in the eye socket.

Care of the Ears

The ears require proper care and attention. The child with running ears is constant danger of deafness or mastoiditis. Wax in ears, sometimes gives rise to partial deafness, so it should be removed by syringing. If dirt is allowed to collect for some time, it may develop into a large hard plug causing earache, boils and even deafness. No attempts should be made to remove wax by prodding any sharp pencil, hairpin or any pointed instrument. Similarly, do not let inexperienced people remove wax by unsterilized instruments or forcibly syringe the ear. The best way is to put a drop of warm oil like olive, mustard, coconut oil or glycerin (if available) for a few days. It will soften the hard wax and bring it the surface, which can be conveniently removed by a lean cotton swab wrapped on the point of a match stick or through syringing. The child with a running ear or perforation is drum should plug in his/her ear with cotton wool before entering a swimming pool for a bath. The infliction of casement by 'boxing' a person's ears should be heavily punished.

The ears are cleansed by the nurse during bed bath. A clean corner of a moistened wash cloth rotated gently into the ear canal works best for cleaning. Also, a cotton-tipped applicator is useful for cleansing the pinna. The nurse should teach patients never to use bobby pins, toothpicks or cotton-tipped applicators to clean the external auditory canal. These objects may damage the tympanic membrane (eardrum) or cause wax (cerumen) impacted within the canal.

Hearing Aids

Hearing loss is a common health problem. The ability to hear enables patients to communicate and react appropriately within their environment. There are several types of hearing aids available. The care of the hearing aid involves routine cleansing, battery care and proper insertion technique. The nurse will assess the patient's knowledge and routines for cleaning, and caring for the hearing aid. The nurse will determine whether the patient can hear clearly with the use of the aid by taking slowly and clearly in a normal voice tone. The nurse should have suggested the patient any additional tips for care of the hearing aid. When not in use, the hearing aid should be stored where it will not be damaged. The hearing aid should be turned off when not in use to prolong the life of the battery. The outside of hearing aid should be cleaned with a dry, soft cloth.

Ears should be kept clean. Outer ear cleaning can be done with soap and water. Remove the wax if the canal is filled with wax, as it can result in hearing difficulty. The wax is removed by using a drop of warm coconut oil, peanut oil, glycerin into ears and later on after a couple of day, wax is removed with a twisted piece of clean muslin. Do not use or put hard instruments into ear. In case an insert enters the ear, a little warm pure oil is put/poured into ear.

Care of the Nose

The patient can usually remove secretions from the nose by gently blowing into a soft tissue. This could be the only daily hygiene necessary; the nurse should teach the patient that harsh blowing causes pressure capable of injuring the eardrum, nasal mucosa and even sensitive eye structure. If the patient is not able to clean his/her nose, the nurse will assist using a saline moistened wash cloth or cotton-tipped applicator. The applicator should not be inserted beyond the cotton tip. If nasal secretions are excessive, suctioning may be necessary. When patients receive oxygen per nasal cannula or have a nasogastric tune, the nurse should cleanse the nares every 8 hours with a cotton-tipped applicator moistened with saline. Because secretions are more likely to collect and dry around the tube, the nurse will also need to gently cleanse the tube with soap and water.

A great care should be taken for nose and mouth. Proper cleaning of nose and mouth can be done in routine; otherwise it can cause health hazards. The nose functions as a filter for microorganism present in air. Presence of small hairs in nose warms the air before it moves to lungs.

Care of External Genitalia

The sexual organs require cleansing even more than other parts of the body. In the case of uncircumcised male penis, the foreskin should be retracted in the bath and the secretion washing away. If this is not regularly done smegma collect and undergoes bacterial decomposition with constant irritation, which may lead to excitement, and unclean habits, e.g. masturbation, etc.

In the case of females, the vulva should be washed in the bath. Commencement of menstruation is not a reason for stopping baths rather calls for their greater frequency. Girls in their childhood should be taught to wipe the anus backwards and not in the reverse direction so as to avoid introducing fecal organisms into vulva or the genital passage. Hygiene of menstruation is also important in girls.

Maintaining Posture

By posture is meant the characteristic form in which the body is maintained during its various activities. There is no single good posture known. Goodness of a posture consists of alignment of parts in relaxation rather than tension and readiness for action. It may be added that the postures of the solider on parade is generally taken as an ideal one, but mistaken concept. Correct mechanical use of body permits the internal organs to function efficiently. Good posture is desirable social assets because of its esthetic value. The vital body functions, i.e. respiration, circulation, exertion, digestion and coordination of body are in perfect physiological balance. The human body makes a poor show when a part of its anatomy is out of alignment. The causes of faulty posture are:

1. Inherited structural irregularities.
2. Malnutrition, which brings with it, insufficient muscular power to balance the body properly against the force of gravity.
3. Tight or constricting garments worn during preadolescent and adolescent ages.
4. Incorrect footwear especially shoes with high heels.
5. Insufficient physical activity, which results in muscular insufficiency and lack of wholesome mental attitude towards life.
6. Occupation, which confines the body in an improper posture for many hours a day.

Incorrect posture may interfere with the functioning of the diaphragm, causing it to sage downwards, thus seriously limiting the action of the diaphragm affects the blood flow in the large veins because the diaphragm does not produce the necessary pumping action to cause rapid return of blood. The sagging of diaphragm displaces the heart and abdominal organs by forcing them downward and forward. This may cause circulatory and digestive disturbances and in women may cause displacement of uterus, ovaries and other pelvic organs.

A common and troublesome fault of postures is an increase of lumbar curvature. This condition known as 'lordosis' or 'swayback' is accompanied by a forward and downward tilt of pelvic organs and protrusion of the abdomen. In this position the last lumbar vertebrae rests at too sharp an angle on the sacrum, producing a weak joint at this place. This results in a general strain on the muscle and ligaments of the lumbar region, producing pain; faulty posture is frequent cause of flow back pain, which is a common ailment of modern mankind.

A common structural change in the spinal column is 'kyphosis' or 'round back', which may result from a stopping posture habitually maintained. In this condition thoracic curve is increased, the shoulders and head are bent forward, and the chest is flat. Later a curvature of spine, known as 'scoliosis' is a condition in which the spine deviates sideways. It usually starts as a simple function lateral deviation. If untreated, it usually progresses to a double curve and finally the vertebrae, and ribs become permanently altered in shape. An individual may have both 'kyphosis' and 'lordosis' at the same time.

Performing Exercise

Exercise is very essential for the normal growth and development of the body, and perfect maintenance of health. It is also required to excite the demand of oxygen required for utilization of food and to promote the repair of worn out tissues. Attainment of bodily strength is essential to achieve success of life. A strong man can work with great vigor and zeal, and withstand cares, and snares of life better than another, who is comparatively weak in constitution.

Effects of exercise

The effects of exercise on various systems are as follows:

Respiratory system: During exercise the number of respiration is increased and breathing becomes deeper. The pulmonary circulation is quickened and brings into use all the air sacs of the lungs. There is a considerable increase in the amount of oxygen inhaled, carbon dioxide and water vapors exhaled. Outdoor exercise plays an important role in prevention of tuberculosis.

Circulatory system: Active exercise increases the force and frequency of the heart. Blood and lymph circulate more freely through the whole body. Oxygenation of the blood is very much increased. Lack of muscular activity tends the blood to stagnate in the abdominal viscera. Exercise is beneficial to the normal heart; for it keeps well-nourished in good tone and prolongs its usefulness.

Muscular system: The nutrition of the muscles is improved, which contributes to their growth and energy. Without exercise, muscles become pale and flabby, and begin to waste and wither away.

Cutaneous system: There is a marked increase of perspiration owing to increased action of the skin.

Alimentary system: Exercise brings about an increased assimilation of food and thus creates a demand for food. The appetite is improved and the actions of bowels are stimulated, it plays an important role in the prevention of constipation.

Urinary system: Quantity of urine is diminished, though the amount of urea remains unaltered. The excretion of uric acid is slightly increased.

Nervous system: The mind is refreshed and the powers of observation, precision and tolerance are developed.

Effects of excessive exercise

Excessive exercise causes either nervous or muscular fatigue or even both. It causes breathlessness, palpitation, hypertrophy of left ventricle, and renders small, frequent and irregular pulse. The voluntary muscles become exhausted due to overexertion, suffer in nutrition and gradually begin to wither away.

Exercise should never be carried on up to a stage, when the body becomes entirely exhausted, this fact of paramount importance, especially when the person taking exercise happens to be raw of untrained. It should not be too strenuous for the age of 40 years, intense exercise may do harm to persons not accustomed to vigorous physical activity. For middle age and old persons, walking is one of the best forms of exercise.

Exercise should be done in early hours of the morning or in the evening. It should not be done within 2 hours of heavy meal. One should not eat too soon either before or after exercise. Games should be encouraged since they combine recreation with exercise.

The risk of getting chill, however increases after exercise and therefore the surface of the body, which is exposed during exercise, required to be covered, and protected from undue loss of heat.

Clothing

Unlike animals, man has not developed natural means of protection from heat, cold and atmospheric phenomena. He/She has neither fur or feathers nor a thick layer of fat under the skin. Thus, he/she has to provide himself/herself with clothing and shelter. Clothing serves as a protective covering. In modern life in the case of civilized man, only about 20% of the body surface is normally exposed to air. The kind and extend of clothing worn have a direct bearing on human well-being:

- To afford protection to the body against effects of heat, and cold, and to protect body from external injuries
- To assist in the maintenance of body heat
- For decency and personal decoration
- Clothing influences metabolic change, if sufficient clothing is used.

CONCLUSION

Hygiene is maintained to preserve the health. It has two aspects such as environmental hygiene and personal hygiene. Environmental hygiene is maintained by maintaining domestic and community environmental hygiene. There are customs, which are associated personal hygiene. Indians are particular about personal cleanliness. Traditionally, people were using neem twigs or ash to do oral hygiene, which is still prevalent in some rural areas of India. But nowadays, tooth brushes are used to do oral hygiene. The bath as a part of personal hygiene is a ritual in India. The women after giving birth to a child have to take two or three ceremonial baths. Other hygiene conditions such as shaving, etc. are still prevalent as a custom in India. For maintaining personal hygiene, practices are adopted to care skin, hands, nails, hair, bowel and bladder, eyes, ears, nose and mouth, i.e. each part of body. A number of factors are associated with hygienic practices such as cultural factors, use of drugs, illness, weather, socioeconomic conditions. Unhygienic conditions lead to several health problems such as scabies, impetigo, diarrhea, cholera, conjunctivitis, dental caries, etc.

CHAPTER 25

Lifestyle: Physical Activity

INTRODUCTION

Physical activity refers to a body movement, produced by skeletal muscles that requires energy expenditure and produces progressive health benefits. Regular physical activity throughout life is important for maintaining a healthy body, enhancing psychological well-being and preventing premature death. Promoting health and fitness in elderly, is important to physical health and mental well-being. If the types of barriers can be identified, then appropriate interventions can be implemented for try to overcome these barriers and safely increase physical activity. Maintenance of physical activity decreases the risk for osteoporosis and falls, decreases peripheral resistance, and insulin resistance and helps to maintain mobility.

BENEFITS OF PHYSICAL ACTIVITY

Physical activity help to provide a means for an outlet for aggression, developing individual from negative influences, enhancing self-confidence and giving several recognition within the community, e.g. sports, games, dance, etc. The education provided to the people.

Physical activity helps to:
- Reduce the risk of overweight, diabetes mellitus and other chronic diseases
- Assist in improving academic program
- People to develop confidence, i.e. feel better themselves that they are healthy
- Reduce the risk for depression and the effects of stress
- The people to be productions and healthy citizen of nation
- Improve overall quality of life.

So, the regular participation in physical activity has been linked to an increased sense of identity and improved self-esteem.

Multiple health benefits or regular physical activity have been identified; regular physical exercise is effective in promoting and maintaining health, and preventing disease. Among the benefits of regular physical activity are increased muscle strength, endurance and flexibility, management of weight; prevention and management of coronary heart disease, hypertension, diabetes, osteoporosis and depression. Families can structure time and activities for family members. It is helpful, when the community in which they live promotes exercise by having accessible parks and walking or biking paths that help families select activities that provide moderate, regular physical exercise, rather than sedentary activities in the home setting.

There are many health and lifestyle benefits of physical activity for older adults. Regular physical activity helps to reduce the effects of aging such as limited mobility, balance, flexibility and muscle strength. Physical activities such as golf, bowels, swimming, tennis, bush, walking, talking, dancing, simply gardening, walking with the dog, all these activities play a vital role in old age, ensuring the old people to look and feel younger, and healthier and to live a better quality of life. Research shows that older adults with active lifestyles are often as healthy as less active people aged 15 years younger.

Physical activity promotes metal and physical health, and helps in the reduction of stress levels. American College of Sports Medicine and the American Heart Association in 2007, 5 days a week or vigorously intense cardio 20 minutes a day, 3 days a week and 8–10 strength-training exercises, 8–12 repetitions of each exercise twice a week. In order to lose weight or maintain weight loss, 60–90 minutes of physical activity may be necessary. The 30 minutes recommendation is for the average healthy adult to maintain health and reduce the risk for chronic disease.

Substance use and abuse is a major contributor to morbidity and mortality. Tobacco use has been identified as the single most preventable cause of death. It has been associated with several types of cancer, coronary heart disease, low birth weight, premature births, sudden infant death syndrome and chronic obstructive pulmonary disease. Furthermore, passive smoke has been linked to disease in nonsmokers and children. Drug use including alcohol is a major social and health problem. Drug use is associated with transmission of human immunodeficiency virus (HIV), fetal alcohol syndrome, liver disease, unwanted pregnancy, delinquency, school failure, violence and crime. The literature consistently identifies the effects of family factors, such as family closeness, families doing activities together and behavior modeled in the family as decreasing the risk of substance use in children.

Although, violence and abuse behavior are not limited to families, the amount of intrafamilial violence is thought to be underestimated. It is difficult to collect data and obtain accurate statistics on family violence because the issue is so sensitive for families. Evidence supports the intergenerational nature of violence and abuse, e.g. abusers were often abused as children.

Regular participation in physical activity during childhood to adolescence, build and maintain healthy bones, muscles and joints; helps to control weight, build lean muscle and reduce fat; prevents or delays the development of hypertension are help to reduce blood pressure (BP), and maintains optimum BP. Along with good nutrition, habits of physical activity provide long-term health benefits for youths. Physical activity is bodily movement of any type and may include recreational fitness, and sports activity such as jumping, rope, playing soccer, lifting weight as well as daily activities such as walking to the store, taking stairs or raking the leaves. Recreation means during the activities in spare time such as watching TV, video games and movies, etc. weekends, holidays and vacations devoted to recreation. It is an integral part of cultural activities. These are carried out for enjoyment and entertainment. There are many benefits, which includes it reduces the heart problems.

Regular physical activity is required regardless of the shape, size, health or age. Physical activity provides energy, strong muscles, less stress, less chance of heart disease, osteoporosis, diabetes and other illness. So one of the best ways to live a long and healthy life is through regular exercise. It might seem like a chore or you may think you do not have time. However, physical activity comes in many ways and forms, including gardening, housework and walking to the shops to buy the milk or newspaper.

The education sector has the potential to reduce the inequalities in health. Educational attainment influences socioeconomic position. Regular participation in physical activity has been linked to an increased sense of identity and improved self-esteem. Physical activity might be an ideal vehicle for engaging the most vulnerable young people is society.

Physical activity provides a mean for:
- An outlet for aggression
- Diverting individuals from negative influences
- Enhancing self-confidence
- Giving social recognition within the community.

EXERCISE

The National Institutes of Health (NIH) defines exercise and physical activity as follows (1995):
1. Physical activity is "bodily movement produced by skeletal muscles that requires energy expenditure and produces progressive health benefits."
2. Exercise is "a type of physical activity defined as planned, structured and repetitive bodily movement done to improve or maintain one or more components of physical fitness."

An activity exercise pattern refers to a person's routine exercise, activity, leisure and recreation. It includes:
1. Activities of daily livings (ADLs) that are required energy expenditure such as hygiene, cooking, shopping, eating, working and home maintenance.
2. The type, quality and quantity of exercise, including sports.

People participate in exercise programs to decrease risk factors for cardiovascular disease and to increase their health, and well-being. Activity tolerance is the type and amount of exercise or daily living activities an individual is able to perform without experiencing adverse effects (Table 25.1).

Table 25.1: Guidelines for physical activity

Features	Description
Frequency	Three times per week
Duration	Cumulative 30 minutes daily (can be divided throughout the day)
Intensity	Moderate intensity as measured by the talk test and perceived exertion scale
Type of exercise	Walking, biking and swimming are recommended for beginners, and older adults; activities that are more strenuous include jogging, running and jumping rope
Safety	Outside of the home, use appropriate safety measures such as checking equipment for proper function, wearing a helmet and other protective gear, using reflective devices at night, carrying identification and emergency information

Types of Exercise

Exercise involves the active contraction and relaxation of muscles. Exercises can be classified according to the type of muscle contraction (isotonic, isometric or isokinetic), and according to the source of energy (aerobic or anaerobic).

Isotonic Exercises

Isotonic (dynamic) exercises are those in which the muscle shortens to produce muscle contraction and active movement. Most physical conditioning exercises are running, walking, swimming, cycling and other such activities are isotonic, as are ADLs and active range of motion (ROM) exercises (those initiated by the client). Examples of isotonic bed exercises are pushing or pulling against a stationary object, using a trapeze to life, the body off the bed lifting the buttocks off the bed by pushing with the hands against the mattress and pushing the body to a sitting position.

Isotonic exercises increase muscle tone, mass and strength, and maintain joint flexibility and circulation. During isotonic exercise, both heart rate and cardiac output quicken to increase blood flow to all parts of the body. Little or no change in BP occurs.

Isometric Exercises

Isometric (static or setting) exercises are those in which there is a change in muscle tension, but there is no change in muscle length and no muscle or joint movement. These exercises involve exerting pressure against a solid object and are useful for strengthening abdominal, gluteal and quadriceps muscles used in ambulation; for maintaining strength in immobilized muscles in casts or traction; and for endurance training. Examples of isometric bed exercise would be extending the leg in supine position, tensing the thigh muscles and pressing the knee against the bed, holding it for several seconds. These are often called quadriceps (or quad) sets.

Isometric exercises produce a moderate increase in heart rate and cardiac output, but no appreciable increase in blood flow to other parts of the body:

1. Isokinetic (resistive) exercises involve muscle contraction or tension against resistance; thus they can be either isotonic or isometric. During isokinetic exercises, the persons moves (isotonic) or tenses (isometric) against resistance. Special machines or devices provide the resistance to the movement. These exercises are used in physical conditioning and are often done to build-up certain muscle groups, for example, the pectorals (chest muscles) may be increased in size and strength by lifting weights.

2. Aerobic exercise is an activity during which the amount of oxygen is taken in the body is greater than that used to perform the activity. Aerobic exercises use large muscle groups are performed continuously and are rhythmic in nature. Examples are walking, jogging, rope, rowing, bicycling, dancing, cross-country skiing, jumping rope, rowing, swimming and skating. Aerobic exercises improve cardiovascular conditioning and physical fitness. The accompanying teaching wellness care feature describes frequency, duration and intensity of exercise recommended for healthy adults.

Intensity of Exercise

Intensity of exercise can be measured in three ways:

1. Target heart rate: With this system, the goal is to work up to and sustain a target heart rate during exercise, based on the person's age. To determine the target heart rate, first calculate the person's maximum heart rate by subtracting his/her current age in years from 220. Then, obtain the target heart rate by taking 60–85% of the maximum. At least 60% of maximum heart rate is the recommended intensity. Because the heart rate are so variable among individuals, the tests that follow are replacing this measure.

2. Talk test: This test is easier to implement and keeps most people at 60% of maximum heart rate or more. When exercising, the person should be able to carry on a conversation even with some labored breathing. However, exercise intensity should be increased if the person can carry on with unlimited unlabored breathing. However, exercise intensity should be increased, if the person can carry on with unlimited unlabored discussion.

3. Borg scale of perceived exertion (Borg, 1998): This scale measures 'how difficult' the exercise feels to the person in terms of heart and lung exertion. The scale progresses are given in Table 25.2.

Table 25.2: Original Borg scale rated perceived exertion (RPE)

Rating	Perception of effort
6	
7	Very very light
8	
9	Very light
10	
11	Fairly light

Contd...

Contd...

Rating	Perception of effort
12	
13	Somewhat hard
14	
15	Hard
16	
17	Very hard
18	
19	Very very hard
20	

'Very very hard' corresponds closely to 100% of maximum heart rate. 'Very light' is close to 40%. Most people need to strive for the 'somewhat hard' level, which corresponds to 75% of maximum heart rate.

Anaerobic exercise involves activity, in which the muscles cannot draw out enough oxygen from the bloodstream and anaerobic pathways are used to provide additional energy for a short time. This type of exercise is used in endurance training for athletes.

Benefits of Exercise

Regular exercise is essential for healthy functioning of major body systems. The benefits of exercise on these systems are given below:
1. **Musculoskeletal system:** The size, shape, tone and strength of muscles (including the heart muscle) are maintained with mild exercise, and increased with strenuous exercise. With strenuous exercise, muscles hypertrophy (enlarge) and the efficiency of muscular contraction increases. Hypertrophy is commonly seen in the arm muscles of a tennis player, the leg muscles of a skater, arm and hand muscles of a carpenter.
   Exercise increases joint flexibility and range of motion. Bone density is maintained through weight bearing. The stress of weight bearing maintains a balance between osteoblasts (bone building cells) and osteoclasts (bone resorption and breakdown cells).
2. **Cardiovascular system:** Adequate exercise increases the heart rate, the strength of heart muscle contraction and the blood supply to the heart and muscles. Cardiac output (the amount of blood pumped by the heart) increases as much as 30 L/min. Normal cardiac output is 5 L/min.
3. **Respiratory system:** Ventilation (air circulating into and out of the lungs) increases. In strenuous exercise, the intake of oxygen increases to as much as 20 times normal intake. Normal ventilation is about 5 or 6 L/min. Adequate exercise also prevents pooling of secretions in the bronchi and bronchioles, decreases breathing effort and improves diaphragmatic excursion.
4. **Gastrointestinal system:** Exercise improves the appetite and increases gastrointestinal tract tone, facilitating peristalsis.
5. **Metabolic system:** Exercise elevates the metabolic rate, thus increasing the production of body heat and waste products, and calorie use. During strenuous exercise, the metabolic rate can increase to as much as 20 times the normal rate. Exercise increases the use of triglycerides and fatty acids, resulting in a reduced level of serum triglycerides and cholesterol. Exercise also enhance the effectiveness of insulin, lowering blood sugar. In diabetics, exercise can reduce their need for injecting supplemental insulin.
6. **Urinary System:** As adequate exercise promotes efficient blood flow, the body excretes wastes more effectively. In addition, of urine in the bladder is usually prevented.
7. **Psychoneurological system:** Exercise produces a sense of well-being and improves tolerance to stress. It may also improve self-concept by reducing depression, and improving one's body image. Energy level increases and quality of sleep is enhanced.

A number of factors affect an individual's body alignment, mobility and daily activity level. These include growth and development, physical health, mental health, nutrition, personal values and attitudes, and certain external factors.

Successful Routine Exercises

Maintaining a successful routine exercise, the following points to be keep in mind:
1. **Begin with a visit to your physician:** Tell your doctor, if you are about to start a new exercise routine, especially, if you have been inactive. He/She will recommend that you have a physical examination to preempt unwanted surprises with your health and ensure that you can exercise safely.
2. **Make good health as your goal:** Although having a smaller waistline or fitting into a smaller size has appeal, remember that your overall health is what matters most. Vow to not make excuses, commit yourself to a lifestyle change and start new habits that will improve the health and outlook.

3. Start slowly and gradually to build your fitness: A gradual approach to fitness will helps to ensure that you maintain your routine and prevent injuries.
4. Eat for balanced energy: Be sure that your overall diet is well-balanced to give you the energy that you need throughout the day and during your workout. Since, eating just before you exercise can lead to cramping, consume and easily digestible food such as a banana at least an hour before you workout.
5. Keep written log of your exercise schedule and set goals: In addition to being a good reminder of what you have done at each workout, a written log will give you a chance to work toward a goal and see what you have accomplished as you progress through the weeks and within a month.
6. Exercise each day: Establishing a routine, often makes it easier to stick with an exercise program.
7. Exercise with a friend whenever possible: Walking or running with a friend will give you the chance to visit as well as ward off boredom. Many exercisers suggest their workout files by when they have a partner.
8. Change your route if you walk or run: Check out new neighborhoods, tracks and parks. Changing the scenery can add interest to your routine and help prevent boredom.
9. Warm up, workout and cool down with each exercise session: Starting slowly and gradually increasing the intensity of the workout in a good way to prevent injuries.
10. Include music in the routine: Music is a good distraction from the monotony of exercise. Use faster tunes to boost the intensity of your workout and calmer music to help you cool down.
11. Consider safely: Choose routes with little traffic. Walk or job on sidewalks, whenever possible. If you exercise outside, schedule your workout during the day. When exercising at dawn, dusk, or at night, wear bright colors and reflectors, so that you can be easily spotted.
12. Keep changing your exercise: Try yoga for stretching and balance. Brisk walking, running, jogging and spinning is useful for enhancing for endurance and weight training to build strength. Cross training or combining a variety of exercise in the weekly routine is the best way to boost the your metabolism, and ensure overall strength and fitness. Make a point of adding extra activities in a day, such as taking the stairs instead of the elevator, and walking instead of driving to lunch.
13. Dress appropriately for activity: Layer clothes in winter for warmth and comfort. Wear fast-drying fabrics, such as polyester blends that wick away moisture and helps to keep you warm. Be sure that your shoes fit well and are made for the activity you have chosen.
14. Focus on a pleasant memory, thought, fantasy or activity, while you workout: Some exercisers find inspiration in positive self-talk as they workout.
15. Have a positive outlook about weather: Exercising outside in light rain, on cloudy days and even cold, windy days can energize you to make feel more in touch with the weather elements.
16. Get plenty of sleep: Sleep is essential for getting a good workout. If you did not have enough sleep, either take a rest day or modify your workout, so that it is less vigorous.
17. Drink at least 2 liters of water per day: Remember that your body content 70% water. If you have not had enough to drink, your workout is likely to fail short of your expectations.
18. Listen to your body: If you are tired or beginning to get a cold, take a break. Your body needs time to rest and repair.
19. For added physical activity and sociability, take a dance class: Dancing provides a terrific aerobic workout and burns up to 300 calories in 1 hour. Remember that increased physical activity of any kind will helps to keep you healthy.
20. Do not let anything come between you and your fitness routine: Since exercise is one of the most important things that you can do to maintain good physical and mental health, be sure to include, it in your daily routine no matter what scheduling complications you encounter. Make exercise as essential as bathing, brushing your teeth, eating and sleeping.
21. Eat a healthy diet: A healthy, low-fat diet, i.e. combined with regular exercise can help guard against obesity, diabetes, high BP, insomnia, depression, anxiety osteoporosis, cancer and heart disease.
22. Reward yourself: Take a hot bubble bath, get a massage or a new outfit to celebrate your hard work.

SLEEP AND REST

Sleep is the most important for maintaining healthy lifestyle. It is process of relaxing. Deprivation of sleep for several consecutive days leads to lack of energy, irritability, blurred vision and memory loss. The need for adequate sleep is very essential:

1. Sleep means a state of altered consciousness, throughout which varying degrees of stimuli produce weakness. It is a recurrent, altered state of consciousness that occurs for sustained periods, restoring energy and well-being. Sleep is an active and complex rhythmic state involving progression of repeated cycles, each representing different phases of body and brain activity.

2. Sleep is a cyclic occurring state of decreased motor activity and perception. Body functions slow and metabolism falls by 20–30%, so the body conserves energy. Sleep is characterized by altered consciousness; a sleeping person is unaware of the environment and responds selectively to external stimuli. For example, an alarm clock, bright light or other 'meaningful' stimuli usually will awaken a sleeper, but everyday background noise and soft light will not.
3. Rest refers to a condition in which body is in a decreased state of activity with the consequent feeling of being refreshed. People at rest feel mentally relaxed free from anxiety and physical calm. Persons at rest are in a state of decreased mental and physical activity that leaves them feeling refreshed, rejuvenated, and ready to resume the activities of the day.
4. Rest is a condition in which body is inactive or engaging in mild activity, after which the person feels refreshed. A person at rest is calm, at ease relaxed, and free of anxiety and stress. People rest by doing things they find calming and relaxing. For example, reading, listening to music, watching television, doing needle work, praying or meditating, gardening, baking, playing golf, walking and camping.

Although necessary and beneficial, rest without sleep is inadequate. At rest, the body is disturbed by all external stimuli, whereas sleep it is screened from them by altered consciousness. Thus, as we discuss next, sleep restores the body; rest alone cannot do this.

Need for Sleep and Rest

People experience fatigue as the energy level goes down and wastes accumulate, and we desire to have rest. Energy is restored during rest and the waste build up is diminished. Rest and sleep are dependent upon our ability to relax. We need more muscular exercise in order to relax, rest and counteract fatigue. Physical activity usually leaves the muscles relaxed, whereas prolonged mental activity alone leaves the muscles tense. Fatigue is protective as it makes the person aware of our need to have rest. Efficiency and performance decreases as fatigue increases. Tobacco, alcohol or other drugs used to relax are not good to use, as they have dangerous side effects and cause the person to borrow excessive amounts of energy from his own emergency reserves. These drug increases the fatigue instead of decreasing it. Sometimes the diseases such as anemia, heart failure, depressed thyroid or adrenal function, cancer or any chronic infection produce fatigue, then it is known as pathological fatigue.

Factors that produce fatigue are:
- Overeating
- Lack of exercise
- Stress
- Stale air
- Not drinking enough of water.

The human body has a 24-hour cycle of wakefulness and sleeplessness regulated by an internal clock. This cycle means that we are naturally wakeful in the morning, when it gets light and naturally sleepy and when it gets dark at night. During sleep at night the central nervous system (CNS) is recharged. The rest is important to life as the vital organs are designed with built-in rest periods, such as the heart rests between each beat, stomach rests between each meal and the lungs between each breath. But rest and relaxation cannot take the place of sleep.

The need for sleep and rest is important in quality of life for all people. All individuals need and receive different amounts, and qualities of sleep and rest, physical and emotional health depend on the ability to fulfill this basic human need, without rest and sleep, the ability to concentrate, make judgments, and participate to activities decrease and irritability increase. It has been relieved then sleep restores well-being; relieves stress and anxiety, and restores ability to cope and to concentrate on ADLs.

Sleep problems may cause clients to seek health care or problem may go unnoticed period. Nurses care for clients who often have pre-existing sleep disturbance and for clients who develop sleep problems as a result of illness, and hospitalization. Ill persons often require more sleep and rest than healthy ones. The environment of a hospital or long-term care facility and activities of healthcare personnel may also make sleep difficult. Identifying and treated sleep disturbances is an important goal of a nurse. Nurse must understand the nature of sleep, the factors influencing the client's sleep habits.

We spend more time in sleeping than engaging in any other single activity; about 8 hours a day or 2,688 hours a yearly nearly one third of our lives. So why is sleep so important? Before you try to answer, think back to the last time you had a poor night's sleep. Remember the mental fogginess, the physical fatigue, the feeling of slight nausea. Missing even one night of sleep can reduce mental performance and long periods of sleep deprivation can result in stress-related illnesses, and injuries (e.g. from an automobile accident). The reason is that sleep and rest are essential for physical, mental and spiritual well-being.

Theorists do not agree on all of the functions of sleep, but studies have shown that adequate sleep restores energy. Despite of the fact that some regions of the brain are more active during sleep than when we are awake, our total energy output is reduced while we sleep, giving the body time for restoration and repair. Research indicates that sleep strengthens the immune system; animals deprived of sleep or more vulnerable to infection. Sleep may also improve learning and adaptation, giving the individual a chance of mentally repeat and rehearse facts; and situations before they are encountered in wakeful life. Some evidence suggests that sleep and dreaming may facilitate the storage of long-term memory, perhaps by assisting brain in reorganizing, and storing information. Sleep also appear to reduce stress and anxiety, improving our ability to cope and concentrate on ADLs.

Sleep/Rest and illness are interrelated. Illness and injury increase the need to sleep and at the same time make it difficult to sleep. In turn, lack of sleep increases the susceptibility to illness by compromising the immune system. People who are ill or injured need more sleep than usual to restore energy needed for tissue repair and healing. However, they often have difficulty resting because of pain and other symptoms of their illness. Lack of sleep and rest increases, our susceptibility to illness, and the pain of illness and injury increases our susceptibility to disturbed sleep.

Because sleep enhances wellness and speeds recovery from illness, promoting sleep is an important independent nursing intervention. In this chapter, learn how to recognize signs of sleep disturbance, as well as factors that interfere with patients' sleep and specific measures to facilitate sleep for each client.

Sleep Requirements

Sleep needs vary widely among individuals. Average sleep requirements based on age are shown in Table 25.3. Even though the accepted standard has been 8 hours per night for adults, there is really not 'correct' amount or pattern of sleep that maintains well-being in all people. In spite of individual variations, however, different sleep patterns are characteristic of different age groups.

Infants have overall greater sleep time than any other age group. Newborns sleep as much as 16-20 hours a day in periods ranging from one to several hours. Sleep time gradually decreases over the next few months, but throughout the 1st year of life, a minimum of 14 hours of sleep per day is recommended. Most infants sleep several hours during one overnight period with a morning and afternoon nap each day.

A baby sleeps throughout the day and need about 16 hours of sleep a day. As one grow older, the frequent napping changed to one long period of sleep. For normal functioning, an adult require 4-8 hours at night, with an average of 7-7½ hours and minimum number of hours of

Table 25.3: Average sleep requirement to age

Age group	Hours/Day
Newborns (birth to 4 week)	16–20
Infants (4 week to 1 year)	14–16
Toddlers (1–3 year)	12–14
Preschoolers (3–6 year)	11–13
Middle and late childhood (6–12 hour)	10–11
Adolescents (12–18 year)	8–9
Young adults (18–40 year)	7–8
Middle age adults (40–65 year)	7
Older adults (65 year and older)	5–7

sleep is 6 hours a night. The elderly (about 80 years and over) may only need about 5 hours sleep a day. According to Chokroverty, Dement, Vaughan, Hauri and Linde, less than 4 hours a night sleep is considered unhealthy and will increase the risk of serious illness such as coronary arterial disease and stroke. Sleep needs changes over the lifespan and with the decreasing age. Nine or more hours also have been associated with poor health status.

After the 1st year of life, sleep duration gradually decreases. In most adults, sleep of 7-8 hours is fully restorative; however, there are wide individual variations. In some cultures, total sleep time is divided into an overnight sleep period and a mid-afternoon nap.

The elderly are more prone to physical conditions that disrupt sleep. These conditions include chronic pain, arthritis, obstructive sleep apnea, sleep movement disorders, frequent urination, gastrointestinal problems, inability to exercise. Alzheimer's disease and Parkinson disease, increased stress and loss of social support may interfere with sleep.

Older adults spend significantly less time sleeping, but need more rest than younger adults. Usually older adults rest or nap during the day, go to bed early and get up early. They take longer falling asleep and their arousal periods during sleep are longer, and more frequent. Frequent waking is commonly due to physical discomfort, anxiety and nocturia. If the sleep is interrupted, the person will need to sleep longer to feel restored. If the older adult does not increase the total time in bed, she may experience fatigue, irritability and impaired cognition.

Physiology of Sleep

Sleep is a set of complete physiological processes. It involves a sequence of state maintained by highly integrated CNS, endocrine, cardiovascular, respiratory and muscular system. Each sequence can be identified by specific behavior, physiological response and pattern of brain activity.

The timing of the sleep-wake cycle and other circadian rhythms such as body temperature is controlled, at least in part by the suprachiasmatic nucleus control the production of melatonin, which is believed to a potent sleep induced. Sleep is a rationally occurring readily reversible altered state of arousal characterized by a decreased responsiveness to the environment. The mediator of arousal and of sensory stimulation is the reticular activity system (RAS). The RAS is located in the brain stem and contains projections to the thalamus and cortex. The diffuse network of neurons in the RAS is in a strategic position to monitor ascending and descending stimuli through feedback loop.

Although, the RAS provides the anatomic framework for arousal it in the neurotransmitters than serve on the chemical messengers. The onset of sleep and each subsequent sleep stage is an active process involving delicate shifts in the balance of several of these transmitters.

The transition from the awake state to non-rapid eye movement (NREM). Sleep is marked by decreases in the concentration of serotonin, norepinephrine and acetylcholine. The later transition to rapid eye movements (REM) sleep is marked by dramatic increases in acetylcholine and further drop in serotonin, norepinephrine. As REM sleep continues the concentration of serotonin and norepinephrine increases eventually stopping REM sleep. Cholinergic activation with release of acetylcholine seems to re-establish REM sleep the continuous interaction of these two system thought to produce the normal alterations between NREM and REM sleep. Other neurotransmitters such as gamma-aminobutyric acid (GABA) and dopamine are also relieved to have part in the reciprocal process involved in shifts in sleep state.

All these neurotransmitters are actively involved and waking processes as well. For example, neurons that produce serotonin and norepinephrine play a role in the modulation of sensory input, mood, energy and information processing including attention, learning and memory. Thus, it can be seen that imbalances in these neurotransmitters induced through sleep pattern disturbances, medications or diseases may reciprocally affect not only sleep but also aspect of sensory processing mood and cognition. REM sleep may be especially important for maintain mental activities such as learning, reasoning and emotional adjustments sleep also serves as an energy-conserving measure for most of the body parts except the brain.

Sleep can be defined behaviorally, functionally and electrophysiologically. The electrophysiologic monitoring of sleep, which is called polysomnography can divide sleep into REM and NREM sleep. NREM further divided into stages 1 through 4. These stages vary in depth, but are characterized by lack of eye movements, low and fragmented cognitive activity.

Factors Affecting Sleep

People vary not only in the amount of sleep they need but also in their sleep patterns. Some people are refreshed after napping for 15–20 minutes; others feel groggy after napping; still others cannot nap at all. Many people routinely waken several times a night and do not report being tried, whereas others report fatigue, and loss of mental clarity if their sleep is even minimally interrupted. In short, sleep quality has both subjective and objective components. It is related to:

1. The total amount of sleep.
2. How well the person slept.
3. Whether the person obtained the needed amounts of NREM and REM. Several factors affect the amount and quality of sleep.

Age

Age is important factor affecting the duration of sleep. But sleep patterns are also affected by age. For example, newborns and young children experienced long REM sleep periods; young adults spend about 25% of their sleep in REM sleep; and older adults experience significantly less REM sleep.

Children and adolescents

Young children experience sleep-related problems a few times a week. The problems included trouble falling asleep, frequent awakenings, nightmares and heavy snoring. Environmental stimuli such as the sounds and lights of older family members activities, may make it difficult for young child to sleep or the child may have difficulty 'winding down' after hectic activities in the late afternoon, and early evening hours. Toddlers and preschoolers are often frightened to go to bed because of imagined monsters or intruders or they may waken frequently at night because of bad dreams, the need to use the bathroom, illness, heavy snoring, tossing off the bedclothes, or falling out of bed. School age children may suffer sleep disturbances because they are anxious about meeting new classmates or having a new schedule, or they may be excited about an upcoming competition, or other activity.

The growth spurt that occurs during adolescence increases the need for sleep. At the same time, teenagers may not sleep well, because of increased demands at school; staying up late to watch television, surf the internet or study; dating or staying out late with friends; or the effect of alcohol or drugs. Some teens consume large amounts of caffeinated colas and other beverages that can delay or disturb sleep.

Young adults

College students may pull 'all-nighters' to cram for exams or experience insomnia because of worries about grades or future career choices. Young adults may drive themselves too hard to succeed, prompting late nights at work or sleep loss due to hectic travel schedules or work-related stress.

Parents of young children often sleep poorly. Breast-feeding mothers typically need to feed their infants one or more times each night until the infant begins take to solid foods. Parents of toddlers often wake to care for a child who is having a nightmare is ill or needs to use bathroom. Studies found that some parents lose as many as 200 hours of sleep a year because of their children's poor sleeping patterns.

Middle-aged and older adults

Middle-aged adults may experience insomnia because of their stress of career demands, the need to care for a parent or martial or financial problems. Menopausal women may be awakened by hot flashes. Older adults may feel displaced in the workforce and worry about their impending retirement. Older adults also suffer sleep disturbances because of nocturia, the side effects of medications and discomfort or pain.

Lifestyle Factors

Lifestyle factors influencing sleep include work, exercise, nutrition, and use of medications and drugs. As noted earlier, a person who changes work shifts frequently may find it difficult to sleep at the right time. Moreover, people who cross time zones frequently because of business travel may experience difficulty falling asleep, early wakening or day time fatigue:

1. Exercise promotes sleep: If it occurs at least 2 hours prior to bedtime. Fatigue from a normal physically active day is thought to promote a restful night's sleep. However, the more tired person is the shorter the first period of REM sleep.
2. Foods can either promote or interfere with sleep. A meal high in saturated fats near bedtime may interfere with sleep. Dietary L-tryptophan, an amino acid found in milk and cheese may help to induce sleep, although some studies indicate that the protein in these foods actually increases alertness, and concentration. Carbohydrates seem to promote relaxation through their effects on brain serotonin levels. In general, satiation induces sleep, whereas many people, especially infants and children have difficulty in falling asleep, when they are hungry.
3. Nicotine and caffeine: Both CNS stimulants and interfere with sleep. Smokers tend to have more difficulty falling asleep and more easily roused than nonsmokers. People who stop smoking often experience temporary sleep disturbances during the withdrawal period. Caffeine blocks adenosine and thereby inhibits sleep. However, individuals vary greatly in their sensitivity to caffeine. Some people can consume coffee throughout the day and evening suffer no loss of sleep, whereas, others cannot consume even small amounts of caffeine without suffering insomnia.
4. Alcohol consumption: If heavy may hasten the onset of sleep; however it disrupts REM and slow wave sleep, and may cause spontaneous awakening with difficulty returning to sleep. In addition, some people heavy alcohol can prompt nightmares during REM sleep. Because alcohol is a diuretic, it can interrupt sleep by inducing nocturia.
5. Medications for sleep: Medications to induce sleep (i.e. hypnotics) tend to increase the amount of sleep, while decreasing the quality. Ambien (zolpidem tartrate) promotes normal REM sleep and appears to influence sleep quality less than do other hypnotics. Amphetamines, tranquilizers and antidepressants reduce amount of REM sleep; barbiturates in addition, interfere with NREM sleep. Opioids such as morphine suppress REM sleep and cause frequent awakening. Beta blockers are reported to cause insomnia and nightmares.

Illness

As we noted earlier, illness increases the need for sleep and rest. At the same time, its associated mental and physical distress can cause sleep problems. Fear of the unknown outcome of an illness and role changes associated with hospitalization can cause anxiety. Disease symptoms such as fever, pain, nausea and respiratory conditions (e.g. shortness of breath, dyspnea and sinus congestion) can also interfere with sleep.

Anxiety increases gastric secretions, intestinal motility, heart rate and respirations. All of these factors contribute to a restless night. Anxiety also stimulates the sympathetic nervous system, increasing the level of norepinephrine. This decreases stage 4 and REM sleep and leads to more awakenings. Depression may be associated either with almost constant sleeping or with insomnia.

Environmental Factors

Environmental factors can promote or inhibit sleep. Some people need a cool room, whereas others need warmth. Some prefer heavy bedclothes and other likes to sleep with just a light sheet. Noise can also inhibit sleep, but a person can become habituated to noise over time and be less affected by it. Some people routinely fall asleep to music or while listening to a radio or television. Usually, loud noises are needed to awaken a person in NREM stages 3 and 4, and REM sleep.

Any change in the usual environmental stimuli can affect sleep. For example, when people who are accustomed to sleeping in a darkroom are hospitalized, they may have trouble falling asleep because of light outside their window or filtering into the room from the hallway. A patient used to falling asleep next to his wife may have trouble sleeping alone in a hospital bed. Equipment noise, the muffled sounds of busy medical surgical unit or the labored breathing, or snoring of a roommate also can interfere with the patient's ability to sleep.

To improve the quality of sleep

The following points are improved the quality of good night sleep:

- Do not take stimulants such as coffee, drugs and the rich spicy food in the late afternoon, and at night before going to bed and also do not watch TV before going to bed
- Do not drink alcohol to induce sleep
- Have a regular sleep and wake schedule
- Do not go to bed on either an empty or a full stomach, as big evening meals interfere will good sleep
- Adopt the ways to relax yourself before going to bed such as:
    - Have a warm bath
    - Listen to music
    - Meditate.
- Do relaxation exercise and avoid household chores, exercise, paperwork and stimulating activities for at least 2 hours before bedtime
- Do breathing exercises
- Maintain comfortable temperature of sleeping room, bedroom
- Sleep in a dark, quiet, well-ventilated room. Leave the windows open to allow fresh air in to the room
- Wear comfortable and light dress, such as pajamas or a nightgown
- Use lighter weight covers instead of heavy blankets
- Take naps before lunch, not in the evening. A 15 minutes rest before lunch is worth about 45 minutes of night time sleep
- Do not cover the head, while sleeping
- Beds should not sag or be too soft
- The pillows should be flat, except the cases where the head should be elevated a few inches such as hiatus hernia and heart failure.

Sleep Disorders

Sleep disorders are classified by their signs and symptoms. The more common disorders fall into two groups:

1. Dyssomnias: Sleep disorders characterized by insomnia or excessive sleepiness. They include insomnia. Sleep-wake schedule (circadian) disorders, sleep apnea, restless leg syndrome, hypersomnia and narcolepsy.
2. Parasomnia patterns of waking behavior that appear during sleep, e.g. sleep walking.

As already the following common sleep disorders, while promoting sleep includes:

1. Insomnia: It is characterized by difficulty in falling asleep, intermittent sleep or early awakening from sleep.
2. Hypersomnia: It is characterized by excessive sleep, particularly during day.
3. Narcolepsy: It is a condition characterized by uncontrolled desire to sleep (force while conversation or while driving, etc.).
4. Sleep apnea: It refers to periods of no breathing between snoring intervals. The person may not breath for longer periods of 10–20 seconds to as long as 2 minutes. Long periods of interval drop oxygen level in blood.
5. Sleep deprivation: It refers to a decrease in the amount consistency and quality of sleep. The symptoms of sleep deprivation are enlisted in Table 25.4.
6. Somnambulism: Sleeping wailing, night terrors and nightmares.
7. Nocturnal enuresis: Bedwetting.
8. Bruxism: Teeth grinding and take measures to induce sleep.

Table 25.4: Symptoms of sleep deprivation

Physiological symptoms	Psychological symptoms
Hand tremors	Moods
Decreased reflexes	Disorientation
Slowed response time	Irritability
Reduction in word memory	Decreased motivation
Decreased reasoning and judgment	Fatigue association
Cardiac dysrhythmias	Sleepiness
Decreased auditory and visual alertness	Hyperactivity

Measures to Induce Sleep

All ailments require a sleep environment with a comfortable room temperature and proper ventilation, minimal sources of noise, a comfortable bed and proper lighting. In a hospital, the nurse can control noise in several ways, which include the following:

- Close doors to a client's room
- Reduce volume of nearly telephone and paying equipment
- Wear rubber, soled shoes, avoid wearing clogs
- Turn off bedside equipment, which is not in use, e.g. oxygen and suction
- Avoid abrupt loud noise such as flushing a toilet or moving a bed
- Keep necessary conversation as low levels, particularly at night
- Conduct discussion or nursing report in a private separate room away from client
- Turn off the TV or radio unless client prefers soft music, and nurse can apply following comfort measures to promote sleep:
    - Administer analgesic or sedatives about 30 minutes before bedtime
    - Encourage clients to wear loose fitting nightwear
    - Remove any irritant against the client's skin such as moist or wrinkled, or drainage tubing
    - Position and support body parts to protect pressure points, and aid muscle relaxation
    - Offer a massage just before bedtime
    - Provide caps and shock for older clients, and those from the cold
    - Administer necessary hygienic measures
    - Keep bed linen clean and dry
    - Provide comfortable mattress
    - Encourage client to void before going to sleep.

Management

1. **Melatonin:** This is widely sold as sleep aid, but remains controversial in medical circles. Melatonin is a hormone produced by the pineal gland.
2. **Herbal sleep aids:** Herbal remedies for sleep problems include Chamomile tea, Valerian root, hops, lavender and passion flower. Like Melatonin, these herbal remedies have not undergone extensive testing for benefits and safety.
3. **Factors affecting sleep** should be assessed as given below:
    a. Physical illness: For example, respiratory disease (asthma and cold), hypertension and cardiac disease (chest pain).
    b. Drugs and substances: For example, hypotonics, diuretics, antidepressant and stimulant alcohol, caffeine, digoxin, beta blockers and narcotics (morphine).
    c. Lifestyle: Night duties, late night, etc.
    d. Sleep pattern: Daytime sleepiness or sleep.
    e. Emotional stress: Worries.
    f. Exercise fatigue.
    g. Calorie intake: Weight loss or gain influence sleep, i.e. less calories and excess calories intake.

Keep in mind the sleep requirement of individuals, i.e. generally 8 hours of sleep every night has been accepted giving no reasons. There is not rigid formula for normal periodicity and duration of sleep. It is important, however that each person follow a pattern of rest that maintains well-being. Usually, on the average infants sleep from 14 to 20 hours each day. Growing children require from 10 to 14 hours of sleep. Adults average 7–9 hours; although 4 hours of range observed in many normal adults.

Recreation

Recreation means undertaking of such activities in spare time, which offer relaxation from work and also stimulate the relaxation. The spare time is neither spent by working nor by sleeping. It includes watching TV, video games, movies, listening to music and the radio or participating in outdoor activities such as fishing, etc. Growing interest and funding via grants and taxation have resulted in an official parks and recreation department, which provides venues and staffing for organized sports, at risk youth activities, arts and craft. There are recreational halls, recreation parks, etc. for carrying out the recreational activities to gain personal satisfaction in free time. As it has become an organized activity of government and for profit organization.

Weekends, holidays and vacations are usually devoted to recreation in many societies. Recreation and leisure are an integral part of cultural activities. Cultural activities are carried out for enjoyment and entertainment as in case of celebration of birthday or marriage, for personal growth and development to learn new skills, to meet new people and to change the mood or behavior. Recreation has the positive benefits for people's physical and mental health. Recreation and leisure are both most important components of a balanced and healthy lifestyle. Leisure time is a time away from work and commitments. During this people can do what they want to do. Everyone feel satisfied, once the recreation activities are carried out in their leisure time.

Advantages of Recreation

1. Recreation provides the people a sense of identity and personal autonomy.
2. Recreation maintains physical and mental health thereby improves the social well-being.
3. Recreation adds meaning to individual and community life.
4. It contributes to people's overall quality of life.
5. Recreation encourages personal growth.
6. It allows self-expression.
7. It provides increased learning opportunities.
8. It satisfies the needs.
9. Recreation helps in reducing the physical health problems. The physical activities such as games, sports, etc. increases the muscle strength and circulation thereby reducing the physical health problems. It increases the productivity at work, especially when combined with a healthy lifestyle and a balanced diet.
10. It has equal benefits for mental health. Several studies have shown that the physical activities during recreation has caused a reduction in the symptoms of mild or moderate depression, stress and anxiety.
11. Participation in recreation activities also have social benefits as it creates opportunities for socialization. It contributes to social cohesion by allowing people to meet, connect and network with others. When families do things together in their leisure time, then it contributes to family bonding.

So people should look for opportunities, which have fun in the leisure time such as:

- Plan family outings and vacations that include physical activity (hiking, backpacking, swimming, etc.)
- Play the favorite music to recreate themself in leisure time
- Dance with someone or by themself
- Join a recreational club that emphasizes physical activity
- Play games or participate in sports in free time
- As picnic do outdoor activities and enjoy the sight with friends and family, and do fun.

SEXUAL LIFE AS A FORM OF ACTIVITY

Sex is most primitive and vital for all expressions. Sex is the term most commonly used to identify biological male or female status. The term sex also used to describe sexual behavior. Sexuality is the collective characteristic that marks the difference between the male, the constitution and life of the individual as related to sex.

Sexual health is the integration of the somatic, emotional, intellectual and social aspect of sexual being, in ways that are positively enriching, and that enhance personality, communications and love (WHO, 1995).

Sexuality is important in developing self-identity interpersonal relationships, intimacy and love. In its broader sense, sexuality involves all aspects of being and behaving. The components that contribute to the development of sexuality are numerous both biological and psychological components exist all ages. Factors that affect sexuality, include development level, culture, religious values, personal ethics, disease processes and medication:

1. The development of sexuality begins with conception and continues throughout the life span. Every society develops expectations about acceptable forms of sexual expressions.
2. Culture: Sexuality regulated by the individual culture. For example, culture influence the sexual nature of dress, rules about marriage, expectation of role behavior and social responsibilities, and specific sex practices.
3. Religions values: Religion influences sexual expressions. It provides guidelines for sexual behavior and acceptable circumstance for the behavior, as well prohibited sexual behavior, and consequences of breaking the sexual rules.
4. Personal ethics: Ethical approaches to sexuality viewed separately from religion. Sexual expressions such as masturbation, oral or anal intercourse and cross dressing are accepted by some groups, and not acceptable to some groups. So, many individual two groups have developed their own written or unwritten codes of conduct based on the ethical principles.
5. Health status: Healthy minds, bodies and emotions are necessary for sexual well-being. Many health factors can interfere with a person's expression of sexuality. For example, common disorders that may alter sexual expression such as heart disease, prostate cancer, hysterectomy, diabetes mellitus, spinal cord injury, surgical procedures, joint disease and chronic pain, sexually transmitted diseases (STDs) and mental disorder.
6. Medications: Many medications have side effects that affect sexual functioning. For example, antidepressants may slow ejaculations, beta blockers and cardio time decreases sexual desire.

Sexual response and love play (recreation) involve people's emotional, psychological, physical and spiritual make-up, which plays a significant role in sexual satisfaction. It is within the role of the nurse to support and facilitate healthy sexual expression and accurate knowledge of the sexual response cycle is important to this role (Table 25.5).

Table 25.5: Physiological changes associated with the sexual response cycle

Phase of the sexual response cycle	Signs present in both sexes	Signs present in males only	Signs present in females only
Excitement/Plateau	Muscle tension increases as excitement increases Sex flush, usually on chest nipple erection	Penile erection; glans size increases the excitement Appearance of a few drops of lubricant, which may contain sperm	Erection of the clitoris Vaginal lubrication Labia may increase two to three times in size Breast enlarge Inner two thirds of vagina widens and lengthens; outer third swells and narrows Uterus elevates
Orgasmic	Respiration may increase to 40 breaths per minute (bpm) Involuntary spasms of muscle groups throughout the body Diminished sensory awareness Involuntary contractions of the anal sphincter Peak heart rate (110–180 bpm), respiratory rate (40/min or greater) and blood pressure (systolic 30–80 mm Hg and diastolic 20–50 mm Hg above normal)	Rhythmic, expulsive contractions of the penis at 0.8 intervals Closing of the internal bladder sphincter just before ejaculation to prevent retrograde ejaculation into bladder Closing of the internal bladder sphincter just before ejaculation to prevent retrograde ejaculation into bladder Orgasms may occur without ejaculation Ejaculation of semen through the penile urethra and expulsion from the urethra, and expulsion from the urethral meatus The force of ejaculation varies from man to man and at different times, but diminishes after the two to three contractions (stage 2 of the expulsive process) A refractory period during which the body will not respond to sexual stimulation; varies, depending on age and other factors from a few moments to hours or days	Approximately 5–12 contractions in the orgasmic platform at 0.8 intervals Contraction of the muscles of the pelvic floor and the uterine muscles Varied pattern of orgasms, including minor surges and contractions, multiple orgasms, or a simple intense orgasm similar to that of the male

Sexual Response Cycle

Commonly occurring phases on the human sexual response are following similar sequence in both females and males regardless of sexual orientation. It does not matter, either, if the motive for being sexually active is true love or passionate lust.

The response cycle starts in the brain with conscious sexual desires called the desire phase. Sexually arousing stimuli, often called erotic stimuli, may be real or symbolic. Sight, hearing, smell, touch and imagination (sexual fantasy) can all invoke sexual arousal. Sexual desire fluctuates within each person and varies from person to person. If people suppress or block out conscious sexual desires, they may not experience any physiological response. Although, psychological causes are the more common cause of a lack of sexual desire, medications, drugs and hormone imbalances can also block sexual desire.

The excitement/plateau phase involves two primary physiological changes. Vasocongestion is an increase in the blood flow to various body parts resulting in erection of the penis and clitoris, and swelling of the labia, testes and breasts. Vasocongestion stimulates sensory receptors within these body parts that in turn transmit messages to the conscious brain, where they are usually interpreted as pleasurable sensations. When stimulation is continued, vasocongestion increases until released by orgasm or fades away. Likewise, myotonia an increase of tension in muscles, may increase until released by orgasm or it may also simply fade away.

The orgasmic phase is the involuntary climax of sexual tension, accompanied by physiological and psychological release. This phase is considered the measurable peak of the sexual experience. Although, the entire body is involved, the major focus of the orgasm is felt in the pelvic region. Male orgasms usually lasts 10–30 seconds, while female orgasms last 10–50 seconds. Men usually have an ejaculation and expel semen as part of their orgasms. Before puberty and in later years, males experience orgasms without ejaculation.

The resolution phase, the period of return to the unaroused state, may last 10–15 minutes after orgasms or longer, if there is no orgasm. This phase in females is quite varied as some women experience multiple successive orgasms followed by a longer period of resolution.

Sex or Love Play

Mention love play and many people think of sexual intercourse of two people caught up in hot passion. Much of our sexual activity, however, does not fit this description.

Over a lifetime, sexual fantasies and solo sex are the most common sexual outlets for women and men, single and coupled persons, and heterosexual, gay/lesbian and bisexual persons. Masturbation is the ongoing love affair that each of us has with ourselves throughout our lifetime. It is the way we discover our erotic feelings and learn about our sexual response. Mutual out hurrying to genital interaction before both partners are ready. Masturbation shared with a partner is a safe alternative to unprotected genital sex.

Male-to-female or female-to-female oral-genital sex is known technically as cunnilingus. This involves kissing, licking or sucking of the female genitals including mons pubis, vulva, clitoris, labia and vagina. Fellatio is oral stimulation of the penis by licking and sucking. 69 position is simultaneous oral-genital stimulation by two persons. Preconceptions and myths are a major deterrent for those who have not tried oral sex.

Anal stimulation can be a source of sexual pleasure because the anus has a rich nerve supply. Stimulation may be applied with fingers, mouth or sex toys such as vibrators. The anus is surrounded by strong muscles and the rectum contains no natural lubrications. The inserting of finger or penis in the rectum requires relaxation and water-soluble lubricants as energy levels, pain and immobility may have an effect.

For older individuals, physical factors such as energy levels, pain and immobility may have an effect. Libido generally diminishes with general ill health, chronic diseases that cause disability or pain and depression. Many prescription medications can also diminish sexual desire.

A common form of sexual activity for heterosexual couples is genital intercourse. Penile-vaginal intercourse can be both physically and emotionally satisfying. There are varieties of positions for this kind of intercourse; the most common is lying face to face (with female or male on top). Side lying, standing, sitting and rear-entry positions are also used. Side lying, female-on-top and rear-entry positions facilitate clitoral stimulation, either by penile or manual contact. The choice of intercourse positions and activities depends on physical comfort, beliefs, values and attitudes about different practices.

During intercourse, the man moves the penis back and forth along with vaginal walls by rhythmic thrusting movements of his hips. At the same time the woman may mover her own body to match the partner's hip movements. Movements continue until orgasm is achieved by one or both partners. Simultaneous orgasm is difficult to achieve. After coitus, caressing, hugging and kissing can increase the shared intimacy, and should be encouraged.

The other form of genital intercourse is anal intercourse, during which the penis is inserted into the anus and rectum of the partner. Anal intercourse most commonly practiced by gay men, but a number of heterosexual couples engage in it as well. Positions for anal intercourse are similar to those for penile-vaginal intercourse, with minor difference due to the position of the anus.

Current practices dictates the use of a condom in both forms of intercourse to prevent the transmission of disease. Because anorectal tissue is not self-lubricating, a lubricant must be used on the condom. Also, since normal bacterial flora from the bowel can produce infection in other parts of the body, the used condom should be removed and another applied before inserting the penis into the other body orifices.

Altered Sexual Function

The ability to engage in sexual behavior is of great importance to most people. Many people experience transient problems with their ability to respond to sexual stimulation or to maintain the response. A smaller percentage of people experience long-standing problems.

Sexual health refers to the integration of somatic, emotional, intellectual and social aspects of sexual being, in ways that are positively enriching, and that enhance personality, communications and love (WHO, 1975). This definition recognizes the biological, psychological and sociocultural dimension of sexuality.

Sexuality and sexual functioning are aspects of health and well-being. The characteristics of sexual health includes:

- Knowledge about sexuality and sexual behavior
- Ability to express one's full sexual potential, excluding all forms of sexual coercion, exploitation and abuse
- Ability to make autonomous decisions about one's sexual life within a context of personal and social ethics
- Experience of sexual pleasure a source of physical, psychological, cognitive and spiritual well-being
- Capability to express sexuality through communications touch, emotional expression and love

- Right to make free and responsible reproductive choices
- Ability to access sexual health care for the prevention and treatment of all sexual concerns, problems and disorders.

Benefits of Healthy Sex

People want to live with love and closeness. Apart from being important for love life, sex also plays a more important role in our healthy life. As healthy sex leads to healthy life, needs to have continued with an active satisfying sex life. Many health benefits of an active sex life includes:

1. Sexuality activity is a form of physical exercise as 7,500 calories are burnt around in a year with making sex three times a week, which is equivalent to jogging 75 miles (Michael Cirigliano).
2. During sexual activity, the amount of oxygen in cells raised thereby helping organs and tissues functioning at optimum level.
3. Programming sexual activity is a kind of physical exercise, which increases testosterone, the testosterone helps to keep mens bones and muscles strong.
4. Sexual activity lowers the levels of the body's total cholesterol.
5. Sexual activity lowers the level of arthritic pain whiplash pain and headache. Where the hormones that are released during sexual excitement and orgasms can elevate pain thresholds (Beverly Whipple).
6. Regular ejaculation, during sex will help washout building fluids within the gland and provide prostrate protection. Sudden changes may also trigger prostrate problems.
7. Sex can be a very effective way of reducing stress levels. Affectionate touch will increase levels of the bonding hormone, i.e. oxytocin, which will help and encourage frequent sexual desire. Sexual activity can increase a woman's estrogen levels that protect her heart.

Sexual Problems

Sexual problems of adults include erectile dysfunction, rapid ejaculation, retarded ejaculation, sexual arousal disorders, orgasmic disorders, vaginismus, dyspareunia and vaginal pain. Female sexual dysfunction (FSD) means the disorders related to sexual desire and/or sexual pain, arousal, orgasm causing significant personal distress. It can be related to age or health problems. According to Janet Casperson, 40–50% of adult women have at least one or more manifestations of sexual dysfunction. These disorders may or may not have a negative effect of the quality of life or the health of the woman, but when they cause enough personal distress then they will seek treatment. Unfortunately, most women with FSD do not seek treatment although there are treatments and options that can help.

Sexual life can be severely affected in patients with health problems. In one of the study it has been seen that sexual life has been affected in patients with psoriasis. Sexual life impairment was investigated in all eligible adults hospitalized with psoriasis in a dermatological hospital from February 2000 to February 2002. The results of study reveal that 35.5 (psoriasis disability index)–71.3% (impact of psoriasis on quality of life questionnaire) reported to have experienced sexual problems because of psoriasis.

A study conducted on 13,882 women and 13,618 men of at least 40 years in 29 countries by Miranda Hitti on Global Gender Gap in sexual well-being reveals that all over the world, men are more satisfied with their sex lives that women. According to this study, sexual well-being was defined as the physical and emotional satisfaction of sexual relationship, satisfaction with sexual health or function, and the importance of sex in one's life.

Nurses have the responsibility to assess the attitudes toward sexuality, including factors that affect attitudes and behavior. An understanding of sexual stimuli and response patterns can help individual to have satisfying sexual relationship. Before assisting clients with sexual problems, nurses must acquire accurate information about sexuality, identify and accept their own sexual values, and behaviors as well as those of others to be comfortable acquiring, and disseminating information about sexuality, responsible sexual behavior that includes prevention of STDs, and unwanted pregnancies, and self-examination of the breasts and testicles. Counseling clients with altered sexual functions can be facilitated.

Sex is the most primitive and vital of all expressions. Its language has remained unchanged. Its craving is till powerful. People want love and closeness. Apart from being important for love life, sex also plays a more important role in the health life. As healthy sex leads to healthy life, but as we grow older, we want to continue an active, satisfying sex life. Making live is good for both body and soul. There are many health benefits of an active sex life.

SPIRITUAL LIFE

The word 'spiritual' derives from the Latin word 'spiritus,' which means 'to blow' or 'to breathe', and has to connect that gives life or essence to being human. Spirituality refers to that part of being human that seeks meaningfulness through intra-, inter-and transpersonal connection. It is generally involves a belief in a relationship with some higher power, creative force, divine being or infinite source of energy.

Spiritual health or spiritual well-being is manifested by feeding of being generally alive and purposeful, and fulfilled (Ellison, 1983). Spiritual wellness is a 'way of living', a lifestyle that views and lives life as a purposeful and pleasurable, that seeks out life sustaining, and life enriching options to be chosen freely at every opportunity, and that sinks its root deeply into spiritual values and/or specific religion beliefs (Pitch, 1998). The characteristics indicative for spiritual well-being includes senses for life, gratitude, appreciation of both unity and diversity humor, wisdom, generosity, ability to transcend the self and capacity for unconditional love.

Concept related to spirituality includes religion, faith, hope, transcendence and forgiveness:

1. Religion is organized system of beliefs and practices. It often a way of spiritual expression that provides guidance for believers in responding to life questions and challenges. Religion rules of conduct, typically influenced concurrently by culture, may also apply to matters of daily life such as dress, food, social intention, menstruation and sexual relationships.
2. Faith is to believe in or be committed to something or someone. It gives life meaning, providing the individual with strength in times of difficulty. For example, individual who is ill, faith, whether in a higher authority (i.e. God) in oneself, in the healthcare team or in combination of all providing strength and hope.
3. Hope is a concept that incorporates spirituality, it is a process of anticipation that involves the interaction of thinking, acting, feeling and relating, and is directed toward a future fulfillment, i.e. personally meaningful.
4. Transcending is the capacity to reach out beyond oneself to extend oneself beyond personal concerns and to take on broader life perspectives, activities and purposes. It is also thought to involve a person's recognition that there is something other or greater than the self and seeking, and valuing the greater other, whether ultimate being force or value.
5. Forgiveness in receiving increased attention among healthcare professional. For many client's illness or disability bring a sense of shame and guilt. The health problem is interpreted as a punishment for past sins, e.g. why having sex before marriage? Why I have breast cancer?

Spiritual Care

To implement spiritual care nurses need to be skilled in establishing a trusted nurse-client relationships. Clients have a right to receive care that respects their individual spiritual and religion values. Since, the spiritual beliefs and practices are highly personal nurses must respect the rights of people to hold their own spiritual beliefs, and to communicate these to others. Nurses need to be aware of their own spiritual beliefs in order to be comfortable assisting others. Nurses cannot rely solely on their own spiritual practices, they need to be aware of the arrays of religion traditions and spiritual expressions to which their clients may subscribe. Example of spiritual needs that need of love, hope, trust, forgiveness to respected and valued, dignity, meaning to the fullness of life, values, creative, connect with high power and need to belong to a community.

Spiritual Distress

The spiritual needs of clients and support persons often come into focus at a time of illness. Spiritual belief can help people accept illness and plan for what lies ahead. Spiritual distress refers to a disturbance on or challenge to a person's belief or value system that provides strength, hope and meaning of life. Possible factors in spiritual distress include physiological problems, treatment-related concerns and situational concerns. Spiritual distress may be reflected in a number of behaviors, including depression, anxiety, verbalization of unworthiness and fear of death.

Nurses can support clients religious practices, if they understand needs related to holydays, sacred writings, sacred symbols, prayer and meditation, dietary practices, dress requirements or prohibitions, healing, birth rituals and death rituals. Nursing interventions that promote spiritual well-being include offering ones presence, supporting the client religion practices, praying with client and referring the client to a religious counselor.

SELF-RELIANCE

Self refers to a person's essential being that distinguishes them from others, especially considered as the object of introspection or reflective action. It is a person's particular nature or personality. It is also one's own interests or pleasure. The term reliance is the dependence on or trust in someone or something. Self-reliance is the reliance on one's own powers and resources rather than those of others. Otherwise self-reliance means one's ability to respond to different life situations faced at different times or occasion. So, the self-reliant person is able to think on himself/herself control his/her life and trust their own judgment.

Self-reliant individuals exhibit competitiveness, self-control and inclination to take interpersonal risks. They are task-oriented cool in interpersonal relationship and inclined to direct others activities.

Definition and Goals

Self-reliant refers to a process by which people make full use of their strength, wisdom, resources, creativity, culture and national heritage, i.e. it is the process by which the person becomes independent.

Self-reliance is the strategy where the people can develop the consciousness of being them matters of their destiny. It is concerned with the attainment of fundamental structural redistribution of world production and trade, control over surplus generation, and allocation of power at local, national and international level. The goals of self-reliance are:

- To make full use of people's strength, wisdom, resources, creativity, culture and national heritage
- To promote social justice, distribution and the utilization of economy's most abundant resources to engender public participation in the development process
- To reduce the concentration of economic power and wealth in few persons
- To establish more egalitarian patterns of international economic relation
- To self-reliant individual must have a plan, which involves in setting his/her own goals. The goals must be written, specific and realistic have a plan for its achievement, and its time.

Health and Self-reliance

People have to be healthy, they should be self-reliant, poverty, hunger and poor health hinders, the self-reliance. Due to this health problems will be emerge. The cost of seeking health care can mean less food for the family, which leads to malnutrition. The malnutrition leads to illness among children as well as others. People, who are suffering with poverty, cannot have the proper capacity to work hard and not taking care of family including their children. For which self-reliance is possible by educating them on preventing and management of illness, provide linkages to local health centers, and clinics. It can help them to have savings account and special funds to pay for medical services by the government and non-governmental organizations educate them for affordable credit, and secure savings immediately improve a family's ability to become self-reliant by launching family-based business. Regular income, savings and assets help hungry families.

So self-reliance means one's ability to respond to different life situations faced at different times. Self-reliance is understanding that you cannot control everything that happens in your life, but you can take charge of your life.

A self-reliant person is able to think for himself. He has control of his life. He trusts his own judgment. A self-reliant have the inner resources required to cope with situations at own. To be a self-reliant you have to work very hard. On becoming self-reliant, one begin to grow and change and see the life as well as oneself differently. Dependence is opposite of self-reliance. Dependence means allowing others to take care of you. It is expecting people to fix your life when you have acted irresponsibly. Dependence demands what you want right now and expecting someone to give it to without any effort on your part.

Self-reliance is an ambiguous concept with no universal definition. Self-reliance forces the members of the society to provide incentives for mobilizing local resources that otherwise would have lain idle and to organize or reorganize domestic, social, economic and political relations in ways that are commensurate with the local values and changes them.

DIETARY PATTERN

Food is a mixture of chemicals, some of which are essential for normal body functions. These chemicals are called nutrients. Nutrients are required for various processes in the body. They serve a source of energy for muscle contraction and cellular function. Some of them are also important to the structure of bones, muscles and all cells. Some of the nutrients also help in regulating bodily processes such as BP, energy production and temperature regulation. In a true sense, a nutrient may be defined as a chemical, whose absence from diet (for a long time) results in specific change in health, i.e. lead to deficiency symptoms. Moreover, its supplementation (before a permanent damage occurs) can reverse such a change. Hence, nutrients are the essential chemicals in food that the body needs for normal functioning and good health. These must come from the diet, because they either cannot be made in the body or cannot be made in sufficient quantities.

Needs of Nutritious Diet

A nutrient, thus may be referred to as any substance in food that the body can use to obtain energy, synthesize tissues or regulate functions. A substance that obtained in the diet, because the body either cannot make it or cannot make adequate amounts of it is referred to as an essential nutrient.

Energy must always be available to the body, if normal life is to continue and it is delivered in the form of food, of which the energy providing nutrients are carbohydrate, fat, protein and alcohol. Energy is required for:

- Tissue maintenance and the internal work of the body, the resting metabolic rate of the body

- Pregnancy or lactation
- Physical activity or muscular work
- Deposition of adipose tissue
- Growth in the young or increasing muscle mass.

The energy required by physical activity or muscular work of any kind depends upon several variables, such as:
- Type of movement
- The muscle masses involved
- Duration of the activity.

Certain types of movement, if they involve relatively small muscle masses such as one are, or if they are performed in an awkward or inefficient manner, may be very fatiguing for the individual, but may require only small amounts of energy expenditure.

It is very important to distinguish clearly and objectively between the different influences of a short strenuous burst of exercise and of long-continued mild activity. The contrast between the vigorous, exhausting exercise on the one hand and the gentle, unhurried routine on the other may tend to deceive us in our assessment of their relative importance for energy expenditure. These values for energy expenditure may be applied, where appropriate to individuals or population groups, but this requires fairly extensive knowledge and experience of the levels, and the variability of energy expenditure.

Pregnancy and lactation may be difficult conditions to assess in relations to energy expenditure. In pregnancy, the theoretical increase in energy intake needed to build-up the maternal and fetal tissues, but in practice this is often counterbalanced, to some extent, by a diminution in physical activity. This change in the pattern of daily life may also occur in lactation, so these are situations that are perplexing to evaluate in general terms and may pose considerable problems in measurement.

Diet is the kind of food that a person, animal or community habitually eats. It is sometime a special course of food to which a person restricts themselves to lose weight or for medical reasons. Individual needs nutritious food and the person cannot eat individual nutrient. They tend to eat nutrients in the combined form of meals. The meal, which is adapting for life is considered as dietary pattern. The dietary pattern will change according to circumstances, i.e. according to age, place of living, season and others. Promoting good nutrition and dietary habits is a key to maintaining child health. The first 6 years are the most important for developing sound lifetime eating habits. The quality of nutrition has been widely accepted as an important influence on growth and development. It is now becoming recognized for an important role in disease prevention.

Factors Influencing Dietary Pattern

Dietary pattern are influenced by many factors, which includes cultural factors, psychological factors, food additives, eating habits and education of the individual, groups and community. It is difficult for a person to achieve a good dietary pattern because of given factors.

Cultural Factors

Culture determines the dietary pattern as the person is brought in that particular culture since birth. An individual learns about the diet from family, i.e. the type of food and vegetables available in the family and eaten by family members. Foods eaten differ from culture to culture such as food eaten by Punjabis differ from the food eaten by Keralite. Depending upon this an idea can be made that which type of disease will be prevalent in particular culture.

Psychological Factors

A healthy diet may be difficult to achieve for a person with poor eating habits. The reason being the tastes acquired in early adolescence and preferences for fatty foods.

Food Additives

Fast foods are now becoming the most popular in young generation. In fast food there are food additives such as artificial sweeteners, colorants, preserving agents and flavorings that influence the persons eating and causes health problems such as cancer or attention deficit hyperactivity disorder (ADHD).

Eating Habits

Eating habits are also associated with the dietary pattern such as eating very frequently, two times, three or more times in a day. Wrong eating habits leads as accumulation of toxins within the system.

Education

Dietary pattern is influenced by the education. If people are made aware of the merits and demerits of eating less nutritive food and inadequate or excess of all nutrients or a specific nutrients will help them to take good meal of appropriate amount.

Individual's health is dependents on the diet they are taking inadequate and unhealthy diet taken can be harmful to individual's health. So, the diet should contain all the nutrients required to maintain health. Healthy diet includes all the nutrients in appropriate amounts from all food groups includes fresh vegetables and fruits. A nutritious diet ensures overall well-being helps to maintain healthy body mass index (BMS), reduces the risk for several debilitating diseases such as cancer, cardiovascular diseases, diabetes mellitus, osteoporosis and smoke, etc.

Nutrition is the sum of all the interaction between an organisms and the food it consumes. In other words, nutrition is what a person eats and how the body uses it. Nutrients are organic or inorganic substances found in foods and are required for body functioning. People require the essential nutrients in food for the growth and maintenance of all body tissues, and the normal functioning of all body processes. An adequate food intake consists of a balance of essential nutrients such as water, carbohydrates, proteins, fats, vitamins and minerals. Food differ greatly in their nutrient value (the nutrient content specified amount of food), and no one food provides all essential nutrients. Nutrients have three major functions; providing energy for body processes and movement, providing structural material for body tissues, and regulating body processes. In other words, nutrients serve three basic purposes forming body structures, i.e. bone and blood, providing energy, and helping to regulate the body's biochemical reactions.

The factor influencing a person's nutrition include development, gender, ethnicity and culture, beliefs about foods, personal preferences, religious practices, lifestyle, medication, and medical therapy, health status, alcohol abuse, advertising, and psychological factors such as stress, isolation and depression. The child and family both provide a range of variables that influence nutritional habits. Ethnic, racial, cultural and socioeconomic factors influence what the parents eat, and how they feed their children. The child brings individual issues to the nutritional arena, such as slow eating, picky patterns, food preferences, food allergies, acute or chronic health problems and changes with acceleration, and deceleration of growth. Parents often have unrealistic expectations of what children should eat.

Nowadays people may because vegetarian for economic health, religion or ecological reasons. There are two base vegetarian diets; those that use only plant foods (vegetarian) and those that include milk, eggs or dairy products. Some people eat fish and poultry, but not beef, lamb or pork, others eat only fresh fruits, juice and nuts; and still others eat plant foods and dairy products, but not eggs.

Vegetarian diets can be nutritionally sound of they include a wide variety of foods, if proper protein, vitamins and mineral supplementation are provided. Because, the proteins found in plant foods are incomplete proteins, vegetarians must eat compulsory protein foods to obtain all the essential amino acids. A plan protein can be complemented by combing it with a different plant protein. The combination produces a complete protein, shown in Table 25.6. Some of the complete protein such as:
- Grains + Legumes = Complete protein
- Legumes + Nuts or seeds = Complete protein
- Grains, legumes, nuts or seeds + milk or milk products (e.g. cheese) = Complete proteins.

Table 25.6: Complete protein

Grains	Legumes	Nuts and seeds
Brown rice	Black beans	Almonds
Barley	Kidney beans	Brazil nuts
Corn meal	Lima beans	Cashews
Millet	Soybeans	Pecans
Oats/Oats meal	Lentils	Walnut
Rye	Tofus	Pumpkin seeds
Whole wheat	Black eyed peas Sunflower seed Split peas	Sesame seeds

Obtaining complete proteins is especially important for growing children, pregnant and lactating women, whole protein needs are high. Generally, legumes (starchy beans, peas and lentils) have complementary relationship with grains, nuts and seeds. Complementary foods must be eaten in the same meal. Diets such as the fruitarian diet do not provide sufficient amounts of essential nutrients and are not recommended for long-term use.

Non-vegetarian diets or foods of animal origin are the best source of vitamin B_{12}. Therefore vegans need to obtain this vitamin from other sources such as brewers yeast, foods fortified with vitamin B_{12} or vitamin supplements. Because, iron from plant sources is not absorbed as efficiently as iron from meat, vegans should eat iron-rich foods (e.g. green leafy vegetables, whole grains, raisins and molasses) and iron-enriched foods. They should eat a food rich in vitamin C at each meal to enhance iron absorption. Calcium deficiency is a concern only for strict vegetarians. It can be provided by including in the diet soybean milk and tofu (soybean curd) fortified with calcium, and leafy green vegetables.

Healthy Diet

Healthy diet means the diet that is arrived at with the intent of improving or maintaining optimal health. It includes all the nutrients in appropriate amounts from all food groups including an adequate amount of water.

It include fresh vegetables and fruits. A nutritious diet ensures overall well-being, helps to maintain a healthy body mass index (BMI), reduces the risk of several debilitating diseases such as cancer, cardiovascular ailments, diabetes, osteoporosis and stroke.

A healthy diet include sufficient amount of proteins, fats, carbohydrates, vitamins and minerals in the diet, which provide sufficient calories to maintain a person's metabolic and activity needs and also the optimum health status. A healthy diet should contain:
- In the diet there should be required amount of fat, including monounsaturated fat, polyunsaturated fat and saturated fat, with a balance of omega-6 and long-chain omega-3 lipids
- Essential micronutrients such as vitamins and certain minerals
- The food should not be exposed directly to poisonous and carcinogenic substance, e.g. heavy metals, benzene
- A good ratio between carbohydrates and lipids, i.e. 4:1 is required in healthy diet
- Foods should not be contaminated by human pathogens, e.g. *Escherichia coli*, tapeworm, etc.

A nutrition diet can rectify underlying causes of disease and restore one to wholeness of mind, and body. On having knowledge of the connection between wholesome balanced diet and good health, then maintaining good health will be matter of making the right food choices, and leading to healthy lifestyle.

There are six classes of nutrients in food designated as carbohydrates, lipids, proteins, vitamins, minerals and water. Though all these regulate body processes and contribute to body structure, carbohydrates, fats and proteins are the sources of energy for the body. Since, these are needed in large amounts in the diet, they are referred as macronutrients. Utilization and conservation of this energy to build, and maintain the body requires the involvement of vitamins and minerals, which function as coenzymes, and cocatalysts. Since, vitamins and minerals are needed in comparatively small amounts in the diet, they are designated as micronutrients. Several mineral functions as buffers in the miraculous watery arena of metabolism, water is the most important amongst all the nutrients.

Carbohydrates

Carbohydrates are the hydrates of carbon, i.e. made of carbon, hydrogen and oxygen. These are major sources of fuel for the body. Dietary carbohydrates are the starches and sugars found in grains, vegetables, legumes and fruits. Carbohydrates are also obtained from dairy products. Body converts most dietary carbohydrates to glucose, a simple sugar. Glucose is found in circulation and provides a source of energy for cells, and tissues.

Carbohydrate foods composed of some combination of starches, sugar and fiber, and provide the body with fuel it needs for physical activity by breaking down into glucose, a type of sugar, our cells use as a universal energy source.

Fiber helps a person to feel fuller faster and longer, keeps blood sugar levels even and maintains a healthy colon. A healthy diet should contain approximately 20–30 g of fiber a day. There are two types of fibers:
1. Soluble fiber: These can dissolve in water and helps to lower blood fats and maintain blood sugar. The primary sources are beans, fruit and oat products.
2. Insoluble fiber: It cannot dissolve in water, so it passes directly through the digestive system and found in whole grain products and vegetables.

Lipids/Fats

Lipids refer to substances such as fat and oils as well as other fat-like substances found in food, e.g. cholesterol and phospholipids. Lipids are organic compounds and contain carbon, hydrogen and oxygen. Fat (triglycerides) is a major fuel for the body. Triglycerides, cholesterol and phospholipids also have other important functions, i.e. they provide structure for body cells, carry fat-soluble vitamins (vitamins A, D, E and K), and provide the starting material for many hormones.

The fats and oil we add to food or cook with, and the naturally occurring fats in meats and dairy products provide dietary lipids. These are less obvious sources in plants such as coconut, olive and avocado.

Proteins

Proteins are organic compounds made of smaller building blocks called amino acids. In addition to carbon, hydrogen, oxygen and amino acids contain nitrogen. Some amino acids also contain sulfur. Amino acids from dietary proteins along with the amino acids made in the body are used to make different body proteins. Proteins can also be used for energy.

Proteins are found in a variety of foods, but meat and dairy products are the most concentrated sources of protein. Grains, legumes and vegetables also contribute protein to the diet.

Protein in food is broken down into the 20 amino acids during digestion. Proteins are required by out body to maintain our cells, tissues and organs. A lack of protein in our diets can result in reduced muscle mass, slow growth, lower immunity and weaken the heart and respiratory system. Protein provide us the energy to keep on going. Following are the different types of proteins required to the body:
1. Complete proteins: These provides all of the essential amino acids. For example, meat, poultry, fish, milk, eggs and cheese.

2. Incomplete protein: These are the proteins low in one or more of the essential amino acid.
3. Complementary proteins: These are two or more incomplete protein sources that together provide adequate amounts of all the essential amino acids, e.g. rice and dry beans.

Vitamins

Vitamins are organic compounds that contain carbon, hydrogen and perhaps nitrogen, oxygen, phosphorus, sulfur or other elements. Vitamins regulate body processes such as energy production, blood clotting and calcium balance. Vitamins also help to keep organs and tissues functioning, and healthy. Vitamins also have vital roles in the extraction of energy for carbohydrates, fat, protein, absorbed and transported in the body, and are stored in different tissues in the body. If taken in large doses, they can be harmful, especially vitamins A and D.

Water, soluble vitamins include vitamin C and B, which include thiamine, riboflavin, niacin, vitamin B_6, pantothenic acid, biotin, folate and vitamin B_{12}. Vitamins are found in a wide variety of foods. Fruits, vegetables, grains and legumes are important sources of water-soluble vitamins whereas meats and dairy products are good sources of fat-soluble vitamins.

Minerals

Structurally, minerals are simple inorganic substances. Several minerals are essential to health, among them sodium, chloride, potassium, calcium, phosphorus, magnesium and sulfur are important. Since body needs these minerals in relatively large quantities compared to other minerals, they are called macrominerals. The remaining minerals are needed in small amounts, hence called microminerals or trace elements. These include iron, zinc, copper, manganese, molybdenum, selenium, iodine and fluoride.

Minerals have diverse functions. They are important in structural roles, e.g. calcium, phosphorus and fluoride in bones, and teeth as well as regulatory roles, e.g. control of fluid balance and regulation of muscle contraction. Animal foods such as meat and milk as well as plant food-like cereals, and grains are important sources of minerals. Excessive intake of some of the minerals can be toxic.

Water

Water, though chemically is the simplest nutrient, but the most important off all the nutrients. We cannot survive longer without water. Body is nearly 60% water. Water has many roles in the body including temperature control, lubricant of joints and transport of nutrients, and wastes. Water is found in beverages, fruits and vegetables.

Recommended Dietary Allowances for Indians

Recommended dietary allowances are important to consume a variety of healthy foods as there is no single food group, which can nourish the body with all the vital ingredients to meet the nutritional needs of the body. There are five main food groups, they are:
- Fruits
- Vegetables
- Cereals and pulses
- Dairy
- Poultry, fish and meat products.

A healthy balanced diet of these five food groups ensures essential vitamins, minerals and dietary fiber. It is also important that one eat a variety of foods from within and across the food groups besides the food variety will make for an interesting meal. As some foods from within a food group provide more nutrients than others.

The recommended daily allowance of energy depend on age, sex, height, weight and physical activity. Some foods have low nutritional value and if consumed on a regular basis will contribute to the decline of human health, and some of foods with adequate nutrients such as fats, if taken in excess can cause the diseases such as heart disease, obesity, etc. In specific individuals ingesting foods containing natural allergens, e.g. peanuts, shell food or drug-induced triggers (tyramine) for a person taking monoamine oxidase (MAO) inhibitor may be life-threatening.

A nutrients diet can rectify underlying causes of diseases and restore one to wholeness of mind and body. On having the knowledge of the connection between a wholesome balanced diet and good health, then maintaining good health will be a matter of making the right food choices and leading a healthy lifestyle.

The Nutrients Advisory Committee of the Indian Council of Medical Research (ICMR) first recommended dietary allowances for Indians for various nutrients in 1944. On the basis of height and body weight patterns, keeping in view the safe allowances of various nutrients as suggested by the expert groups of the Food and Agricultural Organization (FAO) of the World Health Organization (WHO), these recommendations have been revised from time to time. Based on the recommendations of the experts committee of the ICMR who met in 1988, Recommended Dietary Allowance (RDA) for different age and sex groups for Indians are given in (Table 25.7).

Table 25.7: Recommended daily allowance

Group	Energy (kcal/day)	Protein (g/day)	Calcium (mg/day)	Iron (mg/day)	Vitamin A (µg/day)	Thiamin (mg/day)	Riboflavin (mg/day)	Niacin (mg/day)	Vitamin B_6 (mg/day)	Folic acid (µg/day)	Vitamin B_{12} (µg/day)	Ascorbic acid (mg/day)
Infants (units vary from those given above)												
0–6 month	108/kg	2.05/kg	500		350	55 (µg/kg)	65 (µg/kg)	710 (µg/kg)	0.1	25	0.2	25
6–12 month	98/kg	1.65/kg	500		350	50 (µg/kg)	60 (µg/kg)	650 (µg/kg)	0.4	25	0.2	25
Children												
1–3 year	1,240	22	400	12	400	0.6	0.7	8	0.9	30	0.2–1.0	40
4–6 year	1,690	30	400	18	400	0.9	1.0	11	1.6	40	0.2–1.0	40
7–9 year	1,950	41	400	26	600	1.0	1.2	13	1.6	60	0.2–1.0	40
Boys												
10–12 year	2,190	54	600	34	600	1.1	1.3	15	1.6	70	0.21	40
13–15 year	2,450	70	600	41	600	1.2	1.5	16	2.00	100	0.2–1.0	40
16–18 year	2,640	78	500	50	600	1.3	1.6	17	2.00	100	0.21	40
Girls												
10–12 year	1,970	57	600	19	600	1.0	1.2	13	1.6	70	0.2–1.0	40
13–15 year	2,060	65	600	28	600	1.0	1.2	14	2.00	100	0.2–1.0	40
16–18 year	2,060	63	500	30	600	1.0	1.2	14	2.00	100	0.2–1.0	40
Adults												
Males	2,875	60	400	28	600	1.4	1.6	18	2.00	100	1.0	40
Females	2,225	50	400	30	600	1.1	1.3	14	2.00	100	1.0	40
Pregnancy	300	15	1,000	38	600	0.2	0.2	2	2.5	400	1.0	40
Lactation	400	18	1,000	30	950	0.2	0.2	3	2.5	150	1.5	80

Basic Dietary Allowance

Calories
The expert group, taking several factors into consideration has estimated calorie requirement. These are expressed in terms of BMR values for normal healthy individuals.

Fat
Fat provides essential fatty acids as well as in necessary for the absorption of fat-soluble vitamins. Diet should contain at least 15 g fat derived from a vegetable oil-like sesame oil or sunflower oil, which are rich in essential fatty acids. Total calories derived from fat should not exceed 30% of the total calorie intake.

Protein
The protein requirement has been calculated according to the value of net protein utilization (NPU) of dietary proteins. Since, protein requirement varies in the NPU of a dietary protein, it has been calculated by taking the NPU of mixed vegetable proteins contained in Indian diets. This value of NPU is about 65.

Vitamin A
The vitamin A requirements are expressed in terms of retinol equivalents (RE). 1 mg of β-carotene is equivalent to 0.25 mg of retinol. 1 mg of retinol is equivalent to 0.3 IU of vitamin A.

Vitamin D
Vitamin D requirement is calculated taken into considerations that a part of the body needs of vitamin D are met from the vitamin D that is formed in the body, by exposure to sunlight. 1 mg of calciferol is equal to 40 IU of vitamin D.

Thiamin
Requirement of thiamine is directly related to calorie intake. Its requirement has been defined as 0.5 mg/1,000 kcal.

Riboflavin
Requirement of riboflavin is also directly related to the intake of calories. Its requirement has been defined as 0.6 mg/1,000 kcal.

Nicotinic acid
Nicotinic acid requirement is also related to the intake of calories. It has been defined as 6.6–8.0 mg niacin equivalent (NE) per 1,000 kcal. Niacin allowance is calculated by taking into account, the contribution of tryptophan also assuming that 60 mg of tryptophan forms 1 mg of niacin in the body.

Folic acid
The folic acids requirements are expressed in terms of free folic acid present in foods, which is readily absorbed.

Vitamin B_{12}
Vitamin B_{12} is derived entirely from foods of animal origin.

Calcium and phosphorus
The requirement for calcium and phosphorus are expressed taking into account their utilization by the body. A large part of the phosphorus present in cereals, pulses and nuts is in the form of phytin, only a small part of which is available to the human body. Further, phytin also interferes with the utilizations of dietary calcium and iron.

Iron
On an average about 10% of food iron is absorbed. Iron requirement is arrived at by using the factorial approach and taking into account the basal requirement (in man) plus menstrual losses (in women) or the requirement for growth (in children).

Health and Diet

For maintaining a good health, it is very important to have healthy and nutritious food, a balanced diet, good food habits are essential for a healthy life, otherwise we tend to get into many lifestyle diseases.

The health dependents on the diet have taken. Inadequate and unhealthy food taken can be harmful to us. Most of the time we rely too much on certain foods that some important nutrients are completely missed out. Missing out on certain nutrients or consuming too much of nutrients affects our bodies, sooner or later. So, we have to take a diet, which contains all the nutrients required to maintain the health. For example, the goods that contain nutrient are as follows:

- Spinach contains iron and calcium
- Beetroot contains folate, potassium and manganese
- Cauliflower contains folate
- Mangoes contains potassium and antioxidant
- Tomatoes contains lycopene and antioxidant
- Musk melon contains vitamin C
- Avocado contains potassium
- Papaya contains antioxidants, minerals and fiber
- Mushroom contains minerals, vitamin D (ergosterol), thiamin (B_1), riboflavin (B_2), niacin (B_3) and dietary fiber
- Amla or gooseberry contains vitamin C.

To avoid this situation, certain diets such as mineral diets, low-sodium diet, high-calcium diet, fiber diets, high-iron diet can help to give our body what we miss and avoid what we over eat. Minerals play a vital role in our bodies. Sodium controls the fluid equilibrium in the body and even helps transmission of nerve impulses. Calcium makes bones mass and bone structure stronger. Fiber is an essential element in digestive process. The health problems such as high blood pressure, rickets, tetany, constipation, anemia, etc. can occur due to inadequate intake of these nutrients. Following are the list of food stuffs used for some health problems:

- Beetroot used for curing skin problems
- Spinach used for overcome iron deficiency
- Cauliflower used for good for pregnant woman
- Musk melon used for effective in reducing body heat
- Bitter gourd used to cure of diabetes
- Papaya used to helps in skin treatments
- Oats are unique fatty acids and antioxidants, which together with vitamin E slow cell damage
- Watermelon used to helps in eyesight
- Banana is used in the treatment of depression, anemia, blood pressure, brain power, constipation, etc.
- Almond used for lower cholesterol levels
- The egg content lecithin, which prevents the absorption of cholesterol.

Dietary Patterns During Infancy to Childhood

Physical growth severs as an excellent measure of adequacy of the diet. For children younger than 3 years old, height, weight and head circumference, plotted on appropriate growth curves at regular intervals, allow assessment of growth patterns. Good nutritional intake supports physical growth at a steady rate.

A 24-hour diet recall by the parent is a helpful screening toll to assess the amount and variety of food intake. If the recall is fairly typical of the child, the nurse can compare the intake with basic recommendations for the child's age. It is important to ask about parent's concerns regarding diet. It is also helpful to look at the family's meal patterns. An important part of nutrition assessment includes exercise. Behavior problems that occur during meals may also be an issue.

Diet During Infancy

The 1st year of life is critical for growth of all major organ systems of the body. Most of the brain growth that occurs during the life span occurs during infancy. The digestive and renal systems are immature at birth, and during early infancy. Certain nutrients are not handled well. Energy needs are high. Nutrition during this time influences how an infant will grow and thrive.

Types of infant feeding

Breast milk is the preferred method of infant feeding. Breast milk provides appropriate nutrients and antibodies for the infant. Breastfed infants have fewer illness and allergies. If breastfeeding is not chosen, commercially prepared formulas are an acceptable alternative. Although, evaporated milk with added sugar has been used in the past as a low-cost alternative to breast milk, it is now discouraged. Errors in mixing and lacking of vitamins, and minerals have been common problems.

The method of feeding is a choice that parents should make with guidance and education. The advantages and disadvantages of breast, formula, and combination feeding should be discussed with the parents.

Nurses should be prepared to instruct and support parents in the feeding method of their choice. For breastfeeding, teaching topics include comfortable position, appropriate techniques, feeding frequency, the let-down reflex, care of breasts and length of feeding. The mother's feelings about nursing her infant and the presence or absence of family support are important to success. For bottle feeding, parents need instruction about preparation and care of equipment and formula, position, frequency, and amount of feeding. Parents may need to discuss their feelings about the method of feeding.

Supplements

Current recommendations from the American Academy of Pediatrics indicate that the iron in breast milk is highly available to the infant. Breastfed infants do not require iron supplementations. Infants who are not breastfed should be given a commercial formula, i.e. fortified with iron. Addition of iron has reduced the incidence of anemia and does not cause stomach symptoms. After 4–6 months of age, iron needs are further met by the introduction of iron-fortified cereals.

Fluoride at 0.25 mg/day is recommended for infants who drink ready-to-feed formula or formula mixed with water from a supply containing less than 0.3 parts per million (ppm) of fluoride. Fluoride is currently started at 6 months of age and maintained until 16 years of age. Fluoride is not recommended for breastfed infants whose mother have a fluoridated water supply.

Several recent reports have indicated an increase in the occurrence of rickets. Vitamin D supplementation is recommended for breastfed infants at risk for rickets.

Introduction of solid foods and juice

Current trends include the introduction of solids between 4 and 6 months of age and juice at 6 months. There is no nutritional, developmental or psychological advantage to starting earlier. Studies have not shown that cereal helps a baby sleep longer. Parents need to know the risks of feeding solids too early:

- The incidence of constipation is greater, when solid food intake is too high
- Early introduction of solids may lead to overfeeding and obesity
- There is a greater possibility of food allergy because immunoglobulin A (IgA) production is insufficient for solid foods until closer to 6 months
- If the infant lower milk intake because of filling up on solids or juices, there may be an imbalance of nutrients.

Once parents have decided to start solids, nurses can help them plan a schedule for starting appropriate foods. Dry cereal fortified with iron is a useful starter food because of the ease of digestion.

At 1 year of age, the infant may be changed from formula to whole milk. Skim, low fat and 2% milk are not recommended for babies less than 2 years of age because of inadequate fat and caloric content.

Diet During Childhood

The skill and desire to self-feed begins at approximately 1 year of age. The parent's role begins to shift at this time toward providing a balanced, healthy range of foods as the child assumes more independence. Growth rate and caloric needs decrease during this time. Nurses can best assist parents by offering information on daily needs and healthy food choices. Suggestions for children might include the following:

- Frequent, small meals may be better accepted
- Offer a balanced diet incorporating variety and foods that the child likes
- Limit milk intake to the recommendations for the child's age
- Consider the child's development and safety; avoid nuts, popcorn, grapes and similar foods to decrease risk of aspiration in young children
- Encourage children to help with food selection and preparation as appropriate to development skills
- Generally, vitamin and iron supplements are not necessary
- Avoid using food as a punishment or reward.

Fat content in the diet should be restricted to less than 30% beginning at 2 years of age, which is no more than 10% of the total calories coming from saturated fats. Studies show that children as young as 2–6 years of age have diets higher in total fats and in saturated fats than recommended.

In general, the family diet does not contain enough fiber-rich foods or fruits or vegetables. Diet of school age children have been shown to be low in calcium. Children also need regular physical activity. Observations of children indicate that they are too sedentary. The entire family may benefit from suggestions to modify the diet:

- Choose low-fat protein sources: Plant proteins, such as beans, peas and whole grain products or lean cuts of meat chicken or fish, with visible fat trimmed
- Boil, bake, stir-fry or poach foods rather than frying
- Use polyunsaturated and monounsaturated fats found in nuts, seeds, nut butters, wheat germ and vegetable oils
- Decrease salt, sugar and fats
- Increase complex carbohydrates—breads, grain and cereals
- Increase fruits and vegetables to at least five servings per day, especially green and orange vegetables, and citrus fruits
- Use low-fat dairy products
- Increase calcium intake though low-fat dairy products calcium-fortified products and supplements, if necessary
- Maintain regular activity (e.g. exercise, sports, household chores) and limit television viewing.

Remind parents that they are teaching children lifelong strategies to prevent illness and promote good health.

Adolescent Dietary Needs

The preadolescent and adolescent years are a time of increased growth that is accompanied by increases in appetite and nutritional requirements. Caloric and protein requirements increase for boys 11–18 years of age. Girls have an increased protein need, but a decreased caloric need, during the same age span. The iron needed by the adolescent is nearly double that needed by adults.

Adolescent nutritional needs are influenced by physical alterations and psychological adjustments. Teenagers are often free to eat when and where they choose. Eating habits acquired from the family are drooped. Food away from home is a major source of nutrition. Fad foods and diets are prominent. Accelerated growth and poor eating habits make the adolescent at risk for poor nutritional health. Adolescents have the most unsatisfactory nutritional status of all age groups. Deficiencies in iron, vitamins, calcium, riboflavin and thiamin are most common.

Nurses can initiate activities that promote improved nutritional status. Such activities include the following:

- Providing information on good nutrition in individual or group sessions
- Diet assessment

- Educational activities that focus on effects on fad foods and diets
- Supplying a list of 'at-risk' nutrients
- Providing a daily food guide
- Suggesting snacks and 'on the run' foods that supply essential nutrients
- Teaching the relationship of good nutrition to healthy appearance.

In case of health issues, doctors advise the type of diet taken along with medicines. This diet need to be followed carefully, otherwise medicines do not do the complete job. For example, the type of diet in health problems are detailed below.

Diet for cancer: Saturated fats of more harm hence only 55 g of fat intake daily should be taken.

Diet for gout: Rich-carbohydrate diet with limited protein is advised for people who suffer from gout.

For acid reflux: Smaller meals, more than three times a day.

Diet for constipation: The most suggested diet is their diet. Dietary fiber is found in plant foods such as fruit, vegetables and whole grains.

The strategies for healthy eating a healthy diet are:
- Maintain a balance between the calorie intake and calorie expenditure
- Eat a wide variety of foods. Eat plenty of fruits, vegetables, grains and legumes, low in fat and free of cholesterol
- Limit sugary foods, salt and refined-grain products
- Add regular physical activity and exercise to make the eating plan healthy better
- Take time to chew the food and chew the food slowly
- Avoid stress while eating
- Stop eating when you feel full.

EDUCATION

Education plays an important role in health status. Although education is related to income, educational level seems to influence health separately. Higher level education may provide people with more information for making healthy lifestyle choices. More highly educated people are better able to make informed choices of health insurance and providers. Education may also influence perceptions of stressors and problem situations, and give people more alternatives. Education and language skills affect healthy literacy.

Education is an integral part of prevention and the basis of all education is communication. Education helps to increase knowledge and it is believed that knowledge determines the attitude and attitude determines behavior. Health education can bring changes in lifestyle.

There are a number of health problems, which can be prevented through appropriate knowledge of nutrition, physical activity and lifestyle changes.

Health literacy is a measure of patient's ability to read, comprehend and act on medical instructions. Poor health literacy is common among racial and ethnic minorities, older adult persons, and patients with chronic conditions, particularly in public sector settings.

Educational Principles

A variety of educational principles can be used to guide the selection of health information for individuals, families, communities and populations. Three of the most useful categories of educational principles include those associated with the nature of learning, the events of instruction and guidelines for the effective educator.

Nature of Learning

One way to think about the nature of learning is to examine the cognitive (thinking), affective (feelings) and psychomotor (acting) domains of learning. Each domain has specific behavioral components that form a hierarchy of steps or levels. Each level builds on the previous one. Understanding these three learning domains is crucial in providing effective health education, eyesight that is incapable of learning insulin self-injection. The nurse should teach at the level of the learner's ability.

Events of Instruction

To educate others effectively, one needs to understand the basic sequence of instruction. When nurses consider the following nine steps of instructing others, they can systematically plan health education so that learners gain as much as possible from the instruction:

1. Gain attention: Before learning can take place, the educator must gain the learner's attention. One way to this by convincing the learner that the information about to be presented is important and beneficial to the learner.
2. Inform the learner of the objectives of instruction. Before teaching begins, the major goals and objectives of instruction should be outlined so that learners develop expectations about what they are supposed to learn.
3. Stimulate recall of prior learning: The educator should have learners recall previous knowledge related to the topic of interest. This assists learners in linking new knowledge with prior knowledge.

4. **Present the material:** The essential elements of a topic should be presented in as clear, organized and simple manner as possible. The material should be presented in a way that is congruent with the learners strengths, needs and limitations.
5. **Provide learning guidance:** For long-lasting behavioral changes to occur, the learner must store information in long-term memory. With guidance from the educator, the learner can transform general information that the learner can recall.
6. **Elicit performance:** Learners should be encouraged to demonstrate what they have learned. Educators should except that during the educational process, learners will need to correct errors and improve skills.
7. **Provide feedback:** Educators should provide feedback to learners to assist them in improving their knowledge and skills. Learners can then modify their thinking patterns and behaviors, on the basis of this feedback.
8. **Assess performance:** Learning should be evaluated. Knowledge and skills should be formally assessed with the expectation that new information has been understood.
9. **Enhance retention and transfer of knowledge:** Once a baseline level of knowledge and skills has been attained, educators should assist learners in applying this information to new situations.

By using these instructional principles, nurses may help clients to maximize learning experiences. If steps of this process are omitted, superficial and fragmented learning may occur.

Effective Educator

Nurse educators must be effective teachers. Six basic principles guide the effective educator are as follows:
- **Message:** Sending a clear message to the learner
- **Format:** Selecting the most appropriate learning format
- **Environment:** Creating the best possible learning environment
- **Experience:** Organizing positive and meaningful learning experiences
- **Participation:** Engaging the learner in participatory learning
- **Evaluation:** Evaluating and giving objective feedback to the learner.

So, education is an integral part of prevention of illness, promoting of health and health maintenance. Education is the basis for all communications and it help to increase knowledge, which in turns it is believed that knowledge determine the attitude, and attitude determine behavior. Health education helps in increasing the knowledge and reinforces the desired behavior pattern. Health education is a vital part of community health nursing (CHN). The promotion maintenance and restoration of health require that community health clients receive practical understanding of health-related information. Community health clients include individual's families, communities and populations.

Health Education

Community health nurses may educate clients across three levels of illness prevention, i.e. primary, secondary and tertiary. The information that provided by them enables client's to attain optimal health, prevent health problems early and minimize disability. Education allows individuals to make knowledgeable health-related decisions, assume personal responsibility for their health and cope effectively with alternations in their health and lifestyles.

So, health education is a process aimed at encouraging people to want to be healthy, to know how to stay healthy, to do what they can individually and collectively to maintain health, and to seek help when needed.

Objectives

Health education is a process of bringing scientific knowledge on health to the people to bring about changes in their knowledge, attitude and behavior for the betterment of their health, and health of the community in which they live. The main objective of the health educates are:
- To encourage people to adopt healthy lifestyle
- To provide knowledge to the people to adapt health promoting activities and practices
- To create interest among people by education related to the benefits of activities
- To improve skill and to encourage them to change their own health
- To stimulate the people to become self-reliant
- To improve the health of the family and the community at large.

Contents of Health Education

The contents of health education may be human biology, personal hygiene, nutrition, environment, prevention of accidents, prevention of communicable diseases, reproductive health, population control, mental health, etc. depending on the content, the health education is referred to by different names as sex education, population education, safety education, nutrition education, parent crafts education, etc.

Principles of Health Education

There are certain principles, which contribute to the success of health education:

1. **Credibility:** It is the degree to which the message in perceived as trustworthy. Unless the people have trust and confidence in the educator, the message will not be perceived.
2. **Scientific knowledge:** Health education should be based on facts, consistent and compatible with scientific knowledge, and also with local culture, educational system and social goals.
3. **Content/Interest:** Health education should be planned and implemented to meet the real needs of the people. People will listen to those things, which are of interest, meaningful and it should be their felt need. So, the educator should find out their real health needs and educate. Suppose the felt need is not known to the people because of illiteracy, the educator should bring about the recognition of the needs and then educate them.
4. **Context:** The context in which communication is given should be relevant to the receiver.
5. **Clarity:** The message to be given should be in simple terms.
6. **Consistency:** The message must be consistent to penetrate into the minds of receiver.
7. **Channel:** Existing channel or available channels of communications, it should be used for health education.
8. **Capability:** The audience must be capable of understanding, what the communicated message is?
9. **Comprehension:** This means, educating the people is a level, they can understand and preferably in the same language they speak, and avoiding difficult and strange words. Teaching should be done within the mental capacity of the audience/people. So it should be based on understanding, education and literacy of people.
10. **Motivation:** It is the awakening the desire among the people to learn. They can be motivated easily by giving incentives, which may be negative or positive, e.g. obese woman to reduce her body weight help to prevent complication of coronary artery disease and also, her to become slim, beautiful, charming, which is acceptable way of motivation.
11. **Participation:** People must be motivated take part in health education program arranged by health workers and social workers. Thus, participation of people will create opportunity for more effective practically based education.
12. **Learning by doing:** Health education should be based on action process, i.e. learning by doing. Here people should perform activities, which they are learning as learning by doing. Learning is an action-oriented. This makes the man perfect. According to Chinese proverb "If I hear, I forget; if I see, I remember; if I do, I know" illustrates and supports the importance of learning by doing.
13. **Known to unknown:** Health education is given to the people from a level what they known and understand, and then proceeded to new knowledge. Here, health educator must proceed from known to unknown and to concentrate to abstract, and simple to complex.
14. **Reinforcement:** This means repetition of the same message periodically, preferably in different ways, so that audience can understand it better and remember longer. Otherwise they may go back to the pre-awareness stage. So, education provided to people should be repeated at intervals.
15. **Setting an example:** Health educator should set an example in the things, which are taught to people and he/she should act as role, model, i.e. he/she himself/herself should practice, what he/she preaches and he/she should be an ideal example. For example, if he/she is advising the hazards of smoking, he/she should not be found smoking himself/herself.
16. **Good human relation:** Good interpersonal relationship or human relation is very essential to share information, to know the interest, to understand the feelings and ideas of people. Building good relationships with audience, makes the health education successful.
17. **Feedback:** It is most important to achieving good communication. It will provide an idea about the people understanding of the topic related to the health taught to them. Getting feedback or remarks from the audience is paramount important to the health educator so that he/she can improve himself/herself. In communicating next time more effectively.
18. **Leaders:** Involvement of local leaders will make the education more easy and effective, because local leader are respected. If they involve, then people automatically, passively will participate. So that local leaders must be identified and convinced. Health educators should have qualities of good leader such as honest, selfless, impartial, sincere and accessible, knowledgeable, skillful, cooperative, coordinator, etc.

Approaches in Health Education

There are some approaches in health education, which includes regulatory approach, service approach, health education approach and primary healthcare approach:

1. **Regulatory approach:** It is legal approach made by the government to alter the behavior of the people for the betterment of people health. Such regulations may

vary from prohibition to imprisonment, e.g. Child Marriage Restrain Act and all public health acts.
2. **Service approach:** It consists of providing healthcare services to the individual doors, based on the assumption that people would use them to improve their own health, e.g. pulse polio immunization.
3. **Health education approach:** There are many health problems, which can be solved through health education, e.g. prevention of AIDS, accident, etc.
4. **Primary healthcare approach:** The healthcare service is basic, essential, utilitarian, provided by nonmedical persons starting from the people, by the people, of the people and for the people based on the principles of public health ethics (PHE), such as equitable distribution, community participation, intersectional approach and appropriate technology, e.g. role of anganwadi worker, role of traditional birth attendants (TBAs).

Nurses in advanced practice function in several indirect nursing care roles. The educator role includes health education within a nursing framework (as opposed to health educators, who may not have a nursing background) and professional nurse educator (faculty) roles.

The identifies groups at risk within a community and implements, e.g. health education interventions. The CHN increase wellness and contribute to maintaining, and promoting health by teaching the importance of good nutrition, physical exercise, stress management, and a healthy lifestyle. They provide education about disease processes and the importance of following treatment regimens. In addition, they provide anticipatory guidance and educate clients on the use of medications, diet, birth control methods, and other therapeutic procedures. They also counsel clients, families, groups and the community on the importance of assuming responsibility for their own health. This education may occur on an individual, family or group level in an institutional, ambulatory or home setting, or it may occur in the community with vulnerable at-risk populations.

As professional nurse educators, the CHN provide formal and informal teaching of staff nurses, undergraduate and graduate students in nursing, and other discipline. They also serve as role and other instructing (or being a preceptor) students in advanced practice in the clinical setting.

Role of Education in Physical Activity

Regular participation in physical activity during childhood and adolescence build and maintain healthy bones, muscles and joints; helps to control weight, build lean muscle and reduce fat; prevents or delays the development of high blood pressure; helps to reduce blood pressure.

Good nutrition and physical activity habits provide long-term health benefits for young people. Current research indicates the obesity rate amongst Australian children is rising. Higher kilojoule intake and lower levels of physical activity are impacting on the health of many people. Community health nurses, and school teachers can play an important part in promoting physical activity and providing sound nutritional information to students enabling them to make healthier lifestyle choices. The education provided related to the same parents and school teachers as well as all the students help in maintaining the life. In order to provide education related to physical activity, keep following points in mind:

- Engage the people to learn about movement and motor skills
- Promote inclusiveness of all people
- Gradually increase time spent in physical activity
- Assist young people in becoming connected to physical activity
- Decrease TV time and increase moderate and vigorous physical activity.

Education related to physical activity at school, colleges offer the best opportunity to provide physical activity to all students and to teach them the skills and knowledge needed to establish and sustain an active lifestyle. To teach physical activity, physical education teachers can assess student knowledge, motor and social skills and can provide instructions in a safe, supportive environment promotion of physical activity is recommended throughout life. Physical activity is bodily movement of any type and may include recreational, fitness and sport activities such as jumping rope, playing soccer, lifting weights, as well as daily activities such as walking to the store, taking the stairs or raking the leaves.

The education provided to the people on physical activity helps in:

- Reduces the risk for overweight diabetes and other chronic diseases
- Assists in improved academic performance
- Helps people feel better about themselves
- Reduces the risk for depression and the effects of stress
- Helps the people to be productive and healthy members of society
- Improves overall quality of life.

OCCUPATION

Occupation is the action, state or a period of occupying, or being occupied. It is a job or a profession, or a way of spending time.

People have different occupations and they carry out different type of physical activities according to their work. The occupations have been classified as sedentary, moderate active and very active. The sedentary work include—office workers, clerks, drivers, pilots, teachers, journalists, clergyman, lawyers, architects, shop workers, the moderately active work includes light industry and assembly plant workers railway workers, postman, plumber, bus conductor, farm workers, builders, laborers, and very active work, includes coal mine workers, iron and steel workers, forestry workers, army recruits, farm workers, and skilled laborers.

Physical activity is primarily importance, because it is the most fundamental factor affecting energy expenditure. The amount of energy used by the body is called the energy expenditure. This energy expenditure depends upon age, sex, occupation, physical activity and the state of body, i.e. pregnancy or illness. People have different occupations and they carry out different type of physical activities according to their work. The work of a clerk is to do clerical work and the main physical activity is sitting, and the same way of shop owner sitting at counter and having the payments. Skilled workers or the laborer has to do more of work. This energy expenditure is more in case of the work, which require more activity as compare to the work having less activity. So the energy expenditure of the people depends upon the type of physical activity done at the job.

Occupational physical activity is important for epidemiologic studies of physical activity and health outcomes. Moderate-intensity physical activity such as brisk walking is associated with health benefits. Moderate physical activity is typically achieved through leisure-time pursuits; however, some occupations involve high levels of activity during the course of the day. Physical activity may need careful examination in situations where it may appears to excessive as to shorten working life or where the constant fatigue resulting from it may attenuate the enjoying of leisure time.

Occupational physical activity is categorized on the basis of type of physical activity required such as sitting or standing, walking, heavy lifting and physically demanding work. The energy expenditure in different occupations are depend upon the type of work as well as number of hours, the same activity is done. Occupational wellness is the ability to achieve a balance between work and leisure time. A person's belief about education, employment and home influence personal satisfaction, and relationship with others.

Occupational physical activity contribute to overall health and wellness. Moderate intensity, muscle strengthening and flexibility enhancing activity, accrued in occupation contribute to an individual overall activity level, and consequently could promote health. According certain studies increased occupational physical activity decreases the risk of coronary heart disease, heart attack, lowers cholesterol level, higher acrobatic capacity, lower body fat, greater muscular flexibility, etc.

Working population constitutes the major portion of the community, they determine the progress and development of country. In other words, their health status is considered as a sensitive indication for the development of the country. Like home, the place of work is also an important environment for an earning person. Such a person spends nearly 6–8 hours a day in the working place till the retirement for about three decades. Not only the worker should be healthy but also the working environment should be healthy, safe and free from harmful agents of the working environment is healthy, it is not only beneficial for the worker (employee) but also for the employer. There will be mutual benefit for both because there will be increased efficiency, increased production and decreased accidents. For which follow the new concept of occupational health, i.e. ergonomic. It simply means fitting the job to the worker. That means placing the worker in an environment (job), which is adopted to his/her physiological and psychological capacity. Ergonomic has made a significant contribution in reducing the industrial accidents and in overall health and efficiency of the worker.

Characteristics of the Workforce

The workplace has been rapidly changing jobs in the economy continue to shift from manufacturing to service. Longer hours, compressed worksheet, shift work, reduced job security and part-time, and temporary work are realities of the modern workplace with new chemicals, materials, process and equipment are developed, and marketed at an ever-increasing pace. The workforce is the changes going to present new challenges to protecting worker safety and health.

The demographic trends in the workforce describe a changing population aggregate that has implications for the prevention services targeted to that group. Major changes in the working population are reflected in the increasing numbers of women, older individuals and those with chronic illness who are part of the workforce. Because of changes in the economy, extension of lifespan, legislation and society's acceptance of working women, the proportion of the employed population that these three groups represents will probably continue to grow.

In an era, in which the demand for workers is expected to outstrip the available supply, businesses must be concerned about strategies to increase health status, employment longevity and satisfaction of workers. For example, in the 1990s, while nearly 60% of all women were employed (representing 48% of the workforce), it was predicated that women would account for 67% of the increase in the labor force in the 21st century. These workers tended to be married with children and aging parents for whom they were responsible. This aggregate of workers presents new issue for individual and family health promotions, such as child care, and elder that can be addressed in the work environment.

Characteristics of the Work

There has been a dramatic shift in the types of jobs held by workers. Following the evolution from an agrarian economy to a manufacturing society and then to a highly technologic workplace, the greatest proportion of paid employment is now in the occupations of service (e.g. health care, information processing, banking and insurance), professional and technical positions (e.g. managers and computer specialists), and clerical work (e.g. word processors and secretaries). During the 1996–2000 period, service-providing industries accounted for virtually all of the job growth. Only construction added jobs in the goods-producing business sector, offsetting decline in manufacturing and mining. Health services, business services, social services and engineering, management, and related services are expected to account for almost one of every two worker jobs. The occupations have been categorized under sedentary, moderate active and very active.

Sedentary: It includes office workers, clerical task, drivers, pilots, teachers, journalists, clergy, doctors, lawyers, architect and shop workers.

Moderate active: Light industry and assembly plants workers, railways workers, postman, plumber, bus conductors, farm workers, builders and laborer.

Very active: Coal mine workers, steel workers, forestry workers, army recruits, some farm workers and skilled laborers.

Occupational physical activity is categorized on the basis of type of physical activity required such as sitting or standing, walking, heavy lifting or physically demanding work. The energy expenditure in different occupations depend upon the type of work as well as the number of hours, the same activity is done. One example of this is of men doing extremely heavy labor in a steel mill, where work requirements were such that these men needed to be big, muscular, strong individual. The total duration of this very heavy work however, was only about 30–40 min/day and thus total daily energy expenditure of these men was no higher than that of men working at only low-to-moderate levels of activity in a conveyor belt factory. At the other extreme, many jobs necessitate continuous physical activity of moderate intensity for most of the working day, and the energy expended may be high even though the individuals do not need to have a high level of fitness to do this sort of work.

This change in the nature of work has been accompanied by many new occupational hazards, such as complex chemicals, no ergonomic workstation design (requiring the adaptation of the workplace or work equipment to meet the employee's health and safety needs) and many issues related to work organization such as job stress, burnout, and exhaustion. In addition, the emerging of a global economy with free trade and multinational corporations new challenges for health, and safety programs that are culturally relevant.

Work (Health Interactions)

Although occupational physical activity might contribute to overall health and wellness. Moderate intensity, muscle-strengthening and flexibility-enhancing activities accrued in one's occupation might contribute appreciably to a person's overall activity level, and consequently could promote health. Research studies have noted a relationship between increased occupational physical activity levels and a decreased risk of coronary heart disease, fatal heart attack, lower cholesterol levels, higher aerobic capacity, lower body fat, greater muscular flexibility and lower rates of colon cancer. Physical activity during the workday is a practical way to become more active. An active workforce can raise productivity and reduce sickness absence. It can boost morale, improve staff retention and raise the company profile.

A study on physical activity in usual occupation and risk of breast cancer by Patricia F Coogan et al have revealed that women with heavy activity occupations had a lower risk of breast cancer than women with medium activity or light activity and results were consistent with the hypothesis that physical activity reduces the risk of breast cancer.

The influence of work on health or work-health interactions is shown by statistics on illness, injuries and deaths associated with employment. In 2001, 1.5 million reported work-related illnesses and injuries resulted in lost time from work. Of these, approximately 5% were severe enough to result in temporary or permanent disabilities that prevented, the workers from the returning to their usual jobs. Then occupations accounted for nearly one third of the 1.5 million injuries and illnesses involving days from work in 2001. Truck drivers, non-construction laborers and nursing aides, and orderlies were the top three occupations representing days away from work in 2001 with registered nurses being the 10th occupation with lost days from work.

Occupational Hazards

An industrial worker may be exposed to five types of hazards, depending upon his/her occupation:
- Physical hazards
- Chemical hazards
- Biological hazards
- Mechanical hazards
- Psychosocial hazards.

Physical Hazards

Heat and cold

The common physical hazards in most industries is heat. The direct effects of heat exposure cause burns, heat exhaustion, heat stroke and heat cramps; the indirect effects lead to decreased efficiency, increased fatigue and enhanced accidents rates. Many industries have local 'hot spots'—ovens and furnaces, which radiate heat. Radiant heat is the main problem in foundry, glass and steel industries, while heat stagnation is the principal problem in jute and cotton textile industry. High temperatures are also found in mines for instance in the Kolar Gold Mines of Mysore, which is the second deepest mine of the world (11,000 ft), temperatures as high as 65°C are recorded. Physical work under such conditions is very stressful and impairs the health, and efficiency of the workers. For gainful work involving sustained and repeated effort, a reasonable temperature must be maintained in each work room.

The Indian Factories Act has not laid down any specific temperature standard. However, the work of Rao (1952–1953) and Mookerjee et al (1953) indicate that a corrected effective temperature of 69–80°F (20–27°C) is the comfort zone in this country, and temperature above 80°F (27°C) cause discomfort. Important hazards associated with cold work are chilblains, acrocyanosis, immersion foot and frostbite as a result of cutaneous vasoconstriction. General hypothermia is not unusual.

Light

The workers may be exposed to the risk of poor illumination or excessive brightness. The acute effects of poor illumination are eye strain, headache, eye pain, lacrimation and congestion around the cornea and eye fatigue. The chronic effects on health include 'miners' nystagmus'. Exposure to excessive brightness or glare is associated with discomfort, annoyance and visual fatigue. Intense direct glare may also result in blurring of vision and lead to accidents. There should be sufficient and suitable lighting, natural or artificial, wherever persons are working.

Noise

Noise is a health hazard in many industries. The effects of noise pollution are of two types:
1. Auditory effects, which consist of temporary or permanent hearing loss.
2. Non-auditory effects, which consist of nervousness, fatigue, interference with communication by speech, decreased efficiency and annoyance. The degree of injury from exposure to noise depends upon a number of factors such as intensity and frequency range, duration of exposure and individual susceptibility.

Vibration

Vibration, especially in the frequency range 10–500 Hz, may be encountered in work with pneumatic tools such as drills and hammers. Vibration usually affects the hands and arms. After some months or years of exposure, the fine blood vessels of the fingers may become increasingly sensitive to spam (white fingers). Exposures to vibration may also produce injuries of the joints of the hands, elbows and shoulders.

Ultraviolet radiation

Occupational exposure to ultraviolet radiation occurs mainly in arc welding. Such radiation mainly affects the eyes, causing intense conjunctivitis and keratitis (welders flash). Symptoms are redness of the eyes and pain, these usually disappear in a few days with no permanent effect on the vision or on the deeper structures of the eye.

Ionizing radiation

The ionizing radiations are increasingly being used in medicine and industry, e.g. X-rays and radioactive isotopes. Important radioisotopes are cobalt 60 and phosphorus 32. Certain tissues such as bone marrow are more sensitive than others and from a genetic stand point, there are special hazards when the gonads are exposed. The radiation chromosomal hazards comprise genetic changes, malformation, cancer, leukemia, depilation, ulceration, sterility and in extreme case death. The international commission of radiological level of occupational exposure at 5 rem per year to the whole body.

Chemical Hazards

There is hardly any industry, which does not make use of chemicals. The chemical hazards are on the increase with the introduction of newer and complex chemicals.

Chemical agents act in three ways such as local action, inhalation and ingestion. The ill effects produced depend upon the duration of exposure, the quantum of exposure and individual susceptibility.

Local action
Some chemicals cause dermatitis, eczema, ulcers and even cancer by primary irritant action. Some chemicals, particularly the aromatic nitro and amino compounds such as trinitrotoluene (TNT) and aniline are absorbed through the skin, and cause systemic effects. Occupational dermatitis is a big problem in industry. The prevalence of occupational dermatitis due to machine oil, rubber, X-rays, caustic alkalis and lime have been reported from this country.

Inhalation
Dusts
Dusts are finely divided solid particles with size ranging from 0.1 to 150 μm. They are released into the atmosphere during crushing, grinding, abrading, loading and unloading operations. Dusts are produced in a number of industries, i.e. mines, foundry, quarry, pottery, textiles, wood or stone working industries. Dust particles larger than 10 μm settle down from the air rapidly, while the smaller ones remain suspended indefinitely. Particularly smaller than 5 μm are directly inhaled into the lungs and are retained there. These fractions of the dust called 'repairable dust' are mainly responsible for pneumoconiosis. Dusts have been classified into inorganic and organic dusts; soluble and insoluble dusts. The inorganic dusts are silica, mica, coal, asbestos dust, etc. the organic dusts are cotton, jute, etc. the soluble dusts dissolve slowly, enter the systemic circulation and are eventually eliminated by body metabolism. The insoluble dusts remain, more or less permanently in the lungs. They are mainly the cause of pneumoconiosis. The most common dust diseases in this country are silicosis and anthracosis.

Gases
Exposures to gases are a common hazard in industries. Gases are sometimes classified as simple gases (e.g. oxygen and hydrogen), asphyxiating gases (e.g. carbon monoxide, cyanide gas, sulfur dioxide and chlorine), and anesthetic gases (e.g. chloroform, ether and trichloroethylene). Carbon monoxide hazards are frequently reported in coal gas manufacturing plants and steel industry.

Metals and their compounds
A large number of metals and their compounds are used throughout the industry. The chief mode of entry of some of them is by inhalation as dust or fumes. The industrial physician should be aware of the toxic effects of lead, antimony, arsenic, beryllium, cadmium, cobalt, manganese, mercury, phosphorus, chromium, zinc and others. The ill effects depend upon the duration of exposure and the dose or concentration of exposure.

Ingestion
Occupational disease may also result from ingestion of chemical substances such as lead, mercury, arsenic, zinc, chromium, cadmium, phosphorus, etc. Usually, these substances are swallowed in small amounts through contaminated hands, food or cigarettes. Much of the ingested material is excreted through feces and only a small proportion may reach the general blood circulation.

Biological Hazards

Workers may be exposed to infective and parasitic agents at the place of work. The occupational diseases in this category are brucellosis, leptospirosis, anthrax, hydatid disease, psittacosis, tetanus, encephalitis, schistosomiasis and fungal infections. Persons working with animal products (e.g. hair, wool and hides) and agricultural workers are specially exposed to biological hazards.

Mechanical Hazards

The mechanical hazards in industry result from machinery, protruding and moving parts of the machines. About 10% of accidents in industry are said to be due to mechanical causes (accidents).

Psychosocial Hazards

The psychosocial hazards arise from the worker's failure to adapt to an alien psychosocial environment. Frustration, lack of job satisfaction, insecurity, poor human relationships, emotional tension are some of the psychosocial factors, which may undermine both physical and mental health of the workers. The capacity to adapt the different working environments is influenced by many factors such as education, cultural background, family life, social habits and what the worker expects from employment.

Health effects can be classified in two main categories:
1. Psychological and behavioral changes: They comprise hostility, aggressiveness, anxiety, depression, laziness, alcoholism, drug abuse, sickness and absenteeism.
2. Psychosomatic ill health: It comprises fatigue, headache; pain in the shoulders, neck and back; propensity to peptic ulcer, hypertension, heart disease and rapid aging.

Reports from various parts of the world indicate that physical factors (heat, noise and poor lighting) also play a major role in adding or precipitating mental disorders among workers. The increasing stress on automation, electronic operations and nuclear energy may introduce newer psychosocial health problems in industry.

Psychosocial hazards are, therefore, assuming more importance than physical or chemical hazards (Table 25.8).

Table 25.8: List of occupations, which are hazardous to individual with certain diseases/conditions

Occupation as hazard	Undesirable conditions
Lead	Anemia, hypertension, nephritis, peptic ulcer
Dyes	Asthma, skin, bladder and kidney diseases; precancerous lesions
Solvents	Liver and kidney disease, dermatitis, alcoholism
Silica	Healed or active tuberculosis of lungs, chronic lung disease
Radium and X-ray	Signs of ill health, especially any blood disease
Agriculture	
Rye, whole wheat, tofu, black eyed peas, sunflower seed, split peas	Signs of ill health

Role of Nurse in Prevention of Occupational Hazards

Preplacement examination
The foundation of an efficient occupational health service. It is done at the time of employment and includes the worker's medical, family, occupational and social history; a thorough physical examination and a battery of biological and radiological examinations, e.g. chest X-ray, electrocardiogram, vision testing, urine and blood examination, special tests for endemic disease. A fresh recruit may either be totally rejected or given a job suited to his/her physical and mental abilities. The purpose of preplacements examination is to place the right man in the right job, so that the worker can perform his/her duties efficiently without detriment to his health. This is ergonomics. There is a list of some occupations in which it is risky to employ men suffering from certain diseases.

Periodical examination
Many occupational diseases require months or even years for their development. Their slow development, often leads to their nonrecognition in the early stages and this is harmful to the worker. This is the reason why a periodical medical checkup of workers is very necessary, when they handle toxic or poisonous substances.

The frequency and content of periodical medical examination will depend upon the type of occupational exposure. Ordinarily workers are examined once a year. But in certain occupational exposures (e.g. lead, toxic dyes and radium) monthly examinations may be needed such as when irritant chemicals-like chromates are handled. The periodical examinations may be supplemented, where necessary by investigations. Particular care should be given to workers returning from medical leave, tosses the nature and degree of any disability, and to assess suitability or otherwise of returning to the same job.

Medical and healthcare services
The medical care of occupational diseases is a basic function of an occupational health service. In India, the Employees State Insurance (ESI) scheme provides medical care not only for the worker but also his/her family. Within the factory, first aid services should be made available. Properly applied first aid can reduce suffering and disability, and hasten recovery immunizations another accepted function of an occupational health service.

Role of nurse in occupational and industrial disorders to arrange preplacement examination, periodical examination, provided medical and healthcare services to the workers/employees.

The nurse employed in ESI, hospital and dispensaries play an important role in providing medical care for illness as well as to teach the preventive measures to avoid further attacks. The nurse plays an important role in providing immunization and other healthcare services such as counseling.

Health education is a basic health need. It is an important health promotional measures. Health education in the industrial setting should be envisaged at all levels, i.e. the management, the supervisory staff, the worker, the trade union leaders and the community. The content of education varies from personal hygiene and protection to participation of workers in the planning, and operation of the total health program in industry. The nurse must provide health education to the industrial workers/patients attending the ESI dispensary or hospital.

The pregnant women should not be allowed to work in the industries where she is likely to be exposed to toxic substances. The nurse has to take care of such pregnant mothers in antenatal clinics and advises them all the schedules of immunization, nutrition, personal hygiene, and personal care.

The nurse must teach the clients working in industries and attending the ESI dispensaries, the importance of keeping personal hygiene, and measures of hygiene's handwashing, personal cleanliness and cleanliness of clothes. The nurse emphasizes the importance of periodic checkup and follow-up examination.

Nutrition
In many developing countries, malnutrition is an important factor contributing to poor health. Malnutrition may

also affect the metabolism of toxic agents and also the tolerance mechanisms. Under the Indian Factories Act, it is obligatory on the part of the industrial establishments to provide a canteen when the number of employees exceed 250. The aim is to provide balanced diets or snacks at reasonable cost under action with the education of the workers on the value of balanced diet. If the worker carriers his/her own lunch to work, provision should be made for a safe uncontaminated place to store the food before it is eaten to avoid spoilage or contamination. Likewise, some place separate from the workroom should be provided so that the meal may be eaten in sanitary surroundings.

Communicable disease control
The industry provides an excellent opportunity for early diagnosis, treatment, prevention and rehabilitation. It is a general objective everywhere, to detect cases of communicable disease and to render them noninfectious to others by treatment or removal from the working environment, or both. The communicable diseases of special importance in India are tuberculosis, typhoid fever, viral hepatitis, amebiasis, intestinal parasites, malaria and vernal diseases. There should be an adequate immunization program against preventable communicable disease. Anthrax, undulant fever and Q fever are examples of communicable disease, which may be of occupational origin. Their control calls for special sanitary measures in the handling of working materials and substances.

Control of water-and food-borne diseases: By teaching them preparation of food, education regarding food handling to prevent episodes of gastroenteritis.

Notification
National Laws and Regulations (Factories Act, 1976; Mines Act, 1952; Dock Labourers Act, 1948, etc.) require the notification of cases and suspected cases of occupational disease. In the Factories Act, a list of 22 diseases is included, while in the Mines Act 3 diseases and in the Dock Regulations 8 diseases are listed. These diseases are recognized internationally for the purpose of workmen's compensation. The main purpose of notification in industry is to initiate measures for prevention and protection, and ensuring their effective application; and to investigate the working conditions and other circumstance, which have caused or suspected to have caused occupational diseases.

Supervision of working environment by physician
Periodical inspection of working environment provides information of primary importance in the prevention of occupational disabilities. The physician and CHN should pay frequent visit to the factory in order to acquaint himself/herself with the various aspects of the working environment such as temperature, lighting, ventilation, humidity, noise, cubic space, air pollution and sanitation, which have an important bearing on the health, and welfare of the workers. He/She should be acquainted with the raw materials, processes and products manufactured. He/She should also study the various aspects of occupational physiology such weight carried by the workers and render advice to the factory management on all matters connected with the health and welfare of the workers.

Maintenance and analysis of records
Proper records are essential for the planning, development and efficient operation of an occupational health service. The worker's health record and occupational disability record must be maintained. Their compilation and review should enable the service to watch over the health of the workers, to assess the hazards inherent in certain types of work, and to devise or improve preventive measures.

Health education and counseling
All the risks involved in the industry in which he/she is employed and the measures to be taken for personal protection should be explained to him/her. The correct use of protective devices-like masks and gloves should also be explained. Simple rules of hygiene, i. e. handwashing, paring the nails, bodily cleanliness and cleanliness of clothes, should be impressed upon him/her. The employee should be frequently reminded about the dangers in industry through the media or health education such as charts, posters and hand bills. The purpose of health education is to assist the worker in process of adjustment to the working home and community environment.

Classification of Occupational Diseases

Disease Due to Physical Agents

- Heat: Heat hyperpyrexia, heat exhaustion, heat syncope, heat cramps and burns
- Cold: Trench foot, frostbite and chilblains
- Light: Occupational cataract, Miner's nystagmus
- Pressure: Caisson disease, air embolism and blast
- Radiation: Cancer, leukemia, aplastic anemia and pancytopenia
- Electricity: Burns.

Diseases Due to Chemical Agents

1. Gases poisoning: CO, CO_2, NH_3, PH_3 (phosphine), H_2S, SO_3.
2. Dusts (pneumoconiosis):
   a. Inorganic dusts:
      - Coal dust, e.g. anthracosis
      - Silica, e.g. silicosis

- Asbestos, e.g. asbestosis
- Iron, e.g. siderosis.
  b. Organic dusts:
    - Cane fiber, e.g. bagassosis
    - Cotton dust, e.g. byssinosis
    - Grain dust, e.g. farmer's lung.
3. Metals and their compounds:
    - Lead, mercury, arsenic and manganese poisoning.
4. Chemicals:
    - Acid, alkali poisoning and pesticide poisoning.
5. Solvents:
    - Carbon bisulfide, benzene, chloroform, tetrachloroethylene.

Diseases Due to Biological Agents

Diseases due to biological agents are brucellosis, leptospirosis, anthrax, hydatid cyst, tetanus and fungal infections.

Occupational Cancers

Occupational cancers are dermatitis, eczema.

CONCLUSION

Physical activity is required to live a long and healthy life. There are many ways to perform physical activities such as gardening, walking, swimming, golf, etc. Start the physical activity slowly and gradually increase, and consult doctor, if experience chest discomfort, dizziness, severe headache, etc. while doing physical activity. Exercise is a type of physical activity depended as planned, structured and repetitive bodily movement done to improve or maintain one or more components of physical fitness.

Sleep is most important for maintaining healthy lifestyle. It is a process of relaxing. Deprivation of sleep for several consecutive day lead to lack of physical energy, irritability, blurred vision, memory loss and concentration. So it is necessary to have adequate sleep every day. The need vary among individuals. Recreation means doing the activities in spare time such as watching TV, video games and movies, etc. Weekends, holidays and vacations are usually devoted to recreation, it is an integral part of cultural activities. These are carried out for enjoyment and entertainment. There are many benefits and it reduces the health problems. Sex is most vital of all expressions. Sexual activity is a form of physical exercise and it lowers the levels of body cholesterol.

Self-reliance person is able to thinks for himself. For a self-reliant, one has to work hard. By self-reliant, a person become independent. Healthy diet is required to achieve optimum health and include all the nutrients in appropriate amount healthy food groups include fruits, vegetables, cereals and pulses, dairy, poultry, fish and meat product. Various factors are associated with dietary pattern such as cultural, psychological factors, eating habits, etc. Diet requirement is different according to health problem.

Health education helps in increasing the knowledge and reinforces the desired behavior pattern. According to Alma-Ata (1978), health education has been defined as "a process aimed at encouraging people to want to be healthy, to know how to stay healthy, to do what they can individually and collectively to maintain health and to seek help when needed." Health education is the way by which awareness can be created among public. Health education is provided to improve knowledge, the knowledge determine attitude and attitude determine behavior. So health education is a promotional activity that can bring changes in lifestyles. Occupation is the job. Depending on the job, physical activity is done, which determine the energy expenditure. In case of jobs, where less energy expenditure is there, then an individual has to do additional activities. Increased occupational physical activity reduces the risk of coronary heart diseases, cholesterol levels and also lowers the rates of colorectal cancer.

Financial Management

CHAPTER 26

INTRODUCTION

Finance consists of providing and utilizing the money, capital rights, credit and funds of any kind, which are employed in the operation of organization.

It is the branch of economics concerned with resource allocations as well as resource management, acquisition and investment. It deals with matters related to money and the markets. Finance relates to the system, which generates, regulates and distributes the monetary resources needed for the sustenance and growth of health agency. Finance includes planning of financial resources, making of optimum capital structure and effective utilization of financial resources by deep analysis of capital cost and capital budgeting tool.

Finance is the management of large amount of money especially by government or large companies. Finance is the monetary support for an enterprise. It is the monetary resources and affairs of state organization or a person. Finance is an important ingredient of any organization. 'It has been rightly said that money makes the mare go'. It is also regarded as the life blood of the administration, without finance, administration cannot run. Finance and administration has direct correlation with each other. Even though the finance is available, if not administered or managed properly, can go in waste. Hence, finance and administration or management go side by side. Money is a universal lubricant for any organization, man and machine work.

Economic goods are goods or services purchased by consumers from suppliers to provide a benefit to the consumers. Goods and services are acquired through exchange, generally of money. Wealth is the value of the consumer's resources. Increase in additional sources gained over time, consumers does not have the wealth to buy everything they want, so they must make choices about what to purchase. Utility is the benefit consumers get from the purchase of goods and services supply and demand influence costs. Supply is the amount of goods or services that supplies are willing to provide at a given price. Demand is the amount of goods of services the consumers are willing to buy at their price. For equilibrium, the quantity offered and the quantity demanded are same. As supply goes up and demand goes down; the price is likely to go down, as the supply goes down and the demand goes up, the price is likely to go up.

MEANING

Financial management means planning, organizing, directing and controlling the financial activities such as procurement and utilization of funds of the enterprise. It means applying general management principles to financial resources of the enterprise.

Financial administration consists of all those operations, the objective of which is to make funds/money available for the organizational activities, and to ensure the lawful and efficient use of these funds in order to achieve the organizational goals and objectives.

Financial management is that managerial activity, which is concerned with the planning and controlling of organizational financial resources. It was the branch of economics till 1890, but it is important for both academicians and practicing managers, as the most crucial decisions of the organization that relate to the finance and understanding of financial management provides them the conceptual and analytical insights to make those decisions skillfully.

DEFINITION

Financial management is chiefly concerned with maximizing the wealth of owners through wise and rational investment of funds. It involves the application of general management principles to particular financial operations.

— *Harward and Upton*

Financial management is concerned with the proper management of funds. It involves managerial decisions related to procurement of long-term and short-term funds and their proper utilization in the most productive and effective manner and also in framing the dividend policy.

Financial management is concerned with raising the financial resources and their utilization towards achieving the organizational goals. — *Maheshwari SN*

It is the process of putting the available funds to the best advantage from the long term point of view of business objectives. — *Richard A Brealey*

Thus, financial management deals with planning, organizing, directing and controlling the financial activities such as procurement and utilization of funds of the organization. It is concerned with:
- Assessing the need of funds
- Raising required funds
- Effective utilization of funds
- Distribution of surplus
- Financial controls.

OBJECTIVES

1. To implement fiscal policies.
2. To procure the sufficient funds to carry out the organizational activities.
3. To ensure regular and adequate supply of funds to the concern.
4. To ensure the effective and optimum utilization of funds.
5. To ensure the fair and maximum output or health services on capital.
6. To appropriate in the value of funds.
7. To coordinate with different departments of the organization.
8. To ensure effective financial control, i.e. proper utilization of financial resources allocated to the administrative activities of all the departments.
9. To help in increasing the efficiency of the departments by proper distribution of funds.
10. To create good will of the organization.

SCOPE

According to Saxena SC, the following 5 A's are the scopes of financial management:
- Anticipation: To forecast the requirement of the organization based on its estimated needs
- Acquisition: To procure the finances from different sources
- Allocation: Proper distribution of available funds
- Appropriation: Keep a marginal profit in terms to services
- Assessment: Control the finance.

ELEMENTS

Investment Decisions

Investment decisions include investment in fixed assets called capital budgeting investment in current assets, which is also a part of investment decisions called working capital decisions.

Financial Decisions

Financial decisions relate to the raising of finance from various resources, which will depend upon decision on type of source, period and cost of financing, and the returns thereby.

Dividend Decisions

Dividend decisions are the decisions that are taken with regards to the net profit distribution. Net profits are generally divided into two; dividend for shareholders and retained profits that is the amount of retained profits to be finalized, which will depend upon expansion and diversification plans of the organization.

FUNCTIONS

1. Estimation of capital requirements: This is done with regards to capital requirements of the organization. It depends upon expected costs and profits, and future programs and policies of a concern.
2. Determination of capital structure: Once the estimation has been made, the capital structure has to be decided based on short-term and long-term debt equity analysis.
3. Choice of fund sources: For additional funds to be procured, organization has many choices to find out the various sources available.
4. Investment of funds: The utilization of funds is also allocated.
5. Disposal of surplus: The net profit decisions have to be made keeping in mind the expansion and innovational diversification plans of the organization.
6. Management of cash: This is done by the Accounts Officer/Finance Manager. Cash is required for many purposes such as payment of wages and salaries, payment of electricity and water bills, payment to creditors, meeting current liabilities, maintenance of enough stock, purchase of raw materials, etc.
7. Financial controls: The finance administration has not only to plan, procure and utilize the funds but also

has to exercise control over finances. This can be done through many techniques such as ratio analysis, financial forecasting, cost and profit control, etc.
8. Supervision of cash receipts and payments.
9. Safeguarding of cash balances.
10. Safeguarding of securities and papers.
11. Record keeping and reporting.

INCOME

Income is the additional resources gained over time:
1. Household and individual's income is the sum of all the wages, salaries, profits, interest payments, rents and other forms of earnings received in a given period of time.
2. Firms income is a net profit (Income = Revenue – Expenses) for business and for finance accounts, it is revenue. Income may be depending on sum of the market value of rights exercised in consumption and the change in the value of store of property rights. Sometimes, the consumption potential of non-monetary goods such as leisure, cannot be measured, monetary income may be thought of as a proxy for full income.

Income is increase in economic benefits during the accounting period in the form of inflows or enhancement of assets, or decrease of liabilities that result in increases in equity, other than those relating to contributions from equity participations. The national income includes the total income of individuals, corporations and government in the economy. Sometimes income is distributed in uneven manner, then it is called income inequality. Excessive inequality leads to inefficiency and hinder the socioeconomic development including education, health, etc. in all aspects.

The terms used in finance are as follows:
1. Revenue: It is defined as total income produced by a given source.
2. Expenses: Are those items or services necessary for operation that cost the unit, department or organization money, e.g. expenses include salaries, fringe benefits, utilities and office supplies.
3. Variance: The difference between 'the budgeted amount spent and received' and 'the actual amount spent or received':

Variance = Actual income – Budgeted amount

$$\text{Percentage variance} = \frac{\text{(Actual amount} - \text{Budgeted amount)}}{\text{Budgeted amount}} \times 100$$

4. Fiscal year: This is the 12-month accounting period. In India, we have March 1st to 28th February of a year as the fiscal year.
5. Contribution margin: It is the net profit. It is what remains of revenue after the expenses are paid.

Contribution margin = Revenue – Expenses

$$\text{Contribution percentage} = \frac{\text{Contribution margin}}{\text{Revenue}} \times 100$$

Budget

Budget means planning the expenses based on the source of income. A budget is a plan for the allocation of resources and a control for ensuring that results comply with plans. Results are expressed in quantitative terms. Although, budgets are usually associated with financial statements such as revenue and expenses, they also may be non-financial statements covering output, materials and equipment. Budget helps to coordinate the effects of the agency by determining what resources will be used by whom, when and for which purpose. They are frequently prepared for each organizational unit and for each function within the unit.

In family budget, all sources of income are identified and expenses are planned with the intent of making ends to meet. Budget provides support to family in the management of income and the development of family. A personal budget is a finance plan that allocates future personal income towards expenses, savings and debit repayment. It is important to earn the income to fulfill the basic requirement of the family. Additional income can be earned, which will provide the security to person in cases of emergency. The family budget should include all the income from all sources and all the expenses of family. It should be planned in a way that the expenditure should not exceed the income (Table 26.1).

PURCHASING POWER

Purchasing means to buy various materials by paying money or equivalent from supplies or vendors. Purchasing is a process made up of several steps or actions. The key steps of purchasing are request to purchase/requisition, supplier selection, purchase order, fulfillment, order receipts, supplies involved or payment:
1. Purchase requisition in identifying the need, i.e. what to buy and how much of it, and when it is needed for delivery.
2. Supplement selection is identifying the supplier, price and lead time.
3. Purchase order is to raise purchase orders and sent to supplier. The Purchase Officer/Person identifies the items to be procured, the quantity required and price being paid.

Table 26.1: Sample of family budget

Income	Amount	Expenditure	Amount	Percentage count of total income
Salary	₹	Housing	₹	
Rent	₹	Food	₹	
Overtime	₹	Children	₹	
Part time	₹	Education	₹	
Other services	₹	Recreation	₹	
		Entertainment	₹	
		Clothing	₹	
		Medical	₹	
		Insurance	₹	
		Debt repayment		
		Petrol/Fuel		
		Investments		
		Savings		
Total				

4. **Fulfillment:** Here supplier procures the items and sends to buyer.
5. **Order receipts:** Items are checked for quality and quantity as per the order placed.
6. **Supplier invoice/payment:** The supplier sends the invoice, which is processed by the finance department/concerned persons before supplier is paid.

Purchasing is based on needs assessment. The ultimate aim of purchasing is right quality, right quantity, right prices and right sources at right time to the right place with right mode of transportation, right attitude with proper techniques.

Purchasing power is the value of the thing or goods compared to the amount paid with money, i.e. currencies. Having money gives the individual's ability to command others' labor, so purchasing power, to some extent, is power over other people, to the extent that they are willing to trade their labor or goods for money or currency.

The purchasing power of household is declining, while they are saving less and falling increasingly into debt. A sharp rise in the price of housing is the main reason for the raising debt. The purchasing power of households is showing increasing signs of exhaustion, while their savings capacity is also decreasing. These factors are contributing to the slowdown in the national economy. The purchasing power of an individual or family decrease when the price of the commodities increases, but the income remain the same. Purchasing capability of the individual or the family is affected by increase or the decrease in income, the condition, which can occur.

FINANCE SECURITY

Security is an investment, which can be traded in financial markets. Financial security refer to as being debt-free, controlling expenses, increasing savings every month and performing what we like can lead to happiness, fulfillment and provide prosperous lives for human beings. Accordingly, the characteristics of financial security, includes the following:

1. **Free from debt:** When individual is free from debt he/she feels secured.
2. **Control overexpenses:** When an individual has control over his/her expenses, i.e. control over unnecessary expenditure more than their income. That means the spending less amount than actual income, which helps to save money and invest the extra money in some form. This makes the individual to become financially secured.
3. **Increasing savings:** When the individual increases his/her savings on monthly basis or having an asset given greater feeling or financially secured.

Accordingly, the financial security is the ability to meet future needs, while keeping pace with day-to-day obligations, preparing for retirement and potential long-term care costs takes planning, saving and debt control.

Security can be represented by certificate or an electronic book entry. It is fungible, i.e. replaceable by another identical item or mutually interchangeable, or negotiable instrument representing financial values. Securities may be debt securities (bank note, bonds, debentures, etc.), equity shares (e.g. common stocks), certificated securities (e.g. National Saving Certificate) and registered securities, i.e. legal ownership is not acquired by having possession of the certificate, but details of the holder is kept in register by the issuer, and are updated properly.

Effects have been made to control the costs of health care, these costs continue to increases. Employers, legislators, insurers and healthcare providers continue to collaborate in efforts to resolve the issues surrounding how to lessen healthcare costs. Among these, efforts has implemented some cost containment strategies inducing health promotion and illness prevention activities, managed care systems, and alternative insurance delivery systems.

CONCLUSION

Finance is an important ingredient of any organization. Financial management in any organization is compared with circulatory system in the human body. As the blood circulates through the network of veins and arteries is controlled by heart, similarly finance is spread through financial channel throughout the administrative machinery of the organization and is controlled by the top management of that organization through various departments/agencies, by wages and salaries techniques. Finance is needed for households and individual. Income is the sum of all the wages, salaries, profits, interest, payments, rents and other forms of earnings received in a given period of time. Income is increase in economic benefits during accounting period. Income can be improved by improving skills, during overtime, taking more responsibility, searching part time job, etc. Expenditure should be done according to the need. Proper budgeting helps in planning the revenue and expenditure based on previous budget; with the help of budget, expenditure percentage of one item out of total expenditure can be calculated. On the basis of this, modifications in budget can be done by reducing expenditure on unnecessary item. The purchasing power of an individual or family decrease when the price of the commodities increases, but the income remains the same. Purchasing capability of individual or the family is affected by increase or decrease in the income. Family budget can be prepared in simple and understandable forms to keep the simplicity—while making family budget anticipate the expenses for month in advance and make sure the discretion of subcategories such as food, travel, gifts, clothing, shoes, personnel and medical, and other expenses.

Section 3

Concepts of Epidemiology

- Epidemiology

Epidemiology

CHAPTER 27

INTRODUCTION

The term epidemiology is derived from three Greek words—epi means 'upon', 'among'; desmos means 'people' and logos means 'science', 'study'. Thus, it is the science of events that occur (come upon or among) in a community (the people). Epidemiology is a very old word dating back to second century BC. Hippocrates (460–377 BC) regarded as the Father of clinical medicines, gave accurate description of syndromes on the basis of characteristics, symptoms and findings, and dealt epidemiology in three of his books Epidemic I, II and III or air, water and places. Now, epidemiology is viewed by many scholars as:

1. An inductive method applied to a large group.
2. A research method applied to a large group.
3. A research method of public health.
4. The study of statics of disease in population.
5. The quantitative science measures quantities and descriptive terms used to describe groups (Friedman GD, 1980).
6. The measurement of risk of diseases in community.
7. The study of epidemics of hard to large group.
8. A method of diagnosing the conditions of the people (Hill AB, 1965).
9. The study of health of population in relation to their environment and ways of living (Lilliefield AM, 1936).
10. The study of the frequency of distribution, determinants of infectious process:
    - A disease
    - A physiological state and their precursors in a community.

DEFINITIONS

1. The branch of medical science, which treats epidemics.
   —*Perkin, 1873*
2. The science of the mass phenomenon of infectious disease.
   —*Frost, 1927*
3. The study of the distribution and determinants of disease frequency in man.
   —*McMahon and Pugh, 1960*
4. Concerned with the pattern of disease occurrence in human population and of the factors that influence these patterns.
   —*Lillienfield, 1980*
5. The study of the distribution and determinants of health-related states, events in population, and the application of the study to control health problems.
   —*Last, 1983*
6. All these definitions indicate that the scope of epidemiology has expanded over the years. As due of socioeconomic development, the pattern of diseases changes to one predominantly chronic, non-infectious disease; the definition of epidemiology also has been changed and changing from time to time. But the definition of epidemiology by McMahon and Pugh is most widely used for many years. This definition is still closely linked to disease and so fails to take into account the considerably epidemiological interest in nondiseases such as trauma (war, accidents, manslaughters, suicides, etc.) drug addiction, alcoholism, etc. nor does it take into account epidemiology of health, and the provision of health services for which epidemiological methods are used. In general, the science of epidemiology is the methodology of the search required to find answers to the questions posed by Kipling service men "I have six honest serving men they taught me all I knew, their names are what, why, when, how, where and who."
   —*Rudyard Kipling*
7. Epidemiology has been defined as, "The study of distribution and determinants of health-related states or events in specified populations and application of this study to the control of health problems."
   —*John M Last, 1988*

The meaning of 'keywords' need to be explained. The health-related events are all the conditions of the spectrum of health such as disease, injury, disability and death.

These events are with reference to the human population (epidemiology is also studied among animals). The distribution refers to the pattern of occurrence of disease in the community with reference to time, place and person. This part of the study is known as, 'Descriptive epidemiology'. This helps to study the trend of the disease over the years (decades), geographical areas and over different population groups. This study also helps to know the magnitude of the problem gives a clue about the etiology, mode of transmission of the disease and also helps to formulate etiological hypothesis.

The determinant refers the etiological or risk factors related to particular disease. This study helps to test the etiological hypothesis formulated by descriptive study. This aspect of epidemiology dealing with testing the hypothesis is known as 'analytical epidemiology'.

Another important related term is disease frequency, which means measuring the magnitude or extent of the health-related event or health problem in the community, in terms of morbidity rates such as incidence and prevalence, and also in mortality rates. These are expressed in terms of rate, ratio and proportion. This helps to compare with that of other countries or other groups of population in the same country (morbidity means sickness and mortality means deaths). The widely accepted definition is given by 'International Epidemiology Association'. It studies the three components, i.e. disease frequency, distribution of disease and determinants of disease. The first component indicates that the epidemiology is measurement of frequency of disease, disability or death and summarizing this information in the form of rates and ration, i.e. prevalence rate, incidence rate, death rate, etc. The second component is concerned with describing the distribution of health status in terms of age, sex, race, geography, etc. and the third involves interpretation of the distribution in terms of the possible causal factors. Hence, it is a science developed from the study of the unusual to find out an explanation for unusual happenings.

As stated earlier, the word epidemiology is derived from the Greek roots, 'epi' meaning 'upon' and 'emo', meaning 'people' (collectively). Historically, the major focus of the epidemiologist was on analyzing major infectious disease outbreaks (epidemics) so that ways to control and prevent disease occurrence in populations (people, collectively) could be determined. As early as the fifth century, tuberculosis (TB) was a dreaded scourge called 'King's Evil'. King's Evil was thought to have healing powers from God and they held audiences to touch, and supposedly cure their subjects. Today, the definition of epidemiology has been expanded to include the study of variables that affect health and influence disease, and condition occurrence.

There are many variations in the definition of the term epidemiology, but most focus on studying determinants of health and disease states among populations. The following definition, adapted from McMahon and Pugh classic writings is used. Epidemiology is the systematic, scientific study of the distribution pattern and determinants of health, disease and condition frequencies in populations for the purpose of promoting wellness and preventing disease/conditions. Implicit in this definition are two basic assumptions. The first is that patterns and frequencies of health, disease and conditions is populations can be identify. The second is that factors determining or contributing to the occurrence of health, disease or conditions can be discovered through systematic investigation.

Community health nurses (CHN) work with other public health professional using the epidemiological process to carry out their systematic investigation of health, diseases and conditions in populations. This process is similar to the nursing process. The steps are labeled differently, but in essence, they both involve a series of circular, dynamic problem solving actions (Table 27.1). Learning the language of epidemiology gives one distinct advantage, however, because the terminology of epidemiology is used by all community health professionals, the terminology of the nursing processes is not.

AIMS OF EPIDEMIOLOGY

According to the International Epidemiological Association, epidemiology has three main aims:
1. To describe the distribution and size of disease problems in human population.
2. To identify etiological factors in the pathogenesis of disease.
3. To provide the data essential to the planning, implementation and evaluation of services for the prevention, control and treatment of disease, and to the setting up of priorities among these services.

The ultimate aim of epidemiology is to lead to effective action to eliminate or reduce the health problems, or its consequences and to prevent its occurrence in future.

OBJECTIVES OF EPIDEMIOLOGY

- To know the distribution of the disease in the community
- To know the magnitude of the problem
- To identify the etiological and risk factors in the development of disease

Table 27.1: Comparison of the nursing processes and the epidemiological process

Nursing process	Epidemiological process

1. Assessing (data collection to determine) client's problem	1. Determine the nature, extent and scope of the problem:
	  a. Natural life history of condition
	  b. Determinants influencing condition:
	    i. Primary data (essential agent):
	      • Parasite/Bacterium/Virus
	      • Nutritional
	      • Psychosocial
	    ii. Contributory data:
	      • Agent
	      • Host
	      • Environment
	  c. Distribution patterns:
	    i. Person
	    ii. Place
	    iii. Time
	  d. Condition frequencies:
	    i. Prevalence
	    ii. Incidence
	    iii. Other biostatistical measurements

2. Analyzing (formulation of nursing diagnosis or hypotheses)	2. Formulate tentative hypothesis(es)
3. Planning	3. Collect and analyze further data to test hypothesis(es)
4. Implementing	4. Plan of control
5. Evaluating	5. Implement control plan
6. Revising or terminating	6. Evaluate control plan
7. Research	7. Make appropriate report

- To plan for the implementation of prevention and control measures
- To eliminate or eradicate the disease
- To evaluate the control measures
- Ultimate objective is to promote the health and well-being of the people.

EPIDEMIOLOGICAL APPROACH

Epidemiological approach is an approach to achieve the above objectives by collecting the data by asking the following questions and analyzing the data systematically:
- What is the event (Nature of the disease)?
- When did the disease occur (Time distribution of the disease)?
- Where did the disease occur (Place distribution of the disease)?
- Who are the persons affected (Person distribution of the disease)?
- What is the extent of the problem (Magnitude)?
- What is to be done to reduce the problem (Control measures)?
- How can it be prevented in future (Preventive measures)?

In brief, epidemiology is said to be concerned with all health and illness in population groups, and with the factors including health services that affect them. The aims of epidemiology include knowledge of distribution of disease in order to elucidate casual mechanism, explaining local disease occurrence, describe the natural history of diseases, and provide guidance in the administration of health services. Following are human characteristics that are of concern to epidemiologists:

1. Biological characteristics such as biochemical level of blood, including antibodies and enzymes, and measurement of physiological functions of different organ system of the body.
2. Demographic characteristics such as age, sex, race and ethnic group.
3. Social and socioeconomic characteristics such as status, education, occupation and nativity.
4. Personal living habits such as tobacco use, diet and exercises.

Factors other than personal characteristics useful in epidemiology for administrative purpose and for the study of the etiology of disease include place or geography of the existence of an illness, and its time or secularity. The interaction between person, place and time are also important in studying the cause of disease.

USES OF EPIDEMIOLOGY

Epidemiology helps:
1. To study the effects of disease in state a population over a time predicts future health needs. Here, epidemiologists study the history of the health of the population's rise and fall of diseases, changes in their character and predict the future health needs.
2. To diagnose the health the community: Here, the epidemiologists study the condition of the people to measure the distribution and dimension of illness in terms of incidence, prevalence, disability and mortality. To set health problems in perspective and to define their relative importance, and to identify groups needing special attention. New methods of monitoring must be constantly sought. In short, it helps in diagnosing the health status of the community.
3. To evaluate health services: Here, epidemiologists study the working of health services with a view to their improvement by evaluating the healthcare services in the community. Operational research shows how community expectations can result in the actual provision of service. The success with which the services achieve their stated goals and the effect on community health have to be appraised in relation to resources. Action research can lead to future plants for better services, e.g. planning efficient research including drugs trails and new methods of treatment.
4. To estimate the individual risk from group experiences: Here, the work of an epidemiologist is to estimate the risks of diseases, accident and defect and chances of avoiding them. So, it studies the effects of disease state in population over a period of time and predicts the future health needs, and provides the base for preventive measure. Their evaluation also helps in logical planning of facilities for health care.
5. To identify the syndrome: Here, the epidemiologists help to identify syndromes by describing the distribution and association of clinical phenomena in the population or helps in evolving and describing the natural history of disease.
6. To complete the clinical picture of chronic diseases and describe the natural history; it provides complete clinical picture of disease, so the prevention can be accomplished before disease becomes irreversible.
7. To search for causes of health and disease: This can be done by comparing experience of groups that are clearly defined by their composition, inheritance, experience, behavior and environments. So, epidemiology helps in understanding the causation of disease, disability and providing data, which helps to explain the etiology of disease and local disease pattern, which in turn helps to test the hypothesis clinically or experimentally.

The uses of epidemiology encompasses of two main components:
1. The systematic collection of health data (including the utilization of data collected for other purposes):
   a. Identification of health problems and assessment of priorities in allocation of resources, including surveillance.
   b. Detection of new problems or changes in frequency of existing problems.
   c. Identification of risk factors enabling efficient distribution of resources assigned to a particular problem.
   d. Evaluation of effectiveness of control program.
   e. Formulation of hypotheses regarding the reasons for non-random disease distribution (disease etiology).
2. The search for causes of ill health:
   a. Identification of alterable causes.
   b. Identification of susceptible groups for special surveillance.
   c. Identification of disease entities.
   d. Identification of early manifestations of disease or disease syndrome.

SCOPE OF EPIDEMIOLOGY

The scopes of epidemiology are shown in Figure 27.1.

ADVANTAGES OF USING EPIDEMIOLOGY IN COMMUNITY HEALTH NURSING PRACTICE

Epidemiology brings CHN as a dynamic and exciting perspective. The process of epidemiology adds methods of hypothesizing new problem-solving technique to the nursing process for practice in the community.

Epidemiology formulates new relationships and new association between nursing and public health. In today challenging and provocative times, epidemiology assists nurse to meet changing community needs by nursing methods and tools that are held in common with all members of the multidisciplinary team. This common language

Epidemiology

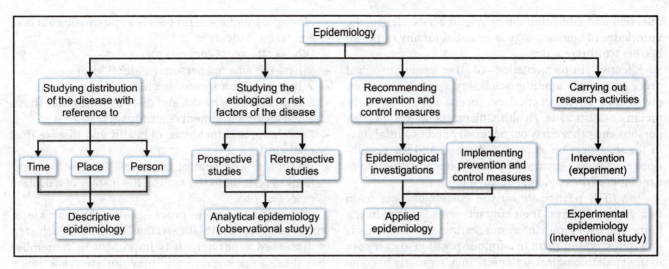

Figure 27.1: Various scopes of epidemiology

improves interprofessional communication and trust. At the same time the unique attributes of nursing as a profession can be maintained and displayed within the framework of epidemiological methods and theory.

The advantages of using an epidemiology perspective for the nursing are as follows:

1. Epidemiology provides a framework within which basic science and behavioral science can be used for community nursing practice.
2. The nursing process extended through applications of epidemiological methods to describe community needs and evaluate nursing services.
3. Public health principle of family is the unit of society. Prevention and control of disease, and health promotion are activated and quantifies through epidemiology approach.
4. Epidemiology provides interdisciplinary language to promote interprofessional communication and trust.
5. An epidemiological perspective provides a method of extending the relationship of family problems to community welfare.
6. The epidemiological model promotes understanding the relationship between the environment and agents that expose susceptible populations at risk of impediments of health.
7. Epidemiology provides time-honored method of quantifying nursing outcomes, i.e. recidivism. Lack of compliance and activities of daily living to promote and improve the quality of nursing care in the community.

Further, the study of the distribution of diseases and health-related problems are not adequate. The fundamental aim of epidemiology is to search for factors, which influence and determine the observed distributors. Illness in individuals is often determined by a selective operation of one or more factors. Further, our environment and our blind destruction of it is so complex that limiting our investigation to individual illness may contribute very little to our efforts to solve community health problems.

The epidemiologist must examine a number of cases of similar diseases or health-related problems as they occur throughout population and subsequently assist in identifying the operational factors in afflicted group of the population. Thus, the discovery of factors causing or contributing to the occurrences of any particular disease or health problem is the most important concern of epidemiology.

The satisfactions of scientific curiosity will lead to a more complete understanding of occurrence of ill health. An increased understanding of the epidemiological approach in turn will enable the providers of health services to plan, implement and assess effective measures of health promotion, the prevention and control of diseases and disabilities.

The use of epidemiology helps the CHN in many ways because he/she is the person in the field, who deals with the people with various settings. So, epidemiology helps the CHN to identify and investigate the problems. Formulatory alternative actions, implements the prevention and control of problem, and also helps to evaluate the effectiveness of actions. For example, nurses in the community have an active role in prevention and control of communicable disease, which includes participation in early diagnosis and treatment notification of certain specific disease to the healthy authority, tracing the contact, keep them under surveillance, identify sources of injection and educating the people in genes. Hence, the knowledge of epidemiology is essential for any nurse for his/her fruitful practice.

Effective implementation of the epidemiological process requires a multidisciplinary approach. Nurses, physicians, environmental engineers, laboratory technicians, statisticians, Health Officer, social workers, lay persons and other carry out necessary and essential roles in the investigation, control of disease, and the promotion of wellness. Any health professional can function as a member of the epidemiological team.

The CHN participate on the epidemiological team in a variety of ways. Their contacts with families in the home and with group in various settings (clinics, schools and industry) put them in a unique position to carry out many epidemiological activities. They regularly become involved in case finding, health teaching, counseling and follow-up essential to the prevention of infectious diseases, chronic conditions and other health-related phenomena. The actions taken by the CHN in the actual case situations how they work to prevent the spread of TB and lower the level of lead in the blood.

The nature, extent and scope of the problem were determined and a conclusion about the problem was reached, treatment was started and resolution of the problem began. The ultimate goal was prevention of additional TB cases in the prison setting and eliminating of lead poisoning in the home setting.

The CHN apply the principle of epidemiology to provide preventive health services to aggregate in the community. For example, nurses serving Asian populations might consider the hidden threat of lead poisoning and implement this potential problem into their screening and education programs. The nurse must understand the significance of expanding epidemiological study from individuals and families to effort with populations. Only in this way the CHN will effectively meet the health needs of the community as a whole.

EPIDEMIOLOGICAL PROCESS

Basic concepts in epidemiology have been discussed to lay a foundation for epidemiological investigation of community health problems. These concepts aid in identifying variables that public health professionals consider when they describe the distribution patterns and determinants of health, disease and condition frequencies in populations. They help to analyze caused relationship in disease or condition outbreaks. To establish these casual relationships, health professional use a scientific process known as the epidemiological process.

The epidemiological process is a systematic course of action taken to identify:
- Who is affected? (Persons)
- Where the affected persons reside? (Place)
- When the persons were affected? (Time)
- Casual factors of health and disease occurrence (host, agent and environment determinants)
- Prevalence and incidence of health and disease (frequencies)
- Prevention and control measures (levels of prevention) in relation to the natural life history of a disease or a condition.

The epidemiological process has eight basic steps, which are graphically illustrated. Although, each step is discussed separately, it is important to remember that these steps overlap and may not always follow a sequential pattern. They are interrelated and dependent on each other. For example, data collected in the initial step provide a foundation for all subsequent steps (Fig. 27.2).

Step 1 (Find out the Nature, Extent and Scope of the Problem)

The primary responsibilities during the initial steps are of two fold:
- To verify the diagnosis by data collection from multiple sources
- To determine the extent and possible significance of the verified problem.

Data gathering begins when an index case is reported or when there is a noticeable change in the incidence rate for a particular disease or condition. The index case is the case that brings a household or other group to the attention of community health personnel. Once this case in known to health professionals, data are collected from various sources to determine if a problem really exists (refer Fig. 27.1).

Clinical observations, laboratory studies and lay reporting assist the epidemiological team in confirming the homogenicity of the current events. For instance, four hospital emergency rooms have reported that several individuals were treated for food poisoning in the last 24 hours, health personnel would want to immediately take the following actions:

1. Interview the affected persons to determine the nature of the symptoms and to identify loci of origin according to person, place and time.
2. Review laboratory studies to confirm common causative organisms. This process could establish that several events are occurring at the same time.

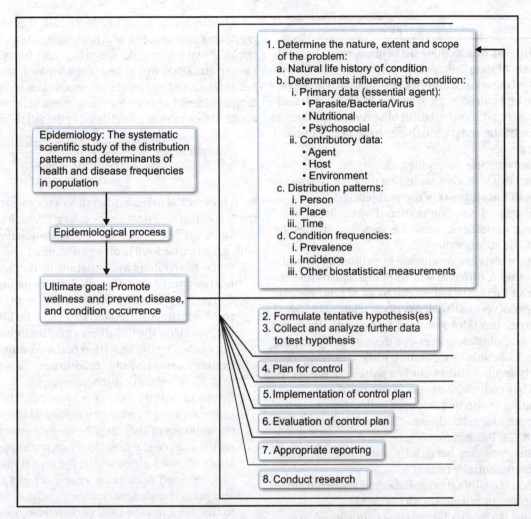

Figure 27.2: Basic steps of epidemiological process

3. Interview friends, relatives and lay acquaintance to discern their description of the vents that led up to the reported illness and to determine if other individuals have symptoms.

Timely, accurate and thorough data collection is critical factor in step 1. Significant data may be destroyed if the data collection process is too slow. In addition, only the most obvious events 'tip of the iceberg' are observed, the extent of the problem will not be identified. The health professional needs to be a detective, beginning by interviewing the affected individual's environment to track down the host, agent and environmental factors that influence disease occurrence. As previously discussed, the measurable variables that facilitate rapid and efficient data collection about host, agent and environment factors are person, place and time.

Analyzing data in terms of person, place and time helps to establish the magnitude of the problem. Data tell the health professional about the proportion of the people affected, the seriousness of the effects on the host and the community, improvement or regression over time, and geographic distribution of the disease or condition. They also help in identifying potential sources of infection and casual relationships.

When prevalence and incidence rates are compared, a word of caution is necessary. If there is a distinct departure from normal, it must be ascertained that a problem really exists. It may be that there is only an improvement in reporting, not an actual increase in disease occurrence. If there is an actual increase in the incidence of a particular disease or condition, the health professionals make an educated guess as to the nature of the causative agent, based on data collected. This formulation of a tentative diagnosis or hypothesis is done to enhance further data collection.

Step 2 [Formulate Tentative Hypothesis(es)]

When dealing with infectious diseases, a rapid preliminary analysis of data is imperative. Disease can spread quickly, affecting a large number of people in a short period of time and can have great ranges in severity. Usually, analysis results in formulation of several hypotheses. Explanation of the most probable source of infection is made in terms of:

1. The agent causing the problem.
2. The source of infection, including the chain of events leading to the outbreak of the problem.
3. Environmental conditions that allowed it to occur. Tentative hypotheses must be tested and may be found to be appropriate.

Laboratory tests are invaluable in validating hypotheses. For example, different strains of *Mycobacterium tuberculosis* can be compared on the basis of their genetic content or genotype, called deoxyribonucleic acid (DNA) fingerprinting. The DNA is cut off into pieces, then the number of size of these pieces are measured by placing them in a gel-like substance across, while a pulsing electrical field is applied. The result is a pattern of bands resembling a bar code, which is the 'fingerprint'.

These patterns can be compared with others to determine the potential relatedness of bacterial strains. The information can be used to:

- Determine, whether bacterial isolates from different clients are potentially related
- Determine, if a clinical isolate matches those obtained from samples implicated in an outbreak
- Determine, if a particular isolate is being found in other states or regions.

Step 3 (Collect and Analyze Further Data to Test Hypothesis)

A basic starting point in this step is to identify the group affected by the disease or problem under investigation. In the previous scenario, the inmates and guards composed the obvious group of concern; however, people out in the community were also at risk for contracting TB. Individual epidemiological histories should be done to classify persons according to their exposure to suspected or causative agents and to identify the clinical data, and bacteriological findings need to substantiate the diagnosis. Significant variation of incidence in contrasted population groups should be noted. These variations can be identified through study of attack rates. In the jail population, longer and frequent incarceration was related to diagnosis.

An attack rate is an incidence rate that identifies the number of people at risk who become ill. In studying a foodborne disease outbreak, the attack rate for persons, who ate certain foods would be compared with attack rate for persons who did not eat certain foods. This is done in an attempt to identify, which food was infected by the causative agent. Attack rates are calculated in the following manner:

$$\text{Attack rates} = \frac{\text{Number of persons affected}}{\text{Number of persons not eating food item}} \times 100$$

It is essential to remember the attack rates do not positively confirm an infective food. Last (1986) has identified the following five reasons, why the association of illness with a particular food is often difficult:

1. Some individuals are resistant to the agent and do not become ill even though they are exposed.
2. The employed definition of an ill person may include some who have unrelated illness, if the illness is one, i.e. prevalent, the ill subjects may include some cases not caused by the ingestion of the common vehicles.
3. Contamination of one food braces of another may take place before or during serving.
4. Errors in history taking may occur. These may be unbiased errors caused by memory lapses or misunderstanding or they may be caused by biases, either on the part of the questioner or the subject. Several kinds of biases are possible; the questioner may have preconceived notices of what food was responsible and press the questions more vigorously with respect to that food in case of ill person than non-ill person; subject may have preconceived notions leading to the same result. The subject may have reasons for wishing to either claim or disclaim illness. Biases may affect the accuracy either of food histories or illness histories and produce spurious association.
5. Finally, biased sampling may also lead to spurious results. All of these factors can affect the validity of an attack rate and thereby the choice of the appropriate infective food. Laboratory studies are necessary to identify the etiological agent and its vehicle or vector. However, identifying the causative agent is not the only step in preventing further spread of disease. Knowing the agent, assists in treating ill individuals, who seek medical care, but does not tell how the disease is being transmitted. The chain of transmission must be broken to stop the spread of disease.

Because one factor alone never causes a disease or condition, it is not sufficient to identify just the causative agent. After the possible agents and the attack group have been identified, the common source(s) to which affected individual was exposed should be investigated. With foodborne diseases, the origin, method and preparation of suspected foods would be primary factors to examine. Concurrently, environmental conditions should be evaluated. These conditions would include such things as the sanitary status of the restaurant, the area where food was served, the water and dairy supply. CHN frequently are responsible for collecting these data during an epidemiological investigation. In some health departments, nurses are also responsible for collecting specimens for laboratory analysis. The epidemiological division of the state or local health department provides information on how to properly collect, preserve and ship specimens for epidemiological analysis.

Completing an epidemiological case history form provides an opportunity for health teaching and case finding. Often the CHN identifies new cases during this process and help clients to learn about the nature of the disease, and how to prevent its spread. Tentative hypotheses must be tested; sometimes, however, none of the origin hypotheses is appropriate. Testing hypotheses helps to determine, if the initial control measures were sufficient to resolve the current outbreak. It also aids in identifying the natural life history of the disease and where further action is needed.

Step 4 (Plan of Control)

When planning for control, it is essential to identify preventive activities based on the knowledge of the natural history of the disease in question, which can be used to control the further spread of disease occurrence. Host, agent and environment factors should be analyzed to determine the following:

1. Population at risk.
2. Primary, secondary and tertiary preventive measures available that would:
   a. Alter the behavior or susceptibility of the host (e.g. health education, case finding, immunization, treatment or rehabilitation).
   b. Destroy the agent (e.g. heat, drug treatment or spraying with insecticides).
   c. Eliminate the transmission of agent (e.g. changes in host's health habits or environmental conditions).
3. Feasibility of implementing the control plan, considering such factors available community resources, time required, cost of control versus partial or no control, facilities, supplies and personnel needs.
4. Priorities in relation to legal mandate, significance of the problem relative to other community needs and the feasibility of implementing the control plan.

Control measures are generally directed toward breaking the chain of transmission. This includes destroying or treating the reservoir of infection, interrupting the transmission of the agent from the reservoir to the new host and decreasing ability of the agent to adapt, and multiply within the host. The concept of multiple causation of disease must be used in breaking the chain of transmission.

When dealing with infectious diseases and establishing a control plan, the concept of herd immunity is important. It is defined as the 'immunity of a group or community'. The resistance of a group to an invasion and spread of an infectious agent is based on the resistance to infection of a high proportion of individual members of the group'. Immunity is 'that resistance usually associated with the presence of antibodies or cells, which have a specific action on the microorganisms concerned with a particular infectious disease or on its toxin'.

If 100% is given group have received measles vaccine, the herd immunity would be 100%. If 80% had received measles vaccine, the herd immunity would be at least 80%. Some people in the group have natural immunity, raising the percentage higher. Herd immunity does not have to be 100% to prevent an epidemic or to control a disease, but is not known just what percentage is safe.

As herd immunity decreases, the chances for epidemic rises. The major concern is that many school-age children are not receiving immunizations for communicable diseases. Immunization coverage levels vary substantially by state and large urban areas, which greatly decreases level of herd immunity, and is a major barrier for maintaining community health.

The CHN are instrumental in helping the public, then need for effective control of disease through active immunization. This will continue to be a major function of the CHN, because immunizing populations at risk is the most effective way to control many childhood communicable diseases.

Case finding the process focuses on early diagnosis and treatment of newly discovered cases of diseases or condition. Case finding may evolve through clinical observation, reviewing records or by mass, or individual screening. TB outbreak in the urban area was found when nurses reviewed records and found high number of them with positive tuberculin skin tests. Other examples of case finding occur with foodborne outbreaks; people, who were part of function where illness is reported are contacted, usually by phone, to ascertain whether or not they became ill after eating specific foods. Careful record keeping assists epidemiologists to quickly spot changing trends in disease or conditions. Health department carry out surveillance of reportable diseases at weekly intervals to track changes in diseases that can quickly involve large number of citizens.

Step 5 (Implement Control Plan)

An active effort should be made to elicit and coordinate the cooperation of the lay public, as well as private and official agencies, when control measures are put into operation. A control program that takes into consideration the beliefs, attitudes and customs of the community is more likely to be accepted by the public than one that ignores community norms.

There are many barriers to the successful implementation of a control plan for both infectious disease and non-communicable conditions. Barriers to control involve factors such as unknown etiology, no known treatment, unavailable community resources, multifaceted etiology, long latency periods and lack of reporting. In the preceding scenario, many of migrants lived in small homes with 15–20 other people. Limited resources gave these folks few other choices; however, it put them all at high risk for exposure to TB and other communicable diseases.

An individual without overt disease symptoms, but who harbors the disease organisms can be a major vehicle in disease transmission. Such individuals are known as carriers. Hepatitis C and salmonellosis are examples of diseases, which are often transmitted by carriers.

With any disease for a variety of reasons, some individuals will delay in confirmation and treatment of the disease can enhance its spread, contamination and impede control plan implementation.

Individuals for whom the diagnosis is not suspected or confirmed are also barriers to the control of disease. Disease may not be confirmed for several reasons. Some people will have atypical symptoms do not fit a disease model, the disease may be missed completely or misdiagnosed. Other individuals are seen too early or too late in the course of the disease process to either suspect or confirm the disease. In these situations, laboratory test may be falsely negative or they may not be done at all because the clinical symptoms do not reflect a need. At other times a diagnosis cannot be confirmed, because specimens (stools, emesis or sputum) inadvertently have been destroyed or handled improperly. Epidemiologists are cognizant that specimens are needed for laboratory testing and often this is the only way that an infectious disease agent is identified. The identical agent often dictates the treatment of the disease and the program of prevention that needs to be instituted.

Step 6 (Evaluate Control Plan)

Evaluation ensures that an epidemiological process can be improved next time, if it is repeated. The first step in evaluation is to determine how well the objectives of the process were met. This implies that before carrying out the process, objectives were clearly and behaviorally written. The next question to be answered is how the current situation compares to the situation before the investigation. Finally, the practical of the control measures should be determined. Feasibility cost in terms of money, time, staff facilities and community support should be analyzed.

Step 7 (Make Appropriate Report)

Prompt, accurate and concise epidemiological reporting provides a basis for further investigations and control measures. Reporting should include what was involved in the epidemiological process diagnosis factors leading to the epidemic, control measures, process evaluation and recommendations for preventing similar situations.

For many reasons under-reporting of epidemiological investigations occur. Completion of necessary forms can be tedious and time consuming, therefore, neglected. There may be one person assigned, the responsibility for seeing that reports are completed, so the responsibility is overlooked. Usually, more effective reporting occurs when one person is designated to coordinate the reporting activities of others.

Accurate reporting is essential for the identification of major community health problems and preventive health action that would correct these problems. Treating only individuals with overt symptoms, rather than collecting and reporting data on population at risk, does very little to prevent future health problems.

Step 8 (Conduct Research)

If health services to populations are to be improved, epidemiological research is essential. Health professionals must be prepared to collect and analyze data systematically, so that the gaps in knowledge relative to disease causation, prevention and control are eliminated. The ultimate goal of epidemiology, 'the prevention and control of infectious diseases, chronic conditions and other health-related phenomena in populations' is far from

CHAPTER 27 — Epidemiology

being realized. It is unfortunate that research in the practice setting is often lacking; it can be exciting and challenging, especially when one discovers significant data that will aid a community to improve its health status.

IMPORTANCE OF EPIDEMIOLOGICAL PROCESS/SURVEILLANCE

Epidemiological surveillance is an essential public health function at all levels of government. Public health surveillance is the ongoing and dissemination of health data, including information on clinical diagnoses, laboratory-based diagnoses, specific syndromes, health-related behaviors and other indicators related to health outcomes. Epidemiologists use these data to detect outbreaks; characterize disease transmission patterns by time, place and person, evaluate prevention and control programs; and project future healthcare needs. As stated earlier, epidemiology helps in many ways, which includes:

1. It helps to study the natural history of a disease, i.e. in relation to agent, host and environmental factors, and further evolution of the disease to its termination as death or recovery in the absence of prevention or treatment. This is a necessary framework for application of preventive measures.
2. It helps to measure the disease frequency in terms of the magnitude of the problem (i.e. morbidity and mortality rates).
3. It helps to make 'community diagnosis' by studying the distribution of the disease with reference to time, place and person. Therefore, epidemiology has been considered as 'diagnostic tool', in community medicine. Community diagnosis also helps in under-standing the social, cultural and environmental characteristics of the community.
4. Descriptive epidemiology helps to formulate an 'etiological hypothesis'.
5. It helps to identify the determinants of the disease and the risk factors.
6. It helps to study historically the rise and fall of the disease in the population, i.e. as old diseases are conquered (e.g. smallpox), new diseases have been identified such as [severe acute respiratory syndrome (SARS), acquired immunodeficiency syndrome (AIDS), etc.]. Similarly, as the quality of life improved in the developed countries, the incidence of diseases such as TB, malnutrition declined.
7. It helps to estimate the individual's risk of a particular disease by using the indices such as absolute risk, attributable risk, relative risk, odd's ratio, etc.
8. It helps to identify syndromes, e.g. AIDS.
9. It helps to formulate the 'plan of action' for providing the health services including preventive and control measures.
10. It helps to 'evaluate' the health services to find out whether the measures undertaken are effective in controlling the disease or not. Further it also helps to find out the cost-effectiveness of different method.
11. It helps to make researches in epidemiology.
12. It contributes to the standardization of biostatistical techniques.

To use the epidemiological process effectively, CHN need to have an understanding of the basic concepts, tool and terms of epidemiology. Because, epidemiology is operationally defined in terms of disease measurements, an understanding of the biostatistical concepts is essential. Biostatistics helps to describe the extent and distribution of health, illness, conditions in the community and aids in the identification of specific health problems, and community strengths. Biostatistics also facilitates the setting of priorities for program planning.

In addition to biostatistics, several basic concepts guide epidemiological study. These aggregates at risk, the natural life history of a disease, levels of prevention, host-agent-environment relationships and person-place-time relationships. In general, these concepts provide the foundation of explaining—how disease develops? How health is maintained? Who is most susceptible to disease? How disease can be prevented and health promoted?

A key concept of epidemiology is that the study of disease in population is more significant than the study of individual's cases of diseases. Epidemiological research has demonstrated that using large sampling groups is essential for formulating valid conclusions about the distribution patterns and determinants of health, disease and condition frequencies in populations. It is by observing large groups that commonalities and differences among people, who have or do not have a particular disease or condition can be identified.

The identification of commonalities and differences among groups focuses attention on the essential or contributory factors that produce illness or promote health. For example, TB has been frequently found in prisons and other settings where there is crowding, thus leading to the conclusion that the disease is spread by respiratory droplets. Examining individual cases would not lead one to that conclusion.

A preventive health philosophy has led professionals in community health to emphasize the study of groups. A goal of epidemiological study is to identify aggregates at risk. Aggregates at high risk are those, who engage in certain activities or who have certain characteristics that increase their potential for contracting an illness or injury, or a health problem. For example, coal miners are daily exposed to dust containing silica, a common mineral. This exposure is known as a risk factor for the development of silicosis, a lung disease.

Risk factors are determined by a risk estimate process. Risk estimates are derived by contrasting the frequency of a disease or health condition in persons exposed to a specific trait, or risk factor and the frequency in another group not exposed to risk factor. Risk factors fall into the three major categories:
- Behavioral or lifestyle patterns
- Environmental factors
- Inborn or inherited characteristics.

These risk factors increase one's susceptibility to death, disease and injury. For example, living in homeless shelters (environmental patterns) may expose men, who abuse alcohol (lifestyle factors) to active TB. Health problems usually result from multiple interacting factors. When these multiple risk factors come together, they form an interrelated web of forces that increases their potential for causing harm.

Many health problems are related to lifestyle patterns and environmental factors such as accidents, child abuse, suicide, domestic violence, alcoholism and sexually transmitted disease (STD). Anticipatory guidance at each stage across the lifespan assists individuals, families and aggregates in developing lifestyle patterns that promote health, reduce the risk of disease and adverse health condition. Health is a part of social, political and economic justice.

The nation has promoted the definition of human rights to include the rights of children, women and youth. The rights to food and environment security; the right to safe water; the right to the highest attainable standard of physical and mental health, including reproductive and sexual health. The values that underlie public health are the values of human rights. In a world where there is such gross inequity in the distribution of resources, a firm belief in those values should give the public health professional cause for concern and introspection.

NATURAL LIFE HISTORY OF DISEASE

In the search for commodities that may produce disease and health-related phenomena in specific aggregates, epidemiological study focuses on determining the natural life history of these conditions. Observing the natural life history of disease and health-related phenomena aids in identifying agent-host-environmental factors that influence their development, characteristic signs and symptoms during their different periods of progression, approaches for preventing and controlling their effects on humans.

The natural life history of disease is defined as the course of a disease from onset (inception) to resolution. Many diseases have certain well-defined stages that taken all together are referred to as the natural history of the disease in question. In their classic textbook, Leavell and Clark (1965) identified two distinct periods in the natural history of a disease—prepathogenesis and pathogenesis (Fig. 27.3).

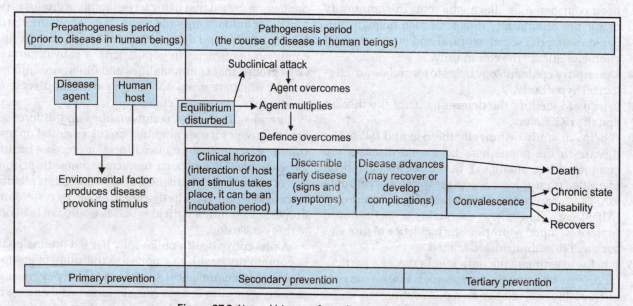

Figure 27.3: Natural history of any disease process in man

In the prepathogenesis period, disease has not developed, but interactions are occurring between the host, agent and environment that produce diseases, stimulus, and increase the host's potential for disease. The combination of human immunodeficiency virus (HIV) infection and substance abused increased the host's potential for developing TB.

The pathogenesis period in the natural life history of disease begins when disease-producing stimuli (TB bacilli) start to produce changes in the tissues of human (development of granuloma). The interrelationship between the prepathogenesis period and the pathogenesis period and how the latter progresses from the presymptomatic stage to advanced clinical disease. It also shows that disease occurs as a result of processes that happen in the environment (prepathogenesis). Preventive interventions can alter the natural life history of many diseases.

The study of the natural life history of disease facilities the achievement of the ultimate goal of epidemiology. The development of the ultimate goal of preventing and controlling disease or conditions in populations. By identifying significant host-agent-environment relationships that influence the progression of the natural life history of a condition, the epidemiologists can identify aggregates at risk and develop ways to prevent disease occurrence among them.

A continuum of preventive activities is essential for the promotion of health in any community. Activities can be grouped under three levels of prevention—primary (health promotion and specific protection), secondary (early diagnosis, prompt treatment and disability limitation) and tertiary (rehabilitation). The Figure 27.4 identifies preventive activities at all three levels that can alter the natural history of disease. The degree to which preventive

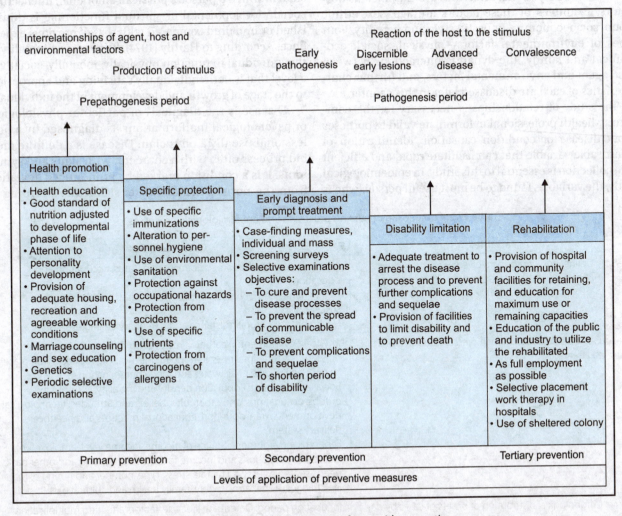

Figure 27.4: Natural history of the diseases of man with preventive measures

activities can be implemented will vary depending on the completeness of knowledge about the disease or health problem in question, the complexity of these conditions and the behavioral and environmental factors influencing the natural life history of the disease.

When epidemiologists analyze the natural life history of disease or a condition for the purpose of identifying preventive measures to eliminate or halt the disease, or condition in question, they study the relationships among three variables—host, agent and environment.

Agents are biological, chemical or physical and include bacteria, viruses, fungi, pesticides, food additives, ionizing radiation and speeding objects. The normal habitat in which an infectious (biological) agent lives, multiplies and/or grows is called reservoir. These habitats include humans, animals and the environment that are discussed in a later section of this chapter.

A wide variety of characteristics are classified as host factors. Examples of these factors are age, sex, ethnic group, socioeconomic status, lifestyle and heredity. Four types of environmental factors—physical, social, economical and family. The dynamic interactions between host, agent and environmental factors, and further characteristics of each are discussed later in this chapter.

The study of relationships is necessary for the community health professional to formulate valid hypotheses about disease or condition causation. Identification of measurable variable that can facilitate rapid and efficient data collection is essential to this study. In epidemiological study, the variables found to be most useful person (who is affected), place (where affected) and time (when affected) relationships. Some of the most frequently analyzed characteristics of these variables are presented in Table 27.2. Timing is a critical factor in disease diagnosis and control. Immediate reporting of a disease outbreak is crucial because the validity of data is often indirectly proportional to the time lapse incurred in obtaining the information. If a significant amount of time is lost in reporting, the ability to formulate valid hypotheses is decreased.

When monitoring incidence of infectious disease, the following terms are used to distinguish relative frequency in time and space.

Disease or Illness

A disease or illness is an alteration in certain areas in the health dimension (Jolsoda, 1956). Illness is an abnormal state in which a person's physical, emotional, intellectual, social, developmental or spiritual functioning is diminished or impaired compared with that of previous experience. According to Hardly (1974), 'Illness is an inability of the individual to function physically, mentally, socially at a level that is both individually satisfying and appropriate to the stage of growth and development of the individual.

Disease is the diagnosis of particular physiological or psychological malformations as diagnosed by a professional usually a physician. Disease is a definite morbid process often with a character with signs and symptoms. It is a condition marked by pronounced deviation from the normal healthy state; sickness. According to

Table 27.2: Comparison of nursing processes and epidemiological processes

Variables	Characteristics
Person: Delineation of group involved	Age, sex, race distribution, socioeconomic status, occupation and education Health habits and behaviors or lifestyle acquired resistance and susceptibility Health history, natural resistance and hereditary characteristics
Place: Geographic distribution in pressure; subdivisions of the area affected	Physical environment: Weather, climate, geography, radiation, vibration, noise, pressure, animal reservoirs, pollutants housing facilities, workplace hazards and source of air, water and food contamination Social environment: Population density and mobility, community groups, occupations, and other roles, beliefs and attitudes, technological developments, transportation, educational practices and healthcare delivery system Economic environment: Source of income, income level, employment status, job frustrations and income for nutrition, housing and other basic needs strategies used to handle stress, type, number and timing of major life changes, home atmosphere, family health and cultural patterns
Time: Chronological distribution of onsets of cases by day, week and month	Incubation period: Determine lifecycle; factors affecting multiplication and virulence of seasonal trends, onset of event and duration of event

dictionary (Oxford English), "A disease is a condition of the body or some part or organ of the body whose functions are disturbed or deranged." Disease is a discomfort, a condition in which bodily health is seriously attacked, deranged or impaired, a departure from a state of health, an alteration of the human body interrupting the performance of vital functions (Webster).

Determinants of Illness Behavior

1. The visibility and recognizability of the illness symptoms.
2. The extent to which the person perceives the symptoms as serious (the person's estimate of the present and future risks).
3. The person's information, knowledge and cultural assumptions, and understanding related to perceived symptoms.
4. The extent to which symptoms disrupt family, work or social activities.
5. The frequency of appearance of the symptoms and their persistence.
6. The extent to which others exposed to the person tolerate the symptoms.
7. The extent to which basic needs are denied, because of illness.
8. The extent to which other need competes with illness responses.
9. The extent to which the person gives other possible interpretations to other symptoms.
10. The availability and physical proximity of treatment resources, the psychological and monetary costs of taking actions (including costs in time and efforts, as well as cost as stigma, social distance and feeling of humiliation).

Epidemiological Triad

The agent, host and environmental factors form epidemiological triad (Fig. 27.5):
1. Agent: Etiological factor.
2. Host: Particular individual or group of immediate concern.
3. Environment: All that is external to the agent and human host.

Natural history of the disease is the process by which disease occurs and progresses in humans involving the interaction of three different kinds of factors; the causative agent(s), a susceptible host (man) and the environment. Without intervention every disease will follow a natural course of event.

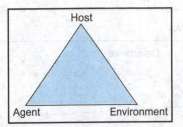

Figure 27.5: Epidemiological triad

Any particular disease or health problem is the result of an interaction between a number of specific or associated risks, which can be classified as agent, host and environment factors. Epidemiological principles are based on the interaction of the host, the causative agent and the environment factors. These interactions can be best understood by visualizing the concepts or positive health and disease.

Positive health is the absence of disease and results from the supremacy of the host over the causative and associated factors. This is possible when the host becomes stronger and/or the agent is removed, and/or the environment becomes unfavorable to the agent.

Disease or disorder, on the other hand, occurs when the agents are more powerful than the host, and/or the host becomes weaker, and/or the environment becomes favorable for growth, multiplication and survival of the agent.

Graphically, the 'triad' may be represented as 'see saw', the fulcrum representing the environment and two seats on the see saw, i.e. the agent and the host.

The state of equilibrium in which the host component exactly balances the agent component, resulting in a person without disease (Fig. 27.6A). This however is similar to a 'tightrope' in that it requires very little change to lose the equilibrium. It is the type of equilibrium met within many children, women and especially pregnant women in the developing countries.

The shift in the equilibrium may be brought about by a change in the weightage of anyone, two or all three components of the triad. Possible triads in developing and developed countries are shown in Figures 27.6B and C.

The developed countries with 'environments behavioral characteristics' and also developing countries with poor sanitation, and hygiene (refer Fig. 27.6B). In both situations, aim is change to Figure 27.6C.

Ill health, which is shown in the diagram as the agent being higher, i.e. stronger than the host; but the opposite is true of good health. This relationship of agent and host is alteration in the environmental condition (refer Figs 27.6B and C).

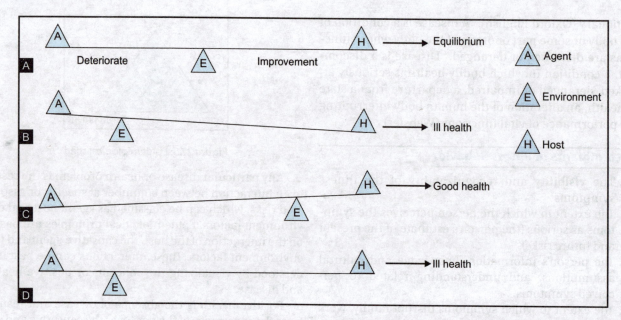

Figures 27.6A to D: See saw model of triad

In Figure 27.6D, the agent is 'bigger', i.e. stronger than the host resulting in ill health. In this situation the environment is not changed. These three elements are closely bound together and each affects the other. The interaction of host, agent and environment determines the mode of transmission, the natural history, occurrence and control of disease, illness or other condition. The health of an individual or community depends upon the state of equilibrium maintained within the triad of elements.

Types of Agent

An agent is a factor whose presence or absence causes a disease. It is a specific factor without which a disease cannot occur. A disease agent may be defined as a substance, living or nonliving, or a force, tangible or nontangible, the excessive presence or relative lack of which is the immediate cause of a particular disease. The disease agents are classified as follows:

1. **Physical agents:** Include various mechanical forces or frictions that may produce injury as well as atmospheric abnormalities such as extremes of heat, cold, humidity, pressure, radiation, electricity sound, etc.
2. **Biological agents:** Include all living organisms, such as bacteria, viruses, *Rickettsia*, chlamydia, spirochetes, *Mycoplasma*, protozoa, fungi, helminths, etc.
3. **Chemical agents:**
   a. **Endogenous:** Some of the chemicals may be produced in the body as a result of deranged function, e.g. urea (uremia), serum, bilirubin (jaundice), ketones (ketosis), uric acid (gout) and calcium carbonate (kidney stones).
   b. **Exogenous:** Agents arising outside the human host-allergens, metals, fumes, gases, insecticides, ingestion or inoculation.
4. **Genetic agents:** Transmitted from parents to child through the genes.
5. **Mechanical agents:** Chronic fiction and other mechanical forces resulting in injuries, trauma, fractures, sprains, dislocations and even death.
6. **Nutrient agents:** Include specific basic dietary components that we need to survive, such as proteins, fats, carbohydrates, vitamins, minerals and water. The excessive or deficient intake of nutrients lead to malnutrition, etc. this in turn leads to susceptibility to any disease. Here, agent is referred to as a seed of the disease.
7. **Absence of insufficiency of excess of factor:**
   a. Chemical hormones, e.g. insulin, estrogen.
   b. Nutrients.
   c. Lack of structure, e.g. congenital defect of the heart.
   d. Chromosome, e.g. mongolism, mental retardation.
   e. Immunoglobulin, e.g. agammaglobulinemia.

Host

Host refers to humans or animals that come in contact with the agent. Since 'agent' has been considered as a 'seed of disease,' the 'human host' is referred to as 'soil'. Host factors influence the interaction with the agent and the environment as follows:

1. Age: Certain diseases are more frequent in certain age group than others. For example:
   a. Childhood: Measles, whooping cough.
   b. Advance age: Diabetes, hypertension and cardiovascular disease.
   c. Old age: Atherosclerosis.
2. Sex: It is fact that are certain anatomical and hormonal differences between two sexes; accordingly there are differences between male and female for occurrence of disease, e.g. disorders associated with pregnancy in females and prostatic hypertrophy in males.
3. Race: Some races also suffer from particular diseases, e.g. Negroes—sickle cell anemia.
4. Genetic factors: Certain diseases are determined by genetic factors such as behavioral disorders and disorders of blood run in the family due to chromosomal factors.
5. Habits: Living habits or lifestyle such as dietary pattern, use of tobacco, alcohol and narcotic drugs are the factors with an influence on susceptibility of disease, e.g. malnutrition, cancer, drug dependence and sexual excesses.
6. Nutrition: The effects of poor nutrition lead to susceptibility to various infections.
7. Customs: Certain traditional systems, i.e. superstitions lead to disease. For example, fixed beliefs in goddess of disease in Hindu society make people not to believe in immunization, which leads to childhood diseases. Certain habits are also followed according to their customs and lifestyles as explained above.
8. Human mobility: Frequent changes in place may cause disease. The convalescent persons are transferred thousand miles in few hours and introduce infection, e.g. malaria, filarial, cholera, aids, syphilis, etc.
9. Immunity: The reaction of human host to infection depends upon his/her previous immunological experience, e.g. infection, immunization. Those who have acquired or natural immunity will not easily be susceptible to disease.
10. Social status: Studies have shown certain diseases occurring according to social class, e.g. low social classes are susceptible to Rh diseases, bronchitis and TB. Usually, upper social classes have lower mortality and morbidity than lower class.
11. Economic status: Person's occupation itself may be cause of certain occupational hazards and infections, e.g. pneumoconiosis, accidents, brucellosis, dermatitis, psychosomatic illness and unemployment also leads to disease.
12. Educational status: Diseases can be easily controlled and managed in the educated class, whereas, it will be difficult in the case of uneducated class.

Environment
The environment refers to the aggregate of all external conditions and influences affecting the life and development of an organism, human behavior and society. The environment may be the external conditions that may enhance or inhibit the interaction between host and agent. The environment includes those external to the host and agent, but they may influence interactions between them. When there is a change in anyone of these components, the balance or equilibrium is disrupted and the possibility of disease occurrence is increased or decreased.

Physical environment
Physical environment includes non-living thing and physical factors such as water, air, soil, heat, light, radiation, noise, housing, climate, geography, etc. Alteration of change in this environment due to various causes leads to water pollution, air pollution, soil pollution, noise pollution, which in turn may cause diseases, e.g. heavy flooding in the village or town can increase the likelihood of that area and the water supply will be contaminated with waste products. This increases the possibility in the residents of that area infected by disease causing organism.

Biological environment
Biological environment includes all living things created in the world. Man lives around the living things, which include bacteria, viruses and other various microorganisms, which may cause disease and maladjustment in the ecological system leading to causative factors of diseases.

Social environment
Man has to live in society and should follow the accepted patterns of particular society such as cultural values, customs, beliefs, attitudes, morals, religion and other psychosocial factors. Any alternations in these factors may lead to conflicts and tensions, which may cause behavioral disorders. The habits such as smoking, alcohol and drug dependence are well known that they are the causes of diseases.

Economic environments
Man and economic position may at times be the factors of disease, e.g. poverty leads to malnutrition, psychological stresses may be the cause of various diseases. Thus, the causative of diseases has been particularly useful in efforts to control infectious diseases. Development of vaccines that increase the immunity of the host, improvement of sanitation and disposal of wastes help to control or prevent the transmission of several infectious diseases. Epidemiological studies of other kinds of disease such as mental illness, cardiac diseases and cancer is not specific cause. Therefore, it is better to have an approach of 'multiple causation' of disease.

Multiple Causation of Disease

In the early days of modern medicine, the cause of disease was visualized in terms of specific germ or agent. This is otherwise known as single cause idea or germ theory of disease. As science and technology advanced in the field of medicine and public health, and many diseases have been controlled or reduced due to antibiotics, chemotherapy and immunization. Also, any single cause for disease is looked for, but other causes are also established, e.g. TB is not merely caused by the tubercle bacillus, and everyone exposed to tubercle bacillus is affected with TB. The other factors that have identified as clearly contributing to the occurrence of TB are poverty, overcrowding, malnutritions, alcoholism and genetic factors. Hence, the factors related to the development of TB include such things as the virulence of the agent, the characteristic of the environments of the host, e.g. genetic makeup, nutritional status and immunity to the disease. Similarly in the case of noninfectious diseases such as coronary heart disease, the various causes include excessive smoking, excessive intake of fats, lack of exercise, obesity and other factors linked with the lifestyle and human behavior.

This concept considers that effects never depend on single isolated causes, but rather develop as the result of chains of causes in which each link itself is the result of a complex genealogy of antecedents. These chains of causations represent only a fraction of reality and the whole complex may be thought of as a web that in complexity, and origin lies quite beyond our understanding. Fortunately, it is not necessary to understand causal mechanisms completely to effective preventive measures.

Thus, the multiple causation approach to the study of disease based on the idea that effects of disease are not results of several improvement and significant factors acting together. This occurs with infection as well as non-infectious diseases. The multifactorial causes may be related directly or indirectly to agent, host and environment. The purpose of having this approach helps us to quantitate and arrange them in priority sequence for modification or amelioration to prevent and/or control disease. Some studies have shown that there is definite relationship between heart disease and lifestyle activities such as smoking, excessive intake of food containing high levels of cholesterols (fats), increased mental and emotional stress, control of diet, regular exercise, and use of effective management techniques have been shown to reduce a person's risk of experiencing myocardial infarction. The agent-host-environment model of health and illness originated in the community health work of Leavell et al (1965) and has been expanded as a model for describing the cause of illness in other health areas. The same model has also been expanded into a general theory of the multiple causes of the disease.

According to this model, there are two stages in the 'natural history of the disease' (Leavell and Clark, 1968).

The first stage of the natural history of disease is the stage of prepathogenesis or stage of susceptibility. In this stage disease has not developed, but factors that favor its occurrence are present.

Within the second stage of the natural history in pathogenesis, there are three substages—presymptomatic disease or early pathogenesis. This individual has no symptoms indicating the presence of illness. Here, the disease provoking stimulus is introduced to the host and the interaction between host and stimulus takes place, the equilibrium is disturbed. At that period the body defends itself through various defense mechanisms to overcome it. When the body fails to defend itself, pathogenic changes begin and lead to second substage of pathogenesis, i.e. discernible easy lesions. Here the interaction of host and stimulus takes place, and stimulus or agent become established. The infectious agent increases by multiplication slowly; the tissues changes and physiologically and clinically the disease be recognized, as the patient develops the early symptoms. In this period, the changes may be detectable through laboratory tests. This may be subclinical case. When the patient is not treated properly or not taken care properly, disease process may move to third substage of pathogenesis, i.e. advanced disease occurs. In this stage, sufficient anatomical and psychological changes have produced recognizable signs and symptoms. This stage includes diseases so advance that death is inevitable. The possible outcomes are complete recovery, a residual defect, therein, may produce some degree of disability or death.

Levels of Prevention

The natural history of disease provides the basis for community health interventions. A disease evolves overtime and pathological changes become less reversible as the disease process continues. The ultimate aim of intervention program is to half or reverses the process of pathological changes as early as possible, thereby preventing further damage. A three-level model for intervention, based on the stages of disease has been developed by Leavell HR and Clark EG (1965) discussed as follows.

Primary Prevention

Primary prevention is true prevention; it precedes diseases or dysfunction, and is applied to patients considered physically and emotionally healthy. It is aimed at interventions before pathological changes have begun during the stage of susceptibility. Activities are directed at decreasing the probability of specific illness or dysfunction. The primary preventive efforts include both general health promotions and specific protection. General health promotion includes all activities that improve the environment and favor healthy living. Health education aimed at educating the public about the good nutrition, the need for rest and recreations, hygiene, etc. The health promotion activities are summarized below:

- Health education
- Good standard of nutrition adjusted to developmental stage of life
- Attention of personality development
- Provision of adequate housing and recreation, and agreeable working conditions
- Marriage and sex education
- Genetic screening
- Periodic selective examinations.

Specific protection refers to measures aimed at protecting individuals against specific agents, e.g. immunization against poliomyelitis or sewage treatment, or pasteurization of milk or chlorination of water. The activities of specific protection will include:

- Use of specific immunizations, e.g. wearing helmets
- Attention to personal hygiene for self-care
- Use of environmental sanitation, e.g. chlorination of well
- Protection from accidents, e.g. wearing helmet
- Use of specific nutrients
- Protection from carcinogens
- Avoidance of allergens.

Secondary Prevention

Secondary prevention focuses on the individuals, who are experiencing health problems or illness and are at risk for developing complications or worsening conditions. Its efforts seek to detect disease early and treat it promptly. The goal is to cure disease at its earliest stage or when cure is impossible to slow its progression as well as prevent complications and limit disability. The activities direct at diagnosis and prompt treatment, thereby, reducing severity and enabling patient to return to normal health at the earliest possible. Thus, secondary prevention is focused primarily on presymptomatic disease or very early clinical disease. Screening test can detect early physiological indicators of disease before the person experiences any symptoms, e.g. cervical cancer tests, hearing tests, TB tests, phenylalanine test, etc.

A large portion of secondary level preventive intervention is taken at home, hospital or skilled nursing facility to prevent complication, which includes activities of early diagnosis, treatment and disability limitation as follows:

1. Early diagnosis and treatment:
    a. Case-finding measures—individual and mass.
    b. Screening surveys.
    c. Selective examinations.
    d. Cure and prevention disease process to prevent spread of communicable disease, prevent complications and shortens the period of disability.
2. Disability limitation:
    a. Adequate treatment to arrest disease process and prevent complications.
    b. Provisions of facilities to limit disability and prevent death.

Tertiary Prevention

Tertiary prevention occurs when a defector disability is permanent. It includes limitation of disability for person in the early stages of illness and rehabilitation for those persons who have already experienced residual damage. Tertiary prevention activities focus on the middle to later phase of clinical disease, when irreversible pathological damages produce disability (e.g. stroke, exercise). Here, the activities of restoration and rehabilitation will include:

- Provision of hospital and community facilities for retaining and education to maximize use of remaining capacities
- Education of the public and industries to use rehabilitation rather persons to the fullest possible extent
- Selective placement
- Work therapy and hospitals
- Use of sheltered colony.

In tertiary prevention, mainly the activities are directed at rehabilitation rather than diagnosis and treatment. Care at this level aims to help the patient to achieve as high level of functioning as possible, despite the limitations caused by illness or impaired functioning.

IMPLICATIONS OF EPIDEMIOLOGY IN COMMUNITY HEALTH NURSING

Epidemiology is the basic science of community health. It is the study of the distribution of states health and of the determinants of deviation from health in populations in a community health science essential to nursing practice. An understanding of the epidemiological concepts and principles are vital for nurse in the community as well as in the hospital setting. Most CHN are employed by authorities that interact directly with individual patient and families. Epidemiology refers to both methods used in the study of disease causations and the body of knowledge that arise from such investigation. Knowledge of the methods of epidemiology is useful to the CHN both as a tool in conducting the investigation to evaluate and explain phenomena observed in the course of work; as a basis for interpreting and evaluating the epidemiological literature. Epidemiological methods such as measures of health serve as tools for assessing community needs and evaluating the impact of community health programs of disease prevention and health promotion. The community health nurse should have knowledge measurement, i.e. calculation of rate, ratio, as in Table 27.3.

The body of knowledge derived from epidemiological studies, including natural history and patterns of disease

Table 27.3: Measurement of rates

Rate	Fraction
Age-specific death rate	$\dfrac{\text{Number of deaths at specified age group}}{\text{Estimated mid-year population of that age group}} \times 1{,}000$
Case fatality rate	$\dfrac{\text{Number of deaths from specified disease}}{\text{Number of persons with the disease (old and new)}} \times 100$
Cause specific rate	$\dfrac{\text{Number of deaths from specified cause}}{\text{Estimated mid-year population}} \times 100{,}000$
Crude birth rate	$\dfrac{\text{Total number of live births}}{\text{Estimate mid-year population}} \times 1{,}000$
Crude death rate	$\dfrac{\text{Total number of deaths during a given year}}{\text{Estimate mid-year population}} \times 1{,}000$
Fertility rate	$\dfrac{\text{Number of live births}}{\text{Estimated number of females aged 15–44 at midyear}} \times 1{,}000$
Fetal death rate (stillbirth rate)	$\dfrac{\text{Number of fetal deaths at 20 weeks or more gestation}}{\text{Number of live births + Fetal deaths of 20 week or more gestation}} \times 1{,}000$
Incidence (crude rate)	$\dfrac{\text{All new cases occurring during a period of time}}{\text{Estimated mid-year population}} \times 100{,}000$
Infant mortality rate	$\dfrac{\text{Number of deaths from puerperal causes (pregnancy, postpartum)}}{\text{Number of live births}} \times 100{,}000$
Maternal mortality rate	$\dfrac{\text{Number of deaths from puerperal causes (pregnancy, postpartum)}}{\text{Number of live birth during that year}} \times 10{,}000$
Neonatal mortality rate	$\dfrac{\text{Number deaths under 28 day of age}}{\text{Number of live births}} \times 1{,}000$

Contd....

Contd....

Rate	Fraction
Perinatal mortality rate	$\dfrac{\text{Number of fetal deaths 28 week or more and infant death under 7 day of age}}{\text{Number of live births and fetal deaths 28 week or more during the same year}} \times 1{,}000$
Postnatal mortality rate	$\dfrac{\text{Number of deaths at age 28 day 1 year}}{\text{Number of live births – Neonatal death}} \times 1{,}000$
Prevalence (crude rate)	$\dfrac{\text{All cases (old and new existing at a given time)}}{\text{Estimate population at that time}} \times 100{,}000$
Proportionate mortality rate	$\dfrac{\text{Number of deaths from specific causes}}{\text{Total number of death from all causes}} \times 1{,}000$
Sex-specific death rate	$\dfrac{\text{Number of deaths of males or females}}{\text{Estimated male or female population at midyear}} \times 1{,}000$

occurrence, and factors associated with high risk for developing disease, serves as an information base for CHN practice. This knowledge provides a framework for planning and evaluating community interventions program aimed at primary, secondary and tertiary prevention. Programs of primary preventions focus on distancing disease agent from susceptible hosts, decreasing agent's viability, increasing host resistance and altering the established agent-host-environment relationship. Screening and risk factor reduction programs are examples of secondary prevention. Vocational retraining and rehabilitative exercises for the disabled are tertiary prevention strategies. For the individual nurse, the body of knowledge derived from the epidemiological research serves as basis for assessing individual and family health needs, and for planning nursing interventions. It also provides tools for evaluating the success of the interventions.

The CHN plays an important role in epidemiological studies. They often may be the one to initiate a study and more frequently assist in the data collection. The CHN often cast in the role of interpreting study findings to families, schools, industries and other. In actual practice, the CHN is considered as the foot soldier in the army of epidemiology. The epidemiologist is dependent on the local CHN for follow-up on various conditions.

It is important to monitor the relative frequency of an event in time and space to determine health and disease patterns in a community. A variety of methods are used to collect data about these patterns and identify aggregates at risk in a population. These methods include such interventions as analyzing all available statistics, carrying out surveys and interviewing key community informants. Basic statistical concepts used in epidemiology and sources of statistical concepts used in epidemiology, and sources of statistical data are as follows.

Epidemiological Studies/Method

Epidemiologist makes use of research strategies to find out the causative factors of diseases. They employ the research design carefully by using the epidemiological methods. The epidemiological methods complement one other. The epidemiological methods are of the following types:
1. Observational methods.
2. Experimental methods.

Observational Methods

In observational methods, observations are made and these type of studies allow the nature to its own course, it is further subdivided into:
1. Descriptive method: It involves the description of the occurrence of a disease in population.
2. Analytical method: In this, the relationship between the health status and other variables is analyzed.

Experimental Method

Experimental method is known as interventional method. Intervention is done so as to make attempts to alter the progress of disease or change in the factor involved in the disease. It is of two types:

1. **Randomized controlled trial:** This study design includes the subjects, who are having health problems or disease, i.e. subjects are the patients.
2. **Non-randomized controlled trial:** In this type of method, the subjects are healthy individual.

Epidemiological approaches to relationship studies fall into two broad categories—observational and experimental. In observational studies, the amount and distribution of disease within a population by person, place and time are noted. In experimental studies, the investigator intervenes and actually changes one variable, and observes what happen to the other, if the investigator controls the condition.

The epidemiologist tries to relate the cases to define population and search for the causes of disease, and modes of transmission with a view to affect prevention and control by asking questions himself that when does the disease occur? Where does the disease occur? Who are the affected people? Why has it appeared? What should be done to prevent, control or eradicate the disease?

Observational Studies

Observational studies fall into two main classifications:
- Descriptive
- Analytical.

Descriptive Epidemiology

Descriptive epidemiology is the study of the amount and distribution of disease or health status within a population by person, place and time. It usually involves the determination of incidence, prevalence and mortality for diseases in large population groups according to characteristics such as age, sex, race and geographical area. For these studies, data on causes and effects in an individual are often not known.

It is the study of factors responsible for distribution of health and disease in human population, such as age, sex, social status, income, occupation, housing, social customs, habits, etc. It provides the body of knowledge for the epidemiological study. It also studies other factors, such as time distribution—when? It gives duration of epidemic and periodicity of the disease.

Time distribution includes the distribution of cases by day, month, year or year of occurrence according to time trends. The trends may be seasonal, cyclic or secular. The seasonal trends mean incidence of certain diseases usually seen in winter season (e.g. gastroenteritis) and other waterborne disease. In cyclic trends, some disease occurs during the course of days, weeks, months or years with certain period of intervals. In secular trends, the changes that occur in disease frequency over periods of many years or decades.

The study of geographic distribution of diseases referred as place of distribution—where? It is used for international, rural and urban comparison. The knowledge of place distribution enables us to make comparison from place to place, variation in disease frequency, which helps us to take proper steps to prevent/control particular disease in particular places.

In person distribution relations of disease with/to characteristics of the person such as age, sex, marital status, ethnic group, occupation, education, diet pattern and habits, e.g. measles usually occur in childhood.

The purpose of descriptive epidemiology is to provide a statistical overview of community health problems and gives clue about the etiological factors involved. This provides information about diseases in terms of incidence, prevalence and mortality rates according to the basic group characteristics, and time of occurrence. All these things provide information for planning, organization and evaluating medical, healthcare services, and also give further directions for research.

The descriptive epidemiology is the first phase of an investigation in which data are obtained from such sources as vital records and vital statistics, census information, survey, and disease reports. The data collected are then presented as percentages or in the form of rates. Rates are fractions, which the numerator (top term) contains the number of people affected by a disease or conditions and the denominator (bottom term) is comprised of population at risk for that specific disease or condition shows rates that are commonly used in community health reports, which are helpful in comparing and consisting the disease frequency in population groups and in measuring the health of the community.

Descriptive method is concerned with observing the distribution of disease in relation to time, place and person. In this method, health-related characteristics are studied and also their distribution in relation to questions such as when (time), where (place) and who (persons) is studied.

Procedure: Various steps involved in descriptive study are:
- Step I: Define the population
- Step II: Define the disease
- Step III: Describe the disease in relation to when, where and who
- Step IV: Measurement of disease
- Step V: Comparison with different or same population
- Step VI: Formulation of hypothesis related to causative factors of disease.

Step I: Define the population

Defined population means the population not only in total number but also its composition in terms of age, sex, occupation and cultural characteristics, etc. The defined population can be:
- Whole population
- Sample population
- A selected group:
  - Hospital patients
  - School children
  - Elderly
  - Female
  - Male.
- Communities.

Criteria for selecting the defined population

Large enough: The defined population should be large enough, so that the conclusion drawn from the study is meaningful.

Stable community: The defined population should be selected on the basis of its stability, i.e. without migration of people into or out of the community.

No migrant or visitor: The visitors should not be included in the defined population.

Access to medical services: The health facilities should be made available nearby to provide medical services to patients who need it.

Step II: Define the disease

The disease, which needs to be studied, should be clearly defined. The definition of the disease should be precise and valid. By this epidemiologists would be able to identify the diseased and non-diseased people, and also be able to get accurate information about the disease in a population the epidemiologists need to keep in mind that the methods used for investigation must be acceptable to the people, who are under study. An operational definition helps the epidemiologists to identify and measure the disease in the defined population.

An operational definition of disease means particular criteria by which the disease is measured. If the valid operational definition is available, then the same can be used by epidemiologists to measure the disease, otherwise own definition can be framed by keeping the objective of study in mind and by which accurate information can be obtained for the study. In such cases, throughout the study, same definition should be used.

Step III: Describe the disease in relation to when, where and who

Describe the disease once the population and disease has been defined, then the next step is to describe the disease in terms of time, place and person.

Time distribution

Describe the pattern of disease in terms of time. A number of questions are raised related to time distribution, these questions are:
- Whether the disease is occurring seasonwise, monthly, weekly or yearly?
- Whether there is periodic rise or fall in the occurrence of disease?
- Whether the disease follows a consistent time trend?

On the basis of time trend or fluctuation in disease occurrence, disease occurs as.

Short-term fluctuation

When the disease occurs in population in epidemic form, then it is short-term fluctuation.

During short-term fluctuations, epidemics are common. When epidemic occurs from the exposure from one common source, is called common source epidemics. This exposure can be for a brief period or prolonged period. Depending on this, it is of two types:

1. Single exposure epidemics: All the individuals, who are exposed to the disease agent for a short period will develop the disease within one incubation period of the disease, i.e. there is one common source, with one exposure for short duration to this common source, the disease will occur among the exposed cases. Simultaneously all cases will go through the same incubation period of disease.

   On exposure to single source for short duration, 50% or more than this, the cases will be developed at a time, which can be seen as a peak in the curve. All this will occur, because of having median incubation period. So, there will be clustering of cases. The common source can be:
   - Contaminated air
   - Contaminated water.

2. Repeated exposure: There is common source and on repeated exposure to this source, the disease will develop among the exposed individuals. This repeated exposure is for prolonged period, which can be continuous or intermittent. The epidemic will be irregular as incubation period for the cases will not be same.

Propagated epidemics

Propagated exposure results from person-to-person transmission of an infectious agent. Propagated epidemics occur where large number of susceptible are aggregated. It also occurs where there is regular supply of new susceptible individuals lowering herd immunity.

Periodic fluctuations

The disease occurs either in season, months, days, weeks, etc. These fluctuations are periodic fluctuations and occur according to:

1. **Seasonal trend:** Many communicable diseases occur in particular seasons. For example, upper respiratory infections occur mostly during winter season and gastrointestinal infections in summer. These seasonal variations are occurring due to following factors:
   - Temperature
   - Humidity
   - Overcrowding
   - Rainfall, etc.
2. **Cyclic trend:** When the disease spread in cycles over days, weeks, months, years, then it is known as cyclic trend:
   - Influenza pandemic occur at an interval of 7–10 years, this is due to antigenic variations
   - Automobile accidents more frequently occur on weekends.

Long-term fluctuations
Long-term fluctuations mean the changes in the occurrence of disease over a long period of time. It can be several years or decades. There can be either an increase or decrease in the occurrence of disease.

In developed countries, during the past 50 years there is consistent upward trend in the diseases such as coronary heart disease and diabetes. There is also a decrease in the occurrence of disease such as diphtheria, polio, etc.

Place distribution
The distribution of disease is studied in different populations. This helps the epidemiologist to compare the variations in disease pattern within countries as well as between countries. Within countries, the distribution of disease among population is different due to culture, standard of living, customs, habits, etc. The changes in the distribution of the disease occur at various levels such as local, rural, urban, national and international. So based upon these, variations are of following types.

International variations
When we study the disease pattern by place, it has been seen that it is not same at all places. It differs from country to country. Due to this difference in disease pattern among countries, cause effect relationship between environment factors and disease can be searched.

National variations
The variations in disease occur within countries. The disease affect some parts of the country more, while some are affected less and even are not affected at all. Leprosy, malaria and guinea worm disease, etc. are distributed with variations in India.

Rural-urban variations
The disease variation can be seen in rural and urban areas. Some diseases occur frequently in urban areas and some in rural areas. It has been seen that accidents and drug dependence occur in urban, while soil transmitted helminths and skin diseases are more common in rural areas.

Local distribution
Local variations can be studied with the help of map. If map shows clustering of cases, it suggests a common source of infection or all cases are having common risk factors.

In 1854, John Snow investigated common water pump in broad streets as the source of cholera in Golden Square district of London.

Person distribution
Person distribution of the disease in relation to person, who develops the disease should be defined. The persons developing the disease need to be defined by:
- Age
- Sex
- Occupation
- Marital status
- Habits
- Social class
- Stress
- Migration
- Behavior.

Age: This is one of the factor, which is related to disease. It has been seen that certain diseases are more frequent in certain age groups. The examples related to age are:
- In old age: Atherosclerosis
- Middle age: Cancer
- Childhood: Measles.

Sometimes there are two separate peaks in the age incidence curve of diseases.

Sex: The epidemiologists study the disease in relation to sex, while describing the disease with respect to person distribution. As studies have shown that certain diseases are found to be more commonly in women than men (Table 27.4).

Table 27.4: Common diseases among males and females

Sex	Common diseases
Males	Lung cancer Prostate cancer Coronary heart diseases
Females	Breast cancer Obesity Diabetes Hyperthyroidism

The reasons for the variations in disease frequency in males and females are:

1. Biological differences: Sex-linked genetic inheritance.
2. Cultural and behavioral differences: Smoking automobile use and alcoholism.

Occupation: It is one of the most important factors, which has bearing on the health status. The people exposed to environment during occupation affect their health. As in coal mines, workers are more prone to silicosis as compared to other individuals because of daily exposures to environment having silicon fibers. Not only this, occupation affect the habit pattern such as sleep, smoking, night shift duties, etc.

Marital status: This can be a risk factor for certain diseases. Cancer of cervix is rare in nuns.

Habits: This is an another characteristic, which is related to disease. An individual who has habit of drinking alcohol or smoking are more prone to diseases such as cirrhosis of liver, lung cancer and coronary heart diseases, etc.

Social class: Such as middle or lower social class have variations in diseases, which has been seen in epidemiological studies. Certain diseases such as coronary heart diseases, hypertension and diabetes are found to have higher prevalence rate in upper classes.

Stress: This increases the susceptibility to diseases. Due to stress, the symptoms exacerbate. So stress is one of the factors, which affect the variations in the disease.

Migration: Means movement of people from one place to another such as from rural to urban or from one state to another, or from one country to another. This movement is either short term, long term or permanent. The migration of people can alter the disease pattern. Migration has resulted the widespread of certain diseases globally, which were earlier present only in certain nations.

Behavior: Epidemiologists study the person in relation to his behavior in order to find out the association between behavior and disease. Certain diseases such as cancer, obesity and accidents are found to be related to the behavior of smoking, eating and carelessness respectively.

Step IV: Measurement of disease

As the epidemiologist wants to have the clear picture about the amount of disease in population. So, they will use the measurements such as rates and ratio in terms of death, disease or disability. The information received is in terms of morbidity, mortality, disability and so on. Descriptive epidemiology uses research design to obtain estimates of magnitude of health and disease in community/population. These designs are:
- Cross-sectional design
- Longitudinal design

Cross-sectional design
In cross-sectional design, there is a single examination of a cross section of population at one point in time. The results of these are projected on whole population. This is done in case the sample chosen is correct or appropriate.

Longitudinal design
In longitudinal design, the observations are repeated in the same population over a prolonged period of time by means of follow-up examinations.

Step V: Comparing with known indices

To arrive at clues to causative factor of disease, comparison is made between different populations and subgroups of the same population.

Step VI: Formulation of hypothesis

Hypothesis can be formulated related to the disease etiology. Hypothesis is a supposition, which is arrived from observations or reflections. It is either accepted or rejected, while formulating hypothesis, the criteria should be met as given below:
- Population
- Specific cause
- Expected outcome
- The amount of cause to effect
- The time period between the exposures to cause the effect.

Keeping these criteria, hypothesis can be formulated as given in following example—the smoking of 30–40 cigarette per day causes lung cancer in 10% of smokers after 20 years of exposure. In this hypothesis:
- Population is smokers
- Specific cause is smoking
- Expected outcome is cancer
- The amount of cause to effect is 30–40 cigarettes per day
- Time period between the exposures to cause effect is 20 years.

Analytic Epidemiology

Analytical epidemiology is concerned with the searching for the underlying causes. Its main purpose is to uncover the source and mode of spread of disease. Here, the epidemiologist seeks to determine the multiple factors that brought the disease and situation into being such as, agent, host and environment. The clue about the origin, nature and size of the problem is discovered, and the factors, which sought the disease are unveiled.

The health administration bases the action and makes programs to control and prevent the disease. Epidemiological method is used to assess the result of work done from time to time.

Data derived from descriptive studies often provide clues of finding about a problem that leads an investigator to make guess or formulate hypothesis for further study. These hypothesis are tested by analytical methods. Analytical epidemiology focuses on the determinants or reasons for the relatively high or low frequency of disease in specific groups. The starting point for any analytical study is often a descriptive finding that raises certain questions or suggests certain hypothesis that requires further investigation. This is often the second phase of investigation in which the investigator has specific question or group of questions that he/she sets about to answer. For analytic study, data on both cause and effect in an individual are known. The study design and the data analysis provide the answers to the specific questions of interest, e.g. smoking related to cancer or forceps delivery related to epilepsy, etc.

The analysis of health, social and economic data, and trends to identify and interpret changes, which have taken place are likely to occur in populations or special group.

Analytical epidemiology goes beyond the descriptive phase to test a hypothesis about the nature of a health problem. The methods of analytical study commonly employed for testing epidemiological hypothesis are:
- Retrospective method (backward survey)
- Prospective method (forward survey).

Advantages and disadvantages of retrospective and prospective study are given in Table 27.5.

Table 27.5: Advantages and disadvantages of retrospective and prospective study

Study	Advantages	Disadvantages
Retrospective	• Relatively inexpensive • Smaller number of subjects • Relatively quick results • Suitable for rare disease • Lack of bias in factor	• Incomplete information • Biased recall • Problem of selecting control group and matching variables • Yields only relative risk • Possible bias in ascertainment of diseases
Prospective	• Yields both relative risk and incidence • Can yield association with additional disease as byproduct	• Requires large number of subjects • Long follow-up period • Problem of attribution • Changes over time in criteria and methods • Very costly

Retrospective method: This is a backward survey. It is economic and time-saving study. This type of study starts from diagnosed cases, who are easily available in hospitals. The sick people are studied and some standard comparisons are obtained. The required knowledge of population is not available or such control is necessary. Retrospective method is called case-controlled study, because it compares cases and controls with regard to the presence of some elements in their past experiences. Here, a group of people who have been definitely diagnosed as having a particular health problem (cases) are compared with a group of people who are free of that particular problem (control). The proportion of the specific characteristics being studied is compared between the two groups. This method is retrospective, because the investigator looks backward at the history of the cause, e.g. the cause of lung cancer is smoking. Here, the investigator looks backward at the history of smoking in both the groups.

As already stated above, the retrospective approach looks backward to analyze the data to see if a disease or other health problem is preceded by or related to some condition more frequently than would be expected to occur by chance. Retrospective studies are relatively inexpensive to carry out are easily repeated, and have advantage of allowing the investigator to study the association of specific diseases or condition with as many characteristics as possible.

Since, it is a retrospective study, the investigator has to depend for information either upon the individual's memory or on the availability of some record and this method allows the investigator to make association between certain characteristics or health practices, and the development of disease, but it cannot give a direct estimate of the risk of developing by an individual.

Case-control study

Retrospective studies are the case-control study and is used to test causal hypothesis. The features of case-control study are:
1. Before the initiation of study, the disease has occurred due to the exposure of infectious agents.
2. The study proceeds backward (effect to cause).
3. The case-control study has one control group. It involves two population:
   - Case: Individuals with particular disease
   - Control: Individuals without particular disease.

The case-control study design is shown by 2 × 2 table, which proves a very useful framework to discuss the various elements from a case-control study:

1. In case-control study, investigation is done by assembling cases (a + c) and control (b + d). The group of controls (b + d) should be suitably matched with cases (a + c).
2. Then the past history of these two groups is studied in relation to smoking, to know, which is the factor responsible for lung cancer.
3. If the frequency of smoking is higher in cases (a/a + c) than in controls (b/c + d). Then, it is said that association exist between smoking and lung cancer.

Steps
The steps for conducting case-control study are:
- Selection of cases and control
- Matching
- Measurement of exposure
- Analysis and interpretations.

Selection of cases and control
The case and control on whom the study is conducted need to be carefully selected. Case and control must be comparable with respect to confounding factors:
1. Selection of cases: Criteria for selecting cases:
   a. There should be a clear definition of a case.
   b. The definition of case should meet two criteria's, i.e. diagnostic and eligibility criteria.
   c. The diagnostic criteria and stage of disease must be specified before conducting the study.
   d. Diagnostic criteria should be same throughout the study.

   For conducting a study on incidence rate of breast cancer stage I among females, the cases included in the study will be females, whose histology report shows the presence of cancer and are in first stage of disease. Another thing is that only those cases, who are newly diagnosed cases within a specified period of time.

   These cases can be taken from hospital or from general population.
2. Selection of control: For selection of control:
   a. The person should be free from disease.
   b. Controls should meet other criteria except disease such as age, sex, occupation, etc. the same as cases.
   c. Controls may be selected from hospitals, relatives, neighbors and general population, etc.
   d. Sometime there is difficulty in selection of control, if the disease under investigation occurs in subclinical form.

For interpretation of the result, there is need to select proper cases and control. Failure to select comparable control can cause 'bias' into the results of case-control study. The bias while selecting the case should be avoided.

Matching
Matching is important to ensure comparability between cases and controls. Matching means a process of selection of control in such a way that they are similar to cases with regard to certain pertinent selected variables, which can influence the outcome of disease if not matched adequately. If the cases and controls are not matched properly, then the result can be distorted or confounded. The factors, which can distort the results are confounding factors.

A confounding factor is one, which is associated with exposure and disease, and is distributed unequally in study and control groups:
- Smoking is confounding factor in the study of role of alcohol in the etiology of esophageal cancer
- In a study of the association between steroid contraceptive and breast cancer, age can be a confounding factor, if the women taking steroid contraceptive were younger than comparison group as disease is common with increasing age.

Matching can be done by:
- Group matching
- Pair matching.

Group matching: Within group, subcategories, i.e. strata can be matched for the purpose of study. The strata's are based on the characteristics such as:
- Age
- Social class
- Sex
- Occupation.

Pair matching: Another way of matching is pair, i.e. for each case, a control is chosen, which can be matched.

Selecting a 40-year-old farmer with a particular disease as a case, a 40-year-old farmer without particular disease as control should be matched.

Measurement of exposure
The information about exposure should be obtained both from cases and controls by using the same method. These methods can be:
- Interview schedule
- Questionnaire
- Records such as hospital records and employment records.

Analysis
The data collected in analytical type of epidemiological study need to be analyzed in order to get the result. Analysis is done to find out:
1. Exposure rate.
2. Estimation of risk.

Exposure rate: This can be determined in case control study. The exposure rate can be calculated from cases and controls.

In cases: Exposure rate is the ratio of the number of individuals who became cases. The exposure to suspected etiological factors to the total number of cases (exposed or not exposed to suspected etiological factor):

$$\text{Exposure rate} = \frac{a}{a+c}$$

In controls: Exposure rate of control can be calculated by the disease even after exposure to suspected etiological factor to the total number in individuals who were without the disease (exposed and non-exposed individuals, who did not get the disease):

$$\text{Exposure rate} = \frac{\text{Controls with suspected factors}}{\text{Total number of controls}}$$

$$\text{Exposure rate of controls} = \frac{b}{a+c}$$

If the frequency rate is higher among exposed than nonexposed, then a statistical association between exposure status and occurrence of disease should be as certain by statistical association, i.e. by calculating P value. P value is the test of significance, which is applied for testing the association depends upon the variable under investigations.

Estimation of risk: The exposure rate of cases in the study group does not mean that all those who exposed to suspected factor will develop the disease. So the estimation of risk is associated with the exposure, which is calculated by relative risk. Odd ratio can be derived from case-control study.

Relative risk: It is defined as the ratio between the incidence of disease among exposed persons to incidence among nonexposed:

$$\text{Relative risk} = \frac{\text{Incidence among exposed}}{\text{Incidence among nonexposed}}$$

$$= \frac{a/(a+c)}{b/(b+d)}$$

Odd ratio: It is a measure of strength of association between risk factor and outcome:

$$\text{Exposure rate} = \frac{\text{Cases with suspected factor}}{\text{Total number of cases}}$$

Odd ratio is closely related to relative risk and is one of the key parameter in the analysis of case-control studies.

The relative risk estimate can increase or decrease as a result of bias, which reflect noncompatibility between the study and control groups. The bias, which can arise in epidemiological studies are due to:
- Confounding factor
- Recalling problem
- Difference in the rates of admission to hospitals
- Prior information about the hypothesis to the interviewer.

Depending upon these factors, the type biases are:
- Bias due to confounding
- Memory or recall bias
- Selection of bias
- Berksonian bias
- Interviewer bias.

Prospective method: This is a forward survey in which host, agent and environmental factors are studied. The study is planned in population group in which frequency and distribution of the disease, etc. are studied.

A prospective method is sometimes called cohort study. The cohort is a specific group of people at a certain time. The study begins with a disease or condition and watches it over a period of time to see what develops. This approach is useful in confirming any association observed from a retrospective study.

In this method, testing of hypothesis on causation of disease starts by defining a population, each individual of which is characteristics by the cause, e.g. smoking free from disease. The whole cohort, as it is called, is then followed to see who developed the disease as defined and how this is associated with smoking habits, the incidence of disease is observed, and compared in smokers and nonsmokers.

The prospective approach is time consuming and fairly expensive to carry out. In this, the investigator selects a group of people for study and gathers information about those who do, and those who do not have the characteristics in question. Thus, in a study about smoking and lung cancer, those who smoke, would be considered the experimental group, and those who do not, would be the control group. This population group or cohort would be followed over a period of time, probably several years, to see how many of the smokers developed lung cancer. Smokers would be compared with nonsmokers as to the incidence of disease.

The prospective method helps us to make estimation of risk of developing particular condition in the presence of certain characteristics. There are two commonly in the used measures of risk—relative risk and attributable risk. The relative risk means the ratio between the incidence or mortality among exposed and incidence or mortality among nonexposed. The formula of relative risk is given below:

$$\text{Relative risk} = \frac{\text{Incidence among exposed}}{\text{Incidence among nonexposed}}$$

An attributable risk means the rate of the disease in exposed individuals that can be attributed to suspected cause. It is simply the difference between the incidence rate or mortality rate among exposed, and the incidence rate or mortality rate among nonexposed.

This method is 'prospective', because it is meant to say looking ahead or they are forward looking. It also enables an investigator to study the relationship of the characteristics to other disease or problem.

Cohort study

Cohort is an analytical study, which provides additional evidence to accept or reject the existing association between suspected cause and disease.

First of all, the concept of cohort should be clear before doing the study. In epidemiology, cohort is a group of people who share common characteristics. It can be a group of people, who experience common characteristics within a defined time period. The cohort can be of marriage, birth, death or exposure.

Types

On the basis of occurrence of disease in relation to time, cohort studies are of three types:
1. Prospective cohort studies.
2. Retrospective cohort studies.
3. A combination of both.

Prospective cohort studies

Prospective studies start from present and continue into future. In this type of study, disease in the individual has not yet occurred at the time investigation starts. The outcome, i.e. the disease result in the future.

In a prospective study on smoking and lung cancer, the study will be undertaken among the individuals, who did not have lung cancer at the time of investigation. But the long-term effect of smoking will be evaluated among a group of individuals who have started smoking and a comparison group, who still do not smoke. In future, the subsequent development of lung cancer in both the groups will be assessed.

Retrospective cohort studies

Retrospective cohort studies are the study in which the outcome (disease) has occurred before the start of investigation. It is the study of going back in time. It can be 10 or 20, or more years of going back. So this study needs the records, from a past date fixed in the records to the present time.

In a retrospective cohort design, an association was picked in relation to angiosarcoma of the liver after exposure to polyvinyl chloride.

Combination of both retrospective

In this type of study, a group is identified from past records and is assessed up to present and is followed up into future for assessment of outcome.

Step of cohort study

Following are the steps of conducting cohort study:
1. Select study subjects.
2. Collect data.
3. Select comparison group.
4. Follow-up.
5. Analysis.

Select study subjects

The study subjects for cohort study can be selected either from general population or special group of population.

General population: Cohort is selected from general population. If the population is too large, appropriate sample should be selected, which is representative of the corresponding segment of the general population.

Special groups: The exposed group, which is readily available is studied. These groups are:
- Select groups
- Exposure groups.

Select groups: These groups can be professional groups and are homogenous in nature. These groups are doctors, nurses, teachers, etc.

Exposure groups: The cohort is selected because of special exposure to physical, chemical and other disease agents. An example of cohort is of radiologist exposed to X-rays.

Collect data

The data can be collected by:
- Personal interview
- Mailed questionnaires
- Review of records
- Medical tests
- Environmental surveys.

Data about demographic variables and the factors relate to the development of the disease should be collected in an appropriate manner, which provides clear information about the exposure of selected factors as well as the degree or extent of exposure.

Select comparison group

A comparison group is selected in order to compare morbidity and mortality rates. The comparison group can be in built or the external group, or the general population depending upon this. There are following ways to assemble comparison groups.

Internal comparison: The cohort on which the study is conducted is classified into several comparison groups based on the degree of exposure of risk factors before the development of disease. The comparison group is in built. For example, a cohort of exposure who are exposed to risk factor smoking. Their degree of exposure is different. On the basis of degree of exposure, the cohort is further subgrouped, which can be compared with each other in order to have outcome.

External comparison: In some cohort studies, outside comparison group is required, the study and control cohorts should be similar in demographic, and other important variable other than those under study.

Smokers and nonsmokers; a cohort radiologist compared with a cohort ophthalmologist are example of external comparison.

Comparison with general population: Sometimes the study group is compared with general population in the same geography area as the study group.

A study on comparison of cancer among asbestos workers with the rate in general population in the same geographic area.

The factors, which limit the use of general population for comparison are nonavailability of required population rates for outcome, and difficulty in selecting the study and comparison groups that are the representative of exposed and non-exposed segments of general population.

The ratio between the observational values and exposed values help in determining the effect of the factors, which are under study.

Follow-up

The study need to be followed up depending upon the type of study. It requires the use of home visits, telephonic talk, observation and mailed questionnaire. Follow-up requires:
- Periodic checkup and investigations
- Reviewing records
- Routine surveillance mortality records.

It is sometimes difficult to achieve 100% follow-up in detail for full duration of study the reason being the death, change of residence and migration, etc.

Analysis

The data collected is analyzed in order to find out the risk rate and frequency of the new cases in terms of incidence rate. In incidence rate, the unit of time should be included, which includes:
- New cases
- Time period
- Population at risk
- Per 1,000 population.

$$\text{Incidence rate} = \frac{\text{Number of new cases of specific disease during a given period}}{\text{Population at risk during that period}} \times 1{,}000$$

How to calculate incidence rate: Suppose, new cases of illness are 600 in a population of 3,000 in a year:

New cases of illness = 600
Time period = 1 year
Population at risk = 30,000

$$\text{Incidence rate} = \frac{600}{30{,}000} \times 1{,}000 = 20/1{,}000 \text{ per year}$$

Estimation of risk: After calculating the incidence rate of disease, next step is to calculate the risk of disease or death. It is done in terms of:
- Relative risk
- Attributable risk.

Relative risk: This is the ratio of incidence of disease among exposed to incidence among nonexposed:

$$\text{Relative risk} = \frac{\text{Incidence of disease among exposed}}{\text{Incidence of disease among nonexposed}}$$

Hypothetically, if the incidence rate of lung cancer among exposed is 30 and incidence rate among nonexposed is 2, the relative risk will be:

$$30/15 = 2$$

It indicates that incidence rate among exposed is higher than nonexposed. This value makes the association between cause and effect.

Relative risk is considered useful at the interval confidence of 95%. An association between cause and effect is included if the relative risk is higher than 2.

Attributable risk: It is calculated by subtracting the incidence of disease rate among nonexposed from incidence rate of exposed and by dividing this by incidence rate of exposed and multiple by 100 in order to get the result in percentage. The attributable risk indicates the percentage of disease among sufferer is due to the causative factor being exposed.

Suppose, the incidence rate of lung cancer among exposed is 30 and among nonexposed is 2:

$$\text{Attributable risk} = \frac{30-2}{30} \times 100 = \frac{28}{30} \times 100 = 93.3\%$$

It indicates that 93% of lung cancer among smokers is due to smoking.

The above explained methods of non-experimental analytical studies in which nature determines the exposure, the investigators do not intervene or control the conditions. The retrospective or case-control studies are similar to cross-sectional studies in that they assess the relationship of the existing disease to other variables or attributes. Selection is on disease that is after initial identification of cases, a suitable control group of persons without disease is identified. The relationship of an attribute to the disease is examined by comparing the diseased and nondiseased with regard to how frequently the attribute is present or what are the levels of the attributes in the two groups.

The essential difference between retrospective and prospective method lies not in the time sequence, but rather in the way the study groups are assembled. The historical retrospective studies are also prospective studies, because such studies consist of the identification of a group at some point in the past and analysis of their subsequent disease experience on the basis of previous recorded information. This method employs previous assembled data, but it is essentially longitudinal, the longitudinal information covers a time interval extending from past to present rather than past to future as in the conventionally termed prospective study.

Thus, the non-experimental analytic studies are designed to determine, if an association exists between a factor and disease, and what the strength of the association is. There are some advantages and disadvantages in the above explained non-experimental analytical studies.

Experimental Studies

In experimental studies, the investigator intervenes and actually changes one variable and observes what happens to the other. In this method, the conditions are under the careful control of the investigator. The experiment follows a study protocol and allows for control of variables, random allocation of subjects, and elimination of bias on the part of the experiments. In these studies, a system is subjected to manipulation, this creates an independent variable whose effect is then determined through measurement of a subsequent event in the system. The subsequent event is the dependent variable.

Experimental studies are undertaken to confirm an etiological hypothesis and to evaluate or assess the effectiveness of the therapeutic or preventive measures before applying them to the community. These experimental studies may be conducted in the laboratory or in the field. In the laboratory, guinea pigs, mice, monkeys and other animals have been frequently used for studying the effects of drugs, vaccines and nutrients. The experiments may be conducted on human beings to investigate the disease etiology or evaluate preventive or therapeutic measures, but it involves medical, ethical and moral issues.

The basic principle involved in the experimental epidemiology includes:
1. Random allocation of subjects to the appropriate subgroups: In this two groups are formed, the experimental or study groups receives a drug or other procedure; the other group often referred to as control group or sometimes placebo receives no treatment.
2. Medical, ethical and moral issues: These are observed, while conducting experiments particularly on human beings.
3. Ability to generalize: If the experiment is conducted on a representative sample of the total population, it is possible to make generalizations. If only a small sampling of persons participate, the results will not be widely applicable.
4. Double blindness: In a double blind study, neither the investigator nor the subjects know who receives the study treatment and who receives control treatment. In addition, the outcome is measured in such a way that the type of treatment is not known. Thus, no bias is introduced by the investigator or subjects. Although, double blindness is desirable in experiments with human subjects, it is not always possible.

Types of Experimental Studies

In epidemiology, there are two types of experiments:
1. Prophylactic trials or clinical trials.
2. Therapeutic trials or community trials.

The clinical trials or prophylactic trials designed to prevent disease or conditions in which the efficacy of a preventive or therapeutic agent, or procedure is tested on individual subjects, e.g. administration of bacille Calmette-Guérin (BCG) vaccine as prophylaxis for TB.

The community trial or therapeutic trail to treat established disease processes in which, a group of individuals as a whole is used to determine the efficacy of a drug or procedure, e.g. the evaluation fluorides in preventing dental caries.

Experimental Studies are International Studies

The approach used is similar to cohort study except that the study is carried out under the direct control of investigator. Experimental study requires the following.

Intervention or action: It means application or withdrawal of suspected case or changing variable in the causative chain in experimental group and no change in experimental group.

Observation: Observing the changes occurring in variable in experimental group.

Comparison: Comparing the findings of experimental group with the control group.

Experimental study is of two types:
- Randomized controlled trial
- Non-randomized controlled trial.

Randomized controlled trial involves the process of random allocation of subjects to be studied. The basic steps of randomized controlled trial include:
- Preparing a protocol
- Selecting target and study population
- Randomization
- Intervention
- Follow-up
- Outcome.

Preparing and protocol
The study is conducted under a strict protocol, which includes:
1. Aims and objective of study.
2. Statement of problem—question to be answered.
3. Criteria for selecting groups, i.e. study and control group.
4. Treatment to be used.
5. Standardization of procedures and schedules.

The aim of preparing the protocol is to prevent the bias and to reduce the errors in the study.

Selecting target and study population
Target population comprises the population of school children, industrial workers or of a whole city depending upon nature of study. This target population is the reference population. The study population is drawn from the target population and this study population participates in the experimental study. The study population has the same characteristics as the target population. The study population should fulfill the criteria:
1. Informed consent should be given by the participants about procedure, purpose and possible complications.
2. Participates should be the representative of the target population.
3. Study population should be eligible for the intervention or trial to be carried out.

Randomization
Randomization is done to eliminate bias and to allow comparison. Participants are grouped under study and control group to receive or not to receive intervention. It ensures that investigator has no control over grouping of participants under study or control group. Randomization is done after the participants has given consent and have qualified criteria of trial.

Types

Randomized control trial
Randomized control trial is of following types.

Clinical trials: These are concerned with the evaluation of therapeutic agents such as drugs.

Preventive trial: These are concerned with primary preventive measures such as vaccines or chemoprophylactic drugs.

Risk factor trials: These are preventive trial in the intervention of risk factors in the development of disease.

Cessation experiments: These are preventive trial by to terminate the habits, which are related to the development of disease.

Evaluation of health services: Assessment of the effectiveness and efficiency of health services.

Trial of etiological agents: In this, trial is made to confirm or refute the etiological hypothesis.

Non-randomized trial
Non-randomized trial (RCT) is approached in studies where randomized controlled trials approach is sophisticated. These type of trials are used when due to some reasons (ethical, administrative) it is not possible to conduct RCT in human beings. In non-randomized controlled trial, there is no randomization. These trials are referred as non-experimental studies.

Epidemiology is the basic science of community health and CHN. The epidemiological methods provide proper understanding of population health and necessary information for improving the plans to prevent disease, and deliver healthcare services. The success of services in reaching stated standards will be assessed and what in fact are the benefits to health, and the relief of suffering in relation to resources consumed. Such a contribution to rationality and fairness is an urgent requirement in the management of health services, and for ordering their priorities. CHN play an important role in epidemiological studies, because they often may be the ones to initiate study and more frequently assist in the data collection. Also, the CHN often cast in the role of interpreting studying findings to families, schools, industries and others. In actual practice, nurses are the major force in the health department to provide all types of services related to health and medical care, and follow-up on various conditions.

Intervention

The intervention is done in the study group by independent variables such as drug, vaccines, etc. The effect of this intervention is measured to have the outcome. The outcome is the dependent variable. The effect of drug in the treatment of a particular disease is either the recovery. This recovery is dependent variable as it depends on the independent variable drug, i.e. application of drug means recovery and absence of drug application, leads to no recovery.

Follow-up

Follow-up means regular observations and assessment of both of the groups, i.e. control and study group till the final assessment of the outcome. This should be done under same circumstances in a standard manner for defined interval of time.

Outcome

The outcome of the trial is assessed. The application of independent variable can either cause positive result or negative results. Positive results means there will be benefits, which will either cause reduction in severity of disease or reduction in the incidence rate, etc.

Negative result means intervention, which will cause more severity of problem and complication. Death opposite to recovery (positive outcome) is the negative results of the intervention.

DYNAMICS OF DISEASE TRANSMISSION

Communicable diseases have affected human life since earlier times. Knowledge of transmission of communicable diseases, current prevention and control measures can assure the CHN in recognizing, treating and changing communicable diseases. In addition, educating the patient and the community regarding potential spread of communicable diseases, and taking suitable measures to reduce them.

Communicable disease is a disease that is primarily infectious in nature, requires interaction between the host and agent, direct or indirect transmission from the agent reservoir in the environment, and a host that can provide adequate living conditions for the infectious agent. In other word, communicable disease is an illness to a specific infectious agent or its toxic products capable of being directly, or indirectly transmitted to man, animal to animal, or from the environment (through air, dust, soil, water, food, etc.).

Communicable diseases are transmitted from the reservoir or source of infection to the host. There are three links in the chain of disease transmission, i.e. reservoir or source, modes of transmission and susceptible host.

Source or Reservoir

The existence of sources or reservoir is the starting point for the occurrence of communicable diseases. The source of infection is defined as the person, animal, object or substance from which an infectious agent passes, or disseminates to the host. A reservoir is the natural habitat in which the organisms metabolizes and replicates. Reservoir can be defined as 'any person, animal, plant, soil or substance (or combination of these) in which infectious agent lives and multiples on which it depends primarily for survival, and where it reproduces itself in such manner that it can be transmitted to a susceptible host'. For example, man is the reservoir of hookworm infection. The terms 'reservoir' and 'source' sometimes used as synonyms', but not always. There are two reservoirs:
- Homologous reservoir
- Heterologous reservoir.

Infection is said to be homologous when it is carried from man to man, e.g. polio. When infection is conveyed to man from animals or plants it is called heterologous.

Homologous Reservoir

Man is the main source of the most infectious diseases. They may be a case or carrier.

A case may be defined as a 'person in the population, identified as having the particular disease, health disorder or condition under investigation'. The presence of infection in a host may be clinical, subclinical or latent.

Cases

The clinical case may be mild or moderate, typical or atypical, severe or fatal. In fact, mild cases are the major sources of infection than severe, because, they can move from place to place in spread infection. Whereas, severe case cannot move. Subclinical cases play a dominant role in maintaining endemicity in the community. Here, agent multiplies in the host, but does not manifest itself by signs and symptoms. Measles, rubella, mumps, polio, hepatitis, Japanese encephalitis B (JEB), etc. are some examples. However, infection can be detected by laboratory tests. In latent cases, the host does not shed the infectious agent, which lies dormant within the host, without symptoms, viral infection (herpes simplex), ancylostomiasis, etc. in man.

Carriers

The carrier is an infected person or animal that harbors a specific infectious agent in the absence of discernible clinical disease and serves a potential source of infection to others. In other words, they are persons who harbor the disease organisms, but do not show any sign or symptoms. They are outwardly healthy, but capable of infecting others.

The carriers may be classified by type, duration and portal exit. Carriers by type are divided into three groups, i.e. incubatory, convalescent and healthy carriers:

1. Incubators carriers are those, who shed the infectious agent during the incubation period, e.g. measles, mumps, polio, pertussis, diphtheria and influenza.
2. Convalescent carriers are those, who continue to shed the disease agent during the period of convalescences, e.g. typhoid fever, dysentery, cholera and meningococcal meningitis.
3. Healthy carriers emerge from subclinical cases, e.g. poliomyelitis, salmonellosis and diphtheria. Carriers by duration may be grouped into two, i.e. temporary carriers and chronic carrier:
   a. Temporary carriers are those, who shed the infectious agent for short period. For example, as in carriers by type.
   b. Chronic carrier is one who exerts the infectious agent for indefinite period, e.g. typhoid, hepatitis B and dysentery.
   c. Carriers by portal exist can be grouped according to the portal exist of the infectious agents. For example, urinary carriers, intestinal carriers, respiratory carriers, nasal carriers, etc. Skin eruptions, open wounds and blood are also considered as portal exit.

Heterologous Reservoir

As stated earlier, infection may be conveyed to man from animals and plants. Lower animals and birds acting as a reservoir of infection, and transferring to man. The diseases in animals and rodents affect the health of man is termed as zoonosis. The risk of infection of zoonotic diseases depend upon the association between man and animal. There are over 100 zoonotic diseases, which may be conveyed to man from animals and birds. The best known examples are listed below:

- Dog: Anthrax
- Goat: Malta fever
- Horse: Glander, equine encephalitis
- Pigs: Tapeworm, trichinosis
- Rats: Plague, Weil's disease, rat bite fever, food poisoning
- Fish: Tapeworm
- Monkey's: Yellow fever, Kyasanur forest disease (KFD)
- Parrots: Psittacosis
- Rabbits: Tularemia
- Birds: Encephalitis.

Modes of Disease Transmission

Communicable diseases may be transmitted from the reservoir or source of infection to a susceptible host in a variety of ways depicted as follows (Fig. 27.7).

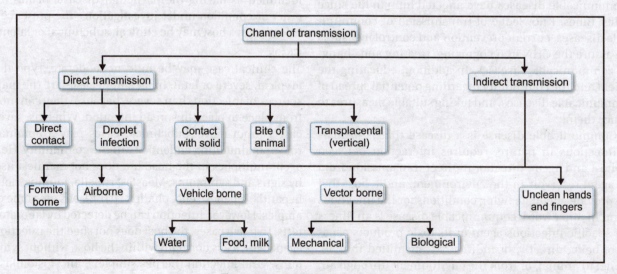

Figure 27.7: Channels of transmission

Direct Transmission

Direct contact: It means contact of diseased part with healthy. This implies direct and immediate transfer of infectious agents from the reservoir and/or source to a susceptible individual, without an intermediate agency. For example, during touching, kissing, sexual intercourse [STD, AIDS, leprosy, skin infections and scratching through fingers (hydrophobia)].

The epidemiological features of direct contact are as follows:
1. It has slow onset and slow progress.
2. It is endemic or may be sporadic. Small number of people are involved.
3. Source easily traced.
4. It can be controlled by personal hygiene and health education (may be difficult due to carries).
5. It is not seasonal.

Droplet infection: It is a direct projection of droplet synergy of saliva and mass-pharyngeal secretions into the mouth during sneezing, coughing, spitting, singing and talking. The larger droplet as projected for 3-4 feet between source and host. Diseases transmitted through droplet are common cold, diphtheria, pertussis, TB, etc. Epidemiological features of droplet infection are as follows:
1. Its outbreak is explosive.
2. It is acute and has short duration.
3. It has distinct geographical distribution.
4. It is favored by overcrowding.
5. It has marked seasonal distribution.
6. It is difficult to trace with certainty.
7. It can be prevented by proper bed spanning, avoidance of overcrowding, proper swabbing and personal hygiene.

Contact with soil: This is a direct exposure of susceptible tissue to a disease agent in soil. Compost or decaying vegetable matter in which it normally leads to saprophytic existence may result in infection, e.g. hookworm larvae, tetanus, mycosis, etc.

Bite of animal: Dog bite leads to rabies. Biting and insects correspondence of the disease prevalence with breeding season.

Transplacental: Transmission in disease through placenta of mother for viral infection, i.e. rubella, AIDS and syphilis and hepatitis B.

Indirect Transmission

Indirect transmission is a transmission of infection by indirect contact, e.g. the agency acts mechanically and organisms survive for a short time only. This embraces a variety of mechanisms including traditional tsetse flies, finger, fomites, food and fluid.

Fomites: Infected feeding bottles, bedpans, urinals, handkerchiefs, etc. are grouped under fomites. Due to infected fomites, they slow onset and progress, long duration and irregular distribution.

Airborne: The direct airborne infections occur by droplet nuclei and indirect airborne infection is by dustborne (certain features explained under direct contact).

Vehicle-borne transmission: Implies transmission of the infectious agent through agency of water, food (including raw vegetables, fruits), milk, blood, serum, plasma or other biological products such as tissues and organs.

Water is the common vehicle, common to largest number of people. Waterborne diseases occur in cities due to breakdown and defect in water supply system, and in rural areas due to scarcity of water. The common waterborne diseases are diarrheal diseases, typhoid fever, polio and hepatitis. Characteristics of epidemiological waterborne disease will include:
- Waterborne infection takes an explosive character
- Geographical distribution is marked
- Resident consumers of water are not affected
- Non-resident consumers are affected
- There is marked seasonal distribution due to chance of water pollution
- All ages are affected expect breastfed infants, who do not drink water
- Both sexes are affected depending upon the use of infected water
- Epidemic waves are explosive, sudden
- Sometimes, food, milk are also contaminated leading to food and milk-borne infections, i.e. food poisoning, brucellosis
- In India, usually people use boiled milk, but an epidemic may breakout in rare cases due to streptococcal infections.

Vector-borne infection: Vectors are intermediate living objects, which may spread the infection from one host to another. Vector is an arthropod or any living carrier that transports an infectious agent to susceptible individual. Arthropod vector falls into seven orders as follows:
1. Diptera—flies and mosquitoes.
2. Siphonaptera—fleas.
3. Orthoptera—cockroaches.
4. Anoplura—sucking lice.
5. Hemiptera—bugs, including kissing bugs.
6. Acarina—ticks and mites.
7. Copepod—cyclops.

Classification

Vector-borne diseases are classified under heterogeneous chain and involve three types:

1. Man and non-vertebrate host:
   - Man-arthropod-man (malaria)
   - Man-snail-man (schistosomiasis).
2. Man and another vertebrate and non-vertebrate host:
   - Mammal-arthropod-man (plague)
   - Bird-arthropod-man (encephalitis).
3. Man and two intermediate hosts:
   - Man-cyclops-fish-man (fish tapeworm)
   - Man-snail-fish-man (clonorchiasis)
   - Man-snail-crab-man (paragonimiasis).

The methods in which vectors transmit agents are biting, regurgitation, scratching of infective feces, contamination of host with body fluids of vectors. The methods in which vectors involved in the transmission and propagation of parasites are mechanical transmission (crawling, flying, passages by excretion) and biological transmission (propagative, cyclopropagative).

Susceptible Host

Host means that human or animal that provides adequate living conditions for any given infectious agent. When an infectious agent wants to enter any host, it must find a portal entry. There are many portals of entry, i.e. respiratory tract, alimentary tract, genitourinary tract, skin, etc. on gaining entry to the host, the organisms must reach the appropriate tissue or site of infection in the body of the host, where it may find optimum conditions for its multiplication and survival. Then, the agent will find a way out of the body, i.e. portal of exit in order to reach a new host and to propagate its species. When there is no portal of exit, the infection continues as the body leads to many complications including death. After leaving human body, the organisms must survive in the external environment for sufficient period till a new host is found.

Disease can occur only in a susceptible human host. The concept of immunity is important for the understanding or resistance of disease caused by infectious agent.

IMMUNITY

Immunity refers to the increased resistance on the part of a host to a specific infectious agent. Immunity can be humoral (antibodies in the blood) or cellular (specific to each type of cell).

Humoral Immunity

Humoral immunity form of immunity comes from the B cells (bone marrow-derived lymphocytes), which proliferate and manufacture specific antibodies are localized in the immunoglobulin fraction of the serum. There are five main classes of immunoglobulins', i.e. immunoglobulin M (IgM), IgA, IgD and a different functional group. The antibodies circulate in the body and act directly by neutralizing the microbe or its toxin rendering the microbe susceptible to attack by the polymorphonuclear leukocyte and monocyte.

Cellular Immunity

Cellular immunity is mediated by the T cells (thymus-derived lymphocytes), which differentiate into subpopulations able to help B cells. The T cells do not secrete antibody, but are responsible for recognition of antigen. On contact with antigens, the T cells initiate a chain of responses, e.g. activation of macrophages, release of cytotoxic factors, mononuclear inflammatory reactions, delayed hypersensitivity reactions, active and passive sensitivity, secretions of immunological mediators, etc.

Active and Passive Immunity

The role of each of these types of immunity varies with the infectious agent and with the immune response of the host. Immunity can also be passive or active acquired, or it may be herd immunity.

Passive Immunity

When antibodies produced in one body are transferred to another, to induce protection against disease is known as 'passive immunity'. Passive immunity is effective almost immediately and includes transplacental, natural passive or artificial passive immunity. Passive immunity is temporary, lasting weeks to months. Inoculation of the host by one of the two routes provide passive immunity:

1. Transplacental immunity is achieved when the mother's antibodies are passed to fetus. The degree to which this protection prevents infections in the infant after birth varies. Human milk also contains protective antibodies, i.e. IgA.
2. Artificial passive immunity can also be administered to the host after exposure to certain disease-causing organisms. Antibodies from the same or different species may be used. An example of antibodies from the same species is immune serum globulin (ISG). Human ISG available for rabies and tetanus.

Serum from animals that increased the allergic reactions to the serum was used. At present, only few diseases require serum of animals, such as diphtheria, botulism or gas gangrene.

Passive immunization is useful for individual, who cannot form antibodies or from the normal host who takes time to develop antibodies following active immunization. Passive immunity differs from active immunity as given in the Tables 27.6 and 27.7.

Active Immunity

Active immunization is achieved by introducing a live/killed or partial component of the invading organism. The host immune system initiates a humoral response to the organisms, recognizing the species the forming antibodies that will identify and destroy the initial, and any subsequent invasion by the identified organism.

Herd Immunity

Herd immunity is the level of resistance of a community or group of people to a particular disease. It provides immunological barrier to the spread of diseases in the human herd. The elements, which contribute to herd immunity are:
- Occurrence of clinical and subclinical infections in the herd
- Immunization of the herd
- Herd structure.

Thus, immunity is the power of resistance of animal body, which it possesses against the infecting organisms and their products. Antigens are the substances, which when introduced into the body of an animal of different species, induce the information of antibodies in that animal.

Immunizing Agents

The immunizing agents may be classified as vaccines, immunoglobulin and antisera.

Vaccines

Vaccine is an immune-biological substance designed to produce specific protection against a given disease. It stimulates the production of protective antibody and other immune mechanisms. Vaccines may be prepared from live modified organisms, inactivated or killed organisms, extracted cellular fractions, toxoids or combination of these. They are used in active immunization. Examples of vaccines are as follows:
1. Live attenuated vaccine:
   - Typhoid, BCG, oral, plague (bacterial)
   - Oral polio vaccine (Sabin), yellow fever, measles, rubella, mumps, influenza (viral)
   - Epidemic typhus (rickettsial).
2. Inactivated or killed vaccine:
   - Typhoid, cholera, pertussis, cerebral spinal meningitis (bacterial)
   - Rabies, inactivated polio vaccine (Salk), influenza, hepatitis B virus (HBV), JEB, KFD (viral).
3. Toxoids: Diphtheria and tetanus (bacterial).
4. Cellular fractions: Meningococcal vaccine and pneumococcal vaccine.
5. Combinations: Diphtheria, pertussis, tetanus (DPT) and measles, mumps, rubella (MMR).

Immunoglobulins

Immunoglobulins are synthesized by the cells of reticuloendothelial system. All known circulatory antibodies are contained in five classes of immunoglobulin such as IgA, IgD, IgG and IgM.

Table 27.6: Differences between active and passive immunity

Active immunity	Passive immunity
Antigen is injected and antibodies are formed in the bodies of a man	Antibodies are prepared in the body of animal or man by injection of antigens. Serum containing immune bodies is injected
In the production of antibodies the tissue of the body takes an active part	Body does not take active part in synthesis of antibodies
The development of antibodies takes time	It does not take time and acts quickly
Antibodies produced give lasting immunity for month and year	Serum containing antibodies give short time immunity for 3–4 week
It is used for prophylactic purposes	It is used for curative purposes mostly and for prophylaxis for contacts

Table 27.7: Resistance to different types of immunity

Types of immunity	How acquired?	Length of resistance
Natural		
Active	Natural contact and infection with the antigen	May be temporary or permanent
Passive	Natural contact with antibody transplacentally or through colostrum and breast milk	Temporary
Artificial		
Active	Inoculation of antigen	May be temporary or permanent
Passive	Inoculation of antibody or antigen	Temporary

Antisera or Antitoxins

Antisera or antitoxins are the solutions of antibodies derived from the serum of animals immunized with specific antigens (e.g. diphtheria, tetanus) used to achieve passive immunity in man.

National immunization schedule and hazards of immunization are dealt in Tables 27.8 and 27.9.

Agent: A biological, physical or chemical entity is capable of causing disease.

DYNAMICS OF INFECTIOUS DISEASE TRANSMISSION

Complex interactions between the host, agent and environment occur before the clinical signs and symptoms of disease observed. The chain of disease transmission (Fig. 27.8) involves a series of events that allow a pathogenic microorganism to come in contact with a host and to invade, multiply and elicit a physiological response to this host. For infection and subsequent disease to occur, the chain of transmission must remain intact. This requires the presence of a pathogenic agent, an appropriate reservoir, a susceptible host with portals of entry and exit, and favorable environmental conditions that support transmission of the agent. Host, agent and environmental factors that influence disease transmission and progression are discussed below in Table 27.10.

Host Characteristics

Host factors affect the ease of contact between the host and agent, and the capability of the host to resist the disease-evoking powers of an agent. Lifestyle patterns can significantly influence the host-agent transmission

Table 27.8: Current national immunization schedule for infants, children and pregnant women (NRHM)

Vaccines	When to be given	Dosage	Routes	Sites
For pregnant women				
Tetanus toxoid (TT)-1	Early in pregnancy	0.5 mL	Intramuscular (IM)	Upper arm
TT-2	4 weeks after TT-1*	0.5 mL	IM	Upper arm
TT booster	One dose if TT is given in last 3 year*	0.5 mL	IM	Upper arm
For infants				
Bacille Calmette-Guérin (BCG)	At birth or as early as possible till 1 year of age	0.1 mL (0.05 mL until 1 month of age)	Intradermal (ID)	Left upper arm
Hepatitis B	At birth or as early as possible within 24 hour	0.5 mL	IM	Anterolateral side of mid thigh
Oral polio vaccine (OPV)-0	At birth or as early as possible within first 15 day	Two drops	Oral	Oral
OPV-1, 2 and 3	At 6, 10 and 14 week	Two drops	Oral	Oral
Diphtheria, pertussis, tetanus (DPT)-1, 2 and 3	At 6, 10 and 14 week	0.5 mL	IM	Anterolateral side of mid thigh

Contd...

Contd...

Vaccines	When to be given	Dosage	Routes	Sites
Hepatitis B-1, 2 and 3	At 6, 10 and 14 week	0.5 mL	IM	Anterolateral side of mid thigh
Measle-1	9 completed month to 12 month	0.5 mL	Subcutaneous	Right upper arm
Vitamin A (first dose)	At 9 month with measles vaccine	1.0 mL	Oral	Oral
For children				
DTP booster-1	16–24 month	0.5 mL	IM	Anterolateral side of mid thigh
OPV booster	16–24 month	Two drops	Oral	Oral
Measles-2	16–24 month	0.5 mL	Subcutaneous	Right upper arm
Japanese encephalitis (JE)**	16–24 month with DPT/OPV booster	0.5 mL	Subcutaneous	Left upper arm
Vitamin A, second dose	With DPT/OPV booster	2.0 mL	Oral	Oral
Vitamin A, third to ninth dose	One dose every 6 month up to the age of 5 year	2.0 mL	Oral	Oral
DPT booster-2	5–6 year	0.5 mL	IM	Upper arm
TT booster	10 and 16 year	0.5 mL	IM	Upper arm

Source: Vipin M Vashishtha. Key statements of IAPCOI and IAP immunization timetable for the year 2012. Pediatric infectious disease. 2012;4(3):112-24.
*Give TT-2 or booster dose preferably before 36 weeks of pregnancy; **JE vaccine in selected endemic districts.
Note: In selected states, pentavalent vaccine [DPT + *Haemophilus influenzae* type b (Hib) + hepatitis B (Hep B)] one, two and three doses replace DPT one, two and three dose and tlib, two and three doses. During the first phase (2011), Kerala and Tamil Nadu states were selected. During 2012–2013 in the second phase, New Delhi, Jammu and Kashmir, Haryana, Gujarat, Goa, Puducherry and Karnataka have been selected. It is proposed to cover the entire country in the next phase. Thus, pentavalent vaccine has been introduced by Government of India in a phased manner.

Table 27.9: Indian Academy of Pediatrics recommended vaccine for routine use

Age (completed week/month/year)	Vaccines	Comments
Birth	Bacille Calmette-Guérin (BCG) Oral polio vaccine (OPV) Hepatitis B (Hep B)-1	Hepatitis B: Administer Hep B vaccine to all newborns before hospital discharge
6 week	Diphtheria, pertussis, tetanus (DPT)-1* *Haemophilus influenzae* type b (Hib)-1* Hep B-2 Inactivated polio vaccine (IPV)-1* Rotavirus-1 Pneumococcal conjugate	*These three are together available as pentavalent vaccine (easy five) Polio: • All doses of IPV may be replaced with OPV, if IPV is unavailable/unaffordable • Additional doses of OPV on all supplementary immunization activities • Minimum age to start IPV is 6 week • If IPV is started at 8 week, only two doses with 8 week interval • IPV catch-up schedule: Two doses at 2 month apart followed by a booster dose after 6 month Rotavirus (RV): Two doses of RV-1 (Rotarix) or three doses of RV-5 (Rotateq); only RV-1 is recommended; maximum age for the first dose is 14 weeks and not to be initiated after 15 week Pneumococcal vaccine minimum age 6 week and 2 year for pneumococcal polysaccharide vaccine (PPSV)

Contd...

Contd...

Age (completed week/month/year)	Vaccines	Comments
10 week	DPT-2 Hib-2 IPV-2 Rotavirus-2 Pneumococcal conjugate vaccine (PCV)-2	DPT and Hib are together available as tetravalent vaccine (easy four)
14 week	DPT-3 Hib-3 IPV-3 Rotavirus-3 PCV-3	
6 month	OPV-1 Hep B-3	Hepatitis B: The third dose of Hep B should not be administered before 24 week of age
9 month	OPV-2 Measles vaccine	
12 month	Hep A-1	Hepatitis A: For both killed and live hepatitis A vaccines, two doses are recommended with 6–18 month interval
15 month	Measles, mumps and rubella (MMR)-1 Varicella-1 PCV booster	Varicella vaccine: Second dose may be administered before age 4 year, provided at least 3 month have elapsed since the first dose
16–18 month	DTP booster IPV booster-1 Hib booster-1	The first booster (fourth dose) may be administered as early as 12 month, provided at least 6 month have elapsed since the third dose
18 month	Hep A-2	
2 year	Typhoid-1	Typhoid revaccination every 3 year, if Vi-polysaccharide vaccine is used
4½–5 year	DPT booster-2 OPV-3 MMR-2 Varicella-2 Typhoid-2	MMR: The second dose can be given at any time 4–8 week after first dose Varicella: The second dose can be given at any time month after first dose.
10–12 year	Combined tetanus diphtheria and pertussis (acellular) vaccine, i.e. Tdap Human papilloma virus (HPV)	Tdap: This is preferred to Td followed by Td every 10 year HPV vaccine: Only for females, three doses at 0, 1–2 (depending upon the brands) and 6 month

Source: Vipin M Vashishtha. Key statements of IAPCOI and IAP immunization timetable for the year 2012. Pediatric infectious disease. 2012;4(3):112-24.

Note:
1. This time table/schedule includes recommendations in effect as April 2012. Any dose not administered at the recommended age should be administered at a subsequent visit when indicated and feasible. Use of a combination vaccine is generally preferred over separate injections of its equivalent component vaccines.
2. The current rotavirus vaccines have been associated with a risk of intussusceptions (about 1–2 per 100,000 infants vaccinated). Therefore, history of intussusceptions in the past is an absolute contraindication for rotavirus vaccine (RV-1 and RV-5) administration.

process. Biological characteristics and the host lines of defense affect how well the host can protect itself against host invasion and dissemination.

Live attenuated (weakened) and inactivated vaccines are used to produce an immune response in a host. The more similar a vaccine is to the natural disease, the better the immune response to the vaccine. The immune response to a live attenuated vaccine is virtually identical to that response to an inactivated vaccine is mostly humoral and little or no cellular immunity results.

CHAPTER 27 — Epidemiology

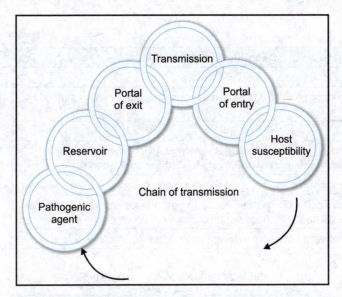

Figure 27.8: Chain of transmission for infection (chain must be intact for an infection to be transmitted to another host; the transmission can be controlled by breathing any link in the chain).

The available vaccines by type are discussed in Table 27.11. Having knowledge of the vaccine type helps predict adverse events, contraindications and immunization schedule. For example, live attenuated vaccines generally produce long-lasting immunity with a single dose and adverse reactions to the vaccine are usually similar to those produced by a mild form of the natural illness (e.g. fever and rash). Inactivated vaccines always require multiple doses, often require periodic boosting to maintain immunity and generally produce mostly localized adverse events (e.g. pain at the injection site) with or without fever.

Agent Characteristics

Agent characteristics influence the likelihood that infection and disease will occur and affect the nature of the disease process. A microorganism, i.e. capable of producing an infection or an infectious disease is commonly referred to as a pathogenic agent. Infection is not synonymous with infectious disease; the result may be in apparent or manifest.

Table 27.10: Factors influencing an infectious disease

Factors	Definitions
Host characteristics	
Lifestyle factors	Factors (e.g. sanitation practices, sexual habits, food storage and cooking practices) that facilitate or inhibit agent-host contact
Biological factors	Factors that decrease or increase a host's resistance to infection (e.g. general health status, nutritional intake, immune response)
General defense mechanisms	External barriers (e.g. skin, nose and digestive system) that prevent the agent from invading the internal organs of the host and the non-specific inflammatory response that fights and destroys pathogens
Specific defense mechanisms	An immune response that creates host immunity to a specific agent
Immunity	Protection from infectious disease associated with the presence of antibodies or cells having a specific action on the pathogens that cause a particular infectious disease
Passive immunity (temporary, short-duration immunity)	Antibody protection transferred from another person either naturally by transplacental transfer from the mother or artificially by inoculation of specific protective antibodies
Active immunity (permanent or long-lasting immunity)	Antibody and cell protection produced by the person's own immune system either naturally by infection with or without clinical manifestations or artificially by inoculation of the agent itself in a killed, modified or variant form
Agent characteristics	
Infectivity	Capability of an infectious agent to invade, survive and multiply in the host
Pathogenicity	Power of the agent to produce clinical disease
Virulence	Degree of pathogenicity of an infectious agent indicated by the severity of disease manifestations (e.g. case fatality rates and tissue damage)
Invasiveness	Capability an infectious agent to spread and disseminate in the host

Contd...

Contd...

Factors	Definitions
Toxigenicity	Capability of an infectious agent to produce poisonous products such as exotoxins
Antigenicity	Capability of an infectious agent to produce an immune response (e.g. production of antibodies or antitoxins)
Environmental characteristics	
Reservoir	Any person, animal, arthropod, plant, soil or substance in which an infectious agent lives, multiplies and reproduces itself in a manner that supports survival and transmission
Mode of transmission	Any mechanism by which an infectious agent is spread from a source or reservoir to another host
Direct transmission	Direct contact transmission to a portal of entry, as a result of a host physically touching an infected reservoir, transplacental transfer or transmission of projected airborne droplet spray
Indirect transmission	Transmission through an intermediate, contaminated vehicle or vector, or an infective vector

When a pathogenic agent invades a host and multiples, an inapparent infection occurs. An infection goes through several stages before it produces clinical disease (Fig. 27.9). The duration and potential outcomes of each stage vary considerably, depending on agent and host characteristics.

Infection in the host proceeds in identifiable stages; the length of each stage varies with the pathogenic agent and host factors. The latent period begins with pathogenic invasion of the body and ends when the agent can be shed (communicability period). The incubation period begins with invasion of the agent during which the organism reproduces and ends when the disease process begins. The communicability period begins when the latent period ends and continues as long as the agent is present. The disease period follows the incubation period and ends at variable times. This stage may be subclinical or produce overt symptoms and it may resolve completely or become latent.

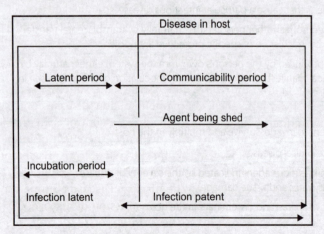

Figure 27.9: Stages of infection

Table 27.11: Available vaccines by type

Vaccines	Disease prevention
Live attenuated vaccines	
Viral	Measles, mumps, rubella, polio, yellow fever vaccine, varicella vaccine
Bacterial	Bacille Calmette-Guérin (BCG)
Recombinant	Typhoid
Inactivated vaccines	
Viral	Influenza, polio, rabies and hepatitis A
Bacterial	Pertussis, typhoid, cholera and plague
Subunit	Hepatitis B, influenza and acellular pertussis
Toxoid	Diphtheria, tetanus
Recombinant	Hepatitis B
Polysaccharide	Pneumococcal, meningococcal and *Haemophilus influenza* type b

The concepts that describe the disease-provoking powers of an agent are infectivity, pathogenicity, virulence, invasiveness, toxigenicity and antigenicity. Disease-provoking powers of an agent influence a pathogenic agent's ability to invade, multiply and survive in a host (infectivity), and to produce clinical disease (virulence, invasiveness and toxigenicity). Agents that lack antigenic properties (antigenicity) have a greater chance of surviving in a host than those agents that possess these properties

The disease-provoking capabilities of an agent vary considerably. While many host-agent-relationships result in varying degrees disease, many others result in inapparent or subclinical infection. From a control perspective, it is important to study asymptomatic individuals exposed to an infectious agent as well as those with visible clinical disease. Individuals with inapparent infection can harbor a specific infectious agent without discernible clinical disease and serve as potential sources of infection. These individuals are carriers of disease. Carriers of disease present considerable danger to other hosts, because they often do not recognize the need to take action to prevent disease transmission. Individuals for example, can have active TB that is capable of being transmitted to others without realizing that they are ill.

Environmental Characteristics

Environmental factors influence agent survival and transmission processes. These factors can determine what type of agents is present in a region and may provide reservoirs, and favorable conditions for the spread of disease. For example, malaria is prevalent in tropical and subtropical areas, because environmental conditions support the breeding habits of the *Anopheles* mosquito, the vector that transmits the disease to human hosts. Human reservoirs are also prevalent in these areas and frequently are carries of the disease. A reservoir is any person, animal, arthropod, plant, soil or substance in which an infectious agent lives, multiples and reproduces mission. The human reservoir may be clinically ill have a subclinical infection or be a carrier.

Environmental factors support or inhibit direct, or indirect transmission of the pathogenic agent from a reservoir to a susceptible host. Direct transmission can occur by actual physical contact with an infected reservoir by transplacental transfer or by host inhalation of projected airborne droplet spray. Indirect transmission occurs through an intermediate vehicle or vector. A vehicle is a contaminated inanimate object or material such as food, water, air, blood, feces, soiled linens or equipment from a diseased person. Objects contaminated by a disease individual are referred to as fomites. A vector is an arthropod or other invertebrate carrier of disease. Vectors may be simple mechanical carriers (flies) or infected non-vertebrate hosts (mosquitoes). Vector-borne transmissions have been responsible for major epidemics of disease (e.g. malaria and yellow fever), and have caused extensive morbidity and mortality.

As discussed earlier in this chapter, a balance between host, agent and environmental factors must be maintained to prevent disease outbreaks. Altering this balance, even slightly, can cause significant spread of disease. For example, day-care worker, who neglects to wash his/her hands one time after changing an infant's diaper can transmit bacterial diseases such as salmonellosis. Astute community health professionals have been instrumental in preventing bacterial and other types of disease by carefully observing for environmental and host factors that facilitate disease transmission.

CONCLUSION

Epidemiology is the study of disease in population and of the factors, which determine its occurrence. With the changing concept of epidemiology a separate area of epidemiology such as infectious disease epidemiology, cancer epidemiology has been formulated. The uses of epidemiology are studying rise and fall of disease, community diagnosis, planning and evaluation, syndrome identification, searching for causes and risk factors, etc. Disease is transmitted from source of infection to susceptible host. The human is the source of infection (as a case or carrier) and acts as a host for infectious agent. The diseased agent from human source of infection is transmitted by direct or indirect contact. Then, it enters the susceptible host. On getting appropriate environment, it multiplies and sufficient density of disease agent is build up to cause disease. The host defenses against infection. If host defense is sufficient to suppress the disease, then recovery and if insufficient to suppress, then disease develop. For investigating an epidemic, first of all find out the incidence of disease in the community. Then, compare this incidence of disease with the usual incidence of disease in the community. On the basis of analysis, conclusion can be drawn for the appropriate line of action. The disease epidemic is controlled at community level by eliminating the factors reducing effective contact, which depends on the spread of disease and increase the resistance of susceptible population by vaccination, drugs and means. Screening is the way to find out undiagnosed cases, i.e. subclinical, clinical cases with or without apparent symptoms, which do not seek medical advice. Periodical health examination is the part of screening. The aim of screening is to cover time lag between the onset of disease and appearance of full-fledged clinical diseases. Screening is the way to bring into limelight the disease, which are mild, untreated, carriers and subclinical cases. It explains the iceberg phenomenon, disease control, elimination and eradication. Disease control is an ongoing process to reduce the incidence, the effect of infection, duration of disease and the risk of transmission of disease. Primary and secondary prevention activities are focused on controlling the disease. Disease elimination means the interruption of transmission of disease. Disease eradication means the termination of all transmission of infection, i.e. taking out the disease by roots.

SECTION 4

Communicable Diseases

- Respiratory Infections
- Intestinal Infection
- Arthropod Infestations
- Zoonoses: Viral
- Zoonoses: Bacterial
- Zoonoses: Rickettsial
- Zoonoses: Parasitic
- Important Surface Infections and Sexually Transmitted Diseases

Respiratory Infections

CHAPTER 28

SMALLPOX (VARIOLA)

Smallpox is an acute infectious disease characterized by severe constitutional disturbances and a single crop of skin eruptions. Previously, every year there was thousands of death due to smallpox in India. The incidence was higher in Indian subcontinent, Indonesia and majority of deaths occurring in 0–10 years of age group.

The meticulous effective preventive measures have succeeded in eradicating the smallpox from the world around 1977. World Health Organization (WHO) declared on 8 May, 1980 that smallpox has been eradicated. Although, as per claims, the disease has been eradicated from the world, preventive measures of the condition still require constant awareness and alertness. Despite the absence of smallpox, surveillance of rumors continue in order to sustain public confidence in the eradication of the disease.

Epidemiological Features

Agent

Smallpox is caused by poxvirus, i.e. variola virus. This virus is antigenically similar to cowpox (vaccinia virus). Growth of virus takes place on chorioallantoic membrane of developing chick. Virus is readily killed by sunlight, but resists drying (Fig. 28.1).

Poxvirus: They are large brick-shaped particle 230–300 nm × 200–250 nm, visible by light microscope. They may cause small pox, vaccinia, molluscum contagiosum, cowpox and milker nodes. Examples of poxvirus are variola, vaccinia, molluscum contagiosum, avian pox, etc.

Reservoir of Infection in Man

Source of infection is a case suffering from the disease. Infective materials are excretion of respiratory tract, droplet infection, lesions of skin, mucosa and scabs. Virus may be recovered from clothing, bedding and articles used by infected person. Even dead bodies are also highly infective. Infective period of the disease is short. It starts from the onset of fever till last scabs are separated. Most family contracts take place during 1st week. Maximum infectivity occurs between 3rd and 8th day after the onset of fever. Incubation period is usually of 11–14 days, but may vary from 7 to 17 days.

Host Factors

1. Age and sex: It occurs in all ages and both sexes, but most victims are children.
2. Occupation: Washerman, travelling population, nomads and persons working in smallpox wards are more susceptible.
3. Immunity: One in 1,000 gets second attack. Neutralizing antibiotics begin to appear on 6th day of illness.
4. Environmental factors: Given below are some of the sociocultural factors associated with the disease:
   - Low socioeconomic group, which is least responsive to vaccination
   - Fear of pain and after effects of vaccination
   - Movement of population from rural to urban areas
   - Concentration of beggars in the urban areas

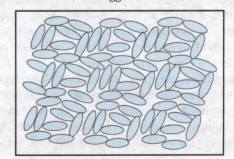

Figure 28.1: Poxvirus

- Infected travelers
- Cultural functions, religious beliefs, misconceptions and superstitions
- Ignorance.

Mode of Transmission

- Airborne transmission—droplet infection, droplet-infected dust
- Direct contact with the infected crusts
- Indirect contact through the linen clothing used by patients.

Pathophysiology

The virus gains entry through mucous membrane of the upper respiratory tract, multiplies in the lymphoid tissue and then viremia occurs. Skin lesion shows localization of virus in the epidermis from the bloodstream, clinical improvement occurs following development of skin eruptions. Localized virus in the cell causes hypertrophy and produces papules. Later degeneration and liquefaction produce vesicles, which are then converted into pustules (Fig. 28.2).

Clinical Features

Pre-eruptive Stage

The onset is gradual or sudden with severe headache, malaise, prostration, nausea, vomiting and diarrhea, and fever. This continues for 1–5 days and falls within 24 hours after the appearance of skin rash.

Eruptive Stage

Main clinical manifestation is rash on 3rd day of illness. The rash is centrifugal in distribution, which appears first on the face and scalp then on the wrists, hands, neck, back, chest, arms, legs and feet (Figs 28.3 and 28.4).

The macules develop into papules in 1–4 days and finally to pustules in 2–6 days. Thereafter, crusts are formed, which fall 2–6 weeks after the first sign of skin lesion. In some case, skin lesions may occur as hemorrhagic. Characteristically all lesions are seen in the same stage of development in any area and at any time.

The condition may produce secondary bacterial infections, pneumonia, encephalitis, blindness and permanent scarring or pitting of the skin as complication. Any preventive and control measure can be effective, following specific treatment such as isolation, rest and symptomatic.

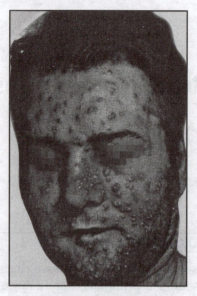

Figure 28.2: Smallpox (variola)

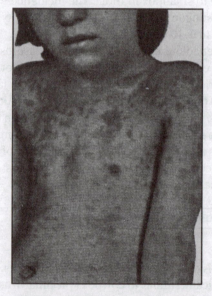

Figure 28.3: Generalized vaccinia

Prevention and Control

- Early diagnosis: Clinically supported by laboratory diagnosis
- Notification: Local, national and international
- Isolation of patient till all scabs fall off (the sole of feet is the last space from where scabs fall off)
- All contacts should be kept under surveillance for 1 day after contact with the case

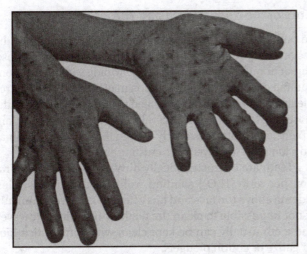

Figure 28.4: Pustules on hand, which is observed in small pox, more rarely in chickenpox

- Restriction against the exposure to the infected persons
- Proper sanitary disposals of the secretion of the patients
- Proper sterilization/disinfection of clothing, etc. of patients
- Mass vaccination—ring vaccination
- Disposal of dead—dead body to be covered with formalin-soaked cloth
- Quarantine for 21 days for persons exposed to infection.

Nursing Management of Smallpox

Isolation

The only known method of preventing smallpox is by vaccination of the non-immune person. Smallpox may not be successfully isolated by the medical aseptic technique. The medical aseptic technique will not prevent the spread of the disease as it is airborne. Even though the patient is isolated in a private room, in a communicable disease hospital it is necessary to vaccinate all other patients, otherwise susceptible will almost surely contract smallpox. The few patients in whom vaccination is contraindicated should be removed from the building in which a smallpox patient is kept.

Every possible effort should be made to keep all infective material confined to the patient's room and so treat it before removal that there will be no possibility of carrying contaminated material to the outside. The outside of bedpans and urinals should be wiped clean with a 1:3,000 Zephiran solution. Soiled linen and clothing should be tightly wrapped into a small compact bundle and carefully placed inside an uncontaminated laundry bag in such fashion that the outside of the bag remains uncontaminated.

Soiled linen and clothing should be sterilized by autoclave before being laundered. The paper bag that contains soiled compact bundle in such a way that no contaminated material escapes. This bag should then be carefully placed into a clean bag before its removal from the room. The diet tray can be slipped into a clean pillow slip that is held by an uncontaminated nurse. It can then be carried safely through the corridor to the sterilizer. After the dishes and the tray are sterilized, they may be washed with other ward dishes.

The floor in the patient's room should be kept free from crusts and other infectious material. A mop moistened with 1:3,000 Zephiran is recommended. When dry, the floor may be kept oiled.

During the period of desquamation, the patient is usually ambulatory. If the following precautions are taken, it will help considerably to keep the floors clean. The male patient should be dressed in pajamas—the pajama coat should be worn inside the pajama pants, socks should be pulled up over the pajama pant legs, the pajama coat sleeves should be folded snugly about the wrists and secured by a rubber band. The patient should be instructed to undress in such fashion that patient will not scatter the crusts (scabs) around the room. Patient should be instructed to place the crusts from the face, hands and scalp into the paper bag at the bedside as they fall off.

The nurse caring for smallpox should be immuned. If there is a slightest question as to the immunity, he/she should be revaccinated immediately. Female nurse should dress in a plain, short-skirted and short-sleeved uniform. Her hair should be completely covered. The uniform should be completely covered with a regulation protective gown. With every possible precaution taken, there still is a possibility that some fragment of infectious material may reach and cling to the upper part of the shoes (shoelaces or hose). There is also the possibility that some invisible fragment be drawn into the nose, while breathing.

Temperature

In the mild or alastrim type of smallpox, temperature may be lower than in a severe case of chickenpox. In fact, it may not exceed 100°F. However, in the severe type of smallpox, the temperature may be very high reaching 110°F. An ice cap to the head is both comforting and helpful. Colonic flushing may be given with good results in reducing temperature. Wet sheet packs and cool sponges are also effective. A cold wet sheet pack of potassium permanganate ($KMnO_4$) will not only reduce temperature but also help keep down the foul odor characteristic of the disease. Fluids are urged.

Diet

A nourishing liquid diet should be given during the acute stage. Water should be urged, forced if necessary. In severe cases, at least four quarts of fluid should be given to an adult. Six quarts are sometimes given with good results. As the temperature returns to normal, a general diet may be given.

Care of the Eyes

In severe cases, care of eyes has been a major nursing problem. Often, the swelling above the head is so severe that the head appears to be much larger than it is almost impossible to see where the eyes are. If it be at all possible to open the eyelids (often lid retractors are necessary) and expose the corneas, the eyes should be gently irrigated with a warm solution (antibiotic), 500 units or more per microliter (µL). Care should be taken not to direct the stream directly against the cornea, but against the conjunctiva then allow it to flow gently over the cornea. The pus from the lesions may seal the eyelids together. This condition will hinder and sometimes prevent drainage. If it is not possible to separate the lids, a dripping cotton pledget saturated with penicillin solution placed over the eye may be helpful. The solution from the pledget may seep in between the lids; if this occurs drainage may be established, even in cases of severe edema. Pus under pressure may cause ulceration of the cornea and ulceration of the cornea may produce blindness. For that reason everyone should be made to keep the cornea clear. If the lids can be seen, antibiotic ointment is usually prescribed to be used along the margin.

If pustules occur on the cornea, vision is impaired and total blindness may result. If pustules occur on the conjunctive of the lids, the cornea may become excoriated by the constant movement of the lids over the cornea. Castor oil is often instilled in the eye to relieve this pain and protect the cornea, and orthoform ointment has been of service. Unquestionably, cortisone will be tried for this condition and may prove of service.

In hemorrhagic smallpox, bleeding from the conjunctive is common. Cold, moist antibiotic compresses may be tried, but patients with this complication usually do not survive.

Care of the Ears

Middle ear infection is not a common complication. However, in severe cases, lesions may appear in the outer ear canal. Gentle swabbing with a moist pledget of cotton or gentle irrigation with a warm antibiotic solution may help to keep the canal open.

Care of the Nose, Mouth and Throat

In both the discrete and the confluent type of smallpox, the lesions may appear in the mucous membranes of the nose, throat or mouth. Frequently, gentle wiping with applications saturated with a penicillin solution may help to keep the area clean. Antibiotic ointment applied to the mucus lining of the nose helps to relieve the discomfort of the patient. In fact, antibiotic given intramuscularly early in the pustular stage may go a long way to prevent this crusting and discomfort.

Teeth are characteristically dirty. About 50% of hydrogen peroxide (H_2O_2) solution will help to relieve sordes. Edema above the face and lips often makes it very difficult, if not impossible, to clean the teeth by brushing. However, the teeth usually can be kept clean with soft applications or gauze or cotton pledgets.

The tongue and mucus lining of the mouth and throat will probably be covered with lesions. Frequent antiseptic mouthwashes, gargles and throat irrigations are helpful. Penicillin ointment may be applied to the lips.

Elimination

The bowels should move well once daily. Laxatives or enemas may be given as indicated. It should be remembered that, however, smallpox lesions may occur in the mucous membrane of the small intestine and colon, and laxatives should be used very judiciously. Urinary retention is not common. The nurse should measure both fluid intake and output, when possible. The nurse should watch for and report abdominal or urinary bladder distention.

General Management of the Disease

There is no disease more repulsive, dirty, foul smelling or more highly infectious than smallpox, which is neither the harder to manage nor more easily preventable.

During the acute febrile stage, the patient is confined to bed. Other cases are inclined to be comatose. With this type of patient, the nurse should see that his/her position is changed every 3–4 hours or often. The head of the bed should be raised and lowered at intervals every 2–3 hours. Bathing presents a problem if the rash is profuse and is usually omitted except in milder cases. In severe cases, the wet permanganate sheet pack is used in place of bathing. Penicillin ointment may be applied during the pustular and crusting stages. This helps to dry up the lesions, so that there is much less trouble from scarring than formerly. However, the intramuscular (IM) use of antibiotic may obviate the need for local treatment with antibiotic ointment and it also helps to shorten the course of the disease to lessen toxicity and facilitate more rapid healing.

The patient remains infectious until all crusts have dropped off and the skin underneath are healed. It is the responsibility of the nurse on the case to see that all crusts on the palms, soles and scalp as well as on the body are completely gone, before the patient is declared convalescent. On the soles, especially, it is frequently necessary to remove the disk from the center of the lesion with a dull, pointed instrument. By soaking the patient's feet in a 1:3,000 Zephiran chloride solution for a half-an-hour or more it is possible to dig into a dried lesion that otherwise could not be removed because of the thickened, tough skin covering the sole of the foot. After all infective disks have been removed, the sole of the foot may present a honeycomb appearance.

After all lesions are removed, and a complete soap, water bath and shampoo have been given, the patient is dressed in clean clothing and is no longer infectious. Very often, patients who are no longer infectious have considerable trouble in public places, because of their appearance. The 'mahogany spots,' dark reddish brown spots that cover the face and hands, give the patient a very alarming appearance, i.e. disconcerting. We have found it necessary, upon occasion, to give our discharged patients a letter stating that they are not suffering from an infectious disease. Later, these lesions whiten and contract, just as other scars do, and they become pitted and very unsightly.

In hemorrhagic smallpox, the ingenuity of the nurse is taxed to the utmost. The patient is prostrated, the fever is high the lesions are a typical and frequently look like rash of toxic scarlet fever. There is constant oozing of blood from all mucous membranes. The care of the eyes, ears, nose, mouth and throat presents unique, if not impossible nursing problems. The nurse should watch for urinary retention. While the skin lesions are a typical, they present more problem to the nurse than the typical pustules that form crusts and drop off. The skin lesions in hemorrhagic, become blebs or large bullae filled with blood. Gangrene areas appear. The skin may crack and slough off. All of the skin of a leg or a thigh may slough off at one time or the nurse may find when he/she turns patient and a large fragment of skin may stick to the sheet. When the skin sloughs off, a bleeding surface remains. Moist dressings in place present a nursing problem. Both pins and adhesive tape are contraindicated. However, bandages and binders fastened with ties are fairly satisfactory.

Convalescence

Convalescence is usually slow. Cardiac damage sometimes result in the severest cases. Toxic psychosis is not uncommon. However, as convalescence progresses, the psychosis usually disappears. In the milder cases, where the patient is permitted to be up during the stage of desquamation, convalescence is usually rapid and uneventful.

CHICKENPOX (VARICELLA)

Chickenpox is a highly contagious disease with mild constitutional symptoms and is characterized by fever, malaise and centripetal distribution of pruritic skin lesions. Its distribution is worldwide.

Epidemiology

Agent

Chickenpox is caused by varicella-zoster virus, morphologically identical with herpes simplex virus. Sources of infection are cases of virus lodges no oropharynx skin mucous membrane and blood. Period of infectivity is usually about a week, 1–2 days before and 4–5 days after the appearance of rash.

Host

1. Age: No age is exempted, but it mostly occurs in children under 10 years.
2. Sex: Both sexes are prone to the disease.
3. Immunity: One attack gives durable immunity, second attack is rare. Maternal bodies protect children up to few months.
4. Environmental: It shows seasonal trend in India, i.e. first 6 months of year. Overcrowding favors transmission.

Mode of Transmission

The infection spreads through droplet infection, droplet nuclei and infected articles. Incubation period is usually of 14–16 days, but may vary from 7 to 21 days.

Pathophysiology

Virus gain entry through the mucosa of the upper respiratory tract followed by viremia and circulation through blood and then becomes localized in the skin. There the virus produces swelling of epithelial cells, ballooning degeneration and accumulation of tissue fluid resulting in vesicle formation. The nuclei of infected cells show eosinophilic inclusion bodies.

Clinical Features

The disease begins with mild headache, backache, moderate fever and malaise (usually 24 hour followed by rash and itching). Later, initially lesions as vesicles appear in the oropharynx, which usually ruptures quickly to form small ulcer. It may cause painful swelling. Cutaneous rash appears in crops over 1–5 days, first appearing in the back, chest, or on the forehead or face, becomes numerous on the trunk and face, and relatively sparse over the extremities. Where the flexor surfaces appear more affected than in extensor.

The skin lesions develop as small, deep pink, slightly raised, ovoid papules, which within few hours become fragile, thin-walled translucent, umbilicated, glistening bleb-like vesicles containing clear fluid surrounded by small red, areola in the super layer of the skin. The vesicles later change to crusts and finally slough out in 7–14 days. The condition, however, can cause secondary bacterial infections, otitis media, pneumonia, myocarditis, hemorrhagic nephritis, encephalitis, etc. Differentiating features of smallpox and chickenpox are given in Table 28.1.

Table 28.1: Differences between smallpox and chickenpox

Smallpox	Chickenpox
Incubation period is 7–17 day	Incubation period is 14–21 day
Rashes are usually present on palms and soles	Rashes seldom present on the palms and soles
Rashes appear on 3rd day of onset of disease	Rashes appear within 24 hour of the onset of disease
Rashes are all over body, but numerous on the face, arms and legs	Rashes are more on trunk and least on extremities
Rashes are in the same stage at the development	Rashes show many stages of development at the same time
Macules, papules and vesicles are not seen together	Macules, papules, vesicles, pustules and scabs may all present together (polymorphism)
Scabs begin to form 10–14 day after the rash appears off 14–28 day after the rash begins	Scabs begin to form 4–7 day after the rash appears off within 15 day after the rash begins

Prevention and Control

The following are the preventive and control measures:
1. Isolation of the patient.
2. Disinfection of oronasal discharge and soiled articles.
3. Terminal disinfection of room.
4. Passive immunization with normal human immunoglobin [varicella-zoster immunoglobulin (VZIG)] given within 72 hours of exposure dose in 0.4–1.2 mL/kg body weight.
5. Active immunization with line-alternated varicella vaccination.
6. Other airborne illness control measures.

Nursing Management of Chickenpox

Isolation

Chickenpox cannot be isolated in an open ward. A private room is necessary. Effective isolation of chickenpox always presents a serious problem. Not only is the disease highly contagious but also difficult to isolate, because it is airborne. The minute scales or crusts may cling to articles removed from the room or be carried in air currents as dust particles.

The causative organisms are in the skin lesions. Everything contained in the patient's room should be considered contaminated and should be cleaned up as soon as possible after use. The patient is infectious until all primary crusts are removed.

Diet

The diet seldom presents a nursing problem. Any diet consistent with the age of the patient usually is prescribed. However, chickenpox occasionally is a very severe disease and then the diet must be fitted to the patient's tolerance and requirements.

Temperature

The temperature seldom is high. However, occasionally it may reach 108°F. Tepid water sponge baths or cool colonic flushing are effective in reducing fever. Both alcohol rubs and fans are contraindicated, because of the irritating effect on the injured skin.

Personal Hygiene

1. A daily warm cleansing bath should be given. However, in order to avoid injuries the lesions baths should be given with a gentle patting motion. The towel should be soft and absorbent.
2. Good oral hygiene should be maintained. Teeth should be cleaned thoroughly at least twice daily. If lesions appear on the mucous membranes of mouth and throat, frequent antiseptic mouthwashes, gargles, irrigations or rinses may be indicated.
3. The nose should be kept clean with cotton pledgets moistened with a prescribed antiseptic solution then dried carefully with sterile cotton.

CHAPTER 28 — Respiratory Infections

4. The eyes should be kept clean. Lesions may appear on either the lid margins or undersurfaces of the lids. Moist, sterile cotton pledgets may be used with good results. However, irrigations may be prescribed, if indicated.
5. If otitis media complicates the disease and the ear is draining, the outer ear should be kept clean. A sterile cotton fluff placed in the outer ear will help, provided it is changed frequently enough, so that it does not become saturated with the drainage. It must not plug the drainage.

Elimination

The bowels should move freely at least once each day. Either laxatives or enemas may be given, if necessary. Catheterization may become necessary if lesions appear in or near the urinary meatus.

General Management of the Disease

The patient should be placed in a warm, well-ventilated room. In uncomplicated cases, the patient usually is ambulatory after the fever has returned to normal for 24 hours.

Itching, which is one of the most distressing symptoms, may be relieved to some extent by the application of calamine lotion with phenol. If lesions are on either the outer or inner surfaces of the lids, cold boric solutions or compresses give some relief. If lesions appear in the vagina, a vaginal douche of sodium bicarbonate gives temporary relief as a rule.

While chickenpox generally is not a serious disease, the nurse should remember that complications may change the entire picture. She/He should note and record any significant symptoms.

Convalescence: As a rule convalescence is rapid and uneventful.

Terminal disinfection: When the patient is no longer able to tolerate the disease, he/she should be given a cleansing bath and shampoo. He/She should be dressed in clean clothes and placed in a clean area. All equipment and material that has come in contact with the patient should be cleaned up or destroyed by burning. The mattress and pillows should be thoroughly aired, preferably in the sunshine for at least 6 hours. The bed, chairs, table and walls should be washed.

MUMPS

Mumps is an acute generalized infectious disease characterized by non-suppurative swelling and tenderness of one or both the parotid glands, of less commonly salivary glands are involved. It is an acute communicable disease caused by a virus called myxovirus parotitis. It has a predilection to the glandular and nervous tissues. Other organs also may be involved. The virus can be demonstrated in the saliva.

Magnitude of the Problem

Mumps is an acute contagious febrile infectious disease characterized by inflammation of the parotid glands and salivary glands. It is less frequent than the other common communicable diseases of childhood. Winter and spring are the seasons of greatest prevalence. Its susceptibility is general and second attacks are uncommon. Generally, lifelong immunity develops after clinical as well as in parent attack. Patient may die due to other complications and not due to mumps, because deaths due to mumps are practically nil.

Epidemiological Features

Geographic Distribution

Mumps occur throughout the world. Although, morbidity rate tends to be high, mortality rate is negligible. It is seen in sporadic form except in large cities, where it is endemic.

Agent

Myxovirus parotitis is the causative agent of the disease (Fig. 28.5).

Source of Infection

Humans are the only reservoir of infection. There are two categories of reservoir:
1. People suffering from mumps.
2. Subclinical cases.

Incubation period is 2–3 weeks. Period of communicability is 4–6 days after the onset of symptoms and a week or more thereafter at the onset of parotitis. Once the swelling of the gland has subsided, the case may be regarded as no longer infectious.

Host Factors

1. Age: Mumps generally occurs in children in the age group of 5–15 years. No age is exempt if there is no previous immunity. The disease tends to be more severe in adults than in children.
2. Sex: Both the sexes are affected.
3. Immunity: One attack of clinical or subclinical is assumed to induce lifelong immunity. Most infants below the age of 6 months are immune, because of maternal

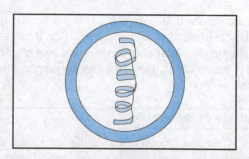

Figure 28.5: Myxovirus

antibodies. A vaccinated child might escape the infection for a time and then might become susceptible after puberty when a more severe infection is likely to appear.
4. Environment: Mumps is largely an endemic disease. It may occur throughout the year. The peak incidence is in winter and spring. Epidemics are often associated with overcrowding.

Modes of Transmission

Mumps is spread directly from person to person, by close contact, by formites, airborne spread and by droplet infection. After an incubation period of 14–21 days, the virus can be isolated from saliva or from swabs taken from the stenosis duct. The virus can be found in the blood, urine, human milk and occasionally in cerebrospinal fluid (CSF).

Pathophysiology

The infection produces desquamation of epithelium in the ducts of parotid gland, interstitial edema, lymphocytic infiltration and polymorphonuclear cells within the lumina. Unilateral parotitis is the commonest mode of preservation of clinical mumps. The gland generally enlarges, displacing the ear lobe outwards and upwards, and occupies the space between the mastoid process and the remains of the mandible in about 1-3 days. The enlargement of the gland is painful and tender, but begins to subside in about 7–10 days. By then the temperature settles down to normal.

The lesions produced by the virus are epithelial necrosis and round cell infiltration of the interstitial tissues of the parotid gland and occasionally of the other glands. The involvement of the organs other than the parotid gland is much more common in adults.

Clinical Features

Mumps is the generalized virus infection with a variety of clinical features. It may affect various organs in the body, e.g. testes, pancreas, central nervous system (CNS), ovaries, prostate, breast, heart, joints, eyes and ears. Although the disease has a predilection for salivary glands.

In parotid mumps, swelling of the parotid gland is the first indication. The patient complains of pain and stiffness on opening the mouth before the swelling of the gland is evident. In severe cases, there may be headache and other constitutional symptoms, which may last for 3-5 days. The swelling subsides slowly over 1-2 weeks period. There may be cervical adenitis in some cases. Fever ranges between 101 and 102°F, and may be present at the onset, often subsides after 48 hours (Fig. 28. 6).

Occasionally, there may be swelling of the submaxillary and sublingual glands. The disease is ushered in after a prodromal phase of fever, sore throat, earache and pain in chewing. Tenderness beneath the angle of the jaw or redness and edema around the mouth of the parotid duct may be noted.

Complications

Complications though frequent are not serious. They are orchitis, oophoritis (but not evidence of sterility), pancreatitis, meningoencephalitis (occurs within 3–10 days after the infection), myocarditis and pericarditis. In some instances, diabetes mellitus occurred in children following mumps infection. Rare complications include nerve deafness, facial neuritis, polyarthritis, hydrocephaly and hepatitis.

Laboratory Data

Virus can be isolated from saliva, urine, pharynx and CSF. The antibodies appear at the end of 1 week and a four-fold rise in titer may be noted by 2 weeks. Serum amylase is elevated and returns to normal in 2–3 weeks.

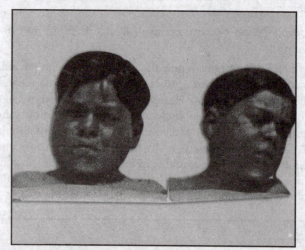

Figure 28.6: Mumps show the uniform swelling in front of the right ear, which has spread to the face and submaxillary region and obliterates the angle of the jaw.

Respiratory Infections

Treatment

Treatment is entirely symptomatic and is carried out under the following heads.

General Measures

In acute stage, the child is isolated and kept in bed till fever and swelling subside. Hot or cold fermentations may help to relieve pain and inflammation. Fluid diet is given when chewing is difficult. Pain is relieved by analgesics.

Passive protection
By means of convalescent immunoglobulin 2.5 mL IM soon after exposure to infection. This is not useful in prevention or to reduce incidence.

Active immunization
Three types of vaccines are available:
1. Mumpsvax: It is a chick embryo adopted mumps virus to which neomycin has been added and is supplied as lyophilized (freeze dried) powder. It is reconstituted and should be used with 7 hours, dosage is 0.5 mL/IM.
2. Inactivated vaccine: Dose is 0.5 mL/IM.
3. Combined vaccine: The mumps vaccine has been combined with measles as well as rubella (MMR) vaccine. The combination appears quite safe and useful.

Preventive Measures

Control of mumps is difficult, because the disease is infectious before the diagnosis is made. The long and variable incubation period and the occurrence of subclinical cases make the control of spread difficult. However, cases should be isolated till the clinical manifestations subside. Steps should be taken to disinfect the articles used by the patient. Contacts should be kept under surveillance. Prognosis is very good. Complications are fortunately rare in children. Even the cases of meningoencephalitis recover completely without sequelae. Unilateral deafness is an infrequent, but an unfortunate complication.

Nursing Management of Mumps

Isolation

Mumps can be isolated in an open ward by the medical aseptic technique. The virus is found in nose and throat secretions. The patient should be isolated until all objective symptoms have subsided.

Diet

The diet in mumps occasionally presents a nursing problem. Both sweet and sour foods may cause pain. This is also true of food that requires much chewing. Therefore, a bland, soft diet usually is prescribed as long as the jaws are sore. Soft-cooked vegetables, gruels, cereals, scraped or finely chopped meat, milk and cream soups are suggested. Citrus fruits and sweetened cooked acid fruits such as apples are contraindicated. As a general rule, it is safe to give whatever the patient tolerates.

Temperature

Temperature in uncomplicated mumps seldom is high enough to present a nursing problem. However, it becomes necessary to reduce fever, it may be done by tepid sponges, alcohol rub or colonic flushing (Fig. 28.7).

Personal Hygiene

The patient should be given a daily cleansing bath. Because of drainage from the affected glands, the mouth of the patient is characteristically dirty. Teeth should be brushed both evening and morning care. Frequent antiseptic mouthwashes may be given if indicated.

Elimination

The bowels should move freely at least once each day. Either laxatives or enemas may be given when needed.

General Management of the Disease

For the comfort of the patient either heat or cold may be applied locally. Heat is usually the patient's choice. For children, aspirin is prescribed for discomfort. For adults, codeine and aspirin are occasionally required. As a rule, children are allowed out of bed and toilet privileges are allowed in the home. Adults with mumps, however, should remain in bed until all swelling has gone for at least 3 days, because of the possibility of developing complications from being on the feet. It has been found over many years of observation that ambulation increases the incidence of orchitis in the male:
1. Orchitis is the common complication in the adult male. It usually develops about a week after onset. A sudden rise in temperature from 104 to 105°F is not uncommon. In all males, past puberty with mumps, the scrotum should be supported by an adequate suspensory from the start, should orchitis develop it may be necessary to use soft packing between the scrotum and the support. Sometimes, an adhesive tape bridge across the thighs and under the scrotum is used. Oophoritis in adult female is rarer than orchitis in the male. However, in women past the age of puberty

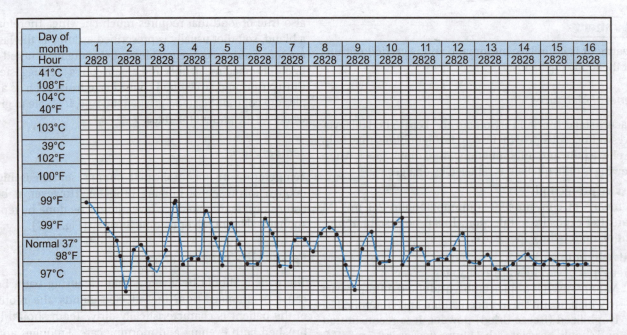

Figure 28.7: Temperature chart of mild case of mumps

bedrest is still advisable, although bathroom privileges may usually be permitted. Symptoms of beginning oophoritis are low abdominal pain, fever, headache, nausea and vomiting.

2. Meningoencephalitis may complicate mumps. Symptoms for which the nurse should watch in this connection are rise in temperature, stiff neck, headache, restlessness, malaise, nausea, vomiting, delirium and double vision. These symptoms usually subside spontaneously within 10–14 days. However, the Doctor may order an electroencephalogram to gauge its severity. If nausea and vomiting persists intravenous (IV), fluids are usually prescribed.

Occasionally, inflammation of the lacrimal glands or conjunctivitis may call for eyewashes. Under such conditions, cold compresses are sometimes used and simple collyria are prescribed. The eyes may require protection from light in which case dark glasses are sufficient.

MEASLES (RUBELLA)

An acute highly infectious disease of childhood caused by a specific virus of the group myxoviruses. It is clinically characterized by fever and catarrhal symptoms of the upper respiratory, i.e. nasal and respiratory mucous membrane followed by a typical maculopapular skin rash and Koplik's spot.

The word 'rubella,' means red spots. The earliest description of measles was given by the noted Arab Physician, Abu Bakr (865–925 AD) known to the west. Phazes Panum did classical studies on the epidemiology of measles in 1846. In 1954, measles vaccine was first used in a clinical trial and in 1963, live measles vaccine was licensed for use.

Magnitude of Problem

The mortality of measles varies greatly in different parts of the world. It is 100–400 times more likely to cause death in preschool children of a developing country than in the United State (US) and Europe. In developing countries, case fatality rates range from 2 to 15% as compared to 2 per 100,000 notified cases in developed countries. Recent estimates by United Nations Internationals Children's Emergency Fund (UNICEF) suggest that measures are responsible for more than 205 million childhood deaths annually.

In India, measles is a major cause of morbidity and a significant contributor to childhood mortality. In 1986, there were 140,827 notified cases and 353 deaths from measles.

Epidemiological Features

Measles is endemic virtually in all parts of the world. It tends to occur in epidemics when the proportion of susceptible children reaches to about 40%.

Agent

Measles is caused by ribonucleic acid (RNA) paramyxovirus, so far as it is known, there is only one serotype. The virus cannot survive outside the human body for any length of time (Fig. 28.8).

CHAPTER 28: Respiratory Infections

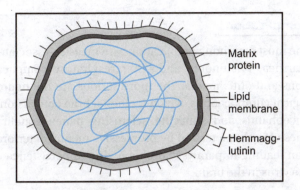

Figure 28.8: Measles virus

Source of Infection

The only source of infection is a case of measles, carriers are not known to occur. Secretions of the nose, throat and respiratory tract of a case of measles during the prodromal period and the early stages of rash are infective materials.

Measles is highly infectious during the prodromal period and at the time of eruption. Communicability rapidly declines after the appearance of the rash. Secondary attack rate is over 80% among susceptible household contacts.

Host Factors

1. Age: It affects in infancy or childhood between 6 months and 3 years of age in developing countries, where environmental conditions are generally poor and older children usually over 5 years in developed countries.
2. Sex: Incidence of infection is equal in both sexes.
3. Immunity: No age is immune, if there was no previous immunity. One attack of measles generally confers lifelong immunity. Second attacks are rare. Infants are protected by material antibodies up to 6 months of age.
4. Nutrition: Measles tend to be very severe in malnourished child, carrying mortality 400 times higher than in well-nourished children having measles.

Environmental Factors

Given a chance, the virus can spread at any season. In temperate, climates, measles is a winter disease, probably because people crowd together in doors. Epidemics of measles are common in India during winter and early spring from January to April.

Mode of Transmission

Transmission occurs directly from person to person mainly by droplet infection and droplet nuclei from 4 days before onset of rash to 5 days; thereafter, the portal of entry is respiratory tract. Incubation period is commonly 10 days to appearance of rash.

Pathophysiology

Measles, which is a generalized infection causes hyperplasia of the lymphoid tissue of the tonsils, adenoids, spleen, appendix and lymph nodes during the prodromal stage of disease. The characteristics feature is the presence of large multinuclear giant cell, which can be observed in the lymphoid tissues and in the inflamed pharyngeal and bronchial mucosa.

There is slight edema and hyperemia with perivascular infiltration of lymphocytes in the superficial portions of the skin, where the rash appears. The mucous membranes of the eyes, nasopharynx, bronchi and lungs are also similarly involved. These changes disappear in about 10 days.

The rash commences in the superficial vessels of the cranium and is associated with perivascular serious exudation and proliferation of endothelial cells followed by vascularization and necrosis of epithelial cells. Finally, it ends in desquamation of the epithelium and endothelium. The skin peels off in small flakes. There is peribronchial inflammatory reaction with mononuclear cell infiltration in the interstitial tissues, where giant cells may occasionally be detected.

Secondary infection may occur in the lungs. In measles encephalomyelopathy, gross evidence of edema, congestion and petechial hemorrhages, and microscopic and lymphocytic cell infiltration are seen in the brain and spinal cord. They are followed by demyelination throughout the CNS. Similar histological changes are found in postvaccinal encephalitis.

Signs and Symptoms

Prodromal Phase

Prodromal phase begins 10 days after infection and lasts until day 14. It is characterized by fever, coryza with sneezing and nasal discharge. Cough, redness of the eyes, lacrimation and often photophobia. There may be vomiting or diarrhea. A day or 2 days before the appearance of the rash. Koplik's spots appear on the buccal mucosa opposite the first and second upper molars. They are small, bluish-white spots on a red base (Figs 28.9 and 28.10).

Eruptive Phase

Eruptive phase is characterized by a typical, dusky-red macular or maculopapular rash, which begins behind the ears and spreads rapidly in a few hours over the face and

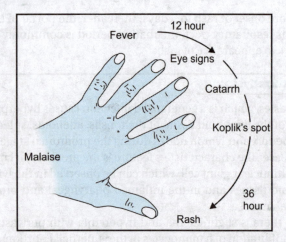

Figure 28.9: Sequence of events during the period of invasion of measles

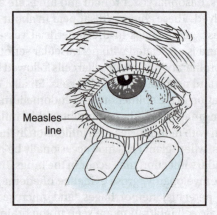

Figure 28.10: Measles line—a sign appearing usually shortly after the onset of fever

Complications

The most common complications are measles-associated diarrhea, pneumonia and other respiratory complications and otitis media. The more serious are the neurological complications, which include febrile convulsions, encephalitis and subacute sclerosing panencephalitis. These are characterized by progressive mental deterioration leading to paralysis, probably due to persistence of the virus in the brain.

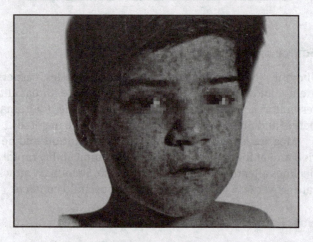

Figure 28.11: Early measles eruption

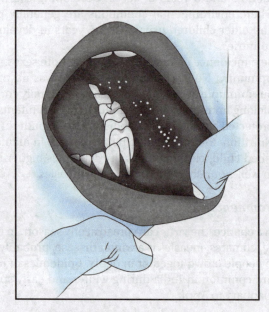

Figure 28.12: Koplik's spots in measles

neck, and extends down the body taking 2–3 days to progress to the lower extremities. The rash may remain discrete, but often it becomes confluent and blotchy. In the absence of complications, the lesions and fever disappear in another 3 days, signaling the end of the disease (Figs 28.11 and 28.12).

Postmeasles State

The child will have lost weight and will remain weak for a number of days. There may be failure to recover and a gradual deterioration into chronic illness due to increased susceptibility to other bacterial and viral infections, nutritional and metabolic effects, and the tissue destructive effects of the virus. There may be growth retardation and diarrhea, cancrum oris, pyogenic infections, candidiasis and reactivation of pulmonary tuberculosis (TB).

Prognosis

Measles causes some deaths among young children every year and must be regarded as a serious disease in infants and debilitated children. Bronchopneumonia is responsible for most of the fatalities, but the death rate has diminished greatly during the past 30 years.

Diagnosis

Pre-exanthematous stage: Common cold, influenza and catarrhal stage of whooping cough.

Exanthematous stage: Two types of exanthematous stage are:
1. Rubella (German measles): No Koplik's spots, small shotty enlargement of suboccipital, posterior cervical and postauricular lymph nodes. In measles, mucous membrane is infected and is dirty.
2. Rubella (measles): Based on the typical rash and Koplik's spots, the diagnosis would normally be incorrect in any febrile exanthema in which red eyes and cough are absent.

Prevention

1. Measles vaccination: Measles is best prevented by active immunization. Only live attenuated vaccines are recommended for use, they are both safe and effective.
2. Immunization is given after the age of 9 months.
3. Administration: Vaccine is administered in a single subcutaneous (SC) dose of 0.5 mL. Vaccine must be kept cold at 4–8°C.
4. Reactions: When injected into the body, the attenuated virus multiply and induces a mild 'measles', 5–10 days after immunization, but in reduced frequency and severity. This may occur in 15–20% of vaccines. The fever may last for 1–2 days and the rash for 1–3 days.
5. Immunity: The vaccine has convincingly demonstrated to provide immunity to even severely malnourished children. Immunity develops 11–12 days after vaccination and appears to be for long duration, probably for life. One dose of the vaccine appears to give 95% protection. Prevention of the infection achieved by isolation of the patient and by avoidance of any close contact with the patient. In addition, adequate disposal of secretions of the patients is needed to following disinfection.

Children are protected against the infection through active immunization with live-attenuated measles virus by SC injection within the age of 9–12 months. SC individuals at risk exposed to the infection can be protected within 2 days since exposure to the infection by IM or IV injection of human immunoglobulins followed by, if not contraindicated, a live-attenuated virus vaccine at any time after 2 months.

Nursing Management of Measles

Isolation

In order to isolate measles, a private room is required. The medical aseptic technique will not prevent the spread of measles, which is airborne. The virus of measles is found in the upper respiratory tract and is usually transmitted from person to person either by direct contact or by droplet infection. However, fomites and indirect contact are capable of transmitting the disease. All articles and materials contaminated by contact with the patient should be removed from the patient's room and cleaned up or sent to the incinerator, as rapidly as possible.

Diet

During the febrile stage, the diet should be limited to nourishing liquids and to a soft, bland diet. Fluids should be urged, forced if necessary. Soup, milk, fruit juices, gruels, jello, custard, ice cream and sherbet are suggested. Karo corn syrup and other easily digested sugars may be used as advantage. Unfortunately, these patients often vomit and food may not be given by mouth. But, hypodermoclysis may be required. If diarrhea is present, fruit juices should be omitted. If the throat is too sore, young or uncooperative patients may refuse fruit juices. However, pineapple juice, grape juice or berry juice may be given to replace the acid citrus fruits. If ice cream or sherbet tends to increase the frequency or severity of the cough, it should be limited or else omitted entirely from the diet. Soda pop or ginger also frequently will be retained and accepted when fruit juices are refused or vomited.

Especially, care should be taken to see that formula babies not only receive sufficient nourishment but also adequate fluids. Frequent dilute feedings are sometimes indicated. During convalescence, a general diet consistent with the age of the patient is given.

Temperature

If the temperature exceeds 103°F or is producing toxic symptoms, it should be reduced by tepid sponge baths or colonic flushing. A sponge may be given every 1–2 hours as indicated. Precautions should be taken, however, to prevent the patient from chilling. Cold water never should be used. To relieve itching, sodium bicarbonate or magnesium sulfate may be added to the bath water. Either an alcohol fan or an alcohol sponge may be contraindicated because of the irritating effect to the skin, while the rash is present.

General Management of the Disease

Care of the Eyes

During the prodromal and acute stage, the eyes are often sensitive to light. For this reason, it is helpful to place the patient so that the patient will not face a direct bright light. An eye shade or dark glasses are sometimes helpful in the care of an older or a cooperative patient. The eyes should be irrigated often enough to keep them clean. Warm boric acid solution is usually prescribed. Boric ointment or liquid petrolatum applied about the eye area adds to the comfort of the patient when eye discharges are profuse.

Care of the Ears

Special attention should be given to the ears. If there is any reason to suspect trouble, the physician should be notified at once. It is the responsibility of the nurse to be on the alert for signs of beginning mastoid involvement. An unexplained, sudden rise in temperature, mastoid swelling, redness or tenderness, complaint of pain in, or above the ear, or a discharging ear should be reported to the doctor as soon as possible.

If the ear is discharging, the hair above the ear should be cut, so short that it will not come in contact with the discharges. While the treatment will be prescribed by the physician, it is the responsibility of the nurse to see that all discharges are kept wiped away using sterile applicators and sterile cotton. A loose fluff of sterile cotton placed in the outer ear will absorb discharges without acting as a plug. A discharging ear should never be plugged. The cotton fluff should be changed as indicated. Petroleum jelly, zinc oxide or cold excoriation of the skin. If sterile cotton fluffs are not applied, sterile swabs should be used often enough to keep the outer ear clean. Sterile ear wicks are inserted and ear swishes or other treatment given as ordered by the physician. Important points for the nurse to remember are never permit a draining ear to become plugged either with cotton or heavy purulent discharges. Do not apply heat without orders from the physician. Hands should be scrubbed and all instruments, cotton and similar items should be sterilized.

Care of the Nose

Since nasal discharge is an outstanding symptom of measles, considerable care is usually necessary to keep the nose clean. Cotton swabs saturated with liquid petrolatum, saline solution or dilute hydrogen peroxide are sometimes used with good results. Cold cream or boric acid ointment or other mild ointments applied about the area will help to prevent excoriation of the skin. Medication and treatment will be ordered by the physician.

Care of the Mouth and Throat

Good oral hygiene is imperative in the nursing care of measles. Antiseptic gargles and mouthwashes used both before and after meals are usually indicated. The teeth should be brushed thoroughly at least twice each day. A patient who is too sick or too young to cooperate should have his/her mouth, tongue and teeth swabbed with antiseptic solution. Sodium bicarbonate and saline solutions are used with good results. Glycerin and lemon mixture is both pleasing and helpful applied to the lips and tongue.

Elimination

Either cleansing enemas or mild laxatives usually are ordered. Milk of magnesia is usually the laxative of choice for children.

Complications

Laryngitis

If laryngitis is severe, it is often relieved by medicated steam inhalations and in severe cases, a croup tent may be used with good results. In milder cases, a croup kettle without a croup tent affords sufficient relief. Hot steam should never be used, if pneumonia is suspected.

Cervical Adenitis

Frequently, mild cervical adenitis develops. It seldom becomes serious. Rest in bed, ice collar and plenty of fluids are usually prescribed.

Bronchopneumonia

Bronchopneumonia is the most dreaded of all complications. It usually develops during or immediately following the height of the disease about 4 days after onset. Both penicillin and sulfonamides are prescribed not only as treatment for bronchopneumonia but often to help prevent its development. While the medication will be prescribed by the physician, good nursing is essential to prevent the development of pneumonia. The patient should be kept warm and out of draughts. Adequate nourishment and fluids should be given. The nurse should see that elimination is sufficient. The patient should have good oral hygiene. The care should be planned to provide adequate rest periods for the patient. An accurate record of the patient's temperature, pulse and respiration must be kept.

Postmeasles Encephalitis

The nursing care outlined under infectious encephalitis is applicable. When caring for measles, the nurse should never lose sight of the fact that uncomplicated measles seldom kills, but that complications frequently develop, which make measles one of the most serious diseases of childhood. Therefore, every effort should be made to prevent complications from developing. Measles patients usually get sick gradually. For that reason often they are neglected during the prodromal stage. Because measles seldom is diagnosed before the rash appears, the child with beginning cold, cough, laryngitis, bronchitis, coryza and slight fever should be put to bed and isolated until the danger of developing measles is past. This precaution not only will prevent contacts from occurring but also goes far toward preventing complications from developing if the case be measles.

When measles develops, the patient should be kept warm and out of draughts. Sudden or prolonged high fever should be reported to the doctor at once. If the cough becomes too annoying or interferes with the patient's rest, a cough medicine is usually given. Small doses of codeine are given to severe cases.

Convalescence

Patients with uncomplicated measles make a quick recovery. About 6 days after the rash is well out, the patient fools well and is anxious to be up and about as usual. However, the danger of developing complications or sequelae is not over. For several weeks, the patient should be protected from cold, draughts and undue fatigue.

RUBELLA (GERMAN MEASLES)

Rubella is a systematic infectious viral disease that runs a mild course and is characterized by maculopapular cutaneous rash, posterior cervical and postauricular lymphadenopathy with little or no constitutional disturbances.

Magnitude of the Problem

The disease is benign in childhood, but when it occurs during pregnancy there is a sever risk of damage to the embryo or fetus, i.e. develops congenital cataract or malformation of heart (during first trimester of pregnancy). The other rubella syndromes, which may occur are microcephaly, deaf-mutism, patent ductus arteriosus, cleft palate and clubfoot.

Epidemiological Features

Agent

The agent is a RNA virus of the togoviridae family.

Source of Infection

The source of infection is a case of rubella or even subclinical cases, infective material being CSF, blood, urine and feces. The virus has been recovered from the nasopharynx and throat of subclinical cases. Period of communicability is 1 week before and 1 week after the appearance of skin rash.

Host

1. Occurs in children and young adults, peak in 5–9 years, but can occur at any age.
2. Sex: Both sexes are susceptible to the disease.
3. Immunity: One attack confers lifelong immunity. Immune mother's transfer antibodies to their offsprings with the protection lasting 4–6 months.
4. Environment: Poor environment is a predisposing factor.

Mode of Transmission

The disease spreads through droplet infection and by direct contact. There may be transplacental transmission (vertical transmission) of the disease. Incubation period lasts 2–3 weeks with an average of 18 days.

Pathophysiology

Virus gain entry through the mucosa of the upper respiratory tract possibly replicates primarily in the cervical lymph nodes. Viremia develops and lasts until the appearance of antibody, which also coincides with the appearance of the skin rash. During pregnancy, the virus infects placenta and fetus. The virus has teratogenic effect on the fetus in utero and continuing a congenital infection can transmit the infections to the susceptible contacts, even though they are born apparently normal.

Clinical Features

There is malaise with low-grade fever (37.2–38.3°C), enlargement of lymph nodes, and superficial cervical and posterior auricular glands. Mild coryza and transient arthralgia may also occur. A fine, pink, slightly raised maculopapular rash, red ears, forehead, face, extends to trunk and extremities appears within 24 hours. Rash may be itchy, but usually subsides within 7 days. It may also lead to otitis media, neuritis, polyarthritis, thrombocytopenia purpura and encephalomyelitis.

Prevention and Control

- Isolation of the patient
- Strict avoidance of close contact with the patients
- Rubella vaccination—live-attenuated rheumatoid arthritis (RA) 27/3 rubella strain for all vaccination of children and women of child caring age
- Passive immunization with human norms immunoglobulin
- Vaccination to girls 11–14 years, duration of immunity offered being 10 years
- Other precautionary measures are needed as applied to airborne infection.

Nursing Care Isolation

Rubella, unlike measles can be isolate in a ward by the medical aseptic technique. The patient usually confined to his/her bed during the febrile stage and until the rash fade. This period usually does not exceed 3–4 days.

Temperature

The temperature characteristically is only slight elevated. In hospitalized cases, it rarely exceeds 101°F, although higher fevers are seen occasionally. Since, complications are rare, it seldom is necessary to reduce the temperature.

Diet

Usually, a general diet consistent with the age of the patient is given. Fluids are taken as desired.

Personal Hygiene

During the febrile or rash period, a daily bath is given. If the skin itches, a loose cupful of sodium bicarbonate may be added to the bath water. An oil rub following the bath adds to the patient's comfort.

INFLUENZA

Influenza is an acute respiratory tract infection caused by influenza virus of which there are three types, such as types A, B and C. Influenza is commonly known as 'flu'. The name 'influenza' is said to be given by Italians during the epidemic of 1358, which they ascribed to the malevolent influence of the heavenly bodies or of inclement weather. The modern history of the disease may be considered to date from the pandemic of 1889–1890 during which Pfeiffer isolated '*Haemophilus*.'

Magnitude of Problem

Influenza occurs in all countries and affects millions of people. Outbreaks of influenza type A occur every year. The first pandemic occurred in 1918–1919, which affected 500 million people and killed more than 20 million. In India, 6 million people died during this pandemic, known as 'swine influenza virus'. Recent pandemics occurred in 1957–1958 and in 1968.

Epidemiological Features

Incidence is higher in temperature climate than in the tropical countries and it outbreaks every year or twice a year. There may be a sudden outburst of the disease and speedily transfers from one human to another.

Agent

Influenza virus is spherical with diameter of 80–120 nm. The virus has ribonucleoprotein in helical symmetry. Single-stranded RNA genome is segmented and nucleocapsid is surrounded by envelope having virus-coded protein layer and lipid layer derived from host cell. Attached to lipid layer are hemagglutinin spikes and neuraminidase peplomers (Fig. 28.13). The virus is inactivated by heating at 50°C for 30 minutes. Ether formaldehyde, phenol and salts of heavy metals and many other chemical disinfectants destroy infectivity.

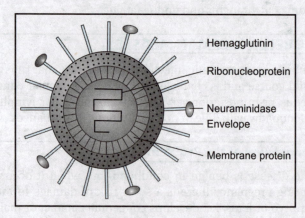

Figure 28.13: Structure of influenza virus

Influenza viruses are classified within the family orthomyxoviridae. There are three viral subtypes, namely influenza type A, B and C. Influenza A and B viruses are responsible for epidemics of disease throughout the world. World Health Organization (WHO) global surveillance activities have identified human infection with avian influenza virus called A (H5N1) in Hong Kong in 1997, where H5N1 stands for hemagglutinin antigen and neuraminidase antigen.

Reservoir of Infection

Many influenza viruses have been found in animals and birds, which are isolated from them, e.g. horses, dogs, swine, wild birds, domestic poultry, etc. Usually a case of subclinical case, the secretions of the respiratory tract is the sources of infection. Period of infectivity, i.e. the period in which it is present in nasopharynx varies from 1 to 2 days before and after the onset of symptoms.

Host Factors

1. Age and sex: Virus affects all ages and both sexes. The attack rate is lower among adults. Children constitute a transmission chain. High-risk groups are old people (over 65 year), infants under 18 months, and people with diabetes, chronic heart disease, kidney and respiratory ailments.
2. Human mobility: It is an important factor in the spread of infection.
3. Immunity: Antibodies are important in immunity against influenza. Antibodies appear in about 7 days after an attack and reach a maximum level in about 2 weeks. After 8–12 months, the antibody level drops to preinfection levels.

Environmental Factors

1. Season: Epidemics usually occur in winter months in the northern hemisphere and in winter or rainy season in the Southern Hemisphere. In India, it often occurs in summer.
2. Overcrowding: This enhances transmission and the attacks are high at closed population groups such as cinema hall, bus station, schools and institutions.

Mode of Transmission

Following are three types of mode of transmission:
1. Direct contact.
2. Droplet infection: Sneezing, coughing and talking.
3. Handling contaminated kerchiefs, articles, etc. Incubation period varies from 18 to 72 hours.

Pathophysiology

In the rather uncommon, fatal, uncomplicated cases, it is found that there is severe inflammation of the trachea, bronchi and bronchioles, hemorrhage in the lungs and marked edema of the lungs. In the usual non-fatal case, it is presumed that the main pathological process is tracheobronchitis of varying severity. Most deaths are due to complicating bacterial pneumonia caused by hemolytic streptococci or staphylococci.

The lesion consists of widespread, patchy and diffuse consolidation in both lungs together with inflammatory changes in the smaller bronchi and bronchioles. Empyema often appears early, while the pneumonic process is at its height. Unlike pneumococcal pneumonia, the disease unless treated early tends to heal by organization and scar formation rather than resolution leading to fibrosis and chronic inflammation of the lung and bronchi. Further, the involved areas may breakdown and suppurate causing multiple abscesses.

Clinical Features

- The virus is airborne and multiplies in the upper respiratory tract, selected invasion of nasal, tracheal and bronchial mucosal cells
- It damages the ciliated epithelium of the tracheobronchial cells
- Sudden onset of fever 39–40°C (102–104°F)
- General malaise
- Sore throat
- Cough
- Rhinorrhea
- Headache
- Myalgia
- Nausea, vomiting
- Abdominal pain
- Diarrhea.

Complications

- Pneumonia
- Chronic bronchitis
- Meningoencephalitis
- Cranial nerve palsy
- Myocarditis
- Heart block
- Peripheral vasoconstriction
- Effects of maternal infection on fetus and neonate
- Increased incidence of abortion and premature labor

- Occasional association of congenital malformation, especially anencephaly and meningomyelocele.

Associated Factor

Active immunization by an attenuated vaccine should not be given during pregnancy for fear of fetal damage.

Preventive Measures

1. Vaccination:
   a. Active immunization consists of a single dose of vaccine (influenza virus vaccine for either primary or annual booster vaccination).
   b. Influenza vaccine should be given during epidemics.
2. Annual vaccination with inactivated influenza vaccine is recommended for the following:
   a. Persons at high risk (i.e. the elderly persons with chronic disorders of cardiovascular, pulmonary or reveal systems metabolic disease, severe anemia and compromised immune function).
   b. Individuals who wish to reduce those chances of acquiring influenza or to reduce severity of the disease.
3. Antiviral therapy: Isolation of the infected person.
4. Provide vaccines to the medical and paramedical members.
5. Type of vaccine:
   a. Killed vaccines are used for protection against influenza, 1.0 mL SC is recommended. Immunity lasts for 3–6 months.
   b. Live vaccine or oiled adjuvant in the form of a live vaccine is given in the dosage of 0.2 mL (IM) immunity for 1 year.
   c. Live vaccine is given intranasally, which was manufactured in Union of Soviet Socialist Republic (USSR).

Control Measures

- Notification of the disease
- Throat pain of Mandie's solution
- Spray the throat with colloidal iodine
- Seek laboratory methods for diagnosis.

Nursing Management of Influenza

Isolation

The medical aseptic technique will not prevent the spread of influenza. The virus is contained in the nose and throat secretions. Because of coughing and sneezing during the onset droplet infection probably plays an important role in the transmission of the disease, although no doubt contact with the fresh secretions that harbor the virus is another way in which the disease is transmitted. We have already pointed out how nefarious indirect contact can be, how unobvious it is, and how it plays a major role in the spread of most communicable diseases.

The patient should be placed in a private room and the medical aseptic technique should be carried out in order to cut down the probability of contact infection. All articles that have come in contact with either the patient or his/her secretions should be cleaned up or destroyed immediately after use. Masking has not proved efficacious in reducing the incidence of the disease.

Diet

During the onset and high temperature stages, diet should be fluid. Fruit juices are most acceptable and citrus fruit juices are taken eagerly. They may be sweetened, but often are preferred without sweetening. Often, the patient craves lemon or lime juice. Because of the foul taste in the mouth most foods are not relished. Milk is taken with difficulty; however, buttermilk with cream added is more acceptable. Hot tea and coffee are sometimes relished. Soups, broths, gruel, ice cream, ginger ale or 7 Up may be given. A more liberal diet is given as soon as tolerated by the patient.

When the disease is complicated with pneumonia, fluids are sometimes limited, because of the tendency to pulmonary edema. Patients tend to drown in their own fluids. Small frequent feedings are taken with less effort than larger amounts at longer intervals. An accurate record of fluid intake and output should be kept.

Temperature

The temperature usually ranges from 101 to 104°F for several days after onset. If high temperature persists, it may be reduced by a cool colonic flushing. Because of the possibility of chilling, neither an alcohol fan nor a temperature sponge should be given. An ice cap may be applied to the head, if it can be kept in place. These patients are very restless. The patient should be kept warm and out of draughts at all times.

Personal Hygiene

The mouth should be kept clean. The heavily coated tongue should be brushed or washed with gauze pledgets. The teeth are covered with sordes (a dark brown accumulation of foul-smelling material). Dilute hydrogen peroxide is an excellent cleaning solution. Frequent mouthwashes of an antiseptic nature are to be given. The nose, which often is partially and sometimes completely obstructed, should be kept as clean as possible with swabs and sprays. Nasal irrigations given with very low pressure are sometimes prescribed and are quite helpful. Liquid petrolatum applied around the nose may help prevent excoriation and relieve the patient of the discomfort caused by dryness.

Very rarely, the eyes may require irrigation or treatment for conjunctivitis. The routine daily bath should be omitted. The face should be washed with warm water two or three times a day. The hands should be washed as often as necessary to keep them clean, at least three or four times each day. Characteristically, these patients sweat in the bed through. They must be kept dry and all linen changed as frequently as necessary. This may be four or five times a day, occasionally more often.

Elimination

The bowels should move freely at least once each day. An enema or cathartic may be given as needed. Nurses should not overlook the possibility of suppression or retention of urine. An accurate record of fluid output should be kept.

General Management of the Disease

Place the patient in a comfortable bed in a quiet, warm (70°F) and well-ventilated room. The bedding should be light in weight, but give adequate warmth. If prostration is great, the weight of the bedding should be kept from the patient by the use of a bed cradle.

The patient should be kept warm and out of draughts. His/Her position should be changed frequently. Small comfort pillows placed at the patient's back may help relieve the rather constant lumbar pain that is a common symptom. Counterirritants sometimes give relief to painful muscles and joints. For sore throat, hot gargles or irrigations are helpful. Tracheitis is relieved by increasing humidity within the room. A croup kettle often relieves patients with a hoarse, dry cough. Tincture of benzoin compound may be added to the kettle.

If the patient is delirious or uncooperative, he/she should have a nurse in constant attendance or else sufficient restraint must be applied to prevent him/her getting from under the covers, falling out of bed or otherwise hurting himself/herself.

Paper tissues should be provided to wipe away nose and throat secretions. The quality of the pulse should be noted at least every 3 hours. In the intestinal form of the disease, the patient frequently is unable to retain either food or fluid, because of nausea and vomiting. When this occurs, IV saline or glucose solutions frequently are given. In the nervous form, the nurse should watch for and report any symptoms referable to the nervous system. A continued high fever, convulsions, muscular twitchings, delirium, stupor and coma are significant symptoms.

Convalescence

Characteristically convalescence is fairly slow and may be very slow. The patient should get up gradually after the temperature, pulse and respirations are normal for at least 2–4 days. He/She should be warned to avoid fatiguing activity for a week or longer. If convalescence is uneventful, the patient may return to normal activity in 10 days to 2 weeks.

Terminal Disinfection

The patient should be given a complete bath and shampoo, dressed in clean clothing and placed in a clean area. All material soiled by contact with either the patient or his/her secretions should be cleaned up immediately or else burned. Bedding should be sunned for at least 6 hours.

ACUTE RESPIRATORY INFECTIONS

Acute respiratory infection (ARI) is sudden onset of infection of any part of the respiratory system from nose to alveoli, including paranasal sinus, middle ear and pleural cavity. Thus, ARIs constitute a complex and heterogeneous group of diseases caused by a great number of etiological agents. It is common among under 5-year children, infants being hit hardest. Thus, contributing significantly for increased morbidity and mortality among infants, more so in the developing countries (about 50 times higher than developed countries) because of increased prevalence of malnutrition, low birth weight (LBW) and indoor air pollution.

Magnitude of the Problem

It has been estimated that 20% of infants born in developing countries fail to survive their fifth birthday and 30% of child mortality is attributable to ARI as an underlying or a contributing cause. In India, in absolute numbers, it is about 2 million deaths among children under 5, every year, i.e. 2,000 deaths/day or 80 per hour, or 1 per every minute.

The ARI constitutes about 40% of total pediatric outpatients and 20% of hospital admissions. About 25% can be managed at home by the mother herself and another 50% can be managed by trained health worker. However, negligence can result in complications. Thus, ARI is a public health problem in India. Timely intervention and correct treatment, and referral service can save many deaths, particularly pneumonia.

Classification of ARI

Etiological Classification

1. Viral: Adenovirus, corona virus, rhinovirus, influenza virus, respiratory syncytial virus, etc.
2. Bacterial: *Streptococcus pneumoniae (S. pneumoniae), Haemophilus influenzae (H. influenzae)* (common causes of community-acquired pneumonia).
3. Fungal.
4. Parasitic.
5. Allergic.

Anatomical Classification

1. First group: Rhinitis, coryza, sinusitis, otitis media, pharyngitis, tonsillitis and quinsy (peritonsillar abscess).
2. Second group: Epiglottitis, laryngitis, tracheitis bronchitis, bronchiolitis, pneumonia and pleurisy.

WHO Classification

1. Acute upper respiratory infections (AURI)—includes anatomical first group.
2. Acute lower respiratory infections (ALRI)—includes anatomical second group.

Etiology

Respiratory tract may be invaded by one pathogen or a variety of pathogens such as viruses, bacteria, fungi, parasites or allergens. Simultaneously one prepares the way for another to invade, i.e. primary infection leading to 10 secondary infection. Usually, viruses cause mild upper respiratory infections and bacteria cause severe lower respiratory infections.

Host Factors

Age
Incidence of ARI is very high among under 5 years children, infants being hit hardest in the developing countries.

Sex
Incidence of ARI is more among male children than among female children in the ratio of 1.7:1. The difference may partly be due to preferential treatment to male children.

Risk factors related to host
Low birth weight: A low-birth-weight child is highly susceptible for any infection, more so for ARI and when ARI occurs in a LBW baby, the infection becomes more severe suddenly than in the healthy counterpart resulting in increased morbidity and mortality. In addition to increased susceptibility, LBW babies have poor respiratory mechanism.

Failure of breastfeeding: This deprives the child of maternal antibodies, more so from colostrum, predisposing the child for a great risk of many communicable diseases including ARI. Studies have shown that the incidence of ARI is high among artificially fed and bottle fed babies than breastfed babies.

Undernutrition: This in general decreases the immune mechanism and vitamin A deficiency in particular decreases the integrity of respiratory epithelium predisposing the child for ARI, which becomes severe and persistent (chronic) predisposing the child for complications and death.

The synergistic action of malnutrition and infection is well recognized. Presence of one predisposes and aggravates the other. The mortality rate of ARI is about 20 times more among malnourished children than among healthy counterpart. Such adverse effect of undernutrition can best be seen in measles.

Lack of primary immunization: Lack of routine primary immunization as per the schedule constitutes a major risk factor for acquiring the respiratory diseases such as TB, measles, diphtheria and whooping cough; pneumonia being the common complication. These are major killer diseases of children in our country.

Young infant age (i.e. neonatal period): During the first 1–2 months after birth, the newborn is extremely vulnerable to ARI. Poor standard of living worsens the situation.

Vitamin A deficiency: This not only decreases the integrity of respiratory mucous membrane but also reduces the secretion of mucus in the respiratory tract, predisposing the bacteria to stick to the mucous membrane easily resulting in the disease.

Antecedent viral infection: This viral infection of respiratory tract not only predisposes the bacteria of oropharynx to invade down resulting in secondary bacterial infection but also impairs the child's immune status and damages the bronchial epithelium as in measles.

Environmental Factors

1. Air pollution: The following industrialization and urbanization, predisposes the people for respiratory infections. Thus, ARI incidence is more among urban children than among rural children.
2. Smoking: Both active and passive smoking predisposes the people for ARI. Thus, the children of cigarette and beedi smokers are more prone for ARI.
3. Season: The incidence of ARI is more in winter season because of indoor living and overcrowding.

CHAPTER 28: Respiratory Infections

Social Factors

There are many social factors responsible for the prevalence of ARI in the community such as poverty, illiteracy, ignorance, lack of personal hygiene, overcrowding, poor standard of living, lack of sanitation, nonutilization of health services, etc. The following are the predisposing factors:

1. Epidemicity of a disease: Most ARIs are endemic. However, some ARI such as measles, pertussis and influenza have potentiality of occurring in epidemics, when the case fatality rate will be very high.
2. Mode of transmission: ARI is primarily transmitted by droplet infection. Epidemics and pandemics occur through airborne route, i.e. by droplet nuclei.
3. Incubation period: This varies according to etiological agents.
4. Neonatal pneumonia: This deserves special mention, because it is highly fatal and it differs from pneumonia of older infants and children in its etiological agents, mode of transmission and non-specific features.

The causative organisms isolated are *Escherichia coli, Streptococcus agalactiae* (group B), *Pseudomonas, Klebsiella pneumoniae, (S. pneumoniae)* and *Staphylococcus aureus*.

The newborn may get infection either transplacentally from the mother during fetal life or by aspiration of amniotic fluid during birth or by droplet infection from others after birth. The clinical features of ARI are not the routine type of cough and fever, but will have signs of toxemia and respiratory distress such as tachycardia, tachypnea and hepatomegaly. Neonatal pneumonia is very common among LBW babies, because of their poor respiratory mechanism.

Prevention and Control of ARI

The measures can be implemented at first three levels of prevention, namely health promotion, specific protection and early diagnosis and treatment. The other two levels of prevention are not implemented, because ARI is an acute condition and not a chronic condition.

Health Promotion

- Efficient antenatal care to reduce the incidence of LBW
- Essential care of the newborn and special care of LBW newborn
- Promotion of exclusive breastfeeding up to first 6 months of life
- Promotion of adequate nutrition of the growing children
- Improvement in the living conditions (housing and sanitation)
- Reduction of parental smoking and smoke pollution indoors
- Limiting the size of family to prevent overcrowding health education of mothers about correct ARI, case management at home with the following points:
  - To increase feeding and to keep the child warm
  - To clear the nose by instillation of breast milk, if runny nose interferes with feeding
  - To relieve cough with homemade decoctions such as tea, ginger, lime juice, etc.
  - To recognize danger signs such as fast breathing (increased respiratory rate) and difficult breathing (chest indrawing).

Specific Protection

- Strengthening the existing routine primary immunization
- Oral vitamin A concentrate, mega doses for children between 9 months and 3 years
- Other vaccines, which can be given are pneumococcal vaccine and *H. influenzae* type B vaccine.

Early Diagnosis and Prompt Treatment

The WHO has recommended the following steps (correct case management).

Assessment of the child

Assessment of the child is done from the following information by asking the mother and by looking and listening to the child for such features as age of the child, duration of cough, wheezing, chest indrawing, stridor, fast breathing, infant stopped feeding well (below 2 months of age), ability to drink (in a child between 2 months up to 5 years of age), antecedent illness (such as measles), fever, malnutrition, excessive drowsiness, convulsions, irregular breathing, cyanosis and any history of (H/O) treatment.

Wheezing is a whistling noise heard during expiration due to narrowing of air passage. Chest indrawing is lower chest wall moving in during inspiration. Stridor is the harsh noise produced during inspiration due to narrowing of larynx and trachea (this is also called croup). Malnutrition is a risk factor and case fatality rate is higher. Cyanosis is a sign of hypoxia.

Fast breathing: This is considered to be present when the respiratory rate is as follows:

- About 60 per minute or more in a child below 2 months of age
- About 50 per minute or more in a child between 2 and 12 months of age
- About 40 per minute or more in a child between 1 and 5 years of age.

Classification of illness

Classification of illness as mild, moderate, severe and very severe:

1. **Mild ARI cases (no pneumonia):** Characterized by cough, cold (runny nose), sore throat, otitis media with or without fever, no chest indrawing and no fast breathing.
2. **Moderate cases (pneumonia):** Characterized by cough, fast breathing and no chest indrawing, with or without fever.
3. **Severe cases (severe pneumonia):** Characterized by cough, fever, chest indrawing, fast breathing (fast breathing may be absent, if the child is exhausted), flaring of alaenasi, grunting (sound made with the voice) and cyanosis. Very severe cases (very severe pneumonia) characterized by all features of pneumonia associated with danger signs such as inability to drink, convulsions, abnormal sleep, stridor and severe malnutrition.

Management (standard treatment)

1. **Mild cases (no pneumonia):** These can be treated at home by home remedies such as ginger tea and lime juice. These cases do not require antibiotics. Most of such cases are self-limiting.
2. **Moderate cases (pneumonia):** These cases require antibiotics orally and can be treated as outpatients. Drug of choice is co-trimoxazole. It is as effective as ampicillin or penicillin with high-cure rates and few side effects and less expensive. This can be used safely by health workers in the field and by the mothers at home. Co-trimoxazole is available in both pediatric tablet and syrup forms (Table 28.2).

Table 28.2: Composition and dose schedule of co-trimoxazole

Tablet	Syrup
Composition	
Sulfamethoxazole (100–200 mg) Trimethoprim (20–40 mg)	Each spoon syrup (5 mL)
Dose schedule	
0–2 month: 1 tablet twice a day (bid) 2–12 month: 2 tablet (bid) 1–5 year: 3 tablet (bid)	0–2 month: Half spoon (bid) 2–12 month: One spoon (bid) 1–5 year: One and half spoon (bid)

Duration of treatment is for 5 days. However, reassessment of the condition of the child should be done after 48 hours. If there is improvement, co-trimoxazole is continued for 3 more days. If there is neither improvement nor worsening of the condition, change the antibiotic and reassessed after 48 hours. If there is worsening of the condition, the child is referred for hospitalization. Along with the antibiotic the child is also given antipyretic and bronchodilator.

Note: For children below 2 months, co-trimoxazole is not recommended routinely. They are treated as severe pneumonia with parenteral antibiotics. However, co-trimoxazole can be initiated before referral. Co-trimoxazole should not be given to premature babies and cases of neonatal jaundice.

3. **Severe cases (severe pneumonia):**
   - Immediate hospitalization
   - Parenteral antibiotics (benzylpenicillin is the drug of choice 5 IU/kg, 6th hourly, IM)
   - Antipyretics
   - Bronchodilators
   - Monitored every day and reviewed after 48 hours for antibiotic therapy
   - If no improvement, then change the antibiotic
   - If there is improvement, continue the same treatment for 3 more days
   - If there is worsening, treated as very severe illness.
4. **Very severe cases (very severe pneumonia):** These cases constitute acute medical emergency:
   - Hospitalization in intensive care unit
   - Oxygen
   - Broad-spectrum antibiotics
   - Maintenance of fluids and electrolytes
   - Steroids as an emergency drug.

Supportive Treatment at Primary Healthcare Level

Supportive treatment is provided by the community health workers. They are trained in making an early diagnosis and giving treatment with co-trimoxazole. They encourage continuation of breastfeeding and intake of liquids to prevent malnutrition. They should refer the following types of ARI cases to the hospital early:

- Neonatal pneumonia (pneumonia below 2 months of age)
- Very severe pneumonia
- Pneumonia among LBW babies
- Pneumonia with measles or following measles
- Children, who do not show signs of improvement after 2 days of treatment with co-trimoxazole.

Nursing Management

Bronchopneumonia usually exists as a complication of some foregoing disease, although this is often nothing, but the common cold. As seen in a communicable disease hospital, it is usually a complication of some other communicable disease. It may be isolated or not isolated as conditions warrant. However, in any event all secretions from the nose and throat should be collected on paper tissues and sent to the incinerator and handled just as in any other communicable disease.

Diet

During the acute stage of the disease, the diet will be that of the underlying primary condition of which bronchopneumonia is a complication. If bronchopneumonia is the sole clinical entity, the patient should be given a nourishing fluid and soft diet. Milk may be given, if well tolerated. Fruit juices sweetened either with honey or sugar usually is acceptable. Gruel, fruit and vegetable purees, cereals, soft-cooked eggs, toast, soups, custard and gelatin may be given. When a more substantial and variable diet is indicated any food consistent with the age and liking of the patient may be given, provided that any food or combination of foods, which tend to produce gas are excluded from the diet. A record of fluid intake should be kept.

Temperature

The temperature usually is high, 103.6–105°F. A warm or tepid sponge bath, or an alcohol fan may be given every 4–6 hours to reduce fever. However, every precaution must be taken to avoid chilling the patient. An ice cap may be placed on the head and cold or cool fluids urged. Sometimes, a colonic irrigation is helpful. However, this procedure is exhausting and should be given only upon the doctor's order. The temperature, pulse and respirations should be taken and recorded every 3–4 hours.

Personal Hygiene

The patient should have a daily cleansing bath. He/She should have a complete change of clothing and bed linen. Good oral hygiene should be maintained. Drainage from either the eyes or the nose may be removed with a cotton pledget moistened with boric solution or saline solution.

Elimination

The bowels should be kept open. There should be at least one good bowel movement each day and either a laxative or an enema usually is prescribed, if needed. Dark scant urine may mean that not sufficient fluids are being taken.

General Management of the Disease

The patient should be placed in a warm room with a high degree of humidity present. The humidity of the room may be increased by placing a croup kettle in the room and tincture of benzoin may be added to the water. If breathing becomes labored and the pulse rate is increased oxygen is usually indicated.

Fluids should be urged. If they are not retained or well tolerated, the doctors may prescribe IV fluids. The patient's position should be changed every 3–4 hours. The head should be lowered and raised at intervals. The nurse should plan his/her work, so that the patient may have as long intervals of rest as possible. Older people in both bronchopneumonia and lobar pneumonia should not be left too long on their backs. They should be kept in a sitting posture even if it becomes necessary to support them. This, of course, is only done at intervals as they must not become tired.

Convalescence

Convalescence is usually slow, there is a tendency to relapse. The patient should be instructed to return to normal activity gradually. Good nourishing food, plenty of fresh air and rest usually are all that are required.

Terminal Disinfection

Terminal disinfection is not required.

DIPHTHERIA

Diphtheria is an acute infectious disease caused by toxigenic strains of *Corynebacterium diphtheriae* and it is characteristically confined to the respiratory tract. Diphtheria bacilli were discovered in 1883–1884 by two German Physicians, Klebs and Loeffler, in bacteriological specimens from the throat of the patients. These bacilli are therefore, sometimes spoken of as Klebs-Loeffler or KL bacilli. This disease was first called diphtheritis by Bretonnean, who recognized it as a distinct malady in 1826.

Magnitude of Problem

Diphtheria is a worldwide problem in most developed countries owing to routine children vaccination. In developed countries such as England and Wales, there were only five cases of diphtheria in 1980 as against 46,281 cases, seen among non-immunized children. In India, it is an endemic disease. The available data indicate a declining of diphtheria in the infectious diseases (ID) isolation hospitals, Mumbai, Chennai, New Delhi and Bengaluru. This may be due to increasing coverage of the child population by immunization. Fatality rate on an average is about 10%, which has changed little in the past 50 years in secreted cases and about 5% in treated cases.

Epidemiological Features

Agent

Corynebacterium diphtheriae is a gram-positive, non-motile organism. It has no invasive power, but produces a powerful exotoxin. Three types of diphtheria bacilli are gravis, mitis and intermedius, all pathogenic to man. Gravis infection is more severe than mitis infection. Not all the strains of the organisms are toxigenic. There is evidence that a non-toxigenic strain may become toxigenic when exposed to a particular bacteriophage, the β phage carrying the gene for toxin production. Diphtheria bacilli are sensitive to penicillin and are readily killed by heat and chemical agents. They may survive for short periods in dust and fomites (Fig. 28.14).

Source of Infection

Nasopharyngeal secretions discharge from the skin lesions contaminated fomites and infected dust are infective materials. The period of infectivity may vary from 14 to 28 days from the onset of the disease. The source of infection may be cases or carriers:

1. Cases: Subclinical to frank clinical cases, mild or silent infections may exhibit no more than a mere running nose or sore throat.
2. Carrier: These are common sources of infection, their ratio is estimated to be 95 carriers for 5 clinical cases. It may be temporary or chronic, nasal or throat carriers. It is more dangerous as source of infections.

The incidence of carriers in a community may vary from 0.1 to 5%. The immunization does not prevent the carrier state.

Host Factors

1. Age: Particularly affects children aged 1–5 years. Schick test surveys in India have shown that about 70% of children are over the age of 3 years and 99% over the age of 5 years.
2. Sex: Both the sexes are affected.
3. Immunity: Infants born of immune mothers during the first few weeks or months of life are immune to infections.

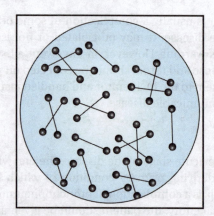

Figure 28.14: *Corynebacterium diphtheriae*

Environmental Factors

Cases of diphtheria occur in all seasons, although winter months favor its spread. In Kolkata, the highest incidence is reported in August in Bombay, Delhi from August to October.

Mode of Transmission

The disease spreads mainly by droplet infection. Portals of entry are:
1. Respiratory route.
2. Non-respiratory routes, e.g. the skin where cuts, wounds and ulcers not properly healed or infected and through infected umbilical cord in the newborn. Incubation period is 2–6 days, occasionally longer.

Pathophysiology

Typically, diphtheria commences as an acute inflammation of pharynx caused by the diphtheria bacillus. The organisms are almost entirely lacking in aggressiveness. They usually remain localized in the tonsils and in the upper respiratory mucous membranes. There, the bacilli secrete an exotoxin comparable in deadlines to the exotoxins of *Clostridium botulinum* and *Clostridium tetani*, all of which are much more poisonous than cobra venom.

The exotoxin irritates the tissues, which give forth a fibrinous exudate that coagulates into a tough, leathery, grayish white pseudomembrane. This is not always present or typical in color or consistency. This membrane along with swelling due to inflammation may occlude the air passages, especially if the larynx is invaded (laryngeal diphtheria). Death may be caused mechanically by asphyxiation in a few hours unless the obstructed larynx is bypassed by inserting an air tube into the trachea from the outside (tracheotomy). Other serious symptoms and often death result from the effect of the toxin on the heart muscle (myocarditis and sudden 'heart failure'), nerves (paralysis), kidneys (nephritis with albuminuria) and adrenal cortex (circulatory failure). In 10–25% of diphtheria patients, exotoxin causes myocarditis, a lethal inflammation of the heart muscles. When bacilli grow on the tonsils and walls of the throat (pharynx) in a susceptive person, they cause the usual (pharyngeal) form of diphtheria.

Clinical Features

In an unprotected population, diphtheria is likely to be seen between the age of 2 and 5 years, immunity being established by the repeated subclinical attacks of low virulence. Three major clinical types have been described as anterior nasal, facial and laryngeal. The skin, conjunctiva, vulva and other parts of the body may be affected. The bacilli, which multiply locally; usually in the throat and elaborate a powerful exotoxin is responsible for:

- The formation of a grayish or yellowish membrane (false membrane), commonly over the tonsils, pharynx or larynx
- Marked congestion, edema or local tissue destruction
- Enlargement of lymph nodes
- Signs and symptoms of toxemia.

Schick Test

Schick test is an intradermal test, which tests:
1. The presence of antitoxin and therefore information regarding the immunity status.
2. The state of hypersensitivity to diphtheria toxin and other proteins of diphtheria cells.

The test is carried out by injecting 0.2 mL of Schick test toxin, intradermally into the skin of forearm, while into the opposite arm is injected as a control the same amount of toxin, which has been inactivated by heat. A better control is to use the fluid toxoid vaccine preparation. This is usually dilated 1–10 and 0.1 mL is injected into the skin. The following reactions may be observed:

1. Negative reaction: If the person is immune to diphtheria, no reaction of any kind will be observed on either arms. In quantitative terms, the test will be negative if the blood serum contains more than 0.03 units of antitoxin per mL.
2. Positive reaction: In the test arm, a circumscribed red flush of 10–50 mm diameter generally appears within 24–36 hours reaching its maximum development by 4–7 days. This slowly fades into a brown patch and the skin desquamates. The control arm shows no change. The person is susceptible to diphtheria.
3. Pseudopositive reaction: A red flush develops equally on both the arms, but much less circumscribed than the true-positive reaction. The reaction fades very quickly and disappears by the 4th day. This is an allergic type of reaction found in certain individuals. The test is interpreted as Schick negative.
4. Combined reaction: The control arm shows a pseudopositive reaction and the test arm a true-positive reaction. The person is susceptible to diphtheria. A person who is proved to be susceptible, but allergic by the Schick test should be greatly reduced and the number of injections increased. About 6 hours after the Schick test, the antitoxin may be given without affecting the result of the test. The Schick test has been largely replaced by measurement of serum antitoxin level by the hemagglutination test.

Control Measurers

Cases and Carriers

1. Early detection: It should be started immediately amongst family and school contracts. Carriers can be detected only by cultural method. Swabs should be taken from both nose and throat for culture and sensitivity methods for diphtheria bacilli.
2. Isolation: All suspected cases and carriers should be isolated in the hospital at least for 14 days or until proved free of infection. At least two consecutive nose and throat swabs, taken 24 hours apart, should be negative before terminating isolation.

Treatment

Cases: In individual cases when diphtheria is suspected, diphtheria antitoxin should be given without delay. IM or IV dosage of diphtheria antitoxin, 10,000–80,000 units depending upon the severity of the cases, after a preliminary test dose of 0.2 mL subcutaneously to detect sensitization to horse serum, should be given. In addition to antitoxin, every case should be treated with:

- Penicillin injection: 2.5 IU every 6 hour
- Tablet: Erythromycin 250 mg every 6 hour for 5–6 days.

Carriers: It should be treated with 10 days course of oral erythromycin. Contacts should be placed under medical surveillance and examined daily for evidence of diphtheria for at least a week after exposure. The bacteriological surveillance or close contacts should be continued for several weeks by repeated swabbing at approximately weekly intervals.

Diphtheria Immunization

The only effective control is by active immunization with diphtheria toxoid of all infants as early in life as possible and scheduled with booster doses every 10 years. The immunization rate must be maintained at a high level in the community.

Current prophylactics
1. Combined vaccines:
   - Diphtheria, pertussis, tetanus (DPT) vaccine: 0.5 mL primary immunization for two to three doses
   - Diphtheria and tetanus toxoid (DT): Three doses from intervals of 4 weeks at 6 months to 2 years followed by another booster at the age of 5–6 years.
2. Single vaccines:
   - Formal toxoid (FT)
   - Alum-precipitated toxoid (APT)
   - Purified toxoid aluminum phosphate (PTAP)
   - Toxoid-antitoxin floccules (TAF).
     Single vaccines are less frequently used. They are all good immunizing agents. Each dose contains 25 Loeffler units of diphtheria toxoid.
3. Antisera:
   - Diphtheria antitoxin prepared in horse serum is still the mainstay of passive prophylaxis and also for treatment of diphtheria
   - Injection antisera in dosage, 500–2,000 U subcutaneously/IM
   - Therapeutic doses are two divided doses IM and 40,000–100,000 U IV.

Side effects
Fever and mild local reaction following DPT immunization are common. Severe complications following DPT immunization are neurological (encephalitis or encephalopathy) prolonged convulsions, infantile spasms and Reye's syndrome.

Nursing Management of Diphtheria

Isolation
Diphtheria can be isolated by medical aseptic technique. The causative organisms usually are found in secretions from the mouth and throat, but may be found on burns or wounds. However, they also occur in discharges from the ears, eyes, vagina and occasionally in skin lesions and in the urine or stool. The nurse should see that material suspected of harboring the causative organism is promptly disinfected or collected in a waste bag at the bedside and sent to the incinerator.

Temperature
Uncomplicated diphtheria seldom runs a fever high enough to cause alarm. However, because of secondary infections such as bronchopneumonia or otitis media, or when diphtheria is present with some other concurrent disease such as measles, the nurse may be presented with a problem of reducing fever.

The method chosen to reduce fever should be the one, which disturbs the patient the least. Never lose sight of the fact that diphtheria patients should be kept as quiet as possible. A tepid sponge bath, carefully given is the most satisfactory method unless contraindicated, because of other conditions. An alcohol rub is effective and refreshing, if carefully given. The patient need not be disturbed too much. Cooling enemas may be used with good effect in a cooperative patient. An ice cap or ice pack to the head and throat may help reduce fever.

Diet
During the acute stage, the diet should be fluid or soft. Frequently, a diphtheritic patient is able to swallow soft or semisolid food with less effort than fluids. However, well-sweetened fruit juices are taken with little trouble. Milk is not easily swallowed. However, gruel with milk, cream soups, custards and eggnogs are usually acceptable. Pureed vegetables and fruits, soft-cooked eggs and soft low-roughage cereals such as cream of wheat are taken with little difficulty. The diet may be increased to a full regular diet as soon as the patient tolerates it. The diphtheria patient should be spared the effort of feeding himself/herself. Even the so-called milder cases should be fed by the nurse. For some of the younger children, we have found that an easy way to increase the carbohydrate content of the diet is to make a homemade lollypop of brown sugar.

Personal Hygiene
The milder cases may have a daily cleansing bath; omit baths for very sick. It is necessary to maintain good oral hygiene. A good nurse usually can secure the patient's cooperation. Teeth should be brushed or washed thoroughly at least twice daily. The throat and mouth may require irrigation. The nose may be kept clean by the use of applicators moistened either with warm boric acid or saline solution. Cold cream or other mild ointments applied around the nose help to prevent excoriation of the skin. Long hair should be parted in the middle and braided securely with a braid on either side. The braids either should be pinned or tied over the top of the head, in such fashion that the patient can lie comfortably on either side or on the back. If the braids are securely tied it is unnecessary to comb the hair oftener than every 3–4 days, thus sparing the patient unnecessary exertion. Alcohol rubs, given at the time, patient's position is changed, are refreshing and comforting.

CHAPTER 28 — Respiratory Infections

General Management of the Disease

Pharyngeal and Tonsillar Diphtheria

Diphtheria patients are strictly bed patients. Even the so-called milder cases should not be allowed up. They must not be permitted to sit up for meals or while their beds are being made. They may have bed baths, but not tub baths or showers. They should be fed by the nurse. Even adult patients, who insist that they feel perfectly well should be spared unnecessary effort until the doctor approves increasing their activity.

Fluids should be urged. Fluid intake records should be kept. If nauseated or if the throat is too sore to swallow, the doctor usually supplements fluids by hypodermoclysis or IV routes. Keep the sick room comfortably warm, 75°F. We have learned by experience that diphtheria patients breathe more easily if the air is warm and not too dry. A croup kettle in the room or 1–10 bed ward, will provide helpful humidity.

Throat irrigations, given only with the patient's cooperation, are helpful. When given, they should be as warm as tolerated in order to ease the pain and clear the throat of mucus and fragments of membrane. A warm throat irrigation given immediately before meals makes swallowing less painful.

Diphtheria patients should not gargle unless specifically ordered by the physician. Small children usually cooperate with the nurse, obey instructions better, if placed in a ward with other patients who have learned to observe the same technique, i.e. to lie flat to be handfed or to have their positions changed when necessary. When placed in a quiet well-disciplined ward, the patient easily adjusts to the new environment and learns to do what is expected without much urging on the part of the nurse.

Septic or bull neck type: Very septic cases are often neglected cases. They are patients, who have been sick 3–5 days or more without specific diagnosis or treatment, due to the fact that patients, their parents or physicians fail to realize the seriousness of the situation, because the patient was believed to have been immunized, or because a diagnosis of tonsillitis was made without taking cultures. Remember that some patients who have been immunized do develop diphtheria, either immunity was not complete or it has worn off without a booster injection having been given. In a few instances, a doctor saw the patient, but awaited a culture report before giving antitoxin or else he/she neglected to take one. There are no cardinal symptoms of diphtheria and severe sore throats with membranes should be cultured.

PERTUSSIS (WHOOPING COUGH)

Pertussis is an acute infectious disease extremely dangerous especially during infancy caused by *Bordetella pertussis (B. pertussis)*. Pertussis is also called whooping cough, which comes with or without whooping. An acute disease of the respiratory tract characterized by paroxysms of cough ending in a whoop upon inhalation.

Epidemiological Features

Agent

The genus *Bordetella* contains three species, *B. pertussis, B. parapertussis* and *B. bronchiseptica*, which were formerly classified under the genus *Haemophilus*. As they do not require the X and V factors for growth, they have been separated into a new genus named after Bordet, who along with Gengou, discovered the most important member of this group.

Bordetella pertussis: It is the causative agent for whooping cough (pertussis) in a large proportion of cases. The members of this genus are small, gram-negative coccobacilli that do not ferment carbohydrates and are strict aerobes. They are hydrogen sulfide (H_2S), indole and Voges-Proskauer (VP) negative. They are parasitic in the respiratory tract of man or animals and grow only on complex media and elaborate exotins and endoriums.

Bordet and Gengou, observed a small ovoid bacillus in the sputum of children suffering from whooping cough and succeeded in cultivating it in a complex medium. This was soon established as a causative agent of whooping cough.

Bordetella parapertussis: It was isolated from mild cases of whooping cough in the United States. This has been reported from other countries also.

Bordetella bronchiseptica: It is originally isolated from dogs, causes bronchopneumonia in animals. It may occasionally infect man producing a condition resembling pertussis.

Magnitude of Problem

Whooping cough occurs in all countries, since the beginning of this century. There has been a marked and continuous drop in deaths from whooping cough. Pertussis is still a clinically serious illness with high mortality and complication rates. Whooping cough occurs endemically and epidemically in tropical countries. Since the reporting of whooping cough is inadequate, reliable information about the incidence of this disease is lacking in most countries. About 10% of all whooping cough cases and about half of the deaths occur in children under 1 year.

Morphology

The *B. pertussis* is a small ovoid coccobacillus. In primary cultures, cells are of uniform size and shape; but on subculture, they may become longer and thread like. It is nonmotile and nonsporing. It is capsulated, but tends to lose the capsule on repeated cultivation. The capsule can be demonstrated by special stains, but apparently does not swell in the presence of the antiserum. In culture films, the bacilli tend to be arranged in loose clumps with clear spores in between giving a 'thumb print' appearance. Freshly isolated strains of *B. pertussis* have fimbriae. Bipolar metachromatic granules may be demonstrated on staining with toluidine blue.

Source of Infection

The *B. pertussis* infects only man. The source of infection is a case of pertussis. The bacilli occur mainly and abundantly in the nasopharyngeal and bronchial secretions, which are infective. Objects freshly contaminated by such discharges are also infective.

Whooping cough is most infectious during catarrhal stage. The infective period may be considered to extend from a week after exposure to about 3 weeks after the onset of the paroxysmal stage. The disease is unlikely to be infectious before the child has developed catarrhal symptoms.

Host Factors

1. Age: Whooping cough is primarily a disease of infants and preschool children. The highest incidence is found below the age of 5 years. Infants below 6 months have the highest mortality. Clinical disease may also occur in adults in whom the disease is often a typical.
2. Sex: Incidence and fatality are observed to be more among female than male children.
3. Immunity: Recovery from whooping cough or adequate immunization is followed by immunity. Second attacks may occur in persons with declining immunity, but these are usually mild. Infants are susceptible to infection from birth, because maternal antibody does not appear to give them protection.

Environmental Factors

Pertussis occurs throughout the year, but the disease shows a seasonable trend with more cases occurring during winter and spring months due to overcrowding, socioeconomic conditions and ways of life playing a role in the epidemiology of the disease.

Mode of Transmission

Whooping cough is spread mainly by droplet infection and direct contact. Each time the patient coughs, sneezes or talks, the bacilli are sprayed into the air. The role of the fomites in the spread of infection appears to be very small, unless they are freshly contaminated. Incubation period is 7–14 days.

Pathophysiology

The mode of infection is either by direct contact with patients or through droplet infection. The disease is most infectious in the early or catarrhal stage of the illness. The patient ejects droplets containing large numbers of *B. pertussis* during each about coughing. There is a congestion of the respiratory tract, principally in the bronchi and bronchioles, but nasopharynx, larynx and trachea may also be affected. Midzonal and basilar epithelium may undergo necrosis and macrophage infiltration. In uncomplicated cases, there is no exudate in the alveoli. Tracheobronchial lymph nodes are swollen.

Secondary atelectasis and localized emphysematous areas are commonly present. In short, the organism liberates toxins, which irritates surface cells and causes marked lymphocytosis. Later, necrosis of epithelium and polymorphonuclear infiltration result. Obstruction of the small bronchioles by mucus plugs results in atelectasis and diminished oxygenation.

Clinical Features

The clinical course of the disease includes three stages:
1. Catarrhal stage: During this stage, which usually lasts for 1–2 weeks, the patient has symptoms of a slight rise of temperature or low fever. The cough, which is troublesome tends to be more severe at night and frequently terminates in vomiting. The cough gradually assumes a paroxysmal character. During this stage, the leukocyte count in the blood is high with relative lymphocytosis. Culture of the coughed material reveals the presence of *B. pertussis*.
2. Paroxysmal stage: Although the fever and catarrhal symptoms improve or disappear, the cough becomes more troublesome and tends to occur in paroxysmal bouts. The paroxysmal cough is usually quite characteristic. After a short, deep inspiration, there is a quick succession of bouts of cough, which continue until it appears as if there is no more air left in the chest. The patient's mouth appears open with the tongue pro-

truded. The child becomes cyanosed and the eyes starts watering. The patient presents a picture of suffocation with protruded eyeballs, congested face, engorged veins in the neck and sweating, because of a laryngeal spasm then suddenly relaxes and there is a long drawn out crowing sound during inspiration referred to as the whoop. Due to refilling of the lungs with air when this phase is over, the child becomes exhausted and may go to sleep. There is copious discharge of mucus secretion from the nose and mouth. During this stage, patient may vomit suddenly, pass urine or stool, bleed from the nose, bite the tongue or get an attack of convulsion. Subconjunctival hemorrhage and rupture of the membrane tympani may also occur. The paroxysms are more often nocturnal than diurnal. This stage lasts for 3 or more weeks.

3. Convalescent stage: The patient tends to improve gradually with the disappearance of the symptoms within 1-3 weeks course.

In mild cases, the disease may last for about only 2 weeks. On the other hand, severe cases may drag on for months before the final cure is achieved, most of the deaths occur in children under 1 year of age.

Complications

The complications of pertussis include:
- Bronchopneumonia
- Massive collapse of the lung
- Pneumothorax, surgical emphysema and spasm of glottis
- Prolapse rectum
- Convulsions
- Right cardiac failure
- Subconjunctival hemorrhages, hemoptysis
- Detachment of the retina
- Inguinal hernia.

Diagnosis

Postnasal swabs for culture and sensitivity in special medium.

Control Measures

1. Cases and contacts early diagnosis, isolation and treatment of cases and disinfection of discharges from nose and throat are the general principles to control whooping cough.
2. Early diagnosis by bacteriological examination of nose and throat secretions within 10-14 days from the onset of illness.
3. The patient should be isolated until considered to be noninfectious.
4. Several antibiotics are effective against B. pertussis. Erythromycin is the drug of choice. Four doses of 30-50 mg/kg of body weight for 10 days have been recommended. Possible alternatives are ampicillin, septran or tetracycline. Antibiotics do not neither reduce the frequency or severity of spasms nor do they shorten illness. They are useful in controlling secondary infection.
5. Infants and young children should be kept away from cases. Those known to have been in contact with whooping cough may be given prophylactic antibiotic treatment for 10 days to prevent the infection.

Prophylaxis

Active immunization

The proper use of vaccine is the most effective way to control pertussis. The vaccines are:
- DPT
- Pertussis vaccine.

DPT

DPT is now common practice to administer, which protects not only against whooping cough but also against diphtheria and tetanus. DPT is generally given in three doses of 0.5 mL each at intervals of 4-8 weeks starting when the infant is about 1½ months old, second dose in 2½ months and third dose in 3½ month. If pertussis is prevalent in the community, immunization can be started earlier at the age of 1 month. At this age, the immune response is poorer, but some feel that the partial protection obtained is better than no protection. Booster doses of DPT are indicated at the age of 18-24 months.

Pertussis vaccine

An effective vaccine is also available against pertussis. Most pertussis vaccines are whole cell preparations prepared from selected, freshly isolated, virulent strains of *B. pertussis*. It contains adequate amounts of major antigens 1, 2 and 3 and as little as possible of the histamine, sensitizing antigen. A good vaccine must contain the serotypes responsible for the disease in the population. Each dose of the vaccine must contain four fifth of the antigen. The vaccine is given intramuscularly in three doses at intervals of 6-8 weeks, starting when the infant is 2-3 months old. Following immunization, a gradual drop in immunity takes place from about 75%, 1 year after vaccination to 33% after 4 years.

In order to step up immunity, two boosters spaced at 3 years intervals should follow primary immunization. The present vaccines do not confer complete or permanent immunity. Reported efficacy varies from 70 to 90%.

Untoward reactions

Occasionally, vaccination against whooping cough causes adverse reactions, viz. prostration, screaming and convulsions. But all these reactions disappear in a few hours, the significance of these reactions is unknown.

Contraindications

The contraindications to pertussis vaccination are a personal or strong family history of epilepsy convulsions, similar CNS disorders, any febrile upset until fully recovered and a reaction to one of the previously given triple vaccine infections.

Pertussis in vaccinated children

Pertussis may sometimes occur in vaccinated children. The reasons maybe it is possible that the vaccine does not contain the serotypes responsible for the disease in the population, lower potency of the vaccine and some of the infections may be due to *B. parapertussis*.

Passive immunization

The merit of hyperimmune globulin in pertussis prophylaxis has yet to be established. So far, there is no evidence of its efficacy in well-controlled trials. The control of pertussis by immunization is still an unsolved problem. Even if the level of immunization reaches 100%, it is possible that the disease would not be entirely eliminated, because whooping cough vaccines have never been claimed to be more than 90% effective.

Transitory protection may be given to highly susceptible children under 5 years of age by the use of serum or beta (β), gamma (γ) globulin from immune persons. Hyperimmune gamma globulin (HGG) is used to hasten recovery, prevent complications and reduce mortality. The children, who need this type of protection are those who have not received pertussis vaccine, those debilitated by other disease or malnutrition and who are likely to be exposed to the infection.

Reactions

1. Pertussis vaccine may give rise to local reactions in the site of infection; mild fever and irritability.
2. A major handicap in developing an improved pertussis is vaccine, it is not known what fraction of the organisms produces reaction.

Contraindications

Not to give vaccine, when having fever convulsions or similar CNS disorders and any other infection.

Health Education

Advise the community people, whenever there is a suspected case to initiate immunization to the contacts. Advise the family members to give vaccine to school children at the entry of school. For as long as 4 weeks from onset, the child with whooping cough expels large number of organisms from the nose and mouth when coughing and sneezing. A susceptible child is almost certain to contract the disease, if he/she spends any time in a closed room with a person who is discharging the organisms by coughing. Even outdoors, close contact should be avoided for at least 4 weeks, after the onset of the disease and for 6 weeks if possible. Adults are not commonly the victims of pertussis, but unless they are known to be immune, they should avoid contact with known cases of the disease. Sometimes, people become infected following a contact with the patient yet manifest only the symptoms of a cold. All somites of the patient contaminated with sputum or vomitus as well as the vomitus itself should be disinfected. *B. pertussis* is a fragile organism and does not live very long in the outer world. Nevertheless, if survives long enough to be effectively transmitted by droplets saliva and so on.

As a medical personnel and as a community health nurse, one has responsibility to control communicable diseases, which are of great importance today in the community. The nurse should know their causative factors, process of transmission and the control measures. The nurse plays a pivot role in early detection reporting and motivating the patients for immediate treatment in relation to communicable diseases. This helps to prevent the individuals and the spread can be minimized in the community.

Nursing Management of Pertussis

Isolation

Whooping cough can be isolated by the medical aseptic technique. The causative organisms are found in the secretions of the nose and throat. Very young children (18 month to 2 year of age) and older children should be taught to cover the nose and mouth with a paper handkerchief white coughing. Also they should be taught to place the used handkerchief into the waste bag at the bedside. All articles used for the care of patient, i.e. the dishes, water pitcher and glass, formula bottles and medicine glasses should be removed from the patient's room and cleaned thoroughly as soon as possible after use.

The patient's clothing and bedding are often grossly soiled with vomitus. They should be rolled carefully into small compact bundles with the soiled part on the inside of the bundle. The bundle then should be placed in a laundry bag, laundry chute or other approved method of disposal. The main point to remember is that contaminated linen should be removed in such a way that there can be no possibility of contaminating a clean area.

Diet

The diet is of utmost importance in the nursing care of whooping cough. Malnutrition is one of the most common and serious complications. This is especially true when the patient is under 5 years of age. When the patient is a formula baby, there are several important points to remember. Several extra formulas should be prepared each day for each baby; the formulas should be given at a tepid temperature; food that is either too hot or too cold may provoke a paroxysm of coughing.

A formula baby should be held in the arms, while taking his/her feeding. He/She should be fed slowly with frequent rest periods. The hole in the nipple should not be large enough to admit more than the baby can swallow without undue haste. The very young or the very sick baby does better as a rule when fed smaller amounts at frequent intervals. Breck feeding or feeding with a medicine dropper is sometimes desirable. If the baby vomits soon after or during a feeding, he/she should be given a rest period of 10-15 minutes and then given an additional formula to equal the amount lost by vomiting. Frequently, sedatives are prescribed to be given before feeding.

An accurate weight chart should be kept. The baby should be weighed daily. After feeding, the baby should be brought to an upright position or turned on the abdomen until the air that has been sucked in with the formula has been eructated. After seeing that the clothing is dry and the baby is comfortable, he/she should be put to bed and should be placed on patient's side. A baby placed on his/her back may vomit and may aspirate vomitus, because he/she is unable to turn his/her head.

Young children should be fed a bland, high-caloric diet. All foods should be finely chopped. The food should be neither too hot nor too cold. Ice drinks and desserts are contraindicated. Highly seasoned foods should be eliminated from the diet. If the patient vomits soon after eating, he/she should have the mouth thoroughly cleaned and should be permitted to rest 10-15 minutes. He/She should then be fed again. A weight chart should be kept on all young children. Older children in whom a sufficient variety of food may be maintained, may do better when milk is eliminated from the diet. Fruit juices at room temperature usually are taken eagerly. High-carbohydrate diets are often prescribed for children, who have difficulty in retaining food.

Temperature

In uncomplicated whooping cough, the temperature seldom is high enough to create a problem. However, the temperature may reach to 102-104°F when complicated with bronchopneumonia, tepid sponges, alcohol rubs, ice caps, plenty of fluids between meals and colonic flushing are effective. Flushing are exhausting to the patient and should be given only upon order of the doctor.

General Management of the Disease

In whooping cough, as in other contagious diseases, nursing care should aim at preventing complications and sequelae. The whooping cough patient should be kept warm and out of draughts. Patients should have plenty of fresh air and sunshine, preferably out doors. The air should be free from dust and smoke, and the patient should be protected from wind. Patients should be warmly, but not heavily dressed. Adequate fluid intake must be maintained. The bowels should move freely at least once each day. There should be no abdominal distention. A tight abdominal binder will help to prevent hernia.

It also helps to prevent vomiting by preventing the full play of the abdominal muscles during a paroxysm of coughing. The binder also affords considerable relief to the patient with these conditions. After a severe and exhausting paroxysm of coughing it is often necessary for the nurse to wipe away mucus that has been forced from the bronchi into the mouth, the patient being too exhausted to do it for himself/herself. Aspiration with mechanical suction is indicated in severe cases.

Whooping cough patients should be kept quiet. Any undue excitement or anything that might provoke either laughter or crying should be avoided. Also a sudden intake of breath due to fright may cause a coughing spell. Older children, 5 years old or older, usually learn how to manage themselves surprisingly well during their paroxysms. However, the nurse may help the very young or the very sick considerably by changing the patient's position, by turning him/her into a small pillow under his/her abdomen and by supporting the head. If the patient suffers from convulsions, oxygen is often prescribed. Watch tongue and mouth for signs of intolerance to antibiotic therapy.

The nurse should remember that many children will continue to cough from habit and also for the purpose of getting attention after the paroxysmal stage has really passed. During convalescence, the nurse should try to get the cooperation of the patient in overcoming any desire to cough. It is a serious mistake to think of whooping cough as a minor disease in childhood.

MENINGOCOCCAL MENINGITIS

Meningococcal meningitis or cerebrospinal fever is an acute communicable disease caused by *Neisseria meningitidis*

(*N. meningitidis*). It usually begins with intense headache, vomiting and stiff neck and progresses to coma within a few hours. The meningitis is part of a septicemic process. The fatality of typical untreated cases is about 50% with early diagnosis and treatment, case fatality rates have declined to less than 10%.

Epidemiological Features

Geographic Distribution

Distribution is worldwide, the disease occurring sporadically and in small outbreaks in most parts of the world. The zone lying between 5° and 15° north of the equator in tropical Africa is called 'meningitic belt', because of frequent epidemic waves that have been occurring in that region. During recent years, several serious outbreaks affecting numerous countries occurred not only in the so-called meningitis belt in Africa but also in both tropical and temperate zones of other continents, e.g. Brazil, Magnolia and Scandinavian countries. Cases of meningococcal meningitis are also reported frequently in India.

Agent

The causative agent *N. meningitidis* is a gram-negative diplococci of which several serotypes have been identified, i.e. group A, B, C, D, X, Y, 29-E, W-135, etc. Groups A and C to a lesser extent and group B meningococci largely are capable of causing epidemics. The incidence of group Y and W-135 strains are increasing in some countries. These delicate, oval or spherical organisms arranged in parts with adjacent sides flattened die readily on exposure to heat and cold. Growth occurs in media enriched with blood serum or ascitic fluid. Meningitis is also caused by *S. pneumoniae* (in adults) and *H. influenzae* (in children and young adults).

Morphology

The *N. meningitidis* is a gram negative, oval or spherical bacteria 0.8–0.6 µ arranged in pairs with adjacent sides flattened (Fig. 28.15). Its considerable variation in size, shape and staining property especially in old culture is due to autolysis. In smear from lesion, the cocci are regular and are intracellular. Sometimes, microcapsule may be demonstrated by quellung reaction.

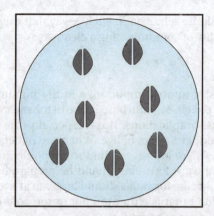

Figure 28.15: Meningococcus

Source of Infection

The organism is found in the nasopharynx and/or the tonsils of cases and carriers. Clinical cases present only a negligible source of infection. More often, the infection causes mild or even unnoticeable symptoms and nasopharyngitis. From nasopharynx, meningococci may spread along perineural sheath of olfactory nerve through cribriform plate to subarachnoid space. Alternatively, spread may be through blood and conjunctiva. On reaching CNS, a suppurative lesion of meningitis is set up involving surface of spinal cord, base and cortex of brain. The cocci are invariably demonstrated from cerebrospinal fluid lying free or intracellular in leukocytes. The organism may be harbored in the nasopahrynx of 5–8% of the normal population. During interepidemic period, carriers are the most important source of infection. The mean duration of temporary carriers is about 10 months.

Host Factors

1. Age: This is predominantly a disease of both adults and children.
2. Sex: Both sexes are affected.
3. Immunity: All ages are susceptible, younger age groups are more susceptible than older age groups as their antibodies are lower. Immunity is acquired by subclinical infection, clinical disease or vaccination. Infants derive passive immunity from the mother.

Environmental Factor

The seasonal variation of the disease is well established. Outbreaks occur more frequently in the drug and cold months of the year. Overcrowding that occurs in schools, barracks, refugee and other camps is an important predisposing factor. The incidence is also greater in the low socioeconomic groups living under poor conditions of housing.

Mode of Transmission

The disease spreads mainly by droplet infection. The portal of entry is the nasopharynx. The germ is spread by direct contact including droplets and discharges of the nose and throat of infectious persons and carriers of those exposed to it. The great majorities do not develop the infection, but become carriers harboring the organism in the posterior nasopharynx for months. Cases rapidly lose their infectiousness within 24 hours of specific treatment. Incubation period lasts usually 3–4 days, but may vary from 2 to 10 days.

Pathophysiology

Predisposing factors include upper respiratory tract infections, otitis media, mastoiditis, sickle cell anemia, certain neurosurgical procedures, head trauma and immunological defects. The venous channels serving the posterior nasopharynx, middle ear and mastoid drain toward the brain and near the veins draining the meninges, this favors bacterial proliferation.

The meningococci enter the bloodstream and cause anti-inflammatory reaction in the meninges, and underlying cortex, which may result in vasculitis with thrombosis and reduced cerebral blood flow. The cerebral tissue is metabolically impaired due to the presence of meningeal exudate, vasculitis and cerebral edema. A purulent exudate may spread over the base of brain and spinal cord. The inflammation also spreads to the membrane lining the cerebral ventricles. In acute cases, however, the patient dies from the toxin of the bacteria before meningitis develops. In these patients, meningococcemia is overwhelming with adrenal damage, circulatory collapse and associated widespread hemorrhages occurring as a result of endothelial damage and vascular necrosis caused by the meningococci.

Clinical Features

The onset may be abrupt of insidious. The symptoms result first from infection and then from increased intracranial pressure. During each epidemic, some patients are scarcely ill, others, at once overwhelmed by the toxemia, develop either high or subnormal temperature with purpura on the skin and die within few hours of the onset. Usually, the persons present with a sudden onset of severe headache, neck pain and stiffness, and fever. There is also resistance to neck flexion. The disease may follow two patterns and the signs include:
1. Positive Kernig's sign: When the patient is lying with the thigh flexed on the abdomen, they cannot completely extend the leg.
2. Positive Brudziński's sign: When the patient's neck is flexed, flexion of the knees and hips are produced.

When passive flexion of the lower extremity of one side is made, a similar movement is seen in the opposite extremity. Convulsions, mental confusion and lethargy may occur. A striking feature is a rash ranging from petechiae to a combination of petechiae and ecchymoses occurring in about 75% of the patients.

Prevention and Control

Cases

Treatment with antibiotics can save the lives of 95% of patients provided that, it is started during the first 2 days of illness. Penicillin is the drug of choice. In penicillin allergic patients, chloramphenicol should be substituted. Treatment of cases has practically no effect on the epidemiological pattern of the disease, because it only reduces the fatality rate according to the treatment efficiency. Isolation of cases is of limited usefulness in controlling epidemics, because the carriers outnumber the cases.

Carriers

Treatment with penicillin does not eradicate the carrier state and more powerful antibiotics such as rifampicin are needed to eradicate the carrier state.

Contact

Close contacts of people with confirmed meningococcal disease are at an increased risk of developing meningococcal illness. Nearly, one third of secondary cases occur in the first 4 days. Chemoprophylaxis has been suggested for close contact. Current recommendations regarding chemoprophylaxis of close contacts are early administration of rifampicin 600 mg twice a day for 2 days for adults. Dosage of sulfadiazine for adults is 19 twice a day for 2 days.

Mass Chemoprophylaxis

Mass chemoprophylaxis is in fact a mass medication of the total population, some of which are not infected. It is recommended that mass chemoprophylaxis has be restricted to close and medically supervised communities. Mass treatment causes an immediate drop in the incidence rate of meningitis and in the proportion of carriers. The efficacy of this preventive measure depends to a large extent on the population coverage.

Immunization

Effective vaccines prepared from purified group A, C, Y or W-135 meningococcal polysaccharides are now available. They may be monovalent or polyvalent. Recent field trials have indicated that immunity lasts for about 3 years, and boosters every 3 years would be reasonable. High-risk population should be identified and vaccinated. The vaccine is not recommended for use in infants and children under 2 years. The vaccine is contraindicated in pregnant women.

Environmental Factor

Improved housing and prevention of overcrowding are long-term measures.

Treatment

Sulfonamides of chloramphenicol are used in the treatment. Immunization with polysaccharide is good, so it is used prophylactically. The various capsular polysaccharide preparations are also available:
- Monovalent, i.e. group A and C
- Bivalent, i.e. group A and C
- Quadrivalent, i.e. group A, C, Y and W-135.

Nursing Management of Meningitis

Isolation

The disease can be isolated by the medical aseptic technique. The causative organisms are found in the nose and throat secretions in drainage from the eyes and ears, and in the spinal fluid. Contaminated articles should be cleaned up immediately or collected in the waste bag at the bedside and sent to the incinerator.

Diet

The diet presents a serious problem. The patient may be wildly delirious or prostrated and comatose. When the patient is uncooperative or comatose high-caloric fluids frequently are given by gavage. Fruit juices, eggnogs, creamed soups, thin gruel and milk are given by tube.

It is often difficult to give even the cooperative patient sufficient calories and fluids. When opisthotonos is present, the position of the patient adds to the difficulty of the feeding problem. Small spoonfuls, fed slowly are advised. A dropper, a Breck feeder or a syringe barrel with a rubber tube may prove helpful.

Elimination

Retention of urine is common. The nurse should be especially careful to note the amount voided and to watch for bladder distention. Overflow of a distended bladder should not be mistaken for true incontinence. The bowels should move freely at least once each day. Either an enema or cathartics may be given as indicated.

General Management of the Disease

While, the patient can be successfully isolated in a ward because of condition, patient should be placed in a warm (70–75°F), quiet, well-ventilated private room. Meningitis patients are sensitive to any sensory stimuli. The eyes should be protected from light. Care should be taken not to jar the bed. Quick, jerky motions in handling the patient and any unnecessary noise should be avoided.

Prevention of pressure sores presents a serious and difficult problem. The patient should be kept clean and dry. The bed should be free from wrinkles under the sheet. The position should be changed every 3–4 hours. This procedure will also help to prevent hypostatic pneumonia. For the continent patient, alcohol rubs are helpful. Oil rubs should be given when the patient is incontinent.

TUBERCULOSIS

Tuberculosis is communicable disease suffered by all ages. It is a problem in community. TB is known to man since ages. Hippocrates called this disease as phthisis, which means, 'to dry of disease accelerated greatly.' In 1882, Robert Koch discovered tubercle bacillus. In 1895, Rontgen discovered X-ray, which proved extremely valuable aid in diagnosis of TB. In 1907, von Pirquet discovered the tuberculin test. Soon after the First World War, the bacille Calmette-Guérin (BCG) vaccine evolved by the French scientists. In India, it was introduced in 1949.

Tuberculosis has had a long and a protracted past. Our Rig Veda has mentioned it as 'Rajayakshma' (king of diseases) and the Chinese literature described it as 'Lao Ping.' Phthisis, consumption, rajrog, the great white plague and the 'captain of all the men of death' has been the other names ascribed to TB in the past.

Pulmonary TB is an infectious disease of the parenchyma of the lung caused by *Mycobacterium tuberculosis (M. tuberculosis)* characterized by the formation of tubercle.

CHAPTER 28: Respiratory Infections

Magnitude of the Problem

Not a single country succeeded in reaching a point of control, i.e. less than 1% tuberculin positive among children of age group 0–14. In the world there are about:
1. About 15 million cases of infectious TB at present.
2. Every year 2–3 million cases are added.
3. Each year 1–2 million people are dying.
4. The problem is acute in developing countries. More than three fourth of total cases of TB and more than three fourth of total tuberculosis deaths occur in developing countries:
   a. Prevalence of infections: It is evinced by tuberculin that testing on an average 50% of population are infected at any one time.
   b. Mortality: About 1 million each year.
   c. Morbidity survey:
      - Prevalence rate of active cases, 1.8% population out 0.4%
      - Prevalence rate in towns, cities and villages are same
      - Prevalence rate showed increase with age.

Epidemiological Features

Geographical Distribution

Worldwide, particularly in developing and underdeveloped countries.

Agent

Mycobacterium tuberculosis: Human and bovine strains of the bacillus are of importance to man and fairly resistant to the action of chemicals and heat. Tubercle bacilli in India are less virulent than those of Europe.

Mycobacterium tuberculosis is a slender, straight or slightly curved bacillus with rounded ends, occurring singly in pairs or in small clumps. It measures $1–4\ \mu \times 0.2–0.8\ \mu m$ (average $3 \times 0.3\ \mu m$) in size. These bacilli are acid-fast, nonsporing, noncapsulated and nonmotile. Ziehl-Neelsen staining is useful to study the morphology of these organisms are stained blue (Fig. 28.16). Tubercle bacilli may also be with the fluorescent dyes (auramine-O, rhodamine) and appear yellow luminous bacilli under frequently seen *M. tuberculosis*. They are gram positive, but are difficult to stain with the Gram stain.

Source of Infection

Human and bovine

Bovine is of no problem in India because people take boiled milk. Infective material is the sputum of the patient suffering from TB bacilli, is also found in pus, pleural and peritoneal fluid. Communicability is as long as the bacilli are excreted by the infected host. The infectiousness is rapidly reduced by chemotherapy.

Host Factors

1. Age: It can occur at any age majority of cases 20–40 years. In India, prevalence is higher in the elder age group.
2. Sex: More in males than in females, more prevalent among males over 40 years. It affects all races and is not a hereditary disease.
3. Nutrition: Studies have shown that diet had no discernible influence on the recovery of patients.
4. Immunity: Man has no inherited immunity against the disease. It is acquired as a result of natural infection or BCG vaccine. There is an infection immunity, but it is not an absolute immunity. It breaks down in the face of heavy superinfection.

Environmental Factors

Standard of living is related factors with occurrence of disease and social factors:
- Overcrowding insanitary and overcrowded, and substandard houses
- Poverty: Low-income group is highly infected
- Education: Low level of education leads to ignorance about health
- Occupation: Silicotics, doctors, nurses and students of medical field
- Large families: Chances of contact are greater
- Industrialization: It is responsible for high incidence
- Malnutrition: Predisposes the disease.

Social customs
- Habits of indiscriminate spitting
- Use of common hookah

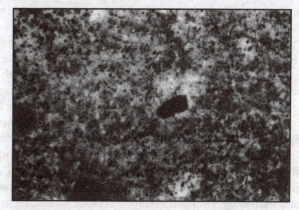

Figure 28.16: *Mycobacterium tuberculosis* in Ziehl-Neelsen stained smear

- Feeding habits in same utensils
- Purdah system, which is common in Muslims and some ladies of Hindus, is also cause of infection
- Early marriages, repeated pregnancies and frequent motherhood
- People hide their diseases due to social stigma.

Economic aspects

Tuberculosis is a chronic disease, which brings a large quantum of human suffering and a great economic loss. Mass treatment by the government is not possible due to high costs.

Mode of Transmission

1. Droplet infection and droplet nuclei generated by an open case.
2. Inhalation of fine dust containing tubercle bacilli from infected sputum.
3. Ingestion of contaminated food and milk.

The period of time from infection to onset of TB, i.e. incubation period may be weeks or months or years depending upon host-parasite relationship and dose of infection. The risk of infection and disease is closely related to the closeness of contact, extent of the disease, sputum positivity of the source case and the host-parasite relationship.

Pathophysiology

The tubercle bacillus requires ready access to oxygen for growth. Under favorable circumstances cell division occurs. In unfavorable circumstances, it may become metabolically dormant and persist in necrotic tissue for years. Initial focus is in the mid or lower fields, where there is greater ventilation. Bacterial multiplication, which proceeds with little or no reaction spreads to regional nodes in the hilum of the lung and gains entry into bloodstream. It is important to emphasize that asymptomatic lymphohematogenous dissemination of the primary infection before acquisition of tuberculin hypersensitivity probably occurs in all instances. In this event, which sets the stage for the development of chronic pulmonary and extrapulmonary TB at a later time.

Metastatic bacterial colonies multiply throughout the body. Circulating bacilli are most efficiently cleared from the bloodstream by reticuloendothelial organs. The development of tuberculin hypersensitivity and cellular immunity greatly alter the balance in favor of the host. Activated macrophages reduce the bacterial population at both initial and metastatic foci and further bacterial growth is inhibited. The lymph nodes are sufficiently large, cellular necrosis may develop and eventually calcify producing the so-called Ghon complex.

Fate of the primary infection is that after the development of tuberculin hypersensitivity, 99% of the infection remains quiescent and is of no further clinical significance. The resemblance of the resulting disseminated tubercles to millet seeds led to the designation miliary TB. The rupture of subependymal foci in brain or spinal cord spread infection into the brain or spinal cord and spread the infection via the subarachnoid fluid and cause tuberculous meningitis.

In progressive pneumonia, large hilar nodes may become necrotic and liquefy discharge into the bronchial tree. Often, partially compress the major bronchi producing bronchial obstruction and collapse of a pulmonary segment or lobe.

Clinical Features

The outset of TB is insidious and early symptoms vary from one individual to other:
- Dry cough, later moist with varying amount of sputum
- There is usually steady and progressive loss of weight and this is associated with general malaise and fatigue
- Persistent pyrexia is present characteristically raised in the evening and lowered in the morning, the evening pyrexia is accompanied by heavy night sweats
- In some cases, cough associated with blood-stained sputum
- At a later state, chest pain
- Dyspnea
- Marked weakness and wasting
- Loss of appetite anorexia
- Wasting of muscles
- Hemoptysis.

Prevention and Control of Tuberculosis

Early Detection of Cases

The case is one whose sputum is positive for tubercle bacilli. All others are termed suspects. Case finding tools are:
1. Sputum examination: It is of two consecutive specimens (e.g. on the spot and overnight sputum) of patients with following symptoms:
   - Cough more than 2 weeks duration
   - Chest pain
   - Hemoptysis—spitting of blood.
2. Mass miniature radiography (MMR).
3. Tuberculin testing: One tuberculin unit (TU) is equal to 0.00002 mg [international standard for purified protein derivatives (PPD)]. Old tuberculin is replaced by PPD. It is given by intradermal route.

4. Mantoux test: The PPD injection 1 tuberculin unit (TU) to forearm results in red papule after 72 hours, palpable edema or induration more than 10 mm in the longitudinal diameter is considered acceptable infection with bacilli. Occurrence of non-specific reaction has lessened the value of tuberculin test.
5. Examination of the chest: It is expensive, but more sensitive and specific like sputum examination.

Chemotherapy

Antitubercular drugs

Thiacetazone 150 mg + Isoniazid isonicotinythydrazine (INH) 300 mg in a single tablet with streptomycin daily for first 2 months yields 100% success. In order to avoid drug resistance, treatment must be complete and regular at least with two to three drugs in combination. Regimens of treatment are as follows:

1. Daily regimens: In rural areas, where medical supervision is not readily at hand, daily oral regimens are ideally suitable number daily regimens:
   - Isoniazid + Thiacetazone
   - Isoniazid + Ethambutol

   For seriously ill, sputum-positive TB patient daily streptomycin 0.75 g may be added in one of the above mentioned regimens for initial 2 months period.

   Note: Isoniazid + para-aminosalicylic acid (PAS) regiment has to be discontinued. INH (300 mg) + Thiacetazone (150 mg) given together in a single dose is most frequently used. It is inexpensive, easy to administer and convenient to patient. In case of toxicity (severe skin eruptions), thiacetazone may be replaced by ethambutol.

2. Biweekly or intermittent regimens: Preferable for sputum positive cases:
   - Streptomycin—0.75 g
   - Isoniazid—600 or 700 mg
   - Pyridoxine—10 mg

   Streptomycin should be cautiously used in elderly patients of 40 years and above, and the patient having kidney diseases. Similarly, ethambutol should be cautiously used in children and in patients having ocular diseases.

Conventional drug

Conventional drug regimen is recommended under the program for sputum positive patient and listed in Table 28.3.

Short-course of chemotherapy

There are two recommended regimens under the program, National Tuberculosis Control Program (NTCP). These regimens have two phases, intensive phase of first 2 months and continuation phase of 4–6 months (refer Table 28.3):

1. Regimen (A): It is a biweekly intermittent supervised regiment. Total duration of treatment is only 6 months. In the first 2 months (intensive phase), patient is given streptomycin (0.75 g), INH (600 mg), rifampicin (600 mg) twice a week for 4 months. Patient has to report to the health institutions and all the drugs are consumed by the patient under the supervision of a doctor or health staff. In case of streptomycin, 1.5 g may be substituted.
2. Regimen (B): Initial intensive phase of four drugs comprises of streptomycin (0.25 mg), INH (300 mg), rifampicin (450 mg) and pyrazinamide (1.5 mg) given daily for 2 months followed by daily administration of INH (300 mg) and thiacetazone (150 mg) for a period of 6 months. Total duration of treatment is 8 months.

Wherever patients cannot tolerate, thiacetazone may be replaced by ethambutol (800 g daily). This regimen is self-administered by the patients at their home (domiciliary). It is as effective as hospital treatment.

Disinfection

Disinfection of sputum and infective articles to avoid spread of infection to other persons.

BCG Vaccination

The aim of BCG vaccination is to induce a benign, artificial primary infection, which will stimulate an acquired resistance to possibly subsequent infection:

1. The BCG vaccine consists of live attenuated bovine strain of tubercle bacilli. Danish 1,331, strain for production of vaccine (after Calmette and Guérin).
2. Type: Liquid or freeze dried.
3. Administration: Intramedullary with a special tuberculin syringe and a 1 cm steel 26 gauge needle.
4. As soon as birth and young adults, hospital nursing staffs, medical students also to be inoculated.
5. Phenomenon after vaccination: About 2–3 weeks after a papule develops, it increases in size, slowly reaches a diameter of about 8 mm in 5 weeks. It then either subsides or breaks into a shallow ulcer, which heals leaving a tiny scar.
6. Complications:
   a. Slight enlargement of regional lymph gland.
   b. Left arm used for BCG vaccination and for 6 months no other injections.
7. Immunity: Protection rate 80% lasting for 10 years. No influence on mortality.
8. Non-specific allergy: It is called natural vaccination. It varies greatly in different parts of India.
9. Direct BCG: 0–20 age groups are covered by prior tuberculin test.
10. Smallpox and BCG combined: They may be given at the same time, but on different arms. It is an adjunct to other methods of control.

Table 28.3: Conventional drug regimens recommended under the program for sputum

Code No.	Drugs and dosage	Mode and rhythm of administration	Instructions
R1	Isoniazid 300 mg and Thiacetazone 150 mg	Both drugs in a single dose or two divided doses orally, daily	Self-administration at home after meals
R2	Biweekly regimen infection streptomycin 0.75 g/1 g and Isoniazid 600–700 mg (15 mg/1 kg body weight) with pyridoaine	Intramuscularly orally	Both drugs given at the same line under supervision of the treating physician twice weekly at intervals of 3–4 day
R3	Isoniazid 300 mg and Para-aminosalicylic acid 10 g	Both drugs in a single dose or in two divided doses orally, daily	Self-administration at home after meals
R4	Isoniazid 300 mg and Ethambutol 20 mg/kg body weight 50 kg and 1,000–1,200 mg	Both drugs in a single dose, orally, daily	Self-administration at home after meals
R5	Biphasic regimen: 1. Intensive phase: Injection streptomycin 0.75 mg/1 g and Isoniazid 300 mg or ethambutol 20 mg/kg body weight, i.e. 800 mg for patients 2 kg and 1,000–1,200 mg for 50 kg body weight or Para-aminosalicylate sodium (PAS) 10 g 2. Continuation phase with R1, R2, R3 or R4	For first 2 month in a single dose orally, daily (PAS and thiacetazine should be given in two divided doses) As per each regimen	Injection given under supervision will rest to be administered at home As per each regimen

11. Duration of TB: Minimum period of treatment is 12 months, optimum is 18 months and treatment beyond 2 years does not have advantage.

Rehabilitation

1. Diversional: Reading, music and indoor games.
2. Occupational: Learning music, knitting, drawing and painting, photography and toy making.
3. Vocational: Clinical job, laboratory job, typing, weaving, carpet making, tailoring and poultry farming.

Chemoprophylaxis

The 1934 expert committee on TB emphasized that preventive treatment is irrational even for special group. In this regimen, BCG has priority over chemoprophylaxis.

Surveillance

Close supervision of particular portion of population for definite period of time. It is used in eradicating TB. Surveillance has two aspects:
1. Surveillance of annual infection rates.
2. Surveillance of control measures applied such as BCG vaccination and chemotherapy.

Role of Hospitals

Main indications are:
- Emergencies such as massive hemoptysis and spontaneous pneumothorax
- Surgical treatment
- Management of serious types of TB (TB meningitis)
- Social indications no one to look after the patient.

Drug-resistant Strains

1. All drugs used in the treatment of TB tend to produce resistant strains:
   a. Primary or pretreatment resistance.
   b. Secondary or post-treatment resistance.
2. Prevention of drug resistance: Since incomplete, inadequate and irregular treatment is the main cause of drug resistance, it can be prevented by:
   a. Treatment with two or more drugs in combination.
   b. Using drugs to which the bacteria are sensitive.
   c. Ensuring that the treatment is complete, adequate and regular.

Health Education

Health education is also an important aspect of the program. More stress to be given on health education of the community to educate them about various aspects of TB for taking timely action in prevention and treatment of TB disease. It should be impressed upon that TB is not a dangerous disease now, provided it is treated timely for the full prescribed period. This will also help in getting early case and to get cooperation of the people.

Improvement of Social Conditions

- Minimum living wage
- Good housing
- Good nutrition
- Open space in town
- Stopping bad customs.

National Tuberculosis Control Program

The NTCP is a centrally sponsored scheme with 50% assistance to the states and 100% to Union territories from central government. The implementation of the scheme is the responsibility of the state governments. The TB program has been included in the Twenty Point Program (TPP). TB is a major health problem. Around 9–10 million people suffer from radiologically active TB out of which 2.2–2.5 million are sputum positive and infectious.

Long-term objective: To reduce the problem of TB in the community sufficiently quickly to the level, where it ceases to be a public health problem.

Main activities, strategies of NTCP: Early detection and treatment of all TB patients out of the symptomatic attending the health and medical institutions giving priority to sputum positive cases:

- The BCG vaccination of susceptible population under Universal Immunization Program (UIP)
- Isolation and treatment of cases
- Setting up of training cum demonstration centers
- Rehabilitations
- Research activities: National institute of communicate disease (NICD) under Director General of Health services (DGHS) is engaged in important epidemiological, sociological, bacteriological and operational research connected with the program and provide suitable technical guidance for improvement of the program.

The services are offered by the state government from all health institutions (integrated program)—urban and rural.

Organization

District Tuberculosis Control Program (DTCP) is the backbone of NTCP. DTCP consists of one District Tuberculosis Center (DTC) and an average 50 peripheral health institutions comprising primary health centers (PHCs), general hospitals, rural dispensaries, etc.

Staffing: The following are the staffing:
- District Tuberculosis Officer (DTO): 1
- Laboratory technician (LT): 1
- Treatment organizer: 1
- X-ray technician: 1
- Statistical assistant: 1
- Health visitors: 2–4.

The DTO is directly responsible for the DTCP.

District tuberculosis program

The DTP is the basic unit of NTCP. It caters to the needs of entire district. An average district (population of 1.5 million) is expected to have about 5,000 sputum positive cases. The functions of the DTP are to plan, organize, implement and supervise in the entire district. The main activities of DTP are:

1. Case finding: This is undertaken by all PHCs and other general institutions in the daily outpatients. Patients with symptoms suggestive of TB are offered sputum microscopy. All sputum positive cases are put under chemotherapy. Repeated sputum positive symptomatic patients referred for X-ray examinations, wherever it is available and radiologically active TB patients are put under treatments.
2. Treatment: Of patients in their homes (domiciliary) has proved effective. Treatment is free and is offered on domiciliary basis.
3. The BCG vaccination included in vaccine preventable diseases (VIP), multipurpose workers (MPWs) to immunize all infants before they are 1 year old, house to house census.
4. Recording and reporting: It should be done on every Saturday. Reports on case finding and treatment activities are submitted to DTC once in a month. DTC registers all cases in district tuberculosis (DTB) case index. The DTO submits quarterly reports on case finding, treatment, supervision and position of the key staff/equipments to state health authorities and National Tuberculosis Institute (NTI) Bengaluru. On receipt of the quarterly report, NTI scrutinizes the reports and gives suggestions for corrective measures to be taken on various deficiencies to the concerned DTO and state health authorities.

In spite of all measures taken, TB still appears to continue as an important communicable disease problem worldwide. This is because of the increased expectation of life, high prevalence of infections, etc.

Revised Strategy

The revised strategy, better known as Revised National Tuberculosis Control Program (RNTCP) was based upon recommendations of above committee and has incorporated the following essentials in its components:

1. Case detection by sputum microscopy than radiology, performing at least three sputum smear examinations for diagnosis and strengthening the sputum microscopy facilities (by ensuring good quality equipment, training of laboratory technicians, establishing sputum microscopy centers per 1 lakh population and appropriate cross-checking mechanisms for quality control assurance).
2. Accordingly the highest priority to treating smear positive patients with directly observed treatment, short-course (DOTS) chemotherapy in the intensive phase and appropriate supervision in the continuation phase through the involvement of most peripheral health functionaries (closest to the patient's residence) such as the MPWs, anganwadi workers, trained dais, Village health guides (VHGs) and community volunteers.
3. Ensuring a regular and an uninterrupted supply of drugs right up to the periphery.
4. Improving the training capabilities of all personnel.
5. Enhancing capabilities of DTCs and state tuberculosis demonstration and training centers (STDCs) for an effective implementation, monitoring and evaluation of the program. Involvement of non-government organizations (NGOs) and private medical practitioners (in view of the fact that a large number of patients visit them).
6. Creation of a subdistrict supervisory level for every 0.5 million population with the team consisting of one Senior Tuberculosis Supervisor (STS) and one senior tuberculosis laboratory technician (STLT) under the supervision of an medical officer (MO), designated as medical officer TB control (MOTC) for registration of cases at the unit instead of a district.
7. Strengthening of the recording and reporting system for ensuring accountability and emphasis on monitoring of treatment outcomes. Encouragement of operational research for the improvement of program efficiency.
8. Establishment of professionally designed information, education and communication (IEC) activities for supporting the program.

Objectives of RNTCP

Operational objectives of the RNTCP are:

1. To provide short-course chemotherapy (SCC) to all detected TB patients for the recommended duration of treatment till they are cured.
2. To treat annually on an average of about 750 sputum positive cases per million population as against the existing rate of 375 per million populations.
3. To cure at least 85% of all newly detected cases of pulmonary TB.
4. To detect at least 70% of the estimated incidence of smear positive pulmonary cases. Efforts targeted at case detection should be made only after achieving 85% cure rates in the already detected cases, which is the prime target of the RNTCP.

Overall objectives of the revised program are:
- To reduce morbidity and mortality from TB
- To interrupt the chain of transmission of infection.

Pilot vs phased coverage and program expansion

The RNTCP was initially implemented in 1993 as a pilot phase (phase I) in five project areas (Delhi, Bombay, Calcutta, Bengaluru and Mehsana district of Gujarat) covering a population of 2.35 million. A sputum conversion rate of around 95% was observed at 2 months and the ratio of sputum positive to negative patients became nearly 1:1 in all project areas (versus the existent 1:4 in rest of the country at that time).

Success of pilot test led to the program extension (phase II), which provided coverage to a 14 million population in 13 states. Again, the results were highly encouraging. Henceforth, with an assistance from World Bank, the Government of India in 1997, formally launched RNTCP in the country (phase III). In the initial years of implementation, about 80% cure rates were obtained and some areas successfully achieved cure rates above 90% consistently. The program began a rapid expansion in late 1998 and early 1999 by the time, the country could boast of having second largest DOTS program in the world. More than 250,000 patients had received treatment by mid 2,000. It provided a regular supply of good quality drugs and state-of the art binocular microscopes to DOTS centers apart from intuiting a vigorous training of the health staff and MOs. Program spanning over 189 districts and 17 states had covered one third of the country till June 2001, with six states being in the 1st year of DOTS implementation. Precisely, a 450 million populations was brought under its purview by December 2001.

Capital of the country witnessed a start of the pilot phase (phase I) of the RNTCP at chest clinic, Gulabi Bagh in 1993. Phase II of the program got commenced in 1995, which also included the clinic at LRS Institute of TB and Allied Diseases, along with two more chest clinics. The entire 10 million populations of the city was covered under the program by 1999 through the distribution of chest clinics and DOTS centers that currently, figure around 20 and 117 respectively. Plans are on-foot to cover half of the country by 2002, 80% by 2004 and the entire country as soon as feasible.

Structural organization

Organization of the RNTCP at various levels is as detailed below.

Central level: The Central Tuberculosis Division located in the Union Ministry of Health and Family Welfare and headed by Deputy Director General (DDG)-TB, is responsible for TB control in the entire country. Its main responsibilities are planning, supervising, monitoring and evaluating the anti-TB activities; coordinating with other governmental agencies; providing drugs, laboratory equipments and the study material related to TB and training of the nodal personnel involved in the program.

State level: An STO trained in RNTCP is responsible for ensuring the performance of above activities within a State and also regularly coordinating with central TB division.

District level: The DTC is the nodal point for TB control activities and the DTO, as its incharge has an overall responsibility for TB control program within the district. For its smooth-functioning, he/she is assisted by an MO, statistical assistant and other paramedical staff. Their responsibilities include implementing the RNTCP through district health staff; maintaining map of the area with details of all health facilities, government organizations and the NGOs involved in TB activities; ensuring a regular supply of drugs, laboratory material and stationary within a district; training of staff; instituting proper treatment; organizing health education; establishing liaison with private practitioners and NGOs in promoting TB services; visiting all subdistrict tuberculosis units (TUs), hospitals, community health centers (CHCs) and PHC blocks (at least quarterly); ensuring a supervisory visit of the subdistrict staff to all microscopy centers (at least once monthly); completing quarterly reports on the notified new and retreatment TB cases along with the results of sputum conversion and treatment; and monitoring performance of the mass and health workers.

Subdistrict level: The TU is constituted by an Medical Officer-TB control (MOTC), Senior Tuberculosis Laboratory Supervisor (STLS) and the STS. Apart from its activities concerning the assurance of supplies, the training of staff, the map-keeping of area and the liaising with private practitioners and NGOs, a TU also carries out the treatment categorization and DOT, supervises the microscopy centers and PHCs (at least monthly), keeps the TB register updated, prepares quarterly reports and acts as the referral point for troublesome patients requiring further investigations/management.

Health unit level: This comprises of the rural hospitals, health centers, dispensaries and other health facilities within a district. Their responsibilities consist of sending TB suspects to the microscopy centers for examination, carrying out the treatment categorization and DOT, tracing and bringing the defaulters back under treatment, maintaining the treatment cards and records, facilitating the follow-up sputum smear examinations, tracing and investigating the contacts and coordinating the patient discharges on completion of their treatment.

Metropolitan cities: In these cities, DOT-cum-microscopy centers are available for catering to a population of 1 lakh. Such centers have a LT (for performing the sputum microscopy) and a TB health visitor (for implementing the DOTS).

DOTS Components

The DOTS is a systematic strategy under the RNTCP comprising of five essential components.

Political and administrative commitment: A political and an administrative commitment from the government, whether at central, state or a district level is an essential component, because the program infrastructure and the operational objectives require a continued availability of a vast variety of items for which the health center requires a substantial financial aid from the government, otherwise the program would only end up as a short-time affair and would be unable to achieve the set target or produce a desirable epidemiological impact.

Good quality diagnosis: Case detection by sputum examination for acid-fast bacilli (AFB) is the best method for diagnosis of pulmonary TB. Similar, smear examinations for AFB can be carried out in pleural, ascitic and pericardial fluids apart from the urine, stool, blood, CSF, pus and tissue samples in various forms of extrapulmonary TB. A good quality microscopy is essential or else the diagnosis of TB could be easily overlooked.

Good quality drugs: Since, the box containing A IT for entire duration of patient's treatment is made at a health center at the very start of treatment itself, therapy can never fail on account of the nonavailability of medicines in the DOTS program. However, an uninterrupted supply of drugs will be required at the center executing this program.

Directly observed treatment (DOT): The 'DOT' is core of the DOTS program and consists of the patient taking secondary drugs directly in the presence of health workers or other trained persons. Achievement of high-cure rates and decline of drug resistance has been demonstrated by the assurance of DOT.

Systematic monitoring and accountability: A patient's progress is monitored during the treatment course by systematic sputum examinations. The monitoring and evaluation also takes place at every level of health system. Thus, the RNTCP shifts responsibility for cure from patient to the health system.

Identification of Suspects

A patient having persistent cough for 3 weeks or more is a suspect of pulmonary TB and should have his/her sputum examined for AFB on 3 consecutive days. There may be associated presence of symptoms such as weight loss, tiredness, fever (with an evening rise), night sweats, chest pain, shortness of breath, loss of appetite and hemoptysis.

A person with the extrapulmonary TB may have weight loss, fever (with an evening rise) and night sweats, along with symptoms of an organ affection. For example, swelling and pus discharge may be observed in a lymph node TB. Headache, neck stiffness and mental confusion may occur in brain or meningeal TB. Symptoms may similarly develop in the tubercular affection of various sites such as pleura, pericardium, intestine, kidney, bone, joint, etc. and investigations therefore need to be conducted accordingly to prove or disprove the diagnosis.

Patients with extrapulmonary TB having pulmonary symptoms of any duration should have three sputum samples examined. The finding of a positive sputum may greatly help to confirm the diagnosis of TB in that individual. Contacts of a smear positive TB must be examined for the presence of disease, in case, they have any of the above mentioned symptoms.

Sputum Collection

Following points need to be considered with regard to the collection of sputum:

1. It is important for a health worker to explain to the patient reasons for sputum examination, prior to the actual collection of sputum.
2. The patient is given a sputum container with a laboratory serial number mentioned on it.
3. The opening and closing of container is properly demonstrated to the patient.
4. The sputum collection is done in an open space away from people.
5. The method of bringing out sputum consists of two to three deep inhalations with an open mouth followed by deep coughing from the chest. The sputum, so obtained by this method is spit into the container, which is then closed with a lid.
6. At least three sputum specimens (spot-early morning-spot) should be collected for microscopic examination in a suspected case of pulmonary TB, ideally within 2 days. The first sputum specimen obtained in front of a health worker is called 'spot specimen'. Thereafter, another sputum container with laboratory serial number written on its external surface is given to the patient for collection of an early morning specimen of the next day. The patient returns with this specimen to the health center and gives a second spot specimen in a different container under the supervision of a staff member.
7. Only one laboratory form need to be filled for all the three sputum specimens collected from patient. The MO generally completes top half of this form, while the results section is filled by LT. The sputum results are reported within 1 day.

Sputum Transportation

If sputum is collected at the microscopy center, transportation is not needed. In case, the center is not being equipped with microscopy, there is a need for the sputum container to be transported to another center with such laboratory facilities. The health worker should put patient's sputum specimens and the laboratory form into a special box, if transportation is being considered immediately. In case of delay, they should be stored in a refrigerator. In general, a specimen should be sent to the laboratory as soon as possible and definitely within a week. However, it should still be examined, even if, received after a week, since the dead bacilli may still be visible on a slide. If the samples of a large number of patients are being transported together in a box, they should be accompanied by their respective laboratory forms and a separate dispatch list of these patients. After taking out the sputum specimen, container must be destroyed.

Diagnosis and Management

On receiving the results section of a laboratory form for sputum examination, an MO would proceed in the following manner:

1. If at least two out of three sputum specimens are positive for AFB, the patient is classified as smear positive and put on appropriate treatment. A thorough education is given about the various aspects of disease, its

mechanism of spread, the treatment being instituted and the need for regular follow-up sputum smear examinations. Treatment details should clearly consist of the required frequency of its administration, the associated unpleasant effects, the treatment duration and the possible occurrence of a drug resistant TB in case of default. It is important to trace the patient contacts and the drug defaulters to put them back on treatment.

2. If one specimen is smear positive for AFB, the patient is referred to MO for an X-ray examination. In case, the radiographic abnormalities determined by them are consistent with active pulmonary TB, the patient is diagnosed as having smear positive TB and put on appropriate treatment. The physician should educate a patient about the disease, the treatment needed for cure and the need for regular sputum smear examinations during follow-up. A responsibility of the contact tracing and the defaulter action also lies with the MO.

3. If all three sputum specimens are negative, the patient gets examined by an MO. If symptoms persist despite giving antibiotics for 1–2 weeks, an X-ray examination is done. In case, the radiographic abnormalities are consistent with active pulmonary TB and the MO decides to treat with antituberculosis treatment (ATT), the patient is diagnosed as having smear negative TB. An appropriate treatment is started and health education imparted to the patient. Various categories of TB cases and their treatment regimens under the RNTCP are specified in Table 28.4. Drug dosages as recommended under RNTCP are mentioned in Table 28.5.

Following the categorization of TB cases, their TB treatment and identity cards are prepared. The entries are done in TB register and TB numbers allotted. The DOT center that is most easily accessible to each case is decided in consultation with him/her. The health education and patient's motivation forming an integral part of program are reinforced prior to the start of therapy and during the subsequent follow-up visits as well.

Drug administration to the patient occurs according to his/her categorization. The treatment in category I consists of an intensive phase of isoniazid (H), rifampicin (R), pyrazinamide (Z) and ethambutol (E) administered under direct supervision thrice weekly on alternate days for 2 months (24 dosage) followed by the continuation phase of H and R thrice weekly on alternate days for 4 months (18 week, 54 dosage) 'appropriately supervised', with first dose of each week given under direct supervision and the patient self-administering next two doses of the week at home. The intensive phase of category II, consisting of streptomycin (S), H, R, Z and E for 2 months followed by 1 month of H, R, Z and E (total 36 dosage) is administered in the same supervised manner as category I. It is followed by an appropriately supervised continuation phase consisting of 5 months (22 week, 66 dosage) of H, R and E. Category III treatment is similar to that of category I, but is executed without an inclusion of ethambutol. For the convenience sake, drugs are dispensed in category wise boxes made at the start of therapy itself. Each box contains drugs in different blister packs. The pack for an intensive phase consists of 1 day medication, while that for the continuation phase contains 1 week's supply.

Table 28.4: Categories of tuberculosis cases and treatment regimens under Revised National TB Control Program (RNTCP)

Categories	Tuberculosis (TB) cases	Treatment regimens	
		Intensive phase	Continuation phase
Category I	New sputum smear positive *Seriously smear negative Seriously ill extrapulmonary	$2^{\dagger}$ (HEZE)$_3$*	4 (HR)$_3$
Category II	Relapse Failure Treatment after default Others	2 (SHREZ)$_3$ Followed by 1 (HRZE)$_3$	5 (HRE)$_3$
Category III	Sputum smear negative Not seriously ill extrapulmonary	2 (HRZ)$_3$	4 (HR)$_3$

*Various definitions under RNTCP may be referred; †A prefix denotes the number of months and the subscript indicates thrice in a week.
Note: H, isoniazid; R, rifampicin; Z, pyrazinamide; E, ethambuto; S, streptomycin.

Table 28.5: Recommended drug dosages under Revised National TB Control Program

Drugs	Dose in mg (thrice a week)	Dose in mg/kg body weight in children (thrice a week)
Isoniazid	600	10–15
Rifampicin	450*	10
Pyrazinamide	1,500	35
Ethambutol†	1,200	30
Streptomycin	750‡	15

*Patients weighing > 60 kg are given an additional 150 mg of rifampicin
†Ethambutol is not given to children < 6 years of age
‡Patients > 50 years of age or weighing < 30 kg are given 500 mg of streptomycin

A patient receives the first dose of medication at the place of diagnosis (DTC/CHC/PHC). Patients' house is visited by the health staff for confirming the address, tracing the contacts and motivating the patient within the 1st week of treatment. The drug administration days are fixed for a particular patient and either Monday, Wednesday, Friday or Tuesday, Thursday, Saturday schedule is followed. If the patient 'misses' a dose during an intensive phase, he/she must be contacted within 1 day of missing the same, so that the missed dose can be administered on the next day. In continuation phase, patients' should be contacted within a week of missing the weekly collection of drugs. Sometimes, a patient is unable to collect medicines from the center located at a place distant from the house.

Reasons for the same may be many, e.g. the loss of job hours, medical disabilities, social beliefs and so on. In such cases, the services of peripheral health workers, who may be either MPWs, anganwadi workers or VHGs are utilized in the delivery of drugs. Both the patient and the peripheral health worker (PHW) may agree on a mutually convenient location for a drug collection/administration. The PHW maintains record of patient's treatment on a duplicate 'treatment card' and collects the medicine box for entire treatment duration from the MO. The MO motivates the patient regularly and refers him/her to the center for sputum microscopy on due dates. A referral to the MO may become necessary, if there is development of drug reaction or intolerance. Occasionally, a home delivery of the drugs may be warranted and carried out through the system of PHWs.

A specialized model exists in certain metropolitan cities, where diagnosis is done in chest clinics. The patient categorization is followed by registration, allotment of TB number and preparation of treatment and identification cards. Thereafter, patient is referred to the area treatment center for DOT, where his/her record is maintained until treatment is completed. A Tuberculosis Health Visitor (TBHV) visits patients' house, motivates toward treatment adherence and gives the first dose. The subsequent dosages are administered during visits to the center on due dates. In case of difficulties in drug collection, the services of community volunteers are utilized in the same way as in a 'general' model. The TBHV retrieves defaulters, refers the patient to MO (in case of drug reaction or intolerance) and provides the health education in manner similar to the staff of 'general' model.

Both the 'general' and 'special' models follow similar patterns in continuation phases of treatment. The 1st weekly dose administered is directly supervised and the next two doses of the week are supplied to patients on the presentation of empty blister pack of the previous week.

Follow-up

As in the diagnosis of pulmonary TB, sputum examination remains method of choice in the follow-up as well. Two specimens are examined at specified treatment intervals. A schedule for the category wise follow-up sputum examinations and therefore, the continuation phase of treatment institution is mentioned in Table 28.6.

Results must be available by the end of intensive phase. For example, a category I patient, who is given a sputum container at the time of 22nd dose, brings an early morning specimen to center at the time of receiving 23rd dose and simultaneously also gives a spot specimen. The results of both sputum examinations are available, when patient turns up to take the 24th dose (which is also the time for switchover of the intensive phase). Thus, the decision regarding treatment to either continue the intensive phase for 1 month more (in case of a positive result) or change to the continuation phase (in case of a negative result) becomes quite easy. Similar, procedure is adopted at the end of treatment as well. All results of the follow-up sputum smear examinations should be recorded on the TB treatment card.

Administration of drugs in the intensive phase on a particular day of the month is recorded on front page of the TB treatment card by ticking (✓) under the 'day' column. In the continuation phase (which is recorded on back page of the treatment card), an 'X' is entered on the day (1–31). Drugs were swallowed under direct observation and a horizontal line (-) is drawn through remaining days of the week to indicate the number of days for which supply was given. A 'missed' entry is indicated by encircling (0) the column. A recording of 'missed' drug entries. Reasons for missing the dose and actions taken to return the patient to treatment should be recorded in the remarks column of TB treatment card.

Table 28.6: Schedule of follow-up sputum examinations

Category	Index	Follow-up
Category I +2	−	Start continuation phase, test sputum again at 4 and 6 month
	+	Continue intensive phase for 1 month, test sputum again at 3, 5 and 7 month
+2	−	Start continuation phase, test sputum again at 6 month
	+	Continue intensive phase for 1 more month, test sputum again at 3, 5 and 7 month
Category II +3	−	Start continuation phase, test sputum again at 5 and 8 month
	+	Continue intensive phase for 1 more month, test sputum again at 4, 6 and 9 month
Category III −2	+	Start continuation phase, test sputum again at 4 and 6 month
	+	Register the patient and begin category II treatment Any patient treated with category I or catergory III, who has a positive smear at 5, 6 or 7 month of treatment should be considered a failure started on category II treatment a fresh

Table 28.7: Symptom-based approach to evaluation of possible side effects of antituberculosis treatment (ATT) used in Revised National TB Control Program (RNTCP)

Symptoms	Drugs	Action to be taken
Gastrointestinal upset	Any oral medication	Reassure patient, give drugs with less water; give drugs over a longer period of time (e.g. 20 minute); do not give drugs on empty stomach; if the above fails, give antiemetic if appropriate
Itching	Isoniazid (H) (other drugs also)	Reserve patients if severe, stop all drugs and refer patient to Medical Officer (MO)
Burning in the hands and feet	Isoniazid	Give pyridoxine 100 mg/day unit symptoms subside
Joint pains	Pyrazinamide (Z)	If severe, refer patient for evaluation
Impaired vision	Ethambutol (E)	Stop ethambutol, refer patient for evaluation
Ringing in the ears	Streptomycin (S)	Stop streptomycin, refer patient for evaluation
Dizziness and loss of balance	Streptomycin	Stop treatment, refer patient for evaluation
Jaundice	Isoniazid (H) Rifampicin (R) Pyrazinamide (Z)	Stop treatment, refer patient for evaluation

At all times in subsequent visits, the communication is done with patients to ensure a regular and correct drug intake to provide remedial measures in case of minor unpleasant drug effects (Table 28.7), to motivate them for treatment adherence and to provide them health education. Management of patients, who interrupt their treatment depends upon the category to which they belong. Patients who are smear negative at diagnosis and interrupt their treatment should be managed as per the protocol. Treatment interruptions of category I and II patients should be dealt, as mentioned underneath in Tables 28.8 and 28.9 respectively. Follow-up is not required for a patient, who has completed treatment and has been declared cured. He/She should be advised to report only if symptoms suggestive of TB recur.

Generally, patients with TB do not need hospitalization. Only extremely ill patients (during the initial phase of treatment) and those having significant hemoptysis, pneumothorax or large pleural effusions should be hospitalized.

While considering special situations, the patients of TB meningitis should be put on early treatment generally in a hospital. Their continuation phases should be carried for 6–7 months (making the total of 8–9 months treatment). Steroids should be given initially to reduce meningeal inflammation and thereafter reduced gradually over 6–8 weeks. During pregnancy, streptomycin should be avoided, while other drugs used in RNTCP are safe. Breastfeeding should be continued regardless of the mother's TB status. In the presence of renal disease; H, R and Z are relatively safe for administration, while S and E are avoided. The vice versa occurs in liver disease, i.e. S and E are considered to be safe, whereas H, R and Z should be stopped. Perform symptom-based approach to evaluate the possible effects (refer Table 28.5).

Preventive Treatment to Children under 6 Years

Children under 6 years of age having a family member of smear-positive TB should be screened for symptoms. If the child has TB symptoms, an MO determines the presence of disease, preferably, in consultation with a pediatrician. A full course of ATT (category III) should be administered to patients'. But, if TB symptoms are not detected, patient should receive preventive chemotherapy (INH 5 mg/kg body weight daily) for 6 months regardless of the BCG vaccination. In case, a tuberculin test is available, it is done after 3 months of preventive chemotherapy. Induration > 6 mm in diameter justifies the need for INH preventive chemotherapy for another 3 months. On the other hand, if it is < 6 mm in diameter. The INH is stopped and BCG vaccination is given (if patient had not received it earlier).

Challenges and Solutions in Implementation

Major challenges that stand in the RNTCP implementation are mentioned below.

Expansion: The country is experiencing a rapid expansion of the RNTCP from early 1999 onwards and has the second largest such program in the world. Although, the overall cure rate achieved in country for the new smear-positive patients stand at around 80%, it is still below the targeted cure rate of 85%. The default rate at many centers continues to be high. Further, the targets have been set to cover four-fifth population of the country by 2004 and the entire country as soon as feasible. An achievement of these goals require a sustained flow of financial and logistic support, and therefore, a high degree of political will at all the times is essential.

Private sector involvement: Nearly 80% of all the qualified doctors, 75% of dispensaries and 60% of hospitals in the country are in private sector. About 80% of patients seek medical attentions from private practitioners for the reasons such as convenient working hours (and easy accessibility), anticipation of better physician attentions, maintenance of confidentiality and an accountability.

Practitioners have largely relied upon the chest skiagram for diagnosis of pulmonary TB (than the sputum microscopy). Further, non-standard regimens are widely prescribed (more so by the quacks). There are no mechanisms in the private setups to ensure defaulter retrievals. Standards of record keeping at the private centers are below the mark. Thus, for assuring the success of RNTCP, it is important to bring the private sector in purview of program. However, it requires gigantic efforts and poses a big challenge to the program implementation, since it needs to be carried out in such a manner that the practitioners not only update themselves about the intermittent DOTS regimens and provide a whole-hearted cooperation in their institution but also do not incur losses in their earnings. Perhaps, it may also require to give them incentives in whatever forms possible. Efforts are already on to develop the models for private sector involvement in DOTS program at various places in the country. Depending upon the results, guidelines may be forthcoming.

Information, education and communication and health education: Religious practices of people such as, the Muslims keeping fasts during Roza days and the Hindus during festivals or on particular days of a week hinder the drug administration to them. At times, the patients are allured into accepting either the nonallopathic, the traditional or the untraditional systems of medicine by the elderly of society. Association of diseases such as chronic obstructive pulmonary disease, etc. continues their symptoms even after the administration of effective ATT, which forces patients to heed to inadvertent advices. Hence, active information, education and communication (IEC) campaigns and health education are necessary to remove superstitions prevalent in the society and bring more and more number of people suffering from TB into mainstream of the program.

Multiplicity of programs: Existence of multiple health programs at a time perplexes the treatment providers. For example, within an institution, all three modes of ATT delivery conventional regimens, daily SCC and DOTS may be operating and even overlapping in a patient. Thus, uniform practices need to be involved in the health programs.

Migratory population: It may constitute about 20–25% of the population in large cities. Difficulties may be experienced in getting it registered under the RNTCP. Policies need to be formulated in respect of this group.

Social stigma: The prevalence of social stigma of TB has led to patient isolations in the past. Although, the concept has been largely done away with notions still prevail in the minds of people that restrict them to accept the TB patients in a way similar to the other diseases. To remove the social stigma attached to TB, an appropriate IEC campaign may be organized often and the subject may be included in the basic school curriculum.

Integration: In a rural setup, it has been observed that the same staff is executing multiple national programs related to the diseases such as malaria, polio, etc. Priorities need to be instituted in respect of the TB control program in minds of the health staff and doctors, so that RNTCP takes a higher status of execution from the present level in comparison to the other diseases of national interest.

Involvement of medical colleges: Initial reservations, expressed by the medical college community in regard to the RNTCP policies were found to exist due to an inadequate communication about the program. Hence, the medical college fraternity needs to be integrally involved in the implementation of DOTS at the national level.

Multidrug resistant TB: The RNTCP as yet does not have much to offer to the chronic cases of multidrug resistant

(MDR) TB, who would otherwise require a prolonged treatment with the costly and toxic second-line drugs. However, efforts are on to introduce the 'DOTS plus' therapy. The relevant subject has been dealt in greater detail in the following section.

Nursing Management in Tuberculosis

In addition to the actual patient care, the nurse handling TB patients must become a public health educator. The patient is usually shocked when first informed he/she has TB. Printed instructions and literature on the disease are given to the patients. It is the nurse, however, who must assist patient in maintaining morale and educate in personal hygiene, never losing sight of the fact that preventing the spread of the disease to other members of the family and community is of the utmost importance. Nurse impresses the patient and his/her family with the necessity of controlling the spread of TB. Unless the complete cooperation of the patient and family is secured efforts of doctor, nurse and modern approach to therapy become valueless. Periodically, films of an educational nature produced by the National Tuberculosis Association are shown.

Tuberculosis Technique

For the nurse, wears gown when doing any bedside nursing. This includes medications and treatments or whenever handling any contaminated or soiled material, or supplies. Do not wear gowns in clean areas. Be sure that the gown completely covers the uniform. See that the gown is in good condition. If the gown needs mending, place it in a container for repair. Do not wear it, do not return it to the gown shelf and do not place it in the soiled linen container unless contaminated. Discard the gown promptly whenever it becomes grossly contaminated or soiled. If several patients are to be taken care of while wearing the same gown, go from the closed case to those with positive sputum, never the reverse. When this procedure for care cannot be followed, the gown must be changed between patients. Nurses and attendants caring for TB patients should keep their bodies in optimum condition at all times. They should have an X-ray of the chest taken every 6 months, and they certainly should observe the tenets of the medical aseptic technique.

Masks

Nurses ordinarily mask whenever working directly with TB patients. The mask must be put on with uncontaminated hands and adjusted for comfort. It should never be touched until removed and the hands should be cleaned before removing it. The nose as well as the mouth must be covered. After removing it from its container with forceps, handle the mask only by the strings. The mask should be changed whenever it becomes damp as it is practically worthless as far as protection is concerned, once it is wet through. Masks should be changed possibly every 45 minutes to hour in some instances more often. The face must be washed before touching the mask.

For the Patient

Upon meeting the patient for the first time, the nurse should introduce herself/himself, inquire as to the patient's comfort and encourage patients to express themself, listening attentively. As diplomatically as possible ascertain, if the patient knows that he/she has TB; if not, considerable tact must be used in acquainting patients' with this definite diagnosis. This is a good time to bring out the part that patients' may be able to play in expediting his/her own recovery. Explain the importance of freedom from worry, bedrest, plain wholesome food, good personal hygiene and the part of patient can play in preventing the spread of the disease. Also explain the patients' about the hospital policies regarding visiting days, special visitors, the rest period, the articles he/she may have at his/her bedside, library service, smoking rules, ward schedules and very important, the mail service. Find out about patients' previous instruction and knowledge regarding TB and the technique of control. Inform patients' that TB is a communicable disease, but it is also a preventable and a curable one. Teach patients' that it can be transmitted directly or indirectly from person to person through contact and by droplet infection such as kissing, sneezing and coughing. Also point out the role that indirect contact plays. Show him/her, how to cover the mouth and nose with at least three thicknesses of tissue when coughing or sneezing or during examination by the doctor or during the bedside care by the nurse. Teach the patient to crush the paper and deposit it in the paper bag at the side of the bed immediately after use. Instruct the patient to expectorate directly into the sputum cup and nowhere else holding the tissue at the side of the mouth, while expectorating and bringing the cup close to the mouth, the lid of the cup to be replaced immediately and kept closed. Explain to the patient, why this is done and impress upon patients its importance. Then have the patient demonstrate their ability to follow the directions.

SEVERE ACUTE RESPIRATORY SYNDROME

There are several communicable diseases that cause mortality and morbidity in the people. Those communicable diseases may be bacterial, viral, fungal and zoonotic diseases, etc. Some of the diseases exist throughout the year in the community, whereas some diseases outbreak occurs in a particular period and threatens the community. Severe acute respiratory syndrome (SARS) is one of the communicable diseases, which draw the attention of the world in the year 2002–2003.

The SARS is a communicable viral disease caused by a new strain of coronavirus, which differs considerably in genetic structure from previous recognized 'coronavirus (CoV)'.

Toward the tail end of 2002, a new syndrome emerged in Southern China. It was named as SARS. The initial outbreak in April 2003. By June 2003, there had been 8,000 cases worldwide and 775 deaths.

The SARS is caused by a novel CoV. It does not appear to be related with three known classes of CoV. It is hypothesized on the basis of available data that animal virus, recently mutated and developed the ability to productively man. Groups 1 and 2 contain mammalian virus, while group 3 contains avian virus. SARS CoV defines 4th class of CoV and it exhibits following features:

1. It has 29, 727 nucleotides in length.
2. It has nine open reading frames that are not found in other CoV and may code for proteins, which are unique to SARS virus.
3. It is large, enveloped having positive stranded (27–30 kb) and may cause respiratory and enteric diseases in man and animal.
4. Its genome is largest found in any RNA virus.
5. Human CoVs are found both in group I (H CoV-229E) and group II (H CoV-OC 43) and are responsible for 30% mild respiratory tract infection (Fig. 28.17).

Magnitude of the Problem

The earliest case was traced to a health worker in China in late 2002 with rapid spread in Hong Kong, Singapore, Vietnam, Taiwan and Toronto. As of early August 2003, about 8,422 cases were reported to the WHO from 30 countries with 916 fatalities. The skeletal report of SARS (Table 28.8) cases with onset of illness from 1st November 2002 to 31st July 2003 are as detailed below.

In May 2005, the disease itself was declared 'eradicated' by the WHO and it became a second disease in mankind to receive this label. The New York Times reported that 'not a single case of severe acute respiratory syndrome' has been reported in late 2004.

Table 28.8: Skeletal report [Severe acute respiratory syndrome (SARS)]

Sl No.	Countries	Cases	Deaths	Fatality %
1.	People's Republic of China	5,327	349	6.6
2.	Hong Kong	1,755	299	17
3.	Canada	432	44	17
4.	Taiwan	34.6	37	11
5.	Singapore	238	33	14
6.	Vietnam	63	5	8
7.	United States of America	27	0	0
8.	Philippines	14	2	14
9.	Thailand	9	2	22
10	India	4	0	0

Epidemiological Factors

Agent Factor

Agent is a new strain or coronavirus (SARS CoV). Initially, electron microscopic examination in Hong Kong and Germany found viral particles with structures suggesting paramyxovirus in respiratory secretions of SARS patients. Subsequently in Canada, electron microscopic examination found viral particles with structures suggestive of metapneumovirus (a subtype of paramyxovirus) in respiratory secretions. Chinese researches also reported that a chlamydia-like disease might be behind SARS.

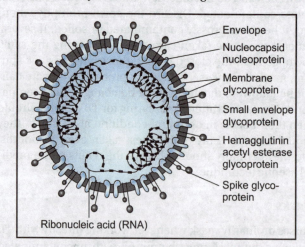

Figure 28.17: Severe acute respiratory syndrome (SARS)-associated coronavirus

The Pasteur Institute in Paris identified CoV in samples taken from six patients. The SARS virus can survive for hours on common surfaces outside the human body and up to 24 hours in human waste. The virus can survive at least for 24 hours on a plastic surface at room temperature and can live for contended periods in cold (Fig. 28.18).

Source of Infection

Respiratory secretions of the case are most infectious. Maximum virus excretion from the respiratory tract occurs on about 10 days of illness and then decreases.

Host Factors

1. Age: Children are rarely affected by SARS, most commonly in adults and aged.
2. Sex: Both sexes are equally affected.

Environmental Factors

The SARS can occur in any season; crowded areas and unhygienic conditions are the high-risk factors, where it can spread easily.

Incubation Period

The incubation period has been estimated to be 2–7 days, commonly 3–5 days.

Mode of Transmission

Mode of transmission is through close contact with the patient and infected material via the eyes, nose and mouth with infections respiratory droplets. Disease transmission is currently not well understood. It is suspected to spread via inhalation and droplets expelled by an infected person, where coughing and sneezing or possibly via contact with secretions on objects. In Hong Kong, the study shows that sewage, feces and cockroaches are suspected transmitters.

Pathophysiology

Pathophysiology description is based on autopsies of eight fatal cases of SARS from Tan Tock Seng Hospital, Singapore. In those individuals with severe disease resulting in death. Transmission is through exposure to infected respiratory droplets during close person-to-person contact and infected fomites. SARS is shed not only in respiratory secretions but also in feces and other bodily fluids as well:

1. The predominant pathology in the lung was diffuse alveolar damage (DAD) in varying phases of organization.
2. In these cases, scattered type II pneumocytes showed marked cytologic changes including multinucleation, cytomegaly, nucleomegaly, clearing of nuclear chromatin and prominent nucleoli. Although these changes were severe, they are within the spectrum of epithelial changes seen in other cases of DAD. Definite viral inclusions were not seen.
3. The DAD is a pattern of acute lung injury characterized in the acute phase by hyaline membranes (photomicrograph left), interstitial and intra-alveolar edema, patchy type II pneumocyte hyperplasia, microthrombi, and scant interstitial infiltrates of mononuclear cells.
4. The acute phase forms a continuum with the proliferative or organizing phase in which proliferation of interstitial fibroblasts and prominent type II pneumocyte hyperplasia are the gold standard hallmarks. The histological correlate of acute respiratory distress syndrome (CARDS), DAD has numerous possible causes including infections, inhalants, ingestants, drugs, shock and sepsis.

Clinical Manifestations

Initial symptoms are flue-like and mimic asthma symptoms and may include:
- Fever sudden in onset and above 38°C
- Chills and shivering
- Myalgia
- Lethargy
- Dry cough
- Sore throat
- Headache, running nose, dizziness and gastrointestinal symptoms.

Later on patient develops:
- Shortness of breath
- Tachypnea
- Rales or auscultation
- In some cases, there is rapid deterioration with low oxygen saturation and acute respiratory distress requiring ventilatory support.

Investigations

1. Chest X-ray: Findings typically begin with a small, unilateral, patchy shadowing and progress over 1–2 days to become bacterial and generalized with interstitial infiltration.
2. Blood for total count (TC) and differential count (DC) shows white blood cell (WBC) and platelet counts are often low is neutrophilia and lymphopenia.
3. Enzyme test shows:

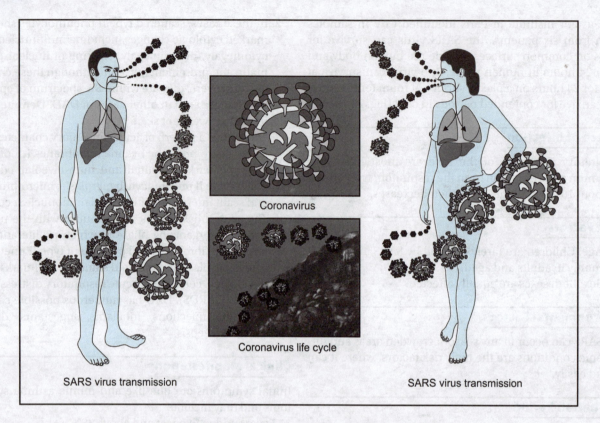

Figure 28.18: Severe acute respiratory syndrome (SARS)

- Increased lactate dehydrogenase (LDH)
- Increased creatinine kinase (CK)
- Increased C-reactive protein (CRP).

Other tests are:
- Enzyme-linked immunosorbent assay (ELISA) test detects antibodies only after 21 days after the onset of symptoms
- Immunofluorescence assay can detect antibodies 10 days after the onset of disease
- Polymerase chain reaction (PCR) test that can detect genetic material of the SARS virus.

Case Detection

By clinical features, which is as follows:
1. Suspected case:
   a. A person presenting after November 1, 2002 with history of:
      - High fever (> 38°C)
      - Cough or breathing difficulty and one or more of the following exposures during 10 days prior to onset of symptoms
      - Close contact with a person, who is a suspect or probable case of SARS
      - History of travel to a SARS affected area
      - Residing in an affected area.
   b. A person with an unexplained acute respiratory illness resulting in death after 1st November 2002, but on when an autopsy has been performed and one or more of the following exposures during 10 days prior to onset of symptoms:
      - Close contact with a person, who is a suspect or probable case of SARS
      - History of travel to an affected area or residing in an affected area.
2. Probable case:
   a. A suspect case with radiological evidence and infiltrate consistent with pneumonia or respiratory distress syndrome (RDS) on chest X-ray.
   b. A suspect case with autopsy finding consistent with the pathology RDS of without an identifiable cause:
      - Treatment and management
      - Medical management
      - There is no specific treatment for SARS, antibiotics are ineffective
      - Supportive treatment with antipyretics
      - Steroids

- The antiviral agent ribavirin given IV in combination with high dose of corticosteroids may have been responsible for some clinical management
- Supplement oxygen and ventilator support may be needed.

Prevention

The preventive measures for SARS control are appropriate detection and protective measures that include:
- Prompt identification of persons with SARS, their movements and contacts
- Effective isolation of SARS patients in hospital preferably in negative pressure rooms and effective barrier nursing precautions must be taken
- Appropriate protection of medical staff treating these patients
- Comprehensive identification and isolation of suspected SARS cases
- Exist screening of international travelers in all airports and shipping ports
- Timely and accurate reporting and sharing of information with other authorities and/or government.

Nursing Management

Isolation of Cases

- Identify the risk population and notification in further investigation
- Check the vital sign, temperature, pulse and respiration (TPR) every 4th hourly
- Follow hypothermic measures to control the fever
- Administer antipyretics and other drugs as per prescription
- Keep ready ventilators for emergency use
- Support the patient and family with explanation
- To be all personal precautionary measures treating the cases.

Health Education

- Education regarding preventive measures
- Advise to hold handkerchief, while coughing, sneezing and laughing
- Advise about sanitary measures
- Educate about high nutrition, which is easily digestible.

AVIAN FLU

The deaths of two young boys in Vietnam were overshadowed by the disastrous Tsunami (2004) that swept across the Indian Ocean. But the boys' death, from a strain of influenza known as influenza A (H5N1) or more simply 'bird flu' could herald a far greater loss of life. In 1918, a pandemic of flu swept the world killing more than 20 million people and many infectious disease experts now believe that another flu pandemic could be imminent. The appearance in humans of a type of flu, which normally only affects birds maybe an important sign that some strains of the virus are changing in way that could threaten people around the globe.

Avian influenza or 'bird flu' is an infectious disease of animals (usually birds and less commonly pigs) caused by type A strains of the influenza virus H5N1 infection may follow an unusually aggressive clinical course with rapid deterioration and high fatality.

Transmission to humans is rare, but there is recent cause for concern. In mid 2003, the largest and most severe avian flu outbreak in history began in Southeast Asia caused by a subtype of the virus called H5N1 and resulting in widespread transmission to poultry and some documented transmission to humans. Transmission of H5N1 to humans is of particular concern, because it mutates rapidly and may therefore change into a form that is highly infectious for humans and more easily spread. In addition, unlike normal seasonal influenza, H5N1 can cause severe disease in humans.

Global

Outbreaks of avian influenza H5N1 occurred among poultry in eight countries in Asia (Cambodia, China, Indonesia, Japan, Laos, South Korea, Thailand and Vietnam). The most number of cases occurred in Vietnam is 93 during late 2003 and early 2004. At that time, more than 100 million birds in the affected countries either died from the disease or were killed in order to try to control the outbreaks. By March 2004, the outbreak was reported to be under control. Since, late June 2004 however, several countries in Asia such as China, Indonesia, Thailand, Russia, Vietnam and Malaysia reported new outbreaks of influenza H5N1 among poultry.

As of July 2006, over 232 human cases have been reported in major part of Southeast Asia; among them, the maximum number of cases was reported from Vietnam, i.e. 93 followed by 54 cases in Iran and 23 cases in Thailand. Egypt reported 14 cases of bird flu. Of the few avian influenza viruses that have crossed the species barrier to infect humans, H5N1 virus has caused the largest number of reported cases of severe disease and death in humans. In the current situation in Asia, more than half of the people infected with the virus have died. Most cases have occurred in previously healthy children and young adults.

However, it is possible that the only cases currently being reported are those in the most severely ill people and that the full range of illness caused by the H5N1 virus has not yet been defined.

India

On 18 February 2006, agricultural authorities in India confirmed the country's first outbreak of highly pathogenic H5N1 avian influenza in poultry. The disease was first detected at several commercial farms in the Navapur subdistrict in the western state of Maharashtra. The government has equipped a Navapur hospital for the management of isolation of possible human cases. WHO was informed that 12 patients with fever and respiratory illness in Navapur subdistrict have been hospitalized for observation as a precautionary measure. However, as of July 2006 statistics in India, there were no human cases of bird flu reported.

Epidemiological Features

Agent

Avian influenza virus usually refers to influenza. Viruses are found chiefly in birds, but infections can occur in humans, the few avian influenza viruses that have crossed tile species barrier to infect humans, H5N1 has caused the largest number of cases of severe disease and death in humans. Unlike normal seasonal influenza, where infection causes only mild respiratory symptoms in most people, the disease caused by H5N1 follows an unusually aggressive clinical course will rapid deterioration high fatality (Fig. 28.19).

All influenza viruses are divided into three types such as A, B or C depending on the virus structure. Type 'A' responsible for lethal influenza pandemics, whereas type B causes smaller, localized outbreaks. Less common and more stable than other strains, type C has milder symptoms. Influenza B and C are usually found only in humans. But type A influenza infects both people and animals including birds, pigs, horses, whales and seals. Influenza A viruses are divided into subtypes based on two surface proteins:

1. Hemagglutinin (HA).
2. Neuraminidase (NA).

Nearly 15 distinct HA subtypes and nine NA subtypes exist, but they can combine to form a number of other subtypes, some of which normally are specific to a single species. For example, subtypes H1N1, H1N2 and H1N3 usually cause influenza in humans, whereas H7N7 and H3N8 viruses cause disease in horses. At least, 15 flu subtypes affect birds, the most virulent of which is H5N1. Until recently, avian subtypes have rarely been found in humans or in animals other than pigs.

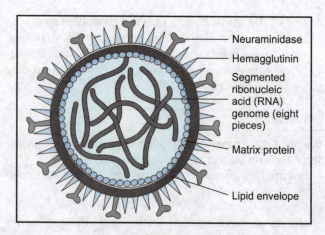

Figure 28.19: Influenza virus

Host

Influenza A viruses naturally occur in wild birds. Although, these birds are not affected by the virus, domestic poultry such as chickens and turkeys may be affected. So far, bird flu is hard for humans to contract, but health officials warn a major flu outbreak could occur in the virus mutates into a form that can spread easily from person to person. The grimmest scenario would be global epidemic to rival the flu pandemic of 1918 and 1919, which claimed millions of lives worldwide.

Age

The pattern of human transmission remains mysterious. Young children seem especially vulnerable to the virus, although some experts note that children are more likely to have contact with sick birds or to play on ground contaminated with droppings as well as, people of all ages have contracted with died of bird flu. At this point, too few people have been infected to know all the possible risk factors for bird flu.

Risk Factors

The two main risks for human health from avian influenza are:

1. The risk of direct infection when the virus passes from the infected bird to humans, sometimes resulting in severe disease.
2. The other risk is that the virus if given enough opportunities will change into a form that is highly infectious for humans and spreads easily from person to person.

Environmental Factors

An attack of influenza is usually seen during winter season. Though it can occur at any time of the year.

Modes of Transmission

Migratory waterfowl and ducks in particular carry the viruses that cause bird flu. Often unaffected themselves, the host birds can spread the infection to susceptible species, especially domesticated chickens, turkeys and geese resulting in severe epidemics that sicken and kill large number of birds sometimes in a single day.

Avian viruses generally do not affect humans, but in 1997, an outbreak of bird flu in Hong Kong infected 18 people, six of whom died. Since, human cases of bird flu have been reported in Asia, Europe and the Middle East. Most were traced to contact with infected poultry or surfaces contaminated by sick birds.

The genetic scrambling that occurs in antigenic shift explains how a disease that normally affects a bird or animal can suddenly turn up in humans. Often, flu viruses that cross the species barrier, originate in areas where people live in close proximity to chickens and pigs. Because pigs are susceptible to infection with both avian and human viruses and so are an ideal 'mixing bowl' for genes.

But at least some bird flu viruses do not need a third party, instead, they shuffle and rearrange their genetic directly in humans, which seems to be the case in most instances of human-acquired bird flu, people after direct contact with infected birds or contaminated surfaces, not from contact with other animals.

Direct Bird-to-human Transmission

Wild birds shed the virus: Infected migratory waterfowl, the natural carriers of bird flu viruses, shed the virus in their droppings, saliva and nasal secretions.

Virus spreads to domesticated birds: Domestic poultry become infected from contact with these birds or with contaminated water, feed or soil. They may also catch the disease, the same way humans contact conventional flu by inhaling the airborne virus. Bird flu spreads quickly and lethally within a domestic flock and is inadvertently transported from farm to farm on tractors and other equipment, on cages and on workers' shoes and clothing. Heat destroys the virus, but it can survive for extended periods in cool temperatures.

Markets provide pathways to humans: Open air markets, where eggs and birds are often sold in crowded and unsanitary conditions are hotbeds of infection and spread the disease into the wider community. Cock fighting, rampant throughout much of Asia, has also been implicated in the spread of bird flu fighting roosters are often trucked long distances and smuggled across borders. At any point along the way, humans may pick up the virus through close contact with sick birds or contaminated surfaces. An ailing bird can shed the virus in its feathers as well as in droppings and some people have contracted bird flu simply by touching an infected chicken or fighting rooster.

Human influenza is transmitted by inhalation of infectious droplets and droplet nuclei by direct contact, and perhaps by indirect (fomite) contact with self-inoculation onto the upper respiratory tract or conjunctival mucosa. The relative efficiency of the different routes of transmission has not been defined. For human H5N1 infections, evidence is consistent with bird to human, possibly environment to human and limited, non-sustained human-to-human transmission to date.

Animal-to-human Transmission

In 1997, exposure to live poultry within a week before the onset of illness was associated with disease in humans, whereas there was no significant risk related to eating or preparing poultry products, or exposure to persons with H5N1 disease. Exposure to ill poultry and butchering of birds were associated with seropositivity for influenza A (H5N1); although, not those who were involved in mass culling of poultry. Plucking and preparing of diseased birds, handling fighting cocks, playing with poultry, particularly asymptomatic infected ducks and consumption of duck's blood or possibly undercooked poultry have all been implicated.

Human-to-human transmission of H5N1 has been suggested in several household clusters and in one case of apparent child-to-mother transmission. Intimate contact without the use of precautions was implicated and nine for no case of human-to-human transmission by small particle aerosols has been identified. In 1997, human-to-human transmission did not apparently occur through social contact.

Environment-to-human transmission

Given the survival of H5N1 in the environment, several other modes of transmission are theoretically possible. Oral ingestion of contaminated water during swimming and direct intranasal or conjunctival inoculation during exposure to water are other potential modes as is contamination of hands from infected fomites and subsequent self-inoculation. The widespread use of untreated poultry feces as fertilizer is another possible risk factor.

The ease of worldwide travel has the potential to spread bird flu around the globe. Now evidence emerged in 2005 that suggests migratory birds are carrying the virus from continent to continent along traditional flyways.

Outbreaks may also spread locally through 'wet markets' contaminated clothing and equipment and smuggled birds.

In the current epidemic, two influenza subtypes have proved dangerous; especially (A) H7N7, which sickened poultry workers in the Netherlands and (A) H5N1, which has been responsible for the majority of human and avian deaths in Asia. Of these, (A) H5N1 is of particular concern for several reasons:

1. Direct transmission: The H5N1 became the first known bird flu strain to jump directly from birds to people when it surfaced in Hong Kong in 1997. It has since infected people in multiple countries. Two other strains have caused illness in humans, but neither is as severe as H5N1.
2. Virulence: The virus is especially lethal, killing close to 100% of susceptible birds and more than half of infected people. Birds, who do survive can shed the virus for at least 10 days, greatly increasing the flu spread.
3. Rapid spread: Since 2003, hundreds of million of birds have died, a loss that is ecologically and economically devastating. It is also alarming from a public health standpoint that view widespread infections among birds may lead to more human disease.
4. Genetic scrambling: The influenza A (H5N1) mutates quickly and is notorious for grabbing large blocks of genetic code from viruses that infect other species, a process called reassortment. For that reason, it has particular potential to combine with a human flu virus creating a new viral strain that spreads rapidly from person to person. The emergence of such a virus would be the beginning of a potentially devastating pandemic.
5. Portal of entry: The influenza virus switches the binding site preferences from the intestinal tract of birds to the respiratory tract of humans.

Incubation Period

The incubation period of avian H5N1 may be longer than for other known human influenzas. In 1997, most cases occurred within 2–4 days after exposure; recent reports indicate similar intervals, but with ranges of up to 8 days. The case-to-case intervals in household clusters have generally been 2–5 days, but the upper limit has been 8–17 days, possibly owing to unrecognized exposure to infected animals or environmental sources.

Pathophysiology

Type A influenza viruses are further divided into strains, which are constantly evolving. It is exactly this, where the ability of influenza viruses change their genetic makeup and swap genes indiscriminately that makes them so unpredictable and potentially deadly. All living things change, but influenza A viruses change quickly, constantly and sometimes cataclysmically. This takes place in two ways:

1. Antigenic drift: These are small, permanent, ongoing alterations in the genetic material of a virus. Because viruses are not able to repair genetic errors that take place as they reproduce, new strains are continually replacing old ones. Once you have a particular strain of flu, you develop antibodies to it, but those antibodies would not protect you from new strains. In the same way, the flu vaccine you received last season would not ward off this year's bug.
2. Antigenic shift: This occurs when influenza A subtypes from different species—a bird and a human, e.g. trade and merge genes. Tile result is an entirely new strait different from either of the parent viruses. Because no natural immunity to the new strain exists it can spread quickly causing widespread illness and death. And when one of the original subtype is a human influenza virus, the new virus has the ability to spread easily from person to person, playing with poultry, particularly asymptomatic infected ducks and consumption of duck's blood or possibly undercooked poultry have all been implicated.

Human-to-human transmission of H5N1 has been suggested in several household clusters and in one case of apparent child-to-mother transmission. Intimate contact without the use of precautions was implicated and nine for no case of human-to-human transmission by small particle aerosols has been identified. In 1997, human-to-human transmission did not apparently occur through social contact. The H5N1 attack a human cell when inhaled, the virus latches on the cells in the respiratory tract and there it takes over the cells to produce new copies' of cells.

The hemagglutinin protein latches on to the receptors on the surface of the host cells, where copies of the virus are produced. The hemagglutinin protein strike on the surface of the virus attaches to a cell in the respiratory system. The virus enters the host cell of the respiratory tract. The RNA of the virus is released in the cell and the RNA enters the nucleus of the host cell. Here, the RNA of the virus hijacks the host cell machinery in order to make new virus protein and RNA. The new virus protein and RNA join together to create new viruses, which then break free into the host cell in search of another. The other subtype neuraminidase protein enables newly formed viruses to burst out of the infected host cells. During the process, the host shows the signs and symptoms of the disease.

Clinical Features

Bird flu viruses are complex with a number of subtypes and strains that vary considerably from one another. In the broadest terms, however, the viruses are classified as having a low or high chance of causing disease (low or high pathogenicity).

Among birds, the effects of low pathogenic viruses are usually minor-ruffled feathers or reduced egg production. But highly pathogenic forms cause severe disease including respiratory distress and almost 100% mortality in susceptible species. In some cases, domestic birds may die, the same day when symptoms appear.

Although, the exact incubation period for bird flu in humans is not clear, illness seems to develop within 1–5 days of exposure to the virus. Sometimes, the only indication of the disease is relatively mild eye infection conjunctivitis. But more often, signs and symptoms of bird flu resemble those of conventional influenza including:
- Cough
- Fever
- Sore throat
- Muscle aches
- Chest pain
- Diarrhea.

People with the most virulent type of bird flu virus [A (H5N1)] may develop life-threatening complications particularly viral pneumonia and acute respiratory distress, which are the most common cause of bird flu related.

Diagnosis

The diagnosis of H5N1 can be considered on the basis of clinical features. In those people, who have touched the ill poultry or poultry that died of illness. The nose and throat swab is taken for virological assay. A more rapid approach was the presence of influenza A specific RNA is detected through the reverse transcription polymerase chain reaction (RT-PCR) and also by ELISA formats.

Common laboratory findings have been leukopenia, particularly lymphopenia; mild-to-moderate thrombocytopenia and slightly or moderately elevated aminotransferase levels. Marked hyperglycemia and elevated creatinine levels also occur. In Thailand, an increased risk of death was associated with decreased leukocyte, platelet and particularly lymphocyte counts at the time of admission.

Treatment

In August 2005, the United State (US) Government announced it would purchase millions of doses of a prototype bird flu vaccine from a French vaccine maker. The announcement came after when the government tests showed that the vaccine promoted an immune system response in healthy adults. The vaccine still needs to be tested over several months in adults older than 65 and in children. The vaccine would not be licensed until late in 2006 and it will take at least 6–12 months to produce useful amounts. Right now, the primary treatment option is the flu drug oseltamivir (Tamiflu), a neuraminidase inhibitor that works by preventing the virus from escaping its host cell. It is not clear how effective Tamiflu will ultimately prove against 'A (H5N1)'. In Southeast Asia, resistance to it seems to be developing quickly. Another antiviral flu drug, Relenza, may be an alternative. But both drugs must be taken within 2 days after the appearance of symptoms, something that may prove logistically difficult on a worldwide scale, even if there were enough to go around. Because, they are in short supply, it is not entirely clear how flu drugs would be allocated, if there were a widespread epidemic.

Prevention and Control

The international effort to prevent the spread of bird flu is multifaceted, focusing on the health of both birds and humans. The measures to help control the virus among domestic poultry include the following:

1. Culling: Since 1997, when the first human cases of bird flu appeared, hundreds of millions of sick or exposed birds primarily chickens have been destroyed. In many cases, affected farms were also quarantined. Although, some have questioned the wisdom of such wholesale slaughter as well as the methods used to cull birds, where many are burned or buried alive and the WHO considers this approach, the first-line defense against avian viruses.
2. Surveillance programs: Some nations have instituted strict vaccination and surveillance programs for poultry farms and markets taken steps to prevent bird smuggling and put in place programs that quarantine new birds until they are proved healthy and that require poultry farmers to disinfect boots and tires.
3. Banned birds: Many countries have banned or restricted the importation of birds and hatching eggs from regions with bird flu epidemics. In February 2004, the Centers for Disease Control and Prevention (CDC) banned the importation of poultry into the US from most Asian nations.

Preparedness and Response Plan

- Stamping out all fowl within 3 km radius from the impact site

- Vaccination of fowl from the periphery of 3–8 km from the impact site
- Prohibition of sale of poultry within 18 km radius from the impact site
- Continuing quarantine of affected areas
- Surveillance of avian influenza in poultry in humans
- Quarantine of infected persons
- Declaration of the area within 3 km to be in state of calamity
- Infection control
- Clinical management of cases
- Manpower pooling
- Vaccines and prophylaxis
- Public information and risk communication
- Managing the psychological aspect of a pandemic.

Recommendations to All Healthcare Workers

- Receive the current seasonal influenza vaccine as soon as possible
- Observe good respiratory and hand hygiene at all times
- Observe all other recommended infection control precaution
- Monitor self for symptoms of influenza-like illness.

Recommendations for Travellers

If one is travelling to Southeast Asia or to any region with bird flu outbreaks, consider these public health recommendations:

1. Avoid domesticated birds: If possible, avoid rural areas, small farms and especially any close contact with domesticated fowl.
2. Avoid open-air markets: These can be colorful on dreadful depending on your tolerance level, but no matter how you see them, they are often breeding grounds for disease.
3. Wash your hands: One of the simplest ways to prevent infections of all kinds, handwashing is also one of the best. When you are travelling, alcohol-based hand sanitizers, which do not require the use of water are an excellent choice. They are actually more effective than handwashing in killing bacteria and viruses that cause disease. Commercially prepared hand sanitizer contain ingredients that help prevent skin dryness. In fact, use of these products can result in less skin dryness and irritation than handwashing. Not all hand sanitizers are created equal, however, some 'waterless' hand sanitizers do not contain alcohol. Use only the alcohol-based products.
4. Watch your kids: Keep a careful eye on young children, who are likely to put their hands in their mouth and who may not wash thoroughly.
5. Steer clear of raw eggs: Because eggshells are often contaminated with bird droppings, avoid mayonnaise, hollandaise sauce, ice cream and any other foods containing raw or undercooked eggs.
6. Ask about a flu shot: Before travelling, ask your doctor about a flu shot. It will not protect you from bird flu, but it may help reduce the risk of simultaneous infection with bird and human flu viruses.

Preparing Poultry

No human cases of bird flu have been linked to eating poultry, although in at least one instance, the H5N1 virus was found in a package of frozen duck. Because heat destroys avian viruses, WHO officials do not consider cooked poultry, a health threat. Even so, it is best to take precautions when handling and preparing poultry, which is often contaminated with *Salmonella* or other harmful bacteria:

1. Wash well: Carefully wash cutting boards, utensils and all surfaces that have come into contact with raw poultry in hot, soapy water. Wash your hands thoroughly before and after handling poultry and dry them with a disposable towel.
2. Cook thoroughly: Cook chicken until the juices run clear and it reaches an internal temperature of 180°F. Avoid eating raw or undercooked eggs or any products containing thorn, including mayonnaise, hollandaise sauce and homemade ice cream.

Vaccine

Currently, available vaccines will not protect against bird flu, as they are not effective against the H5N1 strain of the virus. Although, existing vaccines do not work against the H5N1 virus, they are being used to prevent poultry workers in affected countries from getting ordinary human flu. This reduces the risk that someone might catch human and bird flu at the same time, which would give the viruses the opportunity to merge and create a new virus capable of causing a pandemic. The CDC is taking part in a number of pandemic prevention and preparedness activities including:

1. Providing leadership to the National Pandemic Influenza Preparedness and Response Task Force, created in May 2005 by the Secretary of the US Department of Health and Human Services.
2. Working with the association of public health laboratories on training workshops for state laboratories on

the use of special laboratory (molecular) techniques to identify H5N1 viruses.
3. Working with the Council of State and Territorial Epidemiologists and others to help states with their pandemic planning efforts.
4. Working with other agencies such as the Department of Defense and the Veterans Administration, on antiviral stockpile issues.
5. Working with the WHO and Vietnamese Ministry of Health to investigate influenza H5N1 in Vietnam and to provide help in laboratory diagnostics and training to local authorities.
6. Performing laboratory testing of H5N1 viruses.
7. Starting a $5.5 million initiative to improve influenza surveillance in Asia. Holding or taking part in training sessions to improve local capacities to conduct surveillance for possible human cases of H5N1 and detect influenza H5N1 viruses by using laboratory techniques.
8. Developing and distributing reagents kits to detect the currently circulating H5N1 viruses.
9. The CDC also is working closely with WHO and the National Institutes of Health on safety testing of vaccine candidates and development of additional vaccine virus seed candidates for H5N1 and other subtypes of H5N1 viruses.

Nursing Management

1. Early recognition, isolation and reporting of possible A1 cases (virulent type of bird flu virus):
   a. Make it a facility priority to establish methods to ensure early recognition and investigation of possible A1 cases.
   b. Initiate infection control precautions promptly when A1 infection is suspected.
   c. Link the hospital-based surveillance system to the public health surveillance system and report immediately all available essential.
   d. Use of universal precaution is a must, the mask must be used in conditions of respiratory precaution and the mask should be properly worn, if the mask becomes wet, it should be promptly discarded in biomedical waste.
   e. Gloves should be used when there is contact with body fluids and blood.
   f. Gowns to use when there is activity, which involves holding the patient close specially used in pediatric patients.
   g. Eye protection also should be used to prevent the accidental spraying of secretions into the conjunctiva.
2. Infection control:
   a. Handwashing before and after every patient care.
   b. After removing gloves or any other personal protection equipment (PPE) items.
   c. The PPE based on risk assessment and to avoid contact with blood, body fluids, excretions and secretions.
   d. Handwashing appropriate handling of patient cares equipment and soiled linen. The use of standard precautions is recommended for handling linen and other laundry that may be contaminated with blood, body fluids, etc. The soiled linen is placed in the laundry bag in the isolation room and it should be properly closed. Gloves and aprons to be used, while removing the soiled linen.
   e. Prevention of needle prick.
   f. Appropriate environmental cleaning and spill management: Cleaning of the isolation room and environment is a must. The cleaning always must be predisinfection. The effective disinfectant used is sodium hypochlorite (bleach) for disinfecting the area.
   g. Appropriate handling of waste: All waste generated in the isolation room should be removed in suitable containers or bags that do not allow for spillage or leakage of contents. Outside of the bag should be contaminated, if contaminated two bags should not be used. When transporting waste outside the isolation room, use gloves followed by hygiene. Feces and other liquid waste such as urine should be disinfected and properly flushed in a closed toilet.
3. Respiratory hygiene: Persons with respiratory infection should be educated to:
   a. Cover their mouth and nose with a tissue when coughing and dispose of used tissue in waste containers.
   b. Use mask, while coughing.
   c. Perform hand hygiene.
   d. Stand or sit at least 1 m away from other persons, if possible.
4. Care of patients with infection:
   a. Assess the condition of the client.
   b. Monitor vital signs and for complication such as respiratory distress and observe pneumonia.
   c. Providing symptomatic relief to the patient: Taking measures to bring down temperature. Providing warm saline gargles in case of sore throat, maintaining eye care.
   d. Administer antibiotics or antiviral medication as prescribed.

e. Provide psychological support to the client.
f. Reduce contact with family members, if inevitable the family members should follow strict universal precautions.
g. Providing optimal nutrition and hydration.
h. Providing health education to both patient and family members.

5. Care during patient discharge:
   a. If patient is discharged, while possibly still infectious, family members should be educated in personal hygiene and infection control measures.
   b. Family members should be educated to avoid poultry and other animals that have been ill and to self-monitor their health status.
   c. Terminal cleaning of the patient room should be performed after patient discharge.
   d. Follow-up of the patient's condition by the public health nurse.

6. Care of deceased:
   a. Removal of body from the isolation.
   b. The PPE to be used by the nurse.
   c. The body should be sealed in impermeable body bag prior to removal from the isolation room.
   d. No leaking of body fluids should occur and the outside of the bag should be kept clean.
   e. After removing PPE, perform handwashing.
   f. If the family members wish to see the body, they may do so, if the patient died during infectious process, the family should wear gloves and gown and perform handwashing.

So far, spread of H5N1 virus from person to person has been rare and has not continued beyond one person. Nonetheless, because all influenza viruses have the ability to change, scientists are concerned that H5N1 virus 1 day could be able to infect humans and spread easily from one person to another. Because, these viruses do not commonly infect humans, there is little or no immune protection against them in the human population.

If H5N1 virus were to gain the capacity to spread easily from person to person, an influenza pan (worldwide outbreak of disease) could begin. No one can predict when a pandemic might occur. However, express from around the world are watching the H5N1 situation in Asia and Europe very closely and are preparing for the possibility that the virus may begin to spread more easily from person to person.

Nursing Care

Isolation: The disease may be isolated by the medical aseptic technique. The virus is found in the nose and throat secretions, urine and feces. All articles coming in contact with the patient or his/her secretions should be cleaned up after use as soon as possible. All waste material should be burned.

Diet: This is essentially that of pneumonia. Nourishing fluids should be given during the acute stage. Soft diet is given when tolerated. Fruit juices are usually taken readily, if nausea does not prevent. When fever is high, the patient becomes dehydrated unless fluids are forced. Fluid, 3,000–4,000 mL should be given the average adult patient daily. If stupor, delirious or uncooperative fluid may be given by hypodermoclysis, intravenously or by Levine tube. As a rule, smaller amounts given frequently are better retained than large amounts at less frequent intervals. A intake and output record should be maintained.

Temperature: This is usually high, 104–105°F. It may be reduced in the usual manner with a tepid or warm sponge bath, alcohol rub. A nurse should be careful to avoid chilling the patient. Colonic flushing is effective in reducing temperature. However, it is exhausting and should be given only upon order of the physician. Ice caps or ice packs to the head are comforting to the patient. They also help to reduce temperature. Temperature, pulse and respirations should be taken and recorded every 3 hours.

Personal hygiene: The patient should have a daily cleansing bath. Alcohol rubs should follow each change of position. The teeth should be thoroughly brushed twice daily. The mouth should be rinsed with an antiseptic solution before and after nourishment. The tongue should be washed or brushed, if necessary. Liquid petrolatum, cold cream or other mild ointments should be applied to the lips and area around the nose and mouth. The eyes should be cleaned, when necessary. Sterile cotton pledget warmed with a warm boric solution or with whatever is prescribed usually suffices. However, warm boric acid solution may be given, if necessary to keep the eyes clean. If diarrhea is present, local sponge baths should be given as often as necessary to keep the patient clean. Lanolin or baby oil should be rubbed on the skin around the anus after drying thoroughly.

Elimination: The bowels should be kept open. Constipation is not a problem as a rule. However, cathartics or enemas may be prescribed. The nurse should keep in mind, the possibility of urinary retention if the patient is delirious, stupor or in coma. Fluid intake and output should be recorded.

General Management of the Disease

The patient should be placed in a quiet, warm, well-ventilated room. The bed should be firm, but comfortable. The bedding should be light in weight, but should provide sufficient warmth. If prostration is great, the weight of the bedding should be kept from the patient by use of a bed cradle. The patient's eyes should be protected from light. The position should be changed from side to side at intervals of 3–4 hours. An ice cap may be given to relieve headache. However, headache should persist and be severe, medication may be prescribed by the doctor. If the patient is extremely restless or delirious, he/she should have constant nursing care and observation to keep him/her from falling or otherwise injuring him/herself. Restraints are contraindicated as the patient resists them. Side rails are often necessary.

Oxygen is usually given at or before the first signs of cyanosis. The cough often can be relieved by increasing humidity in the room.

Convalescence

Convalescence is slow. The diet should be increased as tolerated. The patient should get up gradually and he/she should be warned to avoid overactivity and fatigue until convalescence is well established. Relapses are fairly common.

Terminal Disinfection

The patient should receive usual cleansing bath and shampoo. All toilet articles and others that have come in contact with patient or his/her secretions should be cleaned up. Waste material should be burned. The pillows and mattress should be aired for 6 hours. The bed, chairs, table and walls should be washed with soap and water.

Intestinal Infections

29 CHAPTER

POLIOMYELITIS

In Greek polio means 'gray' and muellas means 'marrow'. Poliomyelitis is an acute, highly infectious disease of the children caused by a virus. Basically, it is an infection of the intestine transmitted by fecal-oral route, but in 1% of the cases, it affects the central nervous system (CNS) also (mainly spinal cord).

Clinically, it is characterized by sudden onset of fever associated with constitutional signs and symptoms followed by the rapid onset of lower motor neuron type of paralysis (flaccidity), either of a group of muscles or of a limb.

History

The disease was first described by Heine in 1840 and by Medin in 1890s. Therefore, the disease was also called 'Heine-Medin disease'. The causative virus was identified by Landsteiner and Popper in 1909. Later in 1949, the virus was successfully cultivated by Enders, Robbins and Weller, who got Nobel Prize. In 1955, Salk prepared an effective killed vaccine, which is named after him; in 1957 Sabin prepared a live vaccine, to be used orally, which is named after him as Sabin vaccine. Introduction of Sabin vaccine opened a new avenue in the eradication/elimination of this disease in many countries.

Infectious agents from the external and internal environments may invade the human and set up inflammatory reactions throughout the body. The inflammation of the CNS is diverse and its effects are vast. Some of the most common and most devastating of the group of inflammatory processes include viral encephalitis, meningitis, brain abscess, rabies and poliomyelitis. So, poliomyelitis is an acute viral infection caused by polioviruses. It is one among the six killer diseases or vaccine preventable disease.

Although a disease of antiquity, poliomyelitis came to be recognized as a clinical entity of the description of the disease by Heine in 1840s and Medin in 1890s. The causative agent was identified by Landsteiner and Popper in 1909.

Poliomyelitis is an acute, systemic disease caused by ribonucleic acid (RNA) virus, which replicates mainly in the gastrointestinal tract (GIT). In some cases, the virus may reach the CNS and damage anterior horn cells of the spinal cord, occasionally the medulla, and motor cortex.

Magnitude of Problem

In 1980s, nearly 42,000 cases were notified to World Health Organization (WHO), the data from 136 countries representing 82% of the total population. Now, immunization has brought marked reduction. India plays an important role in the global eradication of poliomyelitis.

Lameness surveys in several Northern India states revealed annual incidence rates of 2–5/1,000 rural preschool children and 1–3/1,000 urban preschool children. Surveys in South India suggest that the prevalence of poliomyelitis lameness among school children is about 3–5/1,000 implying an annual incidence in the whole population of about 15/100,000. At least 70,000 children develop polio each year in India.

The prevalence rate of residual paralysis can be used to estimate annual incidence of paralytic cases for example, if a prevalence rate of 10 cases per 1,000 is found in an age group of 5–10 years, correction for those cases does not involve the lower extremities, it is done by multiplying the prevalence rate by 1.25, which gives a prevalence rate of 12.5/1,000. This can be translated into average annual incidence by dividing the prevalence rate (12.5) by the number of years at risk (i.e. 5).

Epidemiological Features

Geographical Distribution

Poliomyelitis is a worldwide disease affecting people particularly in Africa and Asia. In India, the first reported epidemic of poliomyelitis occurred in 1949 around Bombay city. Since then more epidemics have occurred at various times in Andhra Pradesh, Uttar Pradesh (UP), Gujarat, Maharashtra, Rajasthan, Tamil Nadu, Delhi and more recently (1981) in Kerala.

Agent

Agent factors involved are as follows:
- Type 1: Responsible for 85% of all paralytic cases and major epidemic
- Type 2: Causes sporadic cases
- Type 3: Less frequently implicated.

In India, all the three types of (types 1, 2 and 3) virus have been found to be responsible for causation of polio. Polioviruses are resistant to drying and freezing. They remain viable in the feces at 4°C for months. Exposure to a temperature of 50°C destroys the virus rapidly. In the absence of organic matter, which protects the virus, free residual chlorine at a level of 0.3–0.5 mg/L causes rapid inactivation of the virus. The virus is also rapidly inactivated by formalin, oxidizing agents and ultraviolet rays.

Morphology

Polioviruses are RNA viruses, about 30 nm in size, they are classified as type 1, 2, 3 strains:
- Type I: Brunhilde strain
- Type II: Lansing strain
- Type III: Leon strain.

The poliovirus is a spherical particle, which is 27 nm in diameter. It is the smallest known human pathogen. The virion is in the form of an icosahedral with perhaps, 32 protein capsomeres enclosing an RNA core, which constitutes 25–30% of the particle. Two outstanding characteristics of the virus are its affinity for nervous tissue and its narrow animal host range (Fig. 29.1).

Viability

The poliovirus is one of the most stable virus known. In aqueous suspensions of human feces at 4°C, it survives for many months. It can be preserved for many months or years at –20 or –70°C. In human stools, the virus may survive at room temperature for short time, i.e. 1 day or for as long as several weeks. The virus is readily killed by moist heat at 50–55°C, but milk cream and ice cream exert a protective effect, so that the virus in these food stuffs may survive exposure to heat at 60°C. It is destroyed by the process of pasteurization of milk at 62°C. In infected human spinal cord, the virus is rapidly inactivated at pH values below 2 or over 11. It survives for 10 days at 4°C in 1% phenol, 18 hours at 4°C in ether and in 0.1% sodium deoxycholate. The most active disinfectants are oxidizing agents such as potassium permanganate and hypochlorites.

Type 1 is the common type that causes epidemics. They are resistant to ether, chloroform and bile. They survive in low pH and temperature.

Reservoir of Infection

Man is the only reservoir of infection, i.e. clinical and subclinical cases. There are no chronic carriers. It is estimated that for every clinical case there may be 1,000 subclinical cases in children and 75 in adults. Virus is present in the throat and intestine; feces and oropharyngeal secretions being infectious material. The virus multiplies in the oropharynx and intestinal tract. Patients are most infectious during the acute stage, which is the period of communicability. The virus is found in the throat a week before and a week after the onset of symptoms. In the feces, the virus is excreted commonly for 2–3 weeks, sometimes as long as 3–4 months.

Host Factors

1. **Age:** In India, poliomyelitis is essentially a disease of infancy and childhood. The most vulnerable age is between 6 months and 3 years.
2. **Sex:** The sex differences have been noted as one for the ratio of male to female.
3. **Risk factors:** These include trauma, fatigue, intramuscular injections and operative procedures such as tonsillectomy.
4. **Genetic factors:** A genetic element in the determination of paralytic polio is also suspected.
5. **Immunity:** Infants born of immune mothers escape infection up to age of 6 months. Thereafter, they become susceptible to polio; the susceptibility being the maximum in the age group from 6 months to 3 years.
6. **Environmental factors:** These sporadic cases throughout the year. Seasonal variations in the incidence of paralytic polio are very striking. Approximately, 60% of the cases recorded in India were from June to September. Flies and cockroaches carry the virus from the sewage to food.

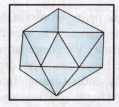

Figure 29.1: Poliovirus

Mode of Transmission

1. Fecal/Oral route: Through contaminated water, food, fingers, milk, etc. where hygiene is poor, spread of virus by fecal-oral route is easier.
2. Droplet infection: Droplet spread from coughing and sneezing is an important route of transmission during the acute stage.
3. Incubation period: The usual range of incubation period is 7–14 days. It may vary from 3 to 35 days.

Pathophysiology

Poliovirus enters GIT by ingestion and then spreads to various organs of the body. Replication of the virus occurs in three phases:

1. Phase 1: Primary replication occurs in the epithelial cells of the oropharynx and intestinal mucosa, and also in subjacent lymphoid tissue.
2. Phase 2: After primary multiplication, virus spreads via the draining lymphatic into regional lymph nodes and undergoes further replication and amplification. It then enters the bloodstream and results in a transient viremia, which clinically manifests as a mild and febrile illness.
3. Phase 3: Following the transient viremia, virus is disseminated into various extraneural tissues. Here, extensive replication of virus occurs, thus producing a persistent viremia. From the blood, the virus passes to the CNS.

The virus attacks the anterior horn cells of the spinal cord, where the motor pathways are located and may cause motor paralysis. Secondary perception is not affected since posterior horn cells are not attacked. Poliomyelitis sometimes takes a somewhat different form and attacks primarily the medullar, and basal structures of the brain including the cranial nerves, the term bulbar poliomyelitis are used for this form.

Signs and Symptoms

The clinical signs and symptoms are grouped under the following headings.

Prodromal Stage

Prodromal stage is the period of onset of the diseases such as:

1. Respiratory infection: Coryza, sore throat or cough.
2. Gastrointestinal tract: Vomiting, diarrhea or constipation.
3. Constitutional: Fever, headache, drowsiness, restlessness, irritability and sweating. Temperature falls to normal in 34–48 hours and rises again as the preparalytic stage is reached.

Preparalytic Stage

The start of neural phase of the infection, signs and symptoms of meningeal irritation are detailed below.

Symptoms include the following:

1. Fever—temperature rises at 39°C and associated pain, and stiffness in the back.
2. Headache—moderate.
3. Nausea is common, vomiting may occur.
4. Pains—spontaneous or provoked by movement of back, neck, limbs and sometimes abdomen.
5. Hyperesthesia—cutaneous may be present, generalized or localized prestaging paralysis of that part.
6. Nuchal and spinal rigidity common and the tests include:
   a. Active tests:
      i. Tripod sign: The child is made to sit up unassisted, the knees flex upward and the child places hands on the bed behind due to spinal rigidity.
      ii. Kiss the knee test: Ask child to sit up and kiss his/her knees. He/She is able to do so only by flexing the knees.
   b. Passive tests:
      i. Positive Kernig's and Brudzinski signs.
      ii. Nuchal rigidity.
      iii. Head drop sign: The head falls backward when the shoulders are elevated.
7. Muscle fasciculation: Flickering movements in muscles may be observed.
8. Micturition disturbances: Difficulty of micturition or retention of urine may occur.
9. Reflexes: Superficial and deep reflexes in early stage are active, and remain so, unless paralysis supervenes.
10. Cerebrospinal fluid (CSF)—clear, pressure increased, protein normal at first rises to 100–200 mg/100 mL during 2nd week, sugar normal, lymphocytes may appear later.

Signs are as follows:
- Pulse is fast
- Excessive perspiration
- Patient is alert.

Paralytic Stage

Usually develops between 2nd and 5th days after onset of signs of involvement of nervous system:
- Paralysis usually appears while there is still fever
- Distribution often asymmetrical
- Paralysis usually begins within 1–5 days after onset of illness.

Distributions of paralysis are follows:
1. The spinal cord—any part of the spinal cord may be involved causing paralysis of group of muscles either upper or lower limbs.
2. Trunk—abdominal muscles, muscles of back, intercostal or diaphragm.
3. Respiratory disturbances—due to paralysis of diaphragm and intercostal muscles or affection of respiratory center in bulbar type; recognized by anxiety, increasing weakness of voice and cough.

Convalescence: Initial paralysis usually diminishes to some extent after a period of 2 or more weeks and improvement may continue for several months. The affected muscles become flaccid, while contraction will tend to produce severe deformities unless these are prevented.

Clinical Features

1. Abortive poliomyelitis: Presumptive diagnosis during epidemic. Brief influenza such as illness with one or more of the following symptoms—malaise, anorexia, nausea, vomiting, headache, sore throat, constipation, localized pain in abdomen and fever more than 103°F, non-specific type of illness, and mild general infection.
2. Non-paralytic poliomyelitis: Subjective symptoms as in abortive type, but headache, nausea, vomiting more intense and soreness, stiffness of posterior muscles of neck, trunk, and limbs. Fleeting paralysis of bladder not uncommon and constipation frequent for 2–10 days.
3. Paralytic poliomyelitis:
   a. Spinal form: Paralysis of flaccid type usually asymmetrical and scattered in distribution. Legs are most frequently involved.
   b. Bulbar form: Muscles supplied by bulbar nuclei involved alone or with spinal musculature. Facial, palatal and sometimes pharyngeal paralysis causes change in voice, difficulty in swallowing, nasal regurgitation, and choking when attempting to drink. Respiratory paralysis is the usual cause of death.

Complications

- Bronchopneumonia develops in severe cases
- Any paralysis occurring in this disease may be regarded as a complication of poliomyelitis
- Atrophy of the muscles, which ultimately results in deformities.

Prognosis

1. Usually, the outcome to the life is good.
2. Mortality rate is between 10 and 20%, which is mainly seen in bulbar and respiratory types of poliomyelitis.
3. About 50% of those cases, who escape death are crippled in various ways and sequelae include permanent muscular paralysis, atrophy of limbs, and deformity of joints.

Laboratory Diagnosis

1. The CSF increased white blood cell (WBC) count often with high polymorph count in first few days followed by predominance of lymphocytes and sugar normal.
2. Isolation of virus poliovirus can be isolated from nasopharyngeal swabs during the first 5 days of illness only, but from stools and rectal swabs containing fecal material up to 5 weeks after onset.
3. Serology a four-fold rise in level of antibody to the strain of virus isolated.

Treatment

There is no specific treatment for polio. Good care from the beginning of illness can minimize or even prevent crippling. Physiotherapy is of vital importance. It can be initiated in the affected limb, immediate helps the weakened muscles to regain strength, very probably the child may have to put on metal calipers.

Special treatment: There is no specific treatment, only supportive and symptomatic treatment is given to the patient:
- Mild analgesics and sedatives may be given to relieve pain, and induce sleep
- For constipation may be mild laxatives
- To prevent respiratory and oral complications give antibiotics—sulfonamides
- Respiratory failure is treated by the use of respirator.

The oral polio vaccine (OPV) is easy to administer and relatively cheap, which is ideally suited for poliomyelitis eradication strategies, because the live vaccine virus by multiplying in the intestine can interrupt the transmission of the wild poliovirus. The simultaneous administration of OPV within a short period of time by mass immunization campaign (Pulse Polio Program) interrupts transmission of wild poliovirus by displacing it from intestine, where the poliovirus multiply. This effect enhanced, if the vaccination coverage is 100% of the population at risk, i.e. children below 3 years of age.

Passive Immunization

Immunization with 5–15 mL, according to age of child, gamma globulin. Some measures of protection are afforded for 6 weeks.

Indications: Newborns in hospitals who are exposed to infection and unimmunized children in hospital wards.

In case if poliomyelitis develops, nurses and medical students who have not been immunized, and who have come in contact with early cases of polio.

Contraindications: For the administration of OPV are acute infectious diseases, fevers, diarrhea and dysentery. Patients suffering from leukemia and its malignancy, and those receiving corticosteroids may not be given OPV.

Management

Since there is no treatment, polio cases require general supportive care and skilled management as follows:

1. Isolation ward.
2. Concurrent disinfection of saliva and excreta in 10% cresol.
3. Absolute bedrest is essential during the acute phase. There should not be any stress on the affected muscles.
4. Expert nursing care with frequent change of postures every 2–3 hours.
5. Symptomatic treatment with paracetamol to relieve pain and fever.
6. Prophylactic oral antibiotics to prevent secondary infection.
7. Massage and injections during the acute phase is absolutely contraindicated (i.e. for about 6 weeks).
8. Supportive treatment with splints is provided to the limbs, to prevent deformity resulting from the action of antagonistic muscles.
9. Maintenance of fluids and electrolyte balance done orally and not by infusion.
10. Physiotherapy is recommended not in the early stage, but only after the acute phase of about 6 weeks, because stress and strain in the acute phase worsens the disease, and also wherever the damage is reversible in the spinal cord, the paralyzed muscles recover within 4 weeks.

Physiotherapy

Physiotherapy is recommended after the residual paralysis persists to regain the muscle power. Maximum recovery takes place in the first 6 months, but slow recovery is continued up to 2 years. However, the residual paralysis remains permanently. Physiotherapy is necessary to prevent contractures and deformities. Muscle stimulators can be used and graded exercises are given.

Hydrotherapy (Treatment in Swimming Pool)

Hydrotherapy is of great benefit to the polio patients. The limbs are bit lighter in water and thereby the patient gets great psychological uplift, but actually there is no muscular recovery. As a part of rehabilitation, the child requires artificial limb, metal calipers or even reconstructive surgery.

Prevention and Control

Since there is no treatment, elimination of reservoir is not possible. Different modes of transmission can be broken by construction of sanitation barrier. However, protection of susceptible by immunization is the only role and most effective method of preventing poliomyelitis. Since, it is a disease mainly of children and the susceptibility being universal, all children must be immunized during their infancy period itself, preferably before 6 month of age. An essential part of the nurses' responsibility is to help to prevent poliomyelitis by encouraging immunizations. It is important to have all children immunized as it is the sole effective means of preventing poliomyelitis. Immunization is carried out under the following heads:

- Report about the case to the health authorities at once
- Patient must be isolated for 1 week from the disease to onset of the disease or as long as the fever
- Proper disposal of urine and feces of the patient
- When there is an outbreak of epidemic, all sources of water must be protected, swimming baths must be chlorinated
- Milk must be pasteurized and fruits should be washed with weak permanganate solution before using
- Avoid overcrowding of the children in schools, cinemas, playgrounds, etc.
- Children must avoid excessive physical strain during an epidemic
- Search of sick persons, investigation of contacts and source of infection must be carried out
- Antifly measures should be adopted
- Active immunization with OPV during an outbreak is of great value
- All suspected carriers must gargle with potassium permanganate solution and take four tablespoon of sulfadiazine in a day
- Educate people about disease and its consequences.

There are two ways of immunization namely active and passive immunization.

Active Immunization (Tables 29.1 to 29.3)

Two types of vaccines are available, namely inactivated polio vaccine (IPV) and OPV.

Table 29.1: Advantages and disadvantages of inactivated polio vaccine (IPV) and oral polio vaccine (OPV)

Vaccine	Advantages	Disadvantages
IPV	Safe, stable, requires no interference by other viruses wide vaccine coverage	More expensive, harder to administer
OPV	Less expensive, easily administered Excellent and strong immunity May provide immediate protection	Less safe (may cause paralytic polio), less stable especially in tropical climates Some interference by enteric viruses

Table 29.2: Comparison of inactivated polio vaccine (IPV) and oral polio vaccine (OPV)

IPV, Salk type	OPV, Sabin type
Route	
It is given subcutaneously	Given orally
Vaccine	
It is killed formalized vaccine	Live, oral attenuated strain of three antigenic types: 1 lakh TCID* 50 of type 1 1 lakh TCID 50 of type 2 3 lakh TCID 50 of type 3
Dosage schedule	
Three to four doses: First dose—4–6 week Second dose—after 4 month Third dose—at 6–18 month Booster (fourth) dose at the time of school entry	Doses of trivalent vaccine for permanent immunity: First dose—1 month Second dose—2½ month Third dose—3½ month
Prevention	
Prevents paralysis, but does not prevent reinfection by wild polioviruses	Prevents not only paralysis but also intestinal reinfection

*TCID, tissue culture infective dose

Table 29.3: Differences between inactivated polio vaccine (IPV) and oral polio vaccine (OPV)

Inactivated polio vaccine (IPV)	Oral polio vaccine (OPV)
A killed vaccine (Salk vaccine)	A live vaccine (Sabine vaccine)
Given intramuscular (IM) only	Given orally
Provides only systemic immunity	Provides both local and systemic immunity
Prevents the disease	Not only prevents the disease but also intestinal reinfection
The reinfection of the gut by wild poliovirus	By wild poliovirus
Does not help in the development of herd immunity	Helps in the development of herd immunity
Neither useful in controlling the epidemic polio nor in the eradication of polio	Not only useful in controlling of the epidemics but also in the eradication of poliomyelitis
Administration is costly	Administration is easy, cheap
Requires the service of a trained person	Does not require the services of a trained person
Immunity is shorter (about 5 year)	Immunity is lifelong with multiple doses
Vaccine associated paralysis does not occur	Vaccine associated paralysis can occur
Stringent conditions are not required to maintain cold chain	Stringent conditions are required to maintain cold chain

Inactivated polio vaccine (Salk vaccine)

The IPV is named after the discoverer Salk as Salk vaccine. It is a liquid-killed vaccine. It contains all the three types of polioviruses, killed by formalin to be administered intramuscularly. Primary course consists of four doses, first three doses are given with an interval of 4–6 weeks, starting from as early as 6 weeks of infancy and the fourth dose is given about 6–12 months after third dose. Immunity lasts for few years. Additional dose is given at the time of school entry and then booster dose is given once in 5 years till the age of 18 years.

An IPV stimulates the production of only systemic (humoral) antibodies, but not intestinal or local immunity. Thereby, the child is protected against poliomyelitis; the wild viruses can still multiply in the intestine and be a source of infection to others.

Merits
- Since, it is not a live vaccine, the vaccine-associated paralysis do not occur
- It is safe for elderly persons and pregnant mothers
- It is also safe for immunocompromised persons such as those who are on steroids or radiotherapy.

Demerits
- Hardly 50% effective
- An IPV is not recommended during epidemics of polio because immunity is not developed with only one dose
- Injections are not advised during epidemics because of provocative paralysis
- Does not provide gut immunity
- Does not provide lifelong immunity
- Booster doses are required once in 5 years.

Modified inactivated polio vaccine: It is more stable and potent vaccine can be combined with diphtheria, pertussis, tetanus (DPT) to prepare a quadruple vaccine to simplify the schedule.

Oral polio vaccine (Sabin vaccine)

Oral polio vaccine is named after the discoverer Sabin as Sabin vaccine. It is a live, liquid vaccine containing attenuated all the three types of polioviruses. It is the vaccine of choice for immunization against polio. So, it is also called 'trivalent vaccine'. Thus, the child is protected against all the three types of viruses, simultaneously, which is of great administrative convenience. The National Immunization Program in India recommends three doses of OPV starting from the age of 2 months. The interval between doses should not be less than 1 month. The OPV is concurrently given with DPT, bacille Calmette–Guérin (BCG) vaccine. One booster dose of OPV is recommended 18–24 months later. The vials of OPV are stored at 20°C in a deep freeze.

Composition
Each dose of two drops contains 300,000 tissue culture infective (TCID50) doses of 50% of type 1 virus, 100,000 TCID50 of type 2 virus and 300,000 TCID50 of type 3 virus.

Route
An OPV is given orally in the form of two drops per dose.

Schedule
Under the National Universal Immunization Program, four doses of OPV are recommended as follows:
1. Zero dose at birth, along with BCG.
2. First dose at 6th week.
3. Second dose at 10th week.
4. Third dose at 14th week; all three along with DPT.

Indian Academy of Pediatrics recommends one more dose at 9th month along with measles vaccine. One booster dose of OPV is recommended during 18th month. Three doses confer 85% protection, four doses confer 90% protection and five doses confer 95% protection. Thus, multiple doses induce higher and lifelong immunity.

The dose given at birth is an optional, but preferable. The option is that it is recommended for institutional deliveries. It is called 'zero dose' because it is given before the recommended first dose and also because it results in the development of gut immunity only and not systemic immunity. The subsequent three doses help in the development of both local gut immunity and also systemic immunity.

Mechanism of protection: After administering the vaccine orally, the live-attenuated viruses multiply in the intestinal epithelial cells. Thus, OPV administration mimics the natural route of infection, the antigenic stimulus becomes much more than what is administered, thereby the production of antibodies will also be more and immunity lasts longer. As long as it is in the intestinal epithelial cells, it helps in the development of intestinal local immunity by the production of immunoglobulin A (IgA) and when it enters the circulation, stimulates the production of humoral, systemic immunity with immunoglobulin G (IgG). Thus, there is double benefit.

Advantages of oral polio vaccine
1. There is development of both local and systemic immunity.
2. When the immunized child drinks contaminated water containing wild poliovirus, it is acted upon by the IgA of the gut and is converted into attenuated, nonpathogenic, vaccine progeny virus, which when enters the mouth of the susceptible child, induces immunity indirectly, thus helps in the development of herd immunity in the community.
3. If all the children are immunized simultaneously and not even a single child is left, the vaccine virus completely replaces the wild poliovirus from the entire nature, thus OPV helps in eradication of the poliomyelitis (unimmunized gut is a must for the wild virus to multiply).
4. It is the vaccine of choice during the epidemics.
5. Administration is simple, easy and given orally its not painful, and inexpensive.
6. Does not require the services of trained personnel.

Associated risk
An OPV being live vaccine, as the viruses are multiplying in the intestine, specially the type 3 virus produces a new mutant strain, which actually results in the disease, it is called vaccine-associated paralytic poliomyelitis. It is rare; one in 1 million vaccines. This risk is more among adults than among children.

Contraindications
Contraindications are acute febrile illness, diarrheal disease, children on steroid therapy, etc. However, mild fever, mild diarrhea are not contraindications. Malnourished children require immunization most. However, there are no contraindications under the National Pulse Polio Program.

Storage

Stabilized vaccine: Oral polio vaccine is stabilized with magnesium chloride ($MgCl_2$), it retains the potency of the vaccine at 4°C for 1 year and for 1 month at room temperature. During transport, the vaccine must be kept either on dry ice or freezing mixture.

Non-stabilized vaccine: This always has to be stored at subzero temperature from the time and place of manufacture to the time and place of its use, i.e. cold chain has to be maintained.

Instructions to the mother
1. Hot fluids such as milk, coffee or tea should not be given to the immunized child for at least half-an-hour after the administration of the vaccine, because it may kill the virus. However, breast milk can be given.
2. Next due date is given.
3. Mother must be educated about the importance of completing the schedule.

Reasons for vaccine failures
- Incomplete schedule
- Use of date-expired vaccine
- Instability of vaccine
- Lack of maintenance of cold chain
- Vaccine-associated paralytic polio, due to multiplicity of strains
- Interference with vaccine uptake by intercurrent enterovirus infection (is not proved).

Passive Immunization

Passive immunization is done by human normal immunoglobulin. It is recommended for those who are at risk such as young and close contacts people who are not immunized before. Doses is from 0.25 to 0.3 mL/kg body weight. But such contacts must be actively immunized after a few weeks. But the current widespread practice of active immunization under the national program has virtually eliminated the need for passive immunization.

Vaccine Vial Monitor

Vaccine vial monitor (VVM) is a small, square shaped, heat sensitive, white-colored material, placed on an outer circle of blue color printed on the label of the OPV vial. Combined effects of time and temperature cause the VVM to change its color gradually from the light color at the starting point and become darker with exposure to heat. The darkening process is irreversible. The outer-colored circle is used as a reference to compare the color of the VVM. The VVM does not directly measure the potency of the vaccine, but definitely it gives information about the potency of the vaccine. Read VVM as mentioned below:

1. Compare the darkness of VVM (inner square) with that of outer circle.
2. If the inner square is lighter than the outer circle and the expiry date has not passed, the vaccine may be used.
3. If the inner square matches with the outer circle or even darker than the outer circle and even if the expiry date has not passed, the vaccine must not be used. It is considered ineffective vaccine.
4. If the inner square is lighter than the outer circle and the expiry date has passed, the vaccine should not be used. Thus, VVM enables the health worker to ascertain, whether the vaccine vials is potent or not. This ensures quality assurance of the immunization program. The use of VVM over the vial has been made mandatory since 1998.

Stages of vaccine vial monitor
1. Start point: Inner square is lighter than outer ring. Use the vaccine, if expiry date not reached. Inner square is darkening, but still lighter than outer ring. Use the vaccine, if expiry date not reached.
2. Discard point: Inner square matches the color of outer ring, do not use the vaccine.
3. Beyond the discard point: Inner square is darker than outer ring, do not use the vaccine.

Eradication of Poliomyelitis

Poliomyelitis is said to be eradicated from a country, when zero incidence is maintained for 3 continuous years with the absence of circulating wild poliovirus in the environment and the people are free from the fear of getting the disease without immunization. Poliomyelitis is amenable for eradication, because of the favorable epidemiological points as follows (epidemiological basis):

1. Human being is the only reservoir of infection.
2. There is no animal reservoir state.
3. There is no chronic carrier state.
4. Half-life of the excreted wild poliovirus in sewage is very short (hardly 48 hour). The spread of infection through sewage can only occur during this period.
5. The available vaccine is a live vaccine, stabilized, highly potent, cheap can easily be administered orally and highly safe.
6. There are no contraindications under National Program Office (NPO).
7. An OPV helps in the indirect immunization of susceptible children in the community.
8. It helps in the replacement of the wild virus from the entire nature by inducing the gut immunity and circulation of the vaccine progeny virus.
9. Correct and complete dosage schedule confers life-long immunity.

Differential Diagnosis of Poliomyelitis

- Guillain-Barré syndrome (Table 29.4)
- Transverse myelitis
- Traumatic neuritis.

Table 29.4: Differences between poliomyelitis and Guillain-Barré syndrome

Poliomyelitis	Guillain-Barré syndrome
Etiology	
Caused by virus	It is a demyelinating disease peripheral nervous system
Age group	
Common among infants, often up to 5 year	Rare among infants, common between 1 and 4 years age group
Onset	
Acute	Chronic
Fever	
Just prior to paralysis (hallmark findings)	2–3 week before illness
Paralysis	
Flaccid and asymmetrical	Flaccid and symmetrical
Course	
Descending starts (lower limbs first followed by upper limbs)	Descending (from the trunk and moves distally down)
Cranial nerve	
Usually uncommon	Usually common (7th and 9th facial and glossopharyngeal nerves)
Sensory deficit	
Absent	Present
CSF* findings	
Cell 20–300 WBCs[†]/mm^3	< 10/mm^3
Protein	
40–65 mg	Up to 200 mg
Electrophysiology findings	
Nerve normal	Reduced
Conduction velocity	
Electromyography usually abnormal	Usually normal

*CSF, cerebrospinal fluid; [†] WBCs, white blood cells.

Transverse Myelitis

The features are:
- Absence of fever
- Symmetrical paralysis of lower limbs usually (paraplegia)
- Marked sensory loss (profound anesthesia)
- Paralysis of legs is followed by loss of control of rectal and bladder sphincters
- Common among children above 4 years of age and adults
- The CSF findings are usually normal.

Traumatic Neuritis

- History of having taken intramuscular (IM) injection
- Paralysis of the limb is accompanied by the pain
- Knee, jerk is present, but ankle jerk is absent (leg is involved below the knee)
- Child walks with a foot drop
- Recovery is gradual with physiotherapy within about 6 months
- Can occur in any age group.

Pulse polio Immunization

The term 'pulse' has been used to describe the sudden, simultaneous, mass administration of OPV to all the children under the age 5. Children in the entire country with a 100% coverage, with two doses on the indicated dates with 6 weeks interval, during the lowest transmission season, October to February, irrespective of their previous immunization status:

1. These doses are supplements and not substitute to the routine immunization.
2. There is no minimal interval between a scheduled dose of OPV and the pulse polio immunization (PPI) dose (that means, even if the child had taken its regular scheduled dose on the previous day of PPI day, it has to be given PPI dose).
3. There are no contraindications for PPI.

This concept of PPI came into vogue, because in spite of correct and complete immunization of the children under Universal Immunization Program (UIP) a small percentage (about 10%) of the children are not completely protected. It is not possible to know, which child is completely protected, which child is not. And also since entry of the wild poliovirus into an unimmunized gut is a must to continue its progeny, it was felt by Government of India to ensure that every child under age 5 in the country is given polio drops, simultaneously on the particular indicated dates, so that not even a single unimmunized gut should be available to the wild poliovirus, thereby the vaccine progeny virus replaces the wild virus from the entire nature, thus helping in the eradication of poliomyelitis.

The PPI was launched on December 1995, when the target age was fixed up to 3 years only. In 1996, the target age was extended to 5 years. Government of India has

CHAPTER 29 — Intestinal Infections

committed to sustain and maintain this massive effort until the disease is eradicated.

VIRAL HEPATITIS

A systematic disorder that primarily involves the liver causing diffuse hepatocellular inflammation and is characterized by fever gastrointestinal manifestations, and jaundice. Virus hepatitis clinically ranging from slight malaise, anorexia, abdominal discomfort, mild fever to severe hepatitis, jaundice culminating in hepatic coma and death.

Epidemiological Features

The distribution of disease is worldwide. It is endemic with frequent reports of minor and major epidemic. In India it broke out in epidemic form. The largest epidemic broke out in Delhi during 1955–1956. Now it is widely prevalent in India.

Agent

The condition is caused by hepatitis A virus (HAV), hepatitis B virus (HBV), hepatitis C virus (HCV) and hepatitis E virus (HEV). All these types possess RNA genome, but HBV with double-shelled particles that contain small circular deoxyribonucleic acid (DNA) molecules and have polymerase activity. The HAV is highly infectious and produces 'infective hepatitis'. HBV causes 'serum hepatitis' or 'epidemic jaundice'. Difference between infective hepatitis and serum hepatitis (type B) are given in Table 29.5. Man is the only reservoir of infection. Injective material includes feces, contaminated blood and other body fluids.

Table 29.5: Differences between infective hepatitis and serum hepatitis

Infective hepatitis (type A)	Serum hepatitis (type B)
Type of onset; acute	Insidious
Agent; hepatitis A virus is resistant to temperature	Hepatitis B virus more resistant killed at 60°C in 4 hour
Incubation period: 15–50 day	50–160 day or more
Fever: 100–101°F common	Not common
Age: Children and adult affected	Can occur at any age
Virus presence in acute stage present on feces and serum	Virus not present in feces at any stage
Immunity: Develops	Doubtful
Mortality: Low in children (1%)	High usually (5%)
Natural immunity: Found	None
Diagnosis: History	Definite history of contaminated needle, blood and products injection
Treatment: Gamma globulin effective	Not effective
Prevention: Gamma globulin useful	Not useful
Route of infection usually oral	Only parenteral

Host

1. Age: Children and young adults are more susceptible; HAV occurs at all ages.
2. Sex: Both sexes are equally affected.
3. Immunity: One attack gives lasting immunity.
4. Environment: Usually a group with low socioeconomic status will be more affected due to lack of clean habits and personal hygiene.

Mode of Transmission

1. Fecal-oral routes, waterborne, foodborne and direct transmissions.
2. Parenteral route: Transmission through blood and blood products transfusion or skin penetration through contaminated needles, syringes and surgical appliances.
3. Transplacental transmission (HBV): Incubation period of HAV lasts up to 15–50 days (usually 28 day), while that of HBV lasts from 6 weeks to 6 months.

Pathophysiology

The infection produces spotty degeneration of parenchymal cells with necrosis of hepatocytes, particularly in the centrilobular areas, diffuse inflammatory reaction and disruption of liver cell cords. There are localized areas of necrosis with ballooning or acidophilic bodies, hyperplasia of Kupffer cells, periportal infiltration with mononuclear cells and cell degeneration. Later, increased number of macrophages continuing a yellow acid-fast pigment and numerous lymphocytes polymorphonuclear leukocytes, and plasma cells accumulate at the base of all necrosis. Bile canaliculi may be disrupted or the excretion of bile may be obstructed due to enlargement of liver cells and necrosis.

Clinical Features

The condition is characterized by jaundice, though many cases may remain nonicterus. Prior to jaundice, the person may complain of chills or chilliness, headache, malaise and influenza-like fever (HAV). There may be severe anorexia, nausea, vomiting, detaste of smoking (nonsmokers), symptoms of upper respiratory tract infection (URI), myalgia and diarrhea. Patient complains pain in right hypochondriac region and may pass dark urine, and pale stool. Spleen may enlarge in children. Signs of toxemia will appear in severe cases. Later on relapsing hepatitis or posthepatitis syndrome may develop.

Treatments

No specific treatment available; rest and diet are symptomatic treatment.

Prevention and Control

Viral hepatitis can be prevented by administering single high dose (1.2 cc/kg body weight) of human normal immunoglobulin before getting infection, it is not effective in case of HBV.

Adopting

Usually measure to control of reservoir and subclinical cases. Control of transmission can be achieved by:
- Personal cleanliness
- Avoid using contamination food, milk and water
- Safe disposed of excreta
- Prevention of contaminated water and milk supplies
- Promotional measures of safe drinking water supply
- Control of flies
- Screening of kitchen, food handlers and latrine.

During epidemic, people are advised to drink boiled water and superchlorination of water sources. Precautionary measure has to be taken to use syringes and needles (need to sterilize properly before use).

In addition HBV, blood containing the Australian antigen should not be used for transfusion. So, identification of infected person including carrier by means of test for Australian antibody is needed prior to drawing the blood for transfusion.

Hepatitis E

Hepatitis E virus (enterically transmitted non-A and non-B hepatitis) was discovered in 1990s, exists in many developing countries including Southeast Asian regions (SEAR), where environmental sanitation is poor. It is essentially fecal-oral-transmitted waterborne disease.

It is RNA virus of about 30 nm size. It is a member of caliciviridae family. The HEV is the most common cause of sporadic hepatitis in adults often resulting in epidemics. First major epidemic was reported from New Delhi, during 1955–1956, due to flooding of river Yamuna, resulting in about 30,000 cases. Other two major epidemics occurred in India were one in Kamal 1987 and Kanpur in 1991. China reported about 100,000 cases between 1986 and 1988. Since then outbreaks have been reported from SEAR countries. Interestingly, young children are often spared in most hepatitis E epidemics.

Incubation period is almost same as that of HAV, i.e. 15–60 days (average of 40 day). Clinically characterized by the same features as those of HAV, followed by recovery, thus proving a self-limiting disease. It lasts for a period of several weeks. No case of chronic disease is reported. Mainly young adults of 15–40 years are affected. Among children, HEV results in inapparent or mild infections (anicteric hepatitis).

Disease severity is higher among pregnant women, resulting not only in abortions, stillbirths and neonatal deaths but also a high fatality of about 80%. The 20% of them are due to development of fulminant hepatic failure. The HEV also enhances the morbidity and mortality in stable cirrhosis.

Though, HEV may cause fulminant hepatitis on its own, the risk of developing severe disease is more with combined infections, e.g. HEV and HAV diagnosis is made by the level of anti-HEV antibodies in the serum. The HEV RNA by polymerase chain reaction is the gold standard for definitive diagnosis, but is available only in few reference laboratories.

Treatment is not necessary, recovery is almost complete. Only supportive treatment for fulminant cases among mothers. Prevention is by sanitation barrier, same as in prevention of HAV. No vaccine or specific immunoglobulin is available. Maintenance of personal hygiene, use of boiled and cooled water protects the individuals. Vulnerable individuals such as pregnant mothers and those with cirrhosis need to be most careful to safeguard against HEV infection.

Hepatitis G

The Hepatitis G virus (HGV) is recently identified in 1996. It belongs to flavivirus group. This has been found to be associated with blood transfusion and intravenous (IV) drug abuse. But it does not appear 10 important causes for liver disease.

CHOLERA

Cholera is an infectious disease characterized by vomiting and severe diarrhea with fluid, and electrolyte depletion.

CHAPTER 29 — Intestinal Infections

It is an acute highly communicable disease caused by *Vibrio cholerae* (*V. cholerae*) and El Tor vibrio (particular strain of the bacterium *V. cholerae*).

It has existed in India since ancient time and has been mentioned in the *'Sushruta Samhita'* (700 BC). Cholera occurred in pandemic form several times. It was the most important cause of morbidity and mortality not only in India, but all over the world till recently.

Epidemiological Features

Agent

Cholera is caused by motile, aerobic, comma-shaped gram-negative rods-like bacteria with a single polar flagellum *'V. cholerae.'* It grows well in peptone water. They are found in stools and vomit of patients. Cases and carriers are the reservoir of bacteria, and cause infection. Stools and vomit from cases, and carriers are sources of infection. Period of infectivity of cases lasts for 3–7 days and convalescent carriers are infection for 2–3 weeks.

Host

1. Age: Cholera affects all ages.
2. Sex: Both sexes are affected, more severe in pregnancy ladies in endemic areas, injection among children predominates.
3. Immunity: Natural infection confers quite effective immunity.
4. Population mobility: Movement of population to pilgrimage, marriages, fairs and festivals, etc. may increase risk of exposure to infection.

Environmental factors: Community with poor environmental sanitation conducive for vibrio transmission is exposed to infection:

1. Season: It has been observed that not a single week in the country is free from diarrheal diseases. Incidence is comparatively high during the summers and post-rainy seasons. In case of cholera, lowest incidence is between February and March. Peak month is August specially in Gujarat, Maharashtra, Orissa and Bihar. So peak month is May in West Bengal, June in UP and January in Southern States.
2. Social factors: It is responsible for spread of infection are ignorance, fairs and festivals, feasts, habits of washing clothes near wells, open air defecation, lack of sanitary latrines, disposal of dead bodies in rivers, and movement of population.

Mode of Transmission

The infection spreads through contaminated water, food and drinks. Eating and drinking utensils washed with contaminated water are the vehicles for transmission of cholera. In short five F's, i.e. food, finger, flies, filths and fomites are the chief modes of transmission. Incubation period varies from a few hours to 5 days, but commonly lasts for 2 days.

Pathophysiology

Cholera is not an invasive infection, but *Vibrio* invades intestinal superficial epithelium. There is mononuclear cell inflammation of the mucosa, vascular congestion and goblet cell hyperplasia followed by atrophy of epithelial cells. The enterotoxin of the *Vibrio* is capable to produce hypersecretion of isotonic electrolyte solution by intact small bowel mucosae alone. Therefore, an outpouring of fluid and electrolytes resulting in diarrhea, dehydration, acidosis, shock, and death.

Clinical Features

After ingestion through food, the cholera germs pass through the stomach to small intestine, where they multiply rapidly producing toxin. This causes intestinal wall to secrete a large quantity of water and salts. This loss of fluid from the bowel leads to severe dehydration and even death.

Signs and Symptoms

- There is abrupt onset of vomiting and purging of large amounts of rice water stools (up to 1 L/h)
- Patient is very thirsty
- Eyes and cheeks are sunken
- Skin is pale, skin of the fingers is shriveled (e.g. washerman fingers)
- Voice husky
- Extremities are cold and blue
- Pulse is rapid and feeble
- Blood pressure (BP) is low
- Urine output is reduced or stopped
- Patient has muscular cramps.

In children, fever, convulsions or coma, loss of muscular tone are seen. It should be noted that stool specimen should not be collected from a bedpan. Quarantine period is 5 Days.

Preventive Measures

Diagnosis

As soon as cholera is suspected, first step is early and accurate diagnosis. Before starting any drugs, collect a stool specimen and send it immediately to the laboratory. There are three methods to collect stool specimen as follows:

1. Rectal swab method:
   a. Prepare a cotton stick swab.
   b. Pass the swab directly into the rectum for 2–4 cm.
   c. Remove the swab and immerse it immediately in the bottle of transport media [(supplied by pregnancy-induced hypertension (PIH)].
   d. Break off the end of the stick and screw on the cap of the bottle.
2. Catheter method:
   a. Use sterile (boiled) soft rubber catheter number 26 or 28.
   b. Lubricate the tip with sterile liquid paraffin and pass it 4–5 cm into the rectum.
   c. Hold the outer end of the catheter over the bottle containing the transport media and allow about 2–3 mL of liquid stool to flow out.
   d. After use, wash the catheter well with soap and water, sterilize by boiling.
3. Blotting paper method:
   a. When transport media is not available, blotting paper method may be used.
   b. Place a strip of dry blotting paper in a plastic packet.
   c. Pour the watery stool onto the blotting paper strip, so that strip becomes soaked.
   d. Seal the plastic packet to avoid the blotting paper from drying during transit.
   e. Educating mothers about diarrhea in children and its prevention at their level.

Treatments

1. Rehydration with prompt replacement of fluids and electrolytes, i.e. sodium chloride (NaCl), sodium bicarbonate (NaHCO$_3$), potassium chloride (KCl) in the proportion of 5:4:1 per liter of distilled water (Ringers lactate IV) or oral rehydration salt (ORS).
2. Tetracycline antibiotics or cephradine 250–500 mg, four times each day (qds) orally—1M, IV as prescribed by the physician.
3. Antidiarrheal kaolin-pectin suspension and its tablet.
4. Nutrition—do not starve the patient, especially children. Give cereals (rice ganji), banana, butter, milk as the patient desires. If the child in breastfed, ask the mother to continue breastfeeding.

Notification

Cholera is a notifiable disease locally, nationally and internationally. The responsibilities of all health workers including nurses are to identity and notify the disease as quickly as possible, i.e. notification about the number of cases, deaths, areas infected, and measures taken for its control to be given to nearest health authorities such as Medical Officer (MO) of primary health center (PHC), District Health and Family Welfare Officers (DH and FWOs), Directorate of Health and Family Welfare Services (DHFWSs), Director General of Health Services (DGHS), and WHO.

Surveillance

Number of reported cases is always less than the actual number including laboratory examination. Investigation of all cases of diarrhea and prompt reporting of all suspected cases.

Isolation

Case should be quickly removed from homely environment, as there is danger of spread of infection. Local schools, community buildings, mobile hospital under tents are the places to be converted into temporary treatment centers. Isolation is necessary till the patient is no longer infectious, which should be confirmed by bacteriological examination.

Vaccination

Cholera vaccine is a killed vaccine, 0.5% phenol is used as a preservative only smooth strain is selected for manufacture because they are fully virulent. Protective value is only 50–60%. Inoculation, 0.5 cc followed by 1 cc, may be administered deep subcutaneous or IM spacing 10–28 days. For adults only one injection of 1 cc during epidemic. For children from 6 months to 5 years 0.1 cc (one dose) and 0.3 cc (two dose), for 5–10 years children 0.3 cc (one dose) and 0.5 cc (two dose). Each cc of vaccine contains 3,000 million organisms. Immunity is brief and lasts for 3 months. It should be remembered that cholera vaccine gives only partial protection.

Disinfection

1. Stools and vomit mix with 2% Lysol or 30% bleaching powder or with 5% cresol (8 ounces to a gallon) for 30 minutes. Then burn, bury or flush down.
2. Clothing, bedding and utensils of the patient should be boiled or soak in 2% Lysol or cresol for 2 hours, before washing, throwing, burning and burying. Washing with soap and water is also practical.

3. Floors, walls and furniture of sick room should be swab with 2% Lysol or 5% cresol, or bleaching powder walls up to 3 ft height should be treated in the same way.
4. Feeding and cooking utensils should be boiled for 15 minutes, then cresol solution for half-an-hour, and final washing in water with soda.
5. Hand may be dipped in 1% cresol solution and washed afterwards with soap, and water.
6. Dead bodies of cholera cases are wrapped in sheet soaked in 2% Lysol before disposal by burying.

Improvement of Sanitation

1. Inspection of sources of water pollution, chlorination of sources and advice people to boil the drinking water.
2. Use of sanitary latrines for proper disposal of human excreta.
3. Supply of safe food, i.e. food is protected from flies, maintaining cleanliness among food handlers.
4. Prevention of the breeding places by proper disposal of garbage.
5. Protection of the host by maintaining personal hygiene and immunization with cholera vaccine.

Health Education

Educating the members of the communities regarding measures for the prevention and control of cholera.

Nursing Management of Cholera

Isolation

Cholera can be isolated by the medical aseptic technique. Nurses are other personnel whose duty is to work with or near cholera patients and should be protected by vaccination. The causative organisms may be found in the nose and throat secretions, stomach contents, stool, and in the urine. All contaminated material should be cleaned up or sent to the incinerator as soon as possible after use.

Diet

Neither fluids nor food taken by mouth can be tolerated during the first 3 days after onset. Vomiting is almost constant. During this stage, IV saline solution is usually given. Fluids by mouth should be given as soon as they can be tolerated. Tea, barley water, whey and boiled milk are given, to be followed by a nourishing soft diet as the patient improves. General diet may be given as soon as it can be retained. A record of fluid and food intake should be kept.

Temperature

Temperature is seldom high. However, there is considerable difference between the surface and rectal temperatures. The surface temperature usually is several degrees below normal, while the rectal temperature may be normal or several degrees above. Mouth or axillary temperatures are not reliable. For this reason two graphic temperature charts should be kept with the temperature, pulse and respiration recorded every 3 hours, one for axillary temperature, and the other for rectal temperature. The prognosis is sometimes determined by variations of the two temperatures. If the temperature is below normal, external heat should be applied.

Personal Hygiene

During the acute stage, the patient should be spared all unnecessary effort. The daily cleansing bath should be omitted and the face, and hands sponged with warm water. A partial bath may be given when the position of the patient is changed from time to time. The buttocks area should be kept clean with warm water and soap sponges, rubbed dry, and baby oil applied. Good oral hygiene should be maintained. The teeth should be cleaned thoroughly at least twice daily. When vomiting occurs an antiseptic mouthwash should be used.

Elimination: Bowel elimination is not a problem, as almost continual diarrhea is a characteristic symptom. The nurse should watch for suppression, which is a fairly common complication. An accurate record of fluid output should be kept.

General Management of the Disease

The patient should be placed in a quiet, private room, which should be warm (70°F), well ventilated and well screened, and kept out of droughts. Dehydration is extreme and fluids should be forced to the point of tolerance. When hypertonic salt solution is given intravenously, the nurse should watch for and report chest pain, cough, headache, unusual restlessness, and cyanosis. Anyone of these symptoms may indicate too much fluid or a too rapid rate of administration.

When morphine or any other toxic drug is given hypodermically, the drug is not absorbed by the circulation during the cold stage. If more than one dose is given during this stage, the cumulative effects of all doses given is felt during the reaction stage with very undesirable results. The patient remains conscious during the course of this disease and restraints are seldom necessary. It is extremely difficult to give an IV injection, because of the collapsed state of the vein. The nurse should be prepared for the doctor to cut down the vein or the femoral vein may be used under such conditions.

Concurrent disinfection should be practiced conscientiously. Contaminated linen should be rolled into small compact bundles with the soiled portion on the inside of the bundle. It should be placed carefully into a clean laundry bag and sterilized by autoclave before it is sent to the laundry. Hands should be scrubbed and disinfected thoroughly immediately before meals, and before coming in contact with any object that may reach the nose or mouth. Flies and all other insects should be excluded from the room.

Convalescence

The duration of the disease is relatively short. Although, the patient usually are extremely sick during the acute stage and recovery is rapid. Frequently, it is difficult to impress upon his/her the necessity for remaining in bed for a week or more after the acute stage has subsided. The nurse should remember that heart failure is a fairly common sequel to cholera. Educating mothers about diarrhea in children and its prevention at their level.

TYPHOID FEVER

Communicable disease is an illness caused due to a specific infectious agent or its toxic products capable of being directly or indirectly transmitted from man to man, animal to animal, or from the environment to man or animal. These diseases are grouped as waterborne, airborne, vector-borne, fomite-borne diseases, etc. Water-borne diseases are many such as diarrhea, cholera, typhoid, etc. Genesis in Britain, enteric fever was the name used for typhoid fever. Until 1890s, typhoid fever was confused with typhus fever. Then, Jenner examined 66 fatal cases of two diseases both clinically and at postmortem examination, and clearly differentiated them. During the First World War, Mary Cook in New York was responsible for at least 50 cases of typhoid fever, many of whom died, before she finally tracked down. By this, it was understood that the contaminated food, water and milk can cause this disease. Typhoid fever is an acute infectious disease caused by *Salmonella typhi (S. typhi).*

Magnitude of Problem

Typhoid fever occurs in all parts of the world and occurs irrespective of climate. Typhoid in the better developed temperate climate, its incidence has steadily decreased and it is now much more prevalent in the tropics than in the colder parts of the globe. Typhoid fever continues to be a significant health problem in developing countries of Africa, Asia, Latin America and some Pacific Islands. In these countries, incidence rate varying from 10 to 1,500 per 100,000 population. Typhoid is not a notifiable disease in India. According to health surveys conducted by the Central Ministry of Health, the morbidity rate varies from 102 to 2,219 per 100,000 population.

Epidemiological Features

Agent

Salmonella typhi is the major cause of enteric fever in India. *S. typhi* has been classified into a number of phage types, the common ones in India are A and E with phage type A predominating.

Morphology

Salmonella typhi organisms are gram negative, motile, rod-shaped bodies provided with numerous peritrichous flagella. *S. typhi* survives intracellularly in the tissues of various organs. On autolysis, the bacilli liberate endotoxin, which plays an important role in the pathogenesis is of typhoid fever. Typhoid bacilli are readily killed by heat. The thermal death point in water or milk is 60°C or 140°F.

Source of Infection

The sole source of infection is the feces or urine of cases and carriers. The bacilli are excreted for varying periods in feces and urine. There is no evidence that the bacilli are excreted in sputum or milk.

Reservoir of Infection

Man is the only known reservoir and natural host of *S. typhi,* and are also detected in the bloodstream of even apparently healthy persons.

Host factors

1. Age: Typhoid fever may occur at any age, but the common age group is between 10 and 30 years. After the age of 30 years, the incidence falls probably due to acquisition of immunity from clinical or subclinical infection.
2. Sex: More cases are reported among males than females, but carrier rate is more in females.
3. Immunity: An attack of typhoid fever gives a fairly lasting immunity. Secondary attacks are not uncommon. Many adults appear to acquire immunity through subclinical infection.

Environmental factors

1. Season: Enteric fever occurs all through the year. The peak incidence is reported in July, August and September. This coincides with the rainy season and increase in fly population in India.
2. Water: Typhoid bacilli do not multiply in water. Many die within 48 hours and do not survive for long in contaminated water.
3. Ice: Freezing does not destroy the bacilli. They may survive for over a month in ice and ice cream.
4. Food: It is a poor conductor of heat and the bacilli may multiply and survive in food for some time.
5. Soil: Research has shown that salmonellae may persist for up to 70 days in soil irrigated with sewage under moist winter conditions and for about half of that period under drill summer conditions.
6. Flies: It carry the bacilli from feces to food. The bacilli have been found to remain viable on the external surface of houseflies for 20 days.
7. Milk: Typhoid bacilli grow rapidly in milk without altering its taste or appearance. Consumption of raw milk is therefore dangerous.
8. Vegetables: These are grown on sewage farms may be infected with typhoid bacilli and enter the host, if eaten raw.

Social factors

The immediate cause of typhoid fever may be *S. typhi*, but the root causes, which perpetuate the disease are many. These may be stated as:

- Lack of safe drinking water
- Open-air defecation and urination leading to dissemination of infection through soil, water, food and flies
- Low standards of personal hygiene, e.g. not washing hands after toilet
- Unhygienic health practices, e.g. washing soiled linen in tanks, rivers and near wells
- Low standards of food and kitchen hygiene illiteracy and health ignorance.

All these factors are responsible for the high endemicity of typhoid fever in India. Unless these social factors are remedied, typhoid hazard in this country cannot be minimized.

Mode of Transmission

1. Vehicle transmission: Typhoid fever spreads chiefly through the medium of contaminated water, food, milk and vegetables. The disease is endemic, where sanitation is poor.
2. Direct contact: Direct transmission of infection occurs from an actual case through contaminated hands. The hands may be contaminated while handling patients, their excreta or infected towels and bed clothes.
3. Flies: Typhoid bacilli are also transmitted through flies. The incubation period of typhoid fever is from 10 to 15 days, with a range from 5 days to 3 weeks. Waterborne infections have a longer incubation period than foodborne infections. Incubation period also depends upon the dose of infection.

Pathophysiology

The normal acid content of the stomach is one of the chief defense against this and other similarly acquired bacillary infections. This physiological barrier is readily broken down by dilution with droughts of fluid by emptiness of the stomach and by other means, and the bacilli then pass into the small intestine.

The bacilli enter the Peyer's patches or solitary lymph follicles, where they rapidly multiply and quickly pass into the bloodstream. The organisms soon reach the bile, either directly from capillaries in the gallbladder wall or indirectly by the liver capillaries into the bile canaliculi and flourish in it. A second and heavier invasion of the intestine through the infected bile takes place. It is this second invasion, which is responsible for extensive lesions in the lymphoid tissue of small intestine, characteristic of the disease and gross clinical manifestations of the disease become evident.

Typhoid is essentially a bacteremia with generalized infection and profound toxemia. It affects the hematopoietic system, especially lymphoid tissue of small intestine, abdominal lymph glands, spleen and bone marrow, but any organ may be involved. In the lymphoid tissue, the organisms cause a peculiar cellular reaction, there are very few polymorphonuclear cells in the lesions, but there is hyperplasia of the lymphoid cells with the appearance of numerous large mononuclear phagocytic cells (typhoid cells), which probably are derived from the reticuloendothelial system.

Clinical Features

The onset commonly is insidious with anorexia, lassitude, a frontal headache, muscular pains, a blurred tongue and often some gastrointestinal discomfort. There is a slight evening fever, which may escape notice (Fig. 29.2).

First Week

Shivering attacks may occur as the temperature with remissions, mounts daily to 103 or 104°F by the end of the week. The pulse rate is 80–100 beats per minute, the pulse remains soft and is dicrotic. There is epistaxis and increase in the respiration rate with signs of catarrhal bronchitis.

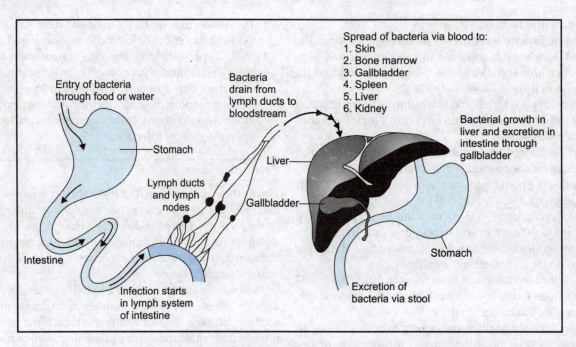

Figure 29.2: Typhoid fever pathogenesis

The abdomen becomes distended and uncomfortable; there may be either diarrhea or constipation and diarrhea at the end of the week. The face becomes drawn and pallid, throat is dry and inflamed rash appears on 6th or 7th day, and lasts for 3–4 days.

Second Week

The temperature is maintained at a high level with slight morning remissions. The toxemia becomes more marked and low muttering delirium is found. Deafness is usual. The tongue becomes dry, glazed and red and sordes collect on the teeth. The pulse rate quickens and BP falls. Spleen becomes palpable. Usually, there is diarrhea and stool mixed with blood.

Third Week

In favorable cases, the symptoms begin to lessen and the remissive temperature slowly declines. In severe cases, the patient does not improve, but becomes delirium or stupor with muscular twitching and picking at the bedclothes. Signs of peritonitis and perforation are seen.

Fourth Week

In favorable cases, convalescence is entered upon. Sometimes lobar pneumonia or thrombophlebitis, especially to left femoral may appear.

Complications

Many structures may become infected in the course of typhoid fever including lungs, pleura, pericardium, heart, kidneys and bones. However, the most common of the serious complications are intestinal hemorrhage and perforation of the bowel with resultant peritonitis.

Intestinal hemorrhages due to erosion of blood vessels in the ulcerated small intestine occur during the 3rd week in about 10% of patients. Some patients have many such hemorrhages. Signs of hemorrhage include apprehension, sweating, pallor, weak rapid pulse, hypotension and bloody or tarry stools. During these episodes, food is withheld and blood transfusion is given.

Intestinal perforation, the most serious complication may happen at any time, but most often occurs during the 3rd week. The perforation usually takes place in the lower ileum. It arises when the ulcer causing the slough involves the entire thickness of the bowel wall. The intestinal content pour into the abdominal cavity, producing peritonitis. The patient may experience a sudden drop in temperature or an increase in pulse rate and complain of acute abdominal pain. There is associated abdominal tenderness and rigidity. However, the pain may only last for few seconds and then stop, with the patient falling sound asleep within a few minutes. If such signs occur, the patient must be ready for intestinal decompression and IV fluids. Surgical intervention may be necessary, if conservative measures do not provide clinical improvement.

Other complications of typhoid fever include thrombophlebitis, urinary infections and cholecystitis. Jaundice may occur from direct infection of the gallbladder by the typhoid bacillus. This is treated conservatively with sedatives, antispasmodics and parenteral fluids.

Convalescence

Since typhoid fever is a very serious disease, the process of recovery may be a slow one. Once a patient has recovered, his/her stools must be checked to see if he/she has become a carrier, as it will be the case in 2–5% of typhoid patients, such carriers harbor the organism and excrete it in their urine and stools. A positive stool culture after 4 months indicates a carrier. Such people must not become food or milk handlers. To abolish the carrier state, ampicillin may be given, although in some instances, ampicillin may prolong the carrier state.

Control of Typhoid Fever

The control or elimination of typhoid fever is well within scope of modem public health. This is an accomplished fact in many developed countries. There are generally three lines of defense against typhoid fever:

1. Control of reservoir.
2. Control of sanitation.
3. Immunization.

Control of Reservoir

The usual methods to control reservoir are their identification, isolation, treatment and disinfection.

Cases

1. Early diagnosis: It is of vital importance as the early symptoms are nonspecific. Culture of blood and stools are important investigations in the diagnosis of cases.
2. Isolation: Since typhoid is infectious and has a prolonged course, the cases are better transferred to a hospital for proper treatment as well as to prevent the spread of infection. As a rule, cases should be isolated till three bacteriologically negative stools and urine reports are detained on three separate days.
3. Notification: This should be done where such notification is mandatory.
4. Treatment: Chloramphenicol remains the drug of choice, if the bacilli are sensitive to it. For adults, the dose is 500 mg (approximately 50 mg/kg of body weight/day), 4 hourly while febrile and thereafter 500 mg 6 hourly for a total period of 14 days. Co-trimoxazole, amoxicillin and trimethoprim are equally effective. Patients seriously ill and profoundly toxic may be given an injection of hydrocortisones 100 mg daily for 3–4 days.
5. Disinfection: Stools and urine are the sole sources of infection. They should be received in closed containers and disinfected with 5% cresol for at least 2 hours. All soiled clothes and linen should be soaked in a solution of 2% chlorine and steam sterilized. Nurses and doctors should not forget to disinfect their hands.
6. Follow-up: Examination of stools and urine should be done for *S. typhi* 3–4 months after discharge of the patient, and again after 12 months to prevent the development of the carrier state. With early diagnosis and appropriate treatment, mortality has been reduced to 1% compared to 30% in untreated cases.

Carriers

Since carriers are the ultimate source of typhoid fever, their identification and treatment are one of the radical ways of controlling typhoid fever, the measures recommended are:

1. Identification: Carriers are identified by cultural and serological examinations. Duodenal drainage establishes the presence of *Salmonella* in the biliary tract in carriers. The antibodies are present in about 80% of chronic carriers.
2. Treatment: The carrier should be given an intensive course of ampicillin (4–6 g/day) together with probenecid (2 g/day) for 6 weeks. These drugs are concentrated in the bile and may achieve eradication of the carrier state in about 70% of carriers.
3. Surgery: Cholecystectomy with concomitant ampicillin therapy has been regarded as the most successful approach to the treatment of carriers. Care rate may be as high as 80%. Urinary carriers are easy to treat, but refractory cases need nephrectomy when one kidney is damaged and the other healthy.
4. Surveillance: The carriers should be kept under surveillance. They should be prevented from handling food, milk or water for others.
5. Health education: Washing of hands with soap and water after defecation or urination, and before preparing food is an essential element of health education. In short, the management of carriers continued to be an unsolved problem. This is the crux of the problem in the elimination of typhoid fever.

Control by Sanitation

The weakest link in the chain of transmission is sanitation, which is amenable to control protection and purification of drinking water supplies, improvement of basic sanitation, and promotion of food hygiene are essential measures to interrupt transmission of typhoid fever.

Typhoid fever is never a major problem, where there is a clean domestic water supply. Sanitary measures not followed by health education may produce only temporary results. However, when sanitation is combined with health education, the effects tend to be cumulative resulting in a steady reduction of typhoid morbidity (refer Chapter 57 'Health Education').

Immunization

Control of typhoid fever must take the form of improved sanitation, domestic and personal hygiene, these are long-term objectives in many developing countries. A complementary approach to prevention is immunization, which is the only specific preventive measure likely to yield the highest benefit for the money spent. Immunization against typhoid does not give 100% protection, but it definitely lowers both the incidence and seriousness of the infection. It can be given at any age upwards of 1 year and is particularly recommended to:
- Those living in endemic areas
- Household contacts
- Groups at risk of infection such as school children and hospital staff
- Travellers proceeding to endemic areas
- Those attending melas and yatras.

Antityphoid vaccines

Although, typhoid vaccine was introduced by Wright in 1896, it was not until the 1960s that its effectiveness was established by controlled field trials. More recently, trials in Egypt have shown that a live-attenuated oral vaccine prepared from a mutant strain gave a clinical protection of 95%. The antityphoid vaccines currently available in India are:

1. **Monovalent vaccine:** Since *S. typhi* is the major cause of typhoid fever in India, the vaccine of choice is naturally the monovalent typhoid vaccine, which is an agar grown, heat killed and phenol-preserved vaccine containing 1,000 million of *S. typhi*/mL. It may also be prepared by inactivation of the organisms with acetone and the vaccine is known as acetone killed and dried (AKD) antityphoid vaccine.
2. **Bivalent vaccine:** It contains *S. typhi* and *Salmonella paratyphi* (*S. paratyphi*) in the proportion of 1,000 million, and 500 million organisms respectively. The organisms are killed and preserved by heating at 54°C for 1 hour and by the addition of 0.5% phenol. The bivalent vaccine may also be prepared by the inactivation of the organisms with acetone in the dried form (AKD vaccine).
3. **Typhoid-paratyphoid A and B vaccine (TAB):** The traditional TAB vaccine contained *S. typhi* (1,000 million), *S. paratyphi* (500–750 million) and *S. paratyphi* B (500–750 million) organisms/mL. The paratyphoid antigens in the vaccine are not only thought to be of doubtful effectiveness, but their presence enhanced reactions caused by extraproteins of paratyphoid A and B components. Therefore, traditional TAB vaccine has fallen into disfavor. The WHO recommended that the TAB vaccine should be discontinued.

Dosage and mode of administration

1. **Primary immunization:** It should consist of two doses (each of 0.5 mL) of the vaccine, given subcutaneously at an interval of 4–6 weeks. Children between 1 and 10 years are to be given smaller doses (0.25 mL). A special diluted vaccine is available for children and should be used when available. The usual site of the injection is the outer aspect of the upper arm, behind the posterior border of the distal part of the deltoid muscle. Immunity develops 10–21 days after inoculation and the protection is maintained for at least 3 years.
2. **Booster doses:** These are recommended every 3 years. If booster is allowed to lapse for more than 3 years, it is necessary to repeat the full primary course. Some individuals do not develop immunity against typhoid fever even though they may have received two or more injections of typhoid vaccine.
3. **Reactions:** Typhoid vaccine generally causes local reactions (pain, swelling and tenderness) and also very frequently constitutional symptoms such as malaise, headache and pyrexia, which however, usually subside within 36 hours. To reduce the severity of reaction, it has been advised that the vaccine be administered late in the afternoon or evening. Aspirin or other antipyretic drugs may be administered to mitigate the unpleasant reactions, women should not be injected during late pregnancy.

Storage

Antityphoid vaccine should be stored in a refrigerator at 2–4°C. They should not be frozen. Under proper conditions of storage, potency is retained for a period of 18 months.

Live oral Ty21a vaccine

Live oral vaccines against typhoid are on scene. Two attenuated strains of *S. typhi*, Ty21a and 541Ty developed by Swiss and United States (US) scientists respectively are being evaluated as live oral vaccines. Extensive trials in Chili and Egypt have demonstrated the safety of Ty21a in more than 500,000 school children. In Egypt, three doses of a liquid formulation gave 96% protection for at least 3 years.

Clinical trials with attenuated *S. typhi* strain, i.e. 541Ty have started only recently, but in these initial studies the vaccine has been safe and highly immunogenic.

Health Education

For prevention of typhoid fever, the following measures should be adopted:
1. Food should be protected from flies. Raw vegetables and fruits should be taken only after washing them in a weak solution of potassium permanganate.
2. Pure and wholesome supply of milk and milk products. Only boiled, pasteurized milk and dairy products including cheese should be taken.
3. Efficient conservancy arrangements, leaving no refuse for breeding of flies, i.e. adoption of adequate antifly measures.
4. Purified and safe water supply. Public water supplies must be chlorinated.
5. Proper supervision of articles of food and places where they are manufactured, and offered for sale. They should be protected from dust and flies.
6. Discovery and proper control of carriers training of convalescents, and chronic carriers in personal hygiene, particularly as to sanitary disposal of excreta.
7. Licensing of food handlers in restaurants and public eating establishments.
8. Education of the public through leaflets, posters, filmstrips and cinema slides, particularly on the role of five F's, viz. fingers, food, flies, feces and fomites.

Nursing Management of Typhoid and Paratyphoid Fevers

Isolation

Typhoid and paratyphoid fevers can be isolated by the medical aseptic technique. The causative organisms are found in urine, stool, nose and throat secretions. If the plumbing leads to a septic tank or is sewer connected, it is not necessary to disinfect deject before they are emptied. However, bedpans, urinals, bath basins, emesis basins and all other equipment, and material contaminated by contact either with the patient or his/her discharges should be sterilized, cleaned up or destroyed as soon as possible after use. Flies and other insects should, of course, be excluded from the patient's room. Thorough screening is a necessity.

All nurses and other hospital personnel should have established immunity through vaccination or by having the disease before caring for typhoid fever patients. Unvaccinated nurses should not be allowed to nurse typhoid patients. The disease has been notorious ill in the past for attacking nurses, doctors and laboratory personnel.

Diet

Diet is of the utmost importance for several reasons:
1. Because of the gradual onset of disease, patient frequently fails to place himself/herself under medical treatment until disease has advanced in 2nd or 3rd week.
2. Because of the onset symptoms of malaise and generalized aching and pains, headache and anorexia, the patient frequently becomes both dehydrated and malnourished before treatment is started.
3. Much of the pathosis of the disease (inflammation and ulceration of Peyer's patches) is in the digestive tract.
4. Because two of the most serious complications are hemorrhage and perforation from the small intestines, the diet must be selected, and prepared very carefully.
5. Chloromycetin, which reduces both the duration and the severity of symptoms when given early in the disease has little or no effect upon complications already present when treatment is initiated.

Because of the many symptoms and complications referable to the GIT, it often taxes the ingenuity of the best nurse to provide sufficient calories, and fluids in a palatable form, and still not have them injurious to the patient. During the high temperature stage, the diet should consist of nourishing fluids, milk, cream, buttermilk, malted milk, eggnogs, fruit juices, cream soups, chicken and beef broth, as well as vegetable juices. It is to be remembered, however some patients are allergic to milk and do not tolerate it. In such cases, milk must be eliminated from the diet.

Later, when the patient can tolerate them, baked potatoes with butter may be given as well as mashed potatoes, beef juice with egg added, cottage cheese, stewed fruit without seeds, soft-cooked eggs, cornflakes, strained oatmeal, cream of wheat or other cereal without rough cellulose, pureed vegetables, gelatin, custards and junket.

The caloric needs of the average adult patient are between 3,000 and 4,000 calories per day, and the fluid intake should be from 3,000 to 4,000 mL/day. Frequently, it is necessary to give fluids by IV injection. The patient can take and retain food better if the feedings are given frequently, every 2–3 hours, and in small amounts. A record of both fluid and caloric intake should be kept.

Temperature

The temperature in typhoid fever is characteristically high, being 104–106°F. It may be reduced by a tepid or cool sponge, or an alcohol rub. An ice bag or ice packs to the head helps to relieve low headache and also to reduce temperature. A small stool, colonic irrigation given without pressure may produce good results. However, a colonic flushing or irrigation should be given only upon advice of the physician.

The nurse should be careful, when giving either a temperature sponge or an alcohol rub, or fan not to permit the patient to become unduly exposed, or chilled. Only a small area of the body should be exposed at one time. The room should be warm (70°F or higher) and the patient should be kept out of droughts.

Personal Hygiene

The patient should have a daily cleansing bath with a complete change of personal linen and bedclothes. Local sponge baths should be given as needed to keep the patient clean, dry and comfortable.

DIARRHEAL DISEASES

Diarrhea is an acute or chronic intestinal disturbance characterized by increased frequency, humidity or volume of lower movement. It has been defined as passing of more than three loose motions in a day or 24 hours. It has been further classified an acute diarrhea, i.e. lasting for less than 21 days and chronic diarrhea, lasting beyond 21 days, while chronic diarrhea is responsible for the serious problem of malnutrition, acute diarrhea is responsible for death due to dehydration.

Magnitude of Problem

According to certain small studies conducted in India, it is assumed as 100 million children (14.1% of the total population) suffer from 300 million episodes of diarrhea per year. About 10% or 30 million may develop dehydration and 1% or 3 million may face death. Diarrheal diseases are a major cause of death and disease among children under 5 years. A child on average suffers 2–3 attacks of diarrhea every year.

Epidemiological Features

Agent

The major pathogens causing diarrhea in India are:
1. Bacteria: *Escherichia Coli (E. coli), Shigella, Salmonella, V. cholerae* (Cholerale EI Tor) *Campylobacter jejuni (C. jejuni), Staphylococcus.*
2. Virus: Rotavirus, adenovirus, astrovirus, calicivirus and noroviruses.
3. Parasites: *Entamoeba histolytica (E. histolytica), Giardia lamblia (G. lamblia), Strongyloides stercoralis (S. stercoralis), Trichuris.*

Host Factors

1. Age: This is the most important disease specially among children particularly under 5 years.
2. Sex: It affects both sexes, male and female.
3. Socioeconomic factors: Poverty, malnutrition, immunodeficiency, low standards of personal hygiene, certain human habits favoring water and soil pollution, lack of education, and poor quality of life are the important socioeconomic factors.
4. Environmental factors: Diarrheal diseases may be easily transmitted in a community with poor environmental sanitation. This includes contaminated water, food and soil pollution.

Mode of Transmission

Most of the enteric pathogens are transmitted primarily by the fecal-oral route, which may be waterborne, foodborne or direct contact:
1. Contaminated water: It is transmitted through drinking of contaminated water from the contaminated water sources, which have been in contact with human excreta.
2. Contaminated food: Ingestion of contaminated food and drink has been associated with diarrheal diseases. Bottle feeding could be a significant risk factor for infants. Fruits and vegetables washed with contaminated water can be a source of infection and food, which has been contaminated by flies or dirty food handlers.
3. Direct contact: Person-to-person transmission readily takes place through contaminated fingers, while carelessly handling excreta, vomit of patients, contaminated linen and eating utensils or dirt, which may be ingested by young children.

Pathophysiology

Wide assortments of organisms cause diarrheal diseases. Viruses (rotavirus), *Shigella* and *Salmonella* pathogens cause an inflammatory reaction in the epithelial layer of intestine cause destruction of cells in the intestine and lead to diarrhea. Organisms such as *E. coli* and *V. cholerae* produce enterotoxin, which consists of 'L' toxin and 'H' toxin. The 'H' toxin stimulates adenylate cyclase in the intestinal epithelial cells and causes a rise in another substance cyclic adenosine monophosphate (cAMP), which provides energy to drive fluid, and ions into the lumen of the intestine. The increase in fluid is the cause of diarrhea.

CHAPTER 29 — Intestinal Infections

Fluid Loss

During diarrhea, large volume of fluids and electrolytes are lost in the stools. As intestinal secretions are isotonic with plasma, there is outpouring of fluid and electrolytes from plasma into the lumen of the intestine to make up the loss. An attempt is made to compensate the plasma volume, in turn, by a shift of fluid and electrolyte from interstitial and intracellular chambers. As the fluid and electrolyte losses continue in the stools, fluid, and electrolyte deficit occur in intracellular, interstitial and intravascular compartments in that order.

Electrolyte Changes

Electrolyte loss, along with the proportionate fluid loss, affects the osmolarity of plasma and many body functions.

Sodium
1. Isotonic dehydration: Where the proportion of the fluid and electrolytes (sodium) is nearly same.
2. Hypotonic dehydration: Where the sodium level is less than normal.
3. Hypertonic dehydration: Here the loss of fluid in proportion to electrolyte is more.

Potassium
1. Hypokalemia: Loss of potassium into the stools leads to hypokalemia.
2. Hyperkalemia: Loss of fixed base bicarbonate into the stools and acidosis occurs.

Clinical Manifestation

Clinical features of the diarrhea depend upon the severity of the disease. When diarrhea is severe, signs of dehydration occur quickly, especially in children:

1. Dehydration:
    - Little to extreme loss of subcutaneous fat
    - Up to 50% total body weight loss
    - Urinary output decreases
    - Poor skin turgor dry skin and dry mouth
    - Sunken fontanels and eyes
    - Low BP and high pulse
    - Collapse imminent.
2. Behavior changes:
    - Irritability
    - Restlessness
    - Weakness
    - Pallor
    - Extreme prostration
    - Stupor and convulsions.
3. Respiration rapid, i.e. hyperpnea stools:
    - Loose and fluid inconsistency
    - Greenish or yellow-green color
    - May contain mucus or blood.
4. Vomiting mild and intermittent to severe vomiting.
5. Fever low grade to 40.1°C (100°F).
6. Anorexia: When the signs of dehydration are present, the patient is in a serious condition and death may occur quickly, if treatment is delayed.

Diagnosis (Table 29.6)

1. Ask and collect the history from the patient, and his/her relatives regarding:
    a. Diarrhea duration of illness:
        - Frequency of stools per day
        - Appearance, consistency, color, smell, presence or absence of blood/mucus.
    b. Vomiting: Present or not.
    c. Thirst: Normal or more than normal.
    d. Urine output normal or decreased in quantity.
2. Look and examine the general conditions of the patient for signs of dehydration:
    a. Presence or absence of tears.
    b. Sunken eye, dry skin and increased skin.
    c. Dry mouth and tongue.
    d. Rapid breathing.
    e. Rapid pulse.
    f. Sunken fontanel.
    g. Temperature of the body.
    h. Loss of weight.
3. Collect the specimen of stool for laboratory diagnosis.

Treatment (Table 29.7)

After assessing, the degree of dehydration treatment can be started depending on the severity. The intervention measures comprise the following.

Oral Rehydration Therapy

Oral rehydration therapy (ORT) is a life-saving measure to combat dehydration, should be started forthwith to prevent the further damages and prevent the death. The oral rehydration therapy is envisaged in three stages:

1. The first stage, is managing diarrheal situation with homemade and home available liquids.
2. In the second stage, ORS packet is to be encouraged to combat dehydration.
3. In the third stage, the primary health centers and hospitals will treat with IV therapy in severe cases.

Preparation of oral rehydration salts at home (Table 29.8)

- Take half a liter of clean drinking water
- Add two finger pinch of salt, stir it

Table 29.6: Diagnosis of dehydration

Diagnosis	Signs of dehydration	Signs of moderate dehydration	Signs of severe dehydration
Ask			
Diarrhea	Less than four loose motions/day	4–10 loose motions/day	More than 10 loose motions/day
Vomiting	None or small amount	Some	Very frequent
Thirst	Normal	More than normal	Unable to drink
Urine	Normal	Small amount, dark	No urine for 6 hour
Look			
Condition	Well, alert	Unwell, sleepy/irritable	Very sleepy, unconscious
Tears, mouth and tongue	Wet	Dry	Very dry
Eyes, dry and sunken	Normal	Faster than normal	Very fast and deep
Breathing	Normal	Faster than normal	Very fast and deep
Feel			
Skin	Pinch goes back quickly	Pinch goes back slowly	Pinch goes back very slowly
Pulse	Normal	Faster than normal	Very fast, weak
Fontanel	Normal	Sunken	Very sunken
Take			
Temperature	–	–	High fever: 38.5°C or in chronic case greater
Body weight	No weight loss	Loss of 25–100 g for each kg of body weight	Loss of more than 100 g for each kg of body weight

Table 29.7: Treatment of dehydration

Mild diarrhea	Moderate diarrhea	Severe diarrhea
Mother should be trained to give plenty of water to prevent dehydration	Health worker to give ORS* packet to correct mild to moderate dehydration	Give ORS and PHC† to give IV‡ drip to treat severe dehydration
ORS packet may be given	Special drink to be prepared, if ORS not available	
Continue feeding	Continue feeding	

*ORS, oral rehydration salts; †PHC, primary health center; ‡IV, intravenous.

- Taste a spoonful of the solution; it should not be more salty than tears
- Add a large fistful of sugar
- Stir the mixture with a clean spoon till the sugar has dissolved
- Give quarter cup to half cup (50–100 mL) of this mixture after every loose motion to a child less than 2 years of age and twice the amount in children above 2 years of age
- Give small sips of the drink if the child vomits, repeat it.

Table 29.8: Composition of oral rehydration salts (ORS)

ORS pack [World Health Organization (WHO)]	Sugar salt solution (at home)
Sodium chloride: 3.5 g	Salt: Three-four tablespoon
Sodium: 2.5 g	Sodium bicarbonate: one-three tablespoon
Potassium chloride: 1.5 g	Lime
Glucose (dextrose): 20 g	Sugar: Five tablespoon
Water: 1 L	Water: 1 L

CHAPTER 29 — Intestinal Infections

Preparation of oral rehydration solution with ORS packet
- Take 1 L of clean drinking water
- Obtain an ORS packet
- Pour the water and the powder from the packet into a large clean vessel
- Stir it with a clean spoon, till it dissolves; there will be about five glasses of the drink
- Give quarter cup to half cup (50–100 mL) after every loose motion to a child less than 2 years of age and twice the amount in children above 2 years.

Keep the rest of the drink covered. Make fresh drink every day. If child vomits wait for 10 minutes, then give it in small amounts sip by sip. The solution should be used within 24 hours. It should not be boiled.

Appropriate Feeding

During episodes of diarrhea, normal food intake such as coconut water, rice water, dal water, mashed ripe banana and weak tea may also be given including breastfeeding. It will help to recover faster and to prevent further infection.

Appropriate Drugs

Administration of appropriate therapeutic agent should be considered where the cause of the diarrhea has been clearly identified as *Shigella, Campylobacter* or *Giardia*:
- Bacterial infection: Ampicillin, chloramphenicol, gentamicin and tetracyclines are used
- Symptomatic treatment for fever, vomiting, etc.
- Protozoan infection—metronidazole can be used.

If the child has blood/mucus in the stool and fever suspect dysentery treat with antimicrobials. If the patient has severe dehydration or high fever, refer the patient to higher medical center for IV therapy and further treatment. The IV infusion is usually required only for the initial rehydration of severely dehydrated patients who are in shock or unable to drink. The solutions for IV infusions are:
- Ringer's lactate solution
- Diarrhea treatment solution
- Normal saline (5% dextrose should not be given).

Recommended dose is 11 mL/kg body weight for adult children. Initially it should be fast and it is maintained until his/her BP and pulse return to normal. When patient's condition improves, change to the oral route should be made.

Control and Preventive Measures

Short-term Objectives
1. Training of medical and paramedical persons.
2. Stream production and distribution of ORS packets.
3. Education of mothers and community in the use of ORT, formulation of proper strategies towards continuous breastfeeding, and weaning practices.
4. Operation/Health services research for identification of a suitable strategy for implementation.

Long-term Objectives
1. Provision of safe drinking water supply.
2. Improvement of sewage disposal system.
3. Improvement of general environmental sanitation.
4. Health and nutrition education of the community.

Plan of Action

Availability of Oral Rehydration Salt

Packets of oral rehydration mixture are freely available at all primary health center (PHC), subcenters and other medical centers. When it is delivered within PHC settings, it is an effective and relatively inexpensive intervention for the reduction of mortality due to dehydration of diarrhea. Every village health guide is supplied with 100 packets of ORS per year. If the ORS mixture of salts is not available, a simple mixture consisting of table salt 5 g and sugar 20 g dissolved in 1 L of drinking water may be safely used until the proper mixture is obtained. In severe dehydration the best form of treatment is IV rehydration such as Ringer's lactate, normal saline available in the hospital.

Training Program

Training program is proposed to include diarrheal management with ORS in the course curricula of multipurpose workers, supervisors, health guides, medical and nursing students, and pediatricians. The medical and paramedical personnel involved at present in PHC at district hospital PHCs/subcenters down to village level have also to be trained. Private practitioners are also to be trained through Indian Medical Association (IMA).

Increasing Host Resistance to Infection

1. Maternal nutrition: Improving pre- and post-natal nutrition will reduce the low birth weight problem, and will improve the quality of breast milk respectively.
2. Child nutrition: Continuing breastfeeding as long as possible is likely to reduce the diarrheal diseases. Improving weaning practices not later than the 6 months and using nutritious, and locally available foods will reduces the diarrheal incidence. Supplementary feeding is also necessary to improve the nutritional status of children.

3. Immunization: Since cases of measles complicated by diarrhea have a high fatality rate, measles immunization is a potential intervention for diarrhea control.

Provision of Safe Drinking Water Supply

All steps must be taken to provide safe water to the community for all purposes such as drinking, washing and cooking, etc. In urban areas, properly treated drinking water containing free residual chlorine should be made available to all families and it should be stored in the household in narrow-mouthed covered containers. In rural areas, water can be made safe by boiling or by chlorination. These emergency measures should be followed by the development of more permanent facilities.

Improvement of Sewage Disposal System

Provision of simple, cheap and effective excreta disposal system (sanitary latrines) is a basic need of all human settlements. With the cooperation of the community, sanitary system should be selected and constructed taking into consideration of the customs, and practices of the population the existing brain, and geology find the available resources. Simultaneously health education is needed to ensure proper use of these.

Improvement of General Environmental Sanitation

An attack should be made on the fly breeding places by improving environmental sanitation, the environmental sanitation program require educational support.

Health and Nutritional Education of the Community

Health education must be actively pursued. Emphasis should be placed on improved practices of the preparation and storage of foods, especially emphasizing the hygienic preparation of weaning foods should be promoted. Health education must stress on the importance of eating cooked hot food and of individual food handling techniques. Cooking utensils should be cleaned and dried after use. Steps should be taken to improve food sanitation, simple hygienic measures such as proper handwashing after defecation and before eating or preparing food should be promoted by appropriate educational campaigns. Health education should stress on proper use and maintenance of new sanitary latrine facilities, and dangers involved in deposition feces on the ground, in or near the water. Health education of the community for the prevention of diarrhea is to be done through mass media.

Research

It is proposed to encourage research activities in relation to the isolation of etiological agents, epidemiological features, preventive and control measures, and drug response.

National Diarrheal Disease Control Program

Since, diarrheal diseases constitute a major cause of mortality and morbidity, especially in children below the age of 5 years, the Government of India in the Ministry of Health and Family Welfare have formulated a National Plan of Action to control diarrheal diseases under PHC. So, National Diarrheal Diseases Control Program started during the sixth plan (1980–1985) through promotion of ORT. The program has been intensified during the seventh plan to cut down diarrhea mortality by 50% by the year 1990s. The program is integrated with PHC at the village/subcenter/PHC/district hospital levels. Every village health guide is supplied with 100 packets of ORS per year. A key activity in this program is oral rehydration supplemented by health education. The National Cholera Control Program has been integrated with this program. During the eighth plan it is intended to print material/booklets on treatment of diarrheal diseases/cholera for distributing free among the states in regional languages.

Primary Health Care

The concept of primary health care involves the delivery of a package of curative and preventive services at the community level. An intersectoral approach centered upon PHC involving activities in the fields of water supply, excreta disposal, communicable disease control, mother and child health, nutrition, and health education is regarded as essential for the ultimate control of diarrheal diseases.

Nursing Management of Diarrhea

Isolation

Epidemic diarrhea of the newborn can be isolated by strict medical aseptic technique. While the cause of the disease is unknown, it is thought to be a virus. The disease is both very serious and highly communicable. Concurrent disinfection during nursing care is most important. All articles contaminated by either direct or indirect contact with the patient must be cleaned up thoroughly immediately after use or sent to the incinerator.

Diet

If the patient is a breastfed, baby he/she usually is taken off breastfeeding and a formula prescribed. All feedings often are withheld for 12–24 hours; however, this must never be done without the direct order of the physician. During this interval of starvation, warm sterile water is given at intervals of 1–2 hours.

If stools are frequent, both the ingenuity and the perseverance of the nurse may be taxed to keep the baby from becoming both malnourished and dehydrated. If the baby is too weak to swallow the formula in the usual manner often it becomes necessary to feed him/her. A Breck feeder or a medicine dropper can be used with good results.

While the baby should be disturbed as little as possible consistent with good nursing, a sick baby frequently can be given feedings with less effort if held in the arms. If vomiting is present small feedings at frequent intervals often are prescribed. Fluids should be urged.

If the baby is unable to take and retain sufficient nourishment and fluid, the physician usually gives supplementary IV feedings. Solutions containing low serum potassium have been found to be the frequent cause of death in these cases. A careful record must be kept of all fluids taken and retained.

Temperature

The temperature is seldom high enough to present a nursing problem. However, it should become necessary to reduce temperature, a warm sponge bath may be given during which every precaution must be taken to prevent the baby from becoming chilled. The temperature should be taken and recorded at least every 4 hours.

Personal Hygiene

Unless prostration is great, the baby should be given a cleansing sponge bath daily. In the case of prostration, less the baby is moved and the more his/her strength is conserved the better for all concerned. The eyes and nose may be kept clean with sterile moist cotton pledgets. The buttocks and anal areas should be sponged carefully with warm water, patted dry with a soft absorbent cloth, and baby oil applied after each bowel movement. It cannot be stressed too strongly that the baby should be kept clean and dry.

Elimination

A careful record of all stools should be kept including the number of stools, the time interval between stools and the consistency, amount, and character of each stool.

General Management of the Disease

Epidemic diarrhea of the newborn always presents an emergency. Prompt recognition of the beginning symptoms and early isolation of a suspect case are most important. More than two watery stools in a 24 hours period should place the baby under suspicion. The baby should be removed immediately from the clean nursery and placed in a separate room. If this is impossible baby should be isolated either in an isolation nursery or in a room with mother.

If the baby has frequent watery stools longer than 48 hours then baby should be removed from the obstetric department. All babies who have been in contact with him/her or in the same.

Diarrheal disease is one of the communicable diseases in which the predominant symptom is diarrhea. Diarrheal diseases are caused by a wide range of organisms. It is one of the important problems among young children. In India, at least 1.5 million under the age of 5 die due to acute diarrhea. This is mainly transmitted by the fecal-oral route may be waterborne, foodborne or direct. Dehydration is the major sign and symptom in this disease. This is treated by rehydration therapy either orally or by IV infusion in severe cases. Control measures include training program, production and distribution of ORS packets, provision of safe water supply, improvement in sewage disposal, environmental sanitation, nutrition and health education of the community. To control diarrheal disease under PHC, a National Diarrheal Disease Control Program was started during Sixth Five-year plan.

BACILLARY DYSENTERY

Dysentery means passing of blood and mucus in stool accompanied by abdominal pain with or without tenesmus (this clinical condition should not be confused with passing of blood per anal canal due to other reasons). The two main forms of dysentery are:
1. Bacillary dysentery (bacterial).
2. Amebic dysentery (protozoan).

Magnitude of Problem

Bacillary dysentery is an acute infection of the bowel, which is characterized by diarrhea. The disease is more common in infants than in adults. The infection is transmitted through contaminated food (especially milk) and water by carriers or patients suffering from dysentery. The disease is prevalent in many parts of the world specially the orients, tropics and subtropics. It is a common disease occurring in all ages and causing many deaths. Death rates are higher in small children, though its susceptibility is general. A relative and transitory strain specific immunity occurs after an attack of this disease. Period of communicability is during acute infection when the feces contain microorganisms.

Epidemiological Features

Agent

There are various species of the genus *Shigella* that causes bacillary dysentery. These are known as *Shigella dysenteriae* (*S. dysenteriae*), *Shigella sonnei* (*S. sonnei*) and others. Some strains of *Shigella* produce few carriers of the disease for 1–2 years and in rare cases even longer.

Shigella: Morphology and straining identical with *S. typhi* except that they do not possess flagella, and are nonmotile. Fimbriae occur only in *Shigella flexneri* (*S. flexneri*) types.

Cultural characters: Resembles the genus *Salmonella* with the exception that *S. sonnei* is a fermenter of lactose thus, colonies of the latter in MacConkey medium become pink when incubation is prolonged beyond 18–24 hours.

Viability: The thermal death point is about 55°C for 1 hour, however, the genus *S. sonnei* is more resistant to adverse environmental factors than other members.

Biochemical reaction: The four groups within the genus *Shigella* display the following biological activities.

Group A: Differ from those in other groups by constantly failing to ferment mannitol.

Group B and C: Comprise species, which are biochemically similar to each other.

Group D: Strain is late fermenter of lactose and never produces indole with the exception of certain strains of *S. flexneri*.

Host

1. Age: The dysentery is most common in children especially those between 6 months and 2 years of age than adults.
2. Sex: Both sexes are affected.
3. Season: It is common in rainy season.
4. General: Low resistance of the body, i.e. when a person is weak and has low resistance then he/she suffers from this disease more than the healthy person.

Environmental Factors

The vibrio transmission is readily possible in a community with poor environmental sanitation, the environmental factors of importance include contaminated water and food. Flies may carry *V. cholerae*, but not vectors of proven importance, numerous social factors have also been responsible for the endemicity of cholera in India. These comprise certain human habits favoring water and soil pollution, low standards of personal hygiene, lack of education, and poor quality of life.

Source of Infection

Main source is feces of an infected person; many mild unrecognized and inapparent cases may become source of infection. Incubation period may be as short as few hours and as long as 7 days, but average period is of 7–14 days.

Mode of Infection

Disease spread by consuming contaminated food, milk or water, etc. by using articles, which are contaminated with the feces of a patient or a carrier. Flies spread the disease mechanically by contaminating food articles. Hand-to-mouth transfer of contaminated food material is the direct mode of infection.

Pathophysiology

The pathology of shigellosis in severe cases consists of organisms reaching the small intestine, where they multiply and release a toxin that initiates secretion of water, and electrolytes from jejunal area. The invading pathogens are capable of initiating an intense inflammatory response in the mucosa followed by small patches of ulceration causes diarrhea with blood and mucus in the stool. The difference between bacillary and amebic dysentery are given in Table 29.9.

Table 29.9: Differences between bacillary and amebic dysentery

Bacillary dysentery	Amebic dysentery
Onset usually acute	Onset insidious
Fever and toxemia commonly present	Fever and toxemia very uncommon
Number of stools more in 24 hour	Number of stools not more than four to six time in 24 hour
Intestinal colic severe	Intestinal colic present, but not severe
Severe tenesmus usual	Tenesmus rare
Stools: Scanty, containing bright red blood and viscid pink-colored mucus	Stools: Copious, mixed with blood and mucus
Stool odorless	Stools offensive
Reaction of stools alkaline	Reaction of stools acidic
Microscopic examination of stools shows polymorphonuclear macrophages, epithelial cells and degenerated endothelial cells	Microscopic examination of stools shows red blood cells, damaged polymorphonuclear cells, many macrophage cells, *Entamoeba histolytica* and Charcot-Leyden crystal

Contd...

CHAPTER 29 — Intestinal Infections

Contd...

Bacillary dysentery	Amebic dysentery
Whole abdomen rigid and tenderness in, especially lower quadrants	Local rigidity and tenderness over sigmoid flexure, transverse colon and cecum
Average type subsides within 10–14 day	Course long or protracted
Complications infrequent in severe infection circulatory failure, renal failure, arthritis and eye complications may occur	Complications may be of hepatitis and lower abscess
Culture of stool reveals dysentery	Culture of stool for dysentery organisms negative
Serological diagnosis by agglutination reaction positive	Serological diagnosis by agglutination
Responds well to sulfonamides and antibodies	Responds well to emotive

Clinical Features

1. Patient has diarrhea, fever and tenesmus.
2. Patient becomes restless, temperature rises up to 103°F and increased pulse rate.
3. Tongue becomes dry and coated.
4. In severe cases have undiagnosed infections, they have only transient diarrhea or no intestinal symptoms.
5. In small children, there is rigidity of the abdominal muscles due to contractions and it becomes tender.
6. Patient starts getting dehydration and starts showing signs of dehydration, and collapse.
7. Due to dehydration, amount of urine diminishes and its specific gravity increases.
8. Patient may have toxemia due to endotoxins and exotoxins, which are produced by the organisms.
9. Severity of degree of collapse depends upon the amount of fluid lost from the body that is the degree of dehydration.
10. Number of stools increase, up to 20 times or more in 24 hours, in severe cases jelly-like substance is seen in the blood. As the severity increases, amount of the fecal matter goes on reducing and ultimately stools do not contain any fecal matter, but the blood and jelly-like substance only.
11. Infants, elderly debilitated persons and person infected with *Shigella* and *Bacillus* most frequently have severe infection.
12. Patient becomes very serious due to toxemia and dehydration.

Assessment

- By signs and symptoms of this disease
- Important sign is presence of blood in the stools with jelly-like substances
- It must be differentiated from other types of diarrhea and dysenteries
- Microscopic examination of the fresh stool, picking out the blood and mucus portion is mandatory in all dysenteries, especially in children above 2–3 years of age
- Rectal swab examination also shows the presence of dysentery bacilli.

Preventive Measures

1. Immunization against measles is a potential intervention for diarrhea control. Rotavirus and improved cholera vaccines are still under development.
2. Sanitation measures to reduce transmission emphasize the traditional improved water supply.
3. Improved excreta disposal and improved domestic, and food hygiene with an adequate supply of clean water close to their homes.
4. Protect and purify public water supply. People should drink boiled water during epidemic season. Chlorine may be used little more without creating danger to safeguard people from this disease.
5. Milk and milk products must be pasteurized or boiled properly before consuming.
6. Special provision should be made for handwashing facilities to those who are engaged in processing, preparing or serving food articles also sanitary supervision of these persons is necessary. All such persons must get themselves thoroughly examined by the physician periodically.
7. Control of flies by using screened doors and windows, protect food from contamination, and eliminate all breeding place of the flies.
8. Infants should be protected from getting any intestinal infection, mothers should be taught to maintain strict cleanliness while feeding babies. They must use boiled milk for children.
9. Report about the patient to the health authorities at once. Reporting about the case, which must be strictly followed in the schools, institutions, colleges, etc.
10. Patient must be isolated during acute illness and until his/her stool report comes as negative.
11. Patient should not be allowed to handle any food articles, until he/she recovers from this disease.
12. All the contacts of the patient must take personal precautions and should not handle any food articles until their stool culture shows no bacilli.

13. Investigations should be made to find out sporadic cases unrecognized and mild cases from the contacts, and contacts of the patient to know the source of infection.
14. Feces of the patient must be collected, disinfected and disposed of properly. All contaminated articles must be sterilized and disinfected. Thorough, cleaning and disinfection of the sick room and contaminated articles is necessary as terminal disinfection.
15. Reduction in the incidence is done by prophylactic administration of chemotherapeutic agents and antibodies under medical supervision to those groups, who are temporarily exposed to the high risk of infection.
16. Health education must be given to the public about practicing personal and environmental hygiene, and dangers of this disease.

Appropriate Clinical Management

Oral Rehydration Therapy

The oral rehydration therapy can be safely and successfully used in treating acute diarrhea in all age groups, in all countries and where domiciliary oral rehydration is not possible, IV rehydration at a medical facility should be resorted to.

Appropriate Feeding

The current view is that during episodes of diarrhea, normal food intake should be promoted to the child, whatever its age is able to eat. This is especially relevant for the exclusively breastfed infants. Newborn infants with diarrhea who show little or no signs of dehydration can be treated by breastfeeding alone, those with moderate or severe dehydration should receive oral rehydration solution alone during the rehydration phase, which lasts less than 8 hours. Once the infant is rehydrated, breastfeeding is continued along with oral rehydration solution given. Not only breast milk helps the infant to recover from an attack of diarrhea both in terms of the nutrients it supplies and its rehydrating effect, but it helps to prevent further infection because it has protective properties.

Specific Treatment

1. Tetracycline antibiotics such as Aureomycin, terramycin and streptomycin, if given parenterally will relieve symptoms rapidly. There is also marked reduction in the bacilli within 24–48 hours and freedom from infection in several cases/days.
2. Streptomycin, especially with sulfadiazine is also effective in these cases.
3. When antibiotics are not available, sulfadiazine may be used alone.
4. Turpentine oil stupes may be given to relieve distension of the abdomen.
5. Starch and opium enema may be given to control pain and diarrhea.
6. To relieve pain morphia injection may be given.
7. Some authorities give antidysentery serum in severe cases of infection caused by *S. dysenteriae*.
8. If all the treatment fails, the urgency may be done to give rest to the large intestines of the patient.

Nursing Management of Bacillary Dysentery

Isolation

Bacillary dysentery can be isolated by the medical aseptic technique. The causative organisms are found in the stool and urine. All contaminated material in the patient's unit should be cleaned up immediately after use.

Diet

In the acute stage, fluids should be forced in order to keep the patient from becoming dehydrated. Fluids are taken eagerly as a rule and fruit juice is contraindicated. Albumin water, thin gruel, barley water, toast water, chicken, lamb or beef broth and tea are suggested. Small amounts at frequent intervals are usually well tolerated. As the patient's condition improves, a more liberal diet is advised. Cottage cheese, soft-cooked eggs, baked or mashed potatoes, dry toast, custard and jello may be added. If fluids are not well retained, IV solutions are given. Formula babies do well as a rule on lactic acid formulas. Both fluid and food intake should be recorded.

Temperature

The temperature often is high, 104°F or more. This is especially true in young children and babies. The temperature may be reduced by warm sponge baths, alcohol rub or fan. The nurse should be careful not to permit the patient to become chilled during the procedure. An ice cap to the head is helpful and fluids should be forced. The temperature should be taken and recorded at least every 3 hours.

Personal Hygiene

The patient should have a daily cleansing bath. The nurse should avoid chilling the patient. The room should be warm 75–80°F and the windows should be closed. Good oral hygiene is essential. The mouth is characteristically dirty.

The teeth should be brushed or washed thoroughly with a gauze pledget at least twice each day, provided a toothbrush if not usable. Hydrogen peroxide 50% is effective for cleansing the teeth. Any good antiseptic mouthwash may be used for frequent mouthwashes. The mouth should be rinsed thoroughly after food is taken and after vomiting. The lips should be kept moist with a bland ointment or oil. The buttocks and anal areas should be washed and dried thoroughly after each stool. Baby oil applied to the area will help to prevent skin irritation.

Elimination

A careful record should be kept on the number and character of the stools passed. The amount and frequency of vomiting is an accurate record of urinary output.

General Management of the Disease

Bacillary dysentery patients get sick suddenly and they are very sick from the onset. For that reason it is recommended that the patient be kept in a quiet, warm, well-ventilated room. If the eyes are sensitive to light, the bed should be placed, so that the patient will not face a window. The patient should be kept warm, especially over the abdominal area. A lightweight woolen pad over the abdomen is recommended, but warm bedding should be provided. An ice cap to the head is helpful, if headache is a problem. It should be remembered that these patients frequently go into shock early in the disease, due to dehydration and toxemia, and treatment for shock must be instituted. The nurse should be on the alert for symptoms of shock.

The patient's position should be changed frequently. Alcohol rubs to pressure points add to the patient's comfort and help to prevent bedsores. See that fluids are taken and the amount recorded. Dehydration is a danger signal and should not be allowed to develop, if it is not at all possible to prevent it.

Soft absorbent diapers should be provided for young children and babies. If the stools are frequent, the nurse can save time and effort for both his/her patient, and himself/herself by placing the diaper in position without pinning it in place.

It is important for the nurse to watch for and report any symptoms of beginning complications or unfavorable reactions to any medication given. A sudden increase in pulse rate, extreme pallor and prostration may indicate impending shock or intestinal perforation. Coryza, urticaria or edema might be due to the patient's inability to tolerate sulfonamides well.

Terminal Disinfection

When the patient is ready for discharge he/she should be given a complete bath and shampoo, dressed in clean clothing and placed in a clean area. Contaminated wall space in the patient's unit, the table, bed and chairs should be washed with soap, and water. The mattress and the pillows should be aired for 6 hours. All treatment equipment should be washed, either boiled or aired. All waste material should be sent to the incinerator and all bedding should be laundered.

Convalescence

Convalescence is slow. The patient should avoid fatigue. Increase food as tolerated and desired by the patient. A high caloric, low residue, high vitamin and mineral diet are usually prescribed during the convalescent period.

AMEBIASIS (AMEBIC DYSENTERY)

Amebiasis is a worldwide parasitic disease, which is responsible for multiple medical-surgical problems. It is caused by the protozoa E. histolytica and is acquired by ingestion of cyst stage of E. histolytica in food or water contaminated by infected human feces.

Magnitude of Problems

Amebiasis is most common endemic infection of man in most regions of the world. In US, it is found in rural areas or in most of the patients who have lived or travelled in the tropics, generally limited to warm regions.

The term 'amebiasis' has been defined as, the condition of harboring the protozoan parasite E. histolytica with or without clinical manifestations. The symptomatic group has been further subdivided into intestinal and extraintestinal amebiasis.

Epidemiological Features

Agent

Amebiasis is a common infection of the human GIT caused by E. histolytica (Fig. 29.3).

Morphology

Amebiasis is caused by potentially pathogenic strains of E. histolytica. Recently, other pathogenic amebae have been identified and include Acanthamoeba, Hartmannella and Naegleria. E. histolytica exists in two forms.

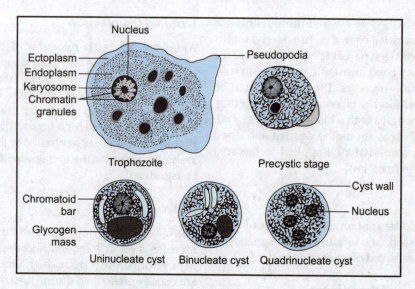

Figure 29.3: Different morphological forms of *Entamoeba histolytica*

Trophozoites: Size varies from 10 to 40 μ. Trophozoite is actively motile, exhibits gliding motility by formation of pseudopodia and is seen in acute amoebic dysentery stools under microscope. Infection is not transmitted from person to person by trophozoites. Trophozoites are demonstrated in feces of acute amebic dysentery and in tissue extraintestinal amebiasis.

Cyst: Trophozoites undergo encystment in the large intestine of the man. Cysts are 10–15 μ in sizes. When mature cysts contaminating food or water are ingested by man, it may result in amebic infection. Cysts are demonstrated in cyst passer. These are never seen in extraintestinal amebiasis. Clinical illness is characterized by mucus diarrhea, steatorrhea epigastric pain and malabsorption. *G. lamblia* lives in the duodenum and upper jejunum of man:

1. Trophozoites: *G. lamblia* trophozoites are 15 μ long, 10 μ wide and 5 μ thick. These are racket shaped, have four parts of flagella and are actively motile.
2. Cyst: It is oval, 12 × 8 μ in size, infection occurs by consuming food or water contaminated by cysts. Cyst and trophozoites can be symptomatic carriers.

Life Cycle

The *E. histolytica* passes its life cycle in only one host (Fig. 29.4). The mature quadrinucleate cysts are the infective forms. Man acquires the infection by ingestion of water and food containing these cysts. When the cyst reaches the cecum or the lower part of the ileum, the excystation occurs. During this process, each mature cyst liberates a single ameba with four nuclei, a tetranucleate ameba, which eventually produces eight metacystic trophozoites by the division of nuclei by binary fission. These metacystic trophozoites ultimately lodge in the submucous tissue of the large intestine and their normal habitat. Here, they grow and multiply by binary fission.

During growth, *E. histololytica* a proteolytic enzyme, which brings about destruction and necrosis of tissue leading to flask-shaped ulcers. A large number of trophozoites are excreted along with blood and mucus in the feces. This condition is called amebic dysentery. Sometimes the trophozoites enter into deeper layers and may gain entry into the radicals of portal vein to be carried away to the liver. In the liver, they multiply and produce amebic liver abscess.

After sometime, when the effect of the parasite on the host is toned down and there is increase in the tolerance of the host, the lesion starts healing. The trophozoites in the lumen of the large intestine transform into precysts and then into mature, quadrinucleate cysts. This process is known as encystation. Cyst formation occurs only within the intestinal tract and not outside the human body.

Host

1. Age: Amebiasis may occur at any age.
2. Sex: There is no sex or racial difference in the occurrence of disease. Amebiasis is frequently household infection. When any individual in a family is infected, other members of the family may also be affected.

Environmental Factors

Amebiasis is more closely related to poor sanitation and socioeconomic status than to climate. The use of night soil

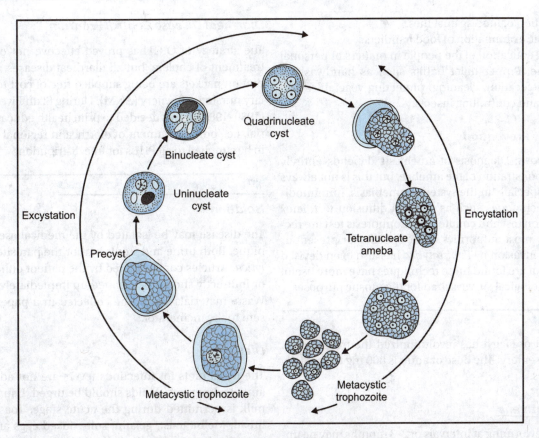

Figure 29.4: Life cycle of *Entamoeba histolytica*

for agricultural purposes favors the spread of the disease. In countries with marked wet-dry seasons, infection rate is higher during rains. Endemic outbreak potential for transmission is thereby increased. Epidemic outbreaks are usually associated with sewage seeping into the water supply.

Modes of Infection

Modes of infection and sources of infection are same as for bacillary dysentery. The incubation period is about 3–4 weeks. In the case of massive infection, the incubation period may be shorter.

Pathophysiology

The amebae gain their way into the intestinal mucosa, where they feed mainly on bacteria. Pus pocket may form with only a small orifice into the bowel from which numerous burrows extend for considerable distances in all directions under the mucous membrane and eventually slough off, exposing an underlying ulcer that may enlarge to size of 1–2 cm in diameter. The large bowel may be so covered by such ulcers that the little normal mucous membrane is left. Usually, the floor of these ulcers is the muscle wall of the bowel, but they may perforate its entire wall and cause fatal peritonitis. In the small intestine, the organism may erode intestinal mucosa, invade the bloodstream and gain an access to the liver through portal.

Clinical Features

May be symptomatic or asymptomatic:
1. Colicky abdominal pain.
2. Diarrhea: Watery and foul-smelling stool containing blood-streaked mucus.

Prevention and Control

Primary Prevention

The measures aimed at the primary prevention are as follows:
1. Sanitary disposal of human excreta.
2. Provision of safe and adequate drinking water, boiling of drinking water is safe preventive measure.
3. Hygienic kitchen practice.
4. Thorough washing or disinfection of uncooked fruits and vegetables.

5. Protection of food against flies.
6. Periodic examination of food handlers.
7. Health education of the people in matters of personal hygiene. Proper toilet habits such as handwashing after defecation, cleaning, protecting vegetables and fruits, and controlling insects.

Secondary Prevention

Early diagnosis: Diagnosis of amebiasis depends entirely on the demonstration of the amebae, but this is not always feasible, especially in the systemic amebiasis. Immunodiagnostic techniques such as agar gel diffusion test, latex agglutination test and counter electrophoresis test are recognized by most authorities, to be specific for present or past tissue invasion by *E. histolytica* has also been devised recently, but are found these techniques have more useful in epidemiological surveys than for diagnostic purposes.

Treatment

The advent of Flagyl has revolutionized the treatment of amebic dysentery. The dose of adult is 800 mg thrice daily for 5-7 days.

Mass Treatment

Periodic deworming at intervals of 2-3 months may be undertaken, this may be needed where parasite and protein energy malnutrition are highly prevalent. Mass treatment will rut interrupt transmission of the disease, but merely reduce the worm load. It would be unrealistic to expect that ascariasis would be eliminated by mass treatment, unless sanitation improvement is combined with treatment. In fact, ascariasis is disappearing spontaneously in certain areas as a result of improved sanitation.

National Program

The amebiasis is mainly caused by ingestion of contaminated water and food, insanitation and lack of health knowledge. So, the National Water Supply and Sanitation Program is effective for eradication of amebiasis.

National Water Supply and Sanitation Program

The program occupies a key position in the health programs of India. It was initiated in 1954 with the object of providing safe water supply and adequate sanitation arrangements for the entire urban and rural population of the country. These efforts of government will help to reduce amebiasis.

Diarrheal Disease Control Program

The strategy of ORT has proved effective not only in the treatment of cholera, but all diarrheal diseases. Oral rehydration packets are being supplied free of cost to all auxiliary nursing midwifery (ANM). During Sixth Five-year plan (1980-1985), it was decided to print health education material, i.e. 'home treatment of diarrhea in regional languages to be supplied to all PHCs for free distribution.

Nursing Management Amebiasis

Isolation

The disease may be isolated by the medical aseptic technique. Both urine and stools harbor the parasite, *E. histolytica*. Articles contaminated by the patient either directly or indirectly should be cleaned up immediately after use. Waste materials should be collected in a paper bag and sent to the incinerator.

Diet

The usual diets for infectious fevers are not advisable in amebic dysentery. Fluids should be urged. Usually boiled milk is permitted during the acute stage. Toasted white bread, Melba toast, gelatin, soft-cooked eggs and tea are given if tolerated. Feedings should be small and frequently given from every hour to every 2-3 hours, depending upon the patient's ability to take, and retain what is offered.

After the acute stage, a high caloric diet rich in vitamins is given. As a rule, fruit juices and raw vegetables are contraindicated. A record of both food and fluid intake should be kept.

Temperature

The temperature as a rule is not high enough to become a nursing problem. However, it should become necessary to reduce fever, a warm sponge bath or an alcohol rub may be given. Care should be taken not to chill the patient, especially over the abdomen, during these procedures. An ice cap should be placed to the head and cool fluids given.

Personal Hygiene

The patient should be given a cleansing bath daily. If diarrhea is present, soiled areas should be washed, dried carefully and anointed with baby oil or bland ointment to prevent irritation. The mouth and teeth should be kept clean. Antiseptic mouthwashes may be given as necessary.

Elimination

If diarrhea is present, the nurse should examine each stool for blood and mucus. If constipation is a problem, enemas may be given as needed. It is important that the nurse record a description of each stool. A record of fluid output should be kept.

General Management of the Disease

During the acute stage, the patient is bedfast. If fluids by mouth increase the frequency of the stools, IV fluids are usually given. The patient should be kept warm. A warm woolen or moist compress over the abdomen frequent relieves abdominal distress. Stool specimens are sent to the laboratory upon the doctor's order. It is important that the nurse should understand that the laboratory usually requires fresh and warm stool specimens, unless otherwise ordered. When the patient's bowels move, the stool should be collected in a sterile bedpan and sent warm to the laboratory, unless other technique is specifically prescribed.

The nurse should watch for any unfavorable reactions to prescribed drugs. He/She should report any increase in pulse rate, especially after emetine. Other unfavorable reactions may be dimmed vision or other visual disturbances, changes in hearing, changes in the pulse rate and quality, fall in BP, unusual pallor, extreme restlessness, cyanosis or coryza. As a rule, the iodine-containing drugs such as Yatren, Anadin, Vioform and Diodoquin are well tolerated.

The temperature should be taken at least every 3 hours. Bedding should be light in weight, but sufficiently warm. The nurse should take advantage of every opportunity to teach patient and family how they may assist in preventing the spread of the disease to others.

Terminal Disinfection

When the patient is discharged, the bedding should be laundered, the mattress and pillow aired for 6 hours or autoclaved, if fecally contaminated. The bed, table, chair and wall space within reach of the patient, and the space where the unit gown hung should be washed with soap and water. All waste material should be sent to the incinerator. All treatment equipment, basins, bedpans and similar objects should be washed and sterilized.

WORM INFESTATIONS

ROUNDWORM INFESTATION (ASCARIASIS)

Ascariasis is a common helminth infection in man characterized by vogue or no intestinal symptoms. It is found in almost all parts of the world even in some parts of United States of America (USA). Some 15–20% of the population has been found infected.

Epidemiological Features

Morphology

Ascaris lumbricoides (*A. lumbricoides*) is the common roundworm (agent) found in the small intestine of man in all parts of the world. It is one of the largest nematode parasites reaching a length of 10–14 inch. It has an unsegmented body with a dull reddish yellow color, long and cylindrical in shape with pointed ends. The posterior end of the female is straight, whereas that of a male is curved ventrally similar to a hook. The mouth lies at the anterior end of the body guarded by three finely toothed lips or oral papillae, one of these is dorsal in position and the other two are ventrolateral. A little behind the anterior end lying ventrally is the median excretory pore. Just before the hind end also ventral in position is the anus in the female. The genital aperture is distinct from the anus and lies ventrally about a third of the length of the body from anterior end, whereas in male there is a single aperture, cloacal aperture, which serves both as anus and genital opening. Two curved spicules can be seen projecting from the cloacal aperture in the male. Four longitudinal lines are present extending from end to end of the worm. One of these is mid-dorsal, one midventral and the other lateral in position (Fig. 29.5).

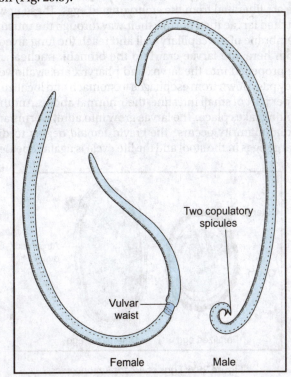

Figure 29.5: *Ascaris lumbricoides* (adult worms)

Host

In India, it is quite common. Children of preschool age are more affected. There is high degree of host parasite tolerance. Roundworms contribute to malnutrition in children and may lead to growth retardation. *Ascaris* is a 'soil-transmitted helminth.' The eggs remain viable in the soil for months or years under favorable conditions. Seeding of the soil by Ascaris eggs (Fig. 29.6) takes place by the human habit of indiscriminate open air defecation. Man is the only reservoir of infection. Infective material is feces containing fertilized eggs. Incubation period, the time required by the worm to reach maturity after entry of eggs in the body is about 2 months.

Life Cycle

Ascaris lumbricoides passes its life cycle in only one host, i.e. man. No intermediate host is required. Man is the only definitive host. Adult worms live in the jejunum of man. Fertilized eggs containing the unsegmented ova are passed in the feces. These eggs are not immediately infective to man. Eggs undergo developed from unsegmented ovum and undergoes first molting within the egg shell. These eggs containing rhabditiform larvae are pathogenic to man. Man acquires infection by ingestion of food, drink or raw vegetables contaminated with eggs containing rhabditiform larvae (embryonated eggs). In the upper part of the small intestine (duodenum), rhabditiform larvae are liberated from the embryonated eggs. These newly hatched larvae then burrow their way through the mucous membrane of the capillary wall and reach the lung alveoli. From here, the larvae crawl up the bronchi, trachea and are propelled into the larynx and pharynx are swallowed. They pass down from esophagus to stomach and localize in upper part of small intestine, their normal abode. Another molting takes place. The larvae grow into adult worms and sexual maturity occurs. The gravid female begins to discharge eggs in the stool and the life cycle is again repeated.

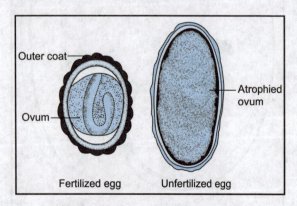

Figure 29.6: Eggs of *Ascaris lumbricoides*

Pathophysiology

It is a common chronic intestinal infection by a nematode. Live worms passed in stools or vomiting are frequently the first sign of infection. Ordinarily, a mild infection, but heavy infestations may result in serious complication.

Roundworm lives usually in the upper portion of small intestine. A female produces an average 200,000 eggs in the life cycle. These eggs develop and become infective within 30–40 days depending upon the temperature, and humidity. These eggs with embryos can live for very long periods and surviving temperatures from 33 to 180°F due to thickness of egg shell. The infection takes place when a man swallows the eggs containing larvae with contaminated food or drink. No damage is caused by small number of migrating larvae within the small intestine or liver. They may become large enough to cause minute hemorrhages at the site of entrance into the alveoli. A large number of larvae during migration may produce hepatitis or pneumonitis.

The normal habitat of the adult worm is the jejunum and here it may cause traumatic or toxic damage. Worms may cause mechanical obstruction or perforation of the bowel, or penetration into the tissues. Toxemia is caused by systemic absorption of the byproducts of the living and dead worms to which many people are sensitive. Large number of worms may rob the infected individual of his/her nutrition (Fig. 29.7).

Clinical Features

- Patient has general weakness and his/her body becomes pale
- There are digestive disturbances such as loss of appetite, occasional vomiting, pain in abdomen, flatulence and few cases may show symptoms of dysentery
- Some patients may have severe stomach ache, which resembles appendicitis
- A live worm may be passed in the vomit or stools
- Sometimes, patient may have an asthmatic attack.

Preventive Measures

1. Provide adequate facilities for night soil collection and disposal.
2. Provision should be made for hand dug well and borehole or any other type of latrines for villagers and persons living in urban areas, where there is no facility of private latrines.
3. Vegetables and fruits must be washed, if possible in running water before using them.
4. Use boiled water for drinking.
5. People must get education about:

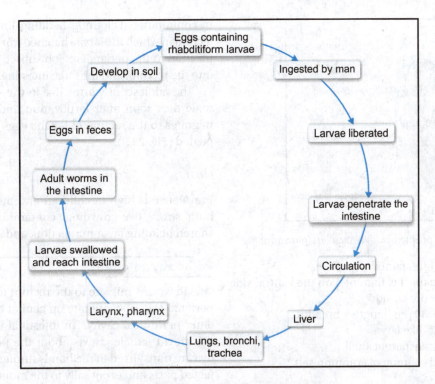

Figure 29.7: Life cycle of roundworm

a. Using latrines or toilet properly.
b. Avoid indiscriminate defecation in the fields, near river banks, tanks or any other water source.
c. Washing hands thoroughly before taking food and after defecation, especially children must follow this rule strictly.
d. Avoid eating raw vegetables without cleaning them.
e. Avoid pollution of the soil and water supply.
f. Avail treatment facilities.
6. Adequate facilities should be made to avoid overflow of *Aascaris* eggs from the drains and latrines, etc.
7. Investigation should be done to find out sources of infection, if any, from person environment and the premises of the patients family.
8. Survey should be carried out in highly endemic area to find out cases.

Specific Treatment

1. Santonin powder is given at bedtime and on the next morning calomel or magnesium sulfate is given to patient.
2. Antipar and elixir also may be given to the patient.
3. Piperazine salts are commonly given.
4. Hexylresorcinol may be given.

PINWORM INFESTATION

Pinworm is very common nematode parasite in the intestine, especially children in all parts of the world. The young and mature forms of the parasites are found in small intestines, whereas they occur in gravid females in colon and rectum. Their presence causes the disease commonly known as 'worms' in children and the parasites can be seen wriggling about in freshly voided feces. The circular alae lobes and the dilated globular or bulbous pharynx are characteristics of the genus. The male has a single terminal spicule.

Epidemiological Features

Agent

Enterobius vermicularis (*E. vermicularis*) is the genus commonly found in young children.

Adult worm: It is small and white in color. It resembles a short piece of thread. Male measures 2–4 mm in length and 0.1–0.2 mm across its girth. The posterior third of the body is curved in male, but straight in female. The size of female is 8–12 mm in length and 0.3–0.5 mm across its thickest part.

Eggs: The characteristics of egg (Fig. 29.8) are as follows:

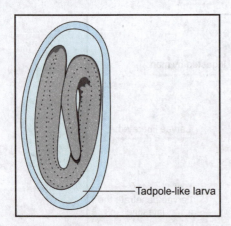

Figure 29.8: Egg of *Enterobius vermicularis* (pinworm)

- Colorless, i.e. not bile stained
- Planoconvex in shape, i.e. flattened on the ventral side and convex on the dorsal side
- They are 50–60 μ × 30 μm (length × breadth)
- Contains a tadpole-like larva
- Surrounded by a transparent shell
- Floats in saturated solution of common salt.

Life Cycle

The gravid females migrate to the perianal region and lay the eggs on the skin. The eggs contain tadpole-like embryos, which are infective. *E. vermicularis* is an intestinal worm infecting only human beings. Eggs are infective within a few hours after leaving the GIT. After ingestion, eggs hatch into larvae in the duodenum and reach the intestine, and become adults within 2 months. Infection of others may be by contaminated clothing, bedding, linen, etc. and retroinfection in which the larvae hatched from eggs after their deposition in the perianal region subsequently migrate back into the rectum, and the large intestine.

The adolescent worms live in the small intestine. The male dies soon after fertilization and the gravid female migrates to the rectum to lay the eggs and the cycle is repeated (Fig. 29.9).

Host

Prevalence is high in children and preschool children of both sexes, overcrowding, contamination clothing and shared bedding favor reinfection, and spread.

Pathophysiology

Gravid worms migrate to the rectum to discharge eggs on perianal skin may migrate up genital tract of females and enter peritoneal cavity. An intestinal itching is caused as the gravid female crawls about the perianal region. The ova are transferred to the hands through scratching the affected parts and eventually to the mouth.

Control Measures

1. Maintenance of clean facilities for defecation.
2. Insistence upon practice of personal hygiene of the toilet, particularly the washing of hands after defecation and always before eating or preparing food.
3. Reduction of overcrowding in living accommodations, adequate provision of toilets and privies.

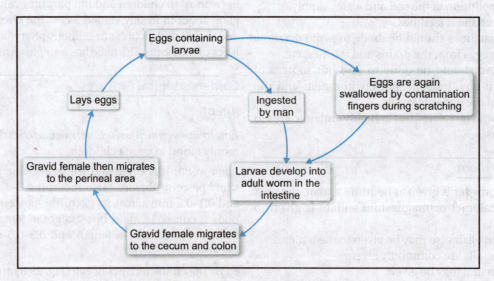

Figure 29.9: Life cycle of *Enterobius vermicularis* (pinworm)

4. Bathing with sufficient frequency to keep the body clean, use of clean underclothing, nightclothes and bed sheets at frequent intervals.
5. Habits of nail biting and scratching bare anal area should be discouraged.
6. Teach diagnosed patient and family by emphasizing importance of sanitary disposal of feces.

HOOKWORM INFESTATION

Hookworm disease is a chronic infestation of small intestine caused by *Ancylostoma duodenale (A. duodenale)* or *Necator americanus (N. americanus)*. It causes anemia, edema, cardiac dilatation and cardiac failure. It retards physical growth and mental development of children, and handicaps the progress of agriculture and industry.

Magnitude of the Problem

A debilitating infection with nematodes, it is prevalent in tropical and subtropical countries, where feces are not disposed of properly. Infective larvae are favored by the temperature, moisture, soil and inadequate disposal of feces. *A. duodenale* is prevalent in Mediterranean countries, Europe, Egypt and India, while *N. americanus* is prevalent in America and throughout tropical East Africa. Its susceptibility is general, but it is more frequent in Whites than in Negroes. Though some immunity develops with infection, the infected persons remain potential spreader of infection, so long as they are infected.

Epidemiological Features

Agent

There are two distinct varieties of the causative organism:
1. *Ancylostoma duodenale*.
2. *Necator americanus* (Fig. 29.10).

Life History of Worm

Hookworm is almost cylindrical in shape, female worm is 8–18 mm and male 6–10 mm in length. Its body is thread-like, head conical shaped, large oval mouth, which is provided with four hook-like teeth (claws) on the ventral side of the buccal cavity and two knob teeth on the dorsal side. By these hooks, the worm fixes itself to the mucous membrane of the intestines.

The patient passes very large number (4,000,000 or over) of ova in the feces and further development takes place in moist earth. In about 5 days after hatching, the larvae move actively in their sheaths and the ensheathed larvae are seen crawling over the blades of the grass.

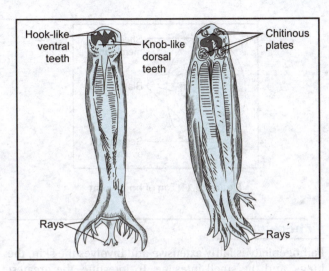

Figure 29.10: Hookworms (adult forms)

These larvae survive in moisture and shade for months together, but die in dry condition. They pass through two molts before they become infective. When these larvae enter into the human body through sweat glands or hair follicles, fix themselves under the skin of the person and give rise to toe itch, ground itch or ground sore.

After reaching subcutaneous tissues, they migrate through the veins or lymphatic vessels to the heart, lungs and then to the bronchial tubes from where they are swallowed into the stomach, where they lose their protective sheath, and pass into the intestine where they develop into adult worm within 4 weeks. The worms attach themselves in the mucous membrane of intestine and cause hemorrhage. During their journey in the body, they molt twice in addition to two outside moltings. From the initial infection of the skin up to first appearance of the eggs (Fig. 29.11) in the stools about 6 weeks interval is necessary (Fig. 29.12).

Host

The common group affected in between 5 and 40 years. The disease is most common in prime of life and less in old age. Worms in agriculture and tea plantation are more prone to the infection. Female suffer more than male, because they choose more segregated place for defecation. Environment favors the hookworm. Temperature, rainfall, humidity and condition of the soil being the most important factors in the spread of this disease, it is commonly prevalent in tropical, and subtropical countries. Porous and sandy soils are more favorable.

Vegetation exerts an influence by providing shades for the development and longevity of the larvae. Mode of transmission is through the skin by infective filariform larvae rarely by oral route, reservoir of infection are cases and carriers, and incubation period is about 74 days.

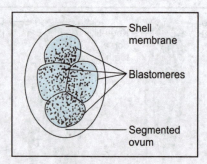

Figure 29.11: Egg of hookworm

hookworms originally feed before shifting to other areas of the intestinal mucosa, there is bloody stool. The infected hosts, because of the anemia and the loss of blood through the stool are never energetic enough to work; ultimately come to be regarded as lazy and shiftless. It affects the economy of the patient and the nation. Women may have sterility, abortions and impaired lactation. There is inevitable epigastric pain, which the hosts will try to ease by eating; they will even eat dirt when they cannot obtain food. If the infection is not checked, fatty generation of the heart, liver and kidney results in death.

Pathophysiology

Pathogenicity is fairly extensive and involves the skin, the lungs, and the small intestine. In intestine, the greatest damage occurs because of the withdrawal of blood from gut, the host suffers a rather severe anemia. It affects adversely the hematopoietic marrow. Further, there is hemorrhage from the intestinal mucosa in the areas, where the

Clinical Features

Signs and Symptoms

1. In the preintestinal phase, infected larvae enter through the skin of barefoot of the person. A variety of vague symptoms occur.
2. After entry through skin, toe itch or ground sores is caused, which causes dermatitis.

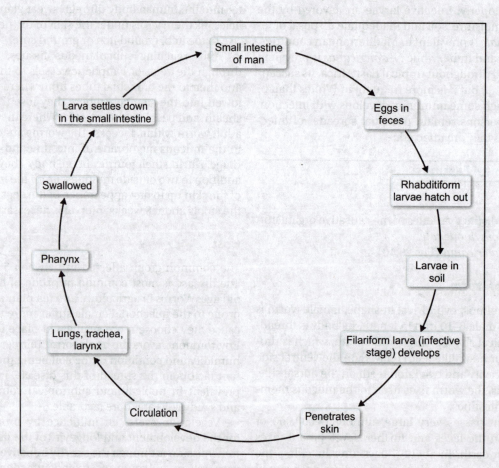

Figure 29.12: Life cycle of hookworm

3. When this worm fixes itself in the intestines, it causes hemorrhage, which give rise to anemia.
4. Patient may have debility or weakness, puffiness of the face, flatulence, constipation with alternate diarrhea and pain in abdomen.
5. Edema of legs and palpation occurs.
6. Marked anemia cause pallor of the whole body, tongue and conjunctiva. Tongue usually appears like a sheet of white blotting paper, which is seen usually in bleeding piles and in no other condition.
7. Patients may have slight fever and loss of appetite.
8. Blood sucking activity of the worm predisposes malnutrition, which leads to hypochromic microcytic anemia.
9. Infected children may have retarded mental and physical development leading to delayed puberty.
10. Affected persons have low body resistance.

Diagnosis

- Patients who have anemia show about 29% eosinophilia in the blood
- Microscopic examination of feces will show presence of the eggs in all infected person's stools
- Patient's stools contain little amount of blood in it.

Complications

- Patient may have allergic reactions
- Lungs are predisposed for pulmonary infection
- If number of larvae is more, patient may have pneumonia or pneumonia-like symptoms
- Microcytic anemia occurs
- Mental and physical development of the child is retarded.

Control Measures

1. In selected endemic areas and not in all parts of the world, it is reportable disease.
2. Source of infection may be isolated, there is no need of isolation and quarantine of the patient, and contacts.
3. Disinfect and dispose off feces (which contain eggs of this worm) carefully, to avoid contamination of water and soil.
4. Investigate the source of infection, because each patient and carrier is the potential or actual spreader of the infection. All the contacts of the patient must be examined.
5. In endemic areas, survey may be done to find out unreported cases, rate of prevalence and source of infection.
6. Follow preventive measures.

Treatment and Prevention

1. People must maintain personal hygiene and cleanliness.
2. People should have habit of wearing chappals, shoes and should not go out barefoot. In the endemic region, people must have habit of washing their feet after coming from outside.
3. Provision of adequate latrines and urinals should be made to avoid indiscriminate defecation, and teach proper use of latrines to the public.
4. In the rural areas, enough number of dug wells or borehole latrines must be provided to the people. Sprinkle salt or lime in the latrines as well as on the soil.
5. Vegetables and fruits must be washed properly before eating. Special care is required when these are taken raw.
6. Educate people about the spread, dangers and prevention of this disease.

Specific Treatment

1. Treatment is replaced by carbon tetrachloride and hexylresorcinol and tetrachloreothylene is given.
2. Tetrachloroethylene and hexylresorcinol can reduce the period of communicability, but they have toxic effects on the person so while giving, care must be taken. It may be repeated if necessary.
3. Carbon tetrachloride may cause toxic manifestations and death of the patient thus it is used rarely with caution.

TAPEWORM INFESTATION

Tapeworm infestation or teniasis is a group of cestode infections, which are important zoonotic diseases. From the stand point of human health, *Taenia solium* (*T. solium*) (pork tapeworm), *Taenia saginata* (*T. saginata*) (beef tapeworm) and *Taenia echinococcus* (*T. echinococcus*) are infective organisms.

Epidemiological Features

Agent

The *T. solium* is prevalent in those places where beef or pork is eaten raw or slightly cooked. Its distribution is cosmopolitan with highest incidence in tropical countries.

Morphology

The male *T. solium* measure about 1½ mm in length, while the female is generally around 3 mm. Each adult has a cuticle, an epidermis and a subepidermal musculature. The digestive system consists of mouth, pharynx and intestine. The pharynx with the exception of a small anterior length extends through a longitudinal row of granular cells called stichocytes. The stichocytes referred to collectively as the stichosome are thought to be glandular pharyngeal cells. The posterior end of the intestine fuses with the ejaculatory duct of the male to form a cloaca. The cloaca, which can be everted in sperm transfer opens through the cloacal aperture at the extreme posterior end between two lobular appendages called bursae.

The male reproductive system consists of a tubular testis, which extends through the pseudocoel to curve back at the level of the caudal end of the pharynx into a vas deferens. This vas deferens posteriorly grades into a seminal vesicle that caudally tapers into an ejaculatory duct. The female reproductive system is composed of one ovary in the posterior part of the pseudocoel. The anterior end of the ovary has a short oviduct, which opens into a rather long swollen uterus. The posterior end of which is differentiated to function as a seminal receptacle. Thereafter, the uterus tapers into a vagina just anterior to the end of the pharynx. The vagina opens out through the genital pore on the ventral surface of the anterior one third of the worm. The females are viviparous, delivering juveniles.

There is no formed excretory system. The central portion of the nervous system is represented in a small circumpharyngeal nerve ring.

Life Cycle

The worm passes its life cycle in two hosts, i.e. the definitive host and intermediate host. Man is the definitive host (which harbors the adult worm) and pig is the intermediate host (which harbors the larval stage). The adult worm lives in the small intestine of man and the eggs or gravid proglottids are passed out with the feces. The animals become infected by swallowing these eggs. After ingestion, oncosphere hatches out from the circulating blood into the muscular tissue. They are transformed into cysticercus stage in the muscle when these are known as cysticercus cellulosae.

Human beings are infected by eating uncooked or partially cooked pork containing cysticercus cellulosae. Inside the alimentary canal of man, the scolex of the cysticercus evaginates and attaches to the gut wall by its suckers and then develops into an adult worm. Life cycle of *T. saginata* is same except that the intermediate host is cattle and the larval stage is named as cysticercus bovis.

Man becomes infected through the ingestion of uncooked pork, which contains the infective juveniles. Since, the juveniles are microscopic, pork cannot be grossly inspected for *T. solium*. Man ingests juveniles along with uncooked pork, which are liberated in the small intestine. Within a short time, the juveniles molt into adult worms and copulation follows; the males dying a short time thereafter. Each female then makes her way into the intestinal mucosa and 4 days later delivers infective juveniles into the mucosa, and frequently into the lymphatic capillaries. Actually, these juveniles hatch out of their 'eggs' in the vagina itself and are delivered either into the mucosal tissues or directly into lymphatic capillaries of the mucosa. The anterior ends of these juveniles incidentally are adapted for burrowing into the lymphatic capillaries. Millions of these juveniles penetrate the lymphatic capillaries and through the lymphatic vessels make their way to the thoracic duct, and finally into the blood circulatory system to be finally transported to the skeletal musculature of the host. Favorite sites of parasitic residence being the musculature of the tongue, diaphragm and orbit. Approximately one third of the infections, the juveniles will end up in the myocardium of the heart. In the skeletal musculature these juveniles mature almost to adulthood. Within 2 weeks each maturing juvenile is walled off by a cyst formed by the host tissue. In the cyst, the juvenile assumes a characteristically spiralized disposition and dies. Indication period is 8–10 weeks (Fig. 29.13).

Pathophysiology

The pathogenicity of *T. solium* expressed in a myositis, which according to the severity of the infection may be severe enough to make low motion temporarily impossible. If the juveniles become enlodged in the laryngeal musculature, speech may be greatly impaired. This disease occurs due to swallowing of the pork worm, which hatch in the small intestines. Grave consequences may ensue when larvae encyst in the tissues, particularly when they localize in heart, eye or CNS. The fatal cases involve the enlodgement of the juveniles in the myocardium and a rapidly ensuing myocarditis. At present, there is no therapeutic agent for the treatment of scoliosis.

Clinical Features

The clinical features are variable, frequently vague or absent and thus some important signs and symptoms are as given below:
- Segments may be seen in the stools
- Abdominal pain or abdominal colic
- Digestive disturbances such as indigestion, either anorexia or vomiting

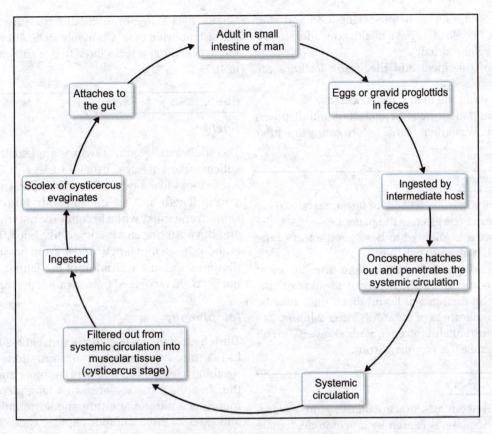

Figure 29.13: Life cycle of tapeworm

- Nervousness and insomnia may be present
- Loss of weight
- Patient may have diarrhea, headache and fits-like epileptic fits due to toxins of the worm infection.

Diagnosis

1. There are no specific signs and symptoms of this disease. So, it is difficult to diagnose only on the basis of signs and symptoms.
2. Segments of the worm may be seen in stools of patient.
3. Then microscopic examination of the infested tissue of the body shows the presence of organism, i.e. worm in any stage of its life.
4. X-ray examination is helpful in locating calcified cysticercus in somatic muscles of body and also in brain of the patient. It also helps in evaluating the intensity and severity of the infection of the patient.

Complications

1. Usually cysticercosis develops in the subcutaneous tissue, striated muscles and other regions. Grave consequences may occur, when they localize in heart, eye or CNS.
2. Patient may have pernicious anemia due to loss of blood in the body.
3. Patient may have epileptic and convulsing.

Preventive Measures

1. Prevent pollution of the soil with human excreta.
2. Proper disposal of human excreta to avoid access of cattle, fish and pigs.
3. People must be taught to eat thoroughly cooked meat and fish.
4. Inspection of cattle, pigs and pork meat in the slaughter houses by the veterinary surgeon.
5. Inspection and control of fish market is also necessary.
6. License should be issued to those who have dogs; stray dogs should be sheltered by concerned municipalities.
7. Deep burial or incineration of dead animals must be enforced by the law.

8. Wash hands thoroughly before taking food and after defecation. People must have health education follow personal hygiene strictly.
9. Provision of treatment and diagnostic facilities are necessary.
10. Environmental sanitation is also necessary.
11. Feces of the patient must be collected and disposed off properly. Wash their hands before eating and after defecation.

Specific Treatment

1. Oleoresin of *Aspidium* is used for intestinal teniasis.
2. Quinacrine may be given to the patient.
3. A long process is followed to have good effect of the drug, which is given to him/her.

In this method, patient's stomach and intestine must be completely emptied for which patient should not take solid or semisolid diet, except liquid diet. Drugs may be given to remove hardness of the stools. After 2 hours, 240 grains magnesium sulfate is given. But never give castor oil in this case, because it is very dangerous.

DRACUNCULIASIS

Synonyms are dracontiasis, dracunculiasis, guinea worm disease. Dracunculiasis is caused by a nematode, female parasite, *Dracunculus medinensis* (*D. medinensis*), transmitted through the vector, *Cyclops*, which in turn is transmitted by drinking contaminated water containing infected *Cyclops*. Clinically, it is characterized by blister in the leg associated with itching, burning and often secondary infection. Later, it may lead to arthralgia and arthritis, disabling the individual temporarily.

Dracunculiasis or guinea worm disease is a vector-borne parasitic disease of public health importance. Man acquires infestation by drinking water containing infected *Cyclops*. It is a non-fatal disease, but can disable its victim temporarily. Its susceptibility is general and multiple, and repeated infection occurs to the same person.

It is an infection with the nematode *D. medinensis*. The adult inhabits the subcutaneous tissues mainly in the legs, but also other parts of the body. The *Cyclops* is another host for larvae, which require a period of 15 days for their development. Reservoir of infection is an infected person harboring the gravida female.

Magnitude

A global problem in the developing countries has been eradicated in the last decade. The disease is now endemic in some countries of Africa such as Sudan, Nigeria and Ghana. Asia is free from the disease since 2000. In India, the last reported case was in July 1996. After 3 years of zero incidence, India was declared free of guinea worm disease in 1999.

Epidemiological Features

Agent

The adult female guinea worms are usually found in the subcutaneous tissues, usually of legs. It is a thin, long worm looks like a twine thread and measuring 60 mm to 1 m in length and 1.5 mm breadth. Body is cylindrical, smooth and milky white in color. The anterior end is round and the posterior end is curved-like hook. The adult male is about 20–30 mm length and 0.4 mm breadth. It dies and disappears after fertilization of the female. Hence, it has not yet been recovered from an adult person.

Morphology

The length of the male guinea worm is 12–20 cm and width is 1–4 mm. Females are enormously longer than males reaching a length of 3 ft (58 cm) or more and width 1 mm, thus bearing a resemblance to a long piece of cord. The mouth is a minute aperture and surrounded by internal and external circles of four papillae each. The esophagus consists of a short anterior muscular part constricted at the middle where the nerve ring is situated. The anus lies in the female a little in front of the posterior extremity. About 10 pairs of genital papillae are present in the male. In the female, the whole of worm is occupied by uterus stuffed with embryos, i.e. about 3 million embryos.

Life Cycle

The guinea worm is found burrowed in the subcutaneous tissues of the leg. The worms attain sexual maturity in the subcutaneous and connective tissues. Copulation takes place and after fertilization the male worm dies, and the gravida female migrates to such surfaces of the body as the ankle, foot and arm, which are likely to be habitually wetted. There, it pierces the skin where a small vesicle is formed. When the affected part of human body comes in contact with water, the vesicle bursts and the loop of uterus extrudes through a small pit in the middle of the ulcer, and millions of tiny larvae are liberated from it. The larvae swim about in the water and ingested by *Cyclops*. In these *Cyclops*, they undergo larval development in 5 weeks.

A healthy person gets infected by drinking water contaminated with the infected *Cyclops*. When these *Cyclops* reach the stomach, gastric juices kill them and the larvae

CHAPTER 29 Intestinal Infections

are set free, which find their way into subcutaneous tissues, where they burry themselves. About a year is required for the worm to mature. Male worm dies after fertilization, but female worm continues above mentioned cycle. The worm passes its life cycle in two hosts, i.e. man and *Cyclops*.

In man

Man constitutes a definitive host. He harbors the parasite in the subcutaneous tissue usually of legs, often in the back. After fertilization in the deeper connective tissues (not in the intestine), the gravid female takes about 6 months to come to the site of its election, i.e. subcutaneous tissue of the leg or back, which is liable to come in contact with water and forms a bleb with its toxin, which later bursts to form an ulcer. When such an infected person gets down in a stepwell or pond, or carries water on the back, the contact with water stimulates the worm to protrude its head through the center of ulcer reflexly discharges milky fluid containing embryos from the prolapsed uterus into the water.

In *Cyclops*

The embryos are coiled bodies measuring about 600 m length and 20 m in breadth. They are ingested by the freshwater crustacean belonging to genus *Cyclops*, if not taken up by the *Cyclops*.

Host factors

The host susceptibility is universal, multiple, repeated infections may occur to the same person. The habit of washing and bathing in surface water, and using stepwells is an important factor in spreading of the disease.

The main link in the transmission of guinea worm disease is water infected with *Cyclops*. Sources are frequented by infected persons. The seasonal variations in the incidence of the disease are marked. Peak transmissions occur during the dry season (March to May), where contact between open cases of guinea worm disease and the drinking water is more. Sometimes when the wells are full during and after rains the larvae develop best between 25 and 30°C and will not develop below 19°C.

Clinical Features/Pathophysiology

When the worms come near the skin, patient shows following signs and symptoms:
1. Patient has blisters and redness. Irritation and urticaria occurs on site.
2. There is burning and itching sensation at the point of exit of the worm.
3. Frequently, patient has nausea, vomiting, diarrhea and sometimes dyspnea.
4. Usually eosinophilia develops.
5. Patient may have generalized urticaria.
6. When the patient keeps their leg in the water, blisters burst and discharge a milky fluid into it, which contains myriads of embryos.

Complications

Aseptic abscesses result through the rupture of immature female worms and die before they reach the skin surface. They are felt cord-like masses under the skin. There may get secondary infection and result in abscesses or become calcified:
- Monoarticular arthritis
- Hydrocele
- Scrotal abscesses.

Diagnosis

Usually there is difficulty in diagnosing until the worm is fully developed:
1. Fully or partially developed worm may be identified by X-ray.
2. Examining eggs under microscope, obtained by sprinkling some water on the wound.

Preventive Measure

1. Prevent pollution of water and soil.
2. Prevent entry to a well or a tank to avoid contamination of the water.
3. Disinfect or purify water with calcium oxide or potassium permanganate, or lime (to kill *Cyclops*).
4. Introduce barbel fish in the wells and tanks for destroying *Cyclops* and larvae.
5. Avoid using stepwells and convert them to draw wells.
6. Strain drinking water with muslin or cloth, or use boiled water for drinking.
7. Freezing of the fish for 24 hours at 100°C.

Treatment

1. Symptomatic treatment may be given to the patient quinacrine or oleoresin of *Aspidium*.
2. Niridazole, mebendazole and metronidazole 200 mg tablets for 7 days.
3. Keeping the local lesion clean, slow removal of the worm by bit and rolling it over a stick. This used to take weeks together to remove entire guinea worm.

Eradication

- Guinea worm disease is amenable to eradication by adopting following measures:

- Provision of safe drinking water
- Control of *Cyclop*s
- Surveillance—active search for new cases
- Disinfect and dispose off feces of the patient carefully
- Educate public relating to boiling or sieving drinking water
- Prevention of water contamination by infected persons
- Educate the people about spread, prevention and dangers of disease, and also teach them above mentioned precautions.

Guinea Worm Eradication Program

A National Guinea Worm Eradication Program in India was established during 1983–1984. The Indian program has mounted its eradication efforts in the context of primary health ethics (PHE). It has concentrated on identifying all affected villages and giving highest priority in provision of safe drinking water resources under the Five-year plan.

It has placed increased emphasis on vector control using emulsion (abate) and health education to promote filtration of drinking water with nylon mesh filters.

FOOD ALLERGY

Aflatoxicosis

Aflatoxicosis is characterized by hepatitis, cirrhosis of liver and/or enteritis caused by the ingestion of food grains such as groundnuts, maize, jowar, etc. mainly groundnuts, infested of certain storage fungi such as *Aspergillus flavus* (*A. flavus*) or *Aspergillus parasiticus* (*A. parasiticus*). These fungi infest the above grains, when they are improperly stored under conditions of high humidity, i.e. moisture levels above 16% and temperature between 11 and 37°C, and produce certain toxins called 'aflatoxins' of which B1 and G1 are the most hepatotoxins in addition to being carcinogenic. It is believed to be associated with childhood cirrhosis. Recently (1975), there was a report of 400 cases including 100 deaths from Banswara and Panchmahal districts of Rajasthan and Gujarat respectively.

Prevention and Control

Proper storage of food grains in dry containers. The moisture content should be kept below 10°C, not to consume the food grains, if it is contaminated by fungi. Health education should be given to the local population about health hazards.

Ergotism

Ergotism is caused by the ingestion of food grains such as bajra, rye, jowar and wheat infested by field ergot fungus called *Claviceps fusiformis* (*C. fusiformis*) or *Claviceps purpurea* (*C. purpurea*), during the flowering stage. The fungus grows as a black mass and the seeds become black, and irregular. Clinically, the condition is characterized by nausea, vomiting, giddiness, drowsiness in acute cases and painful cramps in the limbs, and gangrene due to vasoconstriction of capillaries in chronic cases. The toxin is ergotamine.

Prevention and Control

1. By removal: When immersed in 20% salt water, the infected grains float, hence can be removed.
2. They can also be removed by air flotation or hand picking.
3. By health education.

FOOD POISONING

Food poisoning is an acute inflammatory disease of the GIT caused by the ingestion of food contaminated with either toxin producing bacteria or by their preformed toxins or chemical substances, or other poisonous food substances. Clinically, it is characterized by short incubation period, pain in the abdomen, vomiting and/or diarrhea, with or without fever. Food poisoning differs from foodborne diseases in that it is not transmitted by fecal-oral route. It also differs from food intoxication in that there is neither toxic factor in the food grain nor there is contamination with fungus.

Foodborne Diseases (Table 29.10)

Foodborne are the infectious diseases caused by the pathogens and transmitted through the contaminated food, which acts as a vehicle of transmission

Prevention and Control

The epidemiological features of food poisoning are:
- History of ingestion of common food (as in marriages dinner, hostels, etc.)
- A group of people (ingesting common food) being affected simultaneously
- Similarity of signs and symptoms
- Short incubation period
- Absence of secondary cases.

CHAPTER 29 — Intestinal Infections

Table 29.10: List of foodborne diseases

Diseases	Pathogens	Signs of moderate dehydration
Bacterial		
Anthrax	*Bacillus anthracis*	Contaminated meat
Cholera	*Vibrio cholerae* (El Tor)	Contaminated food or water; houseflies
Bacillary dysentery	*Shigella*	Contaminated food or water; flies
Typhoid	*Salmonella typhi*	Contaminated food or water; milk and milk products; flies
Paratyphoid	*Salmonella paratyphi* A and B	Contaminated food or water, milk, milk products; flies
Streptococcosis, staphylococcosis	*Streptococcus* species, *Staphylococcus* species	Food contaminated from human sources
Parasitic		
Amebiasis and ascariasis	*Entamoeba histolytica, Ascaris lumbricoides*	Contaminated food, water, vegetables eaten raw
Clonorchiasis, diphyllobothriasis	*Clonorchis sinensis, Diphyllobothrium latum*	Improperly cooked freshwater fish
Fasciolopsiasis	*Fasciolopsis buski*	Contaminated vegetables eaten raw
Hydatidosis	*Echinococcus granulosus*	Contaminated food and water
Teniasis	*Taenia saginata*	Infected beef
	Taenia solium	Infected pork
Trichinellosis	*Trichinella spiralis*	Infected pork
Trichuriasis	*Trichuris trichiura*	Contaminated food

Classification of Food Poisoning

They are broadly classified into two types:
1. Nonbacterial.
2. Bacterial (differences of bacterial food poison).

Non-bacterial Food Poisoning

Non-bacterial food poisoning consist of the following types:
1. Mushroom poisoning.
2. Solanine poisoning.
3. Chemical poisoning.

Mushroom poisoning: The two common poisonous mushrooms (fungi), which are eaten in mistake for edible mushrooms are *Amanita pantherina* (*A. pantherina*) and *Amanita muscaria* (*A. muscaria*). Their poisonous effects are due to the presence of muscarine. Symptoms occur within a few minutes or hours. Abdominal pain followed by vomiting and diarrhea occur. Sometimes there may be sweating, twitchings, miosis, diplopia, muscular incoordination and convulsions followed by coma. Atropine is the effective antidote. *Amanita phalloides* (*A. phalloides*) is highly poisonous fungi. It contains amanitin, which is cytotoxic and phallin, in addition to hemolytic action. No antidote for this. Mortality is 50–90%. Both of these are destroyed by cooking. So, the symptoms are produced only when they are improperly cooked or eaten raw. Other poisonous eatables are mussels and sea foods.

Solanine poisoning: It is a toxic alkaloid present in the peelings of potato, specially in sprouts. Symptoms occur within a few hours. There will be fever, headache, pain abdomen, vomiting, diarrhea, weakness and depression. Patient usually recovers within a few days. Since the alkaloid is soluble in water, potatoes are boiled and peeled.

Chemical poisoning: Inorganic chemical substances resulting in poisoning are pesticides, fertilizers, arsenic, zinc, mercury, etc.

Bacterial Food Poisoning (Table 29.11)

Bacterial food poisoning is caused by the consumption of food contaminated with either toxin-producing bacteria or by their preformed toxins. Thus, they are two types namely:
1. Infection type.
2. Toxin type.

Infection type: In this type, organisms enter the body through the food, multiply, produce toxin, cause pathology

Table 29.11: Differentiation of bacterial food poisoning

Types	Causative agents	Reservoirs	Source/Foods	Incubation period	Clinical features
Infection types					
Salmonellosis (caused by *Salmonella*)	*S. gallinarum*, *S. enteritidis*, *S. typhimurium*, *S. choleraesuis*, *S. doublin*, *S. abortus*	Poultry, Pigs, Rats	Milk, milk products, egg, poultry, pork, food contaminated with urine of rats, human carriers	12–48 hour	Mainly diarrhea may be associated with blood, griping pain in the abdomen, usually associated with fever, (gastric flu) and vomiting may occur
Clostridium welchii or *Clostridium perfringens*	*Clostridium perfringens* anaerobic, spore forming organisms there are five strains; type C results in severe form (i.e. enteritis necroticans)	Dust and soil is the reservoir of spores	Reheating the stable cooked foods (meat, poultry, fish, etc.) prior to consumption is the critical factor; the spores germinate	12–24 hour	Moderate diarrhea associated with nagging abdominal pain and prostration; not associated with fever and vomiting
Vibrio parahaemolyticus	Gram negative, non-agglutinating group of *Vibrio*, halophilic (salt-loving organism)	Seafoods such as shellfish, crabs, lobsters, shrimps, prawn, etc.	Improperly cooked seafoods	12–18 hour	Profuse watery diarrhea, often containing blood and mucus, associated with pain abdomen, occasional vomiting with mild fever
Toxin types					
Staphylococcal type	*S. aureus*	Animal—udder of the cattle; Human—cutaneous lesions such as boil, carbuncle, whitlow, burns, etc. nasal and throat carriers	Milk, milk products, salads, ice cream, curds, etc.	1–6 hour	Vomiting is the main feature; vomiting is sudden, severe, violent, associated with abdominal pain without fever and diarrhea
Bacillus cereus type	*Bacillus cereus* are gram positive, aerobic, spore forming, motile bacilli, produces two types of enterotoxins; emetic form and enteric form	Food grains; mainly cereals	Cereal-based diet	8–12 hour	Emetic form results in vomiting and enteric form results in diarrhea; often with abdominal pain
Botulism	*Clostridium botulinum* are strictly anaerobic, blocks the release of acetylcholine	Dust and soil	Canned food, smoked fish, pickled fish, canned vegetables and food	10–12 hour	Features are of parasympathetic paralysis; blurring of vision, ptosis, dysphagia, diplopia, dysarthria, constipation, no vomiting or diarrhea and no fever. Treatment: Guanidine hydrochloride 25–40 mg/kg; reverses the neuromuscular block

and result in clinical manifestations. Incubation period is more than 8–12 hours. The bacteria, which cause this type of food poisoning are *Salmonella* group, *Clostridium perfringens* (*C. perfringens*) and *Vibrio parahaemolyticus* (*V. parahaemolyticus*).

Toxin type: In this type, there is already preformed toxin in the food. Therefore, the incubation period is shorter than that of infection type. It is less than 8–12 hours. The bacteria, which result in this type of food poisoning are *Staphylococcus aureus* (*S. aureus*), *Clostridium botulinum* (*C. botulinum*) and *Bacillus cereus* (*B. cereus*).

Investigation of an outbreak of food poisoning

1. Collection of basic data such as location of the place where the affected people had taken the food.
2. Interrogation of all the participants.
3. Nature of the foods (type) eaten during the previous 2 days.
4. Time of onset of symptoms.
5. Nature of the symptoms in the order of occurrence.
6. Personal data such as total number of participants, number of persons affected their names, age, sex, address, occupation and related information.
7. Number of deaths, if any.
8. Assessment of environmental factors such as inspection of kitchen:
   - To assess sanitation of kitchen and dining hall
   - To know the nature of the storage of food grains and cooked foods
   - To know the presence of rodents
   - Interrogation and examination of food handlers and other employees regarding personal hygiene, habits and illness, if any
   - Laboratory investigations such as vomitus and stools of the patients for culture in aerobic and anaerobic media
   - Sample of suspected food for culture in both media
   - Serological test of the blood of the affected persons for antibody titer
   - Culture of the stools and urine of the food handlers and kitchen employees.
9. Data is analyzed according to the descriptive methods of time, place and person distribution.
10. Food-specific attack rates and case fatality rates are calculated.
11. Etiological hypothesis is formulated.
12. Case control study is undertaken to establish the association between the disease and the particular food.
13. Prevention and control measures undertaken.

Prevention and Control

1. Taking care of food is consists of the following food-hygienic measures:
   - Proper storage of food grains
   - Proper cooking of food
   - Protection of cooked food from rodents, insects and bare hands
   - Eating the food while hot
   - Discouraging caning of food
   - Refrigeration of remaining foods.
2. Taking care of food handlers:
   - They should maintain a high standard of personal hygiene
   - They are educated about the hazards of unguarded coughing and sneezing
   - They are educated to undergo periodical medical check-up
   - They must abstain from the duty, if they develop septic skin lesions, respiratory and intestinal symptoms
   - Carriers should remain absent for the duty till they are cured bacteriologically.
3. Taking care of environment:
   - Kitchen and dining hall must be clean and dry
   - Utensils should be thoroughly washed with soap and hot water
   - Rodents and insects must be controlled.

Arthropod Infestations

CHAPTER 30

DENGUE FEVER

Dengue is an acutely infectious mosquito borne viral disease characterized by episodes of 'saddleback' fever, muscle and joint pain accompanied by an initial erythema and a terminal rash of varying morphology. It is a life-threatening fever and is transmitted through the *Aedes* mosquito, an indoor vector of man. The disease is also called breakbone fever or dandy fever. The disease is endemic in regions where mosquitoes are present throughout the year. Epidemic outbreaks of dengue viral fever have become frequent in recent years in India. In 1980, it was found that there were 4,601 cases and 10 deaths in Uttar Pradesh (UP), Gujarat, Punjab and Delhi. In 1996, it again reappeared in New Delhi and spread to neighboring states, found more than 13,000 cases in seven states of India. The distribution depends upon immigration of susceptible and survival of vector mosquito in larger numbers.

Dengue is caused by group B arbovirus and the virus has four distinct antigenic serotype, i.e. 1, 2, 3 and 4, and is transmitted by certain species of *Aedes* mosquitos, i.e. *Culex fatigans*, *Aedes aegypti* (*A. aegypti*) and *Aedes albopictus*. It can occur at any age. Both sexes are susceptible. No previous immunity. Epidemic usually occurs after rainy season.

The transmission cycle in dengue is direct, i.e. 'man to mosquito to man'. The vector *A. aegypti* acquires the virus by feeding on a patient during the first 3 days (viremic stage) of illness. After an extrinsic incubation period (EIP) of 10–15 days, the mosquito becomes infective and is able to transmit the infection to man. Incubation period is usually 5–6 days, though it may vary from 3 to 15 days after the bite by the mosquito.

Entry of virus causes viremia and the onset of fever and persists for about 3 days. It produces endothelial swelling, perivascular edema and infiltration with mononuclear cells in the small blood vessel leading to varying signs and symptoms.

Definition

The term 'dengue' is a Spanish attempt at the Swahili phrase 'ki denga pepo' meaning cramp-like seizure caused an evil spirit. It emerged during a Caribbean outbreak in 1827–1828. The first case report dates back from 1789, who coined the term 'breakbone fever' (because of the symptoms of myalgia and arthralgia).

Dengue fever is an infectious disease carried by mosquitoes and caused by any of four related dengue viruses. This disease used to be called 'breakbone' fever, because it sometimes causes severe joint and muscle pain that feels like bones are breaking, hence the name. Health experts have known about dengue fever for more than 200 years.

Dengue is an arbovirus disease caused by anyone of four closely related viruses that do not provide cross-protective immunity; a person can be infected as many as four times, once with each serotype.

Clinical Features

The clinical features of dengue fever can be studied under three heading:
1. Dengue viral fever (DVF).
2. Dengue hemorrhagic fever (DHF).
3. Dengue shock syndrome (DSS).

Dengue Viral Fever

The invasive symptom usually starts abruptly with severe pain in a single joint and spreads rapidly to the bone and other joints shifting around from one to another. It presents with fever accompanied abruptly by malaise, chills, severe headache, postorbital pain, backache, pain in the extremities, sore throat and depression. Fever may rise up to 105°F (40.6°C). The fever and other symptoms usually persist for 2–4 days followed by remission with profuse sweating (last few hours to 2 days and reoccurrence of fever, i.e. saddleback).

Dengue Hemorrhagic Fever

Dengue hemorrhagic fever was reported from Calcutta (1963), Madras (1964), Madhya Pradesh (1966) and Pondicherry, following symptoms in addition to features of dengue viral fever. Maculopapular, scarlatiniform or petechial rash appears on 3rd day of illness, i.e. red spots seen all over the body. The lesions first appear on the dorsum of the hands and feet, which spreads on other parts of body. Symptoms usually present are fever, headache, nausea, coffee color vomiting, abdominal pain, pharyngitis, cough and dyspepsia.

Management of DHF
- Management during febrile phase is similar to that of dengue fever
- Antipyretics may be indicated, but salicylates and ibuprofen should be avoided
- Increased fluid intake
- Fluid and electrolyte replacement by intravenous (IV) fluids, isotonics, etc.
- Plasma expanders, if clinically indicated
- Fresh frozen plasma may be indicated in some cases
- Blood transfusion (exceptionally rare cases).

Advice for parents on source reduction in the home
1. Cover all water containers such as pails, urns or drums tightly or add larvicide every 3 months.
2. Add two teaspoons of salt to each ant traps to prevent mosquitoes from breeding.
3. Change the water in flower vases every week.
4. Remove the water and clean the flower pot trays weekly.
5. Check roof gutters weekly and clear leaves or other debris that block the water flow.
6. Clean the surrounding area of the house.
7. Throw all containers, which can collect water such as empty cans and bottles into plastic bags and place them into the appropriate bins.
8. Use an insecticide spray (aerosol) in the house to kill adult mosquitoes.
9. Allow the authorities to fog the interior of the house.
10. Use mosquito repellents and/or mosquito nets to avoid mosquitoes from biting.

Complications
Complications are rare, but may include the following:
- Brain damage from prolonged shock or intracranial hemorrhage
- Myocarditis
- Encephalopathy
- Liver failure.

Prevention and control
Early detection, treatment and notification: The nurses and health personnel working in the hospital and community should be alert and remain always vigilant to observe any clinical features of dengue, which should be monitored carefully and reported to the nearest health authorities. The treatment should be started without waiting for investigation on the basis of symptoms. DVF is controlled by suitable antipyretics; DHF needs immediate hospitalization for maintaining fluid and electrolyte balance and blood transfusion. Transfusion of packed cell and antibiotic therapy may be to prevent shock and further complications. In addition, emotional and spiritual support may be appropriate.

Dengue Shock Syndrome

In addition to signs and symptoms of the above clinical feature, patient may go to shock. DSS usually occurs between 2 and 6 days often with sudden collapse or prostration, cold and clammy extremities, weak thready pulse, circumoral cyanosis along with hemorrhagic manifestation, i.e. petechial, purpura at the site of injection; occasionally with epistaxis, hematemesis, melena or subarachnoid hemorrhage.

Magnitude of the Problem

Global

Dengue fever is found mostly during and shortly after the rainy season in tropical and subtropical areas of:
- Africa
- Southeast Asia and China
- India
- Middle East Caribbean Island and Central and South America
- Australia and South and Central Pacific Island.

An epidemic in Hawaii in 2001 is a reminder that many states in the United States (US) are susceptible to dengue epidemics, because they harbor the particular type of mosquitoes that transmit it. Worldwide, more than 100 million cases of dengue infection occur each year. This includes 100–200 cases reported annually to the Centers for Disease Control and Prevention (CDC), mostly in people who have recently traveled abroad. Many more cases likely go unreported, because some healthcare providers do not recognize the disease.

India

In India, the number of patients diagnosed with dengue is increasing at an alarming rate, which the Dhaka City Corporation (DCC) fears might turn into an epidemic. A survey report of the DCC dengue control section revealed that in the capital at least 230 dengue patients treated in July 09, 2006. Dengue fever, in India 30th October 2003, disease outbreak reported.

From 1st June to 28th October 2003, 1,723 laboratory confirmed cases of dengue fever have been reported in Delhi and surrounding areas. Four deaths among laboratory confirmed cases have been reported on 28th October. Additional information is being sought on possible cases of dengue hemorrhagic fever. Circulating dengue virus serotypes DEN-3 and -2 have been reported to be associated with this outbreak.

Risk Groups

- Residents of or visitors to tropical urban areas
- Increased severe and fatal disease in children under 15 years
- No cross-immunity from each serotype
- A person can theoretically experience four dengue infections.

Epidemiological Feature

Agent Factor

Agent: Dengue fever is caused by four distinct, but closely related dengue viruses called serotypes (DEN-1, DEN-2, DEN-3 and DEN-4) and transmitted to humans through the bites of injected mosquitoes (*A. aegypti* is the primary vector).

Reservoir of infection: Human, mosquitoes (transovarial transmission extremely high levels of infectious particles in salivary glands) and monkey-mosquito cycles are common in West Africa and Southeast Asia.

Vector

Mosquitoes (*A. aegypti* and other *Aedes* species) eggs of *A. aegypti* can withstand long periods of desiccations up to 1 year. *A. aegypti* mosquitoes, which are most active during the day are usually found near human dwellings and are often present indoors. Elevated temperatures significantly shorten the incubation periods for the dengue virus in mosquitoes; this increases the rate of mosquito-human transmission of the virus. *A. aegypti* cannot withstand temperatures below 48°F (9°C) and will die after less than an hour of 32°F. It is currently limited to a range below 35°N latitude.

Host Factor

Age: All ages are susceptible. In endemic areas, a high prevalence of immunity in adults may limit outbreaks to children.

Race: Ethnicity is nonspecific, but the diseases distribution is geographically determined. Fewer cases have been reported in the black population than in other races.

Sex: No predilection is known; however, fewer cases of DHF loss have been reported in men than in women.

Environmental Factor

The mosquitoes that transmit dengue live among humans and the breeding places are:

1. Tropical and subtropical area.
2. Rainy season.
3. Low socioeconomic status and poor sanitation.
4. Discarded tires, flower pots, old oil drums and water storage containers close to human dwellings.
5. Unlike the mosquitoes that cause malaria, dengue mosquitoes bite during the day.

Mode of Transmission

By bite of infectious mosquitoes mainly *A. aegypti*, most bites occur during the 2 hours after sunrise and several hours before sunset. Vertical transmission (infected progeny) does occur, however it is relatively low.

Period of Communicability and Incubation Period

There is no evidence of person-to-person transmission. Incubation period is about 3–14 days, usually 4–7 days.

Pathophysiology

The pathogenic mechanism of DHF is not clear, but two main pathophysiological changes occur:

1. Vascular permeability increases, which results in plasma leakage leading to hypovolemia and shock.
2. Abnormal hemostatic, due to vasculopathy thrombocytopenia and coagulopathy leading to various hemorrhagic manifestations.

The severity of DHF as compared with dengue fever may be explained by the enhancement of virus multiplication in macrophages by heterotopy antibodies results from a previous dengue infection. There are evidences suggesting that cell-mediated immune response may also be involved in the pathogenesis of DHF.

Clinical Manifestation

Dengue occurs in three main clinical forms:
1. Dengue fever is an acute febrile illness with sudden onset of fever followed by development of generalized symptoms and sometimes a macular skin rash. It is known as 'breakbone fever' because of severe muscular pains. The fever may be biphasic (i.e. two separate episodes or waves of fever). Most patients recover after few days and characterized by headache, retro-orbital pain, myalgia and arthralgia.
2. Dengue hemorrhagic fever has an acute onset of fever followed by other symptoms resulting from thrombocytopenia, increased vascular permeability and hemorrhagic manifestations.
3. Dengue shock syndrome supervenes in a small proportion of cases. Severe hypotension develops, requiring urgent medical treatment to correct hypovolemia. Without appropriate treatment, 40–50% of cases are fatal; with timely therapy, the mortality rate is 1% or less.

Laboratory Studies

- Isolation of virus in serum and detection of immunoglobulins (IgM and IgG) by enzyme-linked immunosorbent assay (ELISA) antibody capture, monoclonal antibody or hemagglutination
- Complete blood count
- Hemoconcentration (hematocrit increased 20%)
- Thrombocytopenia (platelet count < 100 x 10^9/L)
- Leukopenia
- Electrolyte imbalances
- Acidemia
- Elevated blood urea nitrogen (BUN).

Epidemiological Surveillance

The epidemiological surveillance should include the following:
- Fever surveillance
- Diagnosis based on standard case definition
- Reporting of dengue fever/DHF cases to state health authorities
- During an outbreak situation, samples of about 5% of clinically diagnosed cases should be tested for confirmation of diagnosis by the laboratory.

Vector Surveillance

Larval surveillance during the pre- and post-monsoon season is important to find out the extent of prevalence of vectors in a locality. Seasonal fluctuation will help to stratify the areas for further control measures. Adult surveillance will indicate the possible infected mosquitoes and may be utilized for virus isolation, susceptibility to insecticides, etc.

Prevention and Control

At present, there is no specific treatment. No vaccine is currently available. The only method of controlling or preventing dengue fever is to combat the vector mosquitoes. Following are some of the control measures:
1. Vector control is implemented using environmental management and chemical methods. Proper solid waste disposal, elimination of stagnant water in domestic environment and improved water storage practices.
2. Aerosol and liquid spray has to be applied directly to the adult mosquito for effective killing, e.g. household pesticides.
3. Mosquito coil and electric mosquito mat/liquid has to be placed near possible entrance such as window for mosquito.
4. Wear long-sleeved clothes and long trousers when going outdoors. Bodies could be protected from mosquito bite by applying insect repellent containing N, N-diethyl-meta-toluamide (DEET) on the clothes and exposed part of the body, especially when you travel to dengue fever endemic areas.
5. Mosquito bed net could be used when the room is not air conditioned. At present, there is no effective vaccine against dengue fever. Therefore, the best way to prevent the disease is to take appropriate personal preventive measures against mosquito bites. Travelers prevent dengue fever during their trip by following ways:
    - Travelers should wear light-colored and long-sleeved clothes and trousers
    - Rest in air-conditioned or well-screened rooms
    - Apply mosquito repellent containing DEET over the exposed parts of the body
    - Avoid staying in scrubby areas
    - Keeping unscreened windows and doors closed.

Treatment

- There is no specific treatment for classic dengue fever and most people will recover completely within 2 weeks
- It is symptomatic and supportive
- Bedrest is advisable during the acute febrile phase
- Antipyretics or sponging are required to keep body temperature below 39°C

- Salicylates and ibuprofen should be avoided
- Paracetamol may be prescribed
- Analgesics or a mild sedative may be required for those with severe pain
- Home available fluids and oral rehydration solution (ORS) are recommended for patients with excessive sweating, nausea, vomiting or diarrhea to prevent dehydration.

Health Education

Health education by nursing personnel is essential to prevent mosquito bites, breeding places of *A. aegypti*:

1. To prevent mosquito bite people are advised to:
   a. Use mosquito nets or repellent at night.
   b. Use mosquito repellent cream on exposed parts both day and night.
   c. Cover whole body parts to avoid exposed arms and legs.
2. To prevent mosquito breeding places, people are advised to:
   a. Clean or remove breeding places of *A. aegypti* usually broken utensils, cigarette tins, etc.
   b. Periodical cleaning or drying of man-made water tanks and water containers.
   c. General antimosquito measures, i.e. using repellents.
   d. Check and inspect the ship for mosquito before leaving a port to prevent immigrations of mosquitoes.
   e. Check and inspect the aircraft before leaving airport.
   f. Aerosol spray, ultra-low volume (ULV) quantities of malathion or sumithion.

Today, dengue control and prevention requires thinking outside the tropical disease box. Many of the affected countries are some of the poorest. Approaches that are realistic for their infrastructure need to be developed. The high frequency of international and regional travel related to tourism, labor, commerce and other activities increases the probability of importation and introduction of dengue virus into our territories.

Nursing Management

Isolation

The medical aseptic technique is not necessary in handling dengue patients. It is not transmissible from person to person only by the bite of a mosquito. The patient should be placed in a mosquito-proof room and dichlorodiphenyltrichloroethane (DDT) spray used to eradicate any insects.

Diet

Because of anorexia, which is practically always present, nausea and vomiting that may be present; the nurse must give considerable time and thought to the diet. During the acute stage of the disease, high-caloric fluids should be given. Small amounts at frequent intervals are fairly well tolerated. As soon as possible, the diet should be increased. The patient preferences should be considered. Ice cream, gelatin desserts, nourishing soups, toast, soft eggs, cottage cheese, pureed vegetables and fruits are suggested. Intravenous glucose, saline, amigen or blood plasma may be given, if nausea and vomiting become too persistent. A return to general diet is indicated as soon as the patient will tolerate it.

Temperature

The temperature is high at the onset, as a rule, ranging from 102 to 105°F. Cool, tepid or warm sponge baths may be given. An alcohol fan is frequently gratefully received and the rash is no contraindication to its use. An ice pack or ice cap to the head and plenty of fluids should be given. A careful record of the temperature should be kept. It should be taken every 3 or 4 hours.

In older men, frequency and strangury is often most distressing. In younger men, orchitis is very common, may occasionally pain and a rise in temperature is seen. The frequency is due to a non-specific prostatitis probably due to the virus of dengue.

Personal Hygiene

The patient should have a daily bath. It should be given without too much pressure on the sore muscles. A good bath is given gently, if the nurse remembers that gentle handling is appreciated by his/her patient. Good oral hygiene should be maintained. The tongue is characteristically dirty. It may be cleaned with a brush or with a gauze pledget. Hydrogen peroxide (50%) is effective. The teeth should be well cleaned at least twice daily. Any good antiseptic mouthwash may be used as a rinse before and after meals and after vomiting. The eyes should be kept clean with warm boric washes or irrigations, if indicated.

Elimination

The bowels should move thoroughly each day. The patient usually is constipated although diarrhea may be present. Enemas may be used as needed. A record of fluid output should be kept. Retention of urine does occur, particularly in older patients and its presence should not be overlooked in any acutely ill patient.

CHAPTER 30 — Arthropod Infestations

General Management of the Disease

The patient should be kept in a quiet room in a comfortable bed. The eyes are sensitive to light and should be protected by turning the head side of the bed away from the light. A good north light is satisfactory, but bright light should be excluded from the room. Ice caps or ice packs help to relieve the more or less constant headache. The rash is rarely bothersome and requires no treatment as a rule. Calamine lotion may be used. These patients are easily depressed and they appreciate a quiet, cheerful manner on the part of the nurse. If delirium is present, a nurse should be in constant attendance or restraint should be applied to prevent the patient from falling. A constant backache may be relieved by small comfort pillows, in addition to prescribed medication. The patient's care should be planned so as to give him/her the longest possible intervals of rest. However, their position should be changed every 3 or 4 hours. The nurse should watch for and report any unusual symptoms. In the majority of cases of dengue, it is a rather mild, self-limited disease, but occasional cases are very severe. Sandfly fever is a very similar disease and the nursing care is similar. Terminal disinfection is not necessary.

Convalescence

Convalescence is usually very rapid. However, in the severe cases it may be slow. In older men, with prostatitis and strangury, it is apt to be prolonged and periods of relapsing prostatitis occur following the acute attack in men over 50.

CHIKUNGUNYA FEVER (EPIDEMIC POLYARTHRITIS)

Chikungunya fever is an acute infectious disease caused by chikungunya virus, transmitted by the bite of infective, female *Aedes* mosquito. Clinically characterized by sudden onset of fever associated with chills, severe myalgia, malaise, polyarthralgia and often associated with rashes with or without mild itching. Case fatality is almost nil. It is an urban disease resembling dengue, seen mainly in Africa, Pakistan, Indian subcontinent, Southeast Asia and Philippines. Chikungunya fever was first described in an epidemic form in East Africa in 1952–1953. In India, epidemic has occurred in Karnataka, Maharashtra, Tamil Nadu and Andhra Pradesh during March 2006 to August 2006. The code according to International Classification of Disease (ICD) is A92.0 chikungunya also called chikungunya virus disease or chikungunya fever, is a viral illness that is spread by the bite of infected mosquitoes and not connected with bird flu, which is spread through chicken. The name chikungunya is from the Makonde language. The name is derived from a word meaning to become contorted and signifies the cause of a contortion or folding. It refers to the stooped posture of patients afflicted with the severe joint pain of this disease.

The disease resembles dengue fever and is characterized by severe, sometimes persistent, joint pass (arthritis), as well as fever and rash. It is a debilitating, but nonfatal, viral illness, i.e. spread by the bite of infected mosquitoes.

Chikungunya occurs in Africa, India and Southeast Asia. It was first detected in 1953 in Tanzania and in India it was detected in 1963 in Kolkata. In 1964, chikungunya was found in Chennai, Pondicherry, Vellore and Visakhapatnam.

Magnitude of the Problem

Global

Chikungunya occurs mainly in Africa, India and Southeast Asia. There have been a number of outbreaks (epidemics) in the Philippines and on islands throughout the Indian Ocean. Because humans act as very efficient reservoirs for the virus, chikungunya is most prevalent in urban areas. Epidemics are sustained by the human-mosquito-human transmission cycle.

The first recognized outbreak of chikungunya occurred in East Africa in 1952–1953. Soon thereafter epidemics were noted in Philippines (1954, 1956 and 1968), Thailand, Cambodia, Vietnam, India, Burma and Sri Lanka, since 2003. There have been outbreaks in the islands of the Pacific Ocean, including Madagascar, Comoros, Mauritius and Reunion Island, with a surge in number of cases after the Tsunami of December 2004. It is suspected that many cases of chikungunya are either misdiagnosed or go unreported.

In February 2005, an outbreak was recorded on the French Island of Reunion in the Indian Ocean. As of May 18, 2006, 258,000 residents have been hit by the virus in the past year (out of a population of about 777,000). About 219 official deaths have been associated with chikungunya. In neighboring Mauritius, 3,500 Islanders have been hit in 2005. There have also been cases in Madagascar, Mayotte and the Seychelles.

India

In 2006, there was a big outbreak in the Andhra Pradesh state in India. Nearly 200,000 people were affected by this disease in the districts of Prakasam and Nellore in this state. Some deaths have been reported, but it was thought to be due mainly to the inappropriate use of antibiotics and anti-inflammatory tablets. As this virus can cause thrombocytopenia, injudicious use of these drugs can cause erosions in the gastric epithelium leading to exsanguinating upper gastrointestinal (GI) bleed (due to thrombocytopenia). There have been reports of large scale outbreak of this virus in Southern India. At least 80,000 people in Kalaburagi, Tumakuru, Bidar, Raichur, Ballari, Chitradurga, Davangere, Kolar and Vijapura districts in Karnataka state are known to be affected since December 2005. A separate outbreak of chikungunya fever was reported from Malegaon town in Nasik district, Maharashtra state, in the first 2 weeks of March 2006, resulting in over 2,000 cases. In Odisha state, almost 5,000 cases of fever with muscle aches and headache were reported between February 27 and March 5, 2006. In Bengaluru, the state capital of Karnataka (India), there was an outbreak of chikungunya (May 2006) with arthralgia/arthritis and rashes also in the neighboring state of Andhra Pradesh. In the 3rd week of May 2006, the outbreak of chikungunya in North Karnataka was severe. All the North Karnataka districts specially Kalaburagi, Koppal, Ballari, Gadag and Dharwad were affected. Stagnation of water, which provides fertile breeding grounds for the vector (*A. aegypti*) should be avoided. In the latest outbreak in Tamil Nadu, India, 20,000 cases were reported in June 2006. Analysis of the recent outbreak has suggested that the increased severity of the disease may be due to a change in the genetic sequence, altering the virus coat protein, which potentially allows it to multiply more easily in mosquito cells. Chikmagalur (1,037), Koppal (5,783), Dakshina Kannada (9) and Mandya (699).

The organism is chikungunya virus (Buggy Creek virus). It belongs to group A arboviruses, family togaviridae, genus alphavirus. It is spherical, enveloped, virion of 60 nm in diameter and single-stranded RNA genome. It is killed by common disinfectants, moist heat and drying.

Reservoir

Chikungunya fever is a disease of human beings only. There is no animal reservoir. There is no carrier state also.

Transmission: The disease is transmitted from person to person by the bite of infective female *Aedes* mosquito. There is no evidence of direct transmission from person to person. Epidemics are sustained by human-mosquito-human transmission, similar to that of dengue and urban yellow fever.

Vector

Chief vector is *A. aegypti* (culicine group).

Breeding place: Aedes aegypti breeds in water collected in containers such as tumbler, coconut shell, bottles, broken tins and cans, tree holes, air coolers and such others in and around the houses.

Biting time: They bite (female *Aedes*) during early hours of the morning 6–9 AM and in the evening 3–6 PM. They are aggressive day biters. They hide underneath the cots, tables and other furniture.

Extrinsic Incubation Period

The extrinsic incubation period (EIP) is the time required for the viruses to undergo multiplication and reach an optimum number, when the infected mosquito is said to have become infective. The EIP is 10–12 days. Since the virus undergoes only multiplication and no cyclical development, it is a propagative type of biological transmission. Once the mosquito becomes infective, it remains infective throughout its life, whomsoever it bites, transmits the disease. This is how several members of the same family are simultaneously affected. The lifespan of the mosquito is about 3 weeks.

The fever is caused by an arbovirus transmitted typically by *Aedes* mosquitoes, although there may be other competent mosquito vectors. The most prominent frequent feature is severe arthritis. The virus is arthropod-borne (it is therefore an arbovirus) and belongs to the family togaviridae, genus *Alphavirus*, which was first isolated from the blood of a febrile patient in Tanzania in 1953. The virus is a positive-sense, single-stranded RNA virus. Human infections are acquired by the bite of infected *A. aegypti* mosquitoes and epidemics are sustained by human-mosquito-human transmission. This epidemic cycle is similar to that of dengue and urban yellow fever. Chikungunya fever is characterized by sudden onset of chills and fever, headache, nausea, vomiting, arthralgia and rash.

Life Cycle

The *Aedes* are temporary pool water breeders. They lay their eggs singly on damp soil near water. Like all mosquitoes they pass through four life stages; egg, larva (four stages or instars), pupa and adult. All mosquitoes live in water continuously from the time of the eggs hatch through the larval (wiggler) and pupal stages until the adults emerge. Multiple generations are possible. They are found in shallow water with abundant vegetation above and/or on the water surface, where there is fluctuating water level and they are protected from wave action. Roadside ditches are common breeding sites. They do not live in running water or deep, open waters of lakes and ponds.

Genetic Sequence of Virus

Scientists have for the first time come out with genetic sequence data of the 'chikungunya viruses,' shedding light on the origin of their outbreak and huge populations of the Indian Ocean countries, most recently in India.

A team of scientists led by Sylvain Brisse of the Paris-based Pasteur Institute has come out with the first molecular data on the viruses involved in the outbreak now published in the international open-access journal Public Library of Science (PLOS) Medicine. The data indicate that the virus strains of this outbreak have distinct molecular features. Whether these features can explain some of the unique characteristics of the current outbreak, leading to developing a remedy to treat the victims, needs to be tested. The causative virus is reported to have undergone genetic mutation by amino acid substitutions. Studies are currently underway to establish whether these substitutions are linked to the neurovirulence of the chikungunya virus on one hand and to greater efficiency of viral multiplication on the other.

Host Factors

Anyone who is bitten by an infected mosquito can get chikungunya.

Age: A survey conducted at Kolkata revealed that the people within the age group of 51–55 years were more affected by chikungunya than the other age groups. Monkeys and possibly other wild animals may also serve as reservoir of the virus.

Environmental Factors

The *Aedes* mosquitoes that transmit chikungunya breed in a wide variety of man-made containers, which are common around human dwellings. These containers collect rainwater and include discarded tires, flowerpots, old oil drums, animal water troughs, water storage vessels and plastic food containers.

Widespread poverty, year-round tropical climate environmental disturbance due to war or natural disaster and lack of public health infrastructure are all factors that promote uncontrolled mosquito breeding and are conducive to outbreaks of chikungunya or other mosquito-borne diseases.

Mode of Transmission

Chikungunya is spread by the bite of an *Aedes* mosquito, primarily *A. aegypti*. The vector longevity is estimated to be between 2 weeks and 1 month, and the time for virus replication in the mosquito (extrinsic cycle) about 10 days, indicating sufficient time for transmission.

Humans are thought to be the major source or reservoir of chikungunya virus for mosquitoes. Therefore, the mosquito usually transmits the disease by biting an infected person and then biting someone else.

An infected person cannot spread the infection directly to other persons (i.e. it is not a contagious disease). *A. aegypti* mosquitoes bite during the day. Mother-to-child transmission of chikungunya virus was a new observation recorded during the French Reunion Islands outbreak in 2006.

Incubation Period

The time between the bite of a mosquito carrying chikungunya virus and the start of symptoms ranges from 1 to 12 days. Incubation period is 1–2 weeks (average = 4–7 day).

Clinical Features

Clinically characterized by sudden onset of chills and fever (103–104°F), headache, nausea, vomiting and severe muscular and joint pains (significant myalgia and polyarthritis). The joints of the extremities in particular become swollen and painful to touch. The person becomes disabled. Fever is followed by maculopapular rash and often buccal and palatal enanthem. Hemorrhage mortality is rare.

It is a self-limiting viral disease. All, but few recover within 5–7 days. Some will have persistent myalgia and arthralgia from several weeks to several months. Children may display neurological symptoms.

The name 'chikungunya' come from the word 'Swahili' meaning 'which bends up,' referring to the stooped posture that victims adopt to relieve the joint pains of this disease. Immunity is long-lasting. Chikungunya usually starts suddenly with fever up to chills, headache, nausea, vomiting, joint pain and skin rash.

Fever and severe arthralgia are accompanied by chills and constitutional symptoms such as headache, photophobia, conjunctival injection, anorexia, nausea and abdominal pain. Migratory polyarthritis mainly the small joints of the hands, wrists, ankles and feet, with lesser involvement of the larger joints. The patient find themself incapable of walking or even talking. Rash may appear at the outset or several days into the illness. The rash is most intense on the trunk and limbs, and may desquamate. Petechiae are occasionally seen and epistaxis is not uncommon. A few patients develop leukopenia.

Frequently, the infection causes no symptoms, especially in children. While recovery from chikungunya is the expected outcome, convalescence can be prolonged (up to a year or more) and persistent joint pain may require analgesic (pain medication), and long-term anti-inflammatory therapy. Infection appears to confer lasting immunity.

Differences Between Chikungunya and Dengue Fever

In contrast to dengue, chikungunya is characterized by a briefer febrile episode, by persistent arthralgia in some cases and by the fortunate absence of fatalities. In case of dengue fever, complications can arise in areas where the disease is endemic and repeated infection is possible. These are DHF and DSS. They are most often found in children, who have been previously had dengue fever. DHS appears first with the child developing internal hemorrhages that lead to the onset of DSS. The condition is fatal in 10–20% of cases.

Complications

Sudden severe headache, chills, fever, joint and muscle pain are the commonest complications.

Laboratory Diagnosis

Chikungunya is diagnosed by blood tests. Since the clinical appearance of both chikungunya and dengue are similar, laboratory confirmation is important, especially in areas where dengue is present.

Detection of antigens or antibody to the agent in the blood (serology); ELISA is available. An immunoglobulin M (IgM) capture ELISA is necessary to distinguish the disease from dengue fever.

Treatment

There is no specific treatment for chikungunya. No vaccine is available. Supportive therapy that helps ease symptoms such as administration of non-steroidal anti-inflammatory drugs (NSAIDs) such as paracetamol, mefenamic acid and getting plenty of rest, may be beneficial. In some cases, administration of chloroquine phosphate is reported to be beneficial. Infected persons should be isolated from mosquitoes in as much as possible in order to avoid transmission of infection to other people.

Management: Is by symptomatic treatment with analgesics, antipyretics, antihistamines and bedrest.

Prevention and Control

Prevention and control is done mainly by the control of *Aedes* mosquitoes (explained under entomology) and health education of the people about the following points:
- To maintain sanitation in and around the house
- To remove the water containers, if any
- To keep the air cooler clean and dry once a week, and to remove the water, if not used
- To use mosquito curtain, if habituated to sleep in the afternoon or apply mosquito repellents.

Preventive Measures

An extensive public education campaign through mass media about protective measures is very essential. Prevention centers on avoiding mosquito bites when traveling to areas where chikungunya occurs. Eliminating mosquito breeding sites is another key prevention measure. To prevent mosquito bites, do the following:

1. When indoors, stay in air-conditioned or well-screened areas; use bed nets, if sleeping in areas that are not screened or air conditioned.
2. When outdoors during times that mosquitoes are biting, wear long-sleeved shirts and long pants.
3. Use mosquito repellents on skin and clothing.
4. Get rid of mosquito breeding sites by emptying standing water from flower pots, buckets and barrels.
5. Change water in pet dishes and replace the water in bird baths weekly.
6. Use insect repellents.
7. For skin, use a product that contains 20–50% DEET; DEET in higher concentrations is no more effective.
8. Use DEET sparingly on children and do not apply to their hands, which they often place in their mouths.
9. Apply DEET lightly and evenly to exposed skin; do not use underneath clothing; avoid contact with eyes, lips and broken or irritated skin.
10. To apply to your face, first dispense a small amount DEET onto your hands and then carefully spread a thin layer.
11. Wash DEET off when exposure to mosquitoes ceases.
12. When using DEET and a sunscreen, apply the sunscreen first; after 30 minutes to an hour, apply the DEET; this allows the sunscreen time to penetrate and bind to the skin and will not interfere with the efficacy of the DEET.

13. For clothing, use an insect repellent spray to help prevent bites through the fabric; use a product that contains permethrin.
14. Permethrin will withstand numerous launderings; it should only be used on clothing, never on skin.
15. When using any insect repellent, always 'follow label directions' do not inhale aerosol formulations.

Nursing Management

1. Imbalanced body temperature (fever) related to the presence of infection:
    - Monitor vital signs [temperature, pulse, respiration (TPR) and blood pressure (BP)]
    - Provide comfortable bed and position
    - Ensure mosquito-free environment
    - Apply cold compress
    - Tepid sponging
    - Administer antipyretics, e.g. paracetamol as per prescription.
2. Arthralgia related to chikungunya infection:
    - Assess the level of pain and subjective changes in pain
    - Provide comfortable bed and position
    - Encourage verbalization of feelings about pain
    - Noise-free environment
    - Protect joints, ease pain with splints
    - Provide adequate rest
    - Massage and position change
    - Diversional therapy
    - Thermal modalities (moist packs, cold applications) and relaxation
    - Administer NSAIDs as per prescription.
3. Fatigue related to increased disease activity:
    - Identify emotional and physical factors causing fatigue
    - Adequate rest
    - Encourage adequate nutrition
    - Relaxation techniques provide emotional rest
    - Psychological support
    - Conditioning exercise such as walking, biking requires gradual progression
    - Encourage adherence to treatment plan.
4. Disturbed sleep pattern related to pain:
    - Sleep-inducing routine (warm bath, relaxation technique)
    - Medication
    - Comfort measures.
5. Impaired physical mobility related to decreased range of motion and pain on movement:
    - Proper body positioning to minimize stress on joints
    - Lie flat on a firm mattress, change position frequently
    - Active range of motion exercise is encouraged to prevent joint stiffness, if not possible, passive range of motion exercises to be done
    - Maintain proper posture, while sitting, self-care deficit related to fatigue and inability to walk
    - Assist patient to identify factors that interfere with activities of daily living (ADL)
    - Develop a plan to meet self-care needs and implement the same
    - Provide appropriate assistive device
    - Allow patient to control timing of self-care activities.
6. Potential for:
    - Epistaxis
    - Leukopenia
    - Stiffness of joints
    - Superinfection
    - Elevated level of aspartate aminotransferases and creative protein due to reduced platelet count.
7. Knowledge deficit regarding:
    - Mode of transmission of disease
    - Preventive measures
    - Diet, medication, exercise, etc.
    - Assess the knowledge and teach about chikungunya infection, mode of transmission and preventive measures
    - No dietary restriction
    - Take medications as per prescription and order
    - Active and passive range of motion exercises are encouraged.

MALARIA

Malaria is a communicable protozoal disease caused by sporozoan of the genus *Plasmodium* and transmitted to man by species of infective female *Anopheles* mosquitoes called vectors or carriers. It is characterized by intermittent fever with rigors, enlargement of spleen and secondary anemia.

Magnitude of Problem

The disease is worldwide, with 143 countries being malarious. In 1950, annual incidence was 250 million with 2.5 million deaths. Now, 100 million cases are reported of which 1 million results into death. Over 1,800 million exposed to the disease. In India, in 1953, 75 million people suffered and 800,000 deaths resulted from malaria. Incidence dropped further to 2 million in 1958, which dropped further to 50,000 cases in 1961 with no death. In 1965 onward a gradual increase was noted and 6.46 million suffered in 1976 was reported.

Epidemiological Features

Agent

As already stated, malaria in man is caused by different species of the genus *Plasmodium*. These are four species:
1. *Plasmodium vivax* (*P. vivax*): Causes benign tertian fever, which recurs every 48 hours. About 65–70% infections are caused by this species. The fever usually lasts for 3 years, if untreated.
2. *Plasmodium falciparum* (*P. falciparum*): Causes malignant tertian fever, which recurs every 48 hours. About 25–30% infections are reported due to the species. This type of malaria is self-limited, lasts about 1 year, if untreated, but it has high mortality.
3. *Plasmodium malariae* (*P. malariae*): Causes quartan type of fever, which recurs every 72 hours. About 4–8% infections reported. It lasts for many years, if untreated. It was found in Tumakuru and Hassan districts of Karnataka.
4. *Plasmodium ovale* (*P. ovale*): Rarely found in man, mainly confined to tropical Africa, Vietnam (Figs 30.1 and 30.2).

Life History of Malarial Parasite

Malarial parasite has two cycles of development:
1. Sexual cycle.
2. Asexual cycle.

Sexual Cycle

Sexual cycle takes place in the definitive host, i.e. mosquito. The cycle begins when some of the merozoites instead of repeating the cycle, grow into male and female gametocytes. These gametocytes are ingested by the mosquitoes during blood sucking and enter the stomach. One of the male gametes impregnated the female gamete and form zygote, which is motionless at the beginning and become motile (ookinete) after 12–18 hours. It starts penetrating the wall of the stomach of mosquito and forms oocyst on its outer surface,

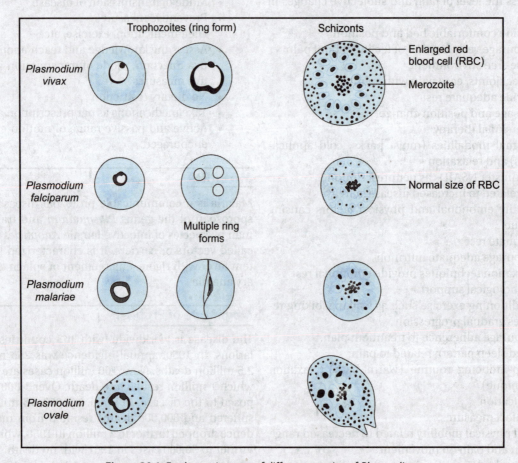

Figure 30.1: Erythrocytic stage of different species of *Plasmodium*

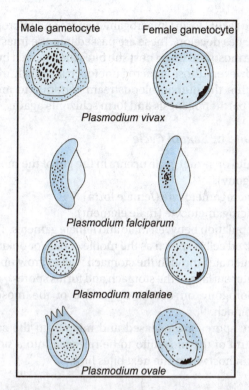

Figure 30.2: Gametocytes of *Plasmodium* species

grows rapidly and ruptures liberating large number of sporozoites into the body cavity of the insect. Many of the sporozoites migrate into salivary glands of the mosquito and become infective to man during its blood meal.

Asexual Cycle

Asexual cycle begins when an infected mosquito bites a person and injects sporozoites. Then sporozoites disappear within an hour from the peripheral circulation. Some of them are destroyed by phagocytes, others reach the liver cells. After 1–2 weeks they become hepatic schizonts, which eventually burst releasing a shower of merozoites, which re-enter the bloodstream (extraerythrocytic phase). Most of these merozoites are destroyed, but some of them penetrate red blood cells (RBCs) and pass through the stage of trophozoites and schizonts (erythrocytes). The erythrocytic phase ends with liberation of merozoites, which infect fresh RBCs, some of them forming gametocytes to be sucked by mosquitoes (Figs 30.3 and 30.4).

Reservoir of Infection

A person harboring both male and female gametocytes, i.e. both the sexes of mature and viable gametocytes in the blood in sufficient density to be sucked by mosquitoes during a bite on the reservoir of infection.

Period of Communicability

Depending on the presence of mature viable gametocytes in sufficient numbers, the period of communicability may be:
1. Infection caused by *P. vivax* infection 4–5 days after appearance of sexual forms.
2. Infection caused by *P. falciparum* 10–12 days.
3. Relapse in borderline tuberculoid (BT)—more than 3 years after first attack.
4. Recurrence usually disappears within 1–2 years *P. falciparum*.
5. In malarial infection, it may last for 30 years or more.

Vectors of Malaria

Among the *Anopheles* mosquitoes, malaria carrying species in India are—*Anopheles culicifacies Anopheles fluviatilis*, subgenus *Anopheles, Anopheles stephensi, Anopheles minimus, Anopheles philippinensis* and *Anopheles sundaicus*.

Mode of Transmission

1. Vector transmission—through the bite of female *Anopheles* mosquitoes.
2. Direct transmission—by hypodermic intramuscular (IM) and IV injections of blood or plasma, e.g. during blood transfusion, drug infections of addicts.
3. Congenital malaria—may occur, but rare.

Factors for Transmission of Malaria

1. Presence of a source of infection (man) with sufficient number of mature, viable male and female gametocytes in their peripheral blood.
2. Presence of sufficient number of anopheline mosquitoes capable of transmitting malaria.

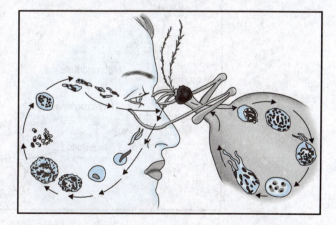

Figure 30.3: Life cycle of the malarial parasite

3. Favorable conditions for mosquitoes and development of parasites and mosquitoes.
4. Presence of susceptible human host.

Incubation Period

The time between the bite of mosquito and first attack of fever in most of the cases is less than 10 days:
- In *P. falciparum*—12 days
- In *P. vivax*—13–15 days
- In *P. malariae*—up to 1 month.

Human or Asexual Cycle

Human or asexual cycle occurs in the human bloodstream (schizogony):
1. Sporozoite.
2. Penetration of the sporozoite into a human RBC.
3. Growth of the schizont.
4. Beginning of nuclear division within the schizont.
5. Division within the schizont completed.
6. Breaking up of the schizont into merozoites.
7. The sexual forms, macrogametocytes and microgametocytes develop. These are passed into the intestine of the mosquito when next she bites the infected human. However, those macrogametocytes, which remain within the human bloodstream continue to multiply by parthenogenesis and form schizonts again.

Mosquito or Sexual Cycle

Mosquito or sexual cycle occurs in the gut of the mosquito (sporogony):
1. Macrogametocyte (female form).
2. Microgametocyte (male element).
3. Copulation between male and female gametes. The fertilized cell is known as the motile copula or ookinete. It penetrates through the stomach wall to grow upon the outer surface of the stomach and forms spores.
4. Sporogony on the outer surface of the mosquito's stomach.
5. The spores are released and migrate to the salivary gland of the mosquito to be released into a new human host when she next bites him.

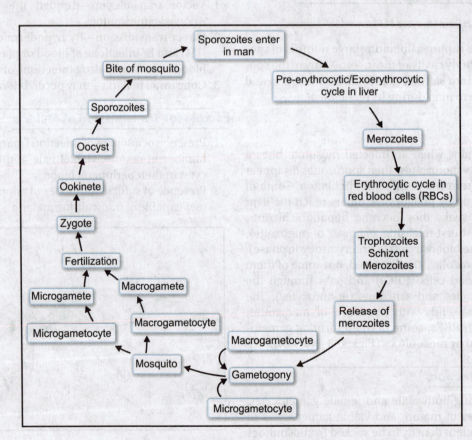

Figure 30.4: Life cycle of malarial parasite

CHAPTER 30 — Arthropod Infestations

Note: An exoerythrocytic stage exists in man in which the infection is latent and the plasmodia exist in tissue cells other than the RBCs. In some strains of *P. vivax* it may be delayed. It is also delayed in persons taking suppressive malarial drugs.

Host Factors

1. Age: It affects all ages.
2. Sex: Men are more frequently exposed than women. Males are more affected as females are clothed better. In India, women cover whole body.
3. Race: Individuals with sickle cell trait have a milder illness, e.g. Negroes with sickle cell trait are immune caused by *P. falciparum* infection.
4. Social and economic factors: More prevalent in underdeveloped countries. Economic depression is associated with epidemic and malaria ill-ventilated and ill-lighted houses.
5. Movement of population: Nomads, laborers and wandering tribes import malarial parasites.
6. Human habits: Sleeping outdoors, sleeping with or without mosquito net, etc.
7. Immunity: Man has no natural immunity.
8. Environmental factors:
   - Season—July to November
   - Temperature: 20–30°C optimum temperature for the development of the malarial parasite in infected vector
   - Humidity: Relative humidity 60% necessary for mosquitoes to live their normal span of life
   - Rainfall: Rain provides opportunities for breeding of mosquitoes
   - Altitude: Mosquitoes are not found at altitude above 2,000–2,500 m (6,000 ft) sea level
   - Manmade: Such as burrow pits, excavations during construction of barrage, railways, roads, irrigation canals, etc. for breeding of mosquitoes due to water collection.

Pathophysiology

The pathophysiology of malarial parasites in the human subjects involves anemia, hemoglobin and urea. The symptoms of malaria appear about 2 weeks after the infection. The anemia is due to the destruction of the erythrocytes. It is also thought that a hemolysin presumably derived from the parasites may bring about the hemolysis of some of the normal erythrocytes during the course of infection. The liver and particularly the spleen become enlarged, there is a thrombosis of the visceral capillaries. The death may result when the capillaries of the brain become plugged with both pigment and parasites. In fatal septicemic form of malignant malaria, there is massive invasion, which enters vascular system by parasites. The cardiac type of subtertian fever, also fatal and, simply involves the plugging of the coronary arteries with both pigment and parasites with the result that the heart is deprived of oxygen and nutrients.

Clinical Features

An attack of malaria consists of three successive stages:
1. Cold stage: Sudden onset of fever and chills, which lasts for 15 minutes to an hour.
2. Hot stage: Temperature rises up to 106°F (41°C) with headache, which lasts for 2–6 hours.
3. Sweating stage: Fever comes down by profuse sweating. It was recognized as early as was described by Charaka and Sushruta.

Usually in malaria cases there is chills, rigor, pallor, cyanosis, nausea, vomiting, headache, which may continue for 15 minutes to an hour and even convulsions in children. The spiking fever, reaching 104°F (40°C) or high, may last for several hours followed by profuse sweating with peripheral vasodilatation and the temperature drops. The patient feels relatively well. The fever comes and goes. As the disease progresses there is splenomegaly. Liver may also be enlarged and tender. In the early stage, paroxysms of fever follow an irregular pattern, but later the paroxysms may occur after every 48 hours in all, but after 62 hours in malariae infection (quartan malaria). The periodicity of chills and fever infection caused by both *P. vivax* and *P. falciparum* infection is however influenced by the immunity of the patient, strain differences and from infection by more than one species of *Plasmodium*. However, in vivax infection (benign tertian malaria) vomiting may be troublesome and the condition tends to relapse after long quiescent intervals. Symptomatically ovale infection (ovale tertian malaria) may stimulate subacute appendicitis or rheumatic fever even though in most cases the condition gives rise to little symptoms. *P. falciparum* infection (subtertian malaria) may resemble influenza, yellow fever or may even simulate typhoid fever and many other diseases when it involves internal organs. Severe *P. falciparum* infection may cause renal damage, while malariae infection is liable to produce nephrosis in children with generalized edema, oliguria, proteinuria and hypoproteinemia.

In *P. falciparum* infection, the fever is irregular and may lack the periodicity or may even occur every day. There may be normocytic anemia, cough, vomiting, diarrhea, jaundice and postural hypotension. The condition may however at any time deteriorate dramatically leading to impaired consciousness and coma.

In severe form of *P. falciparum* infection, there may be cerebral malaria, presenting with high fever, confusion, delirium, seizures, stupor, followed by coma persisting for a few hours. There may also be various paresis and hemiplegia. In addition, there may be renal impairment with low urine output or persistent oliguria, hemoglobinuria, pulmonary edema, hypoglycemia, hypotension and severe anemia. In adults, there may be spontaneous bleeding from the gum, skin bruising, gastrointestinal hemorrhage and oozing from venipuncture. Chronic *P. falciparum* infection, especially in patients treated with quinine can give rise to serious complication, blackwater fever, presenting with intravascular hemorrhage and hemoglobinuria in addition.

Malaria can produce several complications such as hyperpyrexia, algid malaria (resembling acute adrenal insufficiency), pernicious anemia, gastrointestinal disorder, rupture of spleen and abortion in pregnant women.

Diagnosis

Diagnosis is comparatively easy in endemic areas and is confined by detection of characteristic malarial parasites in the erythrocytes in thick and thin blood films.

It is differentiated from several conditions, which cause fever, splenomegaly, hepatomegaly and anemia, though in one of them could malarial parasites be found.

Measurement of Malaria

Prevalence

1. Spleen rate: Percentage of children between 2 and 10 years showing enlargement of spleen.
2. Average enlarged spleen: Denotes the average size of enlarged spleen.
3. Parasite rate: Percentage of children between 2 and 12 years showing parasites in their blood.
4. Parasites density index: Indicates the average degree of parasitemia in a sample of well-defined group of the population. Only positive slides are induced in the denominator.
5. Infant parasite rate: Percentage of infants showing malaria parasite and then blood films. Most sensitive index of recent transmission of malaria. If the infant parasite rate is zero for 3 consecutive years, locally it is regarded as absence of malaria transverse.
6. Proportional case rate: Number of cases diagnosed as clinical malaria for every 100 patients attending the hospitals and dispensaries.

Incidence

The parameters are given below:

1. Annual parasite index (API): It is measured by the following formula:

$$\text{API} = \frac{\text{Confirmed cases during 1 year}}{\text{Population under surveillance}} \times 100$$

2. Annual blood examination rate (ABER) is measured by:

$$\text{ABER} = \frac{\text{Number of slides examined}}{\text{Population}} \times 100$$

Classification of Endemicity

The classification of endemicity is based on World Health Organization (WHO). According to spleen rate, the endemicity may be:

- Hypoendemic—less than 10% spleen rate (SR)
- Mesoendemic—SR 11–50%
- Hyperendemic—SR over 50%
- Holoendemic—SR over 75%.

Vector Indices

Some of the important vector indices are:

1. Human blood index: Proportion of freshly fed female anopheline mosquitoes, whose stomach contains human blood indicates the degree of anthrophilism.
2. Sporozoite rate: Percentage of female anopheles with sporozoite in their salivary gland.
3. Mosquito density: Number of mosquitoes per man-hour catch.
4. Non-biting rate: Average incidence of anopheline bite per day per person.
5. Inoculation rate: The man biting rate multiplied by the infective sporozoite rate is called inoculation rate.

Malaria Survey

Objectives of the malaria survey are:

- To ascertain the extent of malaria prevalence in the area
- To find out factors responsible for malaria in the area
- To devise control program.
  Preliminary survey consists of:
- Territory, slope
- Meteorological factors
- Economic condition
- Study of mosquitoes and their breeding places
- Larval survey
- Spleen index and parasite index, etc.

Prevention and Control
- Elimination of reservoirs
- Breaking the channel of transmission
- Protection of susceptibles.

Elimination of Reservoirs

Elimination of reservoirs consist of making the infectious cases noninfectious by giving treatment.

The treatment consists of presumptive treatment, radical treatment and mass treatment. The current treatment under the National Antimalaria Program since 1999 is as follows.

Presumptive Treatment

All fever cases attending hospitals for the treatment are assumed to be the cases of malaria and treated accordingly depending upon whether that area is a low risk or high-risk area, which is so classified depending upon the following criteria.

Criteria to consider as a high-risk area
- Average slide positivity rate (SPR) of the last 3 years is 5% or more
- *Plasmodium falciparum* proportion is 30% or more provided the SPR is 3% or more during any of the last 3 years
- An area having a focus of chloroquine resistant *P. falciparum*
- Deaths due to *P. falciparum* malaria, during last 3 years.

Doses mentioned for adults

In low-risk areas
Treatment is given irrespective of the type of malaria:
- Day 1, chloroquine 600 mg, single dose, no further treatment.

In high-risk areas
- Day 1, chloroquine 600 mg + primaquine 45 mg
- Day 2, chloroquine 600 mg
- Day 3, chloroquine 300 mg.

Note: No primaquine for pregnant women and infants.
- Presumptive treatment to be given only after taking the blood smears
- Drug to be taken in single dose after food
- Dose is proportionately less for children. 10 mg/kg body weight for chloroquine and 0.75 mg/kg for primaquine.

All fever cases (current or with history) are assumed to be due to malaria and multipurpose workers (MPWs) administer a single dose tablet—chloroquine (4-aminoquinoline) 150 mg or according to age as given below in Table 30.1.

Table 30.1: Doses according to age

Age in years	Dosage (mg and corresponding tablet number)
0–1	75 (1/2)
1–4	150 (1)
4–8	300 (2)
8–14	450 (3)
14 and above	600 (4)

Caution: Chloroquine should not be administered in empty stomach.

Side effects: Toxicity is minimal. Some side effects may occur such as gastric irritation, nausea, vomiting, headache, pruritus, blurring of vision and sometimes dysplasia.

For prolonged use in large doses (300–600 mg dose daily) for weeks or months may produce ocular damage, e.g. neuroretinitis, pigmentation of nail bed, skin and palate. The above symptoms usually disappear soon after withdrawal of chloroquine. More severe side effects may also develop and if given intravenously can cause abrupt fall in BP, which may be fatal.

Radical Treatment

Radical treatment is given for those, whose blood smear report comes as positive for malarial parasites. Dosage depends upon the type of malaria.

In low-risk areas
1. For *P. vivax* malaria—chloroquine 600 mg single dose + 15 mg primaquine on 1 day.
2. Followed by only primaquine 15 mg daily for another 4 days.
3. For *P. falciparum* malaria: Chloroquine 600 mg single dose plus primaquine 45 mg single dose on 1st day followed by chloroquine 600 mg on 2nd day and 300 mg in 3rd day.

In high-risk areas
1. For *P. vivax* malaria: Only primaquine 15 mg daily for 5 days (because chloroquine has already been given under presumptive treatment).
2. For *P. falciparum* malaria: No further treatment is required (because chloroquine and primaquine has already been discussed under presumptive treatment)
3. For resistant cases, i.e. cases resistant to chloroquine (chloroquine and primaquine has already been given discussed presumptive treatment).
4. For *P. vivax* malaria: A single dose combination of sulfadoxine (1,500 mg) plus pyrimethamine (75 mg) is not effective.

5. For *P. falciparum* malaria: Single dose of the combination of sulfadoxine 1,500 mg and pyrimethamine 75 mg on 1st day, followed by primaquine 45 mg on the 2nd day. These drugs are not given on the same day due to precipitation of hemolytic crisis among glucose-6-phosphate dehydrogenase (G6PD) cases.

Cases resistant to above drugs are severe and complicated, and hospitalized for the treatment as under:

1. Quinine dihydrochloride injection, intravenously in 5% dextrose solution, over 4 hours, dose 10 mg/kg body weight. This is continued 8th hourly till the patient regains consciousness. Thereafter, same dose is given orally for 7 days.
2. Other drugs are:
    a. Mefloquine: 750 mg, to be used only in *P. falciparum* cases, only with ring stage in the blood smear report.
    b. Artemisinin: 10 mg/kg body weight, once a day for 5 days.
    c. Artesunate: 2.4 mg/kg body weight, two doses on the 1st day with 6 hours interval, thereafter once a day for 4 days.
    d. Artemether: 1.6 mg/kg body weight, administered similar to artesunate.
    e. Artether: 150 mg intramuscularly daily for 3 days.

Mass Treatment

Mass treatment is recommended in highly endemic areas, where API is more than 5 per 1,000 population. This will be more effective, when supplemented by antimosquito measures.

Antimalarial Measures

1. Prevention of man/vector contact using repellents, protective clothing, use of mosquito nets, mosquito-proof clothing and screening of houses.
2. Destruction of adult mosquitoes: Use of domestic sprays including aerosols, use of insecticides (DDT 5%) emulsion spray or germolene spray, or pyrethrum and DDT in kerosene oil spray. These insecticides are used in a variety of formulations. Spray killing is a major and effective control measure of malaria.
3. Destruction of mosquito larvae:
    a. Physical methods: Peridomestic sanitation, intermittent drying of water containers, clearing the jungle drainage and filling up of water collections.
    b. Use of larvicides: Malarial insecticides (gamma, 2003), Paris green dust against anopheline larvae.
    c. Biological methods: The use of larvicidal fishes has proved very effective to kill the larvae. Most common fishes are khaira and *Gambusia*.
4. Measures against malarial parasites in chemoprophylaxis and chemotherapy:
    a. Proguanil: 100 mg every day.
    b. Chloroquine: 300 mg once a week.
    c. Amodiaquine: 300–400 mg once a week.

It should be taken once a week before arriving in the malarious areas and to be continued for 3–4 weeks after leaving the area.

Chemoprophylaxis

With the development of drug resistance, this has become unreliable. However, it may be recommended for the following groups. Drug recommended is chloroquine:
- Travelers from non-malarious areas to malarious areas
- Military and paramilitary persons moving into malarious areas
- Pregnant women living in endemic and hyperendemic areas.

Revised National Drug Policy (2010) for Treatment of Malaria: Described under National Health Program

In areas of *P. vivax* and *P. malariae*, mixed infection, a single dose of chloroquine will not provide a radical cure. To prevent the relapse primaquine (8-aminoquinoline) must be given to deal with the persistent liver stages of these parasites. Primaquine is administered by MPW as a radical treatment only if the blood smear is found positive for malarial parasite. The agewise dosage of schedule used by field staff under National Malaria Education Program (NMEP) is described in the Table 30.2.

Table 30.2: Agewise dosage schedule

Age in years	Dosage
0–1	Nil
1–4	Single dose of 2.5 mg (1 tablet) + chloroquine 150 mg on 1st day followed by only 2.5 mg primaquine from 2nd to 5th day
4–8	Single dose of 5 mg (2 tablet) + 300 mg chloroquine on 1st day followed by 5 mg primaquine for further 4 days
8–14	Single dose of 10 mg (4 tablet) + 450 mg chloroquine 1st day following only 10 mg for 2nd and 5th day
14 and above	Single dose of 15 mg (6 tablet) + tablet chloroquine (600 mg) 2nd and 5th day primaquine only

Caution: Primaquine should not be administered to infants and pregnant woman on empty stomach.

Side effects: At recommended dosage no symptoms of toxicity are likely. Sometimes anorexia, nausea, cyanosis, epigastric distress, abdominal pain and cramps and passage of dark color urine are reported. Occasionally vomiting, itching, vague chest pain and weakness. In addition, there may be striking effects of bone marrow depression marked by leukopenia, anemia and methemoglobinemia. Tablet recommended is primaquine (2.5 mg base). Antimalarial drugs used in areas where *P. falciparum* is sensitive.

National Malaria Eradication Program

Under NMEP no regular chemoprophylaxis is recommended except in the following situations:
1. In pregnancy and infancy: During malaria infection (*P. vivax*) in pregnant woman and infants, radical treatment with primaquine is not recommended. These cases are put under weekly administration or chloroquine in the following doses:
   a. Infants (0–1 year): Chloroquine 37.5 mg (one fourth of the tablet) weekly once till the children attain 1 year of age then radical treatment is given with primaquine.
   b. Pregnant woman: Chloroquine 300 mg (two tablet) weekly once till the delivery and after that about 45 days. Hemoglobin rises more than 10%, when radical treatment with primaquine should be given.

National Malaria Control Program (1953)

National Malaria Control Program (NMCP) was started in the year 1953 as a joint venture of state and central governments with the assistance from international organizations such as WHO and United State Agency for International Development (USAID). It was the biggest program against a single communicable disease in the world. The main objective of NMCP was to reduce the incidence from massive proportions to such low level that the disease would cease to be a public health problem.

The main strategy of NMCP was indoor residual spraying with DDT dose (100 mg/ft^2 twice) within a year during transmission season. Areas with spleen rate below 10% of population were left out. This program was renamed as 'National Antimalaria Program (NAMP)' in 1999.

Achievements: Before the start of operation, there were 75 million cases with spleen rate of 15.7%, proportional case rate of 10.8%, child parasite rate 3.9% and infant parasite rate of 1.6%. At the end of operations total cases were reduced to 2 million, spleen rate 8.2%, proportion case rate 0.8% and infant parasite rate 0.6%.

National Malaria Eradication Program (1958)

Eradication means putting an end to any problem. Malaria eradication implies elimination of malarial parasite from the human population so that there is no more resumption of transmission even in the presence of vectors. Final aim is total absence of malarial parasite in human population. Success of malaria control was so impressive that it led to concept of eradication. NMEP was first launched in 1958 and by 1965, the annual incidence of malaria was drastically reduced from 75 million to a little over 0.1 million.

The main objective was to root out malaria from the country. The program was divided into four phases:
1. Preparatory phase.
2. Attack phase.
3. Consolidation phase.
4. Maintenance phase.

Preparatory phase: During this phase, an organizational program was planned based on the results of surveys.

Attack phase: The main aim of this phase is to take antimosquito measures, prompt treatment of infected cases and search for malaria cases. Total coverage, by spraying of the area was achieved using insecticide, e.g. DDT. Malathion was used in DDT resistant areas. For about 4 years, surveillance was followed to detect cases. Attack phase is terminated when the incidence of malaria comes down to 0.1/1,000 population in the year.

Consolidation phase: It lasts for 3 years. During this phase, spraying is stopped and surveillance vigorously pursued. The main aim of this phase is to ascertain, whether interruption to transmission has been achieved and to eliminate remaining foci. The main activities undertaken during this phase were active surveillance, passive surveillance, presumption and radical treatment, epidemiological investigation of foci and institutional remedial measures to eliminate foci.

Maintenance phase: It begins when the eradication is achieved. Despite careful search, no case of malaria of indigenous origin for consecutive 3 years of which 2 years must be in consolidation phase. Unless the area has the arrangement of adequate organization capable of preventing re-establishment of endemicity through imported cases.

This phase will last till malaria exists in the world. So, there is no time limit in the phase. In this phase, surveillance is withdrawn and vigilance is introduced. Responsibility of vigilance vested with primary health center (PHC).

Modified Plan of Operation, 1977

The NMEP made satisfactory progress till 1961, the incidence of malaria dropped down from 2 million cases in 1958 to 50,000 cases in 1961 and no death was reported by 1965. There was slow increase in the incidence of malaria up to 1968, but alarming increase was noted after that. During 1975, about 5,200,000 of malaria cases were recorded in India. In some parts of India, a virulent form of malaria caused by *P. falciparum* infection broke out, about 6.46 million cases of malaria and 59 deaths in 1976 being reported. As a result of such focal outbreaks, a number of units in maintenance phase had returned to attack phase.

Malaria has become a public health problem due to some reason for setback. Reasons are administrative, operational and also technical:

1. Failure of spraying DDT according to schedule due to delay in the arrival of DDT and relaxation in program.
2. Failure to give adequate treatment in some areas due to lack of adequate quantities of antimalarial drugs.
3. Failure to stop transmission due to mosquitoes being resistant to insecticides in certain areas.
4. Inadequate transport facilities and basic health services in the maintenance phase.
5. Lack of adequate staff.
6. Import of infected vectors from other infected areas plane.
7. Importation of infected persons from other countries.
8. Poor surveillance and vigilance.
9. Inadequate provisions for coping the problems with the urban malaria, because local bodies fail to provide sufficient resources with the result that antilarval activities lagged behind.

Resurgence of malaria necessitated renewed vigorous antimalarial activities and the program was modified. The modified plan of operation (MPO) was implemented from 1st April, 1977. Since then there has been a gradual downward trend in malaria-positive incidence.

Objectives of MPO (1977)

1. To prevent/elimination of malaria deaths.
2. To undertake intensive antimalaria operators in the areas with high incidence of malaria, reduction in the malaria morbidity.
3. To consolidate the achievements reached. Maintenance of the gains achieved earlier by reducing transmission whenever possible. Flexibility in the policies according to the epidemiological situation and local conditions is an essential feature of MPO program.

Strategy

1. In MPO program, the earlier phasing of antimalarial units as attack, consolidation and maintenance of phase areas was abolished, and reclassification of areas according to annual parasite incidence (API).
2. Areas with API more than two are:
   a. Spraying: Regular insecticidal spray with two rounds of DOT. If the vectors is resistant to DOT, three rounds of hexachlorocyclohexana (HCH) are recommended. If refractory to both DOT and HCH, and three rounds of malathion spray at intervals of 6 weeks. Dosage of DDT, HCH and malathion are 1.0, 0.2 and $2/m^2$ surface respectively.
   b. Assessment: Entomological assessment is done by teams by carrying out susceptibility tests to suggest appropriate insecticides.
   c. Surveillance: Collection and examination of blood smears. Active and passive surveillance carried out fortnightly. Active surveillance done by health workers by visiting houses. Passive surveillance made by hospital, dispensary or heal the center workers (taking blood smears of fever cases).
   d. Treatment of cases: By giving presumptive and radical treatment.
3. Areas with API less than two are:
   a. Spraying: Area not under regular spraying, focal spraying only when *P. falciparum* cases are detected during surveillance.
   b. Surveillance: No regular spraying, so active and passive surveillance operation to be carried out vigorously every fortnight.
   c. Treatment: All detected cases should receive radical treatment as pressures.
   d. Follow-up: Blood smears to be collected from all positive cases on completion of radical treatment and thereafter at monthly intervals for follow-up.
   e. Epidemiology: Epidemiological investigations of all malaria positive cases are to be investigated. This may include mass surveys.

Drug Distribution Centers and Fever Treatment Depots

A wide network of drug distribution centers (to dispense the antimalarial tablets) and fever treatment centers collection of blood slides in addition to distribution of antimalarial drugs. These centers are manned by voluntary workers.

Urban Areas

Intensive antilarval and drug treatment measures are undertaken in the urban areas. Spraying is confined only to the peripheral best of houses to a depth of a mile.

Plasmodium falciparum Containment

An additional component to prevent or control the spread of *P. falciparum* malaria has been introduced from October 1971 with Swedish International Development Agency (SIDA) assistance.

Reorganization

Antimalarial units have been reorganized in conformity with the geographic boundaries of the district making the District Health Officer (DHO) responsible for the program. The existing unit officers have been designated as District Malaria Officers (DMOs) are posted at district headquarters and are assisted by Assistant Malaria Officers. Laboratory services are decentralized, laboratory technicians are posted at each PHC. Entomological teams have been attached to all 72 zones in the country. The Chief Medical Officer (CMO) and the Medical Officers (MOs) (PHCs) have to play a key role in the execution of the program. The program is now horizontal and integrated with the general health services from the district level to periphery.

Technique of Preparation of Blood Smears

In adults this is done by pricking the left middle or ring finger. In babies, capillary blood is collected by pricing left big toe:
1. Hold the finger to be pricked.
2. Clean the tip of the finger with spirit.
3. Dry with another piece of cotton wool.
4. Prick the finger at the side of the tip with Hagedorn needle.
5. Allow the blood to flow freely.
6. Discard the first drop of blood or make the thin film.
7. The new drops should be collected for examination. Rest of the procedure is detailed in Table 30.3.

Nursing Management of Malaria

Isolation

To prevent the spread of malaria it is necessary to screen the patient and eradicate the presence of all insects within the ward. DDT powder or spray may be used with good results.

Table 30.3: Preparation of thin and thick smears of blood

Thin smear	Thick smear
Put a drop of fresh blood on the middle of the slide	Put three drops of fresh blood on the left hand quarter of the slide
Use another slide end and allow the drop blood to spread along it	Note that when the slide is turned over, the drops will be on the right end of the slide
Push the spreader quickly from the center to the left side of the slide, drawing the blood behind it	With the corner of another slide, mix the blood and smear it in a round form about 1 cm in diameter
Leave the film dry, do not blow when film is dried, mark the slide by writing the number given on the thin film using lead pencil	Leave the film dry
Wrap the slide in prescribed form and dispatch	Do not blow on it or shake the slide

Diet

During the acute stage, nourishing fluids should be given. During the cold or chilling stage, hot fluids may be given. Often they are too sick to take anything at this stage. Tea, broth, hot lemon or limeade with honey or sugar added is suggested. During the high temperature or hot stage, cold nourishing fluids are taken eagerly and should be given in large quantities. During the sweating stage it is necessary to urge fluids in order to replace lost fluid content. In order to replace sodium chloride lost in sweating, salt is unusually freely used in the diet and may be supplemented by adding sodium chloride in tablet form. Between paroxysmal episodes, the diet should be liberal, high in calories, vitamins and minerals.

Temperature

During a malarial attack, the fever may go extremely high, 105–106°F being not uncommon. When the temperature exceeds 104°F, the nurse is presented with the problem of reducing fever. Tepid to cool sponges are the methods of choice. An ice cap or pack to the head will help and at the same time be of comfort to the patient. Large amounts of cold fluid should be given, if the patient can swallow sometimes cold IV fluids are given. Their use is not recommended. Fluids given intravenously should not be below 98.60°F. Cool or cold colonic flushings have been used with good results.

During chill the temperature climbs steadily, but the patient feels cold. For this reason, external heat in the form of hot blankets or protected hot water bottles are often applied externally. When available, an electric blanket is the most convenient and satisfactory manner of applying external heat. Heat cradles have been used.

Personal Hygiene

The patient should have a daily cleansing bath. Oral hygiene should be maintained. The teeth should be brushed or washed twice daily. Antiseptic mouthwashes should be given at intervals. The lips that are dry from high fever should be kept moistened with bland ointments or oils.

Elimination

Enemas or laxatives may be given when necessary. However, the enema is the method of choice as a rule. The nurse should watch for both retention and suppression of urine. An abnormal appearance of the urine should be noted and reported at once and also a specimen obtained.

General Management of the Disease

Malarial patients are very sick and abjectly miserable during the three stages of the paroxysm. The nurse need special skill in order to keep the patient comfortable at his/her command. During delirium, a nurse should be in constant attendance, if possible. If not possible, side rails should be applied to the bed or sufficient restraint used to protect the patient. Small comfort pillows can be used to prevent backache, which is common and also relieve pressure on the elbows, heels, and about the shoulders and back. The utmost skill is required on the part of the nurse to sponge the patient and to change both bedding and clothing without chilling him/her. It is of great importance to keep the skin dry and clean. Linen and clothing are necessarily frequently changed when sweating is profuse.

The nurse should chart the time and duration of each stage of the paroxysm. The temperature should be taken at the beginning of the chill, then every hour until it reaches normal; after that, every 3–4 hours or until the beginning of another chill. During the chilling stage, temperature should be taken rectally.

In vivax or tertian malaria, the patient usually falls into a natural sleep after sweating ceases. He/She awakens refreshed and is usually up and about until the beginning of the next paroxysm. In *P. falciparum* or estivoautumnal malaria the duration of chills and sweating is often shorter in duration than in the *P. vivax* type and often not so severe. However, the patient may be completely prostrated and in need of constant care. Indeed, the first symptom may be shock. The urine may be dark and scanty. Gastrointestinal signs may be present. The nurse must watch the patient very carefully for signs of unfavorable reaction to the drugs given. The drugs used in malaria are particularly powerful and are notorious for producing unusual and often alarming side reactions. The nurse should report any dullness of vision, ringing in the ears or deafness, dyspnea, coryza, rashes or urticaria, unusual skin pallor or epigastric pain. Many times the patient may develop an acute psychosis, which usually clears up without treatment. This is particularly true following the use of atabrine. In order to combat anemia, good nutrition should be maintained and the diet should be rich in iron-containing foods. As a rule, paroxysms last from 8 to 10 hours.

Convalescence is slow, attacks recur and anemia in some degree is usually present.

KALA-AZAR

Leishmaniasis are a group of protozoan diseases caused by parasites of the genus *Leishmania* and transmitted man to man by the bite of female phlebotomine sand fly. They are responsible for various syndromes in humans, i.e. kala-azar or vesceral leishmaniasis (VL), cutaneous leishmaniasis (CL), mucocutaneous leishmaniasis (MCL), anthroponotic cutaneous leishmaniasis (ACL), zoonotic cutaneous leishmaniasis (ZCL), postkala-azar dermal leishmaniasis (PKDL), etc. The visceral type of disease kala-azar is by far the most important disease in India. The majority of the leishmaniasis is zoonoses involving wild or domestic mammals (rodents, canines), some forms (e.g. Indian kala-azar) are considered to be non-zoonotic infections.

Magnitude of Problem

1. Visceral leishmaniasis (VL): Occurs widely throughout the world, viz. South America, South Africa, the Mediterranean countries, India and China.
2. Cutaneous leishmaniasis (CL): Occurs in the dry, semi-desert rural areas of Central Asia, Middle East, North and West Africa, and the Highlands of Ethiopia and Kenya. Endemic foci are also found in Central and South America.
3. Mucocutaneous leishmaniasis: The main concentration of this form of leishmaniasis is in Brazil. It is rarely found outside the new world.

In 1979, the WHO estimated that 400,000 new cases of leishmaniasis occurred each year. It is now believed that the disease is severely under-reported and new information suggests that 1.5–2 million new cases occur each year.

In India

Kala-azar

Kala-azar has its home in the plains of the Ganges and Brahmaputra. It has been known to occur epidemically and endemically in well-defined areas in the eastern districts of Uttar Pradesh, foothills of Sikkim, and to a lesser extent in Tamil Nadu and Odisha.

As a result of the massive insecticide spraying campaign for malaria eradication between 1958 and 1964, kala-azar and cutaneous leishmaniasis declined to a point of extremely low endemicity. During this period, some patients with PKDL apparently acted as a reservoir of infection, since periodically, new cases of kala-azar were seen, especially in children. The incidence of kala-azar, however, started gradually rising during the late 1960s and early 1970s. By mid of 1977, the epidemic reached its peak with an estimated 100,000 cases and 4,500 deaths in the Bihar state. This outbreak was mainly confined to the four northern districts of Bihar, viz. Muzaffarpur, Vaishali, Sitamarhi and Samastipur, which accounted for nearly 70,000 cases. Control measures began in 1977 and the number of reported cases declined gradually from 70,000 in 1977 to 17,801 cases and 72 deaths in 1986, as a result of control of measures. While the epidemic was reached a plateau in Bihar with an annual incidence of 12–15 thousand reported cases, it spread to West Bengal in 1980. Currently kala-azar is endemic in 24 districts of Bihar and seven districts of West Bengal, with both the states regularly reporting kala-azar cases.

Another endemic focus has been the state of Tamil Nadu where 53 cases were reported in 1978. A few sporadic cases of VL have been reported from Gujarat, Uttar Pradesh, Madhya Pradesh, Punjab, foothills of Himalayas and also from Jammu and Kashmir.

Cutaneous leishmaniasis

Cutaneous leishmaniasis used to occur in the dry, north-western states of India, bordering Pakistan and extending from Amritsar to Kutch and Gujarat plains. In recent years, one focus of ZCL has been discovered in the Rajasthan area, in the peak year of 1971, 828 cases of ZCL being reported. Recently, cases of ACL have been reported from Bikaner city, where unexpectedly several dogs were also found to be infected with *Leishmania tropica* (*L. tropica*). While both cutaneous (ZCL, ACL) and VL diseases occur in India, kala-azar is by far the most important leishmaniasis in India.

Epidemiological Features

Agents

The members of genus *Leishmania* are intracellular parasites. They infect and divide within macrophages.

At least 19 different *Leishmania* parasites have been associated with human infection. Further, the majority of these offer no cross immunity one against the other. *L. donovani* is the causative agent of kala-azar (VL), *L. tropica* is the causative agent of cutaneous leishmaniasis (oriental sore) and *L. braziliensis* is the causative agent of mucocutaneous leishmaniasis. But this distinction is not absolute, visceral forms may produce cutaneous lesions and cutaneous forms may visceralis. The life cycle is completed in two different hosts, i.e. a vertebrate and an insect. In the former, it occurs in an amastigote form (called 'leishmania bodies') and in the latter as a flagellated promastigote.

Reservoirs of Infection

There is a variety of animal reservoir, e.g. dogs, jackals, foxes, rodents and other mammals. Indian kala-azar is considered to be non-zoonotic infection with man as the sole reservoir. This assumption is based largely on the absence of evidence.

Host Factors

1. Age: Kala-azar can occur in all age groups including infants below the age of 1 year. In India, the peak age is 5–9 years.
2. Sex: Males are affected twice as often as females.
3. Population movement: Movement of population (migrants, laborers, tourists) between endemic and non-endemic areas can result in the spread of infection. The recent resurgence of kala-azar in West Bengal, which is an extension of the epidemic outbreak of the disease in Bihar in 1977 was due to movement of infected persons with either kala-azar or PKDL.
4. Socioeconomic status: Kala-azar usually strikes the poorest of the poor. As a disease, it more often debilitates than kills and makes people become dependents on others.
5. Occupation: The disease is strongly associated with occupation. People who work in various farming practices, forestry, mining and fishing have a great risk of being. There is impairment of cell-mediated immunity, this is reflected in the negative skin reaction to *Leishmania* test.

6. Environmental factors:
   a. Attitude: Kala-azar is mostly confined to the plains, it does not occur in altitudes over 2,000 ft.
   b. Season: In the past epidemics, two peaks; one in November and another in March to April were reported. In the 1977, Bihar epidemic, it was observed that most of the cases occurred between April and September. Generally, there is high prevalence during and after rains.
   c. Rural areas: The disease is generally confined to rural areas, where conditions for the breeding of sandflies readily exist compared to urban areas.
   d. Vectors: In India, *Phlebotomus argentipes* (*P. argentipes*) is a proven vector of kala-azar. Cutaneous leishmaniasis is transmitted by *Phlebotomus papatasi* (*P. papatasi*) and *Phlebotomus sergenti* (*P. sergenti*). Sandflies breed in cracks and crevices in the soil and buildings, tree holes, caves, etc. Overcrowding ill ventilation and accumulation of organic matter in the environmental facilitate transmission. Their habits are primarily nocturnal. Only the females bite.
   e. Development projects: Ironically many development projects are exposing more people to leishmaniasis. Forest clearing and cultivation projects, large water resource schemes and colonization and resettlement programs are bringing human beings into areas of high vector and reservoir concentration.

Mode of Transmission

In India, kala-azar is transmitted from person to person by the bite of the female phlebotomine sand fly, *P. argentipes*, which is a highly anthropophilic species. Transmission may also take place by contamination of the bite wound or by contact when the insect is crushed during the act of feeding. Cutaneous leishmaniasis is transmitted by *P. papatasi* and *P. sergeni*. After an infective blood meal, the sand fly becomes infective in 6–9 days (extrinsic incubation period). This is the time required for the development of the parasite in the insect vector. Transmission of kala-azar has also been recorded by blood transfusion.

Incubation period: The incubation period in man is quite variable, generally 1–4 months range is from 10 days to 2 years.

Clinical Features

1. Kala-azar (VL): The classical features of kala-azar are fever, splenomegaly and hepatomegaly, accompanied by anemia and weight loss. A family history of the disease is also common. Darkening of the skin of the face, hands, feet and abdomen is common in India (kala-azar = black sickness). A typical feature of the disease (e.g. lymphadenopathy) may also occur. Kala-azar, if left untreated, has a high mortality. PKDL caused by *L. donovani* is common in India. It appears one to several years after apparent cure of kala-azar. The lesions consist of multiple nodular infiltrations of the skin, usually without ulceration. Parasites are numerous in the lesion.
2. Cutaneous leishmaniasis: Several forms of cutaneous leishmaniasis (oriental sore) have been described namely ACL, ZCL, diffuse cutaneous leishmaniasis (DCL), etc. The disease may be mistaken for leprosy. The agent is restricted to skin. The disease is characterized by painful ulcers in the parts of the body exposed to sand fly bites (e.g. legs, arms or face) reducing the victim's ability to work.
3. Mucocutaneous leishmaniasis: Ulcers similar to the oriental sore appear around the margins of mouth and nose it can mutilate the face so badly that victims appear to be suffering from leprosy.

Laboratory Diagnosis

Parasitological diagnosis: The demonstration of the parasite *L. donovani* bodies in the aspirates of the spleen, liver, bone marrow and lymph nodes or in the skin (in the case of cutaneous leishmaniasis) is the only way to confirm VL or CL conclusively. The parasite must be isolated in culture to confirm the identity of the parasite.

Aldehyde test: The aldehyde test of Napier is a simple test widely used in India for the diagnosis of kala-azar. From a case of kala-azar 1–2 mL of serum sample is taken and one or two drop of 40% formalin is added. A positive test is indicated by jellification to milk-white opacity like the white of a hard-boiled egg so that in ordinary light newsprint is invisible through it. If it occurs within 2–20 minutes, it is said to be strongly positive. Reaction after 30 minutes is not significant. The test usually becomes positive 2–3 months after onset of the disease and reverts to negative 6 months after cure. Therefore, this test is good for surveillance, but not for diagnosis. The test is nonspecific and demands the use of venous blood. Further, the test is positive in many other chronic infections in which albumin to globulin ratio is reversed.

Serological tests: Of the numerous serological tests available, ELISA and the indirect fluorescent antibody test (IFAT) are considered most suitable. Being a simple test, where blood samples can be collected on a filter paper strip and examined at leisure in laboratory, the ELISA test has a wide potential both for diagnosis as well as for epidemiological field surveys.

Leishmanin (Montenegro) test: The test is based on skin reaction. Leishmanin is a preparation of 106/mL washed promastigotes of *Leishmania*, suspended in 0.5% phenol saline or merthiolate. Sterile and standardized preparations are available commercially. An intradermal injection of 0.1 mL on the flexor surface of the forearm is given and examined after 48–72 hours. Induration is measured and recorded. An induration of 5 mm or more is considered positive. The test is usually positive 4–6 weeks after onset in the case of cutaneous leishmaniasis and MCL. It is usually negative in the active phase of kala-azar and becomes positive in 75% of patients within 1 year of recovery. The test is not species specific. The test remains a valuable tool for distinguishing immune from non-immune subjects. From this information, it may be possible to infer the endemicity or epidemicity of the infection and to identify groups at risk of infection.

Hematological findings: These include progressive leukopenia, anemia and reversed albumin-globulin ratio, with greatly increased IgG. The WBC/RBC ratio is 1:1,500 or even 1:2,000 (normal 1:750) and the erythrocyte sedimentation rate (ESR) is increased.

Control Measures

In the absence of an effective vaccine, the control of kala-azar comprises the following measures.

Control of Reservoir

Since man is the only reservoir of kala-azar in India, active and passive case detection and treatment of those found to be infected (including PKDL) may be sufficient to abolish the human reservoir and control the disease. House-to-house visits and mass surveys may be undertaken in endemic areas for early detection of cases.

Treatment

Pentavalent antimony compounds are the sheet anchor of treatment. The recommended schedule is a daily injection (IV or IM) of sodium stibogluconate, 10 mg/kg body weight (to a maximum of 850 mg) for 20 days adults, and 20 mg/kg of body weight for children. With this dosage and duration, the relapse rate is stated to be virtually negligible (0.05%), as compared to standard 10 days treatment (15%). PKDL responds well to this treatment.

Those who do not respond to the above treatment are given the 'second line' drug, pentamidine isethionate (3 mg/kg of body weight, IV) for 10 days. Since this drug is toxic, the patient should be hospitalized, while the drug is being administered.

The patient in either case should be examined in 3 and 12 months after the treatment course to detect any relapse. If animal reservoirs (e.g. dogs) are involved, appropriate control measures against them should be undertaken. In many endemic countries, extensive dog and rodent control programs have contributed greatly to the reduction in the number of human cases.

Control of Sandflies

The application of residual insecticides has proved effective in the control of sandflies. DDT is the first choice since the vector of kala-azar, *P. argentipes* is susceptible to DDT (*P. papatasi* in North Bihar has been shown to be resistant to DDT, but fortunately it is not the vector of kala-azar in India). Insecticide spraying should be undertaken in human dwellings, animal shelters and all other resting places up to a height of 6 ft from floor level. DDT (two rounds per year) at the rate of 1–2 m² is considered sufficient to control transmission. Spraying should be preceded and followed by an assessment of susceptibility. Any sign of resistance in vector should lead to an immediate change in insecticide. Benzene hexachloride (BHC) should be kept as a second line of defense.

Spraying should be repeated at regular intervals to keep down the density of sandflies. For long-lasting results, insecticidal spraying should be combined with sanitation measures, viz. elimination of breeding places (e.g. cracks in mud or stone walls, rodent burrows, removal of firewood and bricks of rubbish around houses), location of cattle shed and poultry at a fair distance from human dwellings and improvement of housing and general sanitation.

Personal Prophylaxis

The risk of infection can be reduced through health education and by the use of individual protective measures such as avoiding sleeping on floor, using fine mesh nets around the bed. Insect repellents (in the form of lotions, creams or sticks) for temporary protection and keeping the environment clean. There are no drugs for personal prophylaxis.

FILARIASIS

Filariasis is the name given to the group of diseases caused by certain nematodes of the family filarioidea. It is transmitted by certain blood sucking (mosquitoes, gnat, flies)

Culex mosquitoes. The term filariasis is restricted to infections caused by *Wuchereria bancrofti* (*W. bancrofti*) and *Brugia malayi* (*B. malayi*). The disease manifestations range from acute and chronic such as lymphangitis, lymphadenitis, filarial fever, elephantiasis of arms, legs and genitals and the disease is responsible for considerable sufferings, deformity and disability (Table 30.4).

Table 30.4: Human filarial infection

Organisms	Vectors	Diseases produced
Wuchereria bancrofti	Culex	Lymphatic filariasis
Brugia malayi	Mansonia	Lymphatic filariasis
Brugia timori	Anopheles, Mansonia	Lymphatic filariasis
Onchocerca volvulus	Simulium flies	Lymphatic filariasis
Loa loa	Chrysops	Subcutaneous nodules
Tetrapetalonema perstans	Culicoides	Clinical illness
Tetrapetalonema streptocerca	Culicoides	Clinical illness
Mansonella ozzardi	Culicoides	Clinical illness

Magnitude of Problem

Filariasis is a global problem. It affects, in various forms, 300 million peoples throughout the world. *W. bancrofti* and *B. malayi* affect 250 million cases, largely confined to the tropical and subtropical areas occurring in the world, viz. West Indies, South America, Japan, Southern China, Pacific Island, etc.

In India, the disease is endemic throughout except in Jammu and Kashmir, Haryana, Punjab, Himachal Pradesh, Delhi, Meghalaya, etc. Present estimates indicate that about 304 million people are currently living in known filarious zones of which 82 million are living in urban areas and 174 million in rural areas. About 18 million harbor microfilariae and 15 million have filarial disease.

Epidemiological Features

Agent

There are eight species of filarial parasites, but mainly two types of parasites are more prevalent, i.e. *W. bancrofti* and *B. malayi* (Fig. 30.5).

Morphology

These are long, hair-like nematodes, creamy, white in color, filiform in shape with tapering ends. The head is like slightly rounded swelling. Males are 2.5–4 cm in length, 0.1 mm in thickness, the end of tail curved ventrally and contains thick spicules of unequal length. Females are 8–10 cm in length, 0.2–0.3 mm in thickness, the tail end is narrow and abruptly pointed.

Male and female remain coiled together and can only be separated with difficulty. Embryos (microfilariae) passing through the lymph nodes, when unstained they appear bodies with blunt head and rather pointed tail. Embryo measures about 290 mm in length and 6–20 mm in breadth, which is stained with Romanowsky stains. The embryos show a hyaline sheath, a structureless sac beyond the extremities of the embryo. The life span of microfilariae in the human body is as long as 70 days.

Life Cycle

Man is the definitive host and the mosquito is the intermediate host of *W. bancrofti* and *B. malayi* filariasis:

1. **Definitive host:** The both adult parasites are found in the lymphatic system of man. Male measuring about 40 mm and female 50–100 mm in length. Live embryos (microfilariae) are discharged, which find their way into the bloodstream. The embryos are capable of living in the peripheral blood for a considerable time without undergoing any developmental metamorphosis. They are subsequently taken up by the female culicine mosquitoes during their blood meal.
2. **Intermediate host:** It is a mosquito in which the microfilariae undergo further development after which they become infective to man. A large number of species of mosquito belonging to the genus *Culex*, *Aedes* and *Anopheles* act as intermediate hosts for *W. bancrofti* (Fig. 30.6).

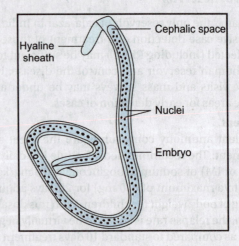

Figure 30.5: Microfilaria of *Wuchereria bancrofti*

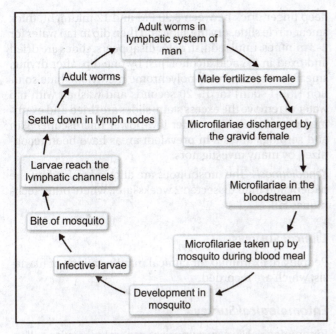

Figure 30.6: Life cycle of *Wuchereria bancrofti*

Development Stages in the Vector (Microfilaria in the Mosquito)

1. Exsheathing: The larva comes out of sheath, it is enclosed in, within 1–2 hours of ingestion. It is called exsheathing, which takes place in the stomach of the mosquito.
2. First stage larva: After exsheathing, it penetrates the stomach wall of the mosquito within 6–12 hours and migrates to the thoracic muscles and develops.
3. Second stage larva: It develops in length and thickness, but it is inactive.
4. Third stage larva: Final stage of inactive larva is found in any part of the insect. It is active and motile when it migrates inside the mosquito. It is ready to be transmitted to the new host. The duration of the mosquito cycle is 10–14 days. In the human host, the infective larva develops into adult worm.

Reservoir of Infection

Infected person or the carrier with circulating microfilaria in their peripheral blood is the reservoir of infection.

Vectors of Filariasis

The main filarial parasites are *W. bancrofti* and *B. malayi*. *Culex fatigans* (*C. fatigans*) is the main vector of *W. bancrofti* filariasis in India and throughout the world, and breed in stagnant water. *Mansonia* are the chief vectors of *B. malayi* infilariasis. The major species involved are *Mansonia annulifera* (*M. annulifera*) and *Mansonia uniformis*. These breeding places are associated with certain aquatic plants such as *Pistia stratiotes*. In the absence of these plants, these mosquitoes cannot breed.

Mode of Transmission

The microfilaria is transmitted by the bite of infected mosquitoes. The parasites, deposited near the puncture site, penetrate the skin on its own and enter the capillaries and reaches the lymphatic system.

Incubation period is 12–18 months. The time interval between inoculation of infective larvae and the first appearance of detectable microfilariae is known as prepatent period.

Host Factors

Man is a natural host. Factors responsible are:
1. Age: All age groups are susceptible. In endemic area, filarial infection is found in infants aged 6 months. But infection rate have been found to rise at the age of 20–30 years.
2. Sex: It does not appear to influence the infection rate.
3. Migration of people: Movement of people from one place to another has led to the extension of the infection.
4. Immunity: Man may develop resistance to infection, but immunological basis of this resistance is not known.

Social Factors

1. Urbanization, industrialization, migration of people, and sleeping habits are some of the social factors associated with filariasis. The disease also carries a social stigma, intimate is very important factor. The maximum prevalence of *C. fatigans* was observed when the temperature was between 22 and 38°C.
2. Drainage: The filariasis is associated with bad drainage. The vector breeds profusely in stagnant waters.
3. Town planning: Inadequate sewage disposal and lack of town planning aggravates. The common breeding places of mosquitoes are soakage pits, illuminated drains, septic tanks, open ditches, burrow pits, etc.

Pathophysiology

The severity of the lesions probably depends on the adult worm load and their site of development and the susceptibility of the host. Light infections are often asymptomatic and microfilariae are detected on incidental blood examinations. Maturing adult in the lymphatics is associated with endothelial thickening, fibrin deposition and infiltration with eosinophils, histiocytes and lymphocytes. Giant cells occur. Fibrotic and inflammatory changes tend to obstruct the lymphatics and this process is exacerbated by death of the worms, which may calcify. There is reactive hyperplasia in the lymph nodes and small granulomas are seen. An eosinophilic endophlebitis of the small veins is present in the lymph nodes. The testicles and epididymis often show similar changes with evidence of chronic inflammation worm may not be present at the site of inflammation. Secretions of the worm, especially after molting are thought to be responsible for some of these changes. A lymphatic obstruction becomes more, extensive, chronic edema develops in the infected areas. Recently, lymphedema has been produced in laboratory animals with long-standing Bancroft's infection.

Clinical Features

There are four stages:
1. Stage of invasion: The infective larva enters into the human host and starts undergoing further development. Diagnosis at this stage rests on the triad of eosinophilia, lymphadenopathy and a positive intradermal test, plus the history of residence in an endemic area.
2. Symptomless or carrier phase: There are no clinical manifestations in this stage. The microfilariae carriers are usually detected by night blood examination.
3. Stage of acute manifestations: In this stage, filarial fever, lymphangitis, lymphadenitis lymphedema of the various parts of the body and of epididymo-orchitis in the male.
4. Stage of chronic manifestation: In this stage, clinical features comprise elephantiasis of the genitals, legs, arms, hydrocele, chyluria, etc.

There are characteristic differences in the clinical manifestations of *W. bancrofti* and *B. malayi* produce elephantiasis of the lower limbs, but rarely affect scrotum or upper limbs. *W. bancrofti* affects not only extremities but also genitals producing hydrocele and elephantiasis of scrotum or penis. The lower limbs are affected more than the upper limbs.

Filaria Survey

Blood Survey

A night blood survey is the most important element. A5 per National Institute of Communicable Diseases (NICD), Delhi, standards 5–7% of the population is to be examined for routine surveys and at least 20% sample for evaluation studies. Blood 20 mm^3 (four to five big drops) collected by deep finger prick between 8.30 PM and 12 midnight, thick smear circle slide, dry the slide and then dip in tap water for 2–3 minutes, until reddish color disappears, slides are dried and fixed in 2% acid alcohol. Just by one dip, after drying, smears are stained with polychrome methylene blue solution (JSB-l stain) for 15–20 seconds and washed with tap water to remove the excess stain; slides are dried and examined for microfilariae under low-power microscope. Skin and serological tests in prevalent areas have been recognized by many investigators.

Xenodiagnosis: The mosquitoes are allowed to feed on the patient and then dissected 2 weeks later, where other techniques fail.

Clinical Surveys

People are examined for clinical manifestations of filariasis, which are recorded.

Entomological Survey

Entomological survey comprises general mosquito collection from houses. A study of the extent and type of breeding places and other bionomics of mosquitoes is conducted.

Filarial Indices

Parasitological Indices

1. Microfilaria rate: It is the percentage of persons showing microfilariae (mf) in their peripheral blood (20 mm^3) in the sample population. One slide being taken from each person.
2. Filarial disease rate: It is the percentage of persons showing visible manifestations of filarial disease in the sample population.
3. Filarial endemicity rate: It is the percentage of persons examined showing mf in their blood or disease manifestations.
4. Microfilarial density: It is the number of mf per unit volume (20 mm^3) of blood in samples from individual persons.
5. Average infestation rate: It is the average number of per positive slide, each slide being made from 20 mm^3 of blood.

Vector Indices

1. Vector density per 10 man-hour catch.
2. Percentage of mosquitoes positive for all stages of development.
3. Percentage of mosquitoes positive for infective (stage III) larvae.
4. Types of larval breeding places, etc.

These indices help to measure the conditions existing before and after control procedures began.

Control Measures

The current strategy as based on:
1. Detection and treatment of human carriers.
2. Recurrent anti-mosquito measures.

Detection and Treatment of Carriers

Diethylcarbamazine (DEC) is the drug of choice. WHO expert committee on filariasis has recommended a total dose of about 75 mg of DEC/kg of body weight for *W. bancrofti* and smaller dose of 30–40 mg/kg body weight for *B. malayi*.

In Indian program, DEC 6 mg/kg of body weight daily for 12 doses to be completed in 2 weeks. Once a week or once a month has also been recommended. Treatment must be given usually for 2 years.

Mass chemotherapy was tried during 1958–1960, but is now restricted to only mf carriers and filaria cases. DEC reactions such as headache, nausea, vomiting, dizziness, etc. are found particularly after 24–36 hours after first dose.

Recently, levamisole hydrochloride is reported having filaricidal properties. DEC and levamisole when used in combination more rapidly decreases mf counts. The recommended doses of DEC are given in Table 30.5.

Table 30.5: Recommended doses of diethylcarbamazine

Age (years)	Doses in mg (single dose)
18 year and above	300
12–17	225
6–11	150
2–5	75
0–1	30

Antimosquito Measures

Vector control must be based on temporary methods, as detailed below.

Antilarval measures

In urban areas, the antilarval measures include an extra 3 km peripheral belt. So that mosquitoes are unable to breed in the vicinity of the population.

The immediate aim is to reduce the transmission of infection reducing vector population. Recurrent antilarval measures have been found very costly and operationally very difficult to apply in the rural areas of the country.

Larvicides currently used in the Indian program are:
1. Mosquito larvicidal oil (MLO).
2. Pyroxene oil-E: This is a pyrethrum-based emulsifiable larvicide, water diluted 1:4 before use.
3. Organophosphorus larvicides Abate, Batex: Abate (temephos) is supplied 50% emulsion concentrate 2.5 mL of Abate in 10 L of water dilution. The doses 170–225 L/ha (15–20 gallons per acre) of water surface, once weekly application on all breeding places.
4. Removal of *Pista* plant reduces mansonoides mosquito breeding.
5. Minor engineering measures filling up of ditches, drainage of stagnant water, adequate maintenance of septic tanks and soakage pits control mosquito population.

Antiadult measures

The mosquitoes causing filariasis have become resistant to BHC, DDT and dieldrin. Therefore, antiadult measures using these compounds like indoor residual spraying of pyrethrum is effective, but costly.

Personal prophylaxis is best achieved by using mosquito nets during night and helping the government in control measures.

National Filaria Control Program

The National Filaria Control Program (NFCP) has been in operation since 1955. According to recent estimates, about 304 million people are exposed to the risk of infection, 15 million manifests the disease and 21 million have filarial parasites in their blood.

In June 1978, the operational component of the NFCP was merged with the urban malaria scheme for maximum utilization of available resources. The training and research components, however, continue to be with the Director, National Institute of Communicable Diseases, Delhi. Under the NFCP, the following activities are undertaken:
1. Delimitation of the problem in hitherto unsurveyed areas.
2. Control in urban areas through:
   a. Recurrent antilarval measure.
   b. Antiparasite measures.

So far, 238–300 districts situated in endemic areas have been surveyed; of these 173 have been found to be endemic for filariasis. Survey work is in progress in other districts. Use of DEC-medicated salt for the control of filariasis was successfully implemented in Lakshadweep during 1976–1978. This method is being carried out in Karaikal district of Pondicherry from 1982. As on December 31, 1985 there was 197 filaria control units, 27 survey units, 148 filaria clinics functioning in the endemic areas. The population protected so far is hardly 83–87 million out of 304 million at risk. Since the 'vertical' approach to the control of filariasis has had a limited success in terms of coverage of the population at risk, it is now the horizontal approach, i.e. making use of the PHC system, which is under consideration. In this case, the VHGs has to be trained and involved in antifilarial activities with local community participation.

Training in filariology is being given at three Regional Filaria Training and Research Centers situated at Kozhikode (Kerala), Rajahmundry (AP) and Varanasi (UP) and National Institute of Communicable Disease, Delhi. Besides, 12 headquarter bureaus are working at the state level.

Zoonoses: Viral

CHAPTER 31

INTRODUCTION

Rabies is a severe viral infection of the central nervous system (CNS) communicated to humans from the saliva of infected animals and commonly transmitted by a bite or by contact of the animal saliva with a mucous membrane or open wound.

Arboviral diseases are the viral diseases, primarily zoonotic in nature, which is transmitted to human beings accidentally by the bite of blood-sucking arthropods.

RABIES

The system of 6 months quarantine for imported canines and felines from 1886 accompanied in the early years by the muzzling of dogs was successful in eradicating rabies from animal life in Britain from 1902 until it was reintroduced in 1918 though illegally imported dogs. From 1922 to 1970, approximately 100,000 imported animals have been quarantined. Of these 27 developed rabies including two dogs retained for more than 6 months for special reasons.

In 1969, a dog imported from Germany, developed rabies about 1 week after release from 6 months quarantine. Another episode occurred in the same year when a dog admitted in Pakistan, developed rabies 3 months after release from quarantine. There were no human or animal cases of infection. Rabies was diagnosed in 675 animals in Europe in 1969. In 1972, the animals were kept in quarantine for 6 months and a dose of an acceptable rabies vaccine on entry and a second dose, 1 month later was administered.

Magnitude of Problem

Rabies is a zoonotic problem of considerable magnitude in India, with an estimated mortality of 25,000 (actual figure may be 50,000) in 1 year, while 3 million people receive post-exposure prophylaxis each year.

Epidemiology

Geographic Distribution

Rabies is an enzootic and epizootic disease of worldwide importance. Some countries have achieved rabies-free status by vigorous campaign of elimination. Australia, China, Cyprus, Iceland, Ireland, Japan, Malta, New Zealand, the United Kingdom (UK) and the islands of Western Pacific are all free of the disease. In India union territory of Lakshadweep, and Andaman and Nicobar Islands are free of the disease.

Agent

Rabies virus are bullet-shaped with one end blunt and other end pointed, 120–200 nm long with cylindrical diameter of 60–80 nm. The core contains ribonucleic acid (RNA) in helical symmetry. The virion is surrounded by lipoprotein envelope from which project hemagglutinin spikes (Fig. 31.1). They are killed by ultraviolet light, heating at 56°C for 1 hour and 60°C for 5 minutes, either by, strong acid, strong alkalis and trypsin. All strains are antigenically similar. They induce formation of fixing, neutralizing and hemagglutination inhibition antibodies.

The causative agent is lyssavirus type I or the rhabdovirus is a bullet shaped with encircled spikes. It belongs to the family rhabdoviridae serotype I (lyssavirus type I) being the causative agent of rabies. Serotype II, III and IV are rabies related, but antigenically distinct viruses, causing rabies-like disease in man and animals. The rhabdovirus is called neurotropic virus because of its preference in affecting the nerve cells in the brain and spinal cord, especially hippocampus and cerebellum in the brain and posterior horn cells in the spinal cord. It also multiplies in salivary glands, secretory glands, corneal cells, kidneys, muscles and lungs. The virus is inactivated by heat, sunlight, formalin, phenol and other disinfectants.

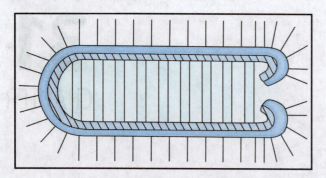

Figure 31.1: Rabies virus

Source of Infection

The source of infection to man is the saliva of rabid animal. In dogs and cats, the virus may be present in the saliva for 3–4 days (occasionally 5–6 day) before the onset of clinical symptoms and during the course of illness till death.

Reservoir of Infection

Rabies exists in three epidemiological forms:
1. Urban rabies.
2. Wildlife rabies (sylvatic).
3. Bat rabies.

Urban rabies: The transfer of infection from wildlife to domestic dogs results in creation of the urban cycle, which is maintained by the dogs and is responsible for 99% of human cases in India.

Sylvan or wildlife rabies: It is maintained in the wild carnivorous animals such as jackals, foxes and wolves, mongoose and skunks (small American animal).

Insectivorous or vampire bats: These small blood-sucking mammals act as carriers in Latin American countries, USA and Canada.

Host Factors

All warm-blooded animals including man are susceptible to rabies. Rabies in man is a dead end infection and has no survival value for the virus. The victims in India belong to the age group of 1–24 years. Laboratory staff working with rabies virus veterinarians, dog handlers, hamsters and field naturalists face bigger risks of rabies than do general public throughout the year.

Modes of Transmission

1. Animal bites: In India most of the human cases of rabies result from dog bites, occasionally from other animal bites such as cat, monkey, horse, sheep and goat.
2. Licks on abraded skin and mucosa can transmit the disease. In rare instances the disease may be caused by accidental injury by the subject contaminated with the saliva of a rabid animal.
3. Aerosols: This (respiratory) transmission has been observed in nature, only in certain cases harboring rabies-infected bats and in the laboratory where aerosols created during homogenization of infected animal brains can infect laboratory workers.
4. Person to person: Man-to-man transmission although rare is possible. There are also reports of transmission of rabies by corneal and organ transplants.

Incubation Period

The incubation period in man is highly variable and depends upon various factors:
1. Site of the wound and the distance of the site of the bite from the brain. Thus the incubation period is short in bites on the head or face.
2. Relation to the nerve and whether the tissue is rich in nerve supply.
3. The virulence of the virus and the quantity of saliva deposited in or on the wound surface.
4. Physical condition of the patient.

The disease generally manifests itself between 1 and 2 months after the bite. The shortest incubation period of less than 15 days is most exceptional. The longest incubation period known is 3 years 2 months and 21 days. The incubation period is somewhat shorter in children than in adults.

Pathophysiology

Rabies virus replicates in muscles or connective tissue cells at or near the site of introduction before it attaches to nerve endings and enters peripheral nerves. It spreads from the site of infection centripetally through the peripheral nerves toward the CNS. It ascends passively through the nerve-associated tissue space. Infection of the CNS is the virus spread centrifugally in peripheral nerves to many tissues, including skeletal and myocardial muscles, adrenal glands and skin. The salivary glands invasion is crucial for the transmission of the virus to another animal or human. There are no naked eye changes apart from congestion of the gray matter of the brain and spinal cord.

Microscopically, there is cell degeneration, phagocytosis of the degenerating cells and collars of inflammatory cells around the small blood vessels. The pathognomonic feature is the presence and of Negri bodies of inclusion bodies 'bf' varying sizes in the cytoplasm of the ganglion cells in the hippocampus major as well as in the cells of the medulla and cerebellum. These are acidophilic bodies with a blue center. The basophilic material probably represents virus, whereas the outer acidophilic material may be a host tissue products when a dog suspected of rabies has bitten a person, the dog's brain must be examined for Negri bodies.

Clinical Features

There are several clinical phases of rabies in humans with eventual complications resulting in encephalomyelitis leading to coma and ultimately death.

Stage I: Prodromal Phase (Invasive Phase)

In prodromal phase, there is abnormal sensation around the site of infection and individual experiences of uneasy feeling and general anxiety accompanied by depression and irritability. The patient may have headache, nausea, sore throat and loss of appetite or may experience unusual sensitivity to sound, light and changes in temperature.

Stage II: Stage of Excitement

There are episodes of irrational excitement alternating with periods of alert calm. The patient is intolerant to noise, bright light or a cold drought aerophobia (fear of air), may be present (Fig. 31.2).

There will be increased reflexes and muscle spasms along with dilatation of the pupil and increased perspiration, hypersalivation and lacrimation. Mental changes include fear of death, anger, irritability and depression. Attempting to swallow or even looking at liquids induces a severe and painful spasm of the muscles of swallowing and respiration. This characteristic hydrophobic (fear of water) symptom is pathognomonic of rabies and is absent in animals. The duration of illness is 2–3 days, but may prolonged 5–6 days in exceptional cases. Death usually occurs in this stage from cardiac or respiratory failure during one of the convulsion or may pass on to the stage of paralysis and coma.

Stage III: Paralytic Stage

Paralysis of muscles causing paraplegia, quadriplegia and patient may go into coma, and eventually death occurs due to respiratory and cardiac failures (Fig. 31.3).

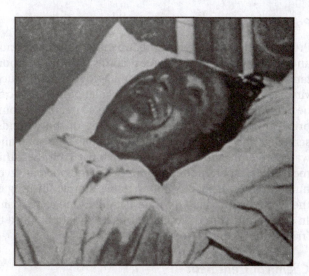

Figure 31.2: Rabies; fright at being asked if he wants a drink

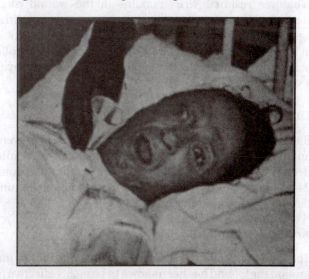

Figure 31.3: Human rabies; facial expression when offered a drink

Preventive Measures

Pre-exposure Prophylaxis

Persons who run a high risk of repeated exposure such as laboratory staff working with rabies virus veterinarians, animal handlers and wildlife officers should be protected by pre-exposure immunization. Such immunization should preferably consist of a dose of cell culture vaccine given either as 1 mL intramuscularly (IM), 0.1 mL intradermally on days 0, 7 and 28, and booster doses of 1 mL/IM or 0.1 mL should be given and should be repeated at intervals of 2 years as long as exposed persons remain at risk.

Postoperative Exposure Prophylaxis

Prompt and adequate local treatment of all bite wounds and scratches is the first request and is of utmost importance. The purpose of local treatment is to remove as much virus as possible from the site of inoculation before it can be reabsorbed on nerve endings. The local treatment comprises immediate flushing and washing of the wounds, scratches and the adjoining areas with plenty of soap and water preferably under a running tap for at 5 minutes. This measure is of paramount importance of the prevention of human rabies. If soap is not available, simple flushing of the wound with plenty of water should done as first aid. In case of punctured wound, catheters should be used to irrigate the wound.

Chemical Treatment

Whatever residual virus remains in the wound after cleansing is inactivated by registration with virucidal agents, either alcohol tincture or 0.01% aqueous solution of iodine or povidone-iodine. Cauterization with carbolic acid or nitric acid is no longer recommended as it leaves a very bad scar.

Suturing

Bite wounds should not be immediately sutured to prevent additional trauma, which may help to spread virus into deeper tissues. If suturing is necessary it should be done 24–48 hours later, applying minimum possible stitches under the cover of antirabies serum locally.

Antirabies Serum

The local application of antirabies serum or its infiltration around the wound has been shown to be highly effective in preventing rabies. The sensitivity of the patient should be tested prior to its use.

Antibiotics and Antitetanus Measure

The application of antibiotics and antitetanus procedures when indicated should follow the local treatment.

Observe the Animal for 10 Days

The biting animal should be observed for 10 days from the day of bite. If the animal shows the symptoms of rabies, it should be humanely killed and its head removed and sent under refrigeration to a qualified laboratory for rabies examination. If the animal remains alive and healthy at the end of 10 days, there is no indication for antirabies treatment.

Immunization

Indications for immunization are:
- If the animal shows signs of rabies or dies within 10 days of observation
- If the biting animal cannot be traced or identified
- Unprovoked bites.

Laboratory Tests

For example, fluorescent rabies antibody test or test for Negri bodies. Laboratory test of the brain of the biting animal are positive for rabies.

All Bites by Wild Animals

Even of the animal that are apparently healthy at the time of inflicting. The bite, appropriately to the degree of exposure should be treated at once. Treatment of the patient may be discontinued after 5 days, if the animal remains healthy during this time.

Antirabies Vaccine

The street virus is responsible for rabies in dogs. It is the natural virus. The virus, which is used in vaccine preparation is fixed virus, which is obtained by the passage of street virus in the brain of sheep or rabbit. The animal is killed when the incubation period is fixed at 8 days. Brain is removed under aseptic conditions. The brain emulsion is made with normal saline in 5% strength and inactivated with phenol. The dose schedule as per the severity of wounds is given in Table 31.1.

Table 31.1: Antirabies vaccine dose schedule

Nature of wound	Adult	Children	Duration	Booster
Class I	2 cc	2 cc	7 day	Nil
Class II	5 cc	2 cc	14 day	3 week after 14th injection
Class III	5 cc	2 cc	14 day	One booster dose 7th day after completion of treatment and second booster 14th day of first booster

Classification of Wounds

Class I (slight or negligible exposure): All cases of licks except those in fresh cuts and scratches.

Class II (moderate exposure): Licks or cuts and scratches. All bites except on head, neck, face, palm and finger. Number of wound less than five.

Class III (severe exposure): Lacerated wounds. All bites on head, neck, face, palm and finger, number of wound five or more.

It is better to give 2,000–3,000 intravenous (IV) of hyperimmune serum after sensitivity test along with 14 days injection. Serum is given in single dose. It is meant for Class III bites due to risk of serum sickness.

The most significant development on rabies vaccine was made in 1972 with the introduction of human diploid cells tissue culture vaccine (HDCV). The vaccine is prepared by growing the virus in human diploid cell fibroblasts and supernatant inactivated by British Pharmaceutical Laboratory (BPL). Several field trials documented the evidence that so for HDCV is the best and safe vaccine to be used for post-exposure therapy in human. Only six subcutaneous injections at spaced intervals offer full protection. The local and systemic reactions are negligible and virus neutralizing antibody titer rises within 7 days post-vaccine therapy.

Very recently a new rabies vaccine has been developed and is known as rhesus diploid-cell-strain rabies vaccine (RDRV). This is an inactivated vaccine intended for use in man. Clinical trials on human volunteers, exposed to rabid animals were done by giving series of five injections at spaced intervals. It has been observed that this vaccine is equally immunogenic as HDCV. This indicates that RDRV perhaps be able to reduce the cost of vaccine.

For the post-exposure therapy for human immunoglobulin, i.e. arginase antibody (Arg) either human or equine has to be along with the vaccine. The dose of antirabies human immunoglobulin 20 IV/kg body weight to be given single intramuscular dose. Repeated dose of Arg is an advocated for the reason that it may suppress the response elicited by vaccination. Local infiltration of avidin-biotin-peroxidase complex (ABC) in and around the wound surface is also recommended to prevent spread of infection from the route of entry.

Mode of Administration of Antirabies Vaccine (Anterior Abdominal Walls)

1. It differs enough space for accommodation of injections. In advanced pregnancy, it is thigh interscapular region.
2. Duration of immunity: Partial immunity is obtained in 3rd week. To achieve maximum, it takes 50 days. Duration of protection is 6 months. Rationale of vaccine treatment is to neutralize the virus before it is fixed in brain.
3. Mortality in treated patients is 3–6%.
4. Mortality in untreated patient is 56–57%.
5. Advice to patient under antirabies vaccine (ARV) treatment:
   - No alcohol during treatment and a month after the course
   - No corticosteroid to be given
   - No undue physical and mental strain.

Complications

- General: Headache and giddiness
- Local: Swelling and infection
- Allergic
- Neuroparalysis.

Health Education to Public

People should be educated regarding the risk of animal bites, hence the domestic dogs should be vaccinated with antirabies vaccine periodically to avoid rabies. The wounds should immediately be washed with running tap water for 5 minutes and health workers should be contacted to seek medical aid and take vaccination according to the dose suggested. They also should be told to keep a close watch on the animal up to 10 days. They also should be told about the signs and symptoms of rabies and if any suspicious case is found, it should be reported immediately to health workers. As home treatment of rabies is not possible, the patients should be shifted to isolation hospitals immediately.

National Program

The government has taken proper measures in control of rabies by eliminating stray dogs. Other methods to control the rabies menace include:

1. Registration and licensing of all domestic dogs.
2. Restrain dogs in public places.
3. Immediate destruction of dogs and cats bitten by rabid animal.
4. Public education through newspapers and mass medias regarding the prophylaxis and treatment.
5. Educating the dog owner to immunize the dog periodically with ARV.

Nursing Management of Rabies

Methods of Control

The patient isolation with a skilled or instructed attendant is desirable. Concurrent disinfection of all articles is required, as well as thorough terminal disinfection.

General Measures

1. Passing and universal enforcement of ordinances requiring dogs to be muzzled, when allowed on the streets or in places to which the public has access.
2. Immunization of animals kept as pets. Vaccination should once a year by competent veterinarians. This measure requires the education of the public concerning its merit before it can ever be accomplished. It has the additional advantage that it is applicable to cats and other pets.
3. Reporting, detention and examination of all dogs or cats, which have bitten people or which are suspected of having rabies.
4. Prompt cleansing with tincture of green soap or cauterization with fuming nitric acid and the institution of prophylactic Pasteur treatment in all persons bitten by any animal known to have rabies or suspected of having it, until proven otherwise.

Isolation

The medical aseptic technic will prevent transmission of the disease. Care must be taken to guard oneself against spitting on the part of the patient. The virus is found in the nose and throat secretions and in the stool and urine. Articles that have come in contact either with the patient or his/her discharges should be cleaned up immediately after use or destroyed by burning. Paper tissues should be provided to wipe. Away the rather profuse drainage of saliva. All used tissues should be placed in the waste bag at the bedside to be burned later.

All persons undertaking the nursing care of a rabid patient should have hands free from skin abrasions. Rubber gloves should be worn when doing anything that may bring the nurse in direct contact either with the patient or his/her secretions.

Diet

The diet is of no great importance. A patient will find it impossible to swallow liquids and very painful to attempt it. Sometimes solids and semisolid food can be swallowed without too much difficulty (Figs 31.4 and 31.5).

Since the patient rarely lives more 2 or 3 days at most the main duty of the nurse is to keep the patient as comfortable and quite as possible. The room should be kept very quiet. There should be no unnecessary conversation, moving of the table or chair, turning on the faucet or flushing the toilet. Do not turn on faucets, omit the bath. The patient should see neither liquids nor containers that associate his/her mind with liquids. We have seen an empty cup throw the patient into a convulsion. Patients are very

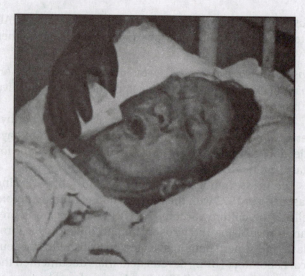

Figure 31.4: Rabies; offering the drink

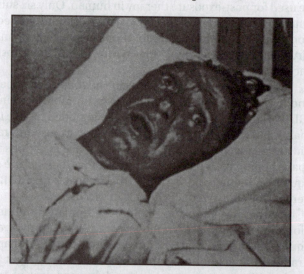

Figure 31.5: Rabies; fearful another drink may be offered

apprehensive and dread to be alone. There should be a nurse in constant attendance. The patient should be in full restraint to prevent him/her from injuring himself/herself and others. The patient usually remains conscious to the last. Laryngeal spasms may occur as the result of any stimulus. Convulsions are common.

While the temperature usually high (103–105°F), there is little that can be done since any stimulus may cause either laryngeal spasm or convulsion. An ice cap to the head, sometimes it is helpful.

Pseudohydrophobia (Lyssophobia)

Pseudohydrophobia is a hysterical manifestation in which a person of neurotic or unstable nervous makeup, so closely simulates hydrophobia after bitten by a dog that a mistaken diagnosis may easily be made. It is believed that all reported cases in which hydrophobia is presumed to have been cured have really been of this pseudohydrophobia type. Tetanus, in one of its forms, may also resemble true hydrophobia, so may the bulbar type of poliomyelitis in very rare instances.

ARBOVIRAL DISEASES

Arboviral diseases are the viral diseases, primarily zoonotic diseases, diseases of vertebrate animals, (except O'nyong-nyong fever), transmitted to human beings accidentally by the bite of hematophagous (bloodsucking) arthropods, such as mosquitoes, *Sandfly*, ticks and mites. Such viruses are called 'arboviruses', which are all RNA viruses, showing varied type of morphology, spherical and cylindrical. They are classified into group A, group B and other groups. Some are named after the place of isolation and some after the clinical features.

Classification of Arboviruses

Group A Viruses (Alpha Viruses)

Chikungunya virus, sindbis virus, eastern equine encephalitis virus, western equine encephalitis virus, Venezuelan equine encephalitis virus, O'nyong-nyong virus, Mayaro virus, etc.

Group B viruses (Flaviviruses)

Yellow fever virus, dengue fever virus, Japanese encephalitis (JE) virus, Kyasanur forest disease (KFD) virus, Omsk hemorrhagic fever virus, Lassa fever virus, Murray Valley encephalitis virus, louping ill virus, Russian spring, summer encephalitis virus, West Nile fever virus, etc.

The arboviral diseases are also classified as febrile group of viral diseases, hemorrhagic group of viral diseases and encephalitis group of viral diseases.

Yellow fever

Yellow fever is an acute communicable disease, caused by an arbovirus belonging to Castle's group B. Primarily, it is a zoonotic disease, specially the monkeys. Man gets the disease accidentally by the bite of infected, female, *Aedes* mosquito. Clinically it is characterized by fever, toxic jaundice and albuminuria followed by hemorrhagic manifestations such as epistaxis, hematemesis and melena. Case fatality rate ranges from 3 to 40%. It will be high up to 8% during epidemics.

Distribution and extent of the problem

The disease is not distributed all over the world. It is endemic only in tropical forests of Central Africa and northern part of South America between the latitude of 15° North and 10° South, and 10° North and 40° South of Equator in Africa and South America respectively. Currently, the disease is maintained enzootically, often resulting in epidemics among human population.

During 1960, an epidemic occurred in Ethiopia affecting 200,000 people resulting in 30,000 deaths. Again during 1978, epidemics occurred in Colombia and Peru in South America, Gambia and Ghana in Africa. The disease is not reported from India.

Agent factors

Agent

The causative agent is a virus, namely flavivirus fibricus. It is a RNA virus. It belongs to arbovirus Castle's group B and family togaviridae. It is a filterable virus and ultramicroscopic, 15–20 nm in size. It has both viscerotropic and neurotropic properties, mainly viscerotropic. It is readily destroyed by heat and chemicals. It resists freezing. So it may be preserved even at 70°F for years together. Lesser the temperature, longer is its duration of life.

Reservoir of infection

Epidemiologically there are two types of reservoirs:
- Sylvan form (jungle form): Wild monkeys are the reservoirs
- Urban/Rural form: Human beings are the reservoirs.

Period of communicability

The person suffering from yellow fever, is communicable (to mosquitoes) during the last 1 or 2 days of incubation period and first 4 days of illness, because the viruses are circulating in the blood during that period.

Host factors

Age incidence

People of all the age group are susceptible to yellow fever. But the incidence is maximum in the age group of 15–40 years.

Sex incidence

People of both the sexes are susceptible to this disease. However, incidence is more among men than among women because of the risk of mosquito bites.

Occupation

Yellow fever is not an occupational disease. But it is high among those in the endemic areas, who work in the forests such as wood cutters, planters, hunters, etc.

Immunity

Immunity is acquired and humoral. One attack confers lifelong immunity.

Environmental factors
Atmospheric temperature of 24°C is favorable for the viruses to multiply in the body of mosquitoes and a relative humidity of 60% is favorable for the mosquitoes to live longer.

Social factors
Deforestation, urbanization, etc. predispose for the extension of the disease from forest to human dwellings.

Vectors
The vectors of yellow fever are hematophagous mosquitoes. In jungle (Sylvan) from, South American forests, the vector is homologous. In Capricorn and in African forests, the vector is *Aedes africanus (A. africanus)*. In urban (rural) form, South America the vector is *A. aegypti* and in Africa, it is *A. simpsoni*.

These vectors are aggressive day biters. The urban/rural forms of mosquitoes are peridomestic mosquitoes. They breed near human habitations. Their breeding places are fresh water collected in artificial containers such as coconut shell, broken pots, broken bottles, empty cans, tree holes, etc.

Mode of transmission
The disease is transmitted from monkeys to monkeys, monkeys to human beings and man to man by the bite of the infective female *Aedes* mosquitoes (species are already mentioned). Man gets the infection, when he enters the forest and once he gets the disease, initiates the urban cycle.

Extrinsic incubation period
It is the period between the successful entries of the viruses into the body of the mosquito (i.e. from the time of bite) till it becomes infective (i.e. till the viruses multiply and reach the optimum number), i.e. about 10–14 days. This type of biological transmission is called 'propagative type'. Once the mosquito becomes infective, it remains infective throughout its life. Whomsoever it bites, transmits the disease.

Pathophysiology
Having entered the body through the percutaneous route, the viruses circulate and later affect liver, heart and kidneys.

Liver
Yellow fever is mainly affected. There will be eosinophilic, hyaline necrosis of hepatocytes, mainly in the midzone of the lobule, which are called 'Councilman bodies', which is pathognomonic. Unconjugated bilirubin gets accumulated in the blood, resulting in hyperbilirubinemia, giving rise to yellow coloration of sclera and urine (jaundice).

Heart
Activity of the heart is suppressed resulting in bradycardia.

Kidney
There is tubular necrosis and resulting in albuminuria. There are hemorrhagic foci under the capsules of the corte, incubation period is varies from 3 to 6 days.

Clinical features
Basically occur in three stages:
1. Stage of infection: Characterized by fever, headache, body ache, flushing of face, photophobia, relative bradycardia (Faget's sign) and pain in the loin. This stage lasts for 3–4 days.
2. Stage of remission: In this stage, the patient is symptom free. This stage lasts for few hours to 1 day.
3. Stage of intoxication: This stage starts from 4th to 5th day. Jaundice gradually develops. Albuminuria and hemorrhagic manifestations are evident. There will be epistaxis, bleeding from the gums, petechial hemorrhages, later hematemesis and malena. Bradycardia progresses to less than 50 per minute. 'Black vomit' is one of the striking features and is always a grave sign. Another grave sign is increase in pulse with fall of temperature. Later hiccups occur. Patient passes onto the stage of delirium, becomes stuporous, develops coma and death supervenes within 6–9 days.

Investigations
- Leukocytosis is followed by progressive leukopenia
- Albuminuria, hyperbilirubinemia
- Liver biopsy is contraindicated because it may result in hemorrhage; if done, shows 'Councilman bodies'.

Management
Hospitalization, symptomatic treatment, blood transfusion, prophylactic antibiotics, maintenance of fluids and electrolytes.

Prevention and control measures
- Elimination of reservoirs
- Breaking the channel of transmission
- Protection of susceptibles.

Elimination of reservoirs
Since it is neither possible to eliminate animal reservoirs such as wild monkeys nor there is treatment for yellow fever, nor it is possible to control the vectors (mosquitoes) in the forests, control of jungle form of yellow fever continues to be an uncontrollable disease. Therefore, control of yellow fever for all practical purposes means control of urban yellow fever, which consists of control of vectors, vaccination of susceptible and surveillance program.

CHAPTER 31 — Zoonoses: Viral

Breaking the channel of transmission
Breaking the channel of transmission consists of control of vectors—antilarval and antiadult measures. Control of vectors reduces transmission.

Antilarval measures: The most important and effective measure is by elimination of breeding places. This is known as 'source reduction' method. This consists of making the water-holding containers (such as broken pots, coconut shell, broken bottles, tins, etc.), topsy-turvy or such things are removed from the human dwellings.

Antiadult measures: Consists of using organophosphorus compounds such as malathion in the form of ultra-low volume (ULV) fogging by using special machines.

Protection of susceptibles
By personal protection and vaccination measures.

Personal protection: This consists of using mosquito repellents mosquito nets, mosquito coils and fumigation mats. But they are not very effective against bites of *Aedes* mosquitoes, because these mosquitoes are day biters.

Immunization: The only very effective measure is by immunization. The internationally approved vaccine is 17D vaccine. It is a live vaccine, freeze-dried and the diluent is sterile normal saline. It contains live attenuated avirulent 17D strain of the virus, grown in chick embryo, to be used within half-an-hour of reconstitution. Dose is 0.5 mL, given subcutaneously, near the deltoid region, irrespective of age and sex. Immunity develops within 1 week and lasts for more than 2 years, probably lifelong. However, World Health Organization (WHO) recommends revaccination once in 10 years for international travelers.

Reactions following vaccination are minimal. But may occur among those who are sensitive to egg protein. Storage temperature is preferably sub-zero degree centigrade (−20°C).

Surveillance program
The WHO has recommended an index for the surveillance of the *Aedes* mosquitoes, called 'A. aegypti index', also known as 'house index', which is defined as percentage of the houses, in a defined area, showing actual breeding of the larvae of these mosquitoes;

$$Aedes\ aegypti = \frac{\text{Index number of houses showing actual breeding of large}}{\text{Total number of houses in the defined area}} \times 100$$

This index should not be more than one, to ensure freedom from yellow fever, in the endemic areas. Thus, this index is also used to evaluate the antilarval control measures. If this index becomes more than one, there is a fear of outbreak.

International certificate of vaccination against yellow fever
This is necessary for those who are traveling from endemic areas of yellow fever to yellow fever receptive area. Yellow fever receptive area is a one, where yellow fever does not exist, but conditions would permit its development, if introduced. The validity of the certificate begins 10 days after the vaccination and lasts for 10 years. If revaccination is performed before the expiry of the validity, renders the certificate valid for a further period of 10 years, from the date of revaccination. On the other hand travelers corning to endemic areas also should receive vaccination for self-protection.

Prevention of yellow fever in India
India is a yellow fever receptive area because:
- People are all unvaccinated and are susceptible
- Monkeys e.g. *Macaca rhesus* (*M. rhesus*) and *M. sinica* are also susceptible
- Vectors (*A. aegypti*) are in abundance
- Climatic conditions are favorable.

But still the disease does not exist because the causative agent virus is not present. Virus can gain entry at any time. Therefore, special precautions have been taken by the Ministry of Health, Government of India, through stringer International Health Regulations. The virus can enter India through travelers and mosquitoes, through aircrafts and ships. So, the aerial and maritime traffic regulations are:

1. For passengers: Travelers must possess valid certificate of vaccination against yellow fever, if not such persons are placed under 'quarantine', in a mosquito-proof ward for a period of 6 days, for observation, from the date of leaving the endemic area. If the traveler possesses the certificate, but arrives before the certificate becomes 'valid', he/she is quarantined till the certificate becomes valid.
2. For mosquitoes: The aircrafts and ships coming from endemic areas are subjected for disinsection for the control of the vectors. In the area of about 400 square meters, near the airport or seaport, the 'A. aegypti index' is kept below one. The ships are also moored about 400 meters away from the shore and disinfected. In spite of these stringent regulations, now it is thought that viruses could have entered in India, at least off and on. But still the disease has not been reported based on the following explanations.
3. Indian *Aedes* mosquitoes may be less efficient vectors than those of Africa and South America.
4. Indians might have developed cross-immunity by suffering from other arboviral diseases such as dengue fever, KFD and JE, which has provided an 'ecological barrier'.
5. Indians might have developed antimosquito antibodies, following bites by *Aedes* mosquitoes.

Nursing management of yellow fever

Isolation
Since, the virus of yellow fever is transmitted from man to man or from animal to man only by the bite of a mosquito, a screened ward is necessary. The virus is known to be in the patient's blood for the first 3 days of the disease.

Diet
Nausea and vomiting usually are present at onset and for the first 3 or 4 days. Usually during this time glucose solution is given intravenously as the patient is unable to retain food. Chipped ice is taken readily. As the patient becomes able to retain food, a low calorie, high-protein diet is given. Thin gruel, albumin water, oyster juice, chicken broth, barley water, rice water and water are acceptable. Milk is not well-tolerated and should not be given. As the condition of the patient improves other foods may be added to the diet. Gelatin, cottage cheese and soft-cooked eggs are suggested.

Temperature
Characteristically the temperature is not high; however, it may reach 103° or 104°F. A cool or tepid sponge and an alcohol rub or fan may be given to reduce fever. An ice cap to the head will add to the comfort of the patient.

Personal hygiene
The patient should be disturbed as little as possible consistent with good care. Partial baths at intervals may be preferable to a complete cleansing bath. Good oral hygiene should be maintained. Bleeding gums and other mucous membranes present a challenge to the nurse. The dirty, furred tongue should be brushed or washed with a gauze pledget. The teeth should be washed and the mouth rinsed at intervals. Hydrogen peroxide is a satisfactory mouth rinse. It is effective in removing dried blood and sordes from the teeth. If drainage from the eyes is present, a warm boric acid pledget may be used to remove secretions.

Elimination
Although constipation is common, a laxative is seldom given except at onset. An enema may be given as necessary. The nurse should remember to disturb the patient as little as possible. Suppression of urine is fairly common and is a grave symptom. It should be watched for and reported to the doctor immediately. The urine usually is dark and scant. A daily specimen should be saved and an accurate record of urine output should be recorded.

General management of the disease
The patient should be placed in a quiet room and disturbed as little as possible. The nurse should plan her work, so that the patient may be permitted long intervals of uninterrupted rest. Fluids should be urged when they can be retained. The position of the patient should be changed every 3–4 hours. Bleeding from mucous membranes should be noted. Specimens of both tarry stools and coffee-ground vomitus should be saved and sent to the laboratory upon order of the physician. The temperature graph will show a characteristic curve. It should be kept carefully and the temperature recorded every 3 hours. Small pillows can be used to advantage for the comfort of the patient. The weight of the bedding should be kept from the patient by a bed cradle.

Convalescence
After the symptoms subside convalescence is rapid. The patient feels well and is anxious to return to normal activity. Within reason, this is usually permitted. However, a return to full diet should be deferred for some time after the acute stage has passed.

Terminal disinfection
Ordinary cleanliness is essential. The mattress and pillow should be aired. The walls, bed, table and chair should be washed with soap and water. The bedding should be sent to the laundry. The treatment equipment, all basins, dishes and similar items should be washed with soap and water.

Japanese encephalitis

Japanese encephalitis (JE) is an acute, viral infection of CNS. It is a zoonotic disease manifested by meningomyeloencephalitis and has a high case fatality rate. Clinical recognition of the disease was first made in Japan in 1924, when it was named as Japanese B encephalitis to differentiate, it from von Economo's disease. However, the disease has now been found to be a distinct entity with different etiological agent and is universally known as JE. To initiate control measures against JE, it is essential to know magnitude of the problem and understand natural cycle of the disease.

Magnitude of the problem

Global distribution
Encephalitis due to JE virus occurs in Eastern Siberia, China, Korea, Japan, Taiwan, Malaysia, Thailand, Singapore and India. An outbreak of JE was reported in 1980 from Madhupur forest area of Tangail district in Bangladesh. Burma reported JE for the first time in 1974. In Nepal, the first outbreak was recorded near the border of India in 1978. In Sri Lanka, virus of JE was isolated from pigs for the first time in 1968 and first outbreak occurred in 1985.

Japanese encephalitis in India
Human disease due to JE virus was first recognized in 1955 in North Arcot district of Tamil Nadu and Chittoor district of Andhra Pradesh. JE virus was also isolated from mosquitoes in the same year. In a 10-year period from 1955 to 1965, 52 proven cases of JE were recognized in these districts. In 1964, a small outbreak occurred in Madurai district of Tamil Nadu.

In 1973, the disease broke out in epidemic form in the districts of Burdwan, Bankura and Birbhum of West Bengal. The number of recorded cases was 96, out of which 325 died with a case fatality of 43%. Since then, outbreaks of JE have been reported from Tamil Nadu, West Bengal, Karnataka, Pondicherry, Andhra Pradesh, Assam, Bihar and Uttar Pradesh. In 1982, for the first time, an outbreak was reported from Manipur. In the same year, Goa, situated in the western coast of India also witnessed the outbreak for the first time. Repeated outbreaks have been reported from almost all these states. The states, which have not reported JE outbreaks, are those of northern and western parts of the country.

During the period from 1979 to 1987, the number of JE cases in the country varied from 1,716 to 7,500. Case fatality rate varied from 29.97 to 41.29%.

Variation of JE incidence within the states
The JE does not occur uniformly all over the affected states. In Tamil Nadu, the districts of North Arcot, South Arcot, Tirunelveli, Madurai, Ramanathapuram have reported outbreaks. In Andhra Pradesh, IE outbreaks have occurred in Anantapur, Chittoor, Cuddapah, Guntur, Prakasam and West Godavari. In Karnataka outbreaks of JE have been reported from the districts of Kolar, Bellary, Tumkur, Mandya and Bengaluru. Cases have been reported from other districts as well. In Assam, most affected districts are Dibrugarh and Lakhimpur. In 1987, however, 10 out of 18 districts were affected. In West Bengal, most affected districts are Burdwan, Bankura and Birbhum. Cases have been reported from other districts as well-except Darjeeling. Most affected districts in Uttar Pradesh are Gorakhpur and Deoria. JE cases have, however, been reported from 45 out of 57 districts in Uttar Pradesh.

The JE is predominantly a rural disease and mainly affects poor sections of the society. Usually, one case occurs in a village. Multiple cases have, however, occurred in some villages.

Case fatality rates in different outbreaks
The rate ranged from 10% in Tamil Nadu to 53.5% in Manipur. In West Bengal, Uttar Pradesh and Andhra Pradesh case fatality rates have been consistently above 30%. In Karnataka, rates were around 25%. In Tamil Nadu, these were relatively low, e.g. 10–23.8%. There might be several reasons for these variations. Care of the patient probably influenced case fatality rate.

Seasonal variation of JE
In South India, JE outbreaks have occurred during the latter half of the year, coinciding with the rainy season and period of high-mosquito density. In West Bengal, during earlier years, outbreaks started in May and continued till October with peak incidence in August. In recent years, the season has shifted September to December. In Assam and Uttar Pradesh outbreaks start in August or September and end in December. It is obvious that outbreaks are associated with rainfall and high-mosquito density. But the exact role of temperature, humidity and rainfall is still not clear.

Age and sex distribution of JE cases
The JE may occur at any age, but children are affected most. In South India most of the cases are among children. In other parts of the country, children (0–10 year) contribute 36–66% of the total cases. It is a common feature of all communicable diseases that, when a disease becomes endemic, children suffer most.

Clinical/Subclinical ratio
Studies conducted in some parts of the country indicated clinical, subclinical ratio as 1:64 to 1:300. For one clinical case of JE many develop subclinical infection.

Natural cycle of JE
Reservoir
Japanese encephalitis is a zoonotic disease having its natural cycle in pigs and certain species of birds. Some of the bird species likely to be involved in natural cycle of the disease are egret pond heron, grey heron, night heron, pigeons, sparrows, chickens and ducklings have also been experimentally infected with demonstration of high titer of viremia. The exact role of these birds in disease transmission requires further studies. Cattle develop antibodies against JE virus. But they do not develop sufficient viremia and thus do not infect mosquitoes. Since vector mosquitoes of JE are zoophilic, cattle provide blood meal and support mosquito population. Cattle thus act as traps for JE infected mosquitoes. Pigs have been incriminated as the most important simple amplifier host in Japan and other countries.

Infection with JE virus in pigs causes abortion and neonatal mortality. Infected adult pigs do not show any manifestation of clinical symptoms. In Japan and other countries population in pigs with short lifespan can continually provide susceptible generations. Pigs attract vector mosquitoes and exhibit viremia for 2–4 days. JE virus has been isolated from pigs in India. Virus transmission from infected pigs to fresh pigs through mosquitoes has also been demonstrated. Serological surveys during epidemics have shown presence of antibodies in large number of pigs.

Infection in pigs precedes human infection by a period of about 3 weeks. Man is the dead end for the transmission of JE. Man is accidentally bitten by vector mosquito. Man-to-man transmission does not occur.

Vector

In India, 11 species of mosquitoes belonging to three genera have been incriminated as the vectors of JE. Maximum number of JE virus isolation has been from members of *Culex vishnui* 'group of mosquitoes', which include *C. tritaeniorhynchus, C. vishnui* and *C. pseudovishnui*. In addition to these, other *Culex* mosquitoes such as *C. biiaeniorhuncus, C. gelidus, C. whitemarei, Cepidesnus* have been incriminated as vector of JE virus. Among the *Anopheles* mosquitoes, i.e. *Anopheles subpictus, A. shyrcanus, A. barbirostris* and among *Mansonia* mosquitoes, *M. annulifera* have also been suspected as vectors of JE virus.

Culex vishnui group of mosquitoes generally breed in rural setting in ground pools, ponds, puddles, rice fields where aquatic vegetation such as grass, paddy crops, water hyacinth, etc. are present in abundance. These vectors are zoophilic in nature. They feed on animals including cattle, pigs and birds. They rarely feed on man and prefer to stay outdoors. They have been collected from cattle sheds during night times, but during day time, they remain outdoors. These mosquitoes may rest indoors, if outdoor condition ceases to be conducive as in peak of summer season. Extrinsic incubation period in vector mosquito is 9–12 days.

Incubation period is not definitely known in man, but it is believed to range between 5 and 15 days. Period of communicability is variable under natural conditions. Virus is not directly transmissible from man to man. Mosquito remains infective for life. Viremia in birds usually lasts 2–5 days.

Susceptibility and resistance

Susceptibility to clinical disease is usually highest in infancy and old age, but varies with type. Inapparent or undiagnosed infection is more common at other ages. Infection results in homologous immunity. In highly endemic areas, adults are largely immune to local strains for reasons of mild and inapparent infections and susceptibles are mainly children.

Ratio of overt desire to inapparent infection varies from 1:300 to 1:1000. Thus cases of encephalitis represent only the tip of the iceberg compared to the large number of inapparent infections. Encephalitis cases due to JE may show a scattered distribution. It was observed in Northern India that the number of cases recorded per village (population 500–5,000) were not more than 1–2.

Clinical features

The course of the disease can be divided into three stages, viz. prodromal stage, acute encephalitis stage, late convalescent and sequelae stage. Prodromal stage is characterized by malaise, headache and fever. Rigors, nausea and vomiting may be present. During acute encephalitic stage, predominant features are confusion, fever, nuchal rigidity, focal nervous system signs and convulsions. Altered sensorium of varying degree occurs in all cases. It is characterized by clouding of consciousness, confusion, delirium, disorientation, stupor and finally progressing to coma in many patients. Motor defects such as palsy, paralysis and involuntary movements are also common during this stage. Sometimes dehydration and features associated with myocardial strain may be observed. Late convalescent stage begins when the temperature and erythrocyte sedimentation rate become normal. Neurological signs may start to improve or remain stationary depending mainly on the degree of severity of acute encephalitis stage. Generally, convalescence is prolonged and residual neurological deficits are not uncommon. Severe emaciation, emotional instability, restlessness, involuntary movements and aphasia are noted during this phase. Some children develop contractures, if spastic limbs are not corrected during this stage.

Ratio between clinical and subclinical infection is between 1:20 and 1:300. Although diagnosis of JE during an epidemic is not very difficult, caution is needed to avoid over diagnosis.

Cases occurring sporadically need to be differentiated from diseases with encephalitis symptoms. These are cerebral malaria, meningitis, encephalitis due to other causes, Reye's syndrome, febrile convulsions, toxic encephalopathies and rabies.

Control measures

As with other viral diseases, there is no specific treatment for JE. However, supportive and symptomatic treatment plays a very important role in recovery of the patient and can greatly reduce the case fatality rate. Control of JE shall include measure against vector mosquitoes, reservoirs of infection and protection of man.

Measures against mosquitoes

1. Action on adult mosquitoes: This involves:
   - Residual sprays
   - Space sprays.
2. Action on aquatic stages of mosquitoes: The measures undertaken are:
   - Elimination of breeding places
   - Chemical methods
   - Biological methods
   - Spraying.

In order to implement adult control measures effectively, the density of the vector mosquitoes has to be monitored throughout the year. The anti-vector measures have to be initiated when the vector density starts building up.

Residual spraying has to be carried out according to resting habits. The vectors are known to rest outdoors, but in some situations they rest indoors also. Spraying should be done in cattle sheds. The susceptibility status of the vectors to different insecticides has to be established.

In affected areas, two rounds of residual spraying with appropriate insecticide should be done in all premises, including cattle sheds. In piggeries, first round of spray is done 1 month before the anticipated JE season, followed by another round after 6–8 weeks.

During JE outbreaks, peridomestic fogging in the affected areas has shown beneficial effect. Aerial spraying of a suitable insecticide in ULV as peridomestic fogging with a cold fogger have been used with varying degrees of success in some countries.

Antislavery measures

Larvicides such as fenitrothion has been found to be effective in control of vector mosquitoes. Biological measures for mosquito larvae are effective. The use of predatory and entomophagous fish, e.g. *Gambusia, Guppy*, etc. has yielded good results. Many viral, bacterial and fungal preparations have been tried with good results. But these measures are still in the experimental stage.

Source reduction

Environmental methods should be the most effective method of vector control, but are difficult to implement. Modification of rice cultivation practice in Japan has helped in bringing down the incidence of the disease. Improved water management and intermittent irrigation should be considered. All development activities such as construction of dams, irrigation channels, etc. which alter the existing ecosystem, should be carried out in consultation with the experts in public health and environment.

Measures against reservoirs

Continuous surveillance should be maintained to detect the virus or seroconversion amongst the possible reservoirs of the disease. This will act as warning signal for the onset of cases in human being. The pigsties may be constructed in a proper way, should be located away from the human habitation and kept well-protected from mosquitoes. It is difficult to build individual pigsties at a distance, but people can be encouraged to adopt cooperative pig farming. Periodic spraying of pigsties with suitable insecticide should be done from beginning of JE season.

Vaccination of pigs with a live attenuated vaccine has yielded encouraging results in Japan. Earlier studies have shown effectiveness of inactivated vaccine. The possibility of vaccinating pigs in JE endemic areas of India should be explored.

Measures for protection of man

To avoid contact with the mosquitoes, various physical and chemical methods such as use of mosquito nets and repellants should be encouraged. Vectors of JE start biting activity at dusk and continue to be active till the early hours of the morning. Health education of the community regarding the mode of transmission of disease and method of its prevention should be imparted. Active participation of the community should be ensured to prevent mosquito growing conditions.

Immunoprophylaxis

Inactivated mouse brain vaccine using Nakayama strain of JE virus has been extensively used in several countries especially in Japan and Taiwan. In Japan, incidence of disease was drastically reduced as a result of use of vaccine. Studies conducted in Taiwan and Thailand with the inactivated vaccine were 80–96%. The inactivated mouse brain vaccine with Nakayama strain is now produced at Central Research Institute, Kasauli. Vaccine is under trial in some states.

In view of the fact that outbreaks of JE have occurred in several states of India, and the present total supply of the vaccine does not exceed 2 million doses, vaccination as a routine measure is not possible. Vaccination may be offered to the population at high risk. Majority of the cases occur in children. Outbreaks usually occur in rural areas.

Vaccination may be limited to the age group of 1–15 years. But in areas where adults are also affected, vaccination for adults should also be considered.

For primary immunization, two doses of 1 mL each (0.5 mL for children less than 3 year of age) should be given subcutaneously at an interval of 7–14 days and a booster dose should be given after 1 year. Subsequent boosters are recommended after 3 years or when an outbreak occurs.

Immunity develops at least 1 month after the second dose. Hence, vaccination should be completed at least 1 month prior to the anticipated outbreak. Vaccine has limited value after the commencement of an outbreak, due to the long period acquired for immunity to develop. It should nevertheless be administered as soon as possible after the commencement of the epidemic, since several outbreaks have been known to continue for 3–5 months.

Surveillance

Surveillance is an integral part of any disease control strategy. Components of surveillance are collection, tabulation and analysis of data, and dissemination of information. Routine reporting of morbidity and mortality from medical institutions is very unsatisfactory. Active surveillance by door-to-door search plays an important role in JE, particularly when an outbreak occurs. Sentinel surveillance should be done by setting sentinel centers in high-risk areas. These centers may serve as early warning system for detection of JE among animals, detection of vector density and infection in man.

Nursing management

All forms of nursing management encephalitis can be effectively isolated by the medical aseptic technic. The room should be kept free of insects. Articles that have come in contact with either the patient or his/her secretions should be cleaned up immediately. Waste material should be burned.

Diet

If nausea and vomiting are not present during the acute stage, the diet should consist of high-caloric fluids. Fruit juices with either honey or sugar added, vegetable juices, gruels, fruit and vegetable purees, soups, ice cream and milk in various forms may be given. Liquids should be urged, forced if necessary. However, if marked intracranial pressure is suspected, fluid intake must be carefully watched under the orders of the physician on the case.

Often it is necessary to tube feed the patient because of his/her inability to swallow or because of lethargy, drowsiness or coma. Intravenous feedings usually are given, if the patient is unable to take and retain a sufficient amount orally. The Levin tube may be used. As the patient improves a more substantial, varied diet is given. The nurse should remember that malnutrition and dehydration usually are considered to be the result of poor nursing care. A record of both caloric and fluid intake should be kept.

Temperature

Temperature is seldom high enough to become a nursing problem. If necessary, warm or tepid sponge baths, an alcohol fan or rub may be given to reduce fever. The temperature, pulse and respirations should be taken and recorded every 4 hours.

Personal hygiene

Because of excessive perspiration and the tendency to incontinence several baths daily may be needed to keep the patient clean and dry.

Because of the difficulty or inability of some patients to swallow, special attention should be given to oral hygiene. It often is difficult and sometimes impossible to secure the cooperation of the patient. It may become necessary to use a mouth gag and swabs to clean the mouth and teeth.

Elimination

The bowels should move once daily. If necessary a cathartic or enemas may be given. Incontinence is a common symptom. However, the possibility of retention of urine must not be overlooked.

General management of the disease

The patient should be kept in a quiet, well-ventilated room. The bed should be firm, but comfortable. The bedding should be light in weight, but should provide sufficient warmth. If prostration is great, the weight of the bedding should be kept from the patient by the use of a bed cradle. The eyes should be protected from too strong light. The lethargic condition of the patient makes prevention of bedsores one of the first considerations in nursing. The patient should be clean and dry. His/Her position should be changed frequently, every 3–4 hours at least. A brisk alcohol rub should be given each time, if the position is changed.

If the patient is unable to swallow, it may be necessary to use suction to remove mouth and throat secretions. Postural drainage has been used with some degree of success. This is done by elevating the foot of the bed to 20° or less. It must be remembered in this connection that measurements with a ventilation meter show that this procedure throws the weight of viscera against the diaphragm and diminishes the amount of tidal air.

Tracheotomy may be ordered. Persistent headache can be relieved to some extent by the use of ice packs or an ice cap. The nurse should watch for and report any eye symptoms double vision, roving or oscillating movement of the eyeballs, or drooping of the eyelids also. Inability to use any muscles, neck rigidity, numbness or muscle twitching. Changes in the mental characteristics of the patient should be noted such as mental dullness, mental depression, melancholia, insomnia, reversed sleep curve and personality changes. Restraints may be needed, if the patient is delirious.

Convalescence

Convalescence usually is prolonged. Some patients make a complete recovery, while many never are able to return to a normal life.

Kyasanur forest disease

Kyasanur forest disease is an acute, communicable disease, caused by an arbovirus, basically a zoonotic disease mainly that of monkeys, transmitted to human beings accidentally by the bite of infected hard ticks. Clinically it is characterized by fever, extreme prostration, red eye followed by hemorrhages. Case fatality is about 5–10%.

History

Kyasanur forest disease was first recognized during 1956–1957, when there was a report of abnormal death of monkeys in Kyasanur forest area of about 800 square miles, of Sagar, Sorab taluks of Shimoga District of Karnataka state, followed by epidemic of this disease among the people living in the villages surrounding the Kyasanur forest, resulting in about 500 cases with a case fatality of 10%. The virus was isolated in 1957. Largest epidemic occurred in 1983, with 2,167 cases and 69 deaths.

In March 1957, there was occurrence of monkey mortality from the forest of Sagar taluk, Shimoga district of Karnataka. The fear that this disease might be yellow fever was fortunately soon dispelled and new disease entity affecting man as well as two species of simians was recognized within the period of 2 weeks. A virus immunologically related to the virus of Russian spring-summer encephalitis (RSSE) complex was isolated from human cases as well as from sick and dead monkeys. Soon they found that the virus was also present in the ticks of the genus *Haemaphysalis* occurring in the forest, more specially in species. Further laboratory experimentation demonstrated the ability of the tick to transmit the disease by bite. The disease is named as KFD because from this place the virus was first isolated.

Magnitude of the problem

From March 1957 to December 1963, 244 human cases were confirmed to be due to KFD either by virus isolation or through serological conversion or both, which have been identified by the surveillance staff, there would certainly be more cases, which had not come to their notice. The disease is now restricted to four districts:

1. Shivamoga.
2. North Kanara.
3. South Kanara.
4. Chikkamagaluru.

According to recent report the disease continues to be active in its endemic foci. During 1983–1984, the largest 2,167 cases and 69 deaths, as against 571 cases and 15 deaths during 1981. Some cases show biphasic course of illness. During second phase of illness, after a febrile period of 1–3 weeks, some patients exhibit symptoms of meningoencephalitis, characterized by high fever, severe headache, vomiting, neck rigidity, tremors, abnormal reflexes and mental disturbances. There are associated hemorrhagic manifestations also. Case fatality rate is 5–10%. Recovery is almost complete in 90% of the cases, but the patient remains asthenic for quite a long time. Convalescence is slow.

Investigations
- Blood for culture of the virus
- Serological tests
- Thrombocytopenia
- Leukopenia
- Urine in positive for albumin.

Management
- Good supportive treatment
- Blood transfusion, if necessary
- Prophylactic antibiotics.

Epidemiological Features

Agent

The agent KFD virus is a member of group B togaviruses (flaviviruses). It is antigenically related to other tick-borne flaviviruses, particularly the Far Eastern tick-borne encephalitis and Omsk hemorrhagic fever. KFD has a prolonged viremia in man for about 10 days or more (Fig. 31.6).

Natural hosts and reservoir

Small mammals such as rats and squirrels are the reservoirs of the virus. Birds and bats are less important hosts. The monkeys are recognized as amplifying hosts for the virus. However, they are not effective maintenance hosts because most of them die from KFD infection. Cattle provide *Haemaphysalis* ticks with a plentiful source of blood meals, which in turn, leads to a population explosion among the ticks. The cattle is important in maintaining tick population, but it will not take part in virus transmission.

Host factors

1. Age: More common in the age between 20 and 40 years.
2. Sex: Greater in males than in females.
3. Immunity: Previous infection gives immunization.
4. Occupation: The attacked people were mostly cultivators who visited forests accompanying their cattle or cutting wood.
5. Human activity: The epidemic period correlates well with the period of greatest human activity in the forest, i.e. from January until the onset of rain in June.

Environmental factors

The highest number of human and monkey infection occurs during drier months particularly from January to June. This period coincides with the peak nymphal activity of ticks.

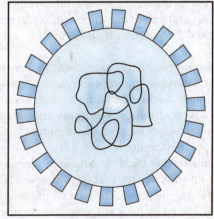

Figure 31.6: Togavirus

Mode of Transmission

The transmission cycle involves mainly monkeys and ticks. The disease is transmitted by bite of infective ticks especially nymphal stages. There is no evidence of man-to-man transmission (as there is very little chance of *Haemaphysalis* ticks). Domestic animal may have an important place in the natural cycle of transmission. There is no indication of any illness among the wild or domestic animals other than monkeys, which could be attributed to the KFD virus. Incubation period of the disease is between 3 and 8 days.

Clinical Features

1. Sudden onset of fever.
2. Headache.
3. Sever myalgia.
4. Low backache and limb pain.
5. Severe prostration often associated with inflammation of the eyes.
6. Diarrhea and vomiting by the 3rd or 4th day of illness.
7. Bleeding from the nose (epistaxis), gum, stomach and intestine might begin as early as the 3rd day.
8. Rarely hemoptysis.
9. The majority of cases, however, run a full course of illness without overt hemorrhagic signs.
10. Mild meningoencephalitis after an afebrile period of 7–21 days.

Physical examination during the early days of illness shows an acutely ill listless and often prostate patient with temperature up to 39.4°C though hyperpyrexia is rare. Some cases show relative bradycardia and hypotension. Congestion of conjunctiva with occasional photophobia, stiff neck due to painful guarding of; spinal and cervical muscle cervical and axillary lymphadenopathy are seen in most cases.

Occasionally, reddish papules or fading macules are noticed in axilla, similar to lesions observed on the skin after manual detachment of nymphal ticks, dryness of skin due to marked dehydration is observed late in the course of illness.

There are no physical sign relevant to any neurological damage. However, mental confusion, drowsiness and rarely treatment disorientation have been seen. There is complete recovery from the syndrome and subsidence of fever, except in those cases, which terminate fatally due to hemorrhagic complications.

Some cases show biphasic course of illness. The second febrile episode occurs 4–21 days after the fall in temperature of the acute phase. The onset is initiated as severe headache followed by neck stiffness, mental disturbance, coarse tremors giddiness and abnormal reflexes, recovery from their symptom is complete.

Vectors

The virus has complex life cycle involving a wide variety of tick species. There are 15 species of hard ticks of the genus *Haemaphysalis* family ixodidae, particularly *H. spinigera* and *H. turturis* are known to transmit the disease. KFD has also been isolated from soft ticks of the family argasidae.

Morphology of Ticks

The body of tick is oval in shape and is not distinctly separated into head, thorax and abdomen. They have four pairs of legs and no antennae. The hard ticks are covered on their dorsal surface by a cutaneous shield, called scutum (Fig. 31.7). This scutum in the male covers the entire back and in the female only small part in front. Hard ticks have a head or capitulum at anterior end. The males are generally smaller than females. The hard tick feeds both night and day, and cannot stand starvation. The hard ticks are always found on their hosts. The common hard ticks, which infest domestic animals such as dogs and cattle in India are *Dermacentor, Haemaphysalis, Hyalomma, Rhipicephalus* and *Boophilus*.

Life History of Hard Tick

There are four stages in the life cycle of tick (Fig. 31.8):
1. Egg.
2. Larva.
3. Nymph.
4. Adult.

Egg: Hard tick lays few hundred or even thousand eggs, all at one time after which the female is exhausted and dies. The eggs are deposited on the ground and hatch in 1–3 weeks.

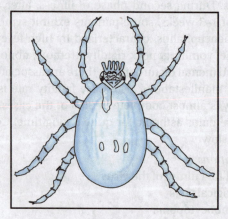

Figure 31.7: Hard tick morphology

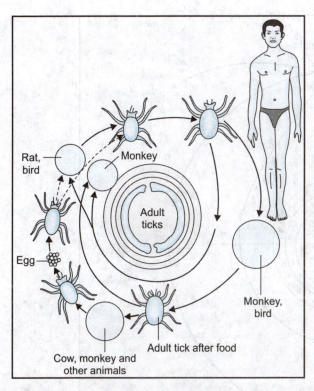

Figure 31.8: Life cycle of tick

Larva: The tick's larva, which comes out of the egg, possesses three pairs of legs. It lies and waits in grass and garbage till a suitable host, rat, squirrel, pig, etc. appears to which it attaches itself and starts feeding by sucking the host's blood.

Nymph: This resembles the adult in having four pairs of legs, but it has no genital pore. The nymph are all blood suckers and they attach themselves to suitable hosts for a blood meal (there are five nymphal stages in the life history of soft ticks).

Adult: The morphology of adult tick has been described earlier. The duration of the life cycle from egg to adult is about 2 months in the hard ticks.

Life Cycle of Haemaphysalis Tick

Life cycle of *Haemaphysalis* tick is similar to hard tick life cycle. Grown up female ticks lay eggs from which comes out the small ticks and search for their food. They suck blood from the rat, squirrel and pig bodies after some time it is covered by a thin layer and becomes encapsulated after few days. It sucks blood from the above mentioned animals and grows to adult stage. These ticks have moustache, which contains the poisonous organisms (Fig. 31.9).

Kyasanur forest disease poisonous organisms have different stages:

1. Young ticks.
2. Encapsulated.
3. Adult ticks.

The eggs will not be affected by poisonous organism. If the young tick sucks blood from the already infected rat or squirrel, then this young tick also gets the KFD disease.

Control Measures

Control of ticks

As KFD is a tick-borne disease, control of ticks should be undertaken. Power equipment or aircraft mounted equipment to dispense carbaryl, fenthion, naked or propoxur at 2.24 kg of active ingredient per hectare can be used. The spraying must be carried out in hot spots, i.e. in areas where monkey deaths have been reported, within 50 meters around the spot of the monkey deaths. Besides the endemic foci, the heavy population of ticks in the forest areas is attributed partly to the free-roaming cattle, restriction of cattle movement is through to bring about a reduction in vector population.

Vaccination

The population at risk should be immunized with killed KFD vaccine.

Prevention and control of KFD

1. Elimination of reservoirs: Since there is no specific treatment, human reservoir state cannot be eliminated and elimination of wild monkeys is not possible. Thus, it is not possible to control KFD by elimination of reservoir.
2. Breaking the channel of transmission: This measure consists of control of ticks. This is done by two ways:
   a. By using insecticides such as carbaryl, fenthion or propoxur. Application can be made by power equipment or aircraft mounted equipment. Spraying is done in 'hot spots' (i.e. areas where monkey deaths are reported).
   b. By restriction of entry of cattle into the forest will also control tick population.
3. Protection of susceptibles.
4. Use of repellants: The people at risk are educated to protect themselves from tick bites by adequate clothing and also application of repellents such as dimethyl phthalate, N,N-diethyl-meta-toluamide (DEET), Replex ointment, etc.
5. Immunization: A killed KFD vaccine is being prepared at Virus Research Center, Pune. It is formalin inactivated, tissue culture vaccine, prepared from chick embryo fibroblasts. Two doses, each of 1 mL is recommended with an interval of 4 weeks for adults and 0.5 mL for children, IM. It is given for those people in that

552 SECTION 4 Communicable Diseases

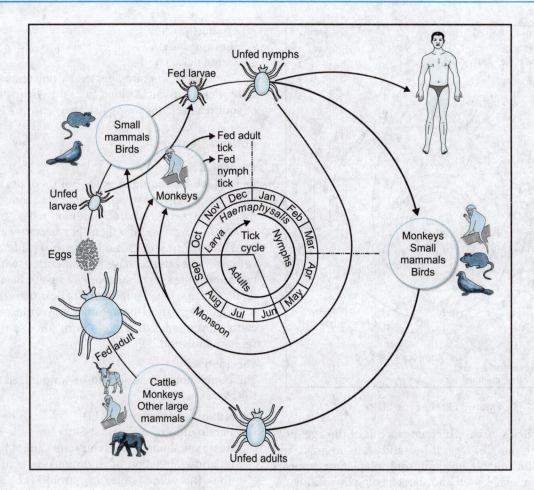

Figure 31.9: Natural cycle of Kyasanur forest disease

area who are at risk. Immunity lasts for 1 year. Booster doses are given every year. It is 50% effective, being a killed vaccine. Storage temperature is 2–8°C.

Personal protection

Protection of individuals exposed to the risk of dimethyl phthalate (DMP), DEET should be encouraged. They should examine their bodies at the end of each day for ticks and remove them promptly. The habit of sitting or lying down on the ground should be discouraged through health education.

Control of ticks in forest by benzene hexachloride (BHC) has been practiced successfully to control ticks is the so called hot spots. Insecticidal treatment of all animals is also a useful measure.

Preventive measures
1. The use of insect repellants should be encouraged.
2. Vaccination against KFD should be carried out.
3. Isolation of KFD patients from others.
4. Avoidance of cattle from roaming specially near to the forest area.
5. Insecticidal treatment for all animals.
6. Keeping the cattle clean and removing ticks from their body.

CONCLUSION

Rabies is a zoonotic disease caused by lyssavirus type I of family rhabdoviridae. It causes signs/symptoms such as fever, headache, paralysis, convulsions and in advanced stages cause difficulty in swallowing, abnormal movement of diaphragm and problem in moving facial muscles. It can be prevented and controlled by adopting appropriate measures such as diagnosis, treatment, isolation, hydration, intensive care and vaccination.

Yellow fever is a zoonotic disease caused by an arbovirus. It is caused by bite of an infective monkey to man or infective man to man. The clinical manifestations of yellow fever are jaundice, black vomit, epistaxis, malaria, agitation and coma. The measures such as vaccination, surveillance, personal protection, etc. can be used to prevent and control yellow fever.

Japanese encephalitis is a mosquito-borne arboviral disease. It occurs most commonly in rainy season. It is characterized by fever, rigors, headache, nausea, vomiting, convulsions, muscular rigidity and behavior abnormalities. It needs early diagnosis, first aid, referral, vaccination, vector control measures, health education, etc. to prevent and control JE.

Kyasanur forest disease affects people between 20 and 40 years of age. It is transmitted by monkeys and infective ticks. The infected case will show the signs/symptoms such as fever, headache, myalgia, mental disturbances, course tremors and abnormal reflexes. It can be prevented and controlled by early diagnosis, treatment, personal protection, controlling the ticks and health education.

Zoonoses: Bacterial

CHAPTER 32

BRUCELLOSIS

Brucellosis is an infectious disease of gradual or insidious onset and prolonged course, characterized by either continuous or wave-like fluctuations in the intensity of symptoms, among India. It may be noted with the appearance of irregular fever of variable intensity, chills or chillness, profuse sweats, muscle and joint pain, progressive prostration and anemia. Brucellosis is worldwide in distribution and is a public health problem. It is an endrome in the areas where there is a large population of cattle, pigs, goats, hogs or sheep. Cases are reported for all states of India, but exact information is not available.

Agent

More generally recognized species in the genus *Brucella* are accepted in the caprine or goat cases. *Brucella melitensis* (*B. melitensis*), micrococcus melitensis, *B. suis* and *B. abortus* are example.

Host

Host is predominantly a disease of adult males. The people, who are at risk are butchers, veterinarians shepherds, farmers and laboratory workers.

Environment

The factors in which disease occurs in the areas of high rainfall, overcrowding of herds, unhygienic milk and meat production practices, lack of exposure to sunlight and the organisms survive in favorable conditions of water, urine, feces and manure.

Mode of Transmission

Brucellosis transmits from infected animal to man by direct contact, such as food and abraded skin, mucosa or conjunctiva with infected tissue, blood, urine or vaginal discharge, strong food, i.e. ingestion of raw material, dairy products from infected animals. Even eating of fresh raw vegetables grown in contaminated soil can cause brucellosis.

Air: By inhaling dust or aerosols containing brucellosis infection, which are found in cowsheds. The incubation period of brucellosis is 1–3 weeks.

Clinical Manifestation

The onset may be gradual and insidious or abrupt, and strong. It is a variable as the subsequent clinical course usually begins with headache, mental depression, muscular aching, excess fatigue and the following:

- Intermittent or irregular fever, or swinging pyrexia (40–41°C)
- Profuse sweating, rigors
- Arthritis involves larger joints
- Enlarged spleen
- Low back pain
- Headache
- Hepatomegaly
- Diagnosis
- Isolating organism from culture of blood and bone marrow
- Serological tests.

Prevention and Control

1. Early diagnosis and treatment: Cases can be identified by clinical manifestations, which are present in man and these cases should be treated with antibiotic tetracycline (500 mg, 6 hourly for 3 weeks). If the patient is having other complications, then along with tetracycline, 1 g of streptomycin injections are given intramuscularly (IM).

2. **Boiling/Pasteurization of milk:** The milk, which is to be consumed should be pasteurized. If pasteurization is not possible, then boiling of milk is required before consumption.
3. **Prevent from direct contact:** The people working with cattle, sheep, goat, swine, buffaloes, horses and dogs should prevent themselves from being in contact with infected tissue, blood, urine and vaginal discharges, if having abraded skin or mucosal membrane. They should exercise proper care while handling and disposing discharges, aborted fetuses or placenta of an infected animal.
4. **Vaccination:** The humans, who are at risk should be vaccinated by human live vaccine of *B. abortus* strain 19-BA and vaccine of *B. abortus* strain 19 is used for animal. So, vaccination is required for animals and humans.
5. **Hygiene of environment:** All the measures should be adopted to keep the environment clean. This requires the proper disposal of urine and feces, proper disposal of discharges, placenta, aborted fetus and veterinary care for animals.
6. **Personal hygiene:** The people, who are at risk should observe high standard of personal hygiene. They should properly wash the skin exposed to infective material. Proper handwashing after touching the infected material.
7. **Testing the animals:** The animals, i.e. cattle, swine, buffaloes should be tested before slaughtering.
8. **Health education:** This regarding safe handling of animals should be provided to the community health education regarding boiling the milk before drinking and not eating raw vegetables, etc. should be provided.

Nursing Management

Isolation

Brucellosis can be isolated by the medical aseptic technique. The causative organisms are found in the nose and throat secretions, urine, feces, and vaginal discharges. Isolation can be maintained in an open ward, but a private room should be provided whenever possible.

Diet

During the acute stage, the diet should consist of high caloric and high-vitamin fluids. Fruit juices, vegetable juice gruels, nourishing soups and eggnogs are suggested. Custards, gelatin, ice cream, pureed vegetables and fruit and cottage cheese may be given as tolerated.

Temperature

The temperature is usually high (103–105°F). It may be reduced by sponge baths, alcohol rub and colonic flushings. Ice caps or ice packs to the head are helpful. Fluids should be forced.

If other methods fail, a wet sheet pack is effective. However, this procedure is contraindicated if the patient's joints are swollen and sore. When chilling is present external heat in the form of warm blankets or a heat cradle may be applied.

Personal Hygiene

The patient should have a daily cleansing bath. Frequent alcohol rubs are refreshing and help to prevent pressure sores. Sweats, which are common should be followed by tepid sponges. The gown and bedding should be changed as indicated.

The mouth, which is characteristically dirty, should be kept clean. The teeth should be brushed carefully and thoroughly at least twice each day. Sore, bleeding or spongy gums should be cleaned carefully with a gauze or cotton pledget. The tongue should be washed or brushed. The mouth should be rinsed with an antiseptic mouthwash before and after taking nourishment.

Elimination

The bowels should move freely once each day. Enemas or cathartics may be given. The nurse should keep an accurate record of fluid intake and output.

General Management of the Disease

The patient should be placed in a pleasant, quiet, well-ventilated room. Bedrest usually is prescribed. The bedding should be light weight, but should provide adequate warmth. A bed cradle may be provided, if the joints are swollen and painful. Counterirritants applied to swollen, painful joints sometimes afford comfort to the patient. External heat should be applied for chills. Hot blankets or a head cradle are recommended. Tepid or warm sponges may be given following sweats. The patient should be kept clean and dry. It may be necessary to bath and change the patient from three to four times in a 12-hour period.

Despondency, irritability, insomnia and mental depression present an outstanding nursing problem. The nurse should have a sympathetic understanding of the patient's condition. Sedatives often are prescribed. The nurse should be especially alert to see that the patient does not injure himself/herself during periods of mental depression.

Convalescence

In an acute case, convalescence is usually very slow. A carefully planned diet, cheerful surroundings and a sympathetic understanding of the patient's mental condition will be beneficial. A skillful, tactful nurse can help the family and understand the patient's need.

Terminal Disinfection

The patient should be given a bath and shampoo, dressed in clean clothing and put into a clean unit. The contaminated unit should be cleaned in the usual way. The bedding should be laundered, the mattress and pillow aired for at least 6 hours, and the walls, bed table and chair washed with soap and water. The waste bag should be sent to the incinerator. The treatment equipment should be boiled or washed and dried in the open air.

Give the Patient these Instructions

1. Not to handle articles used by him/her to visitors, and to avoid handshaking and kissing.
2. To keep such things as pencils, threads and similar objects out of the mouth and to refrain from licking stamps or envelope flaps.
3. To keep the fingernails short and the hands clean, and avoid placing the fingers to the lips or touching anything that has been in his/her mouth.
4. To handle glass drinking tubes or straws at the center or several inches away from the top. The patient should be taught never to cough into his/her bare hands, never to swallow sputum, and to avoid placing thermometers, spoons, toothpaste or anything else that has been in his/her mouth on the bedside table. Place them on a tissue square until proper disposal can be made, oral hygiene should be faithfully carried out and the patient should avoid placing hand on the rim of the medicine glasses or drinking cups.

It is difficult at times to teach a patient, the necessity for remaining in bed. He/she is to be instructed to remain in bed and not get out unless the doctor gives explicit permission. Explain the reason for this precaution. Smoking should be discouraged.

If paper dishes are used they are collected with the leftover food and burned. Serving trays are washed with strong soap solution, rinsed and dried. Drinking tubes are washed and boiled for 20 minutes. Wash basins and emesis basins are thoroughly washed in a solution of saponated cresol, rinsed in hot water and dried. Sputum cup holders are soaked in a similar solution once a day, and then washed and dried.

When a patient is discharged, pillows and mattress are sunned and aired, and the unit washed with soap and water.

Rest

Rest is of prime importance in the treatment of tuberculosis and the patient is constantly reminded of the necessity for rest. The nurse explains the meaning of rest in his/her daily association with the patient. The doctor emphasizes rest in periodic radio talks, as well as during his/her visits. The patient's activity is limited. Everyday afternoon 2 hours are devoted to supervised rest. During rest periods patients are encouraged to close the eyes and relax drawn shades darken the rooms. Open windows allow free circulation of fresh air. Talking, listening to the radio and reading are not permitted. A nurse circulated see that regulations are carried out. All other personnel remain out of the room unless service is required.

Fresh Air

A cool room with plenty of fresh air is maintained at all times. To assure warmth, adequate covering is furnished, covers over the head of the bed and bedside screens serve to ward off undue draft.

Even during the coldest weather, the windows remain open. Only during bath, the windows are closed. However, it is again to be emphasized that these patients are to be kept out of drafts.

Diet

The diet will be worked out by the dietitian, under the direction of the attending physician. Usually a well-balanced high caloric, high-vitamin diet is served three times a day, with additional nourishment at 10 AM, 3 PM and at 8 PM, consisting either of cocoa, milk, fruit juices or eggnogs. The daily diet approximates 2,500 calories. In cases of associated diseases or complications, special diets are prescribed by the physician. The diet may be augmented with specially prescribed vitamins.

Mental Attitude

The patient is encouraged to practice mental relaxation. Every effort is made to relieve from worry. Here, the nurse plays an important part; he/she exercises patient and cheerfulness at all times. It is natural for one confined to bed for a long period to be concerned with the welfare of those near and dear to him/her. Upon recognition of the patient's economic and social problems, the nurse refers him/her to the medical social service worker. Never discuss the case in his/her presence or with unauthorized persons. This is particularly relevant to patients who are getting worse, who have had recent hemorrhages or other bad experiences.

Personal Hygiene

At least once a week, a complete sponge bath is given and all bed linen is changed. Incontinent patients are bathed and changed as frequently as necessary, those who are able to bath themselves; critical and feeble patients are bathed by the attendant. Pressure sores are anticipated. Cod liver oil and lanolin or compound tinctures of benzoin are applied to reddened areas. The back is rubbed twice a day with alcohol or baby oil. Shampoos are given according to doctor's order. Great emphasis is placed on clean hands and oral hygiene. Face and hands are washed twice a day. Alkaline antiseptic mouthwash is also given twice a day.

Exercise

The maximum amount of exercise is the sponge bath. The patient baths himself/herself assisted by the attendant, except patients who are too feeble, critical or hemorrhaging. Turning in bed, eating, getting on and off the bedpan are allowed. Reading, knitting and writing are exercises to be permitted by direction of the physician.

Temperature

The temperature is recorded every morning and afternoon; if over 100°F, it is repeated every 4 hours. Individual thermometers are used and should be left in the mouth for 5 minutes before reading. They are kept in test tubes containing 70% alcohol or other suitable disinfectant. These test tubes are labeled and inserted in a wooden block or container fitted with a handle. Once a week, the test tubes are washed with soap and water, boiled for 20 minutes and refilled with fresh solution. Before the thermometer is placed in the patient's mouth, it is wiped off with a tissue. Weaker patients should not be required to make the physical effort necessary for shaking down thermometers.

Weight

The patient is weighed and his/her weight is recorded as soon as his/her condition warrants, at first monthly, later, weekly. Critical, hemorrhaging and early postpartum, postsurgical or orthopedic cases are not weighed. This applies to children as well as adults.

Sputum Specimens

To obtain a sputum specimen, the patient is instructed to cough and spit directly into the sputum cup. Then the cup is covered with the lid and sent to the laboratory. An early morning specimen is desirable. If a 72-hour specimen is requested, all sputum for that period is saved; the patient expectorates directly into a wide-mouthed glass jar and kept at the bedside. For esthetic and sanitary reasons a paper towel is fastened around the jar. Such specimens may be started at other times during the day. At the end of 72 hours, the jar is sent to the laboratory. When ordered, a fasting stomach contents specimen for tuberculosis is taken in the morning before anything is taken by mouth. A Levine tube, a large Luer syringe, sterile water and a labeled glass container are used for this purpose.

Sputum Disposal

To dispose the sputum, sawdust is poured over the contents in the cup. Cups are securely wrapped in newspaper and placed in the tissue discard bag at the bedside. The bags are collected and dropped into metal cans, which are taken directly to the incinerator. Steam under pressure sterilizes the cans.

Pulmonary Hemorrhage

The care of a pulmonary hemorrhage offers the nurse a fine opportunity to display his/her knowledge of the principles and refinement of tuberculosis nursing. Everything is done for the patient and the patient does nothing. A competent nurse anticipates patient's needs. More than this, nurse skillfully and tactfully obtains their cooperation and confidence. Nurse is cooperative and never raises his/her voice nor speaks in an excited manner. Emesis basin and tissues are placed within easy reach of the patient. When the basin is removed, a clean one is left. Standing orders for hemoptysis are posted on all tuberculosis wards. The charting is important. The time of the hemorrhage, the amount of blood loss and the general condition of the patient are recorded.

The mouth is cleansed with a weak solution of hydrogen peroxide. Crushed ice is given by mouth in small amounts as tolerated. Nourishment consists of cold fluids. The patient is kept warm and in the most comfortable position, usually dorsal recumbent with the head elevated at least a foot; if on the side, remember to keep the good side uppermost to prevent spillover from the bad into the good lung, as well as to exert splinting pressure on the bleeding side. Patient is disturbed as little as possible. For 5 days after the hemorrhage everything is done for them, they are given tremendous doses of reassurance.

PLAGUE

Plague is an acute, communicable disease, primarily a zoonotic disease, disease of rodents, specially of rats, caused by bacilli *Yersinia pestis*. It is transmitted from the rodents to the human beings accidentally by the bite of infected rat flea, an ectoparasite of rats. Clinically, it is characterized by fever, suppurative enlargement of lymph nodes often followed by septicemia (septicemic plague) and pneumonia (pneumonic plague). Pneumonic plague carries high mortality.

History

Plague is not a new disease. It is present from time immemorial. The association of this disease with rats is mentioned in Bhagavata Purana (a book written about 1500–800 BC) stating that as soon as dead rats are seen the residence should be immediately vacated. Down the ages, plague was known as 'mahamari', the great death. Plague has dogged the man's footsteps and it has taken a heavy toll of human lives. Three great pandemics have been authentically recorded. The first was recorded in sixth century (Justinian plague), which resulted in about 100 million deaths. The second was in 14th century and claimed about 25 million lives (Black Death), wiping out half of population of Europe. The third started in China during 19th century and reached all parts of the world by 20th century. It was in this pandemic that Yersin and Kitasato identified the causative organism in 1894. Plague reached India in 1895–1896.

During early part of 20th century in India, plague constituted a serious problem and many epidemics occurred. In the middle of the century, as a result of large scale application of dichlorodiphenyltrichloroethane (DDT) to control malaria, simultaneously rat fleas were also destroyed, thereby plague was brought under control automatically. India became free from human plague during 1966–1967. The incidence was nil till 1994, when an epidemic was reported from Surat and Gujarat. Recently in 2002 cases were reported from Himachal Pradesh. These facts emphasize the need for continued surveillance of plague in India.

One common observation made during these epidemics was that plague following natural calamities such as floods, which results in death of rats. The rat fleas leave their host and seek human beings for their blood meal. The first sign of plague epidemic is the appearance of dead rats. The phenomenon of 'rat fall' occurs, i.e. rat fall from rafters and dies on the floor. 'Rat fall' is a sign of imminent outbreak among human population.

Thus, plague spells disaster and fatality. It sparks off in us a hidden fear and induces us to flee from it. It is a costly national disaster. The rats cause economic avalanche.

Agent Factors

The etiological agent is a bacillus *Pasteurella pestis*, named after Alexander Yersin and Shibasaburo Kitasato, who discovered it in 1894. So, it is also called '*Yersinia pestis*'. It is gram negative, nonmotile, non-spore forming coccobacillus, giving a 'safety pin' appearance and exhibits 'bipolar' staining with Giemsa or Wayson stain. It grows readily on ordinary culture media in 48 hours and is seen as 'beaten copper' appearance. It produces both exotoxin, endotoxin and fraction 1 (F1) antigen, which are not easily destroyed by the body's defense mechanisms.

These bacilli can survive and multiply in the dust or soil of the burrows of the rat, where the microclimate is favorable for them. These bacilli can easily be destroyed by sunlight and disinfectants (5–10% cresol). They can also be easily destroyed by drugs such as sulfonamides, tetracycline and streptomycin.

Reservoir

Reservoir state is found among both rodent animals and human beings.

Animal reservoir: Among the rodent animals, there are two forms, i.e. sylvan form and urban form.

Sylvan form: Wild rodents constitute the reservoirs. They constitute the natural foci and are the sources for epidemics, i.e. epizootic cycle. During epizootic, the susceptible wild rats are all killed (natural focus is an area where disease persists). However, during interepizootic period, the wild rats remain susceptible to infection, but not the disease. Other wild rodents such as squirrel, rabbits and wild carnivores eating infected rodents may also act as a source of infection. It is called 'sylvatic plague'. *Tatera indica* (wild rodent) and *Bandicota bengalensis* are the main reservoirs. They pass the infection to commensal rodents through peridomestic rodents. Those wild rodents, which are immune to plague, act as carriers and maintain enzootic cycle in natural foci.

Urban form: In this type, commensal infected rodents constitute the reservoir. Important genus are *Rattus rattus* and *Rattus norvegicus*. *Rattus norvegicus* is the sewer rat (brown). It is a great traveler. It lives along with rat fleas on cargo ships and thus spreads the disease among rats from one port to another port all over the world, resulting in pandemics. These live close and interbreed with wild rodents and also domestic rodents. Thus, sewer rat gets the infection from wild rodents and spreads to domestic rodents, *R. rattus* (black rat).

Rattus rattus live in human dwellings and result in domestic plague, which in turn has a potential for producing epidemic.

Human reservoir: Only the cases of pneumonic plague constitute the source of infection to other and not the cases of bubonic plague and septicemic plague. There is no carrier state of plague among human population.

Infected rat fleas also act as a source of infection.

Host Factors

Age and sex incidence: No age and sex is bar from the disease. Plague can occur among people of all ages and both the sexes. Susceptibility is universal.

Immunity: There is no natural immunity. Immunity after recovery lasts for a short period. Thus, susceptibility is universal.

Movement of people: In these days of jet travel, it is possible for a person to get the disease thousands of miles away in a place, where plague is not suspected at all.

Occupation: Plague is not an occupational disease, but it often occurs among those who enter forests for hunting, grazing, cultivation, harvesting, deforestation, etc. predisposing for contact with natural foci.

Environmental Factors

1. Season: In North India, 'plague-season' starts from September to May and in South India, there is no definite season, because of topographic and climatic conditions. However, any environmental condition that disturbs the rodent's natural environment such as floods is a potential source of plague in humans.
2. Temperature and humidity: An atmospheric temperature of 30°C and a relative humidity of 60% and above are considered favorable for the spread of plague, because this favors the survival of the vectors and the development of bacilli in the vectors.
3. Rainfall: Heavy rainfall tends to flood the rat burrow and controls plague.
4. Natural calamities: Such as earth quake, floods war, etc. predispose for epidemics.
5. Housing conditions: Poor housing conditions favor the breeding of rats.
6. Vectors: The most common and most efficient vector of plague is rat flea, *Xenopsylla cheopis*. Other less efficient species of rat fleas are *X. astia* and *X. brasiliensis*. Human flea, *Pulex irritans,* may transmit the disease. In South India, styvalius ahale is the efficient vector. Both the sexes of the rat flea bite and transmit the disease.

These vectors are bilaterally compressed, wingless insects, the shape helping the vectors to move easily among the hairs of the rats. They are blood sucking ectoparasites. When the rat dies of plague, the parasites leave the host and go in search of other rodents and bite the human beings accidentally. A flea ingests about 0.5 mm^3 of blood, containing about 5,000 plague bacilli, which multiply in the proventriculus of the gut and are excreted or regurgitated by the bite. Thus, fleas act as 'amplifier vectors'. After reaching an optimum number, the flea aid to have become infective. The time required for the bacilli, from the time of its entrance till it reaches optimum number is called 'extrinsic incubation period' and that is about 10 days. Once the flea becomes infective, it remains infective for the rest of its life. Whomsoever it bites, spreads the disease. The infected flea may live up to an year. There are two types of infected fleas—blocked flea and partially blocked flea.

7. Blocked flea: It is one in which the proventriculus is fully blocked by a mass of plague bacilli, leaving the stomach empty and leading the flea to starvation. Such a blocked flea, facing starvation and death, makes frantic efforts to release the block by biting. While doing so, it regurgitates some plague bacilli into the wound. This is the common mode of transmission. Such a blocked flea is an efficient transmitter of the disease.
8. Partially blocked flea: It is one wherein the proventriculus is only partially blocked with plague bacilli. Bacilli, leaving a canal in the center. From the epidemiological point of view, a partially blocked flea is more dangerous than a totally blocked flea, because it survives longer and can bite more number of persons, and also the blood is regurgitated with greater force and large number of bacilli will enter into the wound.

Flea Indices

Flea indices are the indicators, which not only help in measuring the density of vectors but also to evaluate the control measures of plague in an area:
1. General flea index (total flea index): It is the average number of fleas of all species, found per rat.
2. Specific flea index (species index): For example, *X. cheopis* index is the average number of *X. cheopis* per rat:

a. This is a more significant index than general flea index.
b. The normal general flea index is 4 (3–5). *X. cheopis* index more than one is indicative of possible outbreak of plague and warranting suitable advance antiplague measures to be instituted. After implementing control measures, again *X. cheopis* is estimated. It must be always less than one. Other indicators of less importance are:
   - Specific percentage of fleas: It is the percentage of fleas of different species found on rats
   - Burrow index: It is the average number of fleas per rodent burrow.

Modes of Transmission

1. Commonest method of transmission of plague is by the bite of infective blocked flea from wild rodent to peridomestic rodents and to domestic rodents, and humans. However, humans can get it from wild rodents, when they enter forests and bitten by fleas.
2. Bubonic plague is not transmitted from man to man, because fleas cannot bite and suck the fluid from the buboes, which are in the closed parts of the body. Therefore bubonic plague is a 'dead-end' infection in man.
3. However, pneumonic plague is transmitted from man to man by droplet infection.
4. Domestic cats eat infected rodents, develop pneumonic plague and spread to humans by droplet infection.
5. Contact transmission is possible from handling infected animals (rats) or infected material-like pus from buboes.
6. Percutaneous transmission is possible following scratching over the dried feces of rat fleas, enabling the inoculation of plague bacilli through the abrasions.
7. Aerosol transmission is also possible by inhalation of infected dust (containing plague bacilli), of the burrows of the rodents, resulting in primary pneumonic plague. This is a suggested form of biological warfare (bioterrorism).

Pathophysiology

From the site of bite by rat flea, the bacilli reach regional lymph nodes, where inflammatory reaction occurs resulting in suppurative enlargement. The bacilli are locked up in buboes. If they enter directly into the circulation, bypassing the lymphatic, results in septicemia. The bacilli release exotoxin, endotoxin and F1 antigens. These result in intravascular damage, hemorrhages in almost all viscera with parenchymatous degeneration. When they lodge in the lungs, there will be congestion, hemorrhages in lungs, resulting in pneumonic plague. Associated with that there will be features of toxemia. They often reach meninges, resulting in meningitis plague.

Incubation period: It is 2–8 days in bubonic and septicemic plague and 1–3 days in pneumonic plague.

Clinical Features

The spectrum of plague is of three types, mainly bubonic plague, septicemic plague and pneumonic plague.

Bubonic Plague (Zoonotic Plague)

Bubonic plague is the commonest type and constitutes 75% of the cases. The illness starts with sudden onset of fever often associated with chills, headache, bodyache and extreme prostration. Sordes appear on teeth, lips and nostrils. Thirst is intense and voice is reduced to whisper. Often there is delirium. Vomiting may often occur.

Regional lymph nodes at the site of bite are enlarged, painful and tender (buboes). Since the frequent site of bite is on the lower extremities, inguinal buboes of that side are common. Less often in the axilla or neck.

In favorable cases, temperature falls, buboes burst releasing foul smelling pus followed by contracture and fibrosis of lymphatic tissue. Bubonic plague is not infectious to others.

Septicemic Plague (Pestis Siderans)

Septicemic plague occurs in about 20% of cases, when the organisms enter directly into the circulation. This is severe and dangerous type. There will be features of septicemia such as high fever, palor, prostration, apathy, delirium followed by stupor, coma and death. There are hemorrhages in the viscera.

Pneumonic Plague (Demic Plague)

Pneumonic plague occurs in about 5–10% of cases. Patient will have all features of pneumonia, such as high fever, cough, dyspnea, sputum, frothy and blood-tinged (in lobar pneumonia, the sputum is rusty and viscid). Clouding of consciousness is marked. Most roles are audible at the base of the lungs. Cyanosis is developed later, because of poor oxygenation of blood. Pleural effusion is usually present. Later delirium sets in, patient becomes stuporous, develops coma and thus dies within 4–5 days. This is highly infectious type.

Meningitis Plague

Meninges are involved as a complication in 1% or 2% of case. Patient will have all features of meningitis.

Mortality of plague is very high during epidemics, varying from 60 to 90%. Modern treatment has reduced the mortality.

Laboratory Investigations

- Staining: Smears of bubo fluid or sputum, stained with Giemsa stain
- Wayson stain to look for bipolar stained bacilli
- Culture of sputum, blood or bubo fluid to look for colonies of beaten copper appearance
- Serology test is done for antibody titer
- Leukocyte count: There will be associated leukocytosis (0–20,000 cells/mm^3)
- Animal inoculation: This is done in guinea pigs or mice, died due to plague.

Prevention and Control of Plague

The prevention and control of plague consists of following three major procedures:
- Elimination of reservoirs:
  - Elimination of human reservoirs
  - Human reservoirs and animal reservoirs (rodents).
- Breaking the channel of transmission
- Protection of susceptibles.

Elimination or Control of Human Reservoirs

Elimination or control of human reservoirs (cases) by the following measures:
1. Early diagnosis: 'Rat-falls' (death of rats) provide a warning signal of imminent outbreak.
2. Large number of people suffering from fever and painful enlargement of lymph nodes (buboes) helps to make a clinical (community) diagnosis.
3. Notification: The information of occurrence of cases is notified to the concerned health authorities as early as possible, so that control measures will be implemented.
4. Isolation is necessary for cases of pneumonic plague only, because of its infectiousness. They constitute medical emergency, period of isolation should be at least for 5 full days of chemotherapy.
5. Concurrent disinfection of sputum and patient's belongings must be disinfected; 5% cresol is used.
6. Chemotherapy: Drug of choice is tetracycline 2 g a day for 10 days (500 mg, 6th hourly) sulfonamides is next best.
7. Injection streptomycin is also a very effective antibiotic, but it may result in massive destruction of plague bacilli. Bacilli, release of endotoxin and further complications so not preferred. Dose of 30 mg/kg body weight for 10 days.
8. Chloramphenicol is good in plague meningitis, because it can pass through the blood brain barrier.

Control of Animal Reservoirs (Rodents)

Control of wild rodents is neither practicable nor feasible. Commensal rodents can be controlled as follows.

Trapping of rats: This is done by using poisonous baits containing arsenic, warfarin (an anticoagulant) or zinc oxide, but fleas escape. So, it is not a good method.

Cyanogas fumigation: This is a very effective method. This is done by using cyanogas pump. Calcium cyanide, a white powder, when pumped into the burrows of the rats and closed with mud, comes in contact with moisture, releases hydrocyanic acid, which when inhaled is lethal. This method not only destroys rat but also rat fleas. But the disadvantages are:
- It has to be carried out frequently, because the effect does not last longer
- Rats living in the roof escape
- Persons doing this work are at risk; sulfur dioxide fumigation is also effective.

Use of DDT or benzene hexachloride (BHC): Since DDT is not very effective, 10% be insufflated into the burrows of the rats and sprinkled all along the rat ruins (the passage where usually the rats run). The residual effect lasts for about 3–6 months. Powders containing 1.5% dieldrin or 2% aldrin applied to rat holes and rat remain active for 9–12 weeks. This helps to control rat fleas. Construction of rat-proof godowns:
- The door must be made of metal
- There must be projection of 5 feet called 'ledge' to prevent rats climbing up
- Ventilators must have mesh.

Breaking the Channel of Transmission

- Droplet mode of transmission from cases of pneumonic plague can be prevented by concurrent disinfection of patient's sputum in 5–10% cresol
- Vectors (rat fleas) can be controlled by cyanogas fumigation and insufflation of burrows of the rats with DDT or BHC.

Protection of Susceptibles

Protection of susceptibles is by chemoprophylaxis and immunoprophylaxis.

Chemoprophylaxis

Chemoprophylaxis consists of administration of drugs for those who are at risk of plague such as family contacts, medical and nursing staff attending the patients. Drug of choice is tetracycline 500 mg, 6th hourly for 1 week. Alternative drug is sulfonamide, 3–5 mg daily for 1 week. Susceptible persons also have to be protected by wearing gowns, gloves and masks.

Immunoprophylaxis (vaccination)

Killed vaccine is available, developed by Haffkine (1897) modified by Sokhey. It is a formalin-killed vaccine. Each mL consists of 2,000 million killed, *Yersinia pestis* bacilli. Primary course for adult male consists of two doses, 1.0 mL and 1.5 mL with an interval of 1–2 weeks, given subcutaneously less for children and infants below 6 months do not require vaccination. Vaccination after the outbreak of plague is useless.

However, during the fear of outbreak at least 1 week before, only one dose of double the routine dose (i.e. 3 mL for adult male) is recommended.

Immunity develops after 1 week of inoculation and lasts for 6 months regularly for those, who are at risk such as geologists, biologists and anthropologists. Immunization is also recommended for travelers to hyperendemic areas. It is 50% protective.

Since the vaccine provides only tissue immunity and not humoral immunity, it is not protective against pneumonic plague. Pregnancy is a contraindication, because of its potential risk to result in abortions or fetal damage.

Other measures of control

- Surveillance of susceptible areas
- Health education of the people about the sanitation in and around the houses, not to keep food grains in open containers, not to sleep on the floor, not to go to jungle areas and about their cooperation to inform about ratfalls, so that control measures can be undertaken.

Note: Plague is now no more a quarantinable disease.

Treatment

The cases detected with plaque should be treated with antibiotics. Health education regarding the cause, clinical manifestations, prevention and treatment should be provided to community. With the knowledge of clinical manifestations, people who get infection can be reported by the people to health authority. This is also important to achieve the cooperation of community in achieving prevention and control of plaque.

Nursing Management of Plague

Isolation

Every nurse who undertakes the nursing care of plague should be protected by vaccination against the disease, except under most unusual circumstances. The medical aseptic technique will prevent the spread of plague, in either bubonic or septicemic forms. The bubonic type is not transmissible by contact, unless a bubo is draining. In the septicemic type aseptic technique must be observed, because of the possibility of pneumonia and droplet infection. The pneumonic form presents the greatest problem, because in this type the disease is transmitted from person to person by droplet infection. Formerly almost 100% fatal, the pneumonic form is amenable to treatment with the newer anti-infective drugs, but it is still so deadly that extra precautions must be taken in nursing to safeguard all concerned. The patient should be placed in a quiet, private and well-ventilated room. All attendants, doctor, nurse, maid or porter should wear the completely protective uniform; which was described under the heading 'Isolation', earlier in this chapter. Concurrent disinfection should be rigidly practiced. Everything leaving the room must first be placed inside a container in which it is either cleaned immediately or removed from the ward. Soiled linen and clothing should be placed inside a clean laundry bag in which they can be sterilized before being sent for laundering. Dishes, water pitchers, trays, emesis basins, bedpans and urinals should be sterilized before washing. 'Cedarsweet' or O'Cedar oil will keep the floor reasonably free of flying dust or lint. DDT, used as a spray, will eradicate insects in the room.

Diet

Plague patients are very sick. The temperature is high. Nausea and vomiting are often present. This makes it imperative that the patient receive sufficient food and fluid. Liquids must be supplied by one means or another. If nauseated, small amounts of chipped ice or fluid, offered frequently may be retained. Water, fruit juice with either honey or sugar added, milk in any form, soups, gruels, ice cream or gelatin may be given. Later, as the patient's condition improves, the diet may be increased to meet his/her needs.

Temperature

The temperature is characteristically high in both the septicemic and pneumonic forms, and at times in the bubonic form. The temperature may be reduced by either tepid or cool sponges. Alcohol rubs or alcohol fans may be given. In severe cases, a wet-sheet pack will be less exhausting to the patient. An ice cap to the head is helpful. Fluids should be forced to the point of tolerance. The temperature should be recorded at least every 3 hours.

Personal Hygiene

The patient should be given a daily cleansing bath, alcohol being gently rubbed over all pressure points. If the patient is incontinent, the buttocks area should be washed and thoroughly dried as indicated. Good oral hygiene must be maintained. In pneumonic plague, the mouth is characteristically quite dirty. The profuse bloody sputum must be wiped from the lips and frequent mouthrinses given. If the patient is too sick to cooperate the mouth, teeth and tongue may be cleansed with gauze pledgets or swabs.

Elimination

The bowels should move well once daily. Either laxative or enemas may be used as indicated. Neither retention nor suppression of urine is common; however, this must be watched for in any patient who is acutely ill. A record of fluid output should be kept.

General Management of the Disease

Because of the seriousness of the patient's condition a quiet, private room should be provided. Everything possible must be done for the patient's comfort. The eyes are to be protected from bright light. The bedding is to be light in weight, but sufficiently warm. Frequently, alcohol rubs over pressure points are indicated. The nurse should watch for and report any unusual signs or symptoms, being especially alert for the beginning signs of pneumonia.

Terminal Disinfection

When the patient is removed from the unit all contaminated space, the bed, the table and chairs should be washed with soap and water. The mattress, the pillow, all bedding, the patient's clothing and the nurse's contaminated gown should be sterilized before being laundered. All dishes, basins, pitchers, irrigating cans and tips, bedpans and urinals should be sterilized before washing. All waste material should be sent to the incinerator in a clean paper bag. The floors should be swept with 'cedarsweet' and then mopped with soap and water.

Convalescence

It is slow. The patient should be cautioned to return to normal activity slowly. He/she should be given a good wholesome diet and be provided with some recreational activity, such as radio, games and reading material.

HUMAN SALMONELLOSIS

Human salmonellosis is endemic throughout the world. The disease occurs sporadically in small outbreaks in general population. It usually occurs from contaminated food at source. About 60–80% salmonellosis are found in all food-borne infections.

Agent

The causative organ is salmonellosis, which are commonly found in the feces of household pets, such as dogs and animals, and in most farm animals, particularly in the feces and eggs of domestic food. The organism can survive in food of any kind for years and they are resistant to drying, salting, smoking and freezing. The common ones causing infection are *Salmonella typhimurium*, *S. choleraesis*, *S. montevideo*, *Salmonella newport*, *S. oranienburg* and *S. Paratyphi* A and C. The reservoir of salmonellae is gastrointestinal tract of humans and also present in animals. The primary reason of this disease is commercially prepared food such as meats, poultry and egg products. The predisposing causes consist of infected food handles.

Host

Salmonellosis occurs among any age group of population exposed to contaminated food, animal, man or environment irrespective of sex.

Environment

As stated earlier, the organisms salmonellae are present in environment and can survive in soil for months. The individual came in contact with such environment can be infected as the organisms present in his/her surroundings dust, water, manure, sludge, vegetables, insects and rodents.

Transmission

The disease can be transmitted through by direct contact and/or fecal-oral route. The incubation period is usually 6–72 hours. Whereas, massive infective dose in ingested or in the epidemic cases, the incubation period averages 12 hours, but varies from 4 to 38 hours.

Clinical Manifestation

The onset is characteristically abrupt, with concured nausea and vomiting, severe diarrhea, abdominal cramps, tenderness of the abdomen and dome fever symptoms vary from severe to mild. Depending upon the individual. Diarrhea, the constant symptoms always present. The stools are offensive and putrefactive at first, later becoming watery, greenish and often bloody, nausea is likewise invariably present, but vomiting occasionally absent. Fever varies from 99.6 to 106°F chills or chillness, headache, mental depression or apprehension and restlessness are usually present from the start and are followed by insomnia or delirious and in severe cases coma and death. Diagnosis is made by history of ingestion of food as common source, clinical manifestation and laboratory investigations show as blood culture and stool culture.

Prevention and Control

1. Early diagnosis and treatment: The cases of human salmonellosis should be diagnosed and treated as early as possible.
2. Prevention of food contamination: This can be achieved by initiating preventive measures at farm and embracing all the elements of food chain of processing, handling, preparation, etc.
3. Immunization: All the farm animals should be immunized against salmonellosis.
4. Sanitary environment: The environment should be hygienic where the animals live. It means there is need to ensure a sanitary environment for animals.
5. Pasteurization of milk: The milk should be pasteurized and if not possible, it should be boiled before drinking.
6. Proper disposal of liquid and solid wastes: Liquid and solid waste should be disposed of a proper way, so as to prevent contamination of food, soil, water, etc.
7. Hygienic slaughtering: It is one of the important measures to prevent the human salmonellosis.
8. Health education: The awareness regarding the chain of food preparation, i.e. production, processing, storage, handling and food preparation among the public will reduce the morbidity and mortality associated with salmonellosis:
   - Streptomycin: 30 mg/kg of body weight in two divided doses daily for 7–10 days
   - Tetracycline: 30–40 mg/kg of body weight daily as an alternative or in combination of streptomycin.

Nursing Management of Salmonellosis

Isolation

While in the past it has not been thought necessary to isolate patients suffering from *Salmonella* fever or food poisoning, there is a distinct tendency today to treat them exactly like bacillary dysentery or typhoid fever. Known carriers exist and while the disease is usually of short duration and not severe, at other times it is very severe and death does occur, particularly in children.

Diet

During the acute symptoms, food should be withheld. Usually the patient has nausea, vomiting and diarrhea. Fluids may be given; even though not retained, they act as a stomach lavage. Fruit juices are contraindicated. Hot drinks are preferred; hot water, hot tea, hot coffee, or hot milk may be given. If temperatures are high, these fluids may be given warmed to body temperature. If fluids cannot be retained by mouth, they may be given intravenously or by hypodermoclysis, upon the physician's order. A record of fluid intake should be kept. The patient returns to a normal diet gradually after symptoms subside.

Temperature

As a rule, the temperature is not high enough to become a problem. It ranges from normal to 102°F occasionally; however, it may go so high that it becomes necessary to reduce it. A tepid sponge bath is the method of choice. An ice cap to the head will help. If the patient has a chilly sensation or a true chill, or if the skin is cold and moist, and the pulse thready, the external heat should be applied. In fact, when small children are brought to the hospital in extreme shock due to dehydration and fever, shock therapy will have to be applied. Hot blankets are immediately applied. Hot water bottles may be used, if precautions are taken to avoid burning sensation of the patient. Hypodermic administration of eschaton or adrenaline every 15 minutes until the pulse is reduced and the patient out of shock may be of greatest value, temperature, pulse and respirations should be recorded every 3–4 hours. The quality of the pulse particularly should be noted and recorded. Pulse and respiration should be recorded every 3 hours. The nurse should look for and report a sudden drop in temperature or an increased pulse rate; these may mean internal hemorrhages or perforation. Bloody or tarry stools should be noted and reported to the physician immediately. If the patient complains of abdominal pain or if the abdomen becomes harder and more tender, perforation must be suspected, and the physician should be notified at once.

When hemorrhage is suspected, the foot of the bed should be elevated, pillows should be removed; everything by mouth should be withheld; and current orders should be suspended. The patient should be kept as quiet as possible and a lightly filled ice cap applied to the abdomen.

CHAPTER 32 — Zoonoses: Bacterial

Morphine is usually given to retard peristalsis and also to quiet the patient. This must never be given, however, except upon order of the physician. Transfusions are usually given, if hemorrhage has developed.

If the patient develops symptoms of pneumonia, penicillin may be prescribed. Increased room humidity often helps to relieve the cough. To prevent meteorism, the lower bowel should be kept open and the nurse should exclude from the diet, any food or combination of foods, which the patient does not tolerate well. If tympanitis becomes a problem, relief usually can be obtained by the use of turpentine stupes and gentle low enemas composed of one part magnesium sulfate, two parts glycerin and three parts water. A rectal tube often affords relief. The nurse should be particular in giving an enema in typhoid fever, when the bowel is distended with gas, as the danger of perforation is believed to be greatest at that time.

Elimination

Cathartics should not be used. As a matter of fact, when first seen these patients are usually having diarrhea accompanied by griping abdominal pains. The problem is usually of stopping the dehydration and diarrhea. Dark, scanty urine may indicate that the patient is not retaining sufficient fluid. A record of fluid intake and output should be kept. Either diarrhea or constipation are common symptoms. If constipation is troublesome small enemas usually are prescribed. A small saline or oil enema (one point or less), given slowly and with low pressure, usually is sufficient. A careful record of fluid intake and output should be kept.

General Management of the Disease

The patient should be kept warm and disturbed as little as possible. Abdominal pains often can be relieved by the application of hot and moist packs. If the patient appears to be prostrated, external heat should be applied and hot liquids given.

The patient should be in a comfortable bed in a quiet, well-ventilated room. Special attention should be given to the back and to all pressure points to prevent pressure sores from developing. The position should be changed frequently at least every 3–4 hours. Pressure points should be bathed with warm water and soap several times each day, and rubbed dry after which a brisk alcohol rub should be given. If the skin is thin and dry, a baby oil rub instead of alcohol is helpful. The draw sheet should be kept free from wrinkles, with plenty of talcum in the bed. If a reddened area appears over a pressure point, compound tincture of benzoin painted over the area will give added protection.

Foam rubber pads, air cushions and small comfort pillows prove helpful if used at intervals.

Convalescence

While the acute symptoms usually are of short duration, from a few hours to a day or two, occasionally the last weeks and even months. Also, in many of these cases, relapse sets in after they are apparently on the road to recovery. The convalescent period may be unduly long. While it is usually only a few days to a week before these patients can regain normal activity, at times it is months. Again, depending upon the community in which they live, they may not be released to normal activity until the health department releases them after two or more stools have been found free from the particular causative *Salmonella* organism. Characteristically this is slow. The possibility of relapse is to be kept in mind, particularly since chloromycetin has come to be the method of treatment. Following use of this drug, relapses are much more frequently seen than formerly. The patient should be confined to bed until the pulse rate is normal. He/she should get up gradually, increasing the length of time out of bed each day, provided he/she does not develop an increase in pulse rate or excessive fatigue. Until convalescence has become well-established, the patient should be warned to avoid any exercise sufficiently strenuous to increase his/her pulse rate.

Terminal Disinfection

Terminal disinfection is usually practiced as in typhoid fever or dysentery.

The mouth in typhoid is characteristically dirty. The tongue is heavily coated and the lips and teeth also may be crusted and dry. All tend to develop sordes, a dark brown, tenacious covering of foul smelling material. Sordes may be prevented by an adequate mouth toilet; its presence is always a sign of poor nursing. There probably is nothing that will contribute to the comfort and well-being of the patient more than the proper care of the mouth. The teeth and tongue should be cleaned as often as necessary to keep sordes from accumulating. Equal parts of hydrogen peroxide and water make an excellent solution for cleaning them. Any good antiseptic mouthwash may be used as a mouthrinse both before and after nourishment is taken. Cold cream or other bland ointments may be applied to the lips and help to relieve dryness. When the patient is discharged as noninfectious he/she should be given a complete cleansing bath and shampoo, dressed in clean clothing and placed in a clean area.

All treatment equipment contaminated by the patient should be sterilized and then thoroughly cleaned up. The bedding and contaminated clothing should be sterilized before sending them to the laundry. The wall, bed, table and chairs should be washed with soap and water for better, yet rubbed down with 1:3,000 zephiran chloride solution. The mattress and pillows should be aired, preferably in the sun, for 6 hours.

ANTHRAX

Anthrax is an acute infection disease common to sheep and cattle occurring sporadically in man in three forms, i.e. the cutaneous, the pulmonary and the intestinal in man. The disease occurs only in those, who become infected from material connected with diseased animal.

Agent

Anthracis derived from the Greek word anthrakis, which translates into 'coal' because it causes dark, coal-like structure on affected areas. Anthrax is considered to be the first germ discovered to cause disease in humans.

Bacillus anthracis is a gram-positive, non-acid-fast, nonmotile, large (3–10 μm × 1–6 μm), rectangular, spore-forming bacillus. The spores are refractile, oval and central in position, and are of the same width as the bacillary body so that they do not cause bulging of vegetative cell.

In cultures, the bacilli are arranged end-to-end in long chains. The ends of the bacilli are truncated or often concave and somewhat swollen so that a chain of bacilli presents as a bamboo-stick appearance (Fig. 32.1).

Host

The disease occurs in person, who is hide serapers or tanners as those whose occupation brings them into contact with animals and animal products such as woolsorter and butcher are especially liable to contact the disease.

Environment

The person who living such environment where more sheep and cattle rearing and supplies takes place.

Transmission

Incubation is by accidental wound or scratch, inhalation of spores of the infection of insufficiently cooked infected meat. The period of communicability lasts during the fertile stage of the disease and until lesions have ceased discharging infected hair and hides of infected animals may communicate the disease for many months after slaughter of animals and even after the curing of the hide fur or human discharge.

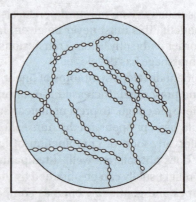

Figure 32.1: Anthrax bacilli

Clinical Manifestation

As studied earlier there are three types of anthrax, such as cutaneous anthrax, pulmonary anthrax and gastrointestinal anthrax.

Cutaneous Anthrax

Cutaneous anthrax usually occurs in arms, hands or face at the site of some abrasions of the skin, which admits infection. A few hours after infection, the site becomes hot and itchy. Occasionally symptoms are delayed for as long as 6 days. In rapid succession a papulae forms, which quickly vesiculated and hardened inflamed area soon surrounds it. The vesicle may appear pustular, but when picked only bloody serum exudes not pus, so the clinical manifestation includes macular or popular, skin lesions, vesicles, which discharge clear or serosanguineous fluid, painless black eschar and painful lymphadenopathy.

Pulmonary or Inhalation Anthrax

The pulmonary form occurs almost entirely in woolsorters and hair handlers or more rarely among rag pickers. The clinical manifestation of this type includes fever, malaria, dyspnea, cough, headache, vomiting, chills abdominal pain, chest pain, diaphoresis, cyanosis and moracie lymphadenitis. This type kills up to 80% of infected persons within 2–4 days. It is 99% lethal in non-vaccination individuals.

Gastrointestinal Anthrax

Gastrointestinal anthrax is enteric form of anthrax, which results from eating infected meat, drinking infected milk or from contamination of food by contact within external form and it is associated with undercooked contaminated meat.

The onset is with chill committing, diarrhea, moderate fever and severe back and leg pain. The breathing becomes difficult, the patient looks very worried and anxious.

Convulsion occurs and death ensues. Petechiae occur on mucous membrane of the mouth and skin, and the spleen is enlarged. The blood is very dark and remains unclotted for some time after death. Death occurs in 24 hours to a week. To sum up, clinical manifestation will appear 2–4 days after ingestion, which will include nausea, vomiting, abdominal pain, bloodstained member, malaise bloody diarrhea, acute abdominal sepsis and ascites. Since it is very difficult to diagnose earlier the mortal rates are high. Intestinal perforation or anthrax toxemia is the usual causes of death. The mortality is due to blood loss, electrolyte imbalance and subsequent stock.

Prevention Measures and Treatment

1. Health education regarding disease and its causes, and advise them to take precautions accordingly.
2. Vaccination consists of six initial doses of 0.2 and 4 weeks and 6, 12 and 18 months followed by a yearly booster.
3. Treatment will be efficacious of initiated during the incubation period. The disease progresses rapidly once symptoms are recognized.

The treatment for bacillus anthracis infection is detailed in Table 32.1.

Nursing Management

Isolation

The medical aseptic technique will prevent the spread of anthrax. The causative organisms are found in the skin lesions in the external form, in the sputum of the pulmonary form, in the spinal fluid of the meningeal form and in the stools of the gastrointestinal form. All articles soiled with discharges suspected of harboring these organisms should be cleaned up or incinerated immediately after use. Remember that these organisms are spore formers. The nurse caring for anthrax should wear rubber gloves when doing anything that brings his/her hands in contact with anything soiled with infectious secretions. A small skin abrasion, a hangnail or a scratch that ordinarily might go unnoticed, may be the means by which one contracts the disease. When nursing the pneumonic type, some hospitals prefer that the nurse be masked. If technique is not most strictly enforced, an impervious mask is preferably worn.

Diet

In average case the diet may be anything that the patient desires. During the stage of high fever, nourishing liquids and soft diets are given. Fluids should be urged.

Temperature

The temperature is usually quite high in the systemic form varying from 103 to 105°F at the onset. In cases of malignant pustule, it is surprising how ugly the lesion may look and how free from fever the patient may be. When fever requires lowering, the usual measures are satisfactory, such as alcohol fans, tepid sponges or colonic flushing. Enemas or colonic hushing should never be given except upon the physician's order.

After treatment is started, the temperature declines rapidly as a rule. In fact, the patient frequently feels so well that it is difficult to get him/her to remain in bed and submit to treatment.

Elimination

The bowels should move at least once a day. Enemas are given when indicated, except in the gastrointestinal form. If retention of urine occurs catheterization may be done.

General Management of the Disease

A quiet, well-ventilated, private room is advisable, because the patient usually is quite sick at the onset; at times, in spite of every effort to control the disease, the patient may remain sick for days. Penicillin or neomycin packs are usually prescribed for the external lesions. If the lesion is on the face, the nurse should report any sudden rise in temperature, severe headache or stiff neck. When the lesion is on the chest, edema may spread to the glottis. This may result in respiratory embarrassment with cyanosis, rapid pulse and extreme restlessness. This condition should be reported immediately, as a tracheotomy may be indicated to the patient's life.

If the patient does not respond favorably to treatment, he/she may remain extremely sick or even get worse, with very high fever delirium and prostration. When this occurs the patient needs constant care, observation and supervision. Usually restraints are necessary, profuse sweating is common. Change of clothing and alcohol rubs, change of position, good oral hygiene and forced fluids are important points in nursing care.

Table 32.1: Treatment for anthrax

Pharmacologic therapy	Dosage for adults	Dosage for children
Penicillin V	200–400 mg orally four times per day	25–50 mg/kg of body weight/day orally in divided doses two to four times/day
Penicillin G	8 million–12 million U total, intravenously in 4–6 h	100,000–150,000 U/kg/day in divided doses every 4–6 h
Streptomycin	30 mg/kg intramuscularly or intravenously per day	
Tetracycline	250–500 mg orally or intravenously four times per day	Tetracycline is not approved for children
Doxycycline	200 mg orally or intravenously as a loading dose, then 50–100 mg every 12 h	Doxycycline is not approved for children < 9 year old
Erythromycin	250 mg orally every 12 h	40 mg/kg/day orally in divided doses every 6 h
Erythromycin lactobionate	15–20 mg/kg intravenously per day	20–40 mg/kg/day intravenously in divided doses every 6 h
Chloramphenicol divided	50–100 mg/kg/day orally or intravenously 6 h	50–75 mg/kg/day in doses every 6 h
Ciprofloxacin	250–750 mg orally twice/ day; 200–400 mg intravenously every 12 h	20–30 mg/kg/day in divided doses every 12 h; oral or intravenous dosing is not approved for patients <18 year old
Prophylaxis		
Doxycycline	100 mg orally twice/day for 4 week	
Ciprofloxacin	500 mg orally twice/day for 4 week, 0.75–0.90 mg/kg/day	
Corticosteroid	Therapy for severe edema orally, intravenously, or intramuscularly in divided every 6 h doses every 6 h 1–2 mg/kg or 5–60	Prednisone 0.5-2 mg/kg/day mg orally/day
Dexamethasone	0.75 mL	

Convalescence

Once started, convalescence is usually uneventful, normal activities should be resumed gradually nursery, at any time after the beginning of symptoms should be considered as contacts, isolated and watched carefully for any beginning symptoms for a period of 2 weeks.

Clean newborn infants should not be admitted to a nursery from which an infected baby has been removed until all other babies have been removed from the nursery, the nursery has been thoroughly cleaned up and a period of 2 weeks has elapsed. To clean the nursery, walls, bassinets, tables, chairs and scales should be washed thoroughly with soap and water. All bedding, blankets, sheets, clothing, basins, formula and water bottles, nipples, breck feeder, medicine droppers, cotton and applicators should be autoclaved. The mattress should be sunned in the open air for at least 8 hours. The mattress cover should be washed with soap and water, and dried in the open air. Thermometers should be washed with soap and water, rinsed in clean water, and immersed in zephiran solution, 1:1,000, for 1 hour, or they may be washed in soap and water, rinsed in clean water, dried, and placed in 70% alcohol for 1 hour.

Medicine bottles, ointment jars and solution bottles should be emptied, washed and autoclaved. Pens, pencils and ink bottles should be washed with soap and water, and dried in the open air. Paper tags, chart forms, record sheets, writing paper and similar objects may be autoclaved. Rubber tubing may be boiled. Oxygen face masks may be washed with soap and water, and dried in the open air. It is important that not one article from the contaminated room shall be overlooked or left as a possible source of infection for the next newly admitted newborn baby. After everything in the room has been cleaned, the floor should be washed with soap and water, and the room aired for 24 hours before admitting any new patients.

After a baby has recovered from epidemic diarrhea of the newborn, he/she should not be returned to a clean nursery. When this disease occurs, the entire ward personnel should be checked for possible sources of infection. The doctors and nurses, who have the care of babies with this disease should not attend clean infants (while this is universally taught, 2 years ago some 60 babies with epidemic diarrhea of the newborn were transferred to our service and handled by the usual medical aseptic technique within the building, the doctors and nurses going about their usual pursuits with no cross infection).

Visitors should be restricted. The baby should be weighed daily and a graphic weight chart kept. The baby's position should be changed at least every 3 or 4 hours. If stools are not too frequent, the buttocks should be exposed to the air or heat lamp for 20–30 minutes every 4–6 hours.

Rectal swabs are sent to laboratory at the first signs of infection to rule out the possibility of diarrhea of bacterial or other origin. If the patient recovers convalescence is uneventful.

Terminal Disinfection

When the patient is ready to be discharged, he/she should be given a complete bath and shampoo, dressed in clean.

LEPTOSPIROSIS

There are various communicable diseases, which are the major cause of mortality and morbidity among human beings in the worldwide, among these diseases, some are zoonotic, mosquito-borne diseases and some are primarily infecting the man himself. Among the zoonotic diseases, leptospirosis is one of the bacterial diseases, which affects humans and animals.

Weil is credited with first describing leptospirosis as a unique disease process in 1886, therefore it is also known as Weil's disease:
- Leptospirosis is essentially animal infection by several serotypes of *Leptospira* (a spirochete) and transmitted to man under certain environmental conditions
- Leptospirosis is a bacterial disease that affects humans and animals
- It is caused by bacteria of genus leptospiraceae and order spirochaetales.

Magnitude of the Problem

- Leptospirosis is a worldwide zoonosis, it is considered to be the most widespread of the disease transmittable from animal to man
- It has high prevalence in warm humid tropical countries
- Hawaii in USA is the state with highest reported incidence of leptospirosis (in 1998–1999 Hawaii reported 405 suspected cases, 61 of those were confirmed)
- Other high-risk areas of the world are Caribbean Islands, Central and South America, Southeast Asia, and Pacific Islands
- Outbreaks mostly occur as a result of heavy rainfall and consequent flooding.

In India

1. It has been known to occur in India since long ago. Reports indicate that it is fairly widespread throughout India.
2. Recently, there was outbreak of leptospirosis in Odisha after the devastating cyclone of 29th October, 1999.
3. Later on in the month of August 2000, there were cases of leptospirosis in Gujarat, Kerala, Maharashtra, and Andaman and Nicobar Islands.

Epidemiological Features

Agent Factors

Agent

Leptospira is a thin, motile spirochete, which is 0.1–0.2 rhm wide and 5–15 rhm long with hooked ends. There are more than 23 different strains of identified types, among them *Leptospira interrogans* are the pathogenic. These are spiral bacteria, 5–20 μm × 0.1 μm with numerous closely set coils and hooked ends (Fig. 32.2). They stain poorly with aniline dyes, but can be observed by fluorescent antibody and silver impregnation techniques. Because of narrow diameter, they are best observed by dark ground, phase-contrast or electron microscopy.

Source of infection

Leptospira is excreted in the urine of infected animals for a long time; humans become infected through contact with water, food or soil containing urine from infected animals.

Animal reservoirs

Leptospirosis affects wild and domestic animals worldwide, especially rodents such as rats and mice, other animal's reservoirs are pigs, horses, cattle, sheep, goats, water buffaloes, dogs, etc. Infection may spread from wild animals to domestic livestock and then to human beings.

Age

Report shows it is more common among children; more than 40% of cases were younger than 15 years. Children acquire infection from dogs more frequently than the adults.

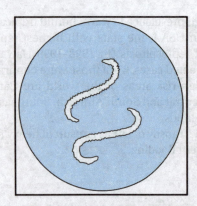

Figure 32.2: *Leptospira* (dark ground illumination)

Host Factors

Sex
Males are more prone, probably resulting from occupational and recreational exposure.

Occupation
Human infections are usually due to occupational exposure to the urine of infected animals. For example, agricultural and livestock farmers; workers in rice fields, sugarcane fields, underground sewers, meat and animal handlers, veterinary workers, etc.

Leisure time exposure such as swimming and fishing may also carry a risk.

Immunity
A solid serovar specific immunity follows the infection.

Environmental Factors
1. Leptospirosis is acquired through contact with an environment contaminated by urine and feces from infected or carrier animals.
2. *Leptospira* can survive in water for as many as 16 days and in the soil for as many as 24 days, so environmental contamination may reach high levels in areas where carrier animals frequently urinate, the other environmental factors such as poor housing, limited water supply, inadequate method or waste disposal all combine to make the disease significant risk for poor population both in urban and rural areas.

Mode of Transmission
1. *Direct contact:* *Leptospira* can enter the body through skin abrasions or through intact mucus membrane by direct contact with urine and tissue of infected animals.
2. *Indirect contact:* Through the contact of the broken skin with soil, water or vegetation contaminated by urine or infected animals or through ingestion of food, or water contaminated with *Leptospira*.
3. *Droplet infection:* Infection may also occur through inhalation as when milking infected cows or goats by breathing air polluted with droplets of urine, direct man-to-man spread of infection is rare.

Incubation period: Usually 10 days with a range of 4–20 days.

Pathophysiology
- Once the organism enters the body, it produces endotoxin and causes hemolysis and multiorgan tissue injury occurs
- Leptospirosis findings show that there will be vasculitis of capillaries, characterized by endothelial edema, necrosis and lymphatic infiltration
- Capillary vasculitis is found in every affected organ, resulting in:
  - Loss of red blood cells (RBCs)
  - Loss of fluids through the edematous capillaries
  - Capillary vasculitis and leakage: Which causes petechiae, intraparenchymal bleeding, bleeding in serosa and mucosa.

In the liver: Vascular congestions, hepatic injury from hemolysis and biliary obstruction causes jaundice.

Pulmonary findings: Alveolar capillary injury causes intraalveolar edema and bleeding by vasculitis in severe cases frank hemorrhage occurs and hemoptysis may also occur.

Renal findings: Tubular necrosis, interstitial nephritis causing decreased glomerular filtration rate (decreased GFR) and leads to renal failure.

Cardiac finding: Petechiae in epicardium and endocardium, and myocardial interstitial edema and myocarditis, and coronary arteritis in 70% cases.

Central nervous system findings: Meningitis and meningeal infection, adrenal gland infiltration may lead to adrenal insufficiency, which further leads to fatal leptospirosis.

Clinical Manifestations
The clinical manifestations may vary from mild febrile illness to severe illness, sometimes may be fatal disease with liver, kidney and brain involvement leptospirosis symptoms may be explained in two phases:
1. First phase: Illness usually begins abruptly with:
   - Fever
   - Chills
   - Headache

- Muscle aches and rashes
- Vomiting or diarrhea.

The patient may recover for a time, but becomes ill again, if not taken proper treatment.

2. **Second phase:** If the second phase occurs, it is more severe with the involvement of liver and kidney failure and meningitis, this phase is called Weil's disease. It is characterized by:
   - Jaundice
   - Abdominal pain
   - Hemoptysis
   - Symptoms of meningeal irritation
   - Decreased urine output and leads to anuria
   - Acute renal failure.

Complications

- Renal failure
- Liver failure
- Meningitis
- Cardiovascular problems
- Anemia
- Vision loss
- Acute respiratory distress syndrome.

Diagnosis

- Blood for culture
- Urine for culture
- Kidney biopsy: All these tests show growth/presence of organisms
- Blood for Hb% to rule out anemia
- Kidney function tests: Blood urea nitrogen and serum creatinine to rule out the abnormality with kidney functions
- Liver function tests: Liver enzymes, serum bilirubin and albumin, urine bilirubin and bile salts assessment
- Bile pigments
- Cerebrospinal fluid for culture to rule out meningitis
- Enzyme-linked immunosorbent assay (ELISA) test is also done for early diagnosis, but expensive, leptodipstick is also available now.

Differential Diagnosis

Since, the leptospirosis is manifested with many symptoms, it may be mistaken for:
- Dengue fever
- Other hemorrhagic fevers
- Hepatitis
- Viral meningitis
- Malaria
- Typhoid fever.

Treatment

Medical Management

Antibiotics: Penicillin is the drug of choice.

Adult dosage: 1.5 million units intravascular (IV) 6th hourly for 7 days.

Pediatric dosage: 100,000 units/kg/day in four divided doses for 7 days.

Other antibiotics: Doxycycline.

Adult dosage: 100 mg bd for 7 days for adults.

Children dose: As follows:
- < 8 years: Not recommended
- > 8 years: 4 mg/kg/day in two divided doses for 7 days.

Ampicillin: It can be given for children as a second line of antibiotic, if patient is less than 8 years in whom doxycycline is contraindicated.

Adult dosage: 750 mg, 6th hourly for 7 days orally.

Children: 75–100 mg/kg/day orally in four divided doses for 7 days.

Amoxicilline: Management as given below.

Adult dosage: 500 mg, 6th hourly for 7 days.

Children dosage: 50 mg/kg/day in four divided doses.

For high-risk adults; as a prophylaxis doxycycline 200 mg, 1 week is 95% effective in preventing leptospirosis, but for children role of prophylaxis has not been studied. Other pharmacological management depends on the symptoms, such as antipyretics to reduce fever. Corticosteroid, in case of severe hemorrhagic effects. Patient may need hemodialysis, if renal failure occurs. Patient may need to be put on ventilator, if acute respiratory distress syndrome (ARDS) persists.

Prognosis

- The mortality rate for patients with severe leptospirosis is approximately 10%, most deaths are from renal failure, massive hemorrhage or ARDS
- Approximately, one third of the patients with meningitis may continue to complain of periodic headaches
- Some patients with leptospiral uveitis have persistent visual acuity loss and blurry vision.

Control Measures

1. Environmental measures:
   - Preventing exposure to potentially contaminated water
   - Reducing contamination by rodent control

- Protection of workers in hazardous occupations
- Measures should be taken to control rodents on proper disposal of wastes and to provide health education to the public in this regard.

2. **Rodent control measures:** Sound environmental sanitation is the most effective weapon. Rats require three basic things for survival such as food, water and shelter. If these are denied, rats will naturally perish and their numbers considerably reduce.
3. **Proper environmental measures:**
    - Sanitation measures:
        - Proper storage, collection and disposal of garbage
        - Proper storage of foodstuffs
        - Construction of rat proof buildings, godowns and warehouses
        - Elimination of rat burrows by blocking them with concrete.
4. **Trapping:** This is a simple measure for rat control, but rats are suspicious animals by nature and will soon become trapwise and avoid traps.
5. **Rodenticides:** These are two main types:
    - Single use (acute)
    - Multiple use (cumulative): An expert committee of World Health Organization (WHO) grouped the acute rodenticides as below, those requiring ordinary care, such as:
        - Red squill
        - Bromide
        - Zinc phosphide.

    Those requiring maximal precautions such as:
    - Sodium fluoroacetate
    - Fluoroacetamide.

    Those, which are too dangerous for use:
    - Arsenic trioxide
    - Phosphorous
    - Thallium sulfate.

    Multi-dose poison use:
    - Warfarin
    - Pindone.

    These are anticoagulants, which cause internal hemorrhage and slow death in 4–10 days and avoid rat carcass within the house nuisance or spread of other diseases such as plague.
6. **Fumigation:** It is an effective method of destroying both rats and rat fleas, it is done by using cyanide gas in a cyanogas pump.
7. **Chemosterilants:** It is a chemical that can cause temporary or permanent sterility in either sex or both sexes of rodents, this technique is still in experimental stage.

Nursing Management

Nursing management mostly focus on prevention of disease and treatment, and control of cases along with considering following aspects:
- Record the vital signs
- Provide all hypothermic measures to control fever
- Observe for urine output
- Administer medications as per prescriptions
- Provide psychological support
- Explain the importance of dialysis, if patient requires
- Watch for meningeal irritation symptoms visual loss
- Gastrointestinal disturbances and take appropriate measures to prevent complications.

Nursing Care

The nursing care is identical with that of typhoid fever. However, in addition, the intense jaundice may produce intense discomfort, which will tax the ingenuity of the nurse to provide relief. Calamine lotion, soda baths, bran baths and soothing lotions or anesthetic ointments each may be tried in turn without avail. Once well established the disease may require sometime to run its course and the nursing care, such as the medical treatment will be purely symptomatic and supportive.

Health Education

- Health education is the strong weapon for the prevention of leptospirosis
- Educate the public regarding how the disease spreads
- Tell them to avoid swimming in water, i.e. contaminated with animal urine such as open ponds
- Protective clothing or footwear should be worn by those exposed to contaminated water or soil, because of their job or recreational activities
- Administration of vaccines for high-risk groups
- Education regarding immunization of pets
- Explain the importance of proper disposal of wastes and rodent control measures
- Tell them to keep the rodenticides out of reach of children.

Leptospirosis is a one of common zoonotic disease found worldwide. Especially in such communities where there is less environmental sanitation, today the health workers from all strata should join hands to educate the people toward the measures that they should adopt to prevent this dreaded disease, which may spread panic through its spread and severity.

Preventive Measures

Immunization of farmers and pets to prevent the disease, but again one should remember that immunity of one genus type of *Leptospira* may not protect against infection by another genus of *Leptospira*.

Doxycycline 200 mg (or a week has been 950/0 effective in preventing leptospirosis among high-risk adults).

Early Detection and Treatment

The cases of leptospirosis should be detected early. All the cases presenting fever with any of the two of following are clinically suspected for leptospirosis. These are:
- Myalgia
- Conjunctival suffusion
- History of contact with animals.

Once the cases are diagnosed, adequate treatment should be given. The presumptive treatment is tablet doxycycline 100 mg bd × 7 days.

All the patients of leptospirosis should be treated at primary health center (PHC) with injection penicillin 20 lakh intrauterine (IU) IV 6 hourly after negative test dose in adults for 7 days. The dose for children should be 2–4 lakh units/kg/day for 7 days.

Protection Against Contagious Material

The people should be protected by using hygienic measures such as avoidance of contact with animal urine. The people working in flooded areas should be protected against contaminated water contact or mud. They should be advised to use protective measures such as gloves or shoes. In case of cuts, the workers should be asked to use Betadine on cuts before entering the fields.

Vaccination

Vaccines provide only limited duration of immunity and booster doses are recommended after everyone or 2 years. The vaccines such as Leptavoid and Spirovac are used for cattle.

Health Education

Health education is one of the main measures to achieve decreased morbidity and mortality associated with leptospirosis. Health education creates awareness and helps in achieving community participation for disease prevention and control.

Control of Rodents

Control of rodents is required to have selective rodent control measures, where large number of leptospirosis cases occur.

Environment Sanitation

Environment sanitation can be maintained by draining the urine of cattle into a pit, instead of draining it to mix with water. By this, water contamination can be prevented.

Chemoprophylaxis

In the areas, from where clustering of cases are reported; there the paddy field workers and canal cleaning workers should be given 200 mg doxycycline once a week during peak transmission.

Zoonoses: Rickettsial

CHAPTER 33

INTRODUCTION

Rickettsial diseases are febrile exanthematous diseases caused by the microorganisms of the family rickettsiaceae. They are small, gram negative, intracellular, parasites of arthropods, exhibit pleomorphic appearance either as cocci or bacilli, seen in singles, pairs and short chains or in filaments.

Basically, all the rickettsial diseases are zoonotic diseases (except Q fever), transmitted through vectors to the human beings. Human infections result from either by bite or contamination with its feces.

In the arthropods, the rickettsiae grow in the gut lining and in the humans they grow in the endothelial cells of small blood vessels, producing vasculitis, cell necrosis and thrombosis of vessels, rashes and organ dysfunction (Table 33.1).

EPIDEMIC TYPHUS

Epidemic typhus is also called louse-borne typhus. It is caused by *Rickettsia prowazekii*, a parasite of the body louse. The parasite is ingested by the louse when feeding on an infected person, multiplies in the gut and passes out in the feces after 5th day. The organisms are capable of living in the dry feces of the louse also. Man gets the infection by three ways:

1. Contamination of the wound or abrasion of the skin (due to itching) by the feces containing the organisms or by the body fluid after crushing the louse.
2. Contact of the conjunctiva of the eye by the dried-infected feces of the louse.
3. Inhalation of the dried, infected feces of the louse.

These organisms can remain viable in the dry feces for about 4 months. The disease transmission is more during famine, wars, overcrowding conditions, etc. The infected louse also suffers and dies on the 10th day. Incubation period is about 12 days.

Clinically, it is characterized by sudden onset of fever associated with headache, malaise and prostration. Macular rashes appear on 5th day, on trunk and axilla spreads to the rest of the body sparing face, palms and soles. Circulatory disturbances such as hypotension, cyanosis can occur.

Diagnosis is confirmed by complement fixation test, Weil-Felix reaction and indirect fluorescent antibody (IFA) test. Treatment is by tetracycline. If not diagnosed early and not treated, fatality rate is as high as 50%. Recrudescence of the disease can occur several years after the primary attack, it is called 'Brill-Zinsser disease'.

Prevention and Control

- Delousing the infected person with application of 10% dichlorodiphenyltrichloroethane (DDT) as dusting powder, to be repeated, weekly for 3–4 weeks
- Stream disinfestations of all the clothes
- High standard of personal hygiene to be maintained by daily bath.

Nursing Management

Isolation

Because the disease is transmitted by the bite of an insect, the rat flea, it is necessary to see that the patient is disinfected before he/she is admitted to the nursing unit. After admission, the medical aseptic technique should be observed because of the possibility that disinfestation may not have been complete. DDT, used either as a spray or a dusting powder, should be applied to both the patient's clothing and their bedding.

Table 33.1: Classification of rickettsial diseases

Diseases	Rickettsial agents	Vectors	Reservoirs
Typhus group			
Epidemic typhus	Rickettsia prowazekii	Louse	Humans
Endemic typhus	Rickettsia typhi	Rat flea	Rodents
Scrub typhus	Orientia tsutsugamushi	Mite*	Rodents
Spotted fever group			
Indian tick typhus	Rickettsia conorii	Tick*	Rodents, dogs
Rocky Mountain spotted fever (RMSF)	Rickettsia rickettsii	Tick*	Rodents, dogs
Rickettsialpox	Rickettsia akari	Mite*	Mice
Others			
Trench fever	Rickettsia quintana	Louse	Humans
Q fever	Coxiella burnetii	Nil	Cattle, sheep, goats

*These vectors also serve as arthropod reservoir by maintaining the rickettsiae through ovarian transmission.

Diet

During the acute stage of the disease nausea and vomiting are present. For this reason, the diet becomes a nursing problem. If vomiting is severe, intravenous (IV) fluids with added vitamins are given; dextrose, amino acids and saline solutions usually are the fluids of choice.

When the patient is able to retain food, high calorie and high-vitamin liquids or soft diets should be given. Fruit juices sweetened either with honey or sugar are taken readily as a rule. Milk in any form, soups, broths, gruels, soft-cooked eggs, custards and gelatin may be given. Nourishment should be offered in small amounts at frequent intervals. After the acute stage of the disease has passed any good nourishing diet is satisfactory. The patient's preferences should be considered. A record of fluid intake and output should be kept.

Temperature

The temperature may be high, 104°F (40°C) or more. When it is necessary for the nurse to reduce the fever, the method recommended is the tepid sponge bath. Alcohol rubs and fans also are effective and refreshing to the patient. An ice cap is usually used and fluids are forced. Colonic flushing may be ordered. The nurse should be careful to see that the patient does not become chilled during any nursing procedure. The room should be warm, i.e. 70°F (21°C) or more, and the patient should be protected from draughts. The temperature, pulse and respiration should be taken and recorded every 3 or 4 hours.

Personal Hygiene

The patient should have a warm, cleansing bath daily. It should be followed by a brisk alcohol rub. It sweating is profuse, a warm sponge bath followed by and alcohol rub, should be given. Both the patient's gown and his/her bed linen should be changed. If the patient is incontinent, local sponge bath should be given sufficiently often to keep the area clean. Baby oil may be applied to protect the skin. Good oral hygiene is essential. The mouth is characteristically dirty. The teeth should be cleaned thoroughly at least twice daily, of tender if necessary to keep sordes from developing. Dilute hydrogen peroxide solution is excellent for removing sordes. The tongue, which usually is heavily coated, should be washed either with gauze pledgets or cleaned with a toothbrush. Mouthrinses should be given. Any antiseptic mouth wash will be satisfactory.

If the patient is unable to take fluids by mouth a small amount of chipped ice may be given; it helps to relieve the characteristic dryness of the mouth.

Elimination

Either diarrhea or constipation may be present. The bowels should be kept open. Cathartics and/or enema may be used when needed. The patient may be incontinent of suffer from retention of urine. The nurse should be especially alert to see that what appears to be incontinence is not actually the overflow of a distended bladder. Frequent specimens of urine usually are requested for laboratory analysis. A record of fluid output should be recorded.

General Management of the Disease

The patient should be placed in a comfortable bed in a warm, well-ventilated, private room. They should be strictly a bed patient. Their position should be changed every 2–3 hours. The change of position not only helps to protect the skin over the pressure points but also helps to prevent hypostatic congestion.

The bedding should be light in weight, but afford sufficient warmth. A bed cradle that will relieve the patient off the weight of the bedding will prove helpful if prostration is great. Restraints are sometimes necessary in delirious patients.

Because of photophobia, the patient's eyes should be protected from bright lights. The bed should be so placed that the patient will not face a window.

During a chill or chilly sensation, external heat should be applied. Headache, which is fairly constant, may be relieved by and ice cap or ice packs. Medication may be ordered for it.

Convalescence

Convalescence usually is uneventful. Generally, the patient recovers within 3–4 weeks.

Terminal Disinfection

Terminal disinfection is not necessary. However, it may be carried out in some hospitals as a routine procedure.

ENDEMIC TYPHUS

Endemic typhus is also known as 'murine typhus'. It is a disease of rats. It is an acute febrile disease, caused by *Rickettsia typhi* transmitted from rat to rat and rat to human beings by the infective rat flea (*Xenopsylla cheopis*). It is mainly transmitted through the contamination of the wounds or abrasions by infected feces of fleas. Infection may also take place through inhalation of dried infected feces.

The infection in the rats is inapparent, long-lasting and nonfatal. Incubation period is about 1–2 weeks. There is gradual onset of fever with mild prodromal symptoms, such as headache, body ache, nausea and vomiting. Rashes appear on 3rd or 4th day on the trunk and fade rapidly. Clinical features resemble those of epidemic typhus, but less severe. Usual course of the illness lasts for about 10–12 days. Rarely, it becomes severe.

Prevention and Control

Weil-Felix reaction with Proteus OX19 becomes positive during 2nd week. Tetracycline is the drug of choice. Dose is 500 mg, three times a day (tid) for 1 week. Vaccine is not available. Control of the disease is by control of rat fleas, by using insecticides [benzene hexachloride (BHC), malathion] and eyanogas fumigation of the rat burrows.

SCRUB TYPHUS

Scrub typhus is the most widespread disease of all the rickettsial disease in India. Basically, it is zoonotic disease, the chief reservoir being certain species of trombiculid mites such as *Leptotrombidium akamushi* (*L. akamushi*) and *Leptotrombidium deliense* (*L. deliense*). The disease is caused by *Rhadinomyia orientalis* (*R. orientalis*). Clinically, the features are the same as that of epidemic typhus. Generalized lymphadenopathy and lymphocytosis are common. Characteristic feature is a punched out ulcer (eschar) covered with a black scab at the site of bite. The Weil-Felix reaction is strongly positive.

Scrub typhus is the most common disease among rickettsial diseases in man. Scrub typhus was reported in China, Japan, India, Indonesia and Malaysia during 1970–1980. Approximately 2% of population sera has shown positive findings among general population, scrub typhus has been found in humans throughout India. It broke in epidemic form in Assam and Bengal during World War II.

The infection is maintained in the nature transovarially from one generation of mite to the next generation. The larva of this mite bites only once during its life time. Rat gets infected with *R. orientalis*. When the infected rat is bitten by the larva, the infection is passed through the nymph and adult (imago) stages. The *R. orientalis* enters the eggs even before they are laid and then goes to the larva of next generation, which transmits the disease. This method of transmission is called transovarial transmission. Man gets the infection accidentally when bitten by the infected larva. Thus, the infection contracted in the larval stage can only be transmitted in the next larval stage. The larva is also called 'chigger'. Thus, the larval stage serves both as a reservoir and as a vector for infecting humans and rodents. The disease is not directly transmitted from person to person. Incubation period is about 1–3 weeks.

Tetracycline is the drug of choice. Dose 500 mg tid for 1 week. Control of vectors is by clearing the vegetation (grass) around the human dwellings and outdoors application of 10% DDT or BHC, dusting powder on grasslands will control larva, nymph and adult stages of this mite.

Personal prophylaxis is by application of repellents such as N,N-diethyl-meta-toluamide (DEET or DET) to the skin and impregnation of cloths and blankets with miticidal chemicals, e.g. benzyl benzoate. Presently no vaccine is available.

Scrub typhus is an infectious disease, which is transmitted to humans from field mice and rats through the bite of mites on animals. Scrub typhus is also known as tsutsugamushi disease. It has been derived from two Japanese words:

CHAPTER 33 — Zoonoses: Rickettsial

- 'Tsutsuga' meaning 'something small and dangerous'
- 'Mushi' meaning 'creature'.

The infection is called scrub typhus, because it generally occurs after exposure to areas with secondary vegetation.

Epidemiological Features

Agent

Scrub typhus is caused by *Rickettsia tsutsugamushi* (*R. tsutsugamushi*), a tiny parasite about the size of bacteria that belongs to rickettsiaceae family. The *R. tsutsugamushi* lives in mites that belong to *L. akamushi* and *L. deliense*.

Environment

Rainy season.

Mode of Transmission

Bite of an infected bite.

Incubation Period

About 10–12 days after initial bite.

Clinical Manifestation

1. Fever with chills (104–105°F).
2. Prostration.
3. Headache.
4. Malaise.
5. Lymphadenopathy.
6. Macular rash.
7. Infection of mucous membrane lining the eyes.
8. A wound at site of chigger bite.
9. In severe cases increased pulse rate, decreased blood pressure, loss of consciousness, enlargement of spleen, twitching of muscles and interstitial myocarditis.
10. Detection of specific antibodies against scrub typhus in blood.
11. Isolation of rickettsiae from blood or other body tissues.
12. Complement fixation test:
    a. Diagnosis and treatment: The scrub typhus cases can be diagnosed on the basis of:
        - Patient's history
        - Physical examination
        - Laboratory.

       Scrub typhus cases should be treated with antibiotics. The drugs of choice are chloramphenicol and tetracycline.
    b. Protective clothing: The people should be instructed to wear protective clothing in the endemic areas.
    c. Use of insect repellents: These containing benzyl benzoate, diethyltoluamide can be used to prevent the chigger bite.
    d. Environmental sanitation: Environmental sanitation such as clearing of vegetation and chemical treatment of soil help in breaking up the cycle of transmission of scrub typhus.
    e. Prophylactic treatment: A single dose of chloramphenicol or tetracycline is given every 5 days for a total of 35 days, with 5 day non-treatment intervals to produce immunity to scrub typhus.

MURINE TYPHUS

Murine typhus is distributed world widely in areas of rat infestation. It is also called flea borne or endemic typhus. It can occur in a variety of environment ranging from hot and humid to cold and semiarid.

Epidemiological Features

Agent

The causative organism of murine typhus is *Rickettsia typhi*. Their feces will often defecate, while biting and feeding.

Environment

Murine typhus occurs during summer months when rats and their fleas are most active.

Mode of Transmission

Rat → Rat flea → Man.

Incubation Period

From 1 to 2 weeks.

Clinical Manifestation

- Headache
- Backache
- High fever (105°F)
- Joint pain
- Nausea
- Vomiting
- Chills

- Abdominal pain
- Rash begins on trunk and then spreads peripherally.

Diagnosis

Blood culture.

Prevention and Control

- The treatment of murine typhus is antibiotic and drugs of choice are chloramphenicol or tetracycline
- Control of fleas: Residual insecticides such as BHC, malathion are effective to control the rat fleas
- Proper disposal of waste: People should be encouraged to properly dump the domestic waste and bulky refuse in fields
- Health education: Educate the public regarding improving the living conditions
- Environmental sanitation: This includes:
  - Remove pet food
  - Cover garbage containers
  - Trim vegetation around buildings
  - Possible complications
  - Pneumonia
  - Central nervous system breakdown
  - Renal insufficiency.

TICK TYPHUS

Tick typhus is also known as Rocky Mountain spotted fever (RMSF), an acute febrile disease caused by *Rickettsia rickettsii* (*R. rickettsii*). It is transmitted by hard-shelled ticks (ixodid). The disease varies in severity from potentially life-threatening to self-limiting.

Epidemiological Features

Mode of Transmission

Bite of an infected tick.

Incubation Period

Varies depending upon disease ranges from 1 to 15 days.

Diagnosis

Blood test.

Clinical Manifestation

- Headache
- High fever chills
- Muscle pain
- Rash
- Vasculitis
- Swollen lymph.

Prevention and Control

- Treat tick typhus with antibiotic, e.g. doxycycline
- Try to avoid tick bites
- Use insect repellents
- Check the skin regularly
- Remove the ticks carefully using tweezers as soon as detected.

INDIAN TICK TYPHUS

The Indian tick typhus is an acute, febrile and exanthematous disease, caused by *Rickettsia conorii* (*R. conorii*). The chief reservoir is the tick. The organisms are maintained in the nature among rodents, dogs and other animals. Man is only an accidental hosts. The disease is transmitted by the bite of infected hard tick. Not only it is a chief reservoir but also a chief vector in transmitting the disease. It is infective in all stages of its life cycle and remains infective for life (about 18 month). Various species of ticks have been incriminated as vectors such as *Rhipicephalus, Ixodes, Boophilus, Haemaphysalis,* etc. The pathogens are also transmitted from one stage of the life cycle to another stage (i.e. transstadial transmission) and also to next generation through ovaries (i.e. transovarial transmission).

Incubation period is about 1 week. Clinically, it is characterized by sudden onset of fever, lasting for about 2–3 weeks. On examination, eschar is seen at the site of bite. Maculopapular rashes appear on 3rd day, first on the extremities (ankles and wrists), spreads centripetally (unlike in other rickettsial diseases) and cover the whole body.

Tetracycline is the drug of choice for the treatment 500 mg, tid for 5 days constitutes the course. Prevention is by disinfection of pet animals to control tick population and by health education of the people about mode of transmission and personal prophylaxis.

Methods of Control

General measures in infected areas

The fumigation of infected premises and the disinfestation of persons and their clothing when coming from infected communities into clean areas is the most single important feature in the control of epidemic typhus. DDT has been found extremely efficient in delousing large masses of people and in preventing infestation of individuals coming into the area. It may be dusted on clothing or the apparel may be treated with a DDT emulsion resulting in louse proofing lasting several weeks. Louse control of this sort has been entirely effective in preventing and stopping typhus epidemics.

Infected individual and environment
The following factors are important:
1. Early recognition of the disease from its clinical picture, the complement fixation test and the Weil-Felix reaction.
2. Isolation: All hairy areas of the body, including the head, should be thoroughly cleaned; shaving has not been found necessary by us to control the endemic type existing in this country. In the European type, the head and hairy portions of the body should be shaved, and all attendants should wear vermin-proof clothes and head coverings.

    Fumigation and disinfestation of the patient's personal effects and clothing should be conducted at once upon admission to the hospital. Destroy all vermin and its eggs. This applies also to the place from which the patient came. Rodent control must be established.
3. Quarantine: A previously uninfected body louse cannot transmit the disease until 9 days elapse after biting a patient. Knowledge of the role played by fleas in spreading disease is incomplete. However, all contents with any patient should be isolated for 2 weeks after their last exposure.
4. Terminal disinfection is not necessary.
5. Vaccination: While not applicable to endemic typhus as it occurs in the United States (US). It is now required by the government for world travelers entering endemic areas of louse-borne typhus fever.
6. General measures: The elimination of rats.

Treatment
Prophylactic
Prophylaxis consists of vaccination when going into epidemic areas of European typhus.

Active therapy
1. Sulfonamide drugs should never be given.
2. Chloromycetin, Aureomycin and Terramycin, in the order named, are the drugs of choice. In adults, the initial doses should be based upon 60 mg/kg of body weight for children. After the temperature falls, which is usually within 72 hours, the same dosage should be maintained for several days after which it may be reduced by half or more but should be continued for at least a week to 10 days, as relapses occur when therapy is discontinued too rapidly. The earlier antibiotic therapy is started, the more dramatic are the results and fewer the complications.

    Other measures required are symptomatic, supportive and meeting conditions as they arise or change.

ROCKY MOUNTAIN SPOTTED FEVER

Rocky Mountain spotted fever is also an acute febrile disease caused by *R. rickettsii*, reservoir being the ticks and rodents. Man is only an accidental host. Disease is transmitted by the bite of tick, all stages in its life cycle is infective. Clinical features are the same as those in Indian tick typhus fever. Control measures are the same as above.

RICKETTSIALPOX

Rickettsialpox is also an exanthematous, febrile disease caused by *Rickettsia akari*, a disease of rats, transmitted by the bite of infective mite. Transovarial transmission occurs in the mite. Clinically, it is characterized by fever lymphadenopathy, eschar at the site of bite and rashes resembling those of chickenpox. Control of the disease is by control of rats.

TRENCH FEVER

Trench fever is also an acute, febrile, exanthematous disease, caused by *Rochalimaea quintana*, reservoir being man, transmitted by the bite of infective louse. Clinically, it is characterized by fever rashes and splenomegaly.

The disease is limited to central Europe. It used to occur among those people who were staying in the trenches for days together during war time. Hence, the name trench fever. The organisms remain viable in the dry feces of the louse for a period of about 2 years. Hence, man gets the infection in the same ways as in epidemic typhus. The infected louse does not suffer from the infection of trench fever unlike in epidemic typhus. Control is by delousing and personal hygiene.

Q FEVER

Q fever is an acute, febrile disease caused by *Rickettsia burnetii* [it is now called *Coxiella burnetii* (*C. burnetii*)]. Primarily it is a zoonotic disease, disease of herbivorous animals such as sheep, goat and cattle, transmitted through the feces, milk and meat. Clinically, it is characterized by fever with chills, associated prodromal symptoms. The infection may result in pneumonia, hepatitis, encephalitis and even endocarditis.

Q fever differs from other rickettsial diseases in that there is no arthropod involved in the transmission of the disease, there are no rashes on the body during illness and Weil-Felix reaction is negative. Man gets the infection from infected herbivorous animals.

Q fever is an acute febrile illness due to *C. burnetii*. It is a zoonotic disease. The first case of Q fever was reported in 1935 in Queensland, Australia. In 1999, Q fever became a notifiable disease in the US, but reported from other countries. Scientists cannot reliably assess how many cases of Q fever actually occurred worldwide. In June 2006, the largest outbreak of Q fever with 138 cases was experienced in Scotland (a slaughter house near Stirling in England).

Epidemiological Features

Agent

- The Q fever is caused by *C. burnetii*
- Primary reservoirs of *C. burnetti* are goat, sheep, cattle and many other animals
- The *C. burnetii* is excreted in milk, urine and feces of infected animals. Organisms are also shed during birthing within amniotic fluid and placenta.

Host

Q fever is an occupational disease of slaughterhouse, animal husbandry and animal research workers:
- Non-productive cough
- Nausea and vomiting
- Diarrhea
- Abdominal pain
- Chest pain
- Weight loss
- Later on can develop hepatitis.

Incubation Period

About 2–3 weeks after exposure.

Mode of Transmission

The animals shed the disease agent in the urine, feces and milk. Placenta also contains pathogen, which create infectious aerosols during parturition. Meat also contains pathogen. Thus, transmission occurs in following ways:
- From inhalation of infected dust from the soil contaminated by the urine or feces of the infected animal
- Through ingestion of contaminated milk or meat
- Percutaneously through the abrasions of the skin
- Tetracycline, 500 mg tid for 5 days cures the disease
- Inhalation of contaminated to organisms dust
- Ingestion of contaminated food
- Tick bites.

Diagnostic Tests

- Blood for platelet count: Person with Q fever may show transient thrombocytopenia
- Serological tests to detect antibodies
- Indirect immunofluorescence assay (IFA).

Clinical Manifestations

- High fever (up to 104–105°F)
- Severe headache
- Malaise
- Myalgia
- Confusion
- Sore throat
- Chills
- Sweats.

Prevention and Control Measures

- Pasteurization or boiling of the milk and meat hygiene
- Sanitation of the cattle shed
- Disinfection and disposal of the wastes of the cattle, sheep and goats
- Inactivated *Coxiella* vaccine is given for those who are at risk
- Treatment: The drug of choice and treatment of Q fever is doxycycline and quinolone; it is effective when initiated within first 3 days of illness; treatment lasts for 2 weeks. Doxycycline 100 mg bid for 14 days
- Pasteurized milk: The community should be advised to use pasteurized milk and milk products
- Vaccination: Vaccinate the people who are involved in research with pregnant sheep or live *C. burnetii*
- The holdings of sheep should be located away from populated areas
- Use appropriate procedures for bagging, autoclaving and washing of laboratory clothing
- Test the animals for *C. burnetii* on routine basis and take preventive measures to prevent the outflow to other occupied areas
- Quarantine the imported animals
- Properly dispose of placenta, birth products; aborted fetuses and fetal membranes at facilities housing sheep and goat
- Restrict the access to laboratories used in potentially infected animals

CHAPTER 33 — Zoonoses: Rickettsial

- Educate the public regarding preventive measures to be adopted to prevent Q fever.

CONCLUSION

Scrub typhus, murine typhus, tick typhus are rickettsial diseases. The mode of transmission of these disease occur by bite of an infected mite to man in scrub typhus, from rat flea to man in murine typhus, bite of an infected tick in tick typhus and inhalation of contaminated dust, ingestion of contaminated food and tick bites in Q fever. Rickettsial disease can be prevented and controlled by diagnosis, treatment, avoiding tick bites and using repellents, etc.

Zoonoses: Parasitic

TENIASIS

Teniasis is a tapeworm infection acquired by ingestion of 'raw or uncooked meat of infected animals'. Two species such as *Taenia saginata* (*T. saginata*) and *Taenia solium* (*T. solium*) causes pathology in humans. *T. saginata* is commonly known as beef tapeworm and *T. solium* as pork tapeworm. The area most affected by teniasis currently is Irian Jaya, Indonesia and the western half of the island of New Guinea, and Island. Infield survey conducted in 2000 and 2001, researchers found that 8.6% of local people and 11% of local dogs living approximately 1 km from local capital city Wamena, in Jayawijaya district, harbored adult tapeworms and cysticerci of *T. solium*.

Because of prevalence of this tapeworm worldwide and increasing immigration and foreign travel, it (*T. solium*) will likely continue to emerge as an important pathogen in the United States (US). Both *T. saginata* and *T. solium* are worldwide distributed, affecting 100 million cases annually.

Taenia saginata (Beef Tapeworm)

Geographical Distribution

The *T. saginata* is worldwide distribution. In India, it is prevalent in Mohammedans who are beef eaters.

Habitat

The scolex of grown-up worm embedded in the mucosa of the wall ileum and rest of worm extends through the lumen.

Morphology (Fig. 34.1)

Adult worm
- It is white, transparent-like tape
- It measures 5–12 m (up to 24 m)
- Scolex is pear-shaped, 1–2 mm in diameter with four round suckers without rostellum and hooks
- Neck is long and narrow
- Proglottids may be up to 2,000 in number, terminal gravid segment 2 × 0.5 cm, genital pore is situated near the margin irregularly in right and left margin, gravid uterus having 15–30 lateral branches
- Gravid segments are expelled singly
- Adult worm is usually single in a host
- Life span of adult worm is nearly 10 years.

Larvae
- It is called cysticercus bovis
- Found only in cattle
- Larva has an elliptical shape (7.5 × 5.5 mm).

Egg
- Spherical and measures 30–40 µ in diameter
- Bile stained
- Thin outer transparent shell
- Embryophore is brown in color, thick walled and radially striated
- Contains an oncosphere with three pairs of hooklets
- Does not float in saturated saline solution
- About 80,000 eggs in a proglottid, which are liberated by rupture of mature proglottid
- Eggs remain viable up to 8 weeks.

Life Cycle

Man is the definitive host, whereas cow or buffalo acts as intermediate hosts.

Eggs are passed out with stools on the ground and cow or buffalo swallow these eggs while grazing in the field. The eggs are not infective to man. In the intestine, eggs rupture with liberation of oncospheres, which penetrate gut wall with the help of hooks, enter bloodstream and are filtered

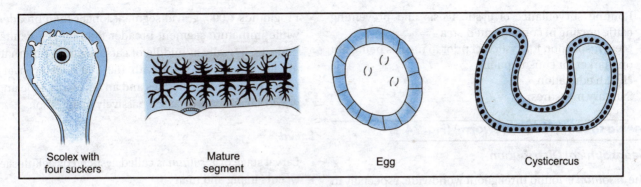

Figure 34.1: *Taenia saginata*

into muscular tissues (tongue, neck, shoulder and cardiac muscles), where they settle and grow. In 8 days, oncospheres are transformed into cysticercus bovis.

Man is infected by eating uncooked beef containing cysticerci (measly beef). In the intestine, scolex exvaginates (stimulation by bile) and anchor to the gut wall by its suckers and slowly grows into adult worm. It attains sexual maturity in 2–3 months and starts producing egg.

Clinical Features

The *T. saginata* is usually asymptomatic. It may cause abdominal discomfort, hunger pain, indigestion, diarrhea alternating with constipation, loss of appetite, pruritusani, intestinal obstruction and appendicitis.

Laboratory Diagnosis

- Demonstration of proglottids or eggs
- Serodiagnosis is done with the help of tests such as indirect hemagglutination, immunofluorescence assay (IFA) and enzyme-linked immunosorbent assay (ELISA).

Treatment

Niclosamide, mebendazole, praziquantel and bithional are the drug used.

Mode of Transmission

- Ingestion of uncooked meat, i.e. beef or pork containing larval cysts
- Intermediate hosts (cow, pigs) get infected when come in contact with worms egg, located in feces of infected humans.

Source of reservoir: Cow for *T. saginata* and pig for *T. solium*.
Incubation period: The period of incubation is 5–12 weeks and T. solium may survive up to 25 years or more.

Diagnostic Test

- Stool examination
- Immunological test detect the presence of cysticerci
- Magnetic resonance imaging (MRI) and computerized axial tomography (CAT) scan, to detect cysticerci in various organs.

Clinical Manifestations

People infected with adult *Taenia* are asymptomatic and those become infected can observe proglottids segments of tapeworm in their feces.

Symptoms

- Nausea
- Gastrointestinal (GI) upset
- Hunger pains
- Diarrhea/Constipation
- Chronic indigestion.

Prevention and Control

- Eggs hatched in small intestine can migrate to various tissues of body and form cysts, so cook meat thoroughly. Freezing at 5°C for 4 days and –15°C for 3 days or –24°C for 1 day, kills the larval as well
- The treatment is use of praziquantel and niclosamide:
  - Praziquantel: 10 mg/kg body weight (single dose)
  - Niclosamide: 2 g (single dose).

  Give the drugs early morning in empty stomach and chew thoroughly, and swallow with water. The eating can be resumed after 2 hours.
- Frequent handwashing is required to avoid ingesting eggs and developing cysticerci in brain
- Surgery (if required to treat cysticerci)
- Proper disposal of feces to avoid contamination of food, soil and water

- Routine surveillance of cysticercosis and preventing cattle grazing in contaminated area
- Meat inspection for cysticerci prior to meat is being put on market for consumption
- Health education
- Sanitary measures.

Taenia solium (Pork Tapeworm) (Fig. 34.2)

Geographical Distribution

The *T. solium* is found throughout worldwide, especially in pork eating persons.

Habitat

Adult worm lives in the small intestine.

Morphology (Table 34.1)

Table 34.1: Differences between *Taenia solium* and *Taenia saginata*

Sl No.	Taenia solium	Taenia saginata
1.	2–3 m	5–10 m
2.	Below 1,000 proglottids	Above 1,000
3.	Non-pigmented suckers	Pigmented
4.	Hooklets present	Absent
5.	Gravid proglottid 1.2 × 0.6 cm	2 × 0.6 cm
6.	Proglottids expelled in the chain of 5–6	Single proglottid crawls out of anus
7.	Uterine branches 5–10 dendritic	15–30 dichotomous
8.	150–200 testicular follicles	300–400
9.	Accessory ovarian lobe	Absent
10.	Vaginal sphincter (absent)	Present
11.	Neck of worm (short)	Long
12.	Life span up to 25 year	10 year
13.	Scolex globular	Quadrate
14.	Rostellum (present)	Absent

Adult worm

- It measures 2–3 m long
- Scolex is pinhead size, globular in outline with four suckers and head is provided with rostellum with two rows (small and large) of hooklets
- Neck is short 5–10 mm
- Proglottids 1,000, gravid segment longer than broader, while immature segment broader than longer, genital pores lie laterally at middle of each segment (alternating left and right), testis with 150–200 follicles, ovary with two symmetrical lobes and an accessory lobe and gravid segments are passed passively in the stool.

Larva

- Larval stage of *T. solium* is called cysticercus cellulosae
- Occurs in pig and man
- It is small, oval, milky white bladder measuring 8–10 mm in breadth and 5 mm in length
- Contains milky fluid rich in albumin and salts
- It lies parallel to muscle fibers as white spot, which represents future head invaginated into bladder
- The pork containing cysticercus is usually named as measly pork.

Egg

Morphological features resemble that of eggs of *T. saginata*.

Life Cycle

Similar to the life cycle of *T. saginata*. However, larval stage (cysticercus cellulosae) occurs in man too. Man acquires infection by eating inadequately cooked pork (containing cysticercus cellulosae) or by ingesting eggs of *T. solium* by consuming contaminated food and drinks.

Clinical Features

As given for *T. saginata*.

Diagnosis

Demonstration of proglottids or eggs.

Treatment

Same as of *T. saginata*.

Cysticercus Cellulosae

Morphology

- Measures 10 mm by 5 mm
- It has opaque invaginated scolex with four suckers, hooks and bladder filled with fluid
- Development to the infective form usually takes 9–10 weeks.

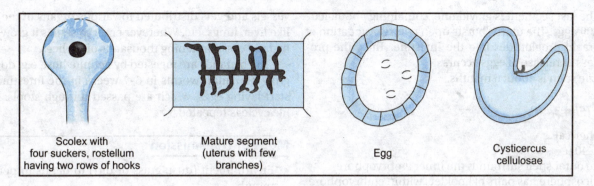

Figure 34.2: *Taenia solium*

Transmission

- By ingestion of eggs of *T. solium*
- By autoinfection (reverse peristalsis)
- External reinfection from anus to finger to mouth.

Clinical Features

- It may be asymptomatic
- Symptomatic picture includes involvement of eye, skin, viscera and muscles. Neurocysticercosis involve central nervous system (CNS) and spinal cord, and presents as epilepsy, hydrocephalus, encephalitis, diplopia, aphasia, amnesia, etc.

Laboratory Diagnosis

- Biopsy of nodule and study of its histological picture
- Radiology
- Serological tests like complement fixation test, indirect hemagglutination, ELISA and immunofluorescence using crude antigen (extracted from pig cysticerci) and purified antigen.

Treatment

Surgical excision or drugs, e.g. praziquantel is quite effective.

HYDATID DISEASE

Hydatid disease occurs due to *Echinococcus granulosus* (*E. granulosus*) and *Echinococcus multilocularis* (*E. multilocularis*). It occurs throughout the world. It emphasizes the global nature of the problem. Maplestone and Sami have reported the endemic nature of hydatidosis. They have described the high frequency of human and animal infections in Southwestern Punjab. In 1968, Reddy et al reviewed the 527 cases of hydatid disease observed in India. The highest prevalence was in Andhra Pradesh and Madras. The endemicity of hydatidosis in or around Delhi and New Delhi in North-West India is described by Prakash et al.

Hydatid disease is a public health problem in Asia, Mediterranean, South America and Africa with immigration. The prevalence of the disease has increased in Europe and North America in recent year.

Echinococcus granulosus is a cosmopolitan parasite and has at least size genetically distinct strains, two of which are relevant to human infection.

Agent: *Echinococcus granulosus* (Dog Tapeworm)

The causative agent is the larval stage of a tapeworm of dogs/sheep.

Geographical Distribution

Worldwide more prevalent in temperate climate than tropical area. It is quite common in cattle and sheep predominating places. From India, West Asia and Mediterranean countries, high incidences of hydatid cyst are reported.

Habitat

Adult worm is found in the small intestine of canines, e.g. dog. Larval form is found most commonly in liver, lungs, etc. of man.

Morphology

Adult Worm (Fig. 34.3)

1. Attached to the wall of intestine of canines, e.g. dogs.
2. It has scolex, neck and three to five segments.
3. It measures about 3–9 mm in length.
4. Scolex is spherical, provided with rostellum carrying 30–40 hooks in two rows. These are four suckers.
5. First one or two segments are immature followed by segment sexually mature.

6. The last segment is gravid one, containing about 400–500 eggs. The uterus bursts open before evacuation of gravid proglottides into the intestine. Thus, the process of release of eggs occurs.
7. Life span is about 6 months.

Eggs (Fig. 34.4)

- Spherical
- 31–40 μ
- The outer shell surrounds the inner embryophore
- Oncosphere has pairs of hooklets within embryophore
- Eggs resemble other taeniid species of dog
- Egg survive in the soil for 6–12 months
- Eggs are infective to man, cattle and sheep.

Life Cycle

Dogs, pigs, fox and jackal are definitive hosts. Intermediate hosts are sheep, goat, cattle horse, pig and man.

As a result of disintegration of gravid proglottids in the intestine eggs are discharged through stools of define host. Ingestion of contaminated food (with eggs of *E. granulosus*) by intermediate host results in hatching out of hexacanth embryo out of eggs (8 hour after ingestion). This liberated oncosphere penetrates the mesenteric blood vessels and gets distributed to various organs of the body like liver, lungs, etc. Wherever embryo settles it grows into hydatid cyst containing thousands of scolices.

The hydatids are ingested by definite host, e.g. dog and grow into adult worms in 6–7 weeks in the intestine and start laying eggs, which are passed through stools. Thus, life cycle is repeated.

Mode of Transmission

- Environment (dust, grass or dirt) to hands to person's mouth
- From dog hairs to hand.

Hydatid Cyst (Figs 34.5 and 34.6)

Hydatid cyst is grows very slowly. At the end of a year, it is about 5 cm in diameter. Hydatid cyst consists of the following compound.

Ectocyst

- It is 1 mm thick
- It is outer cuticular layer, which is as matter of fact laminated hyaline membrane
- It is elastic in nature and resembles the white of a hard-boiled egg.

Endocyst

- It is an inner germinal layer
- It is cellular and consists of a number of nuclei dispersed in a protoplasmic mass
- It is about 1/4th mm
- It has a role in the formation of outer layer, secretion of hydatid fluid and to form brood capsule with scolex.

Hydatid fluid

- It is secreted by endocyst
- It is clear, colorless or pale yellow fluid, weakly acidic, low specific gravity, containing sodium chloride, sodium sulfate, sodium phosphate and calcium salts of succinic acid. It is antigenic, highly toxic and provides nutrition for developing scolex.

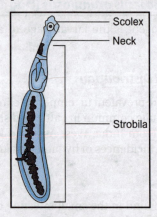

Figure 34.3: *Echinococcus granulosus* (adult worm)

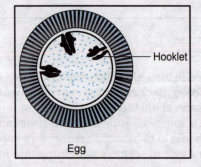

Figure 34.4: Egg of *Echinococcus*

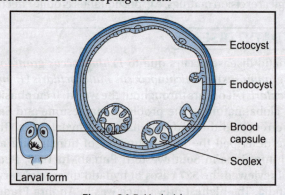

Figure 34.5: Hydatid cyst

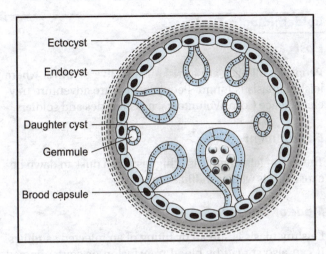

Figure 34.6: Structure of hydatid cyst

Hydatid sand
- It is granular deposit
- It consists of liberated brood capsules, free scolices and loose hooklets.

Formation of daughter cysts
The endogenous daughter cyst develops inside the mother cyst and can also develop from detached fragment of germinal layer. On the other hand, exogenous daughter cyst development results owing to increased intracystic pressure, which may cause either herniation or rupture of germinal as the cyst wall secreted by embryo consists of two layers, i.e. outer layer (ectocyst) and inner or germinal layer (endocyst) (Fig. 34.7).

Ectocyst
Ectocyst is elastic, but when incised or ruptured, it curls on itself thus exposing the inner layer containing the brood capsules and daughter cysts.

Endocyst
Endocyst is inner or germinal layer. It forms the outer layer (endocyst) and gives rise to brood capsules and scolices on inner side. It also secretes hydatid fluid.

Hydatid cyst may involve liver, lung, brain, heart, kidney, spleen, bone, muscles, etc. Liver is the common site. The disease remains symptomless for many years.

Clinical Manifestations

The majority of cysts produce no symptom. The clinical features depend upon:
- Organ involved
- Site of organ involved
- Stage of cyst development
- Viability of cyst contents.

Symptoms of disease are related to expanding mass pressure on adjacent structure, infection and rupture of cyst contents into surrounding body cavities.

Uncomplicated liver cyst usually presents with dull ache in right upper quadrant or a feeling of abdominal pain and distension. On clinical examination, enlarged liver with a rounded mass is felt on its surface. A large cyst in the hilar region can compress the common hepatic duct causing cholestasis. Hepatic vein compression or inferior vena cava compression can cause Budd-Chiari syndrome. Infected hydatid cyst has clinical features of liver abscess. Pressure symptoms of large cyst in lungs are:
- Cough
- Hemoptysis
- Chest pain
- Dyspnea.

Rupture of cyst contents into pleural cavity may cause allergic reactions including anaphylaxis, pleural effusion pleural implantation and empyema. Involvement of other organs causes:
- Soft tissue fluctuant swelling (muscle cyst)
- Raised intracranial pressure and focal epilepsy in case of cerebral cysts
- Segmental portal hypertension in case of splenic cyst
- Acute pancreatitis and jaundice in pancreatic cyst
- Bone pain, swelling and pathological fractures (bone cyst)
- Pericardial effusion and cardiac tamponade (cardiac cyst)
- Loin pain, hematuria (kidney cyst)
- In orbital cyst: Unilateral exophthalmos and blindness.

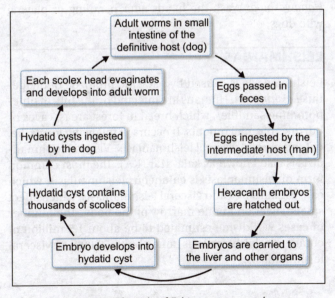

Figure 34.7: Life cycle of *Echinococcus granulosus*

Diagnosis

- Serological tests
- Magnetic resonance imaging
- Ultrasound
- Computed tomography (CT).

Prevention and Control

Identification and treatment of cases: The cases having hydatid cyst should be investigated and proper treatment is required.

Albendazole: About 10–15 mg/kg, 3–4 months courses with an interval of 14 days. Recent studies have shown that uninterrupted drug therapy for 3–6 months have better efficacy with no increase in adverse effects. Other drugs used are mebendazole and praziquantel, pair technique (puncture, aspiration and installation of scolicidal agents can be used for percutaneous drainage of hepatic hydatid cyst). It is the treatment of choice in patients with hepatic hydatid cyst, who refuse surgery or having comorbid disease.

Treatment option for cystic hydatid disease remain the surgery and surgery has the potential to remove cysts, and leads to complete cure.

Deworming all dogs: All the dogs that have eaten uncooked sheep internal organs should be dewormed. There should be adequate disposal of dead sheep and sheep viscera, so that dogs are unable to eat them.

Eliminate stray dogs: Stray dogs should be eliminated from the community. Make sure that the dogs do not defecate in and around children's play areas.

Handwashing: Wash the hands after handling or playing with dogs.

LEISHMANIASIS

Leishmaniasis is caused by parasitic protozoa of the genus *Leishmania*. Humans are infected by the bite of phlebotomine sandflies, which breed in forest areas, caves or burrows of small rodents. It occurs in following forms, i.e. cutaneous and visceral leishmaniasis. Visceral leishmaniasis is also known as kala-azar (KA). The most common form of leishmaniasis is cutaneous leishmaniasis, which causes skin sores and visceral leishmaniasis, which affect spleen, liver and bone marrow of the body. The number of cases worldwide estimated to be about 1.5 million of cutaneous leishmaniasis and about 50,000 of visceral leishmaniasis.

Epidemiological Features

Host

People of all ages are at risk, if they live or travel where leishmaniasis is found. People at risk are adventure travelers, Peace Corps Volunteers, missionaries and soldiers.

Environment

The risk of leishmaniasis is highest from dusk to dawn because this is when sandflies are active.

Mode of Transmission

Leishmaniasis is spread by biting of an infected sandflies. It can also spread by blood transfusion or contaminated needles.

Incubation Period

People who have cutaneous leishmaniasis develop skin sores within a few weeks after being bitten. In visceral leishmaniasis, the people become sick within several months (2–6 month).

Clinical Manifestations

Clinical manifestations of visceral leishmaniasis are:
- High fever
- Substantial weight loss
- Swelling of spleen and liver
- Anemia
- Progressive emaciation
- Malaise
- Hyperpigmentation on forehead, abdomen, hands and feet in light-skinned persons
- Occasional bleeding.

Complications

- Disfigurement of face
- Hemorrhage
- Prone to infections due to damage of immune system.

Treatment

Meglumine antimoniate and sodium stibogluconate are antimony containing compounds used for treatment of leishmaniasis. Other drugs used for treatment are amphotericin B and pentamidine. In case of destructive facial lesions, plastic surgery is required to correct disfigurement and removal of spleen in drug-resistant cases of visceral leishmaniasis:

1. **Use insect repellents:** The people at high risk should use insect repellents in order to prevent leishmaniasis.
2. Other means to prevent leishmaniasis include:
   - Appropriate clothing
   - Screening of windows
   - Mosquito net of 36–42 mesh.
3. **Use of insecticides:** Insecticides such as dichlorodiphenyltrichloroethane (DDT) spraying indoors is effective method to control the sandfly population. Dosage schedule of 1 or 2 g/m^2 or 100–200 mg/ft^2 is effective. Spraying of DDT in indoor human dwellings including the roof structure should be done.
4. **Environmental control:** The main principle behind environmental control is to make it unsuitable for breeding. The crevices of walls should be plastered by mud and lime. Lime has a powerful water absorbing capacity, which makes it unsuitable for sandfly breeding.

Clinical Types

Clinically, mainly there are two types of leishmaniasis:

1. Visceral leishmaniasis, also known as Indian Kala-azar caused by *Leishmania donovani* (*L. donovani*).
2. Cutaneous leishmaniasis are of three types:
   a. Oriental sore caused by *Leishmania tropica* (*L. tropica*).
   b. Espundia or nasopharyngeal leishmaniasis or mucocutaneous leishmaniasis caused by *Leishmania braziliensis* (*L. braziliensis*).
   c. Dermal leishmania (or post-kala-azar dermal leishmaniasis with non-ulcerative skin lesions) a late sequel to visceral leishmaniasis caused by *L. donovani*.

Leishmaniasis is considered to be zoonotic diseases, the infection being maintained in endemic areas in dogs, wild rodents and other mammals. However, visceral leishmaniasis (Indian kala-azar) is considered to be non-zoonotic disease because no animal reservoir of this parasite is known to exist *Taenia*.

The word 'kala-azar' has been derived from two Indian words, kala and azar meaning, 'black sickness', an illness in which the color (pigmentation) of the skin turns black. The word 'kala' also means 'deadly', thereby indicating that it is a fatal illness. Similarly, the parasite *Leishmania donovani* is named after two persons, namely Leishman from London (May, 1903) and Donovan from Chennai in July, 1903.

Visceral leishmaniasis is a chronic parasitic disease caused by the protozoan parasite *L. donovani*, transmitted by the bite of infected female sandfly *Phlebotomus papatasi* (*P. papatasi*). Clinically characterized by fever, malaise, anemia, massive splenomegaly, often hepatomegaly and emaciation. The skin over the entire body becomes dark. Hair tends to be brittle and falls out (Fig. 34.8).

If left untreated, death occurs within 2 years due to complications such as amebiasis, bacillary dysentery, pneumonia, tuberculosis, cancrum oris and other septic infections.

Magnitude of the Problem

Visceral leishmaniasis is a global problem. It is endemic in India, China, Africa, Southern Europe, South America, Mediterranean countries and Bangladesh. About 90% of the cases occur in India, Bangladesh and Brazil.

Globally there are about 13 million cases and every year about 1.8 million new cases are added. KA often occurs as an opportunistic disease in acquired immunodeficiency syndrome (AIDS).

In India, KA is endemic in Bihar, West Bengal, Odisha, Assam, Uttar Pradesh and Tamil Nadu (more along the coasts of rivers Ganges and Brahmaputra). An epidemic occurred in Bihar in 1977 due to migration of infected people. KA, which was almost controlled during National Malaria Eradication Program (NMEP) by DDT spraying, which simultaneously controlled sandflies also, re-emerged during 1986 with 17,806 cases with 72 deaths to 77,102 during 1992 with 1,419 deaths.

Agent Factors

The *L. donovani* parasites are the causative agents. They are intracellular parasites. They infect and divide within macrophages of the host (man). Essentially it is parasite of the reticuloendothelial (RE) system (Fig. 34.9).

Leishmania tropica is the causative agent of cutaneous leishmaniasis (oriental sore) and *L. braziliensis* is the causative agent of mucocutaneous leishmaniasis (espundia).

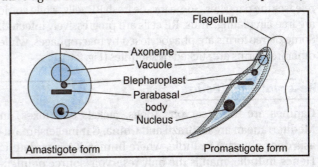

Figure 34.8: *Leishmania donovani*

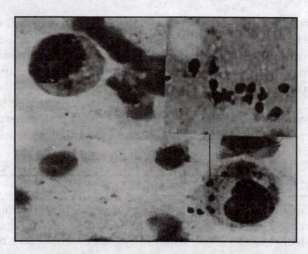

Figure 34.9: Leishman-Donovan (LD) bodies

However, this distinction is not absolute. Visceral form may result in cutaneous form and vice versa. The parasite *L. donovani* exists in two forms—leishmanial form (amastigotes) or aflagellar stage occurring in vertebrate host such as man, dog and hamster. They are found in reticuloepithelial (RE) cells and identified as *Leishmania* bodies. The other form is leptomonad form (promastigote) or flagellar form found in the gut of sandfly.

Life Cycle

The life cycle begins, when a female sandfly bites KA patient, sucks blood containing flagellum or amastigote of leishmanial forms. In the midgut of sandfly, these develop into leptomonad forms, which multiply into enormous number of flagellates. They tend to spread towards the anterior part of the alimentary canal (pharynx or buccal cavity). Salivary glands are not infected unlike in mosquitoes.

After the extrinsic incubation period of about 9 days, the transmission is effected through the bite of the infected female sandfly and inoculating leptomonad forms into the skin. They develop into leishmanial forms, inside the RE cells, multiplies by binary fission, till the cell eventually ruptures and releases the parasites. Some invade fresh RE cells, while some are free circulating. Thus, RE cells are progressively infected. Some of free forms are phagocytosed by macrophages, while other free forms are sucked by sandflies (Fig. 34.10).

Reservoir of Infection

Canines are the reservoirs (dogs, jackals and foxes) in Mediterranean areas, Brazil and China. Canine leishmaniasis does not exist in India, where human KA is endemic. Hence in India, man is the only reservoir/source of infection. In Kenya (Africa), gerbils and ground squirrels are the reservoirs of infection.

Host Factors

- Age incidence: Incidence of KA in India is maximum in the age group of 5–10 years. However, it can occur in any age group
- Sex incidence: It is twice more common among men than among women
- Migration of people: Favors the spread of the disease
- Socioeconomic status: Kala-azar is a disease of the poor, because of the poor living condition.

Environmental Factors

- Attitude: Kala-azar does not occur in high altitudes above 600 m of sea level because sandflies are not found in such height area, so KA is confined to plains
- Season: Incidence is high during and after rainy season
- Area: Usually, KA is a disease of rural areas because of the prevailing predisposing factors
- Project works: The disease is linked to deforestation, dam construction, irrigation, urbanization, migration of laborers and such others.

Miscellaneous Factors

Malnutrition and AIDS are other factors, which predispose to leishmaniasis.

Mode of Transmission

The disease is transmitted by the bite of infected female sandfly of the genus *Phlebotomus*. *Phlebotomus argentipes*

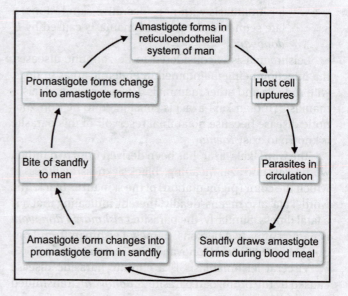

Figure 34.10: Life cycle of leishmaniasis

is highly anthropophilic (cutaneous leishmaniasis is transmitted by *P. papatasi* and *P. sergenti*). Transmission may also take place by contamination of the bite wound, when the insect is crushed by slapping during the act of feeding. Transmission can also occur by blood transfusion.

Incubation Period

Extrinsic incubation period is 6–9 days in sandfly and intrinsic incubation period is about 3–6 months in human beings. It may even extend to 1 year.

Clinical Features

Visceral Leishmaniasis

Fever: This is the early symptoms. It may be continuous or remittent, later becoming intermittent *Taenia*, sometimes it shows double peak in 24 hours.

Splenomegaly: This is progressive and is the most striking feature. It may even fill up the entire abdomen.

Liver: This is often enlarged.

General appearance: When the disease is fully established, the person looks weak and emaciated. The skin all over the body becomes dry and darker. Hence the name 'kala-azar' (black illness). Patient becomes anemic, if left untreated, KA carries high mortality.

Post-kala-azar Dermal Leishmaniasis

Post-kala-azar dermal leishmaniasis occurs after 1 or 2 years of apparent cure of visceral leishmaniasis characterized by nonulcerative, nodular and cutaneous lesions. It develops in about 10% of the KA cases. It is prevalent chiefly in Bengal and less so in Assam and Tamil Nadu. Parasites are numerous in the lesions.

Oriental Sore

Oriental sore type of cutaneous leishmaniasis is caused by *L. tropica*. *L. donovani* and *L. tropica* are never found together in the same locality. *L. donovani* is usually confined to moist eastern part of India, whereas *L. tropica* is limited to dry western part.

Unlike PKDL, oriental sore is characterized by painful ulcers over face, arms and legs, the parts exposed to bites of sandfly. Clinically, it is also called tropical sore (Delhi boil), mistaken for leprosy. Transmitted by infected female *P. sergenti* in India and *P. papatasi* in North Africa and Central Asia.

Espundia or Mucocutaneous Leishmaniasis

Espundia is caused by *L. braziliensis*, transmitted by *Phlebotomus intermedius*, clinically characterized by ulcers similar to oriental sore, but around the nose and mouth.

Prevention and Control of Kala-azar

- Elimination of reservoirs
- Breaking the channel of transmission
- Protection of susceptible persons.

Elimination of Reservoirs

Since human cases are the only reservoir of KA in India, this measure consists of their detection and treatment. Pentavalent antimony compounds are the drug of choice. They are urea stibamine, aminostiburea, neostibosan, etc. Ideal drug is sodium stibogluconate, 10 mg/kg weight, intramuscularly for adults daily for 20 days; 20 mg/kg for children.

Those who do not respond to this drug are given pentamidine isethionate, 3 mg/kg weight for 10 days intraventricularly. This drug is toxic. So, the patient requires supervision.

The patient must be re-examined after 3 months and 12 months to exclude relapse, if any. In the areas where dogs and rodents are the reservoirs, extensive measures are undertaken to control them.

Breaking the Channel of Transmission

This consists of mainly vector control measures, i.e. control of sandflies. Sandflies are best controlled by DDT spraying in the human dwellings (because they live in the cracks and crevices of the walls of the houses) and cattle sheds. Two rounds of DDT spraying is carried out per year, at the rate of 2 g/m². Lindane or benzene hexachloride (BHC) is the next best, if there is development of resistance to DDT.

Insecticidal measure will be more effective when followed by the improvement of sanitation by the following measures:
- Cleanliness in and around the house
- Plastering of walls to close down the cracks and crevices
- Location of cattle sheds and poultry away from human habitation.

Protection of Susceptibles

Protection of susceptibles consists of personal prophylactic measures, such as using mosquito curtains while sleeping, application of repellents, avoiding sleeping on the floor and keeping the house clean.

Important Surface Infections and Sexually Transmitted Diseases

CHAPTER 35

INTRODUCTION

Trachoma, tetanus and leprosy are the surface infections of utmost importance. Some sexually transmitted diseases (STDs) also occur in the form of skin infections. Gas gangrene and yaws are also detailed.

TRACHOMA

Trachoma is a chronic communicable inflammatory disease of the eye, affecting the conjunctiva and cornea. The disease has chronic evolution and is characterized by the development of follicles, formation of granules in upper tarsal regions, papillary hyperplasia, pannus (corneal vascularization) and cicatrization (formation), leading to deformities of the eyelids and in many cases blindness.

Magnitude of the Problem

From this global problem around, 400–500 million people suffer. In India, it is one major public health problem, because it is one of the principal causes of impairment of vision leading to blindness. There are about 9 million blind and 45 million visually handicapped. Trachoma is responsible for five per cell of visual impairments and blindness in India.

Epidemiological Features

Worldwide in distribution, mainly in North Africa and certain regions in Southern Africa, the Middle East and pockets in Latin America, Australia and the Pacific Islands. In India, the distribution is as follows:
- Highly endemic in Punjab, Rajasthan, Uttar Pradesh and Gujarat
- Moderately endemic in Madhya Pradesh, Bihar, Assam and Karnataka
- Low endemic in Jammu and Kashmir, Maharashtra, Kerala, Andhra Pradesh, Tamil Nadu, Odisha and West Bengal.

Agent Factor

A microorganism of the genus *Chlamydia trachomatis* is the specific agent, but other organisms often contribute to the disease process. Eyes of infected individuals, especially children with purulent conjunctivitis, which attract flies are the reservoirs of the infection. Period of communicability is short and disease is of low infectivity and is not communicable after complete cicatrization.

Host Factors

Age: Children below 10 years, mostly children by the age of 1–2 years.

Sex: Prevalence equal in both sexes of younger age groups. In older age group, females affected more than males. Females suffer longer period due to smoke from kitchen.

Community: Higher in Muslims.

Secondary infection: It may facilitate the onset of trachoma, aggravate its course and/or prevent it from healing.

Race: No race is immune.

Predisposing factors: Direct sunlight, dust, smoke and irritants.

Environmental Factors

High incidence is usually associated with two factors:
1. Season: April to May and July to September. High temperature and rainfall are the best environmental factors for the disease to thrive. Increase in fly population has a close relationship with peak seasons of trachoma.
2. Socioeconomic factors: Poverty, bad hygiene, overcrowding, dust and atmosphere. The customs of applying 'kajal' and 'surma' is a positive risk factor.

Mode of Transmission

1. Direct contact: Sleeping together.
2. Direct or indirect: Contact with ocular discharges of infected person or fomites.
3. Indirect contacts:
   - Use of common towels, handkerchiefs, pillows soiled with discharges from active case
   - Housefly: Eye-seeking flies play some role in spreading the disease
   - Kajal or surma: Incubation period varies from 5 to 12 days.

Pathophysiology

In the view of Macallan, the changes in the conjunctival congestion especially in the palpebral and bulbar conjunctiva, formation of papilloma in a tarsal, conjunctiva and fornix leading to the formation of follicles are characteristics of trachoma. Follicle formation is a characteristic lesion of trachoma, the follicles being aggregates of lymphocytes in the adenoid layer. Simultaneously, the changes in the cornea occur and correspond to the changes in conjunctiva. These are epithelium keratitis and trachomatous. Pain is nothing, but vascular infiltration affecting the upper part of the cornea extending from limbus. Epithelial scraping from the conjunctiva shows characteristic inclusion bodies within the cytoplasm of the cells.

The corneal ulcer may develop at the advancing edge of the pannus. The ulcer is shallow, not heavily infiltrated and very irritable, causing much lacrimation and photophobia. Conjunctiva undergoes atrophic causes, the blood vessels get constricted and the normal arrangement of blood vessels is permanently lost.

Lastly, entropion of the upper lid, inspection of the eyelashes, parenchymatous xerosis of the conjunctiva due to obliteration of the ducts of the lacrimal and the accessory lacrimal glands, chalazion formation due to closure of the ducts of the meibomian glands, obliteration of the lower fornix as even symblepharon formation and corneal opacities. Also, there may be pseudoptosis due to thickening of the upper lid.

Clinical Features

- Mild itching, irritation and headache
- After an acute inflammatory process, follicles appear on the conjunctiva
- Blurring of vision and increasing discomfort
- Mild formation of lacrimation, mild foreign body sensation and slight stickiness of the lids due to scanty mucoid discharge
- Acute mucopurulent conjunctivitis
- Minute stained areas are found on cornea
- Photophobia
- Scar formation, atrophy of follicles of conjunctiva and blood vessels get constricted.

Control

Assessment

The blinding lesions are entropion, trichiasis and corneal ulcers. For the purpose of diagnosis in the field, cases must satisfy at least two of the following criteria:

1. Follicles on the upper tarsal conjunctiva.
2. Limbal follicles or their sequelae as Herbert's pits.
3. Typical conjunctival scarring (trichiasis/entropion).
4. Vascular pannus, mostly marked at the superior limbus.

Chemotherapy

Mass treatment: Oral sulfonamide with antibiotics such as Aureomycin, tetracycline, erythromycin and tetracycline eye ointment to apply.

Blanket treatment: All children below 10 years irrespective of sign and symptoms. A prevalence of more than 5% and moderate trachoma in children under 10 years is an indication for mass treatment, continuous treatment for 6 weeks, followed by intermittent family-based self-treatment. The intermittent therapy consists of twice daily application of tetracycline for 5 consecutive days each month and for 6 months each year.

Selective treatment: In communities with low or medium prevalence, the principles of treatment are the same, but treatment should be applied to individual by case finding rather than by community-wide coverage.

The minimum criteria for cure of trachoma are absence of follicles, inactive pannus and absence of hyperemia. The eye to be examined by a biomicroscope for smoothness of conjunctiva even in presence of scar.

Surgical Correction

Individual with lid deformities (trichiasis/entropion) should have surgical procedure and follow-up.

Surveillance

Once control of blinding trachoma has been achieved, provision must be made to maintain surveillance.

Health Education

1. Health education should explain, demonstrate and persuade the people to cooperate in treatment campaign.
2. Handkerchiefs of infected person should not be used by healthy persons; infected children should not be sent to school.
3. The mothers of young children should be the target for education. Measures of personal and community hygiene should be incorporated in program of her education. Good sanitation reduces the chances of infection. Proper disposal of refuse, cattle dung and human excreta reducing fly populations are good sanitary measures. If levels of sanitation and quality of live not improved, reinfection occurs.
4. National program for prevention of infection: The Government of India launched National Trachoma Control Program in 1976, which has been included in the 20-point program.
5. Impairment and National Program for Control of Blindness (NPCB).

Problem of Blindness

The problem of blindness is complex because of gigantic size, multiple causes, shortage of trained ophthalmic personnel and rural-urban imbalance scarce resources. Lack of knowledge towards self-efforts to attain and maintain eye healthy adds to the problem. According to sample survey undertaken by ICM (1971–1973), India has 9 million persons, i.e. 1–4% population who cannot see well at 6 m distance; another 45 million people suffer from visual impairment. The survey assessed the main causes of blindness under the following region:

- Cataract: 55%
- Trachoma: 20%
- Smallpox (old cases): 3%
- Malnutrition: 2%
- Injuries: 1.2%
- Glaucoma: 0.5%
- Other causes: 18%.

Strategy

1. Health education about eye care through all modular eye care (MEC) mass communication with particular emphasis ocular health in children and other vulnerable group.
2. To augment ophthalmic services, so that relief is given to the community in the shortest possible time.
3. Simultaneously establish a permanent infrastructure for community-oriented eye health care.

Goal

To achieve reduction in the incidence of blindness 1.4–0.3% by 2000 AD.

Plan of Action

1. Intensification of educational efforts on eye health through mass communication and extent education methods.
2. Extension of eye care services through mobile units to restore sight and relieve eye ailments by adopting eye camp approach and enlisting participation of voluntary organizations.
3. Establishment of permanent facilities for eye health care as a part of general health services.
4. Peripheral sector includes development of primary eye care services involving block level primary health centers (PHCs) and their subactivities.
5. Intermediate sector includes development of diagnostic and treatment facilities at district and subdivision levels.
6. Control sectors include development of subspecialty services, basic and applied research, and manpower development.

The total infrastructure loped in 1988–1989 has been developed in 1988–1989:

- Strengthening of PHCs: 4,000
- Control mobile units: 80
- Strengthen district hospitals: 404
- Upgradation of department of ophthalmology medical: 60
- Establishment of regional units: 9
- Ophthalmology assessment training centers: 37
- Setting up of district mobile units: 150
- Ophthalmic cells in the states: 18
- Eye banks (including eight in volunteer section): 80.

Nursing Management

Isolation

Trachoma may be isolated by the medical aseptic technique. The virus is found in the eye discharges and nasal secretion. All articles contaminated by the patient should be cleaned up or sent to the incinerator as soon as possible after use.

Diet

The diet in trachoma is important. Poor nutrition may be a predisposing cause of the disease. The diet should be a full general diet, consistent with the age and preference of the patient. It should be rich in minerals and vitamins.

Temperature

The temperature is not significant. It is normal or near normal in this disease.

Personal Hygiene

The patient should receive a cleansing bath daily. The eyes should be cleaned with warm saline or boric solution, or whatever solution the doctor may prescribe, frequently enough to keep the drainage from contaminating the patient's hands, clothing or bed linen. All waste material soiled with eye discharges should be placed in the disposal bag at the bedside. The patient should be taught how to protect others by practicing clean personal habits and the importance of using his/her own personal toilet articles should be stressed, especially with regard to washrags, towels and handkerchiefs. Patient should have own wash basin. Good oral hygiene should be maintained and brush at least twice a day.

Elimination

The bowels should move well once each day. Either enemas or cathartics may be given. However, this should not be necessary and it should be possible to regulate this by diet. The output of urine should be normal, but if sulfonamides are given, a specimen should be saved and sent to the laboratory at the doctor's request.

General Management

The patient is ambulatory. He/She probably will be happier in a ward or room with other patients. If the light is troublesome, the eyes should be protected from bright light. The patient's general resistance should be built up. Coryza or rhinitis tends to aggravate the symptoms of trachoma and increase the virulence of its virus.

In the past, handling of this disease was very discouraging to all concerned—the patient, patient's family, doctor and nurse. With the newer methods of treatment, this has all been changed in the acute cases, but we cannot think that there will be much change in the handling of protracted or chronic cases. A cheerful, helpful manner on the part of the nurse may assist the patients to make better adjustment to affliction. Occupational therapy, the radio, television and visitors; all helps to maintain the patient's morale.

Convalescence

Convalescence is prolonged. The disease tends to become chronic. Each patient soon learns what he/she can do to contribute to patient own well-being. He/She learns to apply medicaments, ointments, irrigate their eyes, make instillations and eyedrops for themselves and generally take care of the eyes when returned from work.

Terminal Disinfection

All contaminated wall spaces, the table and the chair in the patient's unit should be washed in soap and water. The mattress and pillows should be sunned as usual for 6 hours. All treatment equipment such as basins and dishes should be sterilized and then washed. All waste material should be sent to the incinerator. The patient should be bathed, shampooed and dressed in clean clothing before discharge. However, the patient will remain a source of danger to family and close personal friends until disease is cured. He/She should be warned at intervals to continue practicing personal hygiene.

TETANUS

Tetanus is an acute neuromuscular disorder characterized by paroxysms of convulsive tonic and sometimes clonic and contraction of the voluntary muscles. It is produced by the exotoxin of a slender, motile, anaerobic, spore forming gram-positive drumstick bacillus.

Tetanus is an acute disease induced by the exotoxin of *Clostridium tetani* (*C. tetani*). It is clinically characterized by painful muscular contractions of masseter muscle (lock jaw), facial muscle, muscle of the neck and back muscles followed by spsam of other muscles, specially those of the spine, chest and abdomen.

Magnitude of Problem

Tetanus is one of the leading causes of infant mortality. About 5–10% of neonatal deaths in Kolkata were due to tetanus. Geographical variation in incidence has been related to climate, organic content of soil, amount of agricultural activity and prevalence of local customs sending to promote infection. The incidence of the disease in Kolkata during 1971 was 24/100,000 population.

Epidemiological Features

Agent

Clostridium tetani is slender, long, slightly curved gram positive, 4.8×0.5 μ and occurring singly or in chain. It shows iderable variation in length. Spores are spherical, terminal and bulging giving the bacilli drumstick appear. It is non-capsulated and motile (Fig. 35.1).

It is an anaerobe that grows only in the absence of oxygen. It grows fairly well in ordinary media, but growth is enhanced if food is provided. The growth on solid media is characterized by a time film with long branching projections. Spores of *C. tetani* withstand boiling for 15–90 minutes. Autoclaving at 121°C for 20 minutes kills spores. Otherwise, spores can survive in soil for years.

Clostridium tetani inhibit the soil. A hot damp climate together with a fertile soil rich in organic matter are a favorite environment. The spores will survive in soil, street dust, dust, operating room, horse and cow dung for very long periods. On the basis of flagellar antigen there are all types of *C. tetani*, but all these serotypes produce exotoxins. Tetanus organism produces exotoxin (tetanospasmin), which is a powerful poison. It acts in four areas of the nervous system:
1. The motor and plates in skeletal muscle.
2. The spinal cord.
3. The brain.
4. The sympathetic nervous system.

Host Factors

Age: Tetanus is a disease of active period of life 5–40 years of age. Neonatal tetanus occurs due to lead cord hygiene, application of cow dung to the cord stump.

Sex: Prevalence of tetanus is higher in males than in females at all ages except 15–45 years because of criminal abortion and delivery.

Occupation: Agricultural workers are at special risk due to their contact with soil.

Rural-urban differences: Incidence is much lower in urban than in rural areas.

Environmental Factors

- Ignorance about infection
- Religious prejudice
- Traditional unhygienic customs and habits
- Lack of mother and child health services and health education, e.g. delivery conducted by the untrained dais, use of unsterile instruments, application of cow dung to cord stump, etc.

Mode of Transmission

Clostridium tetani is usually found in the soil and feces of animals. It is transmitted through wound contamination. Infection occurs due to a contamination of wounds with tetanus spores, umbilical sepsis and middle ear infection resulting in tetanus is common in India. The spores being introduced by dust, catgut, instruments, plaster of Paris dressing and various powders such as talcum.

The wound may act as a portal of entry for bacilli, pin pick, skin abrasion, puncture wounds, burns, human bites, animal bites and stings, unsterile surgery, intrauterine death, bowel surgery, etc. Spores implanted in wound multiply only if conditions are favorable. Toxin produced is absorbed by motor nerve ending. Toxin travels along the axis cylinders of peripheral nerve and reaches central nervous system (CNS). It is fixed specifically by ganglioside of gray matter of nervous tissue and reaches CNS. It acts at synaptic junctions between anterior horn cells and related internuncial neurons leading to abolition of spinal inhibition. As a result, muscle rigidity and spasm occur. Incubation period varies from 6 to 10 days and it may be as short as 1 day or several months.

Pathophysiology

Tetanus is a disease caused by wound infection with an anaerobic bacillus. The organisms can be seen in the pus from infected wounds. The bacilli remain in the wound, where they produce a toxin that acts on the CNS. It is used to be thought that the toxin was absorbed from the motor end plates, passing along the axis cylinder to reach the spinal cord. The concept of an axonal spread may be acceptable in the case of viral infections, but the relatively rapid rate of travel of the tetanus toxin, sometime less than 24 hours from a peripheral nerve to the lumbar cord

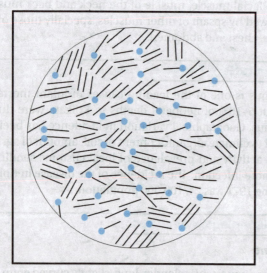

Figure 35.1: *Clostridium tetani*

is quite incompatible with diffusion of such large protein molecules. The axon is highly viscous in texture, semi-solid, but a large proportion of the space inside the epineurium of the motor trunk is occupied by the interstitial fluid. The fluid generated by the high intramuscular (IM) pressure created during contractions is responsible for centripetal spread of the toxin. In support of this view, the fact that injection of a sclerosing solution into a large motor nerve with resulting fibrosis, blocks the absorption of tetanus toxin, although not the transmission of nerve impulses. The toxin is not absorbed when the limb is immobilized and is called 'phenomenon of local tetanus'. When the toxin reaches the cord and brainstem, it become so firmly anchored to the motor nerve cells that it cannot be dislodged. The symptoms are the result of an extreme hypersensitiveness of the motor nervous cells. As a result of this, the most trivial sensory stimuli produces a series of terrible clonic and tonic spasms, and the patient dies because of exhaustion by his/her convulsions or asphyxiated by the tonic spasm of the respiratory muscles. Spasm of the masseter muscles produces 'lockjaw'. No characteristic lesions are found at autopsy.

Types of Tetanus

1. Traumatic: Trauma is a major and important cause of tetanus. Sometimes, it may result from most trivial or even unnoticed wounds.
2. Puerperal: Tetanus follows abortion more frequently than in normal delivery. A postabortal uterus—favorite site for the germination of tetanus spores.
3. Otogenic: Ear may be portal of entry for foreign bodies infected matches, pencils, beds, etc. may introduce the infection. It is usually pediatric problem, but occurs in adult also.
4. Idiopathic: There is no history of sustained injury. Some consider it to be the result of microscopic trauma others think it due to the absorption of toxin from the alimentary tract.
5. Tetanus neonatorum: Cause is infection of umbilical stump. The symptom being seen about the 7th day due to the unsterile way of dressing, the cord stump and use of cow dung and ash, etc.
6. Acute tetanus: In this, incubation period is less than 10 days and the symptoms are acute, progressive and the prognosis is grave.

Signs and Symptoms

1. Early symptoms are difficulty in opening the mouth and swallowing owing to the spasm of masseter and facial muscles (Figs 35.2A and B).

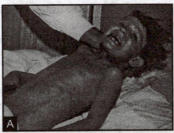
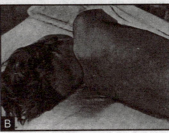

Figures 35.2A and B: Risus sardonicus. **A.** Cannot fully open mouth, case of tetanus; **B.** Opisthotonus during tetanic convulsion of lockjaw, recovery.

2. Risus sardonicus, peculiar grimacing expression may be noted later due to the involvement of jaw muscles.
3. The spasms gradually extend on other skeletal muscles and during the acute spasmodic attack the patient rests on the head and heels a condition of opisthotonus.
4. Spasm of the sphincter muscle of the body reader swallowing defecation and micturition.
5. Spasm of respiratory muscles cause long periods of cyanosis until death.
6. Temperature is elevated.
7. Pulse rate is increased.
8. Death occurs due to asphyxia, physical exhaustion or heart failure.

Diagnostic Measures

1. Clinical picture.
2. Microscopic examination: Smears from wound material after Gram staining show gram-positive bacilli.
3. Culture.

Preventive Measures

1. The main objective is to prevent respiratory and cardiovascular complications, and to promote early recovery.
2. The patient with tetanus should be treated in a calm, quiet, darkroom.
3. Avoid sudden stimulants and light, slightest stimulation may trigger paroxysmal spasm.

4. Adequate airway must be maintained by using endotracheal tube or tracheostomy.
5. Secretion should be removed by frequent suctioning.
6. In case of severe spasm sometimes mechanical ventilation is needed.
7. Muscle relaxants, sedatives and anticonvulsant drugs should be administered to treat muscle rigidity and convulsions.
8. Tetanus immunoglobulin administering will neutralize the toxins.
9. Detrition of necrotic tissue is very essential.
10. Antibiotics are administered to prevent the growth of vegetative organism.
11. Fluid and electrolyte balance must be maintained by nasogastric tube feeding.

Prophylaxis

Prophylaxis is preventable disease. Immunity to tetanus may result from infection or by immunization. There are active and passive immunization and combined immunization.

Active Immunization

Tetanus is entirely preventable disease by means of active immunization with tetanus toxoid. All persons should be immunized regardless of age. Two preparations are available for active immunization:

1. Fluid toxoid.
2. Adsorbed vaccines.

For primary immunization absorbed toxoid recommended, as it stimulates and long-lasting immunizing responses than plain toxoid. Plain toxoid may be employed for booster injections. A complete primary immunization consists of three spaced injections (0.5 mL each dose) for children, from 3 to 9 months along with diphtheria and pertussis, it is given to them in two more doses at 1 month interval intramuscularly:

- First booster dose at 18–24 months
- Second booster dose at 5–6 years
- Third booster dose at 10th year
- Antenatal mothers:
  - First dose at 10–20 weeks
  - Second dose at 20–24 weeks
  - Third dose at 30–38 weeks.

Reactions to tetanus toxoid occur rarely in children. The local reaction consists of excessive pain, redness and swelling around the site of injection for up to 3–4 days.

Indications of tetanus toxoid

- Septic or penetrating injury
- Septic abortion
- Major burns
- Deliveries without adequate care.

Contraindications

- Known hypersensitivity reaction to any of the components of the vaccine to be used
- Active infection with fever
- Active tuberculosis
- Active/Cardiac or pulmonary diseases
- Steroid treatment
- History of convulsions.

Passive Immunization

Antitetanus serum (ATS) is used to impart passive immunity. There are two types:

1. Horse ATS.
2. Human immunoglobulin.

Horse ATS: It is obtained from serum and immunized horses. A dose of 1,500 units subcutaneously used for routine treatment for the wounded. Within 1–3 days, the antitoxin reaches a high level in the blood rapidly eliminating bacteria from the body.

Nursing Management

Isolation

The disease can be isolated by the medical aseptic technic. The causative organisms are found in the wound. All material soiled with secretions should be securely wrapped in paper and sent to the incinerator as soon as possible after use.

Diet

During the acute stage, because of the patient's inability to open their mouth, the diet necessarily consists of fluids. From 3,000 to 4,000 calories are recommended for the adult patient. Sometimes, tube feeding through the nose can be done without disturbing the patient, leaving the tube in place. Frequently intravenous (IV) feeding of fluids high in dextrose, protein and vitamins is necessary.

When the patient is able to cooperate fluids can be given through a drinking tube; however, the patient should never be permitted to put a glass tube between their teeth; as a precautionary measure a short rubber tube should be attached and this end used in the mouth. Milk with cream when tolerated, eggnogs, creamed soups, pureed vegetables and fruit, gruels and fruit juice are suggested for the tube fed patient.

Small amounts given frequently, every 2–3 hours, have been found to be more satisfactory than larger amounts at longer intervals. Food that requires chewing should not be offered until convalescence is well-established. An accurate record of both caloric and fluid intake should be kept.

Temperature

As a rule, the maximum temperature is seldom above 104°F, although occasionally it may be higher. High temperature is exceedingly difficult to combat, as convulsions are apt to ensue after or during any therapeutic procedure. Ice caps to the head are helpful. Fluids should be forced, alcohol rubs, fans or tepid sponge baths, if not contraindicated and given carefully, may be helpful. High fever is not the usual rule.

Personal Hygiene

The patient should have a daily cleansing bath. The water should be comfortably warm. The motions used in giving the bath should be slow, firm and purposeful. Warmed alcohol rubs are not only refreshing but also they help to prevent pressure sores. Oral hygiene is difficult at best. The mouth is characteristically dirty. If not too stimulating, the outer aspect of the teeth can be cleaned with a gauze pledget saturated with a 50% hydrogen peroxide solution or some other antiseptic solution. Fluids by mouth are helpful. Mucus in the throat should be removed by suction when indicated. Do not cause convulsions; use gentle slow movements.

Elimination

The bowels should move freely at least once each day. If necessary, an enema may be prescribed. If too sick, ignore the bowels until the patient is better:
- Retention of urine is not uncommon
- Catheterization may be done when indicated
- An accurate record of fluid output should be kept.

General Management

The patient should be placed in a darkened, quiet, well-ventilated, private room. The room should contain only the furniture and equipment necessary for care of the patient. Bedding should be lightweight, but sufficiently warm. It has been found helpful to cover the patient with a lightweight cotton blanket and use no night gown:
1. For emergency use, a laryngoscope, an endotracheal tube and a suction machine should be readily available.
2. Tracheotomy is frequently performed in severe cases (tracheotomy care should be taken).
3. Oxygen is usually given. Oxygen equipment should be in the patient's room at all times. Light to heavy sedation is necessary depending on the case.
4. The patient's position should be changed every 3–4 hours. The greatest skill and care are required in moving the patient because of the danger of convulsions. There should be as few external stimuli as possible. Loud talking and unnecessary noise should be avoided. Above all, there should be no sudden jarring of the patient's bed. Bright lights should not be turned on.
5. The nursing care should be planned to give the patient long intervals of undisturbed rest.
6. The patient's room should be cleaned only when he/she is under sedation.
7. A nurse should be in constant attendance, until convalescence is well-established. Never leave the patient alone.

Convalescence

Convalescence usually is uneventful, but slow. The patient is quite weakened as a rule by the disease. Nourishing food should be given and patient should resume the normal activities gradually.

LEPROSY

Leprosy as a disease has been known for many centuries and reference to it is found in ancient Hindu scriptures. Until few decades ago, the disease was one of neglect; the affected were interned in leprosariums mainly managed by charitable trusts and voluntary organization.

Leprosy is an infectious disease caused by *Mycobacterium leprae (M. leprae)* and clinically characterized by hypopigmented patches, partial or total loss of sensation, presence of thickened nerves and the presence of acid-fast bacilli in skin smears (Fig. 35.3).

It is a chronic inflammatory disease and displays a wide clinical spectrum related to hosts ability to develop specific cell-mediated immunity (CMI). In high resistant tuberculoid leprosy, the localized signs are restricted to skin and nerves. Low resistant lepromatous leprosy is a generalized

Figure 35.3: *Mycobacterium leprae* stained by Ziehl-Neelsen method

disease involving many systems, with widespread lesions of skin, peripheral nerves, upper respiratory tract, eyes, testis and the reticuloendothelial systems. Common complications include more acute, immunologically-mediated inflammatory episodes (reactions), secondary inflammation in the anesthetic areas, which result from nerve damage and deformity of hands, feet and face.

Magnitude of the Problem

Leprosy is a major health and socioeconomic problem because of long duration of the disease, magnitude of disabilities and socioeconomic consequences. Various social problems results in leprosy loss of employment opportunity, family left destitute and care of infants neglected.

It is a significant public health problem in India and is fairly widespread, though not uniformly. The total number of cases on the basis of 1981 census, was estimated to be around 4 million (now 2.5 million) based on the average prevalence of 5–6 per 1,000 populations. Every year about 3 lakh new cases are detected of which about 60% actually new and 40% are old undetected cases. About 20–25% of these cases are of the infectious type. About 15% of cases are among children below the age of 14 years. It has been estimated that India accounts for about one third of the leprosy cases in the world.

Pathophysiology

Leprosy has two special features; one is slits invasion by *M. leprae* of certain superficial nerves, which may become thickened and firm and the other is the wide range of clinical and histological manifestations, reflecting the intricacies of the host-parasite relationship, skin lesions, which are best seen in good oblique light, may occur, anywhere, some on leathering scalp and perineum. Nervous predilection, which should always be palpated, include the ulnars, at and above the medial, humeral epicondyle, the superficial radials and medians at the wrist, the great auricular at the edge of the sternocleidomastoid muscle and the lateral popliteal at the neck of the fibula. Appropriate muscle weakness and wasting may occur resulting in clean hand (ulnar and/or median), foot drop, clean toes and facial nerve paralysis the last named usually incomplete, but including lagophthalmos, wrist drop is comparatively late (Fig. 35.4).

Clinical Features

Early Signs

1. Hypopigmented or erythematous patches on the skin.

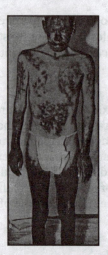

Figure 35.4: Lepromatous leprosy, nodular type

2. Diffuse thickening of the skin with a shiny appearance.
3. Loss of sweating or loss of hair over the skin lesion.
4. Loss of sensation to pain, touch and temperature in the hands and feet.
5. Thickening of cutaneous nerves, especially ulnar, median, lateral popliteal.
6. Nodules in the skin especially of the nose, chin and ears.
7. Thickening of earlobes.
8. Recurrent wounds and ulcers, which do not heal.

Later Deformities

Primary deformities

1. Primary paralytic deformities due to involvement of claw hand, claw fingers, wrist drop, footdrop, claw toes, lagophthalmos, corneal ulcers and facial paralysis.
2. Primary, non-paralytic deformities due to infiltration and damage of the tissue by the *M. leprae* in lepromatous leprosy.

Secondary deformities

Secondary deformities are due to carelessness in protecting anesthetic hands and feet.

Characteristics

Following are the other characteristics of later deformities:
- Depression of the bridge of nose
- Wrinkling of the facial skin
- Loss of eyebrows
- Disfiguration of ear
- Stiffness of joints of fingers
- Shortening and loss of finger and toe.

Diagnosis

Clinical Examination

The cardinal signs of leprosy are pigmented patches, loss of sensation and presence of thickened nerves. At least one cardinal sign must be present. Loss of sensation must be treated for heat, cold, pain and light touch. Nerves ulnar (near the medial epicondyle) involved, greater auricular lateral popliteal and dorsal branch of the radial; presence of pigmented anesthetic patches on skin and thickened nerves.

Areas of Prevalence

High prevalence

There are five or more affected persons per 1,000 population, mostly along east coast of the country, Central and Western India, States of Andhra Pradesh (AP), Tamil Nadu, West Bengal, Odisha, Maharashtra, Karnataka and some parts of Bihar.

Moderate prevalence

About one to five persons per 1,000 populations are affected in foothills of the Himalaya, Bihar, Himachal Pradesh, Jharkhand, Karnataka, Kerala, Madhya Pradesh, Maharashtra, Sub-Himalayan region of Punjab, Western Uttar Pradesh (UP), Gujarat and Rajasthan.

Low prevalence

In these areas, plains of Punjab and Western Uttar Pradesh, Gujarat and Rajasthan, the prevalence is below one person per 1,000 population.

Epidemiological Features

Agent

Mycobacterium leprae, an acid-fast bacilli resembling tuberculosis occurs in clumps or bundles and does not grow in artificial media. Infection is not transmitted to laboratory animals experimentally.

Reservoir of Infection

Men, the active cases of leprosy are the chief resources. Portal of exit from the nose, upper respiratory tract and skin, the bacilli leave the body as indicated below:
- Skin: Ulcers or breach of skin
- Nose: Secretions and ulcers of nose
- Throat: Coughing, sneezing and speaking
- Attack rate: It is 6.8 per 1,000 among contacts as compared to 0.8 per 1,000 without contact.

Host Factors

Age: Person of any age suffers on exposure. Survey shows 70% of cases above 25 years of age and 80% of cases above 20 years of age. A high prevalence of disease among children indicates that the disease is active and spreading.

Sex: More commonly seen in men than in women in proportion of 2:1. Sex difference is due to greater susceptibility than to greater exposure in men compared to women.

Race: All human races are susceptible.

Susceptibility: As follows:
- Contagiousness depends upon genetic susceptibility
- Married partners not more than 5%
- Only small percentage of persons exposed to infection develop the disease, genetic factor have role in leprosy
- Twin study: Identical twin show more similarity
- Blood groups: 'O' group twice as affected as 'B' group, but there is no definite conclusion
- Migration: The trend towards migration and urbanization has greatly increased the spread of disease.

Environmental Factors

- Climate: More common in warm and humid climate
- Social factors: Leprosy is a social disease with a social cause and social consequences
- It is found in persons of:
  - Poor environmental surroundings
  - Low standard of living due to poverty
  - Substandard housing
  - Overcrowding
  - Lack of education
  - Low personal hygiene
  - Unhygienic personal habits
  - Use of common clothing and linen
  - Above all apathetic attitude, prejudices and indifferences to leprosy.

It is most feared disease due to the deformity and ugliness, it imparts to the affected people. Leprosy is not highly contagious. Due to social stigma, the patient conceals the disease in early stage. External manifestations result in the loss of job. Patients are rendered destitute and resort to begging.

Modes of Transmission

1. Contact transmission: Direct or indirect contact between an infectious and healthy, but susceptible person, closeness and duration of contact influence

transmission and also individual susceptibility. Attack rate in household contacts of lepromatous cases is six to eight times higher (close contact with families).
2. Droplet infection is very common. Airborne disease plays any part. Doctors and nurses of leprosy hospital do not get infection in this way.
3. Other routes: Lepra bacilli have been found in human milk.

Incubation Period

Incubation period is not exactly known. Commonly between 2 and 5 years. It ranges from few months to 30 or 40 years. Latent period is used in place of incubation period.

Classification

- Lepromatous leprosy (Fig. 35.5)
- Nonlepromatous:
  - Tuberculoid
  - Maculoanesthetic
  - Polyneuritics.
- Borderline leprosy
- Intermediate type.

Indian Classification

Intermediate type: Early cases with one or two vague hypopigmented molecules and definite sensory impairment.

Lepromatous: Highly infectious skin, mucosa, nerves and internal organs affected.

Tuberculoid type: Which may be flat or raised, hypopigmented or erythematous and are anesthetic. Lesions are bacteriologically negative.

Borderline type: Four or more lesions, which may be flat or raised, well or ill defined, hypopigmented or erythematous and show sensory impairment or loss. Bacteriological positivity is variable.

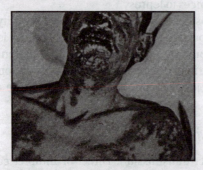

Figure 35.5: Lepromatous leprosy leonine countenance

Lepromatous type: Diffuse infiltration or numerous flat or raised, poorly defined, shiny, smooth, symmetrically distributed lesions and bacteriologically positive.

Pure neuritic type: Cases with nerve involvement, but do not show any lesion in the skin, bacteriologically negative.

Other Types of Classification

1. Lepromatous: Highly infectious skin, mucosa, nerves and internal organs are affected:
   - The ulnar nerve
   - The median nerve over front of the lateral side of wrist joint
   - The popliteal nerve in head of the fibula at the knee joints.
2. Appearance of patch:
   - Flat and reddish with clear cut or ill-defined margin
   - Raised either uniformly or at margin with central flattening.
3. Testing of sensation:
   - Touch: Hold and stiff the part in triangle, touch patch and ask the feeling of tap
   - Temperature: Test tube with hot water mask for heat
   - Pains: Prick a clean pin or needle.
4. Palpation of thickened nerves:
   - Flex the elbow and feel.
5. Identification of complications:
   - Eye: Lagophthalmos, discharge of eyes, conjunctivitis, corneal ulcers
   - Nose: Mucopurulent, foul smelling discharge and nose bleeding
   - Nerve: Neuritis cause severe pains, tingling and numbness trophic ulcer on the feet, and sudden spread of existing lesion
   - Lepra reaction: Fever with flaring up of existing lesions
   - Testis: Orchitis, resulting in swelling and pain.

Bacteriological Examination

1. Skin slit and scrape method: Material from the skin is obtained from an active lesion and also from both the earlobes.
2. Nasal smears of blows: These can be prepared from early morning mucus material or an alternative is to use a nasal mucosal scrapper. The smear is immediately fixed by passing over a spirit lamp and stained with Ziehl-Neelsen method, 5% hydrochloric acid (HCl) is used for decolorization.

3. **Histamine test:** Intradermal infection of 0.1 mL of 1/1,000 solution of histamine phosphate and/or chloral hydrate is injected intradermally into hypopigmented patches or in areas of anesthesia. In leprosy, flare response is lost.
4. **Biopsy:** When the examination stated above, does not yield a diagnosis, a biopsy is required (not routinely done).
5. **Footpad culture:** Inoculate the material into the footpads of mice and demonstrate the multiplication of *M. leprae*.
6. **Lepromin test:** Inject intradermally 0.1 mL lepra antigen or lepromin in the forearm of the patient and examine the reaction at the end of 48 hours and 21 days. There are two types of reactions:
   a. **Early reaction:** Inflammatory response develops within 24–48 hours and remains for 3–5 days. Redness and induration at the site of inoculation. If the red area has more than 10 mm diameter at the end of 48 hours, the test is considered positive.
   b. **Delayed reaction:** The reaction develops late becoming apparent in 7–10 days following the injection and reaching its maximum within 3–4 weeks.

The test is read at 21 days. If there is a nodule more than 10 mm in diameter, the reaction is positive.

Lepromin is a suspension of triturated lepromatous tissue rich in *M. leprae* in an isotonic solution of sodium chloride sterilized by healthy. Two kinds of lepromin are commonly used:
1. The crude antigen of Mitsuda.
2. The refined antigen of Dharmendra.

The early reaction of Dharmendra lepromin test is red at 48 hours. Infiltration greater than 15 mm, but less than 20 mm is considered moderately positive, infiltration greater than 20 mm strongly positive. The early reaction has the same significance as the late reaction.

Bacterial Index

Bacterial index is the only objective way of assessing the benefit of treatment. It should be done every 6 months on all positive cases. Slides are first graded as follows:
- Negative: No bacilli found in 100 fields:
  - One plus (+): One or less than one in each microscopic field
  - Two plus (++): Bacilli found in all fields
  - Three plus (+++): Many bacilli found in all fields.

Add 'G' to the entry if globi are present. Bacteriological index is calculated by totaling the number of '+' given to each smear and dividing this number by the number of smears collected. A minimum of seven sites should be examined, i.e. smears from four skin lesions, one nasal trials and smears from both earlobes.

Morphological Index

Morphological index is the percentage of solid staining bacilli. The criteria for calling the bacilli solid rods are:
- Uniform staining of the entire organism
- Length five times that of the width
- Rained ends
- Parallel sides.

If the index rises after having fallen, it indicates that the patient has not taken or absorbed his/her drugs or that the bacilli have become resistant.

Methods of Leprosy Control

- Survey
- Early detection of cases
- Chemotherapy
- Follow-up of cases
- Selective isolation
- Prevention of contact
- Chemoprophylaxis
- Immunoprophylaxis
- Prevention of disabilities/rehabilitation
- Health education
- Social measures training of medical and auxiliary personnel.

Survey

The size of the problem can be seen by random sample surveys. The survey should bring out not only the prevalence of leprosy but also the age and sex distribution of cases and the various forms of leprosy. A rough estimate of the prevalence can be determined by examining all school-age children, the total prevalence will be about four times the number of cases found.

Early Detection of Cases

Case finding is important because quite often patients do not know they have the disease. Some patients are afraid to disclose themselves. The current recommendation is to involve the primary health workers [village health guard (VHG) multipurpose health workers (MPWs)] in case detection with the active participation of the community. These workers have to be actively trained to make a tentative diagnosis of leprosy. The diagnosis should be confirmed by laboratory methods:
1. **Contact survey/trading:** Examination of household contact, especially children. In areas where the prevalence of leprosy is low (less than one case/1,000), the technique of choice is the examination of all contacts.

2. **Group survey:** When the prevalence is about one per 1,000 population or higher, additional case finding methods should be employed, e.g. surveys in schools, slums and in urban areas, army, labor, industrial areas, etc. for all types of skin diseases.
3. **Mass surveys:** Surveys for examination of each and every individual is recommended in hyperendemic, i.e. in areas where leprosy is about 10 or more per 1,000 populations. Total population (at least coverage of 90%) should be covered in mass surveys.

Chemotherapy

Antileprosy drugs

1. **Dapsone [diaminodiphenyl sulfone (DDS)]:** Till recently dapsone was the only drug of choice available for treatment of leprosy:
   a. *Advantages:* Cheap, effective, given orally, it is completely absorbed from the gut, fairly well-tolerated; rest is needed (11 month treatment + 1 month rest).
   b. *Disadvantage:* The above treatment is required to be prolonged for many years, hence there are chances of dropout.
2. **Clofazimine:** Both antileprosy and anti-inflammatory dose 50 mg daily.
3. **Rifampicin (RMP):** Only drug that is highly bactericidal against *M. leprae*. It is an essential drug in the chemotherapy of leprosy. In a single dose of 600 mg, 99.9% of leprosy bacilli are killed in 3-7 days. It is effective when given at monthly intervals.
4. **Ethionamide and prothionamide:** More expensive and more toxic than dapsone. However, these two drugs remain the only alternative to clofazimine in patients requiring triple drug therapy and who will not accept clofazimine. The dose is 5–10 mg/kg of body weight. The acceptability of these drugs is not yet established.

Recommended treatment: Multidrug therapy regimen
Followed and recommended by National Leprosy Eradication Program (NLEP):

1. **Multibacillary cases (MBC):**
   a. About weeks intensive treatment at the clinic with daily doses are detailed in Table 35.1.

Table 35.1: Intensive treatment (multibacillary cases)

Drug	15 year	10–14 year	6–9 year
Rifampicin	600 mg	450 mg	300 mg
Clofazimine	100 mg	50 mg	50 mg
Dapsone	100 mg	50 mg	25 mg

   b. Continuation phase of multibacillary (MB) treatment regimen, once monthly doses for 24 months at clinic (Table 35.2).

Table 35.2: Continuation of treatment multibacillary cases

Drug	15 year	10–14 year	6–9 year
Rifampicin	500 mg	450 mg	300 mg
Clofazimine	300 mg	150 mg	100 mg
Dapsone	100 mg	50 mg	25 mg

   c. Daily domiciliary dose for 24 hours are detailed in Table 35.3.

Table 35.3: Daily domiciliary dose multibacillary cases

Drug	15 year	10–14 year	6–9 year
Clofazimine	50 mg daily	50 mg (alternate day)	50 mg (twice weekly)
Dapsone	100 mg	50 mg	25 mg

2. **Paucibacillary cases (PBC):** Once monthly doses for 6 months at the clinic (Table 35.4).

Table 35.4: Monthly doses for paucibacillary cases

Drug	15 year	10–14 year	6–9 year	1–5 year
Rifampicin	600 mg	450 mg	300 mg	150 mg
Dapsone	100 mg	50 mg	25 mg	10 mg

3. **Monotherapy** (Table 35.5).

Table 35.5: Monotherapy paucibacillary cases

Drug	15 year	10–14 year	1–5 year
Dapsone	100 mg	50 mg	10 mg daily dose

Criteria for discharge

Multibacillary leprosy: A MB patient, who is clinically inactive and bacteriologically negative at the commencement of multidrug therapy (MDT) should continue treatment for 2 years (24 monthly supervised doses within 36 months). Thereafter, treatment should be discontinued provided the patient continues to remain clinically inactive and bacteriologically negative at the end of 2nd year of this period. MB smear positive patients should continue treatment until they become clinically inactive and bacteriologically negative or for a minimum period of 2 years, whichever is later. If after treatment for more than 36 months, the bacterial count remains the same or increases, the patient should be properly examined again clinically and bacteriologically for deciding the future line of treatment.

Paucibacillary (PB) leprosy patients should continue treatment till supervised monthly doses have been administered. If treatment is interrupted, the regimen should be recommended where it was left off to complete six doses within 9 months. If the lesions show extension or new lesions appear at the end of the prescribed course of treatment, the same schedule must be continued for a further period of 6 months to complete 1 year. Provided the classification is reviewed and found correct. Patients refractory 1 year of treatment should be referred to a specialist for evaluation and advice.

Modified multidrug therapy regimen suggested under NLEP in India

World Health Organization (WHO), Leprosy Elimination Advisory Group (LEAG) met in Geneva on 16th to 17th July, 1997 and strongly supported the recommendations made by 7th WHO Expert Committee on chemotherapy. The LEAG endorsed the technical recommendations of the 7th Expert Committee ill chemotherapy of leprosy and urged all the national governments to implement the same:

1. Leprosy division: The Directorate General of Health Services (DGHS) called meeting of leprosy experts from India on July 28, 1997 to review the development in chemotherapy of leprosy including Elimination Advisory Group on chemotherapy. This Expert Committee concluded as follows:
   a. All the MB cases should be put on 12 months MDT. In absence of improvement or in case of worsening, the period of treatment should be increased to 24 months. After release from treatment, surveillance of patients should be strengthened. MB patients should be put on surveillance once a year for 5 years.
   b. Single skin lesion cases without any nerve trunk thickening should be treated with single dose rifampicin, ofloxacin and minocycline (ROM). If there is worsening of signs and symptoms, such as increase in number and size of the lesion, and appearance of nerve trunk thickening, the treatment should be extended to 6 months PB MDT.
2. In view of the recommendations of the Indian experts decision was taken to modify the present MDT regimen under NLEP as:
   a. Single skin lesion case:
      - Documentation of single skin lesion has to be done in the reporting proforma
      - All the single skin lesion cases will be put on ROM as per above recommendations
      - These patients will be kept on general surveillance after release from treatment (RFT) as per present practice of surveillance once in a year for 2 years
      - In case of worsening (appearing of new lesion or increase in size of patch), the patients will be given 6 months PB MDT.
3. Multibacillary MDI:
   a. All MB patients should be put on 12 months MB MDT.
   b. These MB patients will be kept on general surveillance after RFT for a period of 5 years.

All patients who are already on treatment at present should be treated on the new regimens. The MB patients who have received 12 or more months, MDT treatment will be excluded from the treatment.

Selection of patients for multidrug therapy

Multibacillary patients: The following categories of patients will be considered for MB regimen of MDT:
- All skin smear positive patients irrespective of their classification
- All clinical borderline lepromatous (BL) and lepromatous leprosy (LL) cases whether skin smear positive or negative
- All skin smear positive relapses after dapsone monotherapy or MDT, irrespective of their classification
- All active borderline tuberculoid (BT) cases with six or more skin lesions, irrespective of their skin smear status
- All pure neuritic cases with two or more nerve lesions.

Paucibacillary patients: Following criteria are considered:
- Active LL and BL cases (with less than or equal to five skin lesions)
- Pure neuritic cases with single nerve involvement provided that they are skin smear negative
- All active PB cases on monotherapy
- Newly diagnosed (previously untreated) PB patients.

New multidrug therapy dose schedule

1. Drugs used for PB patients:
   a. Single skin lesion patients:
      i. Adult:
         - Rifampicin: 600 mg
         - Ofloxacin: 400 mg
         - Minocycline: 100 mg.
      ii. Children: Half dose:
         - Duration: Single dose immediately (stat) on confirmation of diagnosis.
   b. Single nerve lesion patients and patients with two to five skin lesions:
      i. Adult:
         - Rifampicin: 600 mg once a month supervised
         - Dapsone: 100 mg daily self-administered.
      ii. Children: Correspondingly lower dose as followed presently:
         - For adults with body weight below 35 kg, the dose of rifampicin should be 450 mg once monthly and dapsone 50 mg daily
         - The dose for children (0–14 year) is given in Table 35.6.

Table 35.6: Doses of children (0–14 year)

Drug	0–5 year	6–14 year
Rifampicin (monthly)	30 mg	450 mg
Dapsone (daily)	25 mg	50 mg

- Duration: Treatment should be continued for a total of six supervised monthly doses to be administered within 9 months.

c. The side effects of antileprosy drugs used under ROM single dose treatment for single skin lesion patients are virtually nil or insignificant. Following side effects have been reported in patients receiving treatment for long period:
   i. Minocycline:
      - Discoloration of teeth
      - Headache, dizziness, vertigo, ataxia, drowsiness, fatigue, blue-green pigmentation of leprosy lesion
      - Pneumonitis, drug-induced esophageal ulceration, acute hepatic failure, black thyroid discoloration, sweat syndrome and toxicity to sperms.
   ii. Ofloxacin:
      - Gastrointestinal system: Nausea, vomiting
      - Central nervous system: Dizziness, vertigo and psychosis
      - Dermatitis or hypersensitive reaction, e.g. exfoliative dermatitis and photodermatitis.
   iii. Rifampicin:
      - Rifampicin is easy to administer and is relatively nontoxic in the recommended doses
      - In case of any untoward side effect reported, expert opinion should be sought before it is labeled as side effect due to ROM
      - Contraindications: In view of single dose therapy of ROM within prescribed dose, there are hardly any contraindication moreover, the children are given half the dose
      - Special precautions:
         - Though there is no need for any special precaution, however, it is suggested that ROM may be avoided when patient has liver or kidney disease, or during early stage of pregnancy
         - Since only half single dose is given for the children, it should be given to children of all age groups.

2. Drugs used for 12 months WHO MDT regimen:
   a. Regimen for MB cases:
      i. Adults: Treatment is to be given for 12 monthly pulses as follows:
         - Rifampicin: 600 mg once monthly supervised
         - Clofazimine: 300 mg once monthly supervised
         - Dapsone: 100 mg supervised and daily self-administered
         - Clofazimine: 100 mg on alternate days or 50 mg daily self-administered.

Note: Adults with body weight below 35 kg should be given rifampicin 450 mg monthly; the self-administered dapsone dosage should be reduced to 50 mg daily.

      ii. Children: In children, the dose shall be proportionately reduced. The following schedule is recommended for children in the age group 6–14 year (Table 35.7).

Table 35.7: Doses of children (6–14 year)

Dose	6–9 year	10–14 year
Rifampicin	300 mg (once monthly)	450 mg (once monthly)
Clofazimine	100 mg (once monthly)	150 mg (once monthly) 50 mg (twice weekly)
Dapsone	25 mg daily	50 mg daily on alternate day

   b. Regularity of treatment: Adequate treatment implies that the patient has taken 12 monthly supervised doses (MDT) of combined therapy within 18 months.

Side effects of antileprosy drugs

Side effects of antileprosy drugs, which are used for MB patients are detailed below.

Rifampicin

Rifampicin is excreted in urine due to which the color of urine becomes orange red. Patients must be explained that it is not due to side effect of medicine so that they do not stop using antileprosy drugs. Rifampicin is easy to administer and is relatively nontoxic in the recommended dose. Adverse reactions occur more frequently with intermittent regimens (once weekly). Reactions are uncommon or trivial when given only once or once monthly. The side effects observed are:

1. Flushing or pruritus with or without rash often on the face and scalp. There could be redness and watering of the eyes in rare cases.
2. Pain in the abdomen and nausea, sometimes accompanied by vomiting and/or diarrhea.
3. Fever, chills, malaise, headache and bone or joint pains—flu syndrome.
4. In rare cases, shortness of breath may occur.

Purpura, acute hemolytic anemia, shock and renal failure are rare. Elevated serum transaminase levels are associated with risk of hepatitis. Most patients with adverse reactions require no modification of the drug regimen, since the symptoms are mild and self-limiting. Symptomatic treatment may be given where the reactions trouble the patients and persist. In patients with respiratory syndrome, caution is necessary. Such cases may require immediate hospitalization. If shock is followed by renal failure, rifampicin should not be given again. This applies also to hemolytic anemia, wherever the reactions persist and bother the patient. The dosage may be lowered to 450 mg besides giving symptomatic treatment. If no improvement occurs, then rifampicin should be discontinued.

Clofazimine
Clofazimine is well-tolerated and virtually nontoxic in the dosage used. The following side effects have been reported:
1. Reversible, dose-related, reddish to brownish black, discoloration of sweat, hair, sputum, urine and feces. General dryness of the skin (xeroderma) ichthyosis and pruritus can be troublesome.
2. Phototoxicity, acneiform eruptions and non-specific skin rashes have also been reported, though rarely.
3. An early abdominal syndrome commencing within a few days of starting treatment and possibly due to direct irritant effect of the drug. Symptoms, however, subside when the dosage is reduced or the drug is discontinued.
4. A late syndrome may commence some months after high-dose therapy with persistent diarrhea, loss of weight and abdominal pain. This syndrome is associated with deposition of clofazimine crystals in the tissues, usually in the submucosa of the small intestine and in the mesenteric lymph nodes.
5. Except for conjunctival pigmentation in the eyes, which does not interfere with visual acuity, no other ocular side effects have been reported.
6. To treat erythema nodosum leprosum (ENL) and reversal reactions and also general ailments, the medical officers must also carry essential supportive drugs.

Dapsone
Side effects are uncommon when the drug is given in recommended doses. However, in rare cases, the following may occur:
- Hemolytic anemia
- Agranulocytosis
- Hepatitis
- Allergic rashes including exfoliative dermatitis
- Psychosis
- Fixed drug eruption or hypermelanosis.

Surveillance
At the time of RFT of patient with ROM treatment, patients should be educated to report when there is extension of pre-existing single lesion and appearance of new skin lesion, fresh nerve involvement and redness of pre-existing skin lesion. Since, ROM treatment is newly introduced, it is advisable to observe such patients once a year up to 2 years.

Surveillance of patients is advised for ME patients after RFT at 12 months once in a year for up to 5 years period. During course of follow-up, worsening cases should be got confirmed by District Leprosy Officer or trained Medical Officer or District Supervisor, wherever they are available.

Reversal reaction after release from treatment should be differentiated from worsening of disease. In case of worsening of MB category, the patient be put on WHO MB MDT for 24 months and worsening of the patient treated on single dose of each should be put on WHO 6 months MDT regimen.

After completion of treatment, mild reversal reaction, neuritis may appear rarely with ROM treatment for single lesion cases, which should be managed with antireaction line of treatment. The follow-up of patient should be without inducing him/her on MDT again. But when worsening is diagnosed, WHO MDT treatment should be given for 6 months. In areas where such differentiation is difficult, MDT can be given along with antireaction treatment. Important difference between signs of reversal reaction and worsening of disease are given in Table 35.8.

Table 35.8: Difference between reversal reaction and worsening of disease

Reversal reaction	Worsening of disease (relapse)
Erythema in pre-existing lesion or appearance of new erythematous lesion	Extension of pre-existing skin lesion or worsening of skin lesion
Onset abrupt and sudden	Demonstration of acid-fast bacilli (AFB) in the skin lesion
Generally occurs during chemotherapy or **within 6 months of stopping treatment**	Fresh nerve involvement with nerve tenderness and nerve thickening
Multiple nerve involvement common, painful and tender	Onset slow and insidious
May have generalized symptoms such as fever, joint pains, malaise	No generalized symptoms
Rapid response to steroids	No response to steroids

Surveillance after completion of chemotherapy as indicated below is essential for detection of relapses as well as the cause of relapse. MB patients should be examined clinically and bacteriologically at least once every 12 months, for a minimum period of 5 years, after completion of treatment, while PB patients require to be examined clinically at least once every 12 months for a minimum period of 2 years after completing treatment. Contact surveillance of households with:
- Lepromatous case should be maintained for minimum of 10 years
- A most non-lepromatous case should be maintained for 5 years.

Prevention of Disabilities

Prevent physical deformities, which occur in 20–25% of cases. With the prevention and treatment of disabilities, physiotherapy and reconstructive surgery, physical rehabilitation has become reality (physical rehabilitation has been achieved through physiotherapy and reconstruct surgery, but psychological and social rehabilitation is still a burning problem).

Health Education

Health education should be directed to the patients and their family, and the general public. Need for regular and complete treatment, repeated examination of contacts, prevention of disabilities, protection of children and family planning—preferably sterilization. Emphasis in education should be to the following aspects:
1. Leprosy is a disease such as other disease.
2. Not a hereditary disease.
3. All cases are not infectious.
4. Children should be segregated from infectious parents.
5. Leprosy is curable.
6. Early diagnosis and treatment are important.
7. About 8% of the deformities are due to neglect.
8. The patient needs sympathy and kindness.

Social Aspect of Leprosy

Regarding human and social consequences of leprosy, it has caused a great reaction in the community and happiness to the patients and their families. It involves an economic factor as the cured patients are not employed and become a burden on the society. There is a need of social assurance to the patients and their families. Physical and mental restoration as far as possible to all treated patients so that they may resume their place in home, society and industry.

The disability from deformities is also a cause of prejudice against leprosy. It is deep rooted. The whole family lives as a social outcast due to social stigma attached to the disease. Leprosy is believed to be a disease due to divine curse or due to sins committed either in this life or in the previous one and is in shape of punishment. Leprosy patient is a source of trouble for the family during social functions. People think it is incurable and a hereditary disease.

If there is any stigma with the leprosy patient in the family or community, the same may be studied. Family and community may be educated accordingly. Leprosy is totally curable disease and is not hereditary. Social factors, which may come in the way of regular treatment should also be explored and adequate counseling may be done to overcome the same.

Several voluntary organizations given below work in the leprosy control measures:
- Indian Leprosy Association, 1950
- Gandhi Memorial Leprosy Foundation, 1951
- Mission of Leprosy
- Ramakrishna Mission.
  The following existing laws relate to the control of leprosy:
- Leprosy Act, 1898
- Railway Act, 1890
- Local Self-Government Act.

These laws do not make any distinction between infection and non-infection leprosy, there is no specific vaccine against leprosy.

Nursing Management

Isolation

Leprosy can be isolated by the medical aseptic technique. Leprosy is a communicable disease, but it is communicated with great difficulty and the means by which it is accomplished remains unknown. However, the appearance of Chinese leprosy patients in the islands of Polynesia, previously entirely free of leprosy and its subsequent spread to the natives of these isolated communities adequately proves the hypothesis of its communicability. To the natives, it has become known as the 'Chinese disease', a case may easily be isolated in an open ward or in a room with other diseases, but because of the fear of leprosy by the public, leprosy patients necessarily are assigned to a private room or to special quarters maintained especially for them, within a communicable disease hospital.

The causative organisms are believed to be the Hansen's bacilli found in the nose and throat secretions, and in the open lesions. All waste material contaminated by the patient should be cleaned up and sent to the incinerator.

Diet

The diet should be a full, wholesome and generous diet. During episodes of high fever and prostration seen in the lepromatous types, the diet and general nursing care should be the same as that in severely ill tuberculous or typhoid patients.

Temperature

In the tuberculoid or indeterminate types, the temperature is rarely a disturbing factor. In the lepromatous type, episodes of fever occur in which the temperature may go quite high, but usually runs from 102 to 103°F in the late afternoon and rarely requires lowering measures. If so, an alcohol rub, fan or tepid sponge may be used.

Personal Hygiene

Special attention must be given to the personal hygiene of the leprosy patient. Patients should have a daily cleansing bath and change of clothing. Oral hygiene should be above reproach.

Elimination

Normal elimination should be maintained. In rare instances cathartics or enemas may be required.

General Management

Most cases of leprosy in the temperate zone of North America are very mild and the patients are ambulatory. All active cases with discharging lesions should be isolated. In cases in which there are no open lesions or in which the nervous system alone appears to present the only visual evidence of disease, parole to the health department and not isolation, should be required and they should make periodic visits to the health department leprologists for inspection and control. There is a growing tendency in this country to turn loose leprosy patients of all types without regard to adequate medical care or inspection, the thought being that any family doctor is perfectly competent to oversee and direct their treatment. Unfortunately, this is not true. The average family doctor in the United States (US) never saw a case of leprosy and has not the faintest idea either of how to treat it or to evaluate its progress. The only way to stamp leprosy out in this country is to control leprosy patients. However, this should be done with justice, with knowledge, with consideration, with kindness, but with firmness, the aim at all times being to accomplish the greatest good for the greatest number, but never unjustly or unduly to abrogate the rights of the individuals or to appear to punish them.

The patient should be assigned to an attractive room with good ventilation and one that admits plenty of sunshine and light. The bed should be comfortable. Leprosy patients are much happier if two or more of them can be placed together so that they have company. For the psychological effect, the patient should be permitted to wear attractive, well fitting, washable clothing and comfortable shoes. Visitors should be permitted, the visitors being protected as circumstances warrant. If conditions are such that friends and relatives are unable to visit, patient should be encouraged to keep in touch with them by letter.

A place for outdoor exercise and recreation should be provided, and the patient should be encouraged to remain outdoors as much as possible. They should be given an opportunity to do useful work such as gardening, weaving, basket making and writing. Magazines and newspapers should be provided, as well as radio, television and other methods of recreation.

If the patient is awaiting transfer to a public health service hospital, the nurse should be able to tell something about the environment there. Everything possible should be done to maintain patient's morale. They should be encouraged to cooperate with the medical staff in all ways and to keep up treatment until discontinued by doctor. An effort should be made to make them feel that society is their friend and that a place in the world will remain for them when their care is completed. However, at present this is very difficult because once the diagnosis becomes known, it is almost impossible to get an employer to hire a healed leper. This leads to secrecy and secrecy leads to suspicion, and this to a furtive demeanor. It is unfortunate that this is true, but until we re-educate the public it will probably remain.

Terminal Disinfection

All bedding and clothing must be sterilized before being sent to the laundry, not that this is necessary from the standpoint of preventing the spread of leprosy, but simply for its psychological effect upon hospital personnel. Mattresses and pillows are sterilized, usually in the autoclave, and then are aired. All contaminated wall space, toilets and bath contacts, bed, table and chairs should be washed with soap and water. In hospital Zephiran disinfectant is also used. The same applies for the treatment of equipment.

SEXUALLY TRANSMITTED DISEASES

Sexually transmitted diseases are a group of communicable diseases that are transmitted predominantly by sexual contact. During past two decades, STDs have undergone a dramatic transformation. The change in name from venereal disease (VD) to STD. There are five classical VDs such as syphilis, gonorrhea, chancroid, lymphogranuloma venereum and donovanosis.

Magnitude of the Problem

The STDs are worldwide, have high prevalence from 1 to 14% in the vulnerable population groups. The trend in gonorrhea and primary syphilis is on the increase, since the late 1970s, which is posing a serious barrier to patient care.

Problems in India

Syphilis: Serological survey is the best source of information on the prevalence of syphilis. The recent survey of 15,762 women attending the antenatal clinics in Aurangabad by Venereal Disease Research Laboratory (VDRL) test showed 2.4% positive cases. Kerala showed seropositivity prevalence of 1.4%.

Gonorrhea: Information of the morbidity of gonorrhea is notoriously lacking as most cases are not reported. It is more widely prevalent than syphilis and 80% of infected women are reported to be asymptomatic carriers.

Chancroid or soft sore: It is reported to be fairly widely prevalent in India.

Lymphogranuloma venereum: It is reportedly more prevalent in the southern states of Tamil Nadu and Andhra Pradesh than in the northern states. But 6% of STDs are seen in Madras.

Donovanosis or granuloma inguinale: It is endemic in Tamil Nadu, Andhra Pradesh, Odisha, Karnataka and Maharashtra along coastal areas reported 6.1% of the total male VD cases and 6.9% of the total female VD cases in 1966.

Epidemiological Factors

Agents

Over 20 pathogens have been found to be spread by sexual contact. A classification of these agents and the diseases caused by them is tabulated in Table 35.9.

Host and Environment

Age: Highest rates of incidence are found between 20 and 24 years.

Sex: Both sexes are prone. Morbidity rate is higher in men than women. Morbidity caused by infection is more severe in women.

Marital status: It is more prevalent in divorced and separated persons, and even in singles.

Table 35.9: Major sexually transmitted diseases (STDs) and their agents

Pathogens	Diseases or syndromes
Neisseria gonorrhoeae	Gonorrhea, urethritis, salpingitis, cervicitis, neonatal conjunctivitis
Treponema pallidum	Syphilis
Haemophilus ducreyi	Chancroid
Chlamydia trachomatis	Lymphogranuloma venereum (LGV), urethritis, cervicitis, neonatal conjunctivitis
Calymmatobacterium granulomatis	Granuloma inguinal, minor STD
Herpes simplex virus	Genital herpes
Hepatitis B virus	Acute and chronic hepatitis
Human papilloma viruses	Genital and anal warts
Human immunodeficiency syndrome (HIV)	Acquired immunodeficiency syndrome (AIDS)
Candida albicans	Vaginitis
Trichomonas vaginalis	Vaginitis

Socioeconomic status: Lowest socioeconomic, strata have the highest morbidity rate.

Social factors: Numerous social and behavioral factors are involved in the spread of STDs are detailed below.

Prostitution: This is a major factor in the spread of STDs. The prostitution acts as a reservoir of infection. In Asia most STDs are contacted from prostitutes, whereas in many developed countries, the professional prostitutes have largely been replaced by the 'good time girls'. The male component of prostitution is equally important.

Prostitution supplies a demand if there were no prostitutes, there would be no prostitution, thus abolishing the factor of STDs.

Broken homes: Social studies indicate that promiscuous women are usually drawn from broken homes, e.g. homes, which are broken either due to death of one or both patients or their separation. The atmosphere in such homes is unhappy and children rated to such an atmosphere are likely to go astray in search of other avenues of happiness.

Sexual disharmony: Married people with strained relations, divorced and separated persons are often victims of STDs.

Easy money: In most of the developing world, prostitution is simply a reflection of poverty. It provides an occupation for earning easy money. It is fostered by lack of female employment and the prospect of a financial return impossible to achieve by other means.

Emotional immaturity: This has been often stressed as a social factor in acquiring STDs.

Urbanization and industrialization: These are conducive to the type of lifestyle that contributes to high levels of infection. Long working hours, relative isolation from the family, geographical and social mobility foster casual sexual relationships.

Social description: Caused by disasters, wards and civil unrest have always caused an increase in the spread of STDs.

International travel: Travelers can import as well as export infection and their important role in the transmission of STDs is exemplified by the rapid *Neisseria gonorhoeae* (*N. gonorhoeae*) and acquired immunodeficiency syndrome (AIDS).

Changing behavioral patterns: In modern society the values additionally set on chastity are in conflict with the more recent ideas of independence, freedom from supervision and equal rights for both sexes. There has been a relaxation at moral and cultural values in present day society. The tendency to break away from traditional ways of life is particularly marked among young people.

Social stigma: It is attached to STDs accounts for the nondetection of cases, not disclosing the sources of contact, dropping out before treatment is complete, going to quacks for treatment and self-treatment.

Alcoholism: The effect of alcohol seems to be more indirect than direct. Alcohol may encourage prostitution and prostitution may boost the sale of alcohol.

Syphilis

Syphilis may be defined as a contagious disease caused by palladium. It may be acquired by sexual contact and occasionally by accidental infection.

Morphology of Treponema pallidum

Treponema pallidum (*T. pallidum*) is 6–8 mm in length, 0.2 mm in diameter with tapering ends. The body is coiled in 8–15 regular, rigid and sharp spirals. It is actively motile rotation around long axis backward and forward movements, and flexion of whole body. It is feebly refractive and so not stained with ordinary staining techniques. It ordinarily reproduces by transverse fission and divided organism may adhere to one another for some time. However, its morphology and motility can be seen under dark ground illumination (Fig. 35.6).

Types

There are two types of syphilis:
1. Congenital syphilis.
2. Acquired syphilis.

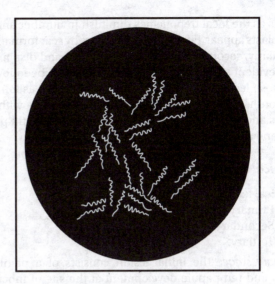

Figure 35.6: *Treponema pallidum* under dark ground microscopy

Congenital syphilis: A pregnant syphilitic women can transmit *T. pallidum* to the fetus through placenta beginning about the 10th week of gestation. Some of the fetuses die and miscarriages result, while others are stillborn. At term some are born live, but develop the signs of congenital syphilis in childhood, e.g. interstitial keratitis, Hutchinson's teeth, saddle nose and periostitis.

Acquired syphilis: It is limited to men only. The organism enters through microabrasions on the skin or mucosa.

Pathophysiology

Treponema pallidum is inoculated into the tissues through a small abrasion usually as a result of sexual contact. Then organisms multiply and the tissues become infiltrated with small lymphocytes and plasma cells, which are concentrated particularly in the perivascular lymphatics and involve the vessel walls as microscopic study shows proliferating small vessels surrounded by traponemous, inflammatory and plasma cells.

The organism seen in capillary endothelium suggested that sites of proliferation. Small blood vessels produce hypertrophic changes in the endothelium, which may obliterate the lumen. Loss of blood supply results in erosion of the surface of lesion before the primary lesion has appeared. Then treponemes reach the regional lymph node by way of the lymphatics and multiply. The tissue response is similar and results in enlargement of the nodes. Sometimes, treponemes find their way into the bloodstream and are disseminated to all the tissues of the body. Multiplication occur producing secondary stage 6–8 hours after the beginning of the primary stage. The primary lesion slowly heals as the local treponemes diminish in number and fibroblasts appear. Finally, healing occurs by scar formation. Similarly, secondary lesions slowly regress and disappear, but evident scarring is rare. They are likely to be followed by fresh lesions. Final disappearance may take as long as 9 months. Now, the patients are in latency stage with no signs and symptoms of diseases yet infection is still present and active.

Clinical Features

Clinical features falls into three stages:
1. Primary.
2. Secondary.
3. Tertiary.

Primary stage: The initial lesion consists of a painless, hard and red papule development at the site of inoculation, which later ruptures and forms an ulcer. This is called chancre. In male this is usually on the penis. In the female, it may be either on the vulva or the cervix. In the latter case it may be symptomless. The neighboring lymph gland becomes enlarged.

Secondary stage: The lesion of secondary stage develops and there are popular spleen rashes, mucous patches in oropharynx and condylomata at mucocutaneous junction. Patient is highly infectious during secondary stage. There may be eye and meningeal involvement. This stage commences about 6 weeks after the onset of the disease and is prolonged to about 2 years.

Tertiary stage: The lesions characteristic of the tertiary stage usually appear within 2–15 years from the onset of infection.

Symptoms of tertiary stage are:
1. The skin and mucous membrane: Ulcers in the legs, palate, face or tongue.
2. The cardiovascular system: Disease of the aortic value or the walls of blood vessels leading to aneurysm.
3. The bones and periosteum, causing osteitis and periostitis.
4. Affections of the central nervous system.

Gonorrhea

Gonorrhea is venereal infection related to its chronicity, latency and multiplicity of localization. Next to measles, it is the most prevalent of the notifiable communicable disease. It is characterized by infection of mucous membrane by *N. gonorrhoeae* an organism more commonly known as the gonococcus. It may occur in both sexes and newborn. Incubation period is 3–10 days.

Morphology of Gonococcus

Gonococcus is strictly a parasite of man. The coccus is gram negative, oval or spherical 0.8–0.6 µ with adjacent sides concave (bean shaped) and arranged to pair. It is found predominantly within the polymorphs.

Pathophysiology

The gonococcus causes a surface infection, ascending in almost all cases by way of the lower genital tract. The primary infection following an incubation period of 3–8 days takes place in or near the urethra. Its drainage is good, subsides spontaneously and cleanses in the course of a few days or weeks. However, infection of the prostatic urethra in the male and also of the female urethral and vaginal glands predisposes to chronic infection with occasionally very serious sequelae. Females are set to contract secondarily a mixed infection of the endometrium and thereafter the tubes constituting pelvic inflammatory disease with resultant pelvic peritonitis.

The ascent of infections is precipitated by the factors such as menstruation, douches and the trauma associated with sexual intercourse or instrumentation.

Clinical Features

1. Urinary frequency.
2. Dysuria.
3. Discharge of a yellowish exudate from the urethra or the vagina.
4. In female tubal infection (salpingitis).
5. Low abdominal and back pain, which is aggravated by defection, dysmenorrhea or menorrhagia.

Chancroid

Chancroid is also called 'soft chancre' and 'ulcus molle'. It is an acute, localized autoinoculable infection of the genitals caused by the streptobacillus of Ducrey [*Haemophilus ducreyi* (*H. ducreyi*)]. First isolated by Ducrey in 1889. *H. ducreyi* is characterized by ulceration at the sites of inoculation and is frequently accompanied by suppuration of the regional lymph nodes. The incubation period is 1–5 days, but it can occasionally last as long as 30 days.

Morphology

Haemophilus ducreyi is a short, slender gram-negative rod with rounded ends. Groups of organisms are often found in chains giving the appearance of a stool of fish. It may be difficult to find the organism in open lesions on the genitalia (Figs 35.7 and 35.8) because of secondary bacterial infection.

Incidence

It is not a common disease in the United Kingdom (UK) or in other western countries. In eastern countries and in tropical and subtropical regions, the incidence is far higher although it is low incidence in women, it appears to be a particular hazard of prostitutes in certain parts of the world.

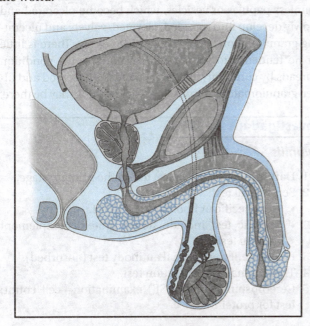

Figure 35.7: Diagrammatic representation of the male genitalia

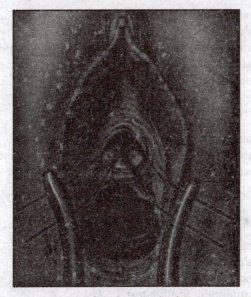

Figure 35.8: External female genitalia demonstrating the openings of Skene's gland

Clinical Types

1. Follicular chancroid: Originates in hair follicles, seen on the vulva and on the hairy surface around the genitals very superficial.
2. Dwarf chancroid: Small lesions.
3. Transient chancroid: Small lesions typical chancroidal type.
4. Popular chancroid: Starts as an ulcer, but latter becomes raised particularly around its edges. It may resemble the condylomata, later, secondary syphilis.
5. Giant chancroid: May start as a small ulcer, but extends rapidly and covers a considerable area.
6. Phagedenic chancroid: May commence as small lesion, but becomes large and destructive with widespread necrosis of tissue. The external genitalia may be destroyed.

Clinical Features

1. There may be only one lesion, but often there are several.
2. Extragenital chancroids as rare.
3. It is small, inflammatory papule surrounded by narrow zone of bright erythema.
4. It soon becomes pustular, if it ruptures forms a painful, sharply circumscribed ulcer.
5. Vascular granulation tissues present, which are tender to touch and bleed easily.

Lymphogranuloma Venereum

Lymphogranuloma venereum (LVG) is transmitted sexually and commences with a transient, primary genital lesion followed by regional suppurative adenitis. After a latent phase, which may last for years, there may be late manifestations due to rectal structure or lymphatic obstruction.

Causative agent, which was first isolated by Hellstrom and Wassan in 1930, belongs to the *Chlamydia* group of agents includes causative organisms of psittacosis and trachoma, e.g. *Chlamydia psittaci* (*C. psittaci*), *Chlamydia trachomatis* (*C. trachomatis*), respectively. These large microorganisms are obligatory intracellular, parasites more related to bacteria, in their structure, mode of reproduction, chemical constitution and susceptibility to chemotherapy.

Incidence

The disease is common in tropical and subtropical climate, but uncommon in temperate countries. In June 30, 1977 about 36 cases were reported in England.

Clinical Manifestations

Lymphogranuloma venereum is usually a small herpetiform is lesion and may be an ulcer, papule, vesicle or pustule appearing on the gland pericoronal sulcus. There are several lesions on prepuce or shaft of the penis. The lesions are small, painless and nonindurated. The conditions rarely found in woman and still very rare urethral discharge (Fig. 35.9)—a rare form of non-gonococcal urethritis accompanied by urethral stricture and fistula.

Granuloma Inguinale

Granuloma inguinale has been called ulcerating granuloma of the pudenda, sclerosing granuloma and granulomatosis in Europe, for the international nomenclature of disease and helps to avoid confusion with LVG.

Causative Organism

Donovania granulomatis (Donovan body) was probably discovered by Donovan in India in 1905. He described bodies seen in epithelial cells of the skin.

Morphology

Donovania granulomatis measure 1.5 by 2.5 mm. With Wright's stain, the capsule is pink and the body of the organism shows bipolar condensation of chromatin material. The nature of the organism is the subject of controversy, but many believe that it is bacterial and related to *Klebsiella* group.

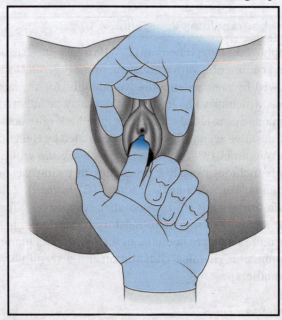

Figure 35.9: Milking the urethra to express pus from Skene's ducts

Incidence

Granuloma inguinale occurs almost exclusively in the colored races. It is found in tropical and subtropical countries. In India, it is much more common in Hindus than in Muslims.

Clinical Findings

The lesions may commence on the genitalia and on the thigh, in the groins or in the perineum. These appear first as painless papules or vesicles, which become ulcerated and slowly develop into rounded, elevated, velvety and ulcerating granulomatous masses that bleed easily. There is little or no tendency to spontaneous healing as the condition spreads by continuity as triable, painless, beefy red and ulcer-granulomatous lesions. Inguinal swelling may be there.

Investigations for STDs

Syphilis

1. Dark ground illumination test in the primary stage.
2. Serological test:
   - Nonspecific or lipoidal test—VDRL
   - Specific test include Reiter protein complement fixation test.
3. Fluorescent treponemal antibody test (absorbed).
4. Treponemal immunization test.
5. Cerebrospinal fluid (CSF) examination—cell count; test for protein.

Gonorrhea

1. Smear stained by Gram stain.
2. Culture enriched media, e.g. chocolate agar.
3. Gonococcal complement fixation test for complicated cases.
4. Fluorescent antibody test.

Chancroid

1. Smear of the pus or unruptured.
2. Culture containing defibrinated rabbit blood; cysteine dextrose and beef infusion agar.
3. Biopsy.

Lymphogranuloma Venereum

1. Smear.
2. Culture.
3. Biopsy.
4. Compliment fixation test.

5. Free test: It is an intradermal test, the antigen is prepared from an infected yolk of chick embryo and injected 0.1 mL into the forearm and the result read after 48 hours, the test is positive for lifelong.

Granuloma Inguinale

1. Staining method.
2. Wright-Giemsa stain.

Chemotherapy of STDs

During the past decades, a standard drug regimen has been worked out, which is effective against all the five major VDs.

In the early phase of the disease, this regimen consists of tetracycline 500 mg orally four times a day for 10 days. As a result of systematically applying this regimen over the decades, the late destruction and disfiguring manifestations of tertiary syphilis have disappeared from the area the regimen was used in. Associated VD will need to be countered by fungicide, antiprotozoal drugs and anthelmintic drugs.

Viral condyloma acuminate (caused by the papillomavirus) has been successfully managed at our center with topical application of podophyllum resin 20% in tincture. Benzoin molluscum contagiosum (caused by a member of the pox group of viruses) is tackled by gauging out the molluscum body and applying tincture iodine to the scalloped are left behind.

Herpes genitalis due to herpes simplex virus (HSV) I and II were tackled initially with smallpox vaccine given by inoculation weekly for 10 weeks. After the vaccine was withdrawn from circulation, it became difficult to test the condition. However, experimental treatment with chloramphenicol 500 mg given orally four times a day for 10 days proved effective and is being used ever since. Recurrence in few cases was traced to untreated contacts (marital and extramarital) and was successfully treated in the contact along with retreatment of the index cases following this finding. It was also found highly effective against the other five VD too, particularly against tetracycline-resistant disease. Even pregnant women with genital herpes were successfully treated and the babies delivered were normal at 6 months follow-up.

Based on these experiences with viral infections, it is felt that chloramphenicol could be effective against human immunodeficiency virus (HIV) in persons detected to be seropositive for HIV antigen. This needs further investigation. Thus, to sum up control of bacterial VD can be accomplished with the broad-spectrum antibiotics tetracycline and viral VD with chloramphenicol.

Preventive Measures

1. People or community must be protected from commercialized prostitution and from clandestine sexual promiscuity. It is done by enforcing law and social force.
2. Community must get sex education. Adolescents and young adults can have it in the school and colleges. They must know about preparation for marriage and premarital examination, and how they contact the disease, etc.
3. Government and owner of industries must provide means of healthy recreations for their workers and public.
4. Provision should be made to improve general health of the community and raise their social, and economic status.
5. Provision should be made for early diagnosis and treatment.
6. All pregnant women must have facility of serological test.
7. Investigation of case is necessary.
8. Survey of selected group should be done to find out cases. This group includes industrial workers, contacts of patients, pregnant women, nurses, doctors, etc.
9. Surveyor case-finding program should be carried on in these areas, where this disease is highly prevalent.
10. Wide publicity and mass education are necessary to prevent people from getting this infection. People must know about personal protection and practice personal hygiene.
11. Sulfonamide or antibiotics may be used to prevent people from getting these infections.
12. Nurses, doctors and such other persons, who are dealing with these patients must protect themselves, while attending these patients.

Control Measures

1. Notify about the case to the health authorities.
2. Isolation of the patients is limited up to 24 hours due to modern therapy. But they should avoid sexual intercourse with their previous partners, who are not under treatment to prevent themselves from reinfection.
3. Discharges from the open lesions must be collected and disinfected daily. Articles, which are contaminated with the discharges of an infected person must be disinfected.
4. If pregnant woman has syphilis, treat her during pregnancy to prevent her baby from getting congenital syphilis.

5. Interviews of patients, their contacts, etc. should be carried out by the trained persons to find out the source of infection.
6. Provision should be made to examine groups of young adults and adolescents, who are moving from areas of high prevalence of infections.
7. Provision should be made for rapid exchange of information internationally about contacts.
8. Provision should also be done for free treatment and diagnosis of these cases. Provision should be made for rapid exchange of information internationally about contacts. Present status of STDs program and future directions much more needs to be done for control of STD than what is currently being done. For example, in Tamil Nadu there are only 20 STD clinics (one in each headquarter town) to cater to a total population of 50 million, which is grossly inadequate, considering that 40% of the population is in the sexually active age group and therefore at risk.

Similarly, in the country we have less than 500 VD clinics to care for 9 million populations. The number of STD clinics as well as number of postgraduate diploma and degree holders in STD must be increased by appropriate expansion of postgraduate seats in this specialty. Even the district level STD clinics are not adequately utilized. This could be either due to lack of awareness or the stigma attached, so that persons who are aware of their risk status or existing disease do not avail the service.

Hence, with the twin objectives of extending services in the rural areas as well as to encourage patients to avail of treatment, STD clinics should be opened at veterinary dispensaries, where people are any way attending for their livestock problems. There are 750 veterinary clinics in Tamil Nadu, alone widely spread out even in interior areas, which can cater to the need of the patients.

Another measure to extend STD control services is to implement the STD control program (including, surveillance treatment and monitoring) through the PHC network. Adequate training should be provided to PHC notify about the case to the health authorities doctors. Training can even be provided at the district hospital to diagnose and treat the disease, as well to tackle the problem with a community approach in the PHC area. They should be linked to the district hospital specialty clinics by two-way referral. The district hospitals should have well-equipped bacteriological, virological and serological diagnostic laboratories.

Lastly, medical personnel should be sensitized to the need for contact tracing and treatment of contacts. As soon as a single case is discovered, this implies a thorough training of the Medical Officers, as well as, health education of the community to participate in the STD Control Program.

Management

Nursing Management of Gonorrhea

The source of infection with the gonococcus is always another human being; the mode is usually by sexual intercourse. While it is possible to carry this infection by indirect contact from one individual to another by means of articles of recent use, intermediary objects probably play a minor role in transmission. The appearance of this disease in one of a married pair is often the occasion for a very serious marital disturbance. In this situation, the nurse may help avert difficulties by casual references to possible sources of the disease outside of sexual contact and may also stress the possibilities of recurrence after a long latent period, if the patient has not had an opportunity for adequate treatment of his/her previous disease or if a previous infection may not have been recognized.

Tactfulness on the part of the nurse in handling patients suffering from gonorrhea is of the greatest importance. During the brief period of infectivity, it is both exemplary and comforting to the patient to see nurse and doctor obviously cleanse their hands by washing both before and after his/her treatment and to see his/her linen and dressings handled with aseptic precautions. A thoughtful nurse will impress the patient with the need for follow-up visits to the doctor until patient is discharged as cured and will find a way to teach the importance of post-treatment examinations including serology tests for syphilis until the danger of an oncoming syphilitic infection, which may have been altered or masked has completely passed.

Nursing Management of Syphilis

Clever and alert nurses rapidly come to realize that when they have to combine professional interest and sympathetic understanding. They will receive the patient's day-to-day confidence to a greater degree than the doctor because they are spending more time with the patient. This is particularly true of the syphilitic patient who returns repeatedly for treatment. At each visit, the syphilitic patients must be prepared for treatment by the nurse, who usually sees them prior to the doctor's visit. The nurse must realize that the syphilitic patients are often frightened out of all proportion to the seriousness of even their very serious illness. Therefore, they need moral support to sustain. Patient's look upon advice from the nurse as being much more impersonal than that of the doctor. The patients are apt to tell the nurse of little subjective sensations of vital importance to their progress. Nurse may thus be the first one to be aware of the beginning of patient's unfavorable physical reaction to therapy of urticaria or little blisters of the hands and feet of dermatitis, or of serum sickness-like reaction, all of which indicate the necessity for immediate present discontinuance of the use of penicillin.

The nurse is often with the patient a much longer time than the doctor. So, nurse should take advantage of the apparently impersonal mechanical duties, which they perform in the preparation of the room and supplies, for the patient, to instill an atmosphere of cheer and confidence. All good nurses, thanks to the elevating leadership of the great Florence Nightingale, find themselves respected leaders in their community. They soon learn the art of guiding conversation into acceptable channels. In dealing with patients suffering from syphilis, the wise nurse will guide the conversation away from the length and kind of treatment, the possible toxic consequences of the drugs used, the failure to cure and the injurious effects of the disease or the possibility of insanity due to syphilitic softening of the brain. They will remember that they are dealing with a patient whose heart is heavy with the burden of trouble. It has a strangely reassuring effect on the patient to be told that many cases of syphilis are innocently acquired.

They may impress upon their necessity for careful oral hygiene, reiterating frequently, the sources and modes of extragenital transmission of the disease. It is also helpful for them to speak in an impersonal manner of the public duty evolving upon each patient infected with syphilis in preventing the transmission of disease to others. A casual word of the amazing 10% incidence of syphilis in the general population will help to re-establish the patient's morale for nearly all syphilitic patients tend to feel themselves social outcasts and in their own minds are benefited by the knowledge of its widespread existence. A competent nurse will find it easily within his/her province to teach the patient, the importance of reporting symptoms of treatment reactions to the physician, the necessity for regular and continuous treatment and long-term follow-up of his/her condition as well as the patient's own responsibility in the control of the spread of the disease during their own period of infectivity. Nurse's may find it easily within their province to teach patients to follow through with post-treatment medical supervision and to assist them to meet other social, economic, personal and family problems, which their confidence in nurse's judgment will lead them to discuss with nurse and that have a direct bearing upon the communicability of this readily communicated infection.

AIDS/HIV Infection

The AIDS sometimes called 'slim disease' is a newly described usually fatal illness caused by a retrovirus own as the HIV, which breaks down the body's immune system, leaving the victim vulnerable, to a host of life-threatening opportunistic infections and neurological disorders or unusual malignancies. Among the special features of HIV infection is that a person once infected will be infected for life. Strictly speaking, the term AIDS refers only to the last stage of HIV infection. AIDS can be called our modern pandemic, affecting both industrialized and developing countries.

Historical Background

Till a decade before, infectious diseases ceased to be a major problem in developed countries, but with the advent of AIDS in early 80s, the situation changed dramatically. Like other viruses, retrovirus cannot replicate without taking over the biosynthetic apparatus of a cell. Retroviruses are unique in their capacity to reverse ordinary flow of genetic information from deoxyribonucleic acid (DNA) to ribonucleic acid (RNA) to proteins. With the help of reverse transcriptase, viral RNA is converted into DNA, which gets integrated into the genome of the host. Once getting established in the host genomes, the viral DNA remains latent, until it is activated to make new virus particles.

Retrovirus and their cancer-causing potential are not new to the scientists. Reverse transcriptase was discovered in 1970. However, up to mid-70s another infectious retrovirus was found in human beings. In 1980, the first human retrovirus, e.g. human T-cell lymphotropic virus type 1 (HTLV-1) was isolated, which causes a rare, highly malignant cancer called adult and T-cell leukemia, i.e. endemic in parts of Japan, Africa and Caribbean islands and spreading to other regions as well 2 years later HTLV-2 was found out. Both these viruses cause immune depressions and therefore, when AIDS cases were first recognized, the initial hypothesis was that the cause of AIDS could be a close relative of HTLV-1. The hypothesis did not prove correct, however, the search in this direction led to finding HIV as the cause of AIDS.

Though HIV has been spreading fast in America, Europe, Australia and Africa. Asia appears to be the continent affected last and fortunately least by HIV infection. The reasons for lesser spread in the Asian countries particularly India, is not very clearly understood though there could be several causes.

Important events in AIDS

- 1981: The first case of AIDS reported in United States of America (USA)
- 1983: Lymphadenopathy associated virus (LAV), i.e. HIV isolated
- 1984: Serological tests developed to identify infected persons

- 1985: Report of in vitro anti-HIV activity of Health Protection Agency (HPA) 23, interferon-α, foscarnet (PFA) and zidovudine (AZT) published
- 1986: Clinical trials of zidovudine show efficacy in AIDS and advanced AIDS-related complex
- 1987: Zidovudine licensed for clinical use in many countries; large scale clinical trials of AZT and other agents began
- 1991: Didanosine is licensed for use by US Food and Drug Administration (FDA) in selected.

Acquired immunodeficiency syndrome is an immunoregulatory disorder that is often fatal because it predisposes the person to severe opportunistic infections or possibly to neoplasms. It happens so because of depletion of helper T cells owing to infection by HIV.

Magnitude of the Problem

Acquired immunodeficiency syndrome knows no geographic, social, racial or cultural boundaries. First described in 1981 in USA, AIDS is now recognized throughout the world. On the basis of available information, the WHO estimates that between 5 and 10 million people are infected with HIV. AIDS is spreading fast and is already a worldwide epidemic. By October 1987, the AIDS epidemic had reached at least 128 countries and a total number of cases reported rose to 60,652. But this is only the tip of the iceberg.

Although, AIDS was first reported in USA in 1981, earlier cases were found by retrospective analysis to have occurred in 1978 in the USA and in the late 1970s in equatorial Africa. Since, the beginning of the epidemic in 1981, the prevalence has increased exponentially with a doubling time of 6–12 months.

Although, the vast majority of reported cases of AIDS have come from USA, AIDS is now seen in several countries throughout the world. According to WHO estimates, between 1 and 2 million Africans may already be AIDS carriers and that 50,000 are now suffering from the disease. Comparatively, Asia has reported a smaller number of cases. The HIV infection appears already infected. The eventual magnitude of AIDS cannot be predicted.

AIDS in India

First confirmed evidence of AIDS infection in India came in April 1986, when six prostitutes from Tamil Nadu were found positive for HIV antibodies. A total of 222 persons have been confirmed to have AIDS infection in the country out of about 80,000 persons belonging to the high-risk group screened up to January 31, 1988.

India has the distinction of having conducted a systemic nationwide serosurveillance for HIV infection from 1986 for defining epidemiology of HIV infection at a very early stage of the epidemic when a few cases of AIDS were reported. Within 2 years, data from the study showed that the magnitude of infection even in high-risk group was low (4 per 1,000) and heterosexual promiscuity is the major mode of transmission of infection in India.

The data from these studies provided the rational basis for evolving rational medium term plan for AIDS control. Serosurveillance among blood donors led to the timely initiation of blood donor screening to ensure safety of transfused blood. The epidemiological data from serosurveillance provided the technical information needed for drawing up appropriate health education material for AIDS control among high-risk and vulnerable groups.

Epidemiological Features

Agent factors

When the virus was first identified, it was called 'lymphadenopathy-associated virus (LAV)' by the French scientists. Researchers in USA called it 'human T-cell lymphotropic virus III (HTLV-III)'. In May 1986, the International Committee on the Taxonomy gives it a new name called HIV, i.e. hemagglutinin-neuraminidase (HN). It now seems that there are two types of HN; the most common HN-I and a more recently recognized virus (in West Africa) called HN-2.

The virus replicate in actively dividing T4 lymphocytes and like other retroviruses can remain in lymphoid cells in a latent state that can be activated. The virus has the unique ability to destroy human T4 helper cells, a subset of the human T lymphocytes. The virus is able to spread throughout the body. It can pass through the blood-brain barrier (BBB) and can then destroy some brain cells. This may account for certain neurological and psychomotor abnormalities observed in AIDS patients. HN mutates rapidly and new strains are continually developing.

It belongs to the lentivirus subgroup of retroviridae family. HIV is an RNA retrovirus. The unique morphologic feature of HIV is its cylindrical nucleoid in the mature virion. The diagnostic bar-shaped nucleoid may be seen in electron micrographs. Under electron microscope it exhibits the characteristic exotic flower appearance (Fig. 35.10). Robert C Gallo discovered HIV in 1984.

The virus is easily killed by heat. It is readily inactivated by either acetone ethanol (20%) or β-propiolactone (1:400 dilution), but is relatively resistant to ionizing radiation and ultraviolet light.

Sources of injection

The virus has been found in greatest concentration to blood, semen and cerebrospinal fluid. Lower concentrations have been detected in tears, saliva, breast milk, urine

CHAPTER 35 — Important Surface Infections and Sexually Transmitted Diseases

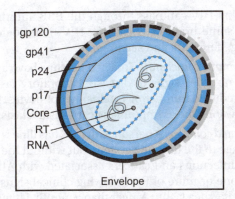

Figure 35.10: Structure of human immunodeficiency virus (gp, glycoprotein; p, protein; RNA, ribonucleic acid; RT, reverse transcriptase).

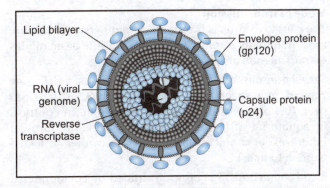

Figure 35.11: Detailed structure of human immunodeficiency virus (gp, glycoprotein; p, protein; RNA, ribonucleic acid)

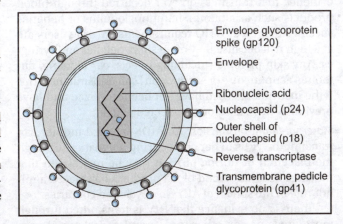

Figure 35.12: Structure of human immunodeficiency virus (gp, glycoprotein; p, protein)

and cervical and vaginal secretions. HN has also been isolated in brain tissue, lymph nodes, bone narrow cells and a skin. To date, only blood and semen have been conclusively shown to transmit the virus.

Human immunodeficiency virus is a spherical enveloped virus, about 90–120 nm in diameter (Figs 35.11 and 35.12). It contains two identical copies of single-stranded RNA genome. In association with viral RNA is the reverse transcriptase enzyme. The virus core is surrounded by a lipoprotein envelope. The major virus coded envelope glycoproteins are the projecting spikes on the surface and the anchoring transmembrane pedicles.

Reservoir of infection
There are cases of carriers. Once a person is infected, the virus remains in the body lifelong. The risk of developing AIDS increases with time, since HN infection can take years to manifest itself, the symptomless carrier can infect other people for years.

Host factors
Age: Most cases have occurred among sexually active persons of age 20–49 years. This group represents the most productive members of society and those responsible for child bearing and child rearing. Children under 15 make up less than 3% of cases. The distribution of AIDS cases by age group and sex in European countries is shown.

Sex: In North America, Europe and Australia about 70% of cases are homosexual or bisexual men. In Africa, the picture is very different, the sex ratio is equal. Certain sexual practices increase the risk of infection more than others, e.g. multiple sexual partners and intercourse and male homosexuality. Higher rates of HN infection are found in prostitutes. High-risk groups are male homosexuals, heterosexual partners (including prostitutes), IV drug abusers, transfusion recipients of blood and blood products, hemophiliacs and clients of STD.

Immunology
Hemagglutinin-neuraminidase virus has a specific tendency to infect and destroy T4 helper lymphocytes. Therefore, majority of AIDS patients have a low number of T helper cells. Whereas, healthy individuals have twice as many 'helper cells'; the 'suppressor cells' in the AIDS patients, the ratio is reversed. A decreased ratio of T helper to T suppressor cells may be an indirect indicator of reduced cellular immunity. One of the most striking features of the immune system of patients with AIDS is profound lymphopenia with total lymphocyte often below 500 mm^3. It is the alteration in T cells function that is responsible for the development of neoplasms, the development of opportunistic infections or the inability to mount a delayed-type hypersensitivity response. The lack of an obvious immunological response by the host to the virus is one of the problems confronting scientists. That is, those with antibodies to HN, usually have too few HN antibodies and these antibodies are also infective against the virus.

Mode of transmission

The causative virus is transmitted from person to person, most frequently through sexual activity. The basic modes of transmission are given below.

Sexual transmission: AIDS is first and foremost a STD. Any vaginal, anal or oral sex can spread AIDS. In the USA, over 70% of the cases were in homosexual. In contrast, in equatorial Africa, AIDS is acquired mainly through heterosexual contact (infected man to women, infected women to man).

Blood contact: AIDS is also transmitted by contaminated blood transfusion of whole blood cells, platelets and factors VIII and IX desired from human plasma. There is no evidence that transmission ever occurred through blood products such as albumin, immunoglobulins or hepatitis vaccines that meet WHO requirements. IV drug users are at a high risk because they often share needles and syringes. Any skin piercing (including injects, ear piercing, tattooing, acupuncture or sacrifice on) can transmit the virus, if the instruments used have not been sterilized and have previously been used on an infected person.

Maternal-fetal transmission: An AIDS-infected mother can transmit the virus to her child during pregnancy (through the placenta) or during birth. It may be mentioned that transfusion of blood and blood products has played a minor role in the spread of AIDS in developed countries.

There is no evidence that HIV is transmitted through mosquitoes or any other insects and casual social contact with infected persons even within households or by food or water. There is no evidence of spread to healthcare workers in their professional contact with people with AIDS. Incubation period, while the natural history of HIV infection is not yet fully known, currently data suggests that the incubation period is long (up to 6 years or more) from HIV infection to the development of AIDS. It is unknown how large a proportion of those infected will subsequently develop AIDS. The virus can be silent in the body for many years.

Clinical Features

The clinical features of HIV infection have been classified into four broad categories:
1. Initial infection with the virus and development of antibodies.
2. Asymptomatic carrier state.
3. AIDS-related complex (ARC).
4. AIDS.

Initial infection: Antibodies of HIV can usually be detected 2–8 weeks after initial infection. All these infected, with or without symptoms can transmit the virus to others. It seems that HIV can pass through the BBB and then can destroy some brain cells causing HIV neurological disease (e.g. dementia and seizures).

Asymptomatic carrier state: Infected persons have antibodies, but no overt signs of disease. Laboratory tasks may show a reduced number of T helper lymphocytes. It is not clear how long the asymptomatic carrier state lasts.

AIDS-related complex: A person with ARC has illness caused by damage to the immune system, but without the opportunistic infections and cancers associated with AIDS, but exhibit one or more of the following clinical signs. Unexplained diarrhea lasting longer than a month, fatigue, malaise, loss of more than 10% body weight, oral thrush, generalized lymphadenopathy or enlarged spleen. Patients from high-risk group who have two or more of these manifestations and who have a decreased number of T helper lymphocytes are considered to have ARC. Some patients with ARC subsequently develop AIDS.

Acquired immunodeficiency syndrome: The AIDS is the end stage of HIV infection. It is characterized by life-threatening opportunistic infection and/or cancers that occur in people with otherwise unexplained defects in immunity. Opportunistic infections vary in the US and UK, is pneumonia. In some parts of Africa, tuberculosis and persistent diarrhea seem to be more common. Death is due to uncontrolled or untreatable infection.

The occurrence of tumors is a major component of AIDS. A frequent form of tumors is Kaposi's sarcoma. Traditionally, Kaposi's sarcoma tends to affect the extremities, but in AIDS patients, it tends to be generalized, scattered purplish lesions over chest and abdomen. Others include Burkitt-like non-Hodgkin's lymphoma and isolated cerebral lymphoma:

- AIDS: Opportunistic organism
- Viruses: Fungi
- Cytomegalovirus: *Candida*
- Herpes simplex: *Cryptococcus*
- Epstein-Barr virus: *Histoplasma*
- Bacteria: Protozoa
- Mycobacterium tuberculosis: *Pneumocystis carinii*
- Atypical mycobacteria: *Toxoplasma gondii*
- Legionella: *Cryptosporidium*.

Diagnosis of AIDS

Clinical

The WHO clinical case definition for adult AIDS envisages the existence of at least two major signs associated with at least one minor sign in the absence of other known cases of immunosuppression such as cancer or severe malnutrition or other recognized etiologies:

1. Major signs:
   - Weight loss (10% of body weight)
   - Chronic diarrhea for longer than 1 month
   - Prolonged fever for longer than 1 month (intermittent or constant).
2. Minor signs:
   - Persistent cough for longer than 1 month
   - Generalized pruritic dermatitis (itching and inflamed skin)
   - Recurrent herpes zoster
   - Oropharyngeal candidiasis
   - Chronic progressive and disseminated herpes simplex
   - Generalized lymphadenopathy.

The presence of generalized Kaposi's sarcoma or cryptococcal meningitis is sufficient by themselves for the diagnosis of AIDS. The above definition was developed by WHO for use in areas where diagnostic resources are limited.

Screening tests
There is now a wide range of screening tasks based on detection of HIV antibodies. To be reliable, a screening test must be specific enough to record few 'false positives'. The ideal test needs both the attributes.

At present, to ensure accuracy, two different tests are commonly applied. At first, a sensitive test is used to detect the HIV antibodies, while a second confirmatory test is used to weed out any false-positive results. The first kind of test is normally the enzyme-linked immunosorbent assay (ELISA), which currently costs ₹50–100 or more per test. The confirmatory test, usually a western blot is a highly specific test. It is based on detecting specific antibody to viral case protein and envelope glycoprotein. This is a more difficult test to protein and requires trained and experienced laboratory workers to interpret the test.

Virus isolation
A test for the virus itself would eliminate the painful uncertainty of AIDS infection. HIV can be recovered from cultured lymphocytes. This type of testing is very expensive and requires extensive laboratory support. The current trend in HIV antibody tests is towards simple, cheap, reliable kits whose results can be read on the spot without much waiting and without the need for laboratory backup.

The WHO has pointed out the danger of compulsory testing programs in their tendency to social rejection of HIV carrier and the resulting social and psychological consequences. Diagnostic testing may be useful in gauging the magnitude and course of the epidemic, but it fails to help break the chain of infection.

New diagnostic test for HIV uses saliva
Saliva samples instead of blood, reports the 'daily laboratory report' in the US. According to the products manufacturer, this test could reduce the risk of exposure to HIV for healthcare workers who must draw blood from patients to test for AIDS. Clinical trials of the HIV saliva test are scheduled to begin soon at five hospitals around the US.

AIDS Control Program

In the context of the foregoing description it is clear that AIDS Control Program activities present a very complex scenario. AIDS Control Program should have the following broad components.

Establishment of a surveillance program
Acquired immunodeficiency syndrome is a new disease. Little information on its epidemiology and spread in the context of our country is available. Therefore, it is imperative to institute good surveillance machinery covering the entire country with more thrust on metropolitan cities and big towns. The surveillance mechanism should address itself to identify and detect AIDS cases/carriers amongst the high-risk groups and follow-up periodically with a sense of human approach and appropriate educational counseling. A good educational program with appropriate approaches will dispel the fear and motivate the high-risk personnel to come forward for screening. Following action points are suggested:
1. Already a network of 40 surveillance centers has been established. The same network could be further strengthened and widened to cover more areas. As a part of community-based surveillance and to work out an estimate of the number of AIDS-infected cases in the country, survey amongst the various high-risk groups such as prostitutes, blood donors and drug addicts should be undertaken periodically in different parts of the country with the assistances of the surveillance centers.
2. Laboratories in blood banks in metropolitan cities may be equipped for AIDS screening for donors. The network could be expanded in phases.
3. In-depth studies of specific population subgroups (in single, nonmonogamous, married persons) are needed in order to derive a more accurate description of levels of risk and risk perceptions and to apprehend how to intervene effectively to reduce the risk. In-depth studies of the sexual behavior and related perceptions in the adult and adolescent population are needed.
4. In-depth studies of opinion of leaders from various fields such as education, industry and media are needed to identify barriers so that appropriate actions could be undertaken, while implementing educational program.

Public opinion, education and behavior
The control measures primarily consist of good educational campaign against AIDS. Therefore, all out efforts need to

be made to institute a good educational campaign to tackle the problems of AIDS. While working out the educational program, the following need to be carefully looked into:

1. All messages directed at the public should be straightforward and people at risk are completely reassured. The messages should redirect the public energy from irrational personal concern to concern for those who are affected or likely to be affected and generating actions for the welfare of the affected victims.
2. Correct scientific information on AIDS should continued to be given as demands for the same will grow. The need for clear specific factual messages regarding transmission of AIDS should be given. Misconceptions regarding AIDS through blood donation should be removed.
3. Confusion regarding AIDS virus, disease progression and testing should be carefully removed. Misconceptions regarding transmission through casual contacts and confusion about HIV testing should be removed. Educational messages should explain what testing can accomplish for an individual and what it can and cannot do to solve the AIDS problem. Messages for anonymous testing for those at risk or concerned about risk should also discuss relevant issues such as allocation for testing sites, anonymity of results, etc. Confusion regarding the meaning of a positive HIV test should be removed. It is important for the public to understand the implication of a positive HIV test result in AIDS. Information about the disease progression, awareness of the probability of the disease progression from HIV infection to AIDS-related complex and finally to AIDS would help.
4. The focus of attention should be shifted away from persons diagnosed with AIDS to persons infected with AIDS virus, which will reinforce gravity of the situation for those engaged in high-risk behaviors.
5. Focus of attention should not be on population subgroups, but on high-risk behaviors. Attention should also be given that reducing risk does not necessarily mean elimination of risk.
6. There is a need for messages targeting perceptions of personal vulnerability. Individuals will not be motivated to change behavior if they do not perceive themselves to be at risk for exposure through actions.
7. Increased number of public forums for discussion of the barriers to risk avoidance and the benefit of changes in risk behavior could conceivably turn risk avoidance into social phenomenon.
8. Messages targeting personal control may help to reduce perceptions that AIDS is someone else problem and reduce the excessive reliance on government's intervention.
9. Motivational message on direct educations programs must attempt to bring about behavioral change. Message must emphasize to maintain behavior changes.
10. A sense of social responsibility and community involvement must be developed. Educational strategies should be built upon current awareness to increase the perception that AIDS is a problem, everyone should feel responsible to do something about providing social support, talk to friends and lovers, abstain from undesirable sex, use condom and avoid high-risk activity.
11. There is a need for messages encouraging community involvement.
12. The specific message targeting subpopulation are needed. HIV negative persons should be encouraged to retail this status and urged when appropriate to donate blood.
13. Intensive educational campaign should be carried out for HIV carriers. They should receive regular periodic counseling and social support, and encounter aged for responsible behavior in sexual relation.

Framing specific guidelines

There is an urgent need to frame specific guidelines for blood banks, blood product manufacturers, import blood products, drug de-addiction clinics, laboratories engaged in AIDS work, etc. Special working groups may be set up to formulate specific guidelines and the same should be implemented in right earnestness.

Training

Acquired immunodeficiency syndrome will continue to remain a problem for sometime to come. A large number of professionals and physical activity leader (PAL) professionals need to be trained in case detected management and their proper follow-up. India is a very large country and therefore, a large number of clinical needs to be trained in case management. AIDS present wide ranging symptom complex involving various organs. Its detection and proper management will be a problem in times to come. Therefore, a suitable training program needs to be chalked out for clinical training of health managers and epidemiologists control is also essential, training of paramedical will also necessitate substantial resource development.

As Indian, experience with AIDS is new, physicians involved in the management of the cases, in our country need to be asked to workout specific guidelines for management of detected cases and their follow-up, so that cases detected in any part of the country could be properly looked after.

Research

Indian Council of Medical Research should sponsor special studies in different parts of the country in the field of AIDS to generate more information on AIDS in Indian situation so that more meaningful control program could be built-up.

Indigenous production of test kits
A large number of test kits will be required for the AIDS Control Program and the surveillance centers.

Presently, it is being procured from outside India, but import of the kits is very expensive. Therefore, there is an urgent need to look into the issue of indigenous production of test kits and make efforts, so that kits could be manufactured in India.

Prostitution issue
Prostitution is illegal in the country, but everybody knows that prostitution continues to flourish in metropolitan cities and big towns and even the rural areas are not very much behind. This trade in human flesh is continuing unabated. Therefore, issue of licensing the prostitutes also needs to be examined and with the concurrence of the other related departments action needs to be initiated. However, till that date, good educational campaign to motivate prostitutes and call girls to come for a periodic medical check-up may pay good dividend. The question of providing free or subsidized consultation to these categories could also be examined.

Legislation
To undertake actions on the above lines, in many of the areas, it is observed that official instructions by various authorities are not implemented because of paucity of funds, paucity of trained manpower, etc. Therefore, the question of legislation comes into the picture. Several countries in the world have taken the help of legislative measures to control the spread of AIDS, because provision of legislative measures ensures that the administrative authorities take punitive actions against defaulters. Legislative measures, particularly with regard to the blood product manufacturers, importation of blood products are no doubt essential, but legislative measures in areas of screening of any specific group of people, etc. needs wider discussions, as initiation of legislative measures without adequate provision of monitoring its implementation, will negate the gains of such measures.

However, there is no denial that if legislative measures are coupled with a good educational prevention program, AIDS spread could be checked to a great extent. Taking into account, the complexity that AIDS presents, it would be worthwhile to bring only those provisions under legislative cover, which need very stern measures, but with regard to the issue such as screening of any specific group, with regard to follow-up measures for the carriers, provision for the blood banks, etc. efforts should be made to handle the situation with strict administrative instructions and follow-up.

Treatment

A number of drugs have undergone clinical trials for the treatment. But all drugs are considered as palliative treatment:

1. Zidovudine popularly known as azidothymidine (AZT) is in longest use:
   - Action: Decreases the frequency of opportunistic infection in advance HN infection and contributes to an increase in the survival time, progress the life span, showed the progression of AIDS
   - Adverse effect: Anemia, nausea, vomiting, headache, etc.
2. Dideoxyinosine (DDI) and dideoxycytidine (DDC) or studies indicate that combination of zidovudine and either DDI or DDC could delay the emergence of resistance and clinical deterioration as well as reduce the incidence of adverse reaction.

YAWS

Yaws is a contagious, non-venereal infectious disease caused by *Treponema pertenue (T. pertenue)*, common among children.

Clinically characterized by a primary papillomatous skin lesion called 'mother yaw', seen on exposed part of the body such as face or trunk, followed by a generalized lesions and a late stage of destruction of skin and bone in an untreated case. The disease is closely linked with standard or living and social customs.

Magnitude

Yaws is a public health problem in Africa, Southeast Asia and central part of South America. In Africa, it is reported from Benin, Ghana and Ivory Coast. In Southeast Asia, it is reported from India, Indonesia, Papua New Guinea and South Pacific. In South America, it is reported from Brazil, Columbia, Ecuador, Guyana and Surinam.

During 1950's, WHO and United Nations International Children's Emergency Fund (UNICEF) launched a concerted program to curb the disease by giving a mass treatment for about 50 million individuals from 46 countries, covering a population of about 400 million people living in the affected areas, resulting in a great reduction in the prevalence of yaws. However, there has been an increasing trend of the disease.

In India, it is mainly a disease of tribal people in Maharashtra, Odisha, Madhya Pradesh, Assam and Andhra Pradesh.

The problem of yaws how is one of either 'residual yaws' or 'recrudescence of yaws', due to continued low levels of transmission.

Epidemiological Features

Agent

The causative agent is *T. pertenue,* which is morphologically similar to *T. pallidum*. It has 10–12 spirals and 20 m in length. It is highly host specific. It occurs in the epidermis of the lesions, lymph glands, spleen and bone marrow. It cannot survive outside the human body (Fig. 35.13).

Reservoir of Infection

There is only human reservoir. Source of infection is the discharges of the cutaneous lesions of yaws. The lesions relapse several times and serve as source for new infections.

Host Factors

Age incidence: It is primarily a disease of children, below 15 years of age; peak incidence is between 5 and 10 years of age. However, it can occur in age group.

Sex incidence: Preponderance is more among males than females.

Immunity: There is no natural immunity. Immunity is acquired slowly over several years. It is suppressed by treatment. However, it offers cross immunity partially against venereal syphilis. The prevalence of yaws is inversely proportional to the prevalence of venereal syphilis, i.e. if the prevalence of venereal syphilis is more that of yaws is less and vice versa.

Social Factors

The disease is endemic among tribal people because of scanty clothing, poor personal hygiene, frequent trauma and wounds, overcrowding, low standard of living, lack of availability of soap and water are responsible for the prevalence of yaws.

Environmental Factors

Warm and humid climate favors the transmission of yaws because it keeps the organisms viable in the discharges from the wound on the ground. Thus, the prevalence is high among tribal living on the top of the hills than among those living in foothills.

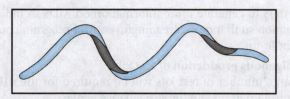

Figure 35.13: *Treponema pallidum*

Modes of Transmission

The disease is mainly transmitted by direct contact with the discharges of cutaneous lesions during holding each other, embracing, sharing bed, mother carrying the child while feeding, etc. that is by close physical contact:
- Indirect contact: The disease is also transmitted indirectly through discharges on ground and the pathogens enter the body through injuries on feet
- Vectors: Houseflies and other small insects have been incriminated as mechanical vectors in the transmission of the disease.

Period of Communicability

May extend for several years, continuously or intermittently. The lesions are infectious as long as they are moist and exudative. The pathogens are usually not found in late, ulcerative lesions.

Incubation Period

Varies from 3 to 6 weeks.

Clinical Features of Yaws

Early Yaws

The primary lesion seen on the exposed part of the body, i.e. face or limb is called 'mother yaws', indicates the route of entry of the pathogen. It is a papillomatous lesion. It is called mother lesion because it is from here, further spread takes place resulting in generalized eruptions, while the mother lesion continues to remain, becomes proliferative, exudative, papillomatous, large, yellow, crusted and granulomatous lesion resembling condyloma lata of secondary syphilis. It goes on spreading. During the next 5 years, waxing and waning or spontaneous healing is a common feature. The early lesions are highly infectious. Local lymph glands are enlarged and the blood becomes positive for serological tests for syphilis (STS).

Late Yaws

Late yaws occur after 5 years, characterized by destructive, deforming and disabling lesions affecting skin and bone. The lesions on the palms and soles are called 'crab yaws', those on the palate (hard and soft) and nose are called 'gangosa', the swelling by the side of the nose due to osteoperiostitis of the maxillary bone is called 'goundu'. These late features occur in about 10% of untreated cases. The late ulcerative lesions are not infectious.

Laboratory Diagnosis

Dark field microscopy of early exudative lesions for treponemal identification.

Medical Treatment

The drug of choice is benzathine penicillin, long-acting penicillin. Dose is 6 lakh units and 12 lakh units for children below 10 years and those above 10 years respectively. It is given deep intramuscularly. Single dose will cure the infection. Those who are sensitive to penicillin are given tetracycline or erythromycin 500 mg four times a day for 2 weeks.

Prevention and Control

Involves the following steps:
- Survey
- Treatment
- Resurvey
- Surveillance
- Improvement of sanitation
- Evaluation.

Survey

A clinical survey is done in the endemic area, covering almost 95% of the total population, to know the magnitude of the problem in terms of prevalence rate of yaws. During the survey, the case and their contacts are listed.

Treatment

The WHO has recommended three treatment policies depending upon the prevalence rate as follows:

1. Selective mass treatment: This is for the area where the prevalence rate is less than 5% (hyperendemic area). In these areas, treatment is given to the cases, family contacts and close extrafamilial contacts.
2. Juvenile mass treatment: This is for the area where the prevalence rate is between 5 and 10% (mesoendemic area). Treatment is given to all cases and to all children below 15 years of age and other extrafamilial close contacts.
3. Total mass treatment: This is for the area where the prevalence rate is more than 10%. Treatment is given to the entire population including the cases because the whole population is at risk.

Resurvey

Since, it is not possible to cover the entire population in a single round of survey, resurvey is undertaken once in 6–12 months to find out and treat all missed cases and new cases.

Surveillance

Surveillance is a technique recommended to detect any new case of yaws (i.e. case detection). Any case detected is investigated epidemiologically to identify the probable source of infection and contacts so as to prevent new cases. The case is given therapeutic treatment and contacts are given prophylactic treatment. Monthly follow-up the family contacts are done for 3–4 months. All these measures help in interruption of transmission.

Improvement of Environmental Sanitation

Since socioenvironmental factors plays a key role in the prevalence of the disease in the community, emphasis has been laid in the improvement of sanitation such as provision of ample water supply, improvement of housing conditions, control of vectors, disposal of the discharges of the lesions, health education of the people to maintain high standard of personal hygiene by using soap and water liberally, avoiding unnecessary close physical contact with others and cleanliness in and around the houses, thus improving the quality of life.

Evaluation

Resurvey is done after implementing the control campaign to find out the prevalence rate. More than the clinical survey, serological studies are done among children borne after the completion of the control campaign. If no antibodies are found among those children that means the disease is under control. Even though there is treatment for yaws and the preventive measures are simple, yaws is not amenable for eradication because:

- The cases are infectious for months and years
- The pathogens remain latent in lymph nodes
- The immunity acquired does not last longer
- There is no vaccine against yaws.

GAS GANGRENE

Gas gangrene or clostridial myonecrosis is a severe infection of skeletal muscle caused by several species of gram-positive clostridia that may complicate trauma, compound fractures, contusions or lacerated wounds by producing exotoxins that destroy tissue. The gas bacilli is an inhabitant of the human intestinal tract, it is likely to be the infecting organism in thigh wounds following amputations, especially if the patient is incontinent. Peripheral vascular disease, gangrene, incontinence and debility often are combined in patients with diabetes.

Magnitude of Problem

Clostridium welchii (*C. welchii*), an anaerobic bacillus was discovered by the American pathologist William Welch in 1891. It is in war wounds that *C. welchii* infection is of the greatest importance. Gas gangrene was found in the war wounds of the soldiers in the First World War. Infection is fatal in approximately 87% of the cases.

Gas gangrene is a disease of muscle, which at first is a dull red and then becomes green or black. Bubbles of foul-smelling gas and blood-stained fluid can be pressed up and down the length of the muscle. The bacilli spread up and down the muscle in the interstitial tissue and the muscle fibers are separated from their sheaths by toxic fluid, as a result of which they are killed and are then invaded by the putrefactive bacteria.

Epidemiological Features

Agent

Several species of clostridia, the *Clostridium perfringens* (also called *C. welchii*), *Clostridium septicum* (*C. septicum*), *Clostridium sporogenes* and *Clostridium histolyticum* produces gas gangrene. The common cause of gas gangrene is *C. welchii* and *C. septicum* ranks second. All these may be present in a given case.

Morphology

Clostridium welchii is a normal inhabitant of the large intestine of man and animals. It is found in feces and contaminates the skin of perineum, buttocks and thigh. It is an anaerobe growing rapidly at 37°C, resistant to heat and antiseptics. The chief characteristic of *C. welchii* is that it produces gas from the muscle sugars, so that it is commonly called 'gas bacilli' and the disease known as gas gangrene. It is a plump, gram-positive bacilli with straight, parallel sides rounded or truncated ends about 4–6 × 1 m. It may occur singly or in chains. Its pleomorphic, filamentous and involution forms are common. Encapsulated and non-motile spores are central or subterminal.

Host Factors

Age: The disease can occur at any age, but more common at the age of 15–50 years.

Sex: Males are more affected than females because they drive vehicles (prone for accident) and fight in the war field.

Environmental factors: Soil, dirt and dead muscle act as a spark, which light the fire. The spores can survive in dry earth for years. The organisms are readily ingested in vegetables and establish themselves in the colon.

Insanitary habits: Improper washing of hands after defecation and open air defecation.

Mode of Transmission

Feces, vegetables and soil are sources of infection, while cases of infected wounds with species of clostridia are reservoirs of infection. Ingestion of vegetables and infection of wounds either by soil containing fecal matter or from contaminated clothing and faulty technique in sterilization are some modes of infection. Improper disposal of soiled dressings also spread the bacteria. Incubation period is from 7 hours to 6 weeks.

Pathophysiology

The bacteria (clostridia) invade the devitalized tissue, especially where blood supply is diminished, lowering of oxygen tension of surrounding tissue and rapid spread of necrotizing process. The bacteria multiply and produce toxins. Toxins cause hemolysis, vessel thrombosis and damage to the myocardium, liver and kidneys.

Clinical Features

1. Sudden and severe pain at site of injury caused by gas and edema in the tissues.
2. Appearance of wound:
   - Skin is white and tense initially, then progresses to bronze, brown or black color
   - Soft tissue crepitus (crackling) produced by gas in the tissue

- Vesicles filled with red, waterery fluid
- Gas bubbles seen emanating from tissues, toxins ferment muscle sugar and produce acid and gas, which digest muscle protein.
3. Rapid, feeble pulse progressing to circulatory collapse, death from toxemia is frequent.
4. Anemia and jaundice from hemolysis, prostration and apprehension.
5. Delirium and stupor.

Preventive Measures

Mixed gas gangrene antitoxin intraperitoneal (IP) injection contains:
- 10,000 units edematous antitoxin
- 10,000 units *C. welchii* antitoxin
- 500 units *C. septicum* antitoxin.

This is given as a prophylactic measure as soon as possible after the injury in the dose of 25,000 units IV/IM.

The dose may be doubled or repeated, if the clinical condition deteriorates or if operative interference is required. The therapeutic dose is 75,000 units IV.

Note: Tetanus and gas gangrene antitoxins may be administered simultaneously, if necessary.

Precaution During Immunization

When antitoxins are given intravenously, the patient should be kept under observation for 20–30 minutes. Symptoms of severe allergic response usually appear within that period.

Treatment

- Surgical debridement and irrigation of the wound
- Strict isolation to avoid infection of others
- Antibiotics, usually penicillin are administered
- Placing patient in hyperbaric oxygen chamber in which the anaerobes are exposed to high-density oxygen
- Intravenous fluids are given to support the cardiovascular system and to maintain fluid and electrolyte balance
- Plasma, albumin and whole blood may be used to restore protein depletion and correcting anemia.

CONCLUSION

Trachoma is a communicable eye disease, which is most commonly found in population living in crowded conditions and having the custom of application of kajal. It can be prevented by giving health education. Tetanus is caused by *C. tetani*. These microorganisms are present in soil and dust. Tetanus bacilli produce soluble exotoxins, which act on spinal cord, brain, sympathetic system and motor plates in skeletal system. It is characterized by paroxymal spasms of voluntary muscles, lockjaw and opisthotonus such as sign/symptom. It is prevented and controlled by immunization, hygienic practices and health education. Leprosy is caused by *M. leprae* and affects the peripheral nerves. The incidence rate is more between 10 and 20 years of age. The cases detected are treated with dapsone (DDS) (chemotherapy). In case of PB, MDT is used. It involves diagnosis, treatment, surveillance, chemoprophylaxis, rehabilitation and health education. The STDs are caused by bacterial (*N. gonorrhoeae*), viral (herpes simplex), protozoal (*Trichomonas vaginalis*), fungal (*Candida albicans*) and ectoparasites (*Phthirus pubis*). There are a number of social factors such as polygamy marriage, prostitution, sexual disharmony, which cause STDs. These can be prevented and controlled by identifying cases, treating, motivating people to use contraceptive methods and by health education. Acquired immunodeficiency disease is caused by HIV. This virus destroys human T helper cells. The mode of transmission of AIDS is sexual transmission, blood transfusion, mother to child, contaminate needles, syringe or any skin piercing instrument. The measures for prevention and control of AIDS involve diagnosis, treatment, use of condom while having sex, avoiding multisexual partners, checking blood before transfusion for HIV/AIDS, etc.

The yaws is a chronic contagious disease caused by *T. pertenue*. It occurs during childhood and adolescence before the age of 15 years. It is characterized by lesions on exposed part of body, enlarged lymph nodes, lesions of soft plate, hard palate and nose. It requires identification of cases, treatment, survey, resurveys, environmental improvement and personal hygiene to prevent and control yaws.

SECTION 5

Non-communicable Diseases

- An Introduction to Non-communicable Diseases
- Malnutrition
- Obesity
- Cardiovascular Diseases
- Cancer
- Accidents
- Diabetes Mellitus
- Mental Illness
- Epilepsy
- Fluorosis

An Introduction to Non-communicable Diseases

CHAPTER 36

INTRODUCTION

All diseases, which are not communicable are called non-communicable diseases (NCDs). Potentially NCDs include:
- Cancers
- Cardiovascular diseases (CVD)
- Blindness
- Renal diseases
- Neurological disorders
- Mental/Psychiatric disorders
- Musculoskeletal disorders such as arthritis and allied diseases
- Chronic respiratory diseases (e.g. chronic bronchitis, asthma and emphysema)
- Accidents and trauma
- Dementia
- Diabetes
- Obesity and various metabolic and degenerative diseases
- Disabilities resulting from communicable diseases
- Orodental diseases
- Disorders of unknown cause.

Many national programs are also qualified to be part of the NCD control program such as:
- The National Iodine Deficiency Disorders Control Program
- National Program for Control of Blindness
- National Cancer Control Program
- Programs Against Micronutrient Malnutrition
- National Mental Health Program
- National Diabetes Control Program
- National Cardiovascular Disease Control Program
- Prevention of Deafness and Hearing Impairment
- Oral Health Programs.

As we can see, NCD control program includes many nutritional programs as well. However, for the purpose of this chapter these have been excluded. Only the following diseases have been included as NCDs:
- Cardiovascular diseases including stroke
- Mental diseases
- Injuries
- Cancers
- Diabetes mellitus
- Orodental problems.

MAGNITUDE OF PROBLEM OF NCDs

The magnitude of problems of NCDs can be considered at three levels such as mortality, morbidity and risk factors. At present, we do not have any regular system for collecting data on all the three levels, which can be at best, said to be of adequate coverage or quality. Thus, most of these estimates at best may be taken as approximation only.

Mortality

The data on the causes of death in the country come mainly from two sources. These are medical certification of deaths in urban areas and survey of causes of deaths in rural areas. While the certification of deaths covers only about 15% of all deaths in the country, the survey of causes of death is based on lay reporting.

Based on these data, it was estimated for 1998 that about 32% of all deaths could be due to the NCDs. This would come to about 3 million deaths in 1 year. Of these 32% deaths, cardiovascular diseases constituted 3%, injuries 8.7%, chronic respiratory diseases 6.7%, cancers with 3.4% and diabetes with 0.2% were the other contributors. However, the above listed limitations of the data on which such estimations are based should be kept in mind.

Morbidity

The major source of information on morbidity comes from ad-hoc surveys conducted by individual researchers. They suffer from small sample size, different methodology, different definitions, etc. The only exception is of cancer for which there is a National Cancer Registry Program.

HYPERTENSION

For hypertension, the few studies in the Indian population are inadequate and the available information cannot be used for national data projection. There are approximately 25 million hypertensive in India and the prevalence of hypertension is 10% among adult population in urban areas and 5% in the rural areas.

RHEUMATIC HEART DISEASE

Rheumatic heart disease (RHD) is prevalent in the range of 5–7 per 1,000 in the 5–15 years age group. There are about 1.9 million RHD cases in India. RHD constitutes 20–30% of hospital admission due to all CVD in India.

CARDIOVASCULAR DISEASES

Cardiovascular diseases comprise of the following disease entities.

Stroke

It has been estimated that there are about 1 million cases of stroke occurring every year in the country. Of these, more than 600,000 die from stroke. This could be an underestimate as not all strokes are recognized and treatment sought for it.

Ischemic Heart Disease

Based on studies conducted, it has been estimated that there are 2.5 million cases of ischemic heart disease (IHD) in the country.

DIABETES

It has been estimated that there are about 32.7 million diabetics in the country. Indians seem to have a genetic predisposition toward diabetes. This becomes manifest on exposure to richer diet and consequent increase in body weight. This is perhaps also borne out by the temporal trends in diabetes prevalence in India. Studies until the early 1970s essentially showed prevalence rates of less than 3%. A study in 1972 showed a prevalence of 2.7% in urban Delhi and 1.9% in rural areas near Delhi. More recent studies (1990–2001) showed significantly higher prevalence than that reported above. Studies in Southern India report an overall prevalence rate of diabetes as 5%. Further, recent studies also indicate rising prevalence in select group belonging to poor socioeconomic status, e.g. urban slum dwellers.

INJURIES

The data on trauma are available from two independent sources in the country, namely:
1. National Crime Records Bureau (NCRB).
2. Registrar General of India (RGI).

Based on these data and some other published studies, it was recently estimated that there are about 0.75 million deaths due to injuries in the country. Of these, 0.14 million were due to intentional injuries and rest due to unintentional injuries. Road traffic accidents accounted for about 85,000 deaths per year in the country.

These figures imply death in India due to trauma every minute or more than 1,800 deaths every day due to injury. For each death due to injury, there are an estimated nine survived patients, who have sustained injuries due to various kinds of trauma.

MENTAL DISORDERS

In India, 10–20 persons per 1,000 suffer from severe mental illness at any given time and at least three to five times that number suffers from distressing and socioeconomically incapacitating emotional disorders. Estimated 20–50% patients have recognizable emotional problems with or without an associated physical illness. Mental subnormality prevalence is 0.5–1% of all children. Approximately, 150 million people in India need ongoing psychiatric and or psychological help. Depression is the most common cause in all age group including geriatric population. An estimated 15–20% of people seeking general health services take help for emotional and psychological problems. Illicit drugs such as alcohol and tobacco are most frequently used. Alcohol use ranges between 24 and 74% among men in different parts of the country. Prevalence of tobacco use ranged between 40 and 75%, and raw opium is used in the northwest region. Heroin prevalence is less than 1%. The general population is mostly free from the use of synthetic drugs, i.e. amphetamines and barbiturates.

CHAPTER 36: An Introduction to Non-communicable Diseases

CANCER

Cancer has become 1 of the 10 leading causes of death in India. It is estimated that there are nearly 1.5–2 million cancer cases at any given point of time. Over 700,000 new cases of cancer and 300,000 deaths occur annually due to cancer. Nearly 1.5 million patients require facilities for diagnosis, treatment and follow-up at any given time. Data from population-based registries under National Cancer Registry Program indicate that the leading sites of cancer have remained unchanged over the years namely oral cavity, lungs, esophagus and stomach among men and cervix, breast and oral cavity among women. Cancers namely those of the oral cavity and lungs in males, and cervix and breast in females account for over 50% of all cancer deaths in India. It has been estimated that 91% of oral cancers in Southeast Asia are directly attributable to the use of tobacco and this is the leading cause of oral cavity and lung cancer in India—World Health Organization (WHO).

ORODENTAL PROBLEMS

About 80% of children and 60% of adults suffer from dental caries. This can be attributed to a shift in diet pattern toward more refined food (fast food) and poor oral hygiene. Similarly, the prevalence of periodontal diseases is also very high to the tune of 90% among people above 30 years.

A large segment of the adult population is toothless due to the crippling nature of dental diseases. Apart from this, about 30% of children suffer from malaligned teeth and jaws affecting proper functioning of the dentofacial apparatus. Oral cancers constitute 35–40% of total body cancers due to wide usage of betel nuts, tobacco, pan masala, etc. Dental and skeletal fluorosis is another endemic problem in many parts of the country.

This is jeopardizing the qualified of life and esthetics of the population of the affected areas. Majority of the population in the country lack knowledge about dental diseases and the relationship between dental problems and general health.

Risk Factors

The data on risk factors are based on the review of different studies done in the 1990s in various parts of the country. The prevalence rates in the rural and urban areas. quoted below are for adults only, though even then they may refer to different age ranges (Table 36.1).

The data on tobacco and alcohol use were estimated in the second National Family Health Survey in 1998–1999. Among males above 15 years, the prevalence of ever smokers was 33.1% and current smokers was 29.4%. The use of oral forms of tobacco was prevalent among 28.3% of them and 16.7% consumed alcohol. Among females in the same age group, ever smokers were 2.8% and current smokers were 2.5%. Of these women, 12.4% used oral forms of tobacco and 2.2% consumed alcohol.

BLINDNESS

Terms such as total blindness, economic blindness and social blindness were in vague. In economic blindness, a person is with less than one tenth of normal vision. Total blindness, as per the International Association for the Prevention of Blindness is one, who has 1/20 of normal vision or when he/she cannot count fingers at 1 m distance. Taking into consideration of existing definitions, WHO proposed a uniform criterion and defined blindness as visual acuity of less than 3/60 or its equivalent. The WHO International Classification of Diseases described the levels of visual impairment in order to facilitate the screening of visual acuity by non-specialized personnel, in the absence of appropriate vision charts, the WHO now added the inability to count fingers in daylight at a distance of 3 m to indicate less than 3/60 or its equivalent.

Magnitude of Problem

The National Survey Organization in 1982 conducted a prevalence study of the blind taking the visual acuity of 3/60 or less in the better eye as baseline. It reported a figure of

Table 36.1: Prevalence of various risk factors for non-communicable diseases (NCDs) in India

Risk factors	Level	Prevalence in urban areas (%)	Prevalence in rural areas (%)
Hypotension	≥ 60/95 mm Hg	10–15	3–8
Hypertension	≥ 140/90 mm Hg	20–30	15–25
Overweight	BMI* ≥ 25	20–40	10
Hypercholesterolemia	≥ 220 mg/dL	20	10
Sedentary physical activity	Activity	50–60 (6)	8–30

*BMI, body mass index

3.47 million blind or 0.5% of the population based on 1981 census. The diseases mainly recognized as responsible for visual impairment and blindness in India are cataract, trachoma and malnutrition. The principal cause of blindness in India today is cataract, which is responsible for 50–70% of all cases. Cataract occurs more frequently with advancing age. Trachoma cases alone are estimated 120 million in India. Trachoma and associated bacterial conjunctivitis are important causes of blindness in India.

In a report of the Indian Council of Medical Research (ICMR) working group on preschool children, it was stated that 14,000 preschool children suffer from vitamin A deficiency-related eye problems at anyone point. Injuries as a cause of blindness account for 1.2% of blindness in India. There is evidence that injuries are on increase due to cottage industry, leg carpentry, blacksmithing, stone crushing, chiseling and hammering, chopping of wood and rapid industrialization in the country. The last group includes congenital disorders such as uveitis, detachment, tumors, diabetes, hypertension disease of the nervous system, leprosy, etc.

Host Factors

Age

About 80% of blindness in India are said to lose their eyesight before they reach 20 years and many under the age of 5 years. Trachoma, conjunctivitis and malnutrition are important causes of blindness among children and the younger age groups. Cataract mucosa and diabetes are causes of blindness among children and in middle age. Accidents and injuries can occur in all age groups, but more importantly in the age group of 20–40 years.

Sex

A higher prevalence of blindness is reported in females than in males in India. This has been attributed to a higher prevalence of trachoma, conjunctivitis and cataract among females than in males.

Malnutrition

As a cause of blindness, malnutrition was hardly recognized a few years ago. It is closely related not only with low vitamin A intake but also with infectious diseases of childhood, especially measles and diarrhea (which precipitate malnutrition). In many cases, protein-energy malnutrition (PEM) is also associated with blindness. Severe blinding corneal distribution due to vitamin A deficiency (e.g. keratomalacia) is largely united to the first from 6 years of life and is especially frequent among those 6 months to 3 years of life.

Occupational

People working in factories, workshops and cottage industries are prone to eye injuries because of exposure to dust, airborne particles, flying objects, gases, radiation (using welding flash), fumes, electrical flush, etc. Many workers including doctors are known to have developed premature cataracts, while exposed to X-rays, ultraviolet rays and heat waves.

Social Class

There is a close relationship between the incidence of blindness and socioeconomic status. It is more prevalent among the poorer class than the rich on account of ignorance, poverty, low personal hygiene and low environmental hygiene and many of these going to quack doctor for treatment. It is more among Muslims. All these form the social factors.

Etiology

The causes are classified as follows:
- Congenital:
  - Congenital abnormalities
  - Hereditary diseases.
- Acquired:
  - Traumatic
  - Infective
  - Neoplastic
  - Nutritional
  - Others.

The percentage of the causes of blindness are as follows:
- Cataract: 55%
- Trachoma and associated infections: 20%
- Smallpox: 3%
- Malnutrition: 2%
- Injuries: 1.20%
- Glaucoma: 0.8%
- Other causes: 18%.

Cataract

Cataract is the opacity of the crystalline lens or its capsules. The rays of light entering the eye must pass through the pupil and lens to reach the retina; any opacity of the lens behind the pupil will produce alterations in vision. Objects may seem distorted to scatter light causing unpleasant glare. The patient experiences no pain and when a cataract develops the pupil, which is normally black, becomes gray and later milky white. It can be cured only by minor surgery.

Trachoma

Trachoma is a highly communicable disease of the eyelids. The symptoms are mild itching and irritation. After an acute inflammatory process, follicles appear on the conjunctiva. Blurring of vision and increasing discomfort occur. The upper palpebral conjunctiva is affected.

Glaucoma

Glaucoma is a disease characterized by increased tension or pressure within the eye and progressive loss of visual field. Symptoms develop slowly. The patient may have mild discomfort such as tired feeling of the eye. Impairment of peripheral vision occurs long before any effect is noted in central vision. The patient may become aware of peripheral visual impairment by bumping into things that he/she did not see at their side. The patient may also note halos around lights.

Prevention

Primary Level of Prevention

Child health care in growing periods

1. Before birth:
   - Nutritious food rich in vitamin A to the mother
   - Regular Venereal Disease Research Laboratory (VDRL) test for all pregnant women to detect syphilis and regimen.
2. During birth:
   - Safe delivery
   - Care of eyes of the newborn by instilling a drop or silver nitrate or penicillin to protect against gonorrheal ophthalmia.
3. Afterbirth:
   - By administrating vitamin A, the xerophthalmia can be prevented
   - Timely vaccination against smallpox and other viral diseases.

Parent care in the home

1. Avoid ill-ventilated rooms, smoke and flies.
2. Insist on children to read in good light.
3. Prohibit games having potential danger in injuring eyes, i.e. bow and arrow, gilli-danda, etc.
4. Avoid access to sharp objects.
5. Keep poisonous drugs such as tincture iodine or any other toxic substance at a height with no access to children.
6. Avoid dangerous fireworks during festivals.

School health care

1. Proper care of eye to be included in the curriculum of education of the school children.
2. Regular eye examination of preschool and school children in detection of diseases leading to partial or total blindness, teachers and volunteers being trained for screening such cases.
3. Teach and practice principles of good posture, proper lighting, avoid glare, keep proper distance and angle between the books and eye.
4. Use of suitable types of letter in the textbooks.
5. Consult the doctor for treatment in case of a red running eye.
6. Health authorities to be informed, if there is large number of cases.
7. Sufficient space for playgrounds and encourage to play games, which are not hazardous to eyes.
8. Prohibit looking at the sun or bright light and so on.

Public care

1. Regular pruning of all trees and shrubs on the roadside and pathways to avoid ocular injuries.
2. School children and public to be taught regarding road sense keeping to the walkways, understand road signals, while crossing.
3. Care, while traveling in speedy vehicles, use of seat belts and helmets.
4. Good road kept properly repaired with no pits, proper directions, good lighting, avoidance of curves, adequate danger signals, speed breakers, priority for school buses and Red Cross vehicles.
5. Enforcement of safety rules and protective glasses in factories and industries.

Health education

At all levels for dissemination of information about eye care through all media of mass communication including newspaper, radio, television, with emphasis on ocular health of vulnerable groups, orienting teachers, social workers and community leaders on problems of eye health care and render first aid.

Secondary Level of Prevention

1. Early treatment will cure trachoma before the eye is damaged.
2. Administration of vitamin A to children will prevent xerophthalmia.
3. Vector control will prevent onchocerciasis.
4. Long-term measures such as better sanitation, abundant clean water, improvement of personal and environmental hygiene will prevent trachoma.
5. Provision of eye protection for certain workers and insistence for the same.

6. Control of dangerous tools in industry.
7. Improvement in safety of toys. Simple and cheap operations to treat blindness caused by cataract.
8. Squint can be cured, if investigated and treated before a child goes to school (5–7 year).

Disability Limitation and Rehabilitation

1. The eye diseases that are tackled by surgery are cataract and glaucoma; cataract is well tackled by organizing eye clinics and eye camps and measures in restoring eyesight to them.
2. Keratoplasty, corneal grafting for persons gone blind due to corneal opacities caused by smallpox or injury. Corneal grafting acts are in force, in many Indian states in establishing eye banks.
3. Special schools for educating the blind in Braille systems and other techniques.
4. Utilization of the services of the blind after training in gainful employment.

Malnutrition

CHAPTER 37

INTRODUCTION

Malnutrition means failure to achieve nutrient requirements, which in turn results in impaired physical and/or mental health. Though, generally malnutrition means undernutrition resulting from hunger, it can be referred to any kind of unhealthy nutritional status including a result of imbalance or excess of the nutrients. The recurrent and involuntary lack of access to food may produce a situation referred to as undernutrition.

In the developing world, about 800 million people do not have enough food to eat. Although, the proportion of the undernourished people has been decreasing, undernutrition is still widespread, particularly in certain regions. About 18% of the people in the developing world still continue to suffer from chronic hunger. Nearly 40% of the children are stunted due to lack of food; about 35% are underweight, while approximately 10% have significant wasting of muscle and fat tissue.

Food supplies, though may not be adequate, factors including poverty, poor sanitation, urbanization and inefficient food distribution contribute to malnutrition and hunger. Infections, rapid population growth, war and environmental degradation worsens the problem. Typically, a malnourished person may have two or more coexisting deficiencies, each worsening the severity of the other.

Some of the common nutritional disorders are shown in Table 37.1. The most critical nutritional deficiencies in the developing world are protein calories, iodine, vitamin A and iron.

PROTEIN-ENERGY MALNUTRITION

The term protein-energy malnutrition (PEM) covers a wide spectrum of clinical stages ranging from the severe forms such as kwashiorkor and marasmus to the milder forms in which the main detectable manifestation is growth retardation. The PEM is due to 'food gap' between the intake and requirement. The average energy deficit in Indian children is 300 kcal/day. The term kwashiorkor was first introduced by Cicely Williams in 1935. This is a local name used by the 'Ga' tribe in Accra, West Africa, which means 'disease of the displaced child.'

The prevalence rate of severe degree of PEM in our community is 3–5%. For every 3–5 cases of severe PEM, we can detect 80–90 cases of mild to moderate PEM and about 10% of well-nourished children.

According to National Nutrition Monitoring Bureau (1988–1990), the prevalence of malnutrition among 1–5 years is high. The underweight (weight/age) children are 68.6%, while stunting (height/age) is at 65.1% and wasting (weight/height) 19.9%.

Table 37.1: Some common nutritional disorders

Nutritional disorders	Causative nutrient
Obesity	Excessive calorie intake, high-carbohydrate and high-fat diet
Marasmus	Low calorie intake
Kwashiorkor	Low protein intake
Night blindness/Xerophthalmia	Vitamin A deficiency
Rickets	Low calcium/vitamin D intake in infants
Osteomalacia	Low calcium/vitamin D intake in adults, particularly in females
Beriberi	Thiamine deficiency
Pellagra	Niacin deficiency
Anemia	Iron and/or vitamin B_{12} (folic acid) deficiency
Scurvy	Vitamin C deficiency
Fluorosis	Excess fluoride intake
Goiter	Iodine deficiency

In more than 50% of deaths in children, malnutrition is the direct or indirect cause. PEM is a silent killer in many children. The PEM refers to a deficiency of protein, energy or both in the diet; since, it is difficult to separate protein and energy intake. Diets adequate in energy, usually, are also adequate in protein; and diets inadequate in energy do inhibit the use of dietary protein by the body for protein synthesis. Though PEM can occur at all stages, it is most common during childhood, when protein is needed to support rapid growth. It is the most common form of malnutrition in the world. It often develops after a child is weaned from the breast. Though people may have symptoms of both, there are two forms of PEM called kwashiorkor and marasmus.

Magnitude

1. The PEM is a type of malnutrition resulting from deficiency of proteins and calories in the food over a long period of time.
2. It is very common among young children, who are in the stage of rapid growth and development. Children below 5 years are usually affected and infants are hit hardest.
3. The most serious forms of PEM are kwashiorkor and marasmus. Nutritional marasmus is more frequent than kwashiorkor.
4. These are the extreme forms (two poles) of a single condition. About 80% of the intermediate ones go unrecognized. Thus, they represent the tip of the iceberg. For every frank case of malnutrition, there are about 10 uses, which are undernourished.
5. The PEM is mainly a problem of all developing countries. In India, the incidence of extreme forms is 1–2%.
6. The adverse effects of malnutrition are growth failure, breakdown of immunity, increased susceptibility to infections, prolongation of the recovery period, impairment of mental capacity and motor skills, decreased alertness and physical capacity.
7. The PEM accounts for 5% of deaths among preschool children. Thus PEM is not only a health problem but also a social and economic problem.

Etiology

Causes of PEM includes:
- Decreased intake of food (i.e. inadequate diet both in quality and quantity)
- Excessive loss of proteins and calories (because of vomiting and diarrhea)
- Increased demand (or requirement), and decreased absorption and utilization (because of infections and infestations).

Infection contributes to malnutrition and malnutrition predisposes to the causation of infection, both acts synergistically. Thus it is a vicious cycle:
- Malnutrition (decreased intake of food)
- Anorexia (loss of nutrient)
- Growth failure lowered immunity
- Infection increased morbidity.

Different Factors Affecting PEM

Social Factors

There are many social causes contributing for the development of malnutrition such as poverty, illiteracy, ignorance, overcrowding, large family size, poor maternal health, failure of lactation, faulty feeding practices, improper weaning practices, food taboos, beliefs, cooking and cultural practices, etc. Thus, PEM is multifactorial in origin.

Cultural Factors

The different cultural factors, which influence the nutritional status are food habits, customs, beliefs, traditions and attitudes. Family plays an important role and many times, the food habits pass from one generation to the other. The cultural factors make the individual to eat or not to eat a particular food item. These factors often affect the vulnerable groups. Some of them are as follows:

1. Papaya is avoided during pregnancy because of the belief that it causes abortion. Mothers restrict diet during pregnancy thinking that if she eats more, then baby will be big and the delivery would be difficult.
2. Disease-oriented cultural factors are restricting certain food items to treat the disease.
3. Religion has a powerful influence on the food habits of the people. Hindus do not eat beef and Muslims pork. Orthodox Hindus do not eat non-vegetarian food and also vegetarian items such as onion and garlic. These are known as food taboos.
4. Cooking practices such as draining away the rice water at the end of cooking, peeling of vegetables, etc. also affect the nutritional status.
5. Childrearing practices such as premature weaning, bottle feeding and feeding artificial foods, etc. also affect.
6. Habits such as alcoholism has got a profound effect.

Socioeconomic Factors

The important socioeconomic factors are income, education and the occupational status. These determine the quality of life, which in turn determines the nutritional status. Thus malnutrition is more among the poor.

CHAPTER 37 — Malnutrition

Food Production

Increased food production should lead to increased food consumption and better nutritional status. An average Indian has 0.6 hectare of land surface compared to 5.8 hectare per head in the developed countries.

Food consumption

It is obvious that the nutritional status of an individual is directly related to the quality and the quantity of the food eaten. Undereating results in PEM and overeating results in obesity.

The food consumption of an individual or a family can be assessed by the following steps:
- Diet survey
- Analysis of the data for the calculation of mean intake of foods, nutrients and calories
- Comparison with the recommended allowances to know the deficiencies, if any.

Classification (Figs 37.1A and B)

The PEM can be classified into two types:
1. Clinical classification: Clinically, malnutrition is classified into two types such as kwashiorkor and marasmus (Table 37.2).
2. Anthropometric methods of grading malnutrition: These are of the following types:
   - Wellcome classification
   - Gomez classification
   - Jelliffe classification
   - Indian Academy of Pediatrics (IAP) classification
   - Waterlow classification.

Marasmus (Fig. 37.2)

Child reacts to the stress of PEM and secretes cortisol, which mobilizes protein from muscle, and subcutaneous tissue to amino acid pool resulting in wasting with no edema and no hepatomegaly. Raised cortisol level lowers growth hormone and so, the child is stunted. Marasmus is said to be well adapted to the stress of deficit in protein and calorie. The signs and symptoms observed in marasmic child are detailed below:
- The eyes appear big because of lack of fat surrounding the eyes
- Severe growth retardation
- Loss of subcutaneous fat
- Severe muscle wasting
- The child looks appallingly thin and limbs appear as skin and bones
- Shriveled body
- Wrinkled skin and thin limbs

Table 37.2: Kwashiorkor versus marasmus

Features	Kwashiorkor	Marasmus
Causes	Deficiency of mainly proteins	Deficiency of mainly calories
General condition of the child	Dull, apathetic, disinterest in hardly moves from the sitting position	Child is alert, but irritable
Face	Bloated, moon-like face	Shriveled monkey face
Growth failure (weight loss)	Less severe (moderate)	More severe (very severe)
Emaciation (muscle wasting)	Masked (present, but not seen because of edema)	Obvious (skin and bone appearance)
Fat wasting	Fat is often retained	Severe loss of subcutaneous fat
Edema	Always present	Absent
Hair changes in texture, thin*	Hairs are lusterless, show 'flag sign' positive, sparse distribution, loss of curliness and easily pluckable	Hair show change in color and silky, show 'flag sign' negative
Skin changes	Skin shows paint-like patches (flaky paint dermatoses)	Skin changes are absent
Mental changes	Present	Absent
Liver enlargement	Often present	Absent
Prognosis	Bad	Good
Serum (total proteins)	Reduced	Normal
Serum (cholesterol)	Reduced	Normal
Urinary nitrogen	Reduced	Raised

*Hairs show alternate white and dark bands, indicating depigmentation and pigmentation, which are the phases of poor and good nutrition respectively.

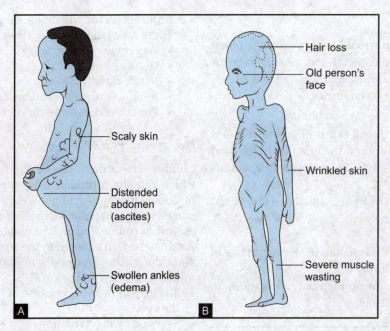

Figures 37.1A and B: Protein-energy malnutrition. A. Kwashiokor; B. Marasmus.

- Bony prominence
- Associated vitamin deficiencies
- Failure to thrive
- Irritability, fretfulness and apathy
- Frequent watery diarrhea and acid stools
- Mostly hungry, but some are anorectic
- Dehydration
- Temperature is subnormal
- Muscles are weak
- Edema and fatty infiltration are absent.

Kwashiorkor (Fig. 37.3)

Sometimes the child is not able to adapt to the stress of inadequate diet, infection and separation from mother due to subsequent pregnancy.

In dysadaptation, the adrenal is unable to secrete cortisol; and the mobilization of protein from muscle is not possible; and the liver cannot synthesize β-lipoprotein and thus fatty liver occurs. When dysadaptation occurs, the child ultimately land up as kwashiorkor and the following symptoms appear:

1. Low bodyweight in spite of edema showing growth failure and some degree of muscle wasting, which is masked by edema.
2. Pitting edema appears first on the feet and legs, and later spreads to the whole body. The face looks puffy with sagging cheeks and swollen eyelids. Puffiness of edema is known as moon face.
3. Mental changes, i.e. apathy and irritability are common.
4. Mental development is affected.
5. Scaly pigmentation of the skin is common and in severe cases, the epithelium peels off leaving behind depigmented patches with oozing fluid, which is described as 'crazy-pavement dermatosis'. There is hypo- as well as hyper-pigmentation with flaky paint appearance.
6. Bulb and root of the hair are distorted unlike marasmus. The hair becomes thin, dry and can be pulled out easily without causing pain. Loss of hair results in diffuse or patchy alopecia (Fig. 37.4). The changes in color, which include brownish or reddish discoloration may be generated or localized with alternate bands of pigmentation and depigmentation described as 'flag sign'. It is the record of nutritional history of the child (Figs 37.5 and 37.6).
7. Anorexia is very common, making it difficult to feed the child.
8. Diarrhea may occur due to defective digestion and absorption or as a result of secondary infection.
9. Other nutritional deficiencies, particularly vitamin A deficiency leading to xerophthalmia and B-complex deficiencies with clinical signs, such as glossitis and angular stomatitis are observed in PEM.

Marasmic Kwashiorkor

The child shows a mixture of some of the features of marasmus and kwashiorkor. This is due to the varying nature of the dietary deficiency and the social factors responsible for the disease, and presence or absence of infections.

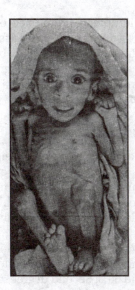

Figure 37.2: Marasmic child

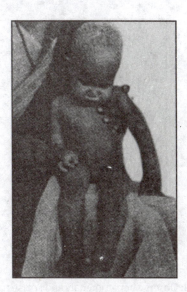

Figure 37.3: Kwashiorkor child (*Note:* Sparse hair, changes in pigmentation of skin and edema. *Courtesy:* National Institute of Nutrition, Hyderabad).

Nutritional dwarfing or stunting

Some children adapt to prolonged insufficiency of food-energy and protein by a marked retardation of growth. Weight and height are both reduced, and in the same proportion, so they appear superficially normal.

Underweight child

Children with subclinical PEM can be detected by their weight for age or weight for height, which are significantly below normal. They may have reduced by plasma albumin. These children grow smaller than their genetic potential and they are at risk of gastroenteritis, respiratory and other infections, which can precipitate frank malnutrition.

Mild to moderate PEM is probably the major reason why the mortality in children is from 1 to 4 years of age in some parts of Africa, Asia and Latin America is 30–40 times higher than in those of Europe or North America.

Electrolyte and water metabolism

1. A deficiency of potassium arises as a result of diarrhea. Losses in the stools can amount to 20–30 mmol/day. Plasma K⁺ is often below normal and have very low values, less than 2.5 mmol/L may be found.
2. A deficiency of magnesium also arises from increased losses in the stools and plasma magnesium concentrations are generally low.
3. Plasma Na⁺ is usually normal. Low values are found, if there have been large losses in sweat of stools and when intake of salt is diminished, but intake of water is large.

Effect on vitamin a status

Protein malnutrition influences vitamin A metabolism by interfering with intestinal absorption of vitamin A and the conversion or β-carotene to vitamin A. Protein malnutrition also affects hepatic storage of vitamin A, and its utilization and transport from the liver to the tissues, and utilization at the tissue level. Vitamin A levels in children suffering from kwashiorkor are lower than normal levels. Mortality in children with PEM increases fourfold when they have xerophthalmia as well. This is due to the irreversible damage caused by vitamin A deficiency to the epithelial cells, which may lead to infections.

Drug metabolism

Malnourished children suffer from infections. Drugs may interfere with nutrition. Streptomycin, chloramphenicol and tetracycline inhibit protein synthesis by interfering with the action of messenger RNA.

Antimalarial trimethoprim is a folate antagonist. They should be used with caution in PEM. Low plasma albumin has a reduced binding capacity for salicylates, digoxin and barbiturate thiopentone. Detoxification in the liver by the microsomal enzyme, oxidizing system and its function may be impaired in PEM. Their half-life of the drug is prolonged and a standard dose may be toxic.

Wellcome Classification (Table 37.3)

Wellcome classification is based on the weight of the child and the presence of edema. The weight (in kg) is compared with the 'reference weight for age', which is 50th percentile

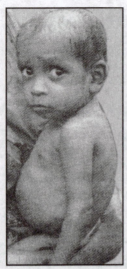

Figure 37.4: Observe hepatomegaly and sparse hair of protein-energy malnutrition (PEM) child

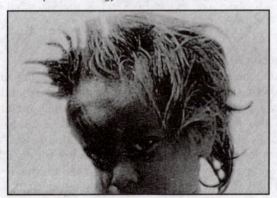

Figure 37.5: Changes in color of hair in protein-energy malnutrition (PEM) child (flag sign)

Table 37.3: Wellcome classification of protein-energy malnutrition (PEM)

Bodyweight (% of reference weight for age)	Edema	
	Present	Absent
80–60	Kwashiorkor	Undernutrition
< 60	Marasmic kwashiorkor	Marasmus

of Harvard standard. Percentile means position of an individual in a grouped series of 100 of the same age and sex, when the recorded weight is arranged in a definite order either ascending or descending. For example, suppose 100 children, all boys, of 1 year age are weighed and recorded in an order, and found to vary from 9 to 11 kg (1st to 100th child); the position of 50th child being 10 kg, then the 50th percentile value of Harvard standard is 10 kg, and that is considered as 'reference standard' (or 100% value) for India.

Because of the widespread prevalence of malnutrition, in India, up to 80% value (i.e. up to 8 kg for 1 year age) is considered as normal nutrition and only below 8 kg (80% value) is considered as malnutrition and graded.

The expected weight of an Indian child is the 50th percentile value of Harvard standard.

Gomez Classification (Table 37.4)

Gomez classification is based on only weight for age and not edema. In this system, the reference child is the 50th percentile of Boston standard. This helps to know the percentage of deficiency in a particular child by comparing with a normal child. Accordingly, malnutrition is graded as follows:

1. Between 90 and 110%: Normal nutritional status.
2. Between 89 and 75%: First degree, mild malnutrition.
3. Between 74 and 60%: Second degree, moderately and severe malnutrition.
4. Below 60%: Third degree and severe malnutrition.

However, this does not help to know whether it is an acute or chronic malnutrition.

Table 37.4: Gomez classification of protein-energy malnutrition (PEM)

Nutritional status	Percentage (%) of height for age (stunting)	Percentage (%) of weight for height (wasting)
Normal	> 95	> 90
Mildly impaired	94–87.5	90–80
Moderately impaired	87.4–80	80–70
Severely impaired	< 80	< 70

Jelliffe Classification

Jelliffe classification is also based on weight for age and is graded as follows:
- Between 90 and 81%: Grade I
- Between 80 and 71%: Grade II
- Between 70 and 61%: Grade III
- Below 60%: Grade IV.

The reference weight is 50th percentile value of Harvard standard.

Indian Academy of Pediatrics Classification

- Between 100 and 80%: Normal nutrition status
- Between 79 and 70%: Grade I, mild malnutrition
- Between 69 and 60%: Grade II, moderate malnutrition
- Between 59 and 50%: Grade III, severe malnutrition
- Less than 50%: Grade IV, very severe malnutrition.

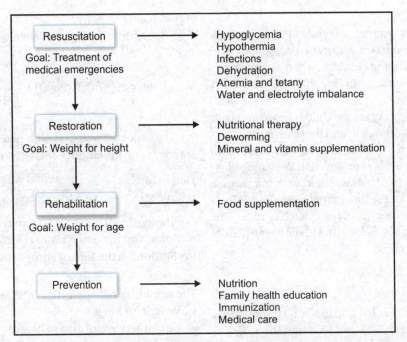

Figure 37.6: Flow diagram for changes in color of hair in protein-energy malnutrition (PEM) (flag sign)

Waterlow Classification

Waterlow classification defines two types of malnutrition, namely stunting and wasting, depending upon 'height for age' and 'weight for height' respectively:

$$\text{Height for age} = \frac{\text{Current height of the child (cm)}}{\text{Expected height for that age}} \times 100$$

A drop in this ratio indicates stunted growth or chronic malnutrition:

$$\text{Weight for height} = \frac{\text{Current weight of the child (kg)}}{\text{Expected weight of the child for that height}} \times 100$$

A drop in this ratio indicates 'wasting' or acute malnutrition. Wasting indicates the nutritional deprivation of shorter duration.

ASSESSMENT OF NUTRITIONAL STATUS

There are three methods of assessment of nutritional status:
- Direct assessment
- Indirect assessment
- Assessment of ecological factors.

Direct Methods of Assessment

Direct methods of assessment includes the following:
1. Clinical examination.
2. Anthropometric examination.
3. Biochemical examination.
4. Biophysical examination.

Clinical Examination

Clinical examination consists of inspection of an individual, clinically, from head to toe for the changes believed to be related to food consumption that can be seen or felt in the superficial tissues such as hairs, eyes, skin, buccal mucosa, tongue, ears, nose, lips, teeth, gums, glands, nails, chest, abdomen and edema. Conglomeration of signs helps in making the diagnosis of a specific disease. If the signs are absent, the subject is declared nutritionally healthy. Thus, clinical examination is the simplest, cheapest, very sound and most practical method of assessing the nutritional status.

Anthropometric Examination

Anthropometric examination is recording the following body measurements, which are although genetically determined, they are profoundly influenced by the nutrition:
- Weight
- Height
- Circumference of head
- Circumference of chest
- Circumference of midarm
- Thickness of the skinfold.

The anthropometric measurements by themselves are of little value, unless they are analyzed with reference to age.

Weight

Weight is the 'key' measurement. 'Weight for age' not only helps in assessing the current nutritional status but also the growth, specially among children, when recorded periodically and plotted in 'Road to Health' card. The weight is employed in two ways:

1. The current weight (in kg) of the child is compared with the expected standard weight and the deficiency in percentage is expressed in terms of degrees of malnutrition.
2. The weight for age is also employed in Wellcome classification to assess PEM, as kwashiorkor or marasmus.

A composite index of the nutritional status of adults is called the 'body mass index' (BMI) or Quetelet index. This is obtained by dividing the weight (in kg) of the individual by the height (in m) squared:

$$\text{Quetelet index} = \frac{\text{Weight (kg)}}{\text{Height (m}^2)}$$

An adult person is regarded nutritionally normal, if his Quetelet index is between 18.5 and 25. More than 25, it is obesity.

Persons having BMI value less than 18.5 are considered to be suffering from chronic energy deficiency (CED) and are further classified as follows:
- 18.5–17: First degree CED
- 17–16: Second degree CED
- < 16: Third degree CED (explained under epidemiology of obesity).

In a child (< 5 year), the ratio of weight/height square below 0.0015 is considered as malnutrition.

Note: Height is recorded in meters in adults and centimeters in children.

Height

Height is a liner dimension. It is a measure of skeletal elongation. Height for age gives an indication of duration of malnutrition.

For preschool children below 3 years, 'crown-heel length' is employed to avoid postural errors, by using infantometer. Height is a stable measurement of growth as opposed to bodyweight; whereas weight reflects the current health status of the child. Height indicates the events in the past also. Low height for age is also known as nutritional stunting or dwarfing. It reflects past or chronic malnutrition (i.e. duration of malnutrition). The cutoff point commonly taken for the diagnosis of stunting is 90% (Waterlow classification).

Indices used to assess the nutritional status of preschool children are grouped into age-dependent and age-independent indices.

Age-dependent indices

Age-dependent indices are 'weight for age' and 'height for age':

$$\text{Weight for age (underweight)} = \frac{\text{Actual weight}}{\text{Expected weight for that age}} \times 100$$

The expected weight is 50th percentile value of Harvard standard and the cutoff point is 80% of 50th percentile value:

$$\text{Height for age (stunting)} = \frac{\text{Actual weight}}{\text{Expected weight for that age}} \times 100$$

The expected height is 50th percentile value of Harvard standard and the cutoff point is 95% of 50th percentile value. Stunting is the sign of chronic malnutrition.

Age-independent indices

The age-independent indices are:
- Weight for height
- Circumference of arm to height
- Circumference of arm to head
- Circumference of chest to head.

Weight for height

Weight for height reflects current nutritional status or acute malnutrition. Only this indicator is more important and practical. Weight for height (wasting) reflects the nutritional deprivation of shorter duration:

$$\text{Weight for height (wasting)} = \frac{\text{Actual weight}}{\text{Expected weight for that height}} \times 100$$

$$\text{Under field conditions} = \frac{\text{Weight}}{\text{Height}}$$

The formula is adopted from Quetelet index. For adults, the normal range is 18.5–25 to assess BMI and for children the cutoff point is 0.0015. Children with a ratio of less than this are considered to have PEM. A child less than 70% of the expected weight for that height is classed as 'severely wasted'.

Circumference of chest to head

Normally, at birth, the circumference of head is little more than that of the chest. Both become same by 1 year of age and crossing over takes after 1 year. This can be calculated using the given formula:

$$\frac{\text{Circumference of chest}}{\text{Circumference of head}} = \text{Ratio is} < 1 \text{ at birth, 1 at 1 year and} > 1 \text{ after 1 year}$$

If the ratio of chest/head circumference is < 1 in a preschool child, it indicates PEM.

Thickness of skinfold (tissue anthropometry)

This gives information about the subcutaneous reserve of calories in the body. Harpenden calipers is used for this. Measurement of skinfold thickness is recorded over triceps of left arm or infrascapular region. For a preschool child, 10 mm is taken is a cutoff point.

Circumference of midarm

Midarm gives information about the muscle mass. Muscle wasting is a cardinal feature of PEM especially during early childhood. Midarm circumference above 13.5 cm means well nourished, between 13.5 and 12.5 cm means mild to moderate malnutrition and below 12.5 cm means severe malnutrition. The limitation is that the child between 1 and 4 years of age will have almost the constant measurement. Therefore, to make this an age-independent indices, it is compared against height and head circumference.

For a quick nutrition survey, a bangle with an internal diameter of 4 cm can be used. If it goes over the child's upper arm, the child is malnourished. Shakir's arm tape can also be employed for quick nutrition survey.

Biochemical Examination

Variations is intake of nutrients in the diet and reflected by their concentration in the blood and urine. Thus, biochemical test helps to detect malnutrition much before the pathology has developed (Table 37.5).

Biophysical Examination

Cytological examination of buccal mucosa is done to study the cornified cells. Percentage of cornified cells increases with the degree of malnutrition. In healthy children, the normal percentage of cornified cells is 30–40%.

Indirect Method of Assessment

Since malnutrition influences morbidity and mortality rates, the three indicators employed are:
- Age-specific death rate among 1–4 years (infant mortality rate and mortality in the age group of 1–4 years)
- Cause-specific death rate among under-fives (due to PEM)
- Proportional mortality rate among under-fives (due to PEM).

Laboratory Investigations

1. Urine for sugar to rule out diabetes, and urine for albumin and microscopic examination to rule out urinary infections, which are common among male children due to pinhole meatus.

Table 37.5: Biochemical examination for nutritional deficiency

Nutritional deficiency	Biochemical test
Proteins	Serum albumin, urinary urea, urinary creatinine
Vitamin A	Serum retinol
Vitamin D	Serum alkaline phosphatase
Ascorbic acid	Serum ascorbic acid
Thiamine	Urinary thiamine
Riboflavin	Urinary riboflavin
Iron	Hemoglobin and serum iron

2. Urine for culture and sensitivity test.
3. Stool for ova and cyst to rule of underlying infestations.
4. Purified protein derivative (PPD) (Mantoux) test, if positive in a child below 2 years, it is considered as a case of primary complex, if negative—does not rule out primary complex.
5. Chest X-ray.
6. Scanning and electrocardiogram (ECG), if necessary.

NUTRITIONAL REQUIREMENT

The rationale behind the dietary management is to provide levels of protein and energy, which will not only meet immediate but also promote 'catch-up' growth. Foods specially rich in protein or protein concentrates are unnecessary. The protein caloric ratio of the most commonly used foods is adequate, when employed in judicious combinations are almost good. The response of children with kwashiorkor is more dramatic and more rapid than in that of children with marasmus who take a much longer time to respond as far as weight gains are concerned (Table 37.6).

Energy

The child should be given 150–200 kcal/kg bodyweight/day for the existing weight. For children less than 2 years, 200 kcal/kg bodyweight and for older children, 150–175 kcal/kg bodyweight should be given. It is very important that there should be enough calories in the diet, otherwise proteins will be utilized for energy purposes and not for building the tissues. Malted cereals can also be given to increase caloric density. 50% of total calories can be from carbohydrate.

Protein

For the existing weight, 5 g of protein/kg bodyweight/day should be given. The calories derived from protein should be 10% of the total calculated calories per day, if the main source is animal protein. If the main and the

Table 37.6: Master chart of classification of protein-energy malnutrition

Grade/Degree	Weight for age in percentage (%)			Waterlow	
	Gomez	Jelliffe	IAP*	Height for age (stunting) (cm)	Weight for height (wasting) (%)
Normal	90–110	> 90	> 90	100–80	> 95
Mild (1°)	89–75	90–81	79–70	94–87.5	90–80
Moderate (2°)	74–60	80–71	69–60	87.4–80	80–70
Severe (3°)	< 60	70–61	70–61	59–50	< 70
Very severe	–	< 60	< 50	–	–

*IAP, Indian Academy of Pediatrics

only source is from cereals and pulses, then the calories derived from protein can be 13–14% of the total calories. This is because the net protein utilization of cereals and pulses is around 60, whereas for milk or egg it is around 90. Through vegetable proteins are as good as milk protein in reversing the acute manifestations of kwashiorkor, they are inferior in their ability to promote regeneration of serum albumin. This can be overcome by giving three parts of vegetable protein to one part of animal protein, i.e. skimmed milk.

Fats

About 40% of total calories can be from fat, which can be tolerated by children. Saturated fats such as butter, milk and coconut oil are preferred because unsaturated fatty acids worsen diarrhea.

Electrolytes

Potassium chloride (2.4 g) and magnesium chloride (0.5 g) should be added daily to the diet for a period of 2 weeks.

Vitamins

If vitamin A deficiency is present, oral administration of a single dose of 50,000 IU of fat-soluble vitamin A should be given immediately, followed by 5,000 U daily. The deficiency symptoms disappear in about 2 weeks.

Management of a Case of PEM

Treatment strategy can be divided into three stages:
- Resolving life-threatening conditions
- Restoring of the nutritional status without disrupting homeostasis
- Ensuring nutritional rehabilitation.

Criteria for Improvement

- Disappearance of mental apathy in 4–5 days
- Disappearance of edema in 7–10 days
- Weight gain in 3–4 weeks
- Rise in serum albumin level in about 2 weeks.

The management scheme described in World Health Organization (WHO) guidelines, when applied, results in lowering death rates to less than 5% in severely malnourished children are detailed below.

Severe cases of malnutrition, especially those with complications such as severe infection or dehydration require intensive care and should therefore be referred to a hospital for initial treatment. Once the life-threatening conditions are controlled, the treatment can be continued outside the hospital. Non-complicated cases can be managed on an outpatient basis in a hospital or primary health care facility.

Dehydration

Patients with mild to moderate dehydration can be treated by oral or nasogastric administration of fluids. The oral rehydration solution (NaCl 3.5 g; $NaHCO_3$ 2.5 g; KCl 1.5 g and glucose 20 g dissolved in 1 L of water) recommended by the WHO can be safely used for correcting dehydration even in malnourished children. Depending on the dehydration 70–100 mL rehydration solution (ORS)/kg bodyweight can be given. This amount should be given in small quantities at frequent intervals over a period of 4–6 hours.

For patients with severe dehydration, intravenous fluid therapy is required to improve the circulation and expand plasma volume rapidly. About 70–100 mL of fluid can be given in the first 3–4 hours. In a majority of cases, after correcting the deficit of body fluid, maintenance therapy can be instituted with oral rehydration solution. As soon as urine flow is established, potassium supplements can be given orally (1–2 g/kg/day).

Infections

Diarrhea and measles are often the immediate cause of death in PEM. When the causative agent of the infection is known or suspected, appropriate antibiotic therapy can be given. For the most frequent infections such as pneumonia, otitis and skin infections, penicillin is the drug of choice. If the infection does not respond to penicillin, broad-spectrum antibiotics must be used. Giardiasis and ascariasis must be treated with appropriate deworming agents.

Hypoglycemia

In mild cases, giving milk feed or glucose in water may be sufficient. If a child develops convulsions or becomes unconscious, glucose should be given intravenously (1 mg of 50% dextrose solution/kg).

Hypothermia

Marasmic children are prone to have low body temperature. If the room is cold, the child should be properly covered with a blanket. The state of shock should be treated with intravenous injection of glucose-saline or blood transfusion. Another person should sleep with the child.

Anemia

Severe anemia is dangerous as it can result in heart failure. If the hemoglobin falls below 5 g/dL, blood transfusion should be given. About 10 mL of packed cells per kg bodyweight should be given over 3 hours.

Congestive Heart Failure

Congestive heart failure can occur as a result of severe anemia or as complication of IV fluid therapy. The main symptoms are rapid pulse and respiratory distress, cold extremities and cyanosis. Treatment must be started urgently with diuretics and digitalis.

Dietary Management

Dietary management is same for all clinical types of PEM. The child should be given a diet providing sufficient quantities of calories and protein in gradually increasing amounts, without provoking vomiting or diarrhea.

Initially, the child may refuse the feeds due to lack of appetite. If necessary, nasogastric tube feeding can be given for a day or two. It is best to begin with a liquid formula with diluted milk. When this is accepted, the strength can be increased and vegetable oil can be added to increase energy content. Most hospitals use milk-based formulae for feeding malnourished children. A formula containing 90 g skimmed milk powder + 70 g sugar + 50 g vegetable oil in 1,000 mL water will provide approximately 100 kcal and 3 g protein/100 mL. The children can be fed 100–150 mL/kg of this formula and the amount can be increased to as much as they can take. If there is milk intolerance, milk formulas can be substituted by buttermilk or cereal foods. In elder children with malnutrition, easily digestible solid foods such as bread, milk and sugar can be given. A mixed cereal-based diet can be given with added oil to increase energy density.

There will be improvement in mental apathy in 3–4 days. There will be increase in appetite and the child gains weight for age. Edema disappears by 7–10 days. Diarrhea and respiratory infection disappear in about 2 weeks. After clinically and biochemically improving in 3–4 weeks, the child is discharged from the hospital.

Suggested Diet During Convalescence

- Increasing the quantity of existing food (idlis, rice and chapatis)
- Increasing the number of meals to satisfy calorie and protein requirement
- Addition of oil or ghee 1–2 tablespoon to increase calories without increasing bulk
- Consumption of sugar and banana can be increased to increase calories in the diet
- The child can be given cereal and pulse mixture in 5:1 proportion
- If the patient can afford, milk, egg and skimmed milk can be included in the diet
- The diet should be locally available, inexpensive and easily digestible.
- Treatment of underlying infection with appropriate antibiotic
- Treatment of underlying infestation with anthelmintic drug
- Adequate diet, as to provide 150 kcal of energy/kg/day, providing 3–4 g of protein/kg weight/day (this much can be fed to the child by giving in small, but frequent feeds)
- Correction of social factors if any.

Advice (instructions) given to the mother for prevention of recurrence of malnutrition in the child:

1. Growth monitoring: The weight of the child is recorded every month and plotted in 'Road to Health' card to monitor the growth curve.
2. Oral rehydration therapy: This is to be given to the child with the onset of diarrhea.
3. Breastfeeding: Exclusive breastfeeding to be given till 6 months, followed by complimentary feeding. However, breastfeeding to be continued up to minimum 2 years.

4. Immunization: This is to be completed.
5. Family planning: Mother is advised to adopt contraceptive method, so that she can take better care of her child.
6. Health education: She is advised to take correct and complete treatment for her child for any illness. She is educated on maintaining personal hygiene and also to take recommended balanced diet for her, specially if she is a lactating mother.

The clinical presentation depends on the type, severity and duration of the dietary deficiencies. The five forms of PEM are given in Table 37.7.

Prevention and Control of PEM in the Community

The PEM is a consequence not only of inadequate food intake but also of poor living conditions, unhygienic environment and lack of health care. It is primarily a disease of socioeconomic inequalities and maldistribution of food and health. There is no simple solution to the problem of PEM. The following steps are suggested by Food and Agriculture Organization (FAO)/WHO Nutrition Expert Committee.

Health Promotion

- Measures directed to pregnant and lactating women (education, distribution of supplements)
- Promotion of breastfeeding
- Development of low cost weaning foods; the child should be made to eat more food at frequent intervals
- Measures to improve family diet
- Nutrition education, promotion of correct feeding practices
- Home economics
- Family planning and spacing of births
- Improving family environment
- Nutritional care of pregnant mothers to prevent low birth weight (LBW)
- Nutritional care of lactating mothers to prevent subsequent malnutrition during infancy and childhood
- Promotion of correct breastfeeding practices
- Frequent feeds to a growing child
- Promotion of health of the mother by family planning and spacing of births
- Improvement in the living condition
- Supplementary feeding program for mothers and children under integrated child development services (ICDS) scheme.

Specific Protection

- The child's diet must contain protein- and energy-rich foods; milk, eggs, fresh fruits should be given, if possible
- Immunization schedule should be followed
- Food fortification may help the child in meeting micronutrient requirements
- Protein- and energy-rich diet for a growing child (i.e. diet containing milk, egg, fruits, etc.)
- Immunization
- Fortification of food.

Early Diagnosis and Treatment of PEM

- Periodic surveillance
- Early diagnosis of any lag in growth
- Early diagnosis and treatment of the infections, and diarrhea
- Development of programs for early rehydration of children with diarrhea
- Development of supplementary feeding programs during epidemics
- Deworming of heavily infested children
- By maintenance of 'Road to Health' card
- By early diagnosis and prompt treatment of infections
- By periodical deworming.

Disability Limitation

- Limiting the development of further disability by giving intensive treatment
- Hospitalization, if necessary
- Follow-up.

Table 37.7: Classification of protein-energy malnutrition (PEM) [Food and Agriculture Organization (FAO)/ World Health Organization (WHO)]

Types of PEM	Bodyweight as percentage of standard	Edema	Deficit in weight for height
Kwashiorkor	80–60	+	+
Marasmic kwashiorkor	< 60	+	++
Marasmus	< 60	0	++
Nutritional dwarfing	< 60	0	Minimal
Underweight child	80–60	0	+

Integrated Child Development Services

Isolated feeding programs will not be effective unless efforts are made simultaneously to improve the environment and to control infections. Supplementary nutrition is therefore integrated with other heath activities such as immunization, treatment of minor illnesses, growth monitoring and health education under the ICDS.

Nutrition Education

Education programs to improve child nutrition should stress the importance of breastfeeding and timely introduction of supplements. Mothers should be advised to give supplements based on the household foods such as cereals and pulses. Addition of oil/sugar increases calorie density. Amylase-rich food prepared from wheat or maize can be used to reduce the bulk of the cereal mixture.

United Nations Children's Funds (UNICEF's) inexpensive measures to prevent PEM is by GOBI (the 'GOBI' stands for 'Growth monitoring, Oral rehydration, Breastfeeding and Immunization') also educate the community regarding recommended dietary allowances (RDA) for nutrients and vitamin as given in Tables 37.8 and 37.9.

Rehabilitation

Nutritional rehabilitation is purely mother oriented. The mother is educated to make simple modifications in the child's diet, with the locally available foods, without external supplement within their economic constraints. This was formulated by Bengoa. This has been modified in various countries and implemented in India. National Institute of Nutrition (NIN), Hyderabad has recommended the following mixture:
- Wheat: 40 g
- Roasted Bengal gram: 16 g
- Roasted groundnuts: 10 g
- Jaggery: 20 g
- Total: 86 g.

This mixture per day provides 11.3 g of proteins and 330 kcal of energy.

VITAMIN DEFICIENCY DISEASES

Nutritional blindness, the blindness occurring due to malnutrition, mainly due to deficiency of vitamin A. It is common among children between 1 and 3 years. It is a permanent blindness and is totally preventable. It is one of the serious public health problems. Younger the child, more serious is the disorder, because a young child is not having sufficient vitamin A reserve in the body unlike adults. It is often associated with PEM.

Extent of the Problem

Nutritional blindness is common among predominantly rice-eating states in India such as Andhra Pradesh, Karnataka, Tamil Nadu, Bihar, West Bengal, because rice is devoid of carotene. Incidence is less in North India.

Nearly, 70,000 children below 3 years are becoming permanently blind only due to vitamin A deficiency every year in India. It is predisposed by many social factors such as poverty, illiteracy, ignorance, etc. Therefore, it is often called 'social disease.'

Etiology

The causes of vitamin deficiency include:
- Low dietary intake of vitamin A
- Infectious diseases, which prevent absorption and utilization of vitamin A and aggravate the condition
- All causes of PEM are also the causes of nutritional blindness.

Clinical Features

Clinical features are described under xerophthalmia.

Prevention and Control of Nutritional Blindness (Xerophthalmia)

Prevention and control of nutritional blindness is now an integral part of primary health care. Nutritional blindness can be prevented by intervening at all the levels in the natural history of the disease as detailed below.

Health Promotion

1. Nutritional care of the pregnant mother, to prevent LBW (i.e. to prevent malnutrition at birth) by promoting the consumption of green leafy vegetables or other vitamin A-rich foods (thus, measures are taken much before the child is born).
2. Promotion of breastfeeding as long as possible.
3. Proper weaning of young infants and feeding of growing children with fruits, carrots and vegetables.
4. Health education (nutrition education) of mothers about hazards of vitamin A deficiency among children and their easy prevention.

Specific Protection

1. Food fortification, i.e. addition of vitamin A to salt, sugar, tea, margarine, dried skimmed milk and vanaspati (Dalda). This helps in covering the people of all the age groups including children.

Table 37.8: Summary of recommended dietary allowances (RDA) for nutrients in Indians

Group	Condition	Bodyweight (kg)	Net energy (kcal/day)	Protein (g/day)	Fat (g/day)	Calcium (g/day)	Iron (g/day)
Man	Sedentary work		2,425	60	20	400	28
	Moderate work	60	2,875				
	Heavy work		3,800				
Woman	Sedentary work		1,875				
	Moderate work		2,225	50	20	400	30
	Heavy work	50	2,925				
	Pregnancy		+300	+15	30	1,000	38
	Lactation						
	< 6 month		+550	+25	45	1,000	30
	> 6 month		+400	+18	45	1,000	30

Table 37.9: Summary of recommended dietary allowances (RDA) for vitamins in Indians

Group	Condition	Body-weight (kg)	Vitamin A retinol	β-carotene (µg/day)	B_1 (mg/day)	B_2 (mg/day)	Nicotinic (mg/day)	B_6 (mg/day)	Vitamin C (mg/day)	Folic (µg/day)	Vitamin B_{12} (µg/day)
Man	Sedentary work				1.2	1.4	16				
	Moderate work	60	600	2,400	1.4	1.6	18	2	40	100	1
	Heavy work				1.6	1.9	21				
Woman	Sedentary work				0.9	1.1	12				
	Moderate work	50	600	2,400	1.1	1.3	14	2	40	100	1
	Heavy work				1.2	1.5	16				
	Pregnancy	50	600	2,400	+0.2	+0.2	+2	2.5	40	400	1
	Lactation										
	< 6 month	50	950	3,800	+0.3	+0.3	+4	2.5	80	150	1.5
	> 6 month	50	950	3,800	+0.2	+0.2	+3	2.5	80	150	1.5

2. Administration of five mega doses of vitamin A concentrate, orally to all children between 9 months and 3 years, under National Vitamin A Prophylaxis Program, which is a component of National Program for Prevention and Control of Blindness. However, it can be extended up to 5 years (Table 37.10).

Thus, the child is 'almost immunized' against xerophthalmia by 200,000 IU (110 mg) of retinol palmitate in oil; one spoon of 2 mL capacity holds 200,000 IU of vitamin A supplied along with the bottle of vitamin A syrup.

Strategy
- Cent percent coverage of children below 3 years with five mega doses of vitamin A orally
- Elimination of blindness and other consequences of vitamin A deficiency.

Early Diagnosis and Treatment of Vitamin A Deficiency (Nutritional Blindness)

1. History of night blindness.
2. Clinical examination of eyes for the manifestations of xerophthalmia.

CHAPTER 37 — Malnutrition

Table 37.10: Vitamin A prophylaxis schedule [under child survival and safe motherhood (CSSM)]

Dose No.	Age of child	Dose (orally)	Remarks
1.	At 9th month	100,000 IU	Along with measles vaccine
2.	At 18th month (1½ year)	200,000 IU	With booster dose of diphtheria, pertussis tetanus (DPT) and oral polio vaccine (OPV)
3.	At 24th month (2 year)	200,000 IU	Nil
4.	At 30th month (2½ year)	200,000 IU	Nil
5.	At 36th month (3 year)	200,000 IU	Nil

3. 'Rose Bengal dye' test: This consists of application of 1% of this dye to conjunctiva. Development of pink-colored stain on conjunctiva indicates conjunctival xerosis.
4. Treatment consists of administration of 200,000 IU of vitamin A concentrate soon after the diagnosis followed by another dose of 200,000 IU on the next day and third dose after 1–4 weeks (WHO). The dosage is same irrespective of age and sex, except among infants and women of the reproductive age group (15–45 year). Infants require 100,000 IU once in 3–6 months till 1 year of age and women (15–45 year) require 100,000 IU daily for 2 weeks.

Children suffering from acute respiratory infection, diarrhea and measles should be given prophylactic dose of vitamin A 200,000 IU orally as soon as the diagnosis is made.

Disability Limitation

Disability limitation means limiting or prevention of further disability by giving intensive treatment with vitamin A injections, when the patient comes in the advanced stage of xerophthalmia (i.e. when there is involvement of cornea as xerosis, ulcer, keratomalacia, prolapse iris, etc.). The intensive treatment prevents the transition from impairment to handicap as shown below:
- Disease → Impairment → Disability → Handicap
- Vitamin A → Corneal xerosis → Inability to see → Loss of job deficiency → Abnormality of structure and blurring of vision or function of blindness cornea.

Rehabilitation

Rehabilitation consists of training and retraining of a blind and handicapped person by the combined and coordinated use of medical (physical), vocational, social and psychological therapies to the highest level of functional ability. For example, schools for the blind, corneal grafting (corneaplasty), vocational training for earning, physical rehabilitation by the supply of walking sticks, etc.

Vitamin A Concentrate Oily Solution

Vitamin A concentrate oily syrup is supplied as a flavored syrup in 100 mL bottle, with a concentration of 100,000 IU/mL. The bottle is always supplied with a spoon of 2 mL capacity. This syrup does not require any storage measures, e.g. cold chain. However, it should be stored in cool and dark place, protected from sunlight.

Once the bottle is opened, it should be used within 6–8 weeks. The shelf life of the sealed bottle is 1 year. The price of the bottle is ₹25, i.e. 25 paise/mL. This is supplied free of cost to the community through primary health center.

Vitamin A is also available in the following forms:
- Capsules: Each capsule contains 200,000 IU
- Tablets: Each sugar coated tablet contains 100,000 IU
- Injectable: Each ampule of 1 mL equivalent to 100,000 IU to be given intramuscularly
- High-risk children for nutritional blindness
- LBW babies
- Newborns deprived of mother's milk (because they do not have sufficient reserve of vitamin A)
- Young children suffering from acute respiratory infection (ARI), diarrhea and measles.

All such high-risk children should be given 200,000 IU of vitamin A orally, as soon as the diagnosis is made (100,000 IU for an infant) and the dose is repeated once in 3–4 months, till the infant completes 1 year and the other children up to 5 years of age. Other vitamin deficiency diseases such as beriberi, pellagra, ariboflavinosis, scurvy, rickets and osteomalacia are explained under vitamins.

MINERAL DEFICIENCY DISEASES

Nutritional Anemia

Nutritional anemia is a health problem, social problem and an economic problem in our country:
1. Nutritional anemia is a condition in which the hemoglobin content/level in the blood is lower than the normal, as a result of deficiency of one or more nutrients, specially iron.

2. Less frequent causes are deficiency of folic acid and/or vitamin B_{12}. It is often associated with malnutrition and chronic infections. The most vulnerable groups are infants, children and women specially during pregnancy.
3. Normal hemoglobin level in the blood is 14 g/dL = 100%.
4. The WHO cutoff criteria for anemia (in venous blood):
   - Adult man = 13 g/dL
   - Adult woman (nonpregnant) = 12 g/dL
   - Adult woman (pregnant) = 11 g/dL
   - Child above 6 years = 12 g/dL
   - Child below 6 years = 11 g/dL

Magnitude of the Problem

Nutritional anemia is a global problem, in the developing countries. Globally, about 3.6 billion people are suffering from this. In India, it is very high among nutritionally vulnerable group such as mothers and children. It varies from 60 to 70%. Among pregnant mothers, it is about 85%.

Causes

Causes of megaloblastic anemia:
- Strict vegetarians, not taking even dairy products.
- Tapeworm anemia, which absorbs vitamin B_{12}
- Increased demand of folic acid, which occurs during pregnancy
- Malabsorption syndrome.

Causes of iron deficiency and the detrimental effects of iron deficiency anemia, and the recommended daily requirement of iron already explained (under minerals).

Clinical Features of Nutritional Anemia (Iron Deficiency)

Since hemoglobin is necessary for oxygen transport and cell respiration in nutritional (iron deficiency) anemia, every tissue cell suffers from lack of oxygen. Thus, there are clinical signs and symptoms related to every organ system of the body. The common features are as follows:

1. General appearance: Pale, plump, person with poorly built and nourishment, and easy fatigability:
   - Head: Headache, giddiness
   - Face: Pale and puffy (edematous)
   - Eyes: Pale conjunctiva
   - Hairs: Dry and lusterless
   - Tongue: Pale, smooth tongue with atrophied papillae
   - Abdomen: Anorexia, acidity, ascites may be present due to associated hypoproteinemia; dysphagia often present.
2. The cutoff points is suggested by WHO to assess the magnitude of iron deficiency anemia given in Table 37.11.

Table 37.11: Cutoff points of iron deficiency by World Health Organization

Prevalence (%)	Public health problem
< 5	Not a problem
5–14.9	Low magnitude
15–33.9	Moderate magnitude
40 and above	High magnitude

3. Thorax and respiratory system: Breathlessness (exertional).
4. Cardiovascular system: Soft systolic (hemic) murmur, best heard over the pulmonary area.
5. Blood pressure (BP): Lower than the normal.
6. Pulse: Rapid and weak.
7. Feet: Edematous.
8. Nails: Koilonychia (spoon shaped), brittle nails.

Edema of the face and feet with or without ascites indicates hypoproteinemia.

Prevention and Control of Nutritional Anemia (Table 37.12)

Health promotion
- Adequate nutrition
- Nutrition education to improve dietary habits
- Health education specially to pregnant mothers about hazards of anemia and their prevention
- Periodical deworming specially among children and at least once during second trimester of pregnancy
- Nutritional supplementation (under ICDS scheme).

Specific protection

1. Food fortification: Recent studies in National Institute of Nutrition, Hyderabad showed that simple addition of ferric orthophosphate to salt, when consumed over 12–18 months was found to reduce the prevalence of anemia.
2. National Nutritional Anemia Prophylaxis Program (NNAPP): This was launched by the Government of India, during the Fourth Five-year plan (1970) in order to prevent and control nutritional anemia among mothers and children (1–12 year).
3. Beneficiaries are pregnant mothers, lactating mothers and children between 1 and 12 years. Benefit is that iron and folic acid (IFA) tablets are distributed free of cost.
4. Eligibility criteria are all those beneficiaries, whose hemoglobin level is between 10 and 12 g/dL. If the hemoglobin level is less than 10 g/dL, such cases are referred to Medical Officer.
5. Dosage: If the pregnant mother has no visible signs of anemia, she is given one large IFA tablet containing

100 mg of elemental iron and 500 mg of folic acid, during the last 100 days of pregnancy, to prevent anemia. If the pregnant mother has visible signs of anemia, but not severely anemic, she is given two large tablets of IFA daily to control anemia. If she is severely anemic, she is admitted to hospital for intensive treatment and blood transfusion. For anemic children (1–12 year) one small pediatric tablet of IFA containing 20 mg of elemental iron and 100 mg of folic acid is given daily.
6. The tablets have to be consumed only after food.

Early diagnosis and treatment
- By history of headache, giddiness, fatigue, loss of appetite, etc.
- By clinical signs
- By laboratory investigations such as hemoglobin concentration (Hb%) peripheral smear and stool examination for ova and cyst.

Iron therapy should be followed by the treatment of the cause including underlying infection, infestation, bleeding piles, bleeding duodenal ulcer, etc.

Disability limitation
Disability limitation consists of limiting the development of further disability when the patient comes in the advanced stage of anemia by giving intensive treatment in the hospital by blood transfusion. If severe anemia is associated with cardiac failure (high output failure), packed cell transfusion is given under the umbrella of digoxin, Lasix and potassium salts.

Rehabilitation
A person with anemia will not become handicapped, if treatment is given correctly and completely. 12 by 12 initiative is launched by Federation of Obstetrics and Gynecology Society of India (FOGSI) Delhi, in collaboration with Government of India, WHO and UNICEF on 23rd April 2007 at All India Institute of Medical Sciences (AIIMS), New Delhi.

Meaning: By the year 2012, every child across the country should have at least 12 g% Hb by 12 years of age.

Table 37.12: Grading and treatment of anemia

Grade (WHO*)	Degree of anemia	Treatment
14–11 g	Normal	Nothing required
11–9 g	Mild	Oral iron therapy
9–7 g	Moderate	Parenteral iron therapy
<7 g	Severe	Blood transfusion

*WHO, World Health Organization

Problem of Iron Deficiency Anemia

Iron deficiency anemia is a global public health problem as harmful as the epidemics of infectious diseases. With a global population of 6.7 billion, about 3.6 billion people have iron deficiency and out of these about 2.0 billion are suffering from iron deficiency anemia. Children and women in reproductive age group are being hit hardest because of their vulnerability. India continues to be one of the countries to have highest prevalence of anemia because of low dietary intake, poor availability of iron and chronic blood loss due to hookworm infestation, and malaria. National Family Health Survey (NFHS-3) estimates reveal the prevalence of anemia to be 70–80% in children, 65–75% in adolescent girls, 70% in pregnant women and 24% in adult men. Compared to the report of NFHS-2, there has been an increased trend.

Adolescents constitute 22% of our country's population. Adolescence, being the phase of rapid growth, has an increased demand for iron requirement in both boys and girls, more so among girls because of menstruation. The adolescent girls constitute potential mothers. Anemia not only affects the present health status of adolescent girls but also has deleterious effects in future specially during pregnancy. The health consequences of anemia in children, adolescents and pregnant mothers are well-documented. Anemia has a serious impact on learning capacity, productivity and survival among children.

Maternal ill effects include reduced physical capacity and work performance, impaired immune response predisposing for infections, decrease in peripartum reserve, risk of cardiac failure, and increased need for blood transfusions; thus anemia can result in negative reproductive, consequences and endangering her life. Anemia during pregnancy is the result of uncared anemia during adolescence.

Fetal effects include LBW baby, who subsequently suffers from impaired psychomotor and cognitive function. Infants born to severely anemic mothers have a higher risk of irreversible brain damage, lower school achievement, a reduced physical and exercise tolerance, and poor immune response.

Anemia during pregnancy puts the woman at three times greater risk of delivering LBW babies and nine times higher risk of perinatal mortality, thus contributing significantly for increased infant mortality rate (IMR) and maternal mortality rate (MMR) 30% of maternal deaths are due to anemia.

The consequences of anemia extend over generations. Girls born underweight are at risk of producing premature infants themselves.

Thus, anemia is a silent epidemic. It is a critical health concern. However, it is a preventable condition. In order to reduce LBW, IMR and MMR, there is a need to combat anemia during adolescence, a motive behind '12 by 12 initiative', so that women enter pregnancy and motherhood free of anemia, and that newborns and infants are assured of good health. The IMR, MMR are reduced in a life cycle approach.

This initiative is an implementable, effective and sustainable nation-building exercise with far reaching benefits in terms of safe motherhood and healthier future generations.

This initiative will contribute immensely to the achievement of the Millennium Development Goals 4 and 5, to reduce high rate of global child and maternal deaths by the year 2015.

Goals of 12 by 12 Initiative

- To decrease the prevalence of anemia among adolescents to ensure healthy parenthood
- To increase the awareness among adolescents regarding anemia and appropriate nutrition.

Objectives

- To determine the prevalence of anemia among children between 10 and 14 years of age
- To create awareness about anemia among children
- To provide the nutritional guidelines for the anemic children
- To treat those detected to be anemic
- To vaccinate all children against tetanus and all girls against rubella
- To deworm all children and treat malaria, if present.

Iodine Deficiency Disorders

Iodine deficiency disorders (IDDs) are the spectrum of disorders that occur due to deficiency of iodine and associated hypothyroidism, commencing from intrauterine life, and extending through infancy, childhood, adolescence to adult life with serious implications. Till recently, iodine deficiency was equated with goiter only. But now, it has become very clear that iodine deficiency not only results in goiter but also affects all stages of human growth and development resulting in varied manifestations, coined under the term 'iodine deficiency disorders'. This term was introduced in 1983.

The various disorders are abortions, premature births, growth failure, mental retardation, cretinism, myxedema and neurological defects. Iodine deficiency is the most common cause of preventable mental retardation in the world today.

Extent of the Problem

Global: About 190 million people are suffering from goiter and nearly 800 million people in developing countries are at risk.

South East Asia: In this region, eight countries have significant IDD problems. These countries are India, Indonesia, Bangladesh, Bhutan, Myanmar, Nepal, Sri Lanka and Thailand. Out of these eight countries, 102 million people have goiter, 277 million are at risk, 1.5 millions are cretins and more than 35 million are physically or mentally disabled.

India: In India, the major geographical focus is the Sub-Himalayan region. It is estimated that about 55 million people are suffering from endemic goiter and about 150 million are at risk, about 2.2 millions are cretins, and 6.6 million are having neurological deficits. The Sub-Himalayan region extending over 2,400 km from Kashmir to Naga Hills is called 'Himalaya Goiter Belt', which is the biggest goiter belt in the world.

In addition, pockets of endemic goiter have been reported from almost all states of India. These are called 'Extra Himalayan' foci of endemic goiter. No state in India is said to be entirely free from goiter.

The prevalence of goiter in India is 7.3% of the total population. Endemic goiter is said to be present and considered as significant public health problem, when the prevalence of goiter (total goiter rate) exceeds 10% among school children, aged 6–11 years.

In fact with every passing hour, 10 children are born in the country without attaining optimum, physical growth and mental development due to neonatal hypothyroidism. This has been going unnoticed as a 'silent epidemic'. The endemicity of goiter is graded as depending upon 'total goiter rate' (i.e. prevalence rate) Tables 37.13 and 37.14.

Table 37.13: Goiter prevalence rate

Goiter prevalence rate (%)	Grade of endemicity
< 20	Mild
20–30	Moderate
43	Severe

The other indicators of iodine deficiency are prevalence of cretinism, prevalence of neonatal hypothyroidism and urinary iodine excretion.

Spectrum of Iodine Deficiency Disorders

It is seen that the problem is of greater magnitude than that of goiter alone. It is a national problem with grave socio-economic consequences, affecting the human resources development. People become less vigorous and productive in their work, and domestic animals also suffer in the same way resulting in decreased production of wool, meat, eggs, etc. Abortions and sterility can also occurs.

Table 37.14: Goiter prevalence rate according to age group

Age group	Disorders
Fetus	• Abortion, stillbirths, congenital anomalies • Neonatal cretinism: Mental deficiency, deaf mutism, spastic diplegia, squint psychomotor defects, neonatal goiter and neonatal hypothyroidism
Neonate	• Goiter, juvenile hypothyroidism and dwarfism, cretinism, impaired mental functions (low IQ), educational backwardness, personality problems
Child/Adolescent	• Goiter, juvenile hypothyroidism, dwarfism • Cretinism, impaired mental functions (low IQ), educational backwardness, personality problems
Adult	• Goiter (cosmetic effect and pressure effect) hypothyroidism impaired mental functions myxedema

Thus IDD is not only a health problem but also a social and economic problem. Iodine sources, physiology, pathophysiology and daily requirement are detailed under trace elements.

Prevention and Control of Iodine Deficiency Disorders

There are four methods of iodine supplementation namely iodized salt, iodized oil, iodized water and Lugol's iodine.

Iodized salt

Iodized salt consists of incorporation of iodine in the common edible salt. It is an example of fortification of salt. Edible salt is an ideal vehicle for iodine fortification because everyone consumes salt, thus easily distributable to entire population in an inexpensive way. More than all, the added iodine does not affect the appearance and taste of salt, and is well-accepted by the consumer. Since, excess consumption of salt is not possible, it eliminates the danger of overdosage. Iodized salt should be added to the food after cooking to have the maximum benefit.

Therefore, iodization of salt is now the most widely used prophylactic public health measure against endemic goiter. In India, the level of iodization is fixed under the Prevention of Food Adulteration Act (PFA Act). The iodine concentration in the salt should not be less than 30 ppm at the production point and not less than 15 ppm at the consumer level. Thus iodization of salt is the most economical, convenient, safe, feasible and effective means of mass prophylaxis in endemic areas.

There are three processes of iodization of salt:
1. Dry mixing: This consists of mixing salt with potassium iodide.
2. Spray mixing: This consists of spraying the aqueous solution of potassium iodate (KIO_3) on salt and then mixing in a blender.
3. Submersion process: This consists of mixing the salt with a solution of potassium iodate in a tank and then drying.

Iodization

About 50 kg of potassium iodate are added to 100,000 kg of salt. This provides 50 ppm of KIO_3, which is equivalent to 30 ppm of iodine, because only 60% of KIO_3 contains elemental iodine at the production point. Since, iodine is unstable, it comes to 15 ppm at the consumer level:

$$\frac{60}{100} \times 50 = 30 \text{ kg of elemental iodine}$$

Recently the National Institute of Nutrition (NIN), Hyderabad has recommended 'double fortification' of salt with iodine and iron ('two in one' salt). Community trials are going on. The NIN has also recommend addition of stabilizers to increase the stability of salt such as calcium carbonate in iodized salt and sodium hexametaphosphate in double fortified salt. Stabilizers are found to be not hazardous.

Hazards of iodization

A mild increase in the incidence of thyrotoxicosis has now been described following iodized salt programs. An increase in lymphocytic thyroiditis (Hashimoto's disease) has also been reported. Excess of food consumption results in the following conditions:
- Hypervitaminosis A and D: These are explained under vitamins A and D respectively
- Obesity: Explained under epidemiology of obesity
- Fluorosis: Explained under trace elements and fluorine.

Iodized oil

Iodized oil consists of incorporation of iodine into vegetable oil (poppy seed oil). The NIN, recently have successfully used sunflower oil for iodization. Most widely used is Lipiodol. About l mL of Lipiodol oil containing 480 mg of iodine, given intramuscularly has proved to correct severe iodine deficiency for a period of over 4 years. The effective protection rate is 80% against neonatal hypothyroidism. A repeat injection may be required in 3–5 years. High cost of iodized oil is a limiting factor in its widespread use in India and lot of manpower to meet individual persons for giving injections. Sodium iodate oral tablets or oral iodized oil has been found to have half of the effects of injectable oil, i.e. for about 2 years. Oral intake is not popular. Moreover, oral intake is costlier than injections.

The use of iodized oil is preferred in those areas, where the problem is large and iodized salt is not available. China has developed iodized walnut oil and iodized soybean oil for use in community programs.

Iodized water

Iodized water consists of incorporation of I_2 or KI or KIO_3 to drinking water in a concentration as to achieve a daily intake of 150 mg of iodine. This method is practiced in Northern Thailand.

Lugol's iodine

Lugol's iodine solution can also be taken directly, but the effect is considerably shorter than that of iodized oil. The advantages are its easy availability and low cost. Repeated applications are necessary because of shorter duration of action.

Out of all the four methods, use of iodized salt is the most rational and feasible approach in our country.

CONCLUSION

Malnutrition is a health problem especially among children under 5 years of age. It occurs due to relative or absolute deficiency, or excess of nutrients in human body. It is of four types. It occur due to various causes such as infectious disease, food habits, food taboos, cooking practices, etc. Malnutrition can be assessed using parameters such as weight, height, chest circumference, midarm circumference, etc. Deficiency of proteins, minerals and vitamins cause deficiency/disease disorders. Appropriate steps can help in prevention and control of malnutrition.

Obesity

38 CHAPTER

INTRODUCTION

Obesity is a pathological condition characterized by an accumulation of fat much more than is necessary in the body. This form of overnutrition is more common in developed countries. The degree of obesity can be assessed by comparing the patient's weight with standard weights for heights. A man, whose body fat amounts more than 20% of his total weight is considered obese. For a woman, it is 30% and above.

Obesity, which makes a person bulky and overweight, may be a result of genetic endocrine and behavioral factors. Apart from genetic factors, hypo or lowered activity of the pituitary, thyroid and gonads lead to decreased secretion of hormones of these endocrine glands, which results in obesity. Behavioral factors such as eating, sleeping and activity are generally responsible for the regulation of body weight. Overconsumption of carbohydrate foods, concentrated high-calorie foods, i.e. fried foods coupled with inactivity and oversleep make a person prone to obesity. Emotionally disturbed individuals who feel lonely, often find consolation and pleasure in overeating. Emotional trauma is associated with such overeating. An obese person is self-conscious and therefore, may develop psychological problems.

Obesity is a disease of civilization. The provision for storing excess energy as fat was a useful biological mechanism for primitive man who could not get a steady supply of food. A person overeats, when food was available and starved, when it was not. This was the pattern even in civilized societies, until recently as feast days were often preceded by fast days. Now, the fasts have gone, but not the feasts. What is more in affluent countries? One can have feasts everyday if one chooses to. Food has become plentiful for people who coupled with labor-saving devices, which reduce physical activity has become a major problem.

In addition to psychological and emotional disturbances, obesity often leads to social humiliation and other complications. The human skeleton is not adapted to carrying of an extraload and this may lead to flat feet, problems with the knees, hip and lumbar spine. The work of the heart is increased owing to the extra energy needed to move the overweight body.

Obese people are more prone to diabetes, tuberculosis, cardiovascular irregularities, hypertension, arthritis and respiratory problems. Normal heat loss by the skin tends to be restricted and there is excessive perspiration often leading to rashes and inflammation of the skin. Vitamins A and D toxicosis is commonly observed in the obese. Children of young mothers suffer from toxicosis, when given large doses of vitamin drops.

Obesity increases the risk of complications during surgery, pregnancy and childbirth. Obese women appear to be more prone to menstrual irregularities and infertility. There is impaired glucose tolerance and in many cases, hyperglycemia leads to diabetes.

Obesity is more common in men and women after the age of about 30 years and could be associated with the reduction in basal metabolic rate and inactivity apart from other factors mentioned earlier. Every kilogram increase in weight is liable to increase the workload of the heart up to 5 kilometers. Obesity is a type of nutritional disorder, characterized by the abnormal growth of the adipose tissue, resulting in an increase in the body weight to the extent of 20% or more of the standard weight for the person's age, sex and height.

INDICATORS OF OBESITY

Obesity is expressed by four indicators namely corpulence index, body mass index (BMI), waist circumference and waist-to-hip ratio (WHR).

Corpulence Index

Corpulence index is based on only weight of the individual;

$$\text{Corpulence index} = \frac{\text{Actual body weight (ABW) of the individual}}{\text{Expected body weight (EBW)}}$$

Corpulence index of 1.2 or more is considered as obesity. Expected body weight can be calculated by two methods:
1. Broca's method:
   EBW = Height (cm) – 100

   For example, a person who is 160 cm tall, his/her ideal weight is 160 – 100 = 60 kg.
2. Lorentz method:
   - EBW (males) = {Height (cm) – 100 – [Height (cm) – 150]/4}
   - EBW (females) = {Height (cm) – 100 – [Height (cm) – 150]/2}.

Body Mass Index

Obesity means increase in weight due to excess of fat contents. World Health Organization (WHO) defines obesity as increase in BMI > 30 kg/m². BMI is calculated as:

$$BMI = \frac{\text{Weight (kg)}}{\sqrt{\text{Height (m}^2)}}$$

Normal BMI of adults is 18.5–24.9 kg/m². BMI between 25–30 kg/m² is taken as overweight (Table 38.1). According to current estimate, 23% of US population is obese and 55 people are overweight. Two phenotypes of obesity are depicted in Figures 38.1A and B, and the risks associated with weight gain (overweight/obesity) are given in Table 38.2. Visceral fat is more dangerous than subcutaneous fat, therefore, truncal obesity is associated with more risk than generalized obesity.

The BMI is based on weight and height of the individual.

$$BMI = \frac{\text{Weight (kg)}}{\text{Height (m}^2)}$$

This is also called 'Quetelet's index' named after Lambert Adolphe Jacques Quetelet, a Belgium scientist. For example, an adult who is 80 kg in weight and 1.7 m in height will have a BMI of 27.7.

BMI = 80/(1.7)² = 27.7.

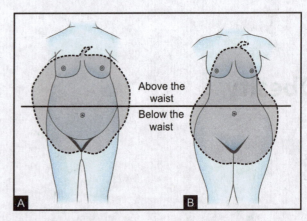

Figures 38.1A and B: Two phenotypes of obesity. **A.** Abdominal/Central obesity; **B.** Generalized obesity.

Classification

Classification of the obesity according to BMI (refer Tables 38.1 and 38.2) helps in comparison of weight status within and between population, helps in identification of at risk groups, for implementation of intervention programs and also for evaluation of the program. The BMI values are age independent and it is same for both the genders. Higher the BMI above 25, greater is the risk of morbidity according to grades.

Limitations

1. The BMI does not distinguish between the weight associated with muscle and weight associated with fat. As a result, the relationship between BMI and body fat content may vary according to body built and proportion. Therefore, a given BMI may not correspond to the same degree of fatness across the populations. For example, Polynesians tend to have a lower fat percentage than Caucasians.

Table 38.1: Classification of obesity according to body mass index (BMI)

Classification	BMI (kg/m²)
Underweight	< 18.5
Normal range	18.5–24.9
Overweight	> 25
Preobese	25–29.9
Obese class I	30–34.9
Obese class II	35–39.9
Obese class III	> 40

Table 38.2: WHO* classification of overweight and obesity, and associated risk of comorbidities based on BMI†

Class	BMI (kg/m²)	Risk of comorbidities
Overweight	25–30	Mildly increased
Obese	> 30	Mildly increased
Class I	30–35	Moderate
Class II	35–45	Severe
Class III	> 40	Very severe

*WHO, World Health Organization; †BMI, body mass index

2. Australians are at an identical BMI. In addition, the percentage of body fat mass increases with age up to 60–65 years in both sexes and is higher in women than in men of equivalent BMI.

In spite of the limitations, BMI is considered to be the most useful, albeit crude, population level measure of obesity and the risks associated with it.

Waist Circumference

Waist circumference helps to measure abdominal fat. It is measured at a midpoint between the lower border of the rib cage and the adipose crest. It is an approximate index of intra-abdominal adipose tissue and total body fat. It is a convenient and simple measurement, not related to height and correlates closely with BMI and WHR. Furthermore, changes in waist circumference reflect the changes in risk factors for cardiovascular diseases and other forms of chronic diseases, i.e. diabetes mellitus.

The risk of metabolic complications of obesity (waist circumference) is observed to be high among men with a waist circumference greater than 102 cm and among women greater than 88 cm.

Waist-to-hip Ratio

It is accepted that WHR of more than 1.0 in men and 0.85 in women indicates abdominal fat accumulation.

Magnitude of the Problem

Prevalence of overweight and obesity is increasing worldwide at an alarming rate, affecting children and adults alike in both developed and developing countries. It is more among urban population. The increasing prevalence is due to changes in the lifestyle of the people. In India, about 8% of population is estimated to have a BMI of more than 25.

Public Health Importance

Obesity is a risk factor in the natural history of other non-communicable diseases such as diabetes, cardiovascular diseases, hyperlipidemia and their consequences. In simple terms, obesity is a consequence of an energy imbalance, where energy intake is greater than the energy expenditure, resulting in positive energy balance and an increase in the energy stores and body weight.

RISK FACTORS OF OBESITY

Risks associated with obesity are:
- Metabolic, e.g. metabolic syndrome, type 2 diabetes mellitus (DM), hyperlipidemia
- Cardiovascular system (CVS), e.g. hypertension and coronary artery disease
- Gastrointestinal (GI) tract, e.g. gall stones and reflux esophagitis
- Joints, e.g. degenerative joint diseases
- Cancer, e.g. colorectal, prostrate in men, breast and genital tract in women
- Thromboembolic, surgical and obstetric risks
- Increase in mortality and morbidity
- Psychological upset.

Risk factors of obesity are classified into two, i.e. non-modifiable and modifiable.

Non-modifiable Risk Factors

Age: Obesity can occur in any age group. Generally, it increases with age. Obese children usually will have a tendency to remain obese in future adult life.

Sex: The prevalence of overweight is more among men, but obesity is more among women, specially during the menopausal age, between 45 and 49 years. Many physiological processes contribute to an increased storage of fat in females.

Studies have shown that woman's BMI increases with successive pregnancies. On the other hand in developing countries, successive pregnancies with short spacing is associated with weight loss rather than weight gain, due to depletion of maternal reserve.

Genetic factors: Obesity is a complex multifactorial phenotype with a genetic component that includes both polygenic and major gene effects. Obesity therefore tends to run families, with obese children frequently having obese parents.

Modifiable Risk Factors

Physical Activity

The physical activity pattern (including occupational work, household work and leisure time activity such as sports and exercise) determines the food intake and fat balance. The physical activity level (PAL) of a physically active individual is 1.75 and that of sedentary individual is 1.4.

The likelihood of becoming overweight is reduced at a PAL of 1.8 and 1.6, in men and women respectively. To elevate PAL by 0.5, it requires 1 hour of moderate activity such as brisk walk of 6 km/h or running at a speed of 12 km/h or cycling at a speed of 15 km/h. Thus, regular physical activity burns the fat and is protective against obesity, whereas sedentary lifestyle constitutes a risk factor. Sedentariness is an account of factors such as affluence, motorized transport, mechanical aids for work (e.g. washing machine), too much television (TV) viewing, internet surfing, etc.

Socioeconomic Status

High socioeconomic status correlates positively with obesity in the developing countries. Interestingly, this association is reversed in the developed countries, specially among women.

Literacy Level

The relation has been observed to be reverse, i.e. higher the literacy level, lesser is the prevalence of obesity.

Body Image

Traditionally, it is considered that an increased body weight is a sign of prosperity. But this concept is now changed. Thin and slim body symbolizes competence, success, control and sexual attractiveness, while obesity represents laziness, lack of will power and self-indulgence.

Eating Habits

Overnutrition is responsible for 95% cases of obesity. This is known as 'regulatory obesity'. Non-nutritional causes such as genetic, endocrinal, metabolic, etc. account for the remaining 5%. These are known as 'metabolic obesity', e.g. Cushing's syndrome, hypothyroidism, hypogonadism, etc. The capacity for storage of fat in human beings is highly efficient and unlimited compared to protein and carbohydrate. Therefore, weight gain occurs primarily due to high-fat intake leading to anomalous fat balance.

Fat makes the food more palatable and pleasurable resulting in increased consumption. Consumption of sugars also leads to excess energy balance. Food habits of relevance are eating between the meals, frequent consumption of sweets, chocolates, toffees, ghee, butter, fried foods, fast foods, etc. Often the foundation of adulthood obesity is laid in infancy. If a growing child is overfed, the number of adipose cells increase. In later life, these abundant cells store excessive fat and cause obesity.

Thus the composition of diet, the periodicity of eating and the amount of energy obtained are relevant to the development of obesity, as far as eating habits are concerned. This is predisposed by heavy advertisements of fast foods and beverages in TV.

Alcoholism

Every gram of consumption of alcohol provides 7 kcals of energy. Since the body is unable to store alcohol, it is oxidized first thereby allowing the greater proportion of energy to be stored obtained from other foods. Thus alcohol intake is associated with increased risk of abdominal fat. However, the controversial report is that heavy alcohol intake tend to be thinner, later resulting in paradox, i.e. such people eat less and drink alcohol more to get their energy requirement. A recent report is that the relationship between alcohol consumption and development of obesity is positive among men and negative among women.

Smoking

Smoking increases the metabolic rate and decreases food consumption. Thus, smoking and obesity are inversely related. Smokers often gain body weight after giving up the habit.

Psychological Factors

People who are under constant emotional strain, find satisfaction in eating food. Another motive for overeating is the yearning for companionship. This forces the individual to spend much time in the company of friends and foods.

Drugs

Use of certain drugs such as corticosteroids, oral contraceptive pills, insulin, adrenergic blockers, etc. can promote weight gain.

Environmental Factors

Fast process of industrialization and urbanization has resulted in the modernization of standard of living, affecting the physical activity pattern contributing to the development of obesity, such as using liquefied petroleum gas (LPG) for cooking purpose, washing machines for washing clothes, vacuum cleaners for cleaning purpose, elevators, escalators and automatic door. Watching TV, using vehicles for traveling short distances rather than going by walk or cycling, etc. are other factors. The relative risk data of various health hazards associated with obesity are enumerated in Table 38.3.

Table 38.3: Relative risk (RR) of health problems associated with obesity

Greatly increased	Moderately increased	Slightly increased
RR > 3	RR 2–3	RR 1–2
Non-insulin-dependent diabetes mellitus (NIDDM)*	Coronary heart disease	Cancer*
Gallbladder Disease*	Hypertension*	Impaired fertility
Dyslipidemia	Osteoarthritis	Low back pain
Insulin resistance	Hyperuricemia and gout	Fetal defects associated with maternal obesity, breathlessness and sleep apnea

*Life-threatening chronic health problems; others are nonfatal, but debilitating health problems.

PREVENTION AND CONTROL MEASURES

It is difficult or not possible to control obesity, caused by non-modifiable factors such as age, sex or genetic factors. The preventive measures should start early in childhood, because once obesity is developed, it is difficult to treat and the health consequences associated with obesity may not be fully reversible by weight loss.

Aims

- To maintain BMI between 18 and 25 throughout the adulthood
- To prevent the development of overweight
- To prevent the progression of overweight to obesity
- To prevent regain of weight among those obese patients, who have already lost some weight.

Strategies

Diet and Prevention of Risk for Disease

Fat-rich diet is associated with risk for coronary artery disease and a variety of cancer (e.g. colon, rectum, breast, prostate, etc.). Similarly, a low fiber diet is associated with GI tract disorder and risk for cancer. The American Cancer Society (ACS) recommends that low fat and high fiber diet rich in fruits and vegetables reduce the risk for cancer and other health problems. To maintain a good health, the person should choose items from plant sources rather than animal source, eat frequently (four to five times) rather than a large meal, use whole grains and reduce consumption of meat and meat products.

For clients who are at increased risk of coronary artery disease due to identifiable and modifiable risk factors, such as borderline or elevated serum cholesterol levels, the National Cholesterol Education Panel recommends dietary intervention (Table 38.4). If diet modification is not successful, then patient/client may be referred to a dietician.

Table 38.4: Risk stratification and diet modification*

Nutrient	Recommended intake
Total calories (energy)	Balance energy intake and expenditure to maintain a desirable body weight and prevent weight gain; daily energy expenditure of moderate physical exercise (e.g. about 200 kcal/day) may be included
Saturated fat†	< 7% of total calories
Polyunsaturated	Up to 10% of total calories
Monounsaturated fat	Up to 20% of total calories
Total fat	25–35% of total calories
‡Carbohydrate	50–60%
Fiber	20–30 g/day
Protein	About 15% of total calories
Cholesterol	< 200 g/day

*From 3rd Report of the Expert Panel on detection, evaluation and treatment of high-blood cholesterol in adult (adult treatment panel III);
†Saturated fat (trans fatty acids) raise LDL, hence to be kept low;
‡Carbohydrate should be mainly derived from food rich in complex carbohydrate (whole grain, fruits and vegetables).

Dietary changes

Refrain from overconsumption of fats and carbohydrates:
- Diet should contain suitable proportion of cereals, legumes and vegetables, fiber content should be increased
- Food energy intake should not be greater than what is necessary for energy expenditure.

Healthy Physical Activity

To remain active, one has to perform physical activity. People who remain active throughout life, live longer than their inactive or less active counterparts. Physical activity is a therapeutic boon to healthy life. On the other hand, physical inactivity or sedentary lifestyle is a serious health problem and gives birth to many diseases such as hypertension, metabolic syndrome, type 2 DM and coronary artery disease. The most common cause of obesity is physical inactivity. More than 60% obese adults do not achieve the recommended level of regular physical exercise, while 40% adult obese do not find time to perform activity due to the busy life schedule.

Advantages of physical exercise
1. It reduces weight and reshapes the body (Fig. 38.2).
2. It reduces weight and helps to maintain the weight.
3. Improves mood and relieves depression.
4. It improves lipid profile, decreases low-density lipoprotein (LDL) (bad cholesterol) and increases high-density lipoprotein (HDL) (good cholesterol).
5. Improves sense of well-being and longevity as well as quality of life.
6. Improves joint mobility and increases bone mass.
7. It increases stamina and muscle strength.

Keeping these benefits in mind, the nurse should encourage the clients to take physical activity so as to reduce the population of obese persons.

Management of physical inactivity
Current recommendation to maintain weight for every adult is to engage for 45–60 minutes in moderate exercise every day. Persons who are fit and engaged in high intensity activity, can achieve health benefits within 30 minutes of high-level activity on most of the days in a week. To the beginners, simple walking is a good initial activity that requires no equipment and can be performed anywhere. Care providers or nurses can advise this level of activity to every client they encounter, should ensure them that they can derive health benefits through modest amount of daily physical activity/exercise.

Assessment of client for exercise
Before advising the client for any physical exercise, one must assess the client's current physical activity pattern. Two effective tools are—the 24-hour recall and a 3-day activity schedule. The 24-hour recall identifies the form of activities performed during that day. The nurse must focus attention to find out time spent in moderate or heavy exercise per day.

While making recommendations for physical exercise, the nurse must consider benefits and risks involved. Before starting an activity program, all clients must be screened for risk that contraindicate the unsupervised activity. All patients with known cardiac risk factors (e.g. hypertension, diabetes, hyperlipidemia, cigarette smoking family history of early heart attack) must be evaluated for exercise/activity tolerance.

Activity Program Advice (Intervention)

In clients with no evident risks, chart out a plan for physical activity. The activity plan chart/pyramid is an excellent tool to begin with exercise/activity program. The activity pyramid or chart is a pictorial representation of principles of healthy activity (Fig. 38.3). The minimum goal for an exercise program is moderate activity (intensity) performed at least for 60 minutes (duration), most of the days in a week (frequency). Many activities performed by the client during daily routine work can be used as mode of physical activity program (Box 38.1).

Box 38.1: Moderate physical activity program

Activities around the house
• Washing the floor
• Climbing the stairs
• Washing or waxing the car
• Digging and weeding in the garden
• Walking or running with children
• Washing the clothes
Sports and leisure activities
• Playing volleyball or basketball
• Fast dancing
• Cycling
• Swimming

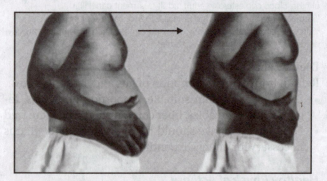

Figure 38.2: Health promotion; reshape the body with diet and physical exercise, and reduce cardiovascular and all mortality risks.

To make the activity program successful, seek social support within community as well as within client's circle. Simple strategies can increase the likelihood of success in implementing activity program, such as advising the client

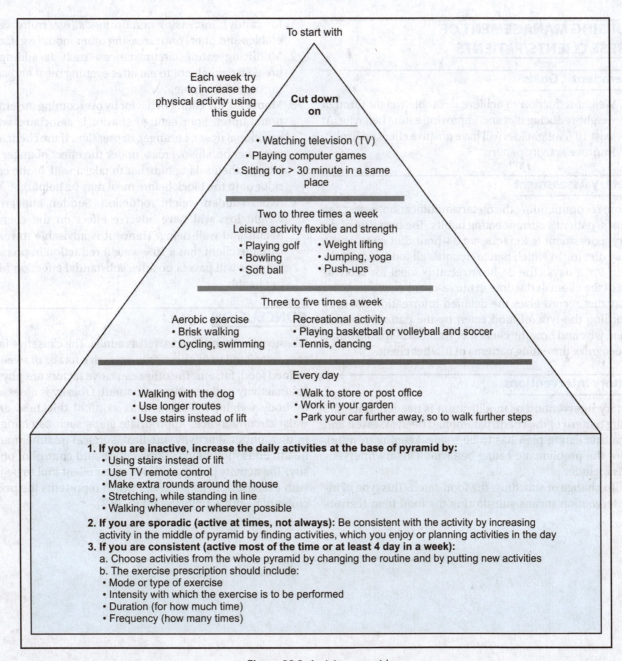

Figure 38.3: Activity pyramid

to increase the time spent in moderate activities, asking the client to incorporate pleasurable activities into current routine and encourage the client to identify the friends or family members who can support him/her by joining the activity program.

Physical activity
Regular physical activity helps in increasing the energy expenditure. So, sedentary lifestyle should be discouraged. Leisure pursuits such as gardening, dancing, cycling and swimming should be encouraged. Walking should be preferred to other means. Exercises should be encouraged; yoga exercises should also be encouraged.

Health education
People are educated about hazards of obesity and its prevention by healthy diet and lifestyle, to be promoted from early age.

NURSING MANAGEMENT OF OBESE CLIENTS/PATIENTS

Therapeutic Goals

1. Weight reduction to achieve desirable weight through weight-reducing diet and improving eating behavior. At least 10% weight loss will have positive effect on health.
2. Improve activity pattern.

Dietary Assessment

Before recommending the dietary modification, assess the client's/patient's current eating habits. The best way of dietary assessment is to request a 24-hour diet chart and a 3-day diet log in which patient records all food and drinks taken for 3 days. The 24-hour recall is ideal for motivation of the client at the time of nurse-client encounter. The 3-day diet record gives the detailed information not only regarding the type of food eaten by the patient but also when, why and how the client ate. This tool helps the nurse to recognize the eating patterns of his/her client.

Dietary Interventions

Dietary intervention or modification is needed, once the eating pattern of the client/patient had been assessed and a realistic eating plan has to be made, keeping in mind, about the problematic eating behavior. Dietary interventions include:

1. To change or substitute the food eaten. This type of intervention means substituting the food item (carrots for candy), increasing certain foods (e.g. fruits, vegetables and fiber) or decreasing other foods (e.g. fats).
2. Modifying eating circumstances, such as adding a breakfast, meal, not to eat after evening meal and eating only at the table.
3. Modifying the eating behavior by overcoming the emotional upset. Poor eating behavior is associated with emotional upset, i.e. anger, depression. If the client admits that he/she overeats under the effect of anger or fatigue, then asking him/her to take a walk in the corridor or in the block before meal may be helpful.
4. Avoid sudden weight reduction. Sudden and great weight loss will have adverse effect on the client's health and well-being. Hence it is advisable to reassure the client that a 10% weight reduction in phased manner will have a positive substantial effect on his/her health.

CONCLUSION

Obesity affects children as well as adults. The causative factors associated with obesity are excessive intake of sweets, refined food, fat, etc. The other causative factors are physical inactivity and genetic component. Obesity is assessed by body weight, waist/hip ratio, skinfold thickness and waist circumference. Appropriate steps such as changes in diet, physical activity, medical, surgical treatment and health education helps in prevention and control of obesity. The activity plan pyramid is an excellent tool to begin with exercise activity program, which represents the principles of health activity (refer Fig. 38.3).

Cardiovascular Diseases

CHAPTER 39

INTRODUCTION

Survival, growth, reproduction and productivity of the human organism depend upon a balance between movement of nutrients to the cells and of wastes away from the cells. In health, this is accomplished by the efficient functioning of the three factors—a pump (heart), a circulatory circuit and a fluid medium (blood).

Diseases or structural alterations in any of these three may hinder the transport system and ultimately affect the survival of the organism, and thus causes many of the cardiac diseases. More people are affected directly or indirectly by cardiac diseases than by any other single disease. Deaths caused by cardiac disease vary with age. Congenital, malformations of the heart and closely related vascular system are the causes, over 90% of the deaths. From these causes, children in 5 years of age and of more than one third of people of 5–24 years get affected.

CLASSIFICATION OF HEART DISEASES

1. Congenital heart disease (CHD): The heart diseases follow an abnormality of structure caused by error in fetal development.
2. Acquired heart disease: These diseases may affect the heart either suddenly or gradually.

Congenital Heart Disease

Congenital heart diseases are of two types cyanotic and acyanotic.

Cyanotic Heart Diseases

Tetralogy of Fallot
Tetralogy of Fallot consists of four defects:
1. Ventricular septal defect.
2. Pulmonary stenosis.
3. Right ventricular hypertrophy.
4. Overriding of aorta.

This combination produces cyanosis in infant who is often referred to as a 'blue baby'.

Transposition of great vessels
In transposition of the great vessels, the aorta arises from the right ventricle instead of the left and blood is pumped back into circulation without having received oxygen from the lungs.

Tricuspid atresia
In case, complete congenital atresia of the tricuspid valve is present, there is no ductal communication between the right atrium and the right ventricle. The right atrial blood is shunted through a foramen ovale or an atrial defect into the left atrium, where it is mixed with pulmonary venous blood.

Acyanotic Heart Disease

Coarctation of aorta
Coarctation of aorta is a localized structure just below the origin of the left subclavian artery blood pressure (BP) in blood vessels above the constriction to become lower than the pressure above the commissures of aortic valve, which obstruct the flow of blood from left ventricles.

Intra-atrial septal defect
The foramen ovale or normal opening in the atrial septum, fails to close shortly after birth as it should and blood returning from the lungs to left atrium shunts over to the right atrium.

Intraventricular septal defect
Intraventricular septal is an abnormal opening between the right and left ventricles; blood is shunted into the right ventricle and circulated through the pulmonary artery and lungs.

Pulmonary stenosis

Pulmonary stenosis is the narrowing of pulmonary valve, which decreases the amount of blood flowing into the lungs.

Patent ducts arteriosus

In patent ducts arteriosus, the blood vessels does not remain patent (open) resulting in regular transmission of blood between two of the most important arteries close to the heart and aorta.

Prevention

Heart disease can be prevented in many people and many of them who have heart disease, can be helped to live happy, useful and long lives:

1. Immunization against acute infectious diseases such as diphtheria, scarlet fever and measles, and control of infection through selective antibiotics to decrease the incidence of infectious complications.
2. Immune serum globulin (ISG) for women with the first trimester of pregnancy who have been exposed to German measles in an effort to prevent coronary heart disease (CHD) or other malformation of their babies.
3. Children are the major source of rubella infection in the community. The best method for preventing rubella in pregnant women is to vaccinate children; this decreases the incidence of German measles among pregnant women and thus reduce congenital anomalies.

Acquired Heart Diseases

Pericarditis

Pericarditis is an inflammatory process of the pericardium, characterized by fever, chills and fatigue. More common in children of both sexes. Acute pericarditis may be caused by viral or bacterial infection. Prevention is best achieved by avoiding infection with proper antibiotics.

Treatment: Surgical drainage of the pericardial fluid may be necessary.

Myocarditis

Myocarditis is an inflammatory disease of the myocardium, which may occur with a wide variety of systemic disease. Causative organisms are virus and bacteria. Clinical features involve antibiotics and corticosteroids, and management of the arrhythmias to prevent heart failure and cardiogenic shock.

Subacute Bacterial Endocarditis

The endocarditis is a serious complication of heart disease. Organisms in the bloodstream invade the heart. The valves are most often involved, being covered with vegetations or product of bacterial degenerations. Causative organism is *Streptococcus* and predisposing causes are diseased teeth and gums. It affects males of all ages. Clinical features include fever with malaise, petechiae in the conjunctiva, mouth, legs and fingers, and clubbed fingers. Complication may lead to heart failure. Prevention involves a strict oral hygiene before and after the tooth extraction. Patient can be treated with massive doses of penicillin.

Rheumatic Fever and Rheumatic Heart Disease

Rheumatic fever (RF) and rheumatic heart disease (RHD) is a problem in all parts of the world especially in the developing countries. The reported prevalence rates in school age children in various parts of the world range from very low to high as 33 cases per 1,000. The incidence of RF and the prevalence of mortality from RHD have fallen during the last two decades. Acute RHD is an acute inflammatory reaction. It may involve:

1. Lining of the heart or endocardium including valves.
2. Muscle of the heart or myocardium.
3. Outer covering of the heart or pericardium.

Males of urban areas of low economic families suffer most in the age group of 8–10 years. Causative organisms are group A *Streptococcus* bacteria. Clinical features include anorexia, fever, weight loss, weakness, skin changes, fatigue and joint involvement.

Treatment involves administration of salicylate, avoidance of athletics and bedrest. Advice to do salt gargle to avoid sore throat and injection penicillin to be given, and smoking has to be in control. Advice patient to take regular treatment without fail.

Mitral Stenosis

Mitral valve is an important landmark in the history of echocardiography. Mitral valve echo is the earliest to be recorded and recognized due to the characteristic pattern of motion. First, it has been described the typical findings in mitral stenosis and subsequently various co-workers contributed a lot on this subject. Following repeated attacks of RF, rheumatic nodules grow on the mitral valve at the line where the valves meet. The valves thicken and fuse together. Causative organism involves is *Streptococcus* as the disease is an extension of RF. It affects people of the age group of 30–50 years.

Clinical features are dyspnea, orthopnea, pulmonary edema and hemoptysis. Prevention involves in decreasing the cardiac workload and treating infection, low sodium, and calcium intake. Treatment with digitalis and diuretics along with surgical treatment in the form of mitral commissurotomy and valvotomy complications are atrial fibrillation, subacute endocarditis and thrombi formation. As a follow-up measure educate the patient to observe any sign and symptom of mitral stenosis; to attend the clinic immediately and advice to adhere to low calcium and salt intake.

Ischemic Heart Disease

Ischemic heart disease (IHD) is the most widespread health problem in the west and an important problem in our country. In USA, more than 675,000 people die each year from arteriosclerotic coronary artery disease and an additional 1.3 million sustain a non-fatal myocardial infarction. The death rate of IHD has not been sufficiently influenced for the last few years despite various attempts. Coronary heart disease is caused by a narrowing or obstruction of the coronary arteries, resulting in a reduction of blood supply to the myocardium. The causes of IHDs are hypertension (HTN), increasing in the level of blood lumen, cholesterol, diabetes, obesity, smoking and sedentary lifestyle.

Clinical features

Temporary anoxia of myocardium, obstruction of coronary arteries, angina pectoris and myocardial infarction. Complications include congestive cardiac failure, arrhythmias and death.

Prevention

The nurse has real responsibility to contribute to the prevention of coronary artery diseases by general health education to the people. Education to the people about good health practices regarding diet, exercise and not to smoke.

ANGINA PECTORIS

Heberden provided the classic and widely quoted description of angina pectoris, but made no mention of the associated hemodynamic alterations. Bruston and Morgon first reported clinically observable hemodynamic changes accompanying spontaneous angina pectoris. In United States 600,000 people die of angina pectoris. It is a serious cardiac disorder, caused by atherosclerosis of the coronary vessels in people usually above 40–45 years of age. Males are more prone. Causes include hypertension, diabetes, thromboangiitis obliterans, polycythemia vera and periarteritis nodosa.

Clinical Features

Substernal pain often radiating down the inner aspect of the left arm. Pain is often associated with exertion and is relieved through vasodilation of the coronary arteries by means of medication or by rest. Complications include myocardial infarction and cardiac standstill follow-up.

Prevention

1. If the attacks of angina pain are precipitated by eating, six small meals taken at evenly-spaced intervals, rather than three average meals may give relief. If the patient is overweight a low-caloric diet may be prescribed and low-fat diet to be given. Advice not to smoke.
2. Patients with angina pectoris can tolerate mild exercises, such as walking and playing golf. But they should avoid running, climbing hills or stairs rapidly and lifting heavy objects, which cause pain.
3. Since the pain is more evoked in cold weather, they should not be exposed to the cold and walking against the wind.
4. Advice not to get excited.

Treatment

Nitroglycerin tablets placed under the tongue and allowed to dissolve in the saliva often relieve the pain by causing vasodilation of the coronary artery.

Follow-up

1. Explain the avoidance of nosocomial infection.
2. Strictly instruct the patient to follow instructions after discharge.
3. Continuity of rest, drugs, diet and any sign of discomfort is reported at once, irrespective of the date given for attending regular follow-up care.
4. Inform the patient about the factors, which contribute to further complications, e.g. obesity, highly-saturated fat and cholesterol, low sodium and sedentary lifestyle.

CARDIAC ARRHYTHMIAS

Cardiac arrhythmias of whatever cause influence the performance and the metabolic efficiency of the heart, and almost always for the worse. Many arrhythmias only have a depressant effect on myocardial function. Cardiac arrhythmias are the result of disturbance in the conduction of electrical impulses within the heart. Predisposing causes are anemia, pulmonary tuberculosis, RF, hyperthyroidism, myocardial infarction, congestive heart failure, etc.

Clinical Features

Arrhythmias do not cause any symptoms, but they are noticeable to the patient, who presents for sensation, flutter fusing over, pounding, palpitation and skipping of the heart.

Prevention

1. Immediate resuscitation may be maintained until the dysrhythmias have been corrected.
2. Steps should be taken to minimize the risk of accidental poisoning, particularly in young children and of deliberate self-poisoning, particularly seen in patients with a psychiatric illness.
3. It is also recommended that patients receiving cardioactive medication should be given a full explanation of potential changes.
4. Arrhythmia's causes are identified and instructions given to them, and to their families, friends and colleagues on the necessity of summoning immediate help in a potential emergency situation.

Treatment

Cardiac resuscitation by intravenous (IV) fluids, oxygen inhalation, injection. Epinephrine and sodium bicarbonate.

Follow-up

- Ask the patient to withhold the digitalis
- Advice to take rest
- Advice to take low-saturated diet
- Ask them to attend the clinic regularly.

CONGESTIVE HEART FAILURE

Heart failure is a state in which the cardiac output is inadequate to meet the peripheral needs of the body. Failure may occur when there is inadequate ventricular filling. In this state, the heart will initially try to compensate with an increased rate, dilation and hypertrophy, when this fails the blood supply becomes inadequate and decomposition exists. The congestive heart failure is often classified according to the side of the heart at fault that is left sided or right sided.

Clinical Features

1. Edema and dyspnea: In excessive amount of fluid in the extracellular tissue and body cavities, are common symptoms of congestive failure. It may occur in the legs, liver, abdominal cavity and lungs, plural spaces or other parts of the body. As edema becomes more pronounced, it progresses up the legs into the thighs, external genitalia and lower trunk. If the tissues become too engendered, the skin may crack and fluid may 'weep' from the tissue.
2. Ascites.
3. Pulmonary edema and plural effusion.
4. Hyperpnea.
5. Fatigue.

Prevention

1. The prevention of heart failure and pulmonary edema will depend on the detection and adequate treatment of HTN.
2. While awaiting for drugs we can use the rotating tourniquet. This may be applied to limbs to reduce venous return to the heart, while awaiting the full effect of drug therapy.
3. Well-ventilated place to be provided.
4. In severe cases physical activity should be restricted.
5. During acute stages the diet should be soft and liquid.

Treatment

1. Provide rest to the patient.
2. Checking patient's daily.
3. Administration of sedation, if needed.
4. The nurse should be guided by the patient's habit patterns and his/her symptoms in finding a position. Head of the bed should be elevated in a high Fowler's position. A pillow may be placed lengthwise behind the shoulder and back that provides proper and comfortable position to the patient.
5. Provide oxygen inhalation.
6. Activity: Some patient's are not even permitted to turn or to feed themselves and bathe themselves, special attention to be given to the back and body prominence.
7. Self-care: Provide personal care, massage the bony prominence in circular movement, nurse should have a careful watch on elbows and sacrum. Lubricant should be applied to the skin since irritation often occurs. Right plastic waterproof material should be used for protecting the matters.
8. Nutrition: During acute stage, soft and liquid diet to be given. Resuscitation of sodium intake and supplemented with vitamins.
9. Elimination: During the acute stage, one should not strain, while passing motion so it should be soft, provide privacy to pass stool. Administer milk of magnesia.
10. Ambulation: The usual procedure for ambulation is to have the patient dangle his/her legs from the side of the bed for 15 minutes twice a day; and gradually according to the condition of the patient, the movements to be increased.

CHAPTER 39 — Cardiovascular Diseases

11. Digitalization to be administered such as digoxin, lanatoside, deslanoside and digoxin.
12. Diuretics should be administered, which reduces the pulmonary edema.

Follow-up

1. Educate the patient and his/her family about the nature of disease process treatment.
2. Teach the patient to observe signs and symptoms of recurrence, and to inform doctor immediately.
3. Explain the patient, about the importance of medication in controlling the disease.
4. Advice patient not to change the brand of digitalis, which he/she is taking.
5. Ask the patient to take medicine in proper time.
6. Teach the patient to record his/her pulse rate.
7. Advise to keep a check on weight of himself/herself daily.
8. Advise to take oral potassium dilated with juice and taken after a meal.
9. Advise to take in diet low sodium.
10. Advise not to expose to extreme heat or cold, it increases heart activity.
11. Ask to avoid excessive eating and drinking.
12. Advise to stop smoking and taking alcohol.
13. Advise to avoid sexual activity when usual fatigue.
14. Advise to attend the clinics regularly.

CORONARY ARTERY DISEASE

Coronary artery disease (CAD) is the impairment of the function of heart due to inadequate blood flow to the myocardium, as a result of obstruction in the coronary circulation. It is manifested in any of the following forms:
- Angina pectoris of effort
- Myocardial infarction
- Irregularities of the heart
- Cardiac failure
- Cardiac arrest.

Coronary artery disease is the leading cause of death in all the developed countries, accounting for 25–30% of total deaths. In developing countries such as India, there has been an increasing trend in the incidence of CAD because of changes in the lifestyle and behavior pattern of the people; it is so important that CAD counts for nearly 15% of all deaths. Therefore, CAD is considered as 'modem epidemic'. This trend is increasing in India.

The incidence is two to three times greater in urban areas than rural areas. It is one and half times more among men than among women. Incidence is maximum in the age group of 50–60 years.

The CAD is a local manifestation of progressive and generalized disorder of the arteries, namely atherosclerosis. The disease is produced from the blockage of the lumen of the coronary arteries. A plaque is formed inside the arteries, which gradually grows to form a thrombus that fills up the lumen and causes obstruction to the flow of blood.

Predisposing Factors

There are many factors associated with CAD. They are grouped into nonmodifiable and modifiable risk factors, which includes the following:

1. Age: Incidence of CAD is high above 50 years and maximum between 50 and 60 years of age.
2. Sex: It is more among men than women.
3. Family history: The CAD has been seen to run in the families.
4. Genetic factors: It plays a role indirectly by determining the total cholesterol and low-density lipoprotein (LDL) level.
5. Cigarette smoking: This has been considered as a major risk factor, because of the following mechanisms involved:
    a. Carbon monoxide, induces atherosclerosis.
    b. Nicotine stimulates the release of adrenaline resulting in HTN.
    c. Nicotine also increases myocardial oxygen demand and decreases high-density lipoprotein (HDL) level.

    The risk of developing CAD is directly proportional to the number of cigarettes smoking per day and the duration of exposure (i.e. earlier the smoking is started, greater is the risk). Smoking acts not only independently, but also synergistically with other factors such as HTN and elevated serum cholesterol. The risk however comes down once smoking is given up, but after a few years.
6. Hypertension: It increases the risk of CAD by accelerating the atherosclerotic process.
7. Serum cholesterol: It is proved beyond doubt that increases in serum cholesterol level increases the risk of CAD. The threshold level is 220 mg/dL beyond, which the risk increases. The risk increases progressively with higher levels of LDL cholesterol. On the other hand, very low density lipoprotein (VLDL) cholesterol is associated with the atherosclerosis of peripheral vessels resulting in intermittent claudication rather than CAD.

However, the risk of CAD decreases with higher levels of HDL cholesterol. The ratio of LDL to HDL more than five indicates the risk.

Recent studies indicate that the level of plasma apolipoprotein A-1 (a fraction of HDL protein) and apolipoprotein B (a fraction of LDL protein) are better predictors of CAD than HDL and LDL cholesterol respectively. Thus, apolipoproteins are replacing lipoproteins.

8. Serum homocysteine: High serum levels of this amino acid more than 15.5 mol/L, damages the intima of the arteries, thus correlating positively with the presence of CAD. Such levels are related to a diet low in pyridoxine and folates.
9. Diabetes mellitus: The risk of CAD is two to three times higher among diabetics than among nondiabetics.
10. Obesity: It increases the risk of CAD because of its association with LDL cholesterol level, HTN and diabetes.
11. Exercise: Regular physical exercise increases the concentration of HDL, a protective factor and decrease both body weight (obesity) and BP, which are beneficial to cardiovascular health.
12. Hormones: Hyperestrogenemia favors the development of CAD. Women on oral contraceptives are more to develop CAD than those not using them.
13. Type A personality: Such people with type A behavior are characterized by competitive drive, restlessness, impatience, irritability, short temper, sense of urgency, overthinking, etc. are at a higher risk of CAD than the calmer type B personality people.
14. Alcohol: The CAD is common in heavy drinkers.
15. Soft water: Incidence of CAD has been found to be higher among those consuming soft water than those consuming hard water. The salts in the latter are protective to the cardiac muscle.
16. Noise: Chronic exposure to noise over 110 dB increases serum cholesterol level and thus the risk of CAD.
17. Drugs: Misuse of fenfluramine and phentermine used for reduction of weight can also be damaging to the heart.

Prevention

Primary Prevention

Primary prevention consists of elimination or modification of 'risk factors' of disease with the following approaches:
- Population strategy
- High-risk strategy.

Population strategy (mass primary prevention)
Population strategy is directed towards the whole population focusing mainly on the control of underlying risk factors, irrespective of individual risk levels. This is based on the principle that a small reduction in the BP or serum cholesterol level in a population would go a long way in reducing the incidence of CAD. This requires a large community-wide efforts to alter the lifestyle practices, as given below.

Dietary changes
- Consumption of saturated fats should be less than 10% of total energy intake
- The average intake of cholesterol should be less than 300 mg/day for adult
- Serum cholesterol level should be less than 200 mg/dL
- Consumption of carbohydrates must be proportionately increased
- Smoking changes
- Goal is to achieve 'smoke-free' society and many countries are at it. To achieve this, it requires educational activities, legislative measures and other programs.

Blood pressure
Studies have shown that a small reduction in the BP in the population would produce a large reduction in the incidence of CAD. This involves a multifactorial approach based on prudent diet (reduced salt intake and avoidance of high alcohol intake), regular physical activity and control of weight.

Physical activity
Regular physical exercise will go a long way in preventing obesity, HTN and thus indirectly CAD.

High-risk strategy
High-risk strategy consists of identifying the 'at-risk' group of people for CAD and providing preventive care. The at-risk, or high-risk group of individuals can be identified by simple screening tests, such as recording BP estimation of serum cholesterol, history of smoking, strong family history of CAD and history of taking oral pills among women, and estimation of fasting blood sugar to detect diabetics.

Having identified such high-risk people, preventive care is taken by motivating them to take action against the risk factors individuals with HTN are given treatment, smokers to give up smoking, people with hyperlipidemia are treated. Sometimes this strategy will not help, for instance the treatment of hypertension does not reduce the risk of CAD.

Primordial Prevention

Primordial prevention consists of prevention of the emergence or development of risk factors among the population groups, in whom they have not yet appeared. Since, many adult health problems such as HTN, obesity have their early origins in childhood. Efforts are directed towards discouraging the children from adapting harmful lifestyle such as smoking, eating pattern, physical exercise, alcoholism, etc. The main intervention is through mass education.

Secondary Prevention

Secondary prevention is the action, which stops the progress of the disease in its early stage and prevents complications. With reference to CAD, this consists of prevention of recurrence of CAD by cessation of exposure to risk factors as mentioned in high-risk strategy, e.g. giving up smoking after an attack of myocardial infarction followed by bypass surgery, prompt treatment with antihypertensive after detecting HTN, similarly starting antidiabetic drugs after detection of diabetes mellitus, etc.

CONGENITAL HEART DISEASES

Congenital heart disease is a defect in the structure and function of the heart, developed during fetal growth, present at birth, often detected during later life. These malformations occur as a result of a complex interaction between genetic and environmental system. The CHD constitute an important cause of infant morbidity and mortality. The prevalence of CHD is estimated to be about 5–9/1,000 children below 10 years.

Congenital heart diseases are grouped into acyanotic and cyanotic heart diseases:

1. Acyanotic heart diseases (left-to-right shunt):
   - Atrial septal defect (ASD)
   - Ventricular septal defect (VSD)
   - Patent ductus arteriosus (PDA)
   - Persistent truncus arteriosus
   - Acyanotic heart diseases without a shunt:
     - Congenital aortic stenosis
     - Coarctation of aorta
     - Congenital aortic incompetence; mitral incompetence.
2. Cyanotic heart diseases (right-to-left shunt):
   - Tetralogy of Fallot
   - Complete transposition of great arteries
   - Tricuspid atresia
   - Coarctation of aorta
   - Ventricular septal defect with reversed shunt (Eisenmenger's complex)
   - Patent ductus defect with reversed shunt
   - Atrial septal defect with reversed shunt.

A child with CHD is suspected, if there is history or apnea, growth failure and repeated attacks of respiratory infections. The child is physically retarded and often cyanotic. Cardiac murmurs are common. Anomalies of other organs in the body may coexist.

The etiology of CHD is multifactorial. The intrinsic agents are chromosomal aberration, defects of T lymphocytes, systemic lupus erythematosus. The external agents are rubella virus, X-ray, alcohol and drugs acting on women during pregnancy. Often CHD occur themselves or be a part of syndrome such as Down syndrome, Trisomy 13 syndrome, Turner's syndrome, Marfan syndrome, etc.

Other determinants (influencing factors) are altitude at birth, prematurity, maternal age, sex of the child, consanguineous marriage as detailed below:

1. Altitude at birth: Persistence of the ductus arteriosus is six times more frequent among the children born at high altitudes than those born at sea level.
2. Prematurity: The VSD and PDA are relatively common among premature infants; maternal age, late maternal age seems to increase the risk of Fallot's tetralogy.
3. Sex of the child: The bicuspid aortic valve is predominantly a male disease:
   - Aortic atresia is almost exclusively a disease of male infants
   - The PDA and ostium secundum, atrial septal defect are higher among females
   - Congenital aneurysm of sinus of Valsalva carry a male-to-female ratio of 4:1.

Prevention

About 90% of CHD, the cause is not known clearly. Therefore, prevention is possible only in about 10% of cases by the following measures:

1. Health education: People are educated to avoid consanguineous marriages. Women are advised not to postpone marriages and first pregnancy beyond 30 years. Pregnant women are advised to avoid infections, alcohol, smoking, X-ray, drugs and chemicals. They should consume only iodized salt. Diabetic women should keep the disease under control during pregnancy.
2. Rubella vaccine to be given to all potential mothers before becoming pregnant.
3. Genetic counseling is offered to the parents who have given birth to a child suffering from CHD.
4. Detected cases of CHD are referred to pediatric surgeons for the corrections by surgery, if any.
5. Efficient antenatal care to be taken to prevent the prematurity.
6. Deliveries at high altitudes are avoided.

RHEUMATIC HEART DISEASE

Rheumatic heart disease (RDH) is the ultimate, sequelae and crippling stage of RF, which in turn is the result of streptococcal pharyngitis. Rheumatic fever is an acute febrile disease, affecting the connective tissues particularly in the heart and joints, which occurs following the infection of throat (pharynx) by group A β-hemolytic streptococci. Thus, although RF is a non-communicable disease, it results from communicable pharyngitis.

The RDH is a major public health problem in India. About 20% of all sore throats among children are due to streptococcal infection and of these about 2% results in rheumatic fever (RF). Almost 80% of those who get RF, end up with RHD. Thus, RHD is the commonest and most widely prevalent heart disease (30–50% of all cardiac cases) among children in India. Its prevalence is about 611,000 among children in the age group of 5–15 years. In absolute numbers, about 6 million children in India are suffering from RHD. It is responsible for about 30% of all cardiovascular deaths.

It is estimated that about 2–3 lakh of the overall population in the country, including people of all the age group and both the sexes are suffering from RHD.

In the last two decades, the incidence of RF fever and the prevalence of RHD have fallen remarkably as the living conditions improved, indicating relation between the prevalence of the disease, and the socioeconomic factors. Thus, it indicates that RHD is one of the most readily preventable chronic disease.

Epidemiological Features

Agent Factor

Agent: An RHD is the late sequel of RF, which in turn is the result of the infection of tonsils, pharynx, adenoids, etc. caused by group A β-hemolytic streptococci (also called *Streptococcus pyogenes*) particularly of the serotype 'M type 5' has been incriminated as the causative agent, because of its rheumatogenic potential. They are gram positive, nonmotile, non-spore forming, spherical bacilli, 0.5–1.0 m in diameter arranged in the form of chains.

They are called hemolytic streptococci because they cause lysis of red blood cells (RBCs) due to the presence of a heat-stable toxin called 'streptolysin O.' They also have a heat labile mildly antigenic toxin called 'streptolysin-S.'

Because of the presence of many strains of the streptococcal to cocci, it has not been possible to prepare an effective vaccine.

Reservoir of infection: All the cases and the carriers of streptococcal pharyngitis are the reservoirs. Among the carriers, both temporary and chronic carrier state occurs. Cases of streptococcal pharyngitis are at a greater risk of developing RF than the carriers.

Host Factor

Age incidence: Incidence is maximum among school children in the age group of 5–15.

Sex incidence: It is equal in both the sexes.

Immunity: There has been an immunological basis for the development of RF and RHD. According to toxic immunological hypothesis, the streptococci have certain toxic products leading to immunological process, resulting in RF.

Another concept is that it requires repeated exposure to precipitate the illness. Another belief is that RHD is an autoimmune disease.

Predisposing Factors

The RF and RHD is considered as 'social disease' because many social factors are responsible for the prevalence of this disease, such as poverty, poor housing, undernutrition, illiteracy, ignorance, large families, overcrowding, etc. This disease is therefore common among slum dwellers and inmates of barracks. Prevalence declines sharply as the standard of living improves.

Pathogenesis

Aschoff nodule is the pathognomonic sign of RF. The nodule is a perivascular aggregate of lymphocytes and plasma cells surrounding a fibrinoid core.

So, the basic disease process is that of an inflammatory vasculitis. In the heart, mitral valvulitis is the most common lesion. Later, as the fibrosis of valve takes place results in mitral stenosis and incompetence.

Clinical Features

Fever: Usually low-grade fever lasts for about 3 months.

Polyarthritis: This occurs in 80–90% of the cases. The arthritis is asymmetrical, migratory and non-deforming type. Large joints such as knees, ankles, elbows and wrists are affected. Rarely, smaller joints of hands and feet are affected. There will be painful swelling of these joints, which later subside spontaneously after about 1 week. There is no residual damage to the joints. The movements of the affected joints are limited because of the pain. As it subsides, it appears in another joint (migratory).

Carditis: Heart is affected in 60–70% of the cases of RF. All layers of the heart such as pericardium, myocardium and valves are affected. The damage is permanent. The manifestations are tachycardia, cardiomegaly, pericarditis and heart failure. The common cardiac murmur indicating the involvement of mitral valve is soft, mid-diastolic murmur called Carey Coombs' murmur. The most common electrocardiography (ECG) finding is prolonged PR interval and first-degree atrioventricular (AV) block. Thus in RF the organisms 'lick the joints and bite the heart' involvement of the heart is the last stage of RF.

Subcutaneous nodules: These are round, firm and painless nodules appearing below the skin, over the bony prominences such as occiput, elbow, ankle or wrist joints, about 4 weeks after the onset of RF. The skin over the nodules moves freely and is not inflamed. The nodules last for a variable period of time and then disappear, leaving no residual damage. This is also called 'erythema nodosum.'

Chorea: This is a late manifestation occurring due to involvement of brain, which can occur alone or with carditis, characterized by purposeless, abnormal, jerky movements of arms often associated with muscular weakness and/or behavioral abnormalities. It is seen in about 10% of cases. It disappears gradually leaving no residual damage.

Erythema marginatum: It is a nonpruritic, pink-colored skin rashes, appearing in about 5% of the cases of RF. They appear for a transient period of time over the trunk and extremities, but never on the face, the center being pale and margin being serpiginous, and they blanch on pressure. They disappear later without any damage.

Thus, except carditis all other manifestations of RF do not cause permanent damage. According to Duckett Jones I, the clinical feature of RF are grouped into major and minor manifestations:
1. Major manifestations includes carditis, polyarthritis, chorea, erythema nodosum (nodules) and erythema marginatum.
2. Minor manifestations includes fever, polyarthralgia, past history of RF raised erythrocyte sedimentation rate (ESR), leukocytosis and raised C-reactive protein.

Diagnosis

The World Health Organization (WHO) criteria (2002–2003) for the diagnosis of RF and based on revised Jones criteria RHD (Table 39.1).

Prevention

Health Promotion

Measures necessary for primordial prevention are:
- Improvement in the living conditions
- Improvement of sanitation in and around the house
- Prevention of overcrowding
- Prevention of malnutrition among children
- Improvement in the socioeconomic condition
- Health education of the people regarding dangers of sore throat
- 'Health-fair' should be conducted in the schools to make the children health conscious.

Specific Protection

1. No vaccine is available.
2. Chemoprophylaxis of the contacts of a case of pharyngitis or scarlet fever with benzathine penicillin.

Table 39.1: Diagnosis criteria of rheumatic fever and rheumatic heart disease

Category	Criteria
Primary episode of rheumatic fever (RF)	One or two major and two minor manifestations plus evidence of preceding group A streptococcal infection [such as prolonged PR interval in electrocardiography (ECG), rise in antistreptolysin O titer, a positive throat culture]
Recurrent attack of RF in a patient with established rheumatic heart disease (RHD)	One or two major and two minor without manifestations plus evidence of preceding group A streptococcal infection
Recurrent attack of RF in a patient without established RHD	Two minor manifestations plus evidence of preceding group A streptococcal infection

3. 'Secondary prophylaxis' is given for all cases of RF to prevent RHD with 1.2 million units of benzathine penicillin, once in 3 weeks, regularly for 5 years or until the age of 18 years, whichever is later; if they have developed RHD, prophylaxis is continued for life.

Early Diagnosis and Treatment

- By conducting periodical 'school health survey', to detect the causes of sore throat
- By surveillance of 'high-risk' groups such as slum dwellers
- Detected cases of sore throat (or acute pharyngitis) are treated by one dose of 1.2 million units of benzathine penicillin, a long acting one; this essentially prevents the subsequent development of RF and RHD.

Disability Limitation

Disability limitation consists of limiting the development of disability in an individual who has already developed RHD. This consists of giving intensive treatment with aspirin for joint pains and prednisolone for carditis, lifelong benzathine penicillin 1.2 million units, once in 3 weeks, and balloon valvotomy or valve replacement.

Rehabilitation

By social, vocational and psychological measures of those who are suffering from RHD.

HYPERTENSION

Hypertension is a condition characterized by an increase in the arterial pressure of the individual. It is the commonest cardiovascular disease all over the world and constitutes an important risk factor for the cardiovascular deaths. Higher the BP, higher is the risk of complications such as stroke, myocardial infarction and renal failure.

'Isolated systolic hypertension' is defined as a systolic pressure of 140 mm Hg or more and a diastolic BP of less than 90 mm Hg.

The WHO expert committee has also recommended that:
- The BP should be recorded in the sitting position of the patient
- Only one arm (either right or left) to be used consistently
- The reading at which 'Korotkoff sound' is first heard is considered as systolic pressure and at which the K-sound disappears as diastolic pressure
- At least three readings should be taken over a period of 3 minutes and the lowest reading is recorded.

The HTN is a disorder of elevated systolic and/or diastolic blood pressure at a level above the generally accepted norm, and is characterized by non-specific symptoms. It is a common cardiovascular disease frequently occurring both in the developing and developed countries. It is an ubiquitions health problem and 8–18% of adults suffer from it in most countries.

Hypertension in adults is defined, as a systolic pressure equal to or greater than 160 mm Hg and/or diastolic pressure equal to or greater than 95 mm Hg WHO, 1978.

Classification (Table 39.2)

There are two types of HTN; primary or essential and secondary as detailed below:
1. The primary or essential HTN is a most common form of hypertension, usually occurs in 90% of the populations and a high-risk factor for coronary heart disease, stroke, heart failure and renal disease. Essential hypertension is more frequent among elderly persons between 25 and 55 years. It is common where there is high intake of sodium.
2. The secondary HTN occurs from several conditions such as coarctation of aorta, narrowing of one or both renal arteries, glomerulonephritis, diabetes glomerulonephritis, glomerulosclerosis, pheochromocytoma, Cushing's syndrome, Conn's syndrome, systemic lupus erythematosus, toxemia of pregnancy, from oral contraception and estrogen therapy—obesity might have a significant influence in its causation and so is consumption of alcohol.

Table 39.2: Classification of blood pressure (World Health Organization)

Category	Systolic (mm Hg)	Diastolic (mm Hg)
Normal	< 130	< 85
High normal	130–140	85–90
Mild (stage I)	140–159	90–90
Moderate (stage 2)	160–179	100–100
Severe (stage 3)	> 180	> 110

Hypertension varies between communities and might have an association with socioeconomic background, old age. To sum up a number of factor responsible, increasing level of BP are heredity, weight increase, increased salt intake, stress and serum in physical inactivity, long-term exposure to adverse psychosocial factors, etc.

Blood Pressure in Normotensive and Hypertensive Subjects

- Normal: Systolic less than 130 mm Hg; diastolic then 85 mm Hg
- High normal: Systolic 130–139 mm Hg; diastolic 85–89 mm Hg
- Mild HTN (stage 1): Systolic 140 mm Hg; diastolic 90–99 mm Hg
- Moderate HTN (stage 2): Systolic 160 mm Hg; or diastolic 100–109 mm Hg
- Severe HTN (stage 3): Systolic 180 mm Hg; diastolic 110–119 mm Hg
- Very severe hypertension (stage 4): Systolic 210 mm Hg or above diastolic 120 mm Hg or above.

The people with other than normal BP should be adviced to seek medical check-ups periodic according to the physicians.

Clinical Features

The pathological changes, the conditions are widespread inflammation, swelling of small arteries and arterioles, thickening of intima leading to arteriolar narrowing, hypertrophy of muscular coats, hyaline degeneration. Usually, essential hypertensic symptomatic until its complications develop secondary HTN most cases do not usually show any specific symptoms. The usual symptoms encountered are suboccipital headache, dizziness, flushed face, trembling, nausea, vomiting, epistaxis, muscle weakness, tinnitus, palpitation, nervousness and irritability polyuria. Long-standing cases give rise to signs and symptoms of left ventricular hypertrophy, a pectoris and myocardial infarction and centred involvement producing hemiplegia, aphasia or hemorrhage from rupture of renal intracerebral aneurysms. The condition can produce stroke, malignant HTN, subarachnoid hemorrhage, cerebellar hemorrhage, hypertensive encephalopathy, retinopathy such as papilledema, atherosclerotic heart disease, cardiac failure and renal failure as complication.

Magnitude

Hypertension is a global problem. In India, it is estimated to range from 4 to 8% and the trend is increasing due to changes in lifestyle.

Rule of Halves

Hypertension is an 'iceberg disease' and constitutes the tip of the iceberg. The submerged portion corresponds to undiagnosed cases, asymptomatic cases and inadequately treated cases, etc. that are all represented diagrammatically as rule of halves:

- Whole community
- Normotensive subjects
- Hypertensive subjects
- Undiagnosed HTN subjects
- Diagnosed HTN subjects
- Diagnosed, but untreated
- Diagnosed and treated
- Inadequately treated
- Adequately treated.

First rule: About half of the cases of HTN are aware of their condition.

Second rule: About half of those who are aware are under treatment.

Third rule: About half of those who are under treatment are receiving adequate treatment.

Tracking of Blood Pressure

Suppose the BP recordings in a group of children are followed up over a period of several years, it will be observed that those individuals, whose BP was initially high would probably continue in the same track as they grow older and those with low BP would continue in the same track as they grow older. This phenomenon of persistence of the rank order of BP has been described as 'tracking' of BP. This knowledge helps to identify the 'at-risk' group of children and adolescents, who can develop hypertension in the future period, so that preventive care can be provided for them.

Risk Factors

Hypertension itself is a risk factor for cardiovascular diseases, stroke and renal failure. But still, it has its own risk factors, which are grouped into two groups, i.e. nonmodifiable and modifiable.

Non-modifiable Risk Factors

Age: The prevalence of hypertension rises with age and the rise is greater in those, who had higher initial BP. Usually as the age advances, there will be cumulative effect of environmental factors. Thus, usually the prevalence is high above 40 years of age.

Sex: During young age, there is no difference in BP in both the genders. But in the middle age, there is male preponderance. However, in later life, the pattern is reversed and it is more among women, may be because of postmenopausal changes.

Genetic factors: A polygenic type of inheritance has been postulated based on twins and family studies. However, no genetic markers have been identified. If both the parents are hypertensive, offsprings have 45% possibility of developing hypertension and if parents are normotensives, the possibility is only 3%.

Ethnicity: Studies have shown higher BP levels among black people than among whites.

Modifiable Risk Factors

1. Occupation: It involves stress and strain including tension predisposes for the development of hypertension as in professional group of people such as doctors, lawyers, engineers, business executives, etc. The stress and strain, which is made up of psychosocial factors operate through mental processes, consciously or unconsciously, result in hypertension, through sympathetic nervous system and noradrenaline.
2. Socioeconomic status: Prevalence of hypertension is usually higher among people of higher socioeconomic status than the people of lower status. However, in the

fast developing countries, it has been observed to be higher among lower class also, because of the changes in the lifestyle, as it is seen in India nowadays.
3. Physical activity: Physically inactive and those leading a sedentary way of life are more susceptible for hypertension.
4. Obesity: Greater the weight gain, higher the risk of acquiring hypertension. Specially central obesity (increased waist to hip ratio) has been positively correlated with hypertension. Thus, obesity has been identified as a risk factor.
5. Diet:
   a. Higher the salt intake in the daily diet, greater the risk. However, potassium antagonizes the biological effects of sodium, thereby reduces BP. Other cations such as calcium, cadmium and magnesium have also been suggested is of importance in reducing BP levels.
   b. Foods rich in saturated fats are a risk factor for hypertension and serum cholesterol.
   c. Foods rich in fats and sweets predispose for obesity, which in turn predisposes for hypertension.
   d. Consumption of dietary fibers is associated with reduced risk of hypertension, because it reduces LDL cholesterol level.
6. Diseases: Diabetes mellitus predisposes the patient for hypertension.
7. Lifestyle (habits): High alcohol intake raises systolic pressure more than diastolic pressure. However, it returns to normal level on stopping the consumption of alcohol. This indicates that alcohol-induced elevation is not fixed.

Other Factors

Consumption of oral contraceptive pills over a long period for several years, constitutes the risk of hypertension because of estrogen component. However, the role of other factors such as noise, vibration, humidity, etc. require further investigations.

Clinical Manifestations

The most consistent symptom is headache. It is early morning, suboccipital pulsating headache. It is often associated with the stiffness of the neck, awakening the patient from sleep and gives relief after vomiting. Other features are dizziness, palpitation, easy fatigability, epistaxis, blurring of vision, breathlessness and personality changes. Complications are angina pectoris, myocardial infarction, stroke (cerebral thrombosis and hemiplegia, cerebral hemorrhage) and renal failure. Ocular manifestations are blurring vision, scotoma, unilateral or bilateral papilledema and exudates on the retina. Hypertensive patients are grouped into three groups:
- Those who do not have any symptoms, but are detected during the routine check-up
- Those who come with specific complaints as explained above
- Those who come with complications.

Prevention

Primary Prevention (Primordial Prevention)

Primary prevention consists of modification or elimination of the risk factors by two approaches, population strategy and high-risk strategy.

Population strategy

Population strategy is directed at the whole population based on the fact that even a small reduction in the average BP of a population would produce a large reduction in the incidence of HTN and its complications. This involves health promotive measures as follows:
1. Nutrition: The dietary changes should be:
   a. Average consumption of the salt to be reduced to less than 5 g/day caput (to avoid pickles, salted nuts, etc.).
   b. Moderate fat intake (avoiding fats of animal origin, except fish as well as coconut oil and vanaspati).
   c. Prudent diet (rich in fruits and vegetables) to be encouraged.
   d. Consumption of alcohol to be discouraged.
   e. Energy intake to be restricted to body needs.
2. Dietary approach to stop hypertension (DASH) diet: It is a now recommended, as an important step in controlling BP. This diet is not only rich in important nutrients and fiber, but also includes foods that contain two and half times the amounts of electrolytes, potassium, calcium and magnesium. It makes the following recommendations:
   a. To avoid saturated fats.
   b. To include monounsaturated fatty acids (MUFA), also known as omega 9 and MUFA, such as olive or canola oils.
   c. To include polyunsaturated fatty acids (PUFA), e.g. omega 3 and 6 PUFA present in sunflower, cottonseed, fish oils, which have anti-inflammatory and anti-blood clotting effects is significantly beneficial to heart; omega 3 is further categorized as α linolenic acid (ALA) and docosahexaenoic acid (DHA); the DHA appears to have specific benefits on BP.
   d. To choose whole grains over white flour.

e. To include fresh fruits and vegetables daily, specially potassium-rich fruits such as bananas, oranges and vegetables such as carrot, spinach, mushrooms, beans and potatoes (grape fruits boost the effect of calcium channel blocking drugs used for hypertension).
f. To include nuts, seeds or legumes (dried beans or peas daily).
g. To choose modest amount of protein preferably fish or poultry; oily fish may be particularly beneficial; a combination of DASH diet and salt restriction is very effective in reducing BP.
h. Weight: Reduction of weight is done by diet control and promotion of physical activities, specially by the obese people; regular physical activity leads to fall in body weight, blood lipid and BP maintain normal body weight.
i. Behavioral changes: Modification in the personal lifestyle, reduction in the stress, practicing yoga and meditation goes a long way in controlling BP; abstain from alcohol and smoking.
j. Health education: People are made health conscious about hypertension and its consequences, and encouraged to practice health promotive measures as explained above.
k. Self-care: All hypertensive patients are educated to take self-care by maintaining a log book of the BP readings, which will be helpful for follow-up.
l. Recreation: The establishment of recreation clubs, involving in hobbies such as gardening, music, periodic excursions, cultural shows and the like will help to relieve the stress.

High-risk strategy

High-risk strategy consists of screening of all high-risk cases (such as obese people, individuals above 50 years of age, alcoholics, diabetics, sedentary workers, pregnant mothers, individuals having family history, etc.) by recording BP. The aim is to prevent the attainment of levels of BP at which treatment has to be started. This constitutes 'specific protection' of primary prevention.

Secondary Prevention

Secondary prevention consists of the following measures:
- Identification of hypertensive individuals (early diagnosis)
- Instituting non-pharmacological management of hypertension in all
- Use of appropriate drugs to control the BP
- Regular follow-up to ensure control of BP and compliance of management, because the drugs have to be taken lifelong.

Tertiary Prevention

1. Disability limitation: If the patient comes with very high BP, treatment is given intensively to limit the development of disability.
2. Rehabilitation: This is given for those who have become handicap due to complications of hypertension such as hemiplegia (following stroke), blindness (due to retinopathy), etc.

Role of Nurses in Prevention and Control of Hypertension

Control of HTN is possible through control of psychological overactivity and of obesity; diagnosis and adequate management of the condition, which eventually predispose to the disorder, preprevention include weight reduction and charges in the lifestyles of people, i.e. the people are adviced to avoid smoking, alcohol intake and vigorous work or labor, and they must be encouraged for regular exercises, according to their age. Every effort is made to control obesity and it is better to advise low-sodium diet.

A community appearance to the control of hypertension is feasible, because it can be easily identified and the benefit of adequate control can be established by giving health education regarding minimum knowledge concerning the promotion, and preservation of cardiovascular health.

The responsibilities of the health services in hypertension control program include:
- Appropriate training of the health personnel and volunteers
- Preparation of the technical information required for health education
- Detection, treatment and follow-up of HTN patients
- Maintenance of referral links
- Monitory and insulation program.

The role of community health nurses and prevention and control of HTN includes:
1. Monitor BP and weight.
2. Educate above nutrition and antihypertensive drugs.
3. Teach stress management techniques.
4. Promote an optimum balance between rest and activity.
5. Establish BP screening program.
6. Assess the patients lifestyle and promote lifestyle changes.
7. Promote dietary modification by using techniques scan and diet diary.
8. Teach about simple classification of HTN and recommend for referral to a source of medical care.

It has been found that hypertensive persons benefits from diet, low in sodium. The normal diet contains about 3–6 g of sodium. Low-sodium diet ranges from 200 to 300 mg right up to 2,000–3,000 mg depending on the degree of restriction, can be advised to the hypertensive patients. Food rich in sodium can be restrictive, i.e. milk, eggs, cheese, meat, carrot, poultry, fish, best green turnips and spinach. In addition hypertensives are also recommended, high potassium, low-cholesterol diets and unsaturated fat.

CEREBROVASCULAR ACCIDENT (STROKE)

Cerebrovascular disease (CVA) is the third commonest cause of death after heart disease and cancer in the developed countries. The incidence of stroke is 1–2 per 1,000 population per annum in Europe and USA. It is uncommon below the age of 40 years and slightly more common in males. The stroke remains the major cause of morbidity and mortality in old age.

Definitions

Stroke: It is defined as focal neurological deficit due to a vascular lesion. It is usually of rapid onset and by definition, lasts longer than 24 hours if the patient survives. Hemiplegia is a common manifestation.

Stroke-in-evolution: When signs and symptoms of neurological injury are getting worse within 24 hours of onset, it is called stroke-in-evolution.

Transient ischemic attack (TIA): This is a focal neurologic deficit lasting less than 24 hours. There is complete recovery. The platelet-fibrian clot formed over an atheromatous plaque within produces TIA in 90% cases.

Ischemic stroke: With cerebral infarction/ischemia due to cerebral thrombosis and embolization produces TIA in 90% cases.

Hemorrhagic stroke: It is caused by an intracerebral hemorrhage. Ruptured aneurysm is the cause in the young and hypertension in the elderly.

Stroke (or apoplexy) is an acute, focal or global disturbance of cerebral function, lasting for more than 24 hours or leading to death with no apparent cause. Other than vascular origin, such as stenosis, occlusion or rupture of the arteries, resulting in various neurological signs and symptoms such as convulsions, paralysis, speech and visual disturbances, coma, etc. The commonest manifestation being hemiplegia. This excludes transient ischemic attack, if the duration is less than 24 hours.

Stroke includes the following syndromes:
- Cerebral hemorrhage
- Subarachnoid hemorrhage
- Cerebral thrombosis or embolism
- Occlusion of precerebral arteries
- Transient cerebral ischemia, lasting for more than 24 hours
- Ill-defined cardiovascular disease.

Problem: Stroke is a global problem. It is responsible for increased disability, morbidity and mortality all over the world. Cerebral thrombosis is the most frequent form occurring all over. The incidence varies from 0.2 to 2.5 per 1,000 population per year at the global level. But in India it is 2–5% population.

Etiology

The causes of cerebrovascular disease are given below:
1. Ischemic stroke:
   - Cerebral thrombosis, cerebral embolism, TIA
   - Lacunar infarct, cerebral arteritis
   - Blood diseases, i.e. polycythemia, disseminated intravascular coagulation (DIC)
   - Dissecting aneurysm of aorta or shock
   - Cardiac arrhythmias, i.e. atrial fibrillation
   - Cerebral malaria
   - Hyperviscosity and antiphospholipid syndrome
   - Hypercoagulable states (pregnancy, puerperium).
2. Hemorrhagic stroke:
   - Hypertension, trauma
   - Ruptured aneurysm (saccular, mycotic, etc.) angiomatous malformations
   - Blood dyscrasias such as purpura, leukemia and bleeding diathesis
   - Anticoagulants
   - Bleed in a brain tumor.

The predisposing conditions and risk factors of cerebral vascular disease are given below:
- Hypertension
- Oral contraceptives
- Old age
- Obesity
- Alcohol
- Smoking
- Puerperium
- Diabetes mellitus
- Hyperlipidemia
- Sedentary lifestyle.

Progressive atherosclerosis: With narrowing of carotid and vertebrobasilar arteries is the common cause of TIA and stroke.

Low cardiac output and low cerebral perfusion: May cause TIA. The massive gastrointestinal (GI) bleed, hypotension, cardiac arrhythmias may evoke TIA and thrombosis.

Microembolization into the brain: The principal sources of embolic stroke are atheromatous plaques within the great vessels (the carotid and vertebral systems) or from the heart (e.g. atrial fibrillation, valvular heart disease especially mitral stenosis with left atrial thrombus or mural thrombi formed after myocardial infarction).

Epidemiology

1. Age and sex incidence: The incidence rate rises steeply as the age advances, specially after 40 years of age. It is twice as common in men as in women.
2. Preexisting diseases: In more than 75% cases of stroke, there is usually associated preexisting disease such as hypertension, diabetes, ischemic heart disease or other cardiovascular (atherosclerosis) disease. This supports the view that in most cases stroke is merely an incident the slowly progressive course of a generalized vascular disease.

Risk Factors

- Hypertension is considered as a main risk factor for cerebral thrombosis and cerebral hemorrhage
- Obesity and smoking constitute the next important factors
- Other factors are diabetes left ventricular hypertrophy, cardiac dilatation, oral contraceptives, hypercholesterolemia, disorders of blood coagulation, etc. also constitute the risk factors.

Recurrence of TIA characterized by episodes of focal, reversible, neurological deficit and constitute a warning sign of stroke.

Management

The management of a patient with cerebrovascular accidental is done with following aims:
1. To save life and to speed-up recovery.
2. Rehabilitation by physical and occupational therapies for a gainful employment.
3. To prevent recurrence.
4. To remove the cause, if possible.

Medical Treatment

General Measures

In acute stroke CVA or hemiplegia, maintenance of vital signs (pulse, BP, temperature, respiration), patent airway, fluid and electrolyte balance, and prevention of complications such as pulmonary aspiration, seizures, thrombophlebitis, bedsores, etc. are mandatory. Health management includes healthy diet, weight control, regular exercise, no smoking, limited alcohol consumption, routine health assessment and control of risk factors. The steps to be taken to the following.

Ventilation: Cerebral hypoxia predisposes to cerebral edema, raised intracranial pressure and brain herniation. Patent airway must be maintained to prevent accidental aspiration by continued suction of tracheobronchial secretions.

Oxygen administration (4–6 L/min): Oxygen through a nasal catheter or venturi mask is advocated. Ventilatory support in a comatosed patient is necessary in case of hypoxia or rising $PaCO_2$. Long-term ventilatory support warrants tracheostomy.

Blood pressure: In acute stage of cerebral ischemia/infarct, BP should not be lowered unless there is moderate to severe hypertension. Keep the diastolic BP between 90 and 100 mm Hg with decongestive therapy and diuretics. On the other hand, in hypertensive CVA with encephalopathy, or malignant hypertension, parenteral calcium channel blockers or parenteral beta blockers and diuretics may be employed to reduce the BP, but not below 100 mm Hg. Hypotensive episode may be treated by vasopressors (dopamine) or by IV fluids and corticosteroids.

Cardiac arrhythmias: Frequent ventricular premature beats may be treated with phenytoin (100 mg three times a day). Bradyarrhythmias due to raised intracranial pressure will disappear with decongestive therapy.

Fluid and electrolyte balance: Restriction of fluid intake during first 2–3 days or even a negative balance is beneficial to reduce cerebral edema.

Reduction of cerebral edema and increased intracranial pressure: IV mannitol or glycerol or dexamethasone is used to reduce the vasogenic cerebral edema.

Lipid-lowering agents: Statins and fibrate for the hyperlipidemia.

Nursing Management

Emergency management: Nurse posted in accidental and emergency is involved in the emergency management of stroke. The nurse first of all makes nursing assessment by observing the altered state of consciousness, weakness or paralysis of the part involved, speech disturbance, vital signs (pulse, BP, heart rate, respiratory rate) size and reaction of pupil, seizures, cranial nerve paralysis, head injury and bladder or bowel disturbance. The nurse takes following emergency measures:

1. To make the patient lie comfortably in bed.
2. Ensure patent airway and O_2 therapy.
3. Remove the dentures and clothing.
4. Procure IV line and start normal saline infusion. Monitor the BP.
5. Elevate head end of the bed to 30°. Railing be is provided if patient has seizures.
6. Institute anticonvulsant therapy if patient has seizures.
7. Obtain computed tomography (CT) head. In ischemic stroke, anticipate thrombolytic therapy.
8. Emergency decongestive therapy, e.g. mannitol or glycerol if there is raised intracranial pressure.
9. Monitoring of vital signs, O_2 saturation, electrocardiography (ECG), Glasgow coma scale for pupil size and reaction.
10. Take all the measures of coma management if patient is in coma.

Subsequent Nursing Management

Subsequent nursing management is done when patient is admitted in intensive care unit (ICU) or shifted in medical ward. The nursing assessment is again done in details to find out the etiology of sudden CVA, i.e. thrombosis, embolism or hemorrhage. Assessment includes the same parameter as detailed neurological examination is done to find out the net neurological deficit, cranial nerve involvement, speech, bowel and bladder involvement. The risk factors or predisposing conditions, e.g. hypertension, diabetes, hyperlipidemia, CAD and TIA are explored to know the present status. Assessment is further made regarding emotion or anxiety, coping abilities, family and social support network, financial and insurance status, etc. The investigations done are collected and interpreted in the light of history and physical examination so as to make a clinical nursing diagnosis and plan the further management.

Prevention and Control

- Control of hypertension in the community
- Detection and treatment of TIA attack
- Prevention and control of other risk factors such as diabetes and smoking
- Creation of treatment facilities for stroke, controls the complications
- Community health education.

CONCLUSION

Hypertension has relation with cardiovascular disease. The higher the BP, higher the risk of coronary disease. Hypertension occur due to high fat intake, alcohol, oral contraceptives, stress, tension, etc. There are various ways to prevent and control hypertension such as early case detection, treatment, health education.

The RHD, occur due to the causative agent hemolytic streptococci. There are a number of environmental factors such as poverty, overcrowding, poor housing conditions and inadequate health services, which can lead to RHD. It can be prevented and controlled by early diagnosis, treatment, health promotion activities, surveys and non-medical measures.

Coronary artery disease is also known as ishemic heart disease occurs due to smoking, high BP, elevated serum cholesterol, diabetes, obesity and sedentary habits. It can be prevented and controlled by early diagnosis, treatment, dietary modification, physical activity, regular checkup and health education.

Stroke contributes to morbidity and mortality. According to WHO, stroke is rapidly developed clinical signs of focal disturbance of cerebral function, lasting more than 24 hours or leading to death. The prevention and control of stroke include lifestyle changes and health education.

Cancer

CHAPTER 40

INTRODUCTION

The terms cancer, neoplasm, malignant neoplasm and tumors are used interchangeably by professionals and the lay public, but actually these denote different meanings. Tumor simply means a lump, mass or swelling, which can be neoplastic. The word 'neoplasm' ('neo' stands for 'new', and 'plasm' stands for 'molding') is defined as a new growth or mass of tissue, which can be harmless (benign) or harmful (malignant). The benign neoplasms are non-invasive, remain localized, while malignant neoplasm is aggressive, invades the other tissues and metastasize to distant organs.

The term 'cancer' denotes malignant neoplasm in which normal mechanism of cell growth and differentiation has been altered leading to abnormal proliferation. It is invasive and spreads directly to nearby tissues as well as distant sites.

Cancer may be best regarded as a group of diseases characterized by:
- Abnormal growth of cells
- Ability to invade adjacent tissues and even distant organs
- The eventual death of the affected patient, if the tumor has progressed beyond that stage, when it can be successfully removed.

Cancer can occur at any site or tissue of the body and may involve any type of the cells. It may be defined as active and uncontrolled proliferation of cells of epithelial tissue of the body.

Cancer cells have a great invasive property and can be classified into two major categories:
1. Solid tumors.
2. Leukemias and lymphomas.

The latter are often disseminated diseases from the very beginning.

MAGNITUDE OF PROBLEM

The cancer is becoming a more challenging problem in industrially developed countries. Cancer is the second leading cause of death in ageing population. This may be due to increasing number of carcinogens, skilled diagnosis and more people seeking medical care.

PROBLEMS IN INDIA

With the control of communicable diseases and increase in life expectancy, the incidence of cancer in the country is rising. Jussawalla observes that "cancer is one of the 10 leading causes of death today in India and is advancing in rank year by year." The incidence of cancer is about 70 in 100,000 population as against 289 in 100,000 population in developed countries. This is almost one fourth of the reported incidence from the industrialized countries of the west.

In India 370,000 suffer annually and 200,000 die every year. Oropharyngeal cancer alone accounts for 30–35% of all malignancies in India. Improved method of technology is now available, which detects a good number of cases hitherto remaining undiagnosed. With an average survival of 3 years after diagnosis, nearly 1,500,000 patients require facilities for diagnosis, treatment and follow-up at any given time. At the beginning of this century, cancer was the sixth cause of death in industrialized countries; today, it is the second leading cause of death. The three main reasons for this is being a longer live expectancy, more accurate diagnosis and the rise in cigarette smoking, especially among males since World War I. The overall rates do not reflect the different trends according to the type of cancer. For example, there has been a large increase in lung cancer incidence since 1930; the stomach cancer has shown a declining trend in most developed countries for reasons not understood.

ETIOLOGY OF CANCER

The cause and development of each type of cancer is multifactorial in origin. Certain individuals are genetically predisposed to cancer. Carcinogens are the factors associated with cancer etiology. The carcinogens are:
- Radiation
- Chemicals
- Viruses
- Other physical, environmental and immunologic agents.

Each factor plays a role and accumulation of two or more factors increases the risk of cancer:

1. **Radiation:** Exposure to radiation (ionizing radiation from radioactive materials or ultraviolet radiation from sunlight and tanning beds) induces cancer. Radiation exposure from diagnostic procedure or radiation therapy is safe in lower doses given for short periods. Higher doses for prolonged periods can induce carcinogenesis.
2. **Chemicals:** Smoking is injurious to health; this reminds us that tobacco is a proved chemical carcinogen and can leads to lung cancer. There is linear relationship between the amount and number of years of smoking, and cancer risk. Chewing tobacco or tobacco used as snuff is associated with mouth cancer.

    Occupational and industrial exposure causes 2–8% of all human cancers. For example, asbestos, arsenic, chromium, nickel, polycyclic hydrocarbons can lead to lung cancer, while aflatoxin and *Aspergillus* can lead to liver cancer. Benzidine compounds are associated with bladder cancer.
3. **Viruses:** A large number of viruses, i.e. hepatitis B, hepatitis C, Epstein-Barr virus (EBV), human T-cell leukemia virus type-1 (HTLV-I), herpesvirus-8, the human papillomavirus (HPV) and *Helicobacter pylori* are associated with cancer risk. These viruses, at some point, infect the cells and cause damage to deoxyribonucleic acid (DNA) of the cell, thus leading to the development of cancer.
4. **Drugs and hormones:** Alkylating agents such as chlorambucil, cyclophosphamide, melphalan, nitrosourea are capable of interacting with DNA and have the potential to cause acute and chronic myeloid leukemia. Cyclosporine, an immunosuppressive drug, increases the risk of non-Hodgkin's lymphoma and Kaposi's sarcoma.

    Certain hormones, i.e. non-steroidal estrogens increase the risk of vaginal cancer, breast cancer and testicular cancer. Steroidal estrogens, oral contraceptive pills and tamoxifen increase the risk of endometrial cancer. Androgens and anabolic steroids can lead to liver cancer.
5. **Age, gender, genetics and ethnicity:** Cancer can occur in young (acute leukemias) and older persons (cancer of colon, prostate and chronic lymphoid leukemia). Females have generally lower risk of cancer incidence, but women are susceptible to cancer cervix and breast cancer.

    Heredity plays a role in colorectal cancer, developing from familial adenomatous polyposis, which is governed by four genes, the mutations of these genes lead to transformation of adenoma to carcinoma. Metastatic colorectal cancer develops only if all the four mutations take place.
6. **Diet and lifestyle:** May be a factor in the development of cancer. A balanced healthy diet, limited intake of fat, balanced caloric intake, physical activity, limited consumption of alcohol and high-fiber intake can reduce cancer risk, and maintain healthy weight throughout life. On the other hand, high fatty food, excessive consumption of alcohol, obesity and less intake of dietary fibers are associated with cancer risks.
7. **Lowered immunity:** Immunosuppression is associated with cancer. Human immunodeficiency virus (HIV)-related tumors (non-Hodgkin's lymphoma, Kaposi's sarcoma) are as a result of profound immunosuppression associated with HIV infection.
8. **Precancerous lesions:** Certain lesions such as leukoplakia and benign adenomas or polyps of the colon, run the risk of transformation into carcinoma. It is the transformation of normal cells into cancer cells.

Stages of Carcinogenesis

There are four identified stages of carcinogenesis:
1. **Stage 1 (initiation):** The event sets, when a carcinogen damages DNA and changes in the structure and function of the cell at the genetic or molecular level. This damage may be reversible or may lead to genetic mutations, if it does not get reversed.
2. **Stage 2 (promotion):** This stage of the event occurs, where there is additional assault to the cell resulting in further genetic damage. The stage transforms the initiated cell to precancerous cell.
3. **Stage 3 (conversion):** Further genetic events result in malignant conversion or transformation leading to the development of full-fledged cancer cell.
4. **Stage 4 (progression):** This event leads to malignant behavior of cancer cells. The cells become invasive and spread to nearby tissue and metastasize to distant body parts.

Clinical utility of this process helps in health promotion, programs and policy making. Smoking cessation program can help to reduce lung cancer through prevention.

Precancerous colon polyps can be removed by colonoscopy before these progresses to malignancy.

EPIDEMIOLOGICAL FEATURES

Agent Factors

There is no single cause. Of the hundreds of causes, some are known and some are unknown:

1. Oral cancer is related to tobacco smoking and chewing; reverse smoking, betel and zarda chewing.
2. Lung cancer death rate is higher among smokers than nonsmokers.
3. Exposure to radiation produces cancer. Watchmakers in factory, farmers, sailors and X-ray operators are more prone to radiation.
4. Air pollution in urban areas causes lung cancer.
5. Chemicals in coal tar and in chimney sweeping, tar, pitch, soot, chromium, nickel and petroleum products are carcinogenic.
6. Cancer of penis is common. Muslims and Jews were done circumcision after birth; cancer of penis is virtually unknown.
7. Hindus suffer more from cancer of penis. Cancer in cervix is commonly found in early marriage and absence of circumcision in male partner.
8. Some viruses are believed to cause cancer in animals and human also. However, work is going on to pin down the agent, which is responsible for causing cancer.

Host Factor

1. Age: After the age of 50, carcinoma in breast, if first child at 30 years.
2. Sex: Cancer of lung and esophagus are more in males. Cancer of cervix and breasts in females.
3. Marital status: Breast cancer lower in early maternity.
4. Race: Cancer of skin, face and neck are more common in white race.
5. Heredity: Genetic influences very much to cancer. Napoleon died of stomach cancer and so died his grandfather, father and brother too.
6. Environmental factors: These are generally held responsible for 80–90% of all human cancers, they are:
   a. Tobacco: In various forms of its usage (e.g. smoking and chewing), tobacco is the major environmental cause of cancers of the lung, larynx, mouth, pharynx, esophagus, bladder, pancreas and probably kidney. It has been estimated that, in the world as a whole, cigarette smoking is now responsible for more than one million premature deaths each year.
   b. Alcohol: Excessive intake of alcoholic beverages is associated with esophageal and liver cancer. Some recent studies have suggested that beer consumption may be associated with rectal cancer. It is estimated that alcohol contributes to about 3% of all cancer deaths.
   c. Dietary factors: Smoked fish is related to stomach cancer, dietary fiber to intestinal cancer, beef consumption to bowel cancer and a high-fat diet to breast cancer.
   d. Occupational exposures: These include exposure to benzene, arsenic, cadmium, chromium, vinyl chloride, asbestos, polycyclic hydrocarbons, etc. The risk of occupational exposure is considerably increased, if the individuals also smoke cigarettes. Occupational exposures are usually reported to account for 1–5% of all human cancer.
   e. Viruses: The hepatitis B virus is usually related to hepatocellular carcinoma. The EBV is associated with two human malignancies, viz. Burkitt's lymphoma, nasopharyngeal and carcinoma. The HPV is a chief suspect of cancer in cervix. The HTLV is associated with adult T-cell leukemia in United States of America (USA) and other parts of Japan.
   f. Parasites: Infections may also increase the risk of cancer. For example, schistosomiasis in Middle East producing carcinoma of the bladder.
   g. Other: There are other numerous environmental factors such as sunlight, radiation and water pollution, medications (e.g. estrogen) and pesticides, which are related to cancer.
   h. Customs, habits and lifestyles: To the above causes must be added customs, habits and lifestyles of people, which may be associated with all increased risk for certain cancers. The familiar exemplary cures are demonstrated as associated between smoking and lung cancer, tobacco and betel chewing and oral cancer, etc.
7. Genetic factors: Genetic influences have long been suspected. For example, retinoblastoma occurs in children of the same parent. Mongols are more likely to develop cancer (leukemia) than normal children. However, genetic factors are less conspicuous and more difficult to identify. There is probably a complex interrelationship between hereditary susceptibility and environmental carcinogenic stimuli in the causation of a number of cancers.

PATHOPHYSIOLOGY OF CANCER CELLS

Cancer cells histologically show inadequate maturation of cells and its structure. There is variation in size and shape—bizarre type of cells. Enlargement of nuclei and cytoplasmic ratio, hyperchromatism, clumping of chromatin and hyperplasia, lack of differentiation and loss of cellular organization and differentiation, frequency of mitotic figures.

Cancer comprises of a group of cells that are altered or transformed in some way due to any cause, but are able to grow, multiply and spread. Cancer development begins at molecular level with mutations or damage to one or more genomes. Cancer cells differ from normal cells in appearance, growth and function. Two major dysfunction that occur in cancer are defective cellular differentiation and defective cellular proliferation.

In normal cell growth, immature cells derived from embryonic cells, mature and differentiate into a specialized particular line and committed to that special function. This process of differentiation is under the influence of cellular oncogenes or proto-oncogenes, which remain suppressed with the result that mature cells differentiate into specialized cell lines performing specific function. Genetic mutations can alter the genetic products and activate proto-oncogenes to oncogenes, resulting in inhibition of this cellular differentiation process. Thus, one can say that proto-oncogenes act as a genetic lock that keeps the cells in mature functioning state. Any condition that can break this lock, such as viruses, genetic mutations can lead to abnormal cell differentiation and transform normal cells into malignant cells with abnormal functions.

CLINICAL FEATURES

According to American Cancer Society (ACS), early signals of cancer are as follows:
- Unusual bleeding and discharge
- A lump or thickening in the breast or elsewhere
- A sore that does not heal
- Persistent change in the bladder or bowel habit
- Persistent indigestion or difficulty in swallowing
- Sudden change in wart or mole
- Hoarseness of persistent change in voice.

If any of the above signs continue for 2 weeks, a doctor must be consulted for final diagnosis. Delay lessens chance of recovery.

LUNG CANCER: SPUTUM CYTOLOGY

Uterine Cancer: Pap Test

Papanicolaou (Pap) test is the direction and identification of malignant cells in the secretions from the walls of the uterus.

Control Measures

Cancer control consist of a series of measures based on present medical knowledge in the fields of prevention, detection, diagnosis, treatment aftercare and rehabilitation, aimed at reducing significantly the number of new cases, increasing the number of cures and reducing the invalidism due to cancer.

Primary Prevention

Cancer prevention until recently was mainly concerned with early diagnosis of the disease:
1. Control of tobacco and alcohol consumption: Primary prevention offers the greatest hope for reducing the number of tobacco-induced and alcohol-related cancer deaths.
2. Personal hygiene: It can reduce cancer, e.g. cancer in the cervix.
3. Radiation: Special efforts should be made to reduce the amount of radiation (including medical radiation) received by each individual to a minimum without reducing the benefits.
4. Occupational exposures: The occupational aspects of cancer are frequently neglected. Measures to protect workers from exposure to industrial carcinogens should be enforced in industries.
5. Immunization: In the case of primary liver cancer, immunization against hepatitis B virus presents are existing protect.
6. Foods, drugs and cosmetics: These should be tested for carcinogen.
7. Air pollution: Control of air pollution is another preventive measure.
8. Treatment of precancerous lesions: Early detection and prompt treatment.
9. Legislation.
10. Cancer education: An important area of primary prevention is cancer education. It should be directed at 'high-risk' groups. The aim of cancer education is to motivate people to seek early diagnosis and early treatment. Cancer organizations in many countries remind the public of the early warning signs ('danger signals') of cancer.

Secondary Prevention

Cancer Registration

Cancer registration is a registration of all cases for a cancer control program. It provides a base for assessing the magnitude of the problem and for planning to necessary services.

Hospital-based registries
Hospital-based registries include all patients treated by a particular institution whether inpatients or outpatients.

Population-based registries
The aim is to cover the complete cancer situation in a given geographic. An early detection of cancer screening is the main weapon for early detection of cancer at a preinvasive (in situ) or premalignant stage. Effective screening programs have been developed for cervical cancer, breast cancer and oral cancer. Primary prevention and early diagnosis has to be conducted on a large scale, however, it may be possible to increase the efficiency of screening programs by focusing high-risk groups. Clearly, there is no point in detecting an early stage, unless facilities for treatment and aftercare are available. Early detection programs and development of a cancer infrastructure starting at the level of primary health care, ending with complex cancer cell or institutions at the state or national levels.

Treatment facilities should be available to all carcinoma patients. Certain forms of cancer are available to surgical removal, while others respond favorably to radiation or chemotherapy, or both. Since most of these methods of treatment have complementary effect or ultimate outcome of the patient, multimodality approach to cancer control has become a standard practice in cancer centers all over the world. In the developed countries, today, cancer treatment is geared to high technology. For those who are beyond the curable stage, the goal must be to provide relief from pain. A largely neglected problem in cancer care is the management of pain. 'Freedom from cancer pain' is now considered a right for cancer patients.

NURSE'S ROLE IN CANCER PREVENTION

The incidence and mortality of all cancer patients have changed over time. The downward trend in the mortality rate is due to prevention and early detection of cancer. The nurse plays a prominent role in cancer management and prevention at all levels, starting from screening, counseling, early detection, prevention, treatment with chemotherapy and final outcome. It is not possible to prevent all types of cancer, but certain cancers have modifiable factors, which, if removed, can prevent cancer, i.e. smoking and dietary items.

Primary Prevention

Primary prevention aims at preventing occurrence or reducing the risk of cancer in healthy persons before its development. The primary prevention measures include alterations of lifestyle behaviors that eliminate or minimize exposure to carcinogens. There are certain modifiable factors associated with cancer risk, such as smoking, poor dietary habits, alcohol consumption, exposure to radiation, and environmental and occupational carcinogens; their removal or avoidance can reduce the risk of cancer development.

Role of Nurse in Primary Prevention

Nurse stresses the activities that promote health and reduce the risk of cancer. The nurse's capabilities in convincing people that change in the lifestyle behavior will have positive impact on health promotion and cancer prevention:

1. Dietary changes: Nurses advise increased intake of high-fiber foods such as fruits, vegetables and whole grain cereals, which are rich source of antioxidants and vitamins. They further advise reduced intake of salt-rich and nitrate-rich foods, fats and oils. Smoking and alcohol should be avoided.
2. Education to public: Regarding reduction in exposure or avoidance of exposure to known carcinogens, i.e. radiation, environment and occupational exposure.
3. Role of physical exercise: Nurse educates the public regarding the role of exercise in the prevention of cancer. They promote regular exercise programs in public.
4. Intermittent rest: The nurse explains the importance of intermittent rest during activity and good sound sleep at night (restful night).
5. Regular health check-up: The nurse promotes regular health check-up for early detection.
6. Eliminate stressors: Avoid stressors or stressful activities. Enjoy consistent period of relaxation and leisure.

Secondary Prevention

Secondary prevention aims at early detection of cancer before manifestations appear, so as to plan prompt treatment. Screening of the public for early detection of cancer includes physical examinations to identify lesions/lump/nodule and use of test or procedures. For example, mammograms (for breast cancer), Pap smears (for cervical cancer), occult blood testing and endoscopy, etc. As a result of early detection, premalignant lesions may be excised, arrested or reversed, or cancer treatment is instituted earlier for better prognosis.

Screening identifies high-risk groups of people more likely to have cancerous/precancerous lesions; therefore, the ACS has recommended screening for prevention because of the following reasons:

- The disease is detectable at the presymptomatic stage
- Prognosis is good, if diagnosis is made early
- Create awareness among public; the population to be screened has a high incidence of the disease
- Effective treatment is available for the disease if diagnosed early
- There is an effective method for screening
- Benefits of screening are more than its risk.

Role of Nurse in Secondary Prevention

Nurse plays an effective role in secondary prevention by educating the people regarding early detection of cancer by screening. The nurse stresses that cancer can be treated effectively, if detected early and he/she can motivate the high-risk groups for screening by telling them that screening does not have any risk.

High-risk Patients and Screening Procedures

The screening procedure for high-risk patients of different cancers can be followed as per protocol.

Chemoprevention

Chemoprevention means use of drugs for prevention of cancer. Beta-carotene and retinoic acid have been shown to cause regression of leukoplakia. Tamoxifen reduces the incidence of contralateral breast cancer in patients on adjuvant chemotherapy.

NATIONAL CANCER CONTROL PROGRAM

Evolution of National Cancer Control Program

During 1975–1976, National Cancer Control Program was started. At that time, priorities were given for equipping the premier cancer hospital/institutions. Central assistance at the rate of ₹250,000 was given to each institution for purchase of cobalt machines. In 1984–1985, the strategy was revised and stress was laid on primary prevention and early detection of cancer cases. During 1990–1991, District Cancer Control Program was started in selected districts (near to the medical college hospitals). In 2000–2001, Modified District Cancer Control Program was initiated.

Objectives

The National Cancer Control Program, started in 1975, was revised in 1984 to strengthen it with the objectives of:

1. Primary prevention: By health education, specially regarding hazards of tobacco consumption and necessity of genital hygiene for prevention of cervical cancer.
2. Secondary prevention: Early detection and diagnosis of common cancer such as cancer of cervix, mouth, breast and tobacco-related cancer by screening self-examination methods.
3. Tertiary prevention: Strengthening of the existing institutions for comprehensive therapy, including palliative care.

Schemes under National Cancer Control Program

Assistance to Regional Cancer Centers

The existing Regional Cancer Centers are being further strengthened to act as referral centers for complicated and difficult cases at the tertiary level. About ₹7.5 million each year are provided to Regional Cancer Centers besides providing assistance to the Institute Rotary Cancer Hospital (AIIMS), New Delhi and Chittaranjan National Cancer Institute (CNCI), Kolkata.

Development of Oncology Wings in Government

Medical college hospital
The scheme had been initiated to fill up the geographical gaps in the availability of cancer treatment facilities in the country. Central assistance is provided for purchase of equipment, which include a cobalt unit besides other equipment. The civil works and manpower are to be provided by the concerned state government/institution. The quantum of central assistance is ₹20 million per institution under the scheme.

Cobalt therapy installation
Efforts are being made to further strengthen the program. Financial assistance for cobalt therapy units is provided up to ₹10 million per unit to non-government charitable organization and ₹15 million for government institution. Financial assistance for mammography units up to ₹3 million can be availed by institutions having cobalt machine.

District Cancer Control Scheme
District Cancer Control Scheme is well-known that a large number of cancer cases can be prevented with suitable health education and early case detection. Accordingly, the scheme for district projects regarding prevention, health education, early detection and pain relief measures were started in 1990–1991. Under this scheme, one time

financial assistance of ₹1.5 million is provided to the concerned state government for each district, project selected under the scheme with a provision of ₹1 million every year for the remaining 4 years of the project period.

Financial assistance to voluntary organizations

Financial assistance to voluntary organizations scheme is meant for information, education and communication (IEC) activities, and early detection of cancer. Under the scheme, financial assistance up to ₹500,000 is provided to the registered voluntary organizations recommended by the state government for undertaking health education and early detection activities in cancer.

Regional cancer centers

The number of regional cancer centers (RCCs) has now been raised to 17. The list is given below. The functions of the regional centers are:

1. Cancer diagnosis, treatment and follow-up.
2. Survey of cancer mortality and morbidity.
3. Training of personnel, both medical and paramedical.
4. Preventive measure with emphasis is on screening health education and individual hygiene.
5. Research (fundamental and applied).
6. Rehabilitation.

Linkages and referral system between RCC medical college and other institutions need to be developed. Referral system (regionalization) can be availed by states for optimal utilization and also for availing services from grantee institutions.

Assistance for Regional Research and Treatment Centers

A recurrent expenditure of ₹7.5 million is being given to these RCC and medical colleges. These centers are considered as the tertiary level of cancer care as far as cancer control program is concerned.

List of Regional Cancer Centers

The following are the list of 17 RCCs in the country:

- Kidwai Memorial Institute of Oncology, Bengaluru (Karnataka)
- Gujarat Cancer and Research Institute, Ahmedabad (Gujarat)
- Cancer Hospital Research Institute, Gwalior (Madhya Pradesh)
- Cancer Institute, Chennai (Tamil Nadu)
- Regional Cancer Centre, Thiruvananthapuram (Kerala)
- Regional Centre for Cancer Research and Treatment Society, Cuttack (Odisha)
- Dr B Borooah Cancer Institute, Guwahati (Assam)
- Chittaranjan National Cancer Institute, Kolkata (West Bengal)
- Institute Rotary Cancer Hospital (AIIMS), New Delhi
- Tata Memorial Hospital, Mumbai (Maharashtra)
- Rashtrasant Tukdoji Regional Cancer Hospital, Nagpur (Maharashtra)
- Kamala Nehru Memorial Hospital, Allahabad (Uttar Pradesh)
- MNJ Institute of Oncology, Hyderabad (Andhra Pradesh)
- Indira Gandhi Institute of Medical Science, Patna (Bihar)
- Acharya Tulsi Regional Cancer Centre, Bikaner (Rajasthan)
- Indira Gandhi Medical College, Shimla (Himachal Pradesh)
- Postgraduate Institute of Medical Sciences, Rohtak (Haryana).

National Cancer Registry Program

The National Cancer Registry Program (NCRP) is functioning under a de-escalating budgeting scheme, wherein the entire financial support for individual registries is provided by the Indian Council of Medical Research (ICMR) for the first 5 years and thereafter the quantum of financial support reduces by 25% every 5 years with a corresponding increase in inputs from the host institute. After a period of 20 years, the registries would remain under the network, with a 25% support for contingencies from ICMR. The current network of registries consists of six population-based and five hospital-based cancer registries. This is quite small considering the sociocultural differences in the country. It is proposed to expand the network of the registries, especially in rural areas.

TOBACCO-RELATED HEALTH PROBLEMS AND EDUCATION

Tobacco has been seen to be related to many health problems, especially cancers and one third of the cancers in India are tobacco related. An ICMR study on cost of management of tobacco-related cancers revealed that in the year 1990, the average cost due to cancers of tobacco-related sites, was ₹134,449 per case, which discounted to the current level, would amount to approximately ₹350,000 per case. This cost included the expenditure by patients or their relatives/friends on diagnosis, consultation, treatment, travel and additional expenditure on food during treatment, loss of income due to the disease and loss due to premature death. Adopting similar methodologies, the average annual cost (if management of coronary artery disease for 1992 was estimated at ₹14,909 per case, whereas average annual cost of managing a case of chronic obstructive lung diseases was ₹11,952. The magnitude of diseases caused by tobacco use in the country during 1999 was estimated as 163,000 incident cases of cancers; 4.45 million prevalent cases of coronary artery disease; and 3.92 million cases of chronic obstructive lung diseases. Using discounting methodology, the cost of diseases caused by tobacco in the country during the year was estimated at ₹277.61 million.

A multicenter project to study the feasibility of involving existing infrastructures in anti-tobacco community education was carried out at Bengaluru, Thiruvananthapuram (both through healthcare services), Goa (through schools) and Agra (through community volunteers). The primary health workers also examined the oral cavity to identify and classify lesions. Pretested health education material was prepared by the project staff and used by the existing infrastructure personnel. Pre- and post-intervention surveys on knowledge, attitude and practice of tobacco use, measured the effect of intervention. The overall reduction in the prevalence of tobacco usage in Goa was 11.8% among men and 9.1% among women in intervention zone 1; 13.4% among men and 13.3% among women in intervention zone 2; and 2.0% for men and 10.2% for women in control zone. Based on the experience of this project, Ministry of Education, State of Goa, included an 8-hour course on tobacco as a part of co-curricular activities for standard five and above. The intervention through community volunteers at Agra center showed that 26.3% males and 10.5% females left tobacco and another 10.1% males and 4.3% females are likely to be quitters (6 months have not passed after leaving tobacco). The project at Thiruvananthapuram center could not achieve optimum participation of healthcare workers. The nine workers, who worked on the project, referred 408 patients out of which 258 reported, giving a compliance of 63.2%. Intervention at Bengaluru center achieved a reduction of tobacco habit in experimental area, amounting to 5.7% in the males and 6.9% in the females. The control area I, showed an increase of 3.8% among male and 8% among female, while in control area II, among men there was a 2.9% increase in tobacco habit and 4.6% decrease among females.

GUTKA AND ORAL CANCER

The popularly use of pan masala and gutka has increased tremendously over the last decade. Gutka has been hypothesized to be an etiological agent for oral cancers. Studies on association of gutka with oral cancers and understanding the process of carcinogenicity due to gutka, pan masala would be taken up. The studies would utilize modern biological techniques including role of genetic factors to understand cellular changes involved in the pathogenesis. Study of behavioral factors associated with initiation and quitting of tobacco use would help in development of control strategies. A study on prevalence rate of tobacco use at national level would help in providing the national perspective and thus dwelling upon control of tobacco-related cancers.

PROJECTS FOR CONTROL OF CERVICAL CANCER

The twin center project (in Gujarat and Karnataka) aimed at assessing the efficacy of clinical downstaging with selective cytology for control of cervical cancer. The project was carried out in three primary health center (PHC) areas, with intervention in one PHC area being provided at the subcenter level; while in the second PHC area, the strategy of imparting health education to the women and advising the eligible women to attend the PHC for a clinical examination was adopted. After 18 months intervention, the proportion of women covered for health education at Karnataka was 8.3% in the area with clinical examination in the field and 22.0% in the area with only health education in the field. The coverage for health education at Gujarat was carried out in the field (28.3%). The coverage for clinical examination was poor. The major reasons being, monetary difficulties, feeling of no obvious problem and domestic responsibilities. A total of 147 dysplasia cases were detected out of total of 2,044 women screened in the area with clinical examination in the field in Gujarat.

Transformation of Precancerous Lesions to Invasive Disease

Many common cancers of the country, especially oral and cervical cancer, are associated with a precancerous stage, which may last for several years. Studies have indicated that such patients are at higher risk of development of invasive disease, although many of them are known to regress spontaneously. The current management protocols tend to follow-up early lesion and treat late lesions with various modalities. It would be useful, if one could identify specific features of precancerous lesions that are associated with their progression to cancers. The study would assess the role of genetic and other biological markers for identifying the lesions with potential of transformation. Identification of relevant predictive parameters, including mutation, would also be attempted.

CANCER OF GALLBLADDER

Cancer of gallbladder is one of the five common cancers of North India, especially among women. Studies on understanding the etiological factors of cancer of gallbladder, biological processes associated with pathogenesis, and identification of better modalities for its early detection and treatment are proposed to be initiated.

BREAST CANCER

The data from NCRP indicate that its incidence may be increasing in certain registry areas. It is proposed to initiate studies on etiology of breast cancer and identify the role of genetic, environmental, hormonal and lifestyle factors, which may help in evolving cost-effective strategies for its early detection and control.

OPERATIONAL RESEARCH TO CONTROL CANCER

National Cancer Control

As elements related to control of cancers have still not been integrated in the health services, operational research projects would provide important leads in optimal implementation of National Cancer Control Program. Operational research projects on control of cervical cancer with focus on search for alternate strategies and project on control of cancer through multiorgan approach are expected to start within Ninth Five-Years Plan Period. These projects would continue with forthcoming plan period.

Chemoprevention

Scientific literature indicates that progression of precancerous lesions can be retarded/arrested by use of certain chemical substances, including commonly used substances such as turmeric. It is proposed to initiate studies aimed at chemoprevention of common cancers similar to that of oral cavity and cervix, using less expensive, indigenous Indian products.

Breast Cancer

- Study of telomeric dynamics and cyclins in inducing immortalization/senescence in human mammary epithelial cancer cells in vitro
- Propagation and characterization of cell lines from primary breast and prostate tumors.

Genitourinary Malignancies

Expression and application of *cyclin* genes in prostate cancer.

Lymphoma

To correlate cellular survival, cell death and drug resistance with probability of obtaining complete remission in patients with hematopoietic-lymphoid malignancies. In vitro evaluation and comparison of cytotoxicity to standard chemotherapeutic agents on freshly isolated malignant T or B lymphocytes.

Comparison of in vitro cytotoxicity assays with the clinical response of the patients to standard chemotherapeutic regimes. Flow cytometric analysis of all leukemia/lymphoma cases for immunophenotyping. In addition, flow cytometric analysis and intracellular expression of *p53*, Bcl-2, multiple drug resistance (MDR) protein and apoptotic index will be evaluated by immunofluorescence staining of fixed and permeabilized leukemia/lymphoma cells.

The future program in tumor biology is aimed at a better understanding of the basic cellular process in cancer, elucidation of the genetic basis for breast cancer in Indian women and attempt to design a model for in vitro cytotoxicity of hematopoietic lymphoid malignancies.

CONCLUSION

Cancer is a chronic non-communicable disease caused by smoking, alcohol intake, radiations, chewing of tobacco, etc. Identification of persons having danger signs of cancer and appropriate treatment can prevent and control cancer.

Accidents

CHAPTER 41

INTRODUCTION

Accident is an unintended event occurring in a sequence of events, which usually produces unintended injury, death or property damage. Among the many causes of death, accidents constitute a serious epidemic in the developed countries. Accidents are part of the price we pay for technological progress and are no longer considered accidental, because majority of them are preventable.

According to World Health Organization (WHO), accident is defined as an event, independent of human will caused by an outside force acting rapidly, which results in bodily or mental injury.

Accident occurs, independent of human will power, by a rapidly acting external force, resulting in physical with/without mental damage or injury. If death occurs at once or within a week after the accident, it is called fatal accident; if death occurs after a week, but within a month, it is called death due to accident or killed in accident; and if death occurs after 1 year, it is called sequel of accident.

Accident rank third in order among the leading causes of death. It is more in developed countries. Currently, road traffic accidents rank ninth among the leading causes of deaths in the world. It is projected to be second leading cause of death by the year 2020, next to coronary artery disease. For every accidental death, there are about 10–15 serious injuries. Injuries in turn are responsible for about 9% of all causes of death and about 16% of disabilities, i.e. respectively it corresponds to about 5 million deaths and about 9 million disabilities every year. Road traffic accidents constitute the primary cause. More than 25% of these deaths occur in South East Asia only.

ACCIDENTS IN INDIA

In India, the trend of accidents is on the increasing rate, which is not only due to population explosion but also due to industrialization and urbanization including mechanization in agricultural industry, predisposed by lack of awareness and safety precautions. Out of 5 million accidental deaths occurring in the world, about half million occur in India alone every year.

Measurements of Accidents and Injuries

Mortality Indicators

- Proportional mortality rate, i.e. percentage of total deaths due to accidents (this can also be estimated per 1,000 total deaths)
- Number of deaths per million populations
- Number of deaths per 1,000 (or 10,000) registered vehicles per year
- Ratio of number of accidents: Number of vehicles (or passengers) per kilometer.

Morbidity Indicators

Morbidity is measured in terms of 'serious injuries' and 'slight injuries', assessed by a scale known as 'abbreviated injury scale'.

Disability rate: Since the outcome of the accident is death or disability, it is measured in terms of 'disability-adjusted life years' (DALY), which is the number of healthy years lost due to disability. This depends upon the severity of the accident and the duration of disability.

Types of Accidents

Accidents are grouped into following major types:
- Road traffic accidents
- Railway accidents

- Domestic accidents
- Industrial accidents
- Other accidents include violence, homicide, suicide, air accidents, drowning, poisoning, field accidents, fire accidents, etc.

Road and Traffic Accidents

In the 20th century, the epidemic of road accidents has become a great problem. In India, the major cities such as Mumbai, Bengaluru and Delhi lead in the number of casualties per 1,000 vehicles. India has the highest accident rate in the world, in spite of the fact that the road traffic density is quite low.

Motor vehicle accidents contribute highest in the total deaths due to accidents. For every fatal accident, there are about 10–15 serious injuries and about 50 minor injuries. The accident rate in India is about 8/1,000 registered vehicles. It is highest in USA (80% fatality).

In India, there has been unprecedented increase in the number of motor vehicles in this decade. Death rate is more among men than women. Among men, it is more among children and adults. It is more with two wheelers than four wheelers. Pedestrians are affected most compared to vehicle riders. The important reasons for this type of distribution of accidents are:

- Pedestrians and animals share the roadway
- Poor maintenance of vehicles
- Large number of vehicles
- Overloading of the vehicles
- Low-driving standard
- Poor road conditions, poor street lighting and speed checkers (humps)
- Lack of traffic knowledge
- Overspeed
- Alcoholism by the drivers
- Diversion of attention, while driving due to advertisements on the roadside, etc.

Railway Accidents

There has been an increase in the number of trains and the passengers. Proportionately, casualties are also increasing. This is mainly due to human failure including antisocial activities of the terrorists.

Domestic Accidents

Domestic accident means an accident, which takes place in the home or in immediate surroundings and more generally, all accidents are not connected with traffic, vehicles or sport.

The most frequent accidents are:
- Poisoning (by drugs, insecticides, rat poisons, antiseptics, mushrooms and plants)
- Burns (by a flame, hot liquid, electricity, chemicals, crackers or fireworks)
- Drowning
- Falls
- Bites and other injuries from animals.

Domestic accidents are a frequent cause of death or disability at the extremes of life, throughout childhood and after the 1st year of life. They are an outstanding cause of death in most developed countries. The majority of home accidents (60%) are attributed to carelessness of parents and about 20% to poor maintenance. People who are subjected to attacks of unconsciousness have an increased risk of domestic accidents (e.g. epilepsy, vertigo). These are the accidents occurring in and around the house. These include burns, drowning, poisoning, falls, injuries and from animals.

Burns: By flame, hot liquids, electricity, crackers and chemicals (acids). It is more among women due to dowry problems.

Drowning: This takes place in ponds, rivers and oceans especially during floods and cyclones. It is more among children. It can also occur, while crossing the waterways by boats.

Poisoning: This is often caused by pesticides, kerosene and drugs. Organophosphorus compounds are often used to commit suicide.

Falls: These occur from trees, while picking fruits, coconuts, tapping toddy, from construction of buildings, children falling from rooftops while flying kites, etc.

Injuries: These can occur from any of these above and also from sharp instruments. Injuries can also result from animal bites.

Industrial Accidents

Agricultural industry being the largest industry in India, the agriculturist workers are at risk caused by mechanized equipment, tractors, use of fertilizers, pesticides, etc.

Miscellaneous

Violence: This has been increasing very rapidly caused by war, terrorists and antisocial activities. The predisposing factors are availability of weapons, as a means to solve problems, consumption of alcohol, political unrest, ethnic and communal violence, and such others.

Suicides: It have also been increasing. It is more among women due to ill treatment by the husband and/or family members, dowry harassment, among students due to failure in the examination, among certain people due to depression, heavy economic loss, etc. Common methods adopted are hanging, poisoning and drowning. It is more in males than in females.

Causes

Road Accidents

- Excessive speed
- Defective roads
- Poor street lighting
- Defective layout of cross roads and speed breakers
- Defective vehicles
- Disregard of road signs
- Fatigue
- Alcoholism
- Unusual behaviors of men and animals.

Domestic Accidents

- Keeping the poisons within the reach of the children
- Not labeling them properly
- Constructing the platform to the wells
- Lighting the stove on the floor
- Keeping away the sharp or pointed instruments
- Not to play with animals
- Defective floors
- Bad lighting
- To be careful about the persons who are at risk.

Railway Accidents

- Faulty railway lines
- Negligence of the personnel
- Becoming a victim of terrorist, etc.
- Agent factors are vehicles in road accidents, machines in industries.

Host Factors

Age: Accidents are high in the extremes of age, but due to road traffic accidents, it is high in the age group of 15–34 year.

Sex: Usually accidents are more among men than women. However, in case of bombs, suicides, falls, females are the usual victims.

Medical conditions: Existence of medical conditions such as epilepsy, vertigo, refractive errors, etc. contributes to accidents.

Experience and training: Industrial accidents are more common among inexperienced, untrained and unskilled workers associated with lack of protective devices to the machines.

Habits: Certain habits such as drugs, alcoholism, smoking, etc. play a significant role in accident causation.

Other Factors

Other factors such as fatigue, boredom, anxiety, fantasy also predispose to accidents. 'Accident proneness' is a condition that drives the person subconsciously to take unnecessary risk. In industries, 75% of accidents repeatedly occur among the same 25% of workers. Curiosity (as among toddlers), haste and negligence (e.g. to wear safety gadgets) also contribute to accidents.

Environmental Factors

- Relating to road:
  - Accidents are more common in urban than rural areas
  - Defective, narrow roads, too many curves and slippery roads
  - Presence of cross roads and poor lighting
  - Acute humps, etc.
- Relating to vehicles:
  - Overspeed
  - Poorly maintained
  - Overload
  - Low-driving standard
  - Season
  - Due to fog and bad weather conditions as in winter and rainy season (so more from July to December).
- Mixed traffic:
  - By pedestrians and animals
  - Children playing on the streets.
- Legislation:
  - Ignoring the traffic rules
  - Paucity by the traffic police in enforcing traffic regulations
  - Fraudulent issue of driver's license
  - Traveling on footboard of buses.
- Domestic environment:
  - Greasy floor
  - Vegetables and fruits peelings on the floor
  - Badly lit staircase
  - Dark comers
  - Faulty electrical connections (improper earthing)
  - Hanging of electrical wires
  - Smoking in the bed
  - Keeping burning candles near window curtains

- Forget fullness to switch off liquid petroleum gas (LPG) cylinders
- Use of soft pillows for infants, etc.

Prevention of Accidents

Safety Education

People are educated to impress that accidents are not inevitable, they are caused; so, they can be prevented also. 'If accident is a disease, education is its vaccine.' Safety education is related mainly to prevent road, domestic and industrial accidents. So, the target groups are school children, housewives and industrial workers. They should also be trained in first aid. Parents are educated to take care of their young children, especially if they are naughty.

Safety Measures

Road safety: Roads are made broader, free from curves and intersections properly illuminated during nighttimes, self-luminescent sign boards are set up along the highways, multitrack roads, being ideal preferably with a separate pedestrian traffic. Attention should be given to accident prone areas.

Vehicle safety: Vehicles are fitted with seat belts, shoulder traps, indoor locks and with radial tires.

Personal protection: By the following gadgets:
- Protective device: Class of persons
- Seat belt: Motor drivers
- Crash helmet: Motorcyclists, scooterists and mine workers
- Lead aprons: Persons working in radiology department
- Rubber gloves: Electricians
- Steel capped shoes: Persons engaged in lifting and carrying heavy objects
- Life jacket: Crew of ships.

Machine safety: In industries, the machines must be properly installed, and periodically serviced and maintained. There should not be loose moving parts.

Legislative measures: Following rules must be enforced strictly:
- Wearing of helmets by two wheeler drivers
- Use of seat belts by the drivers and passengers of cars
- Prohibition of consumption of alcohol and drugs such as sedatives, antihistamines, barbiturates and such others
- Prohibition of overload of trucks and buses
- Regular inspection of vehicles and imposition of speed limits
- Periodic medical examination of drivers

- Similarly, Indian Factories Act provides many compulsory safety rules for industrial workers.

Since accidents have assumed the proportion of an epidemic, measures appropriate to control an epidemic should be undertaken. The various measures comprise the following.

Survey: Accidents do not just happen, they are caused. The causes must be determined by a survey, which will indicate the appropriate measures needed in a given situation.

Education: There is widespread belief that accidents are inevitable, this fatalistic attitude must be curbed. It has been aptly said that if accident is a disease, education is a vaccine. Safety education should be part of general education. It should be imparted in schools and factories.

Elimination of factors: The factors, which tend to cause accidents must be sought and eliminated, e.g. reduction of electric voltage, improvement of roads, imposition of speed limits, marking of danger points, provision of fire guards; use of safety equipment in industries, improvement of housing, safe storage of drugs, poisons and weapons, etc.

Emergency care: The care begins at the accident site, continues during transportation and is concluded in the hospital emergency room. At any of these stages, a life may be saved or lost, depending upon the skill of the attending and the availability of needed emergency equipment. To achieve this, there should be an accident services organization at least in all major cities.

Enforcement: Legal and regulatory measures are enforced by the state to prevent accidents such as enforcement of speed limits, compulsory wearing of seat belts and crash helmets, checking of blood-alcohol concentration in drivers and regular inspection of vehicles. In addition, there are factory and industrial laws to ensure safety of the people at work.

Accident research: The future of accident is in research. Such research will be concerned with gathering precise information about the extent, type and other characteristics of accidents, correlating accident experience with personal attributes, and the environment in which accidents occur. Investigating new and better methods of altering human behavior, seeking ways to make environments safer and evaluating more precisely the efficiency of control measures are also included. Accidents are complex phenomenon of multiple causations. The etiological factors may be classified into two broad categories—human and environment. Up to 90% of the factors responsible for accidents are attributed to human errors.

DOMESTIC ACCIDENTS

'Domestic accidents' is meant an accident, which takes place in the home or in its immediate surroundings, and more generally, all accidents are not connected with traffic, vehicles or sport. The most frequent causes of domestic accidents are:

1. Drowning.
2. Burns (by a flame, hot liquid, electricity, crackers or fireworks and chemicals).
3. Falls.
4. Poisoning (e.g. drugs, insecticides, rat poisons and kerosene).
5. Injuries from sharp or pointed instruments.
6. Bites and other injuries from animals.

Drowning

Drowning is the process of experiencing respiratory impairment from submersion/immersion in liquid.

Victims of drowning have a very slim chance of survival after immersion. The victim loses consciousness after approximately 2 minutes of immersion and irreversible brain damage can take place after 4–6 minutes. Therefore, prevention strategies are very important.

Risk Factors of Drowning

The risk factors of drowning are:

1. **Age:** It is one of the major risk factor for drowning. This relationship is often associated with a lapse in supervision. In general, children under 5 years of age have the highest drowning mortality rates worldwide. Canada and New Zealand are the only exceptions, where adult males drown at higher rates.
2. **Gender:** Males are especially at risk of drowning with twice the overall mortality rate of females. They are more likely to be hospitalized than females for non-fatal drowning. Studies suggest that the higher drowning rates among males are due to increased exposure to water and riskier behavior such as swimming alone, drinking alcohol before swimming and boating.
3. **Access to water:** Increased access to water is another risk factor for drowning. Individuals with occupations such as commercial fishing or fishing for subsistence, using small boats in low-income countries are more prone to drowning. Children who live near open water sources, such as ditches, ponds, irrigation channels, or pools are especially at risk.
4. **Other risk factors:** There are other factors that are associated with an increased risk of drowning, such as:
    a. Infants left unsupervised or alone, or with another child in a bathtub.
    b. Unsafe of overcrowded transportation vessels lacking flotation devices.
    c. Alcohol use, near or in the water.
    d. Medical conditions, such as epilepsy.
    e. Tourists unfamiliar with local water risks and features.
    f. Floods and other cataclysmic events, e.g. tsunamis.

Prevention of Drowning

Drowning prevention strategies should be comprehensive and include engineering methods, which help to remove the hazards, legislation to enforce prevention and assure decreased exposure, education for individuals and communities to build awareness of risk and to aid in response, if a drowning occurs.

Engineering methods to eliminate exposure to water hazards are the most effective strategy for drowning prevention. Examples include:

1. Development and implementation of safe water systems such as drainage systems, piped water systems and flood control embankments in flood-prone areas.
2. Building four-sided pool fences or barriers preventing access to standing water.
3. Creating and maintaining safe water zones for recreation.
4. Covering of wells or open cisterns.
5. Emptying buckets and baths, and storing them upside down.

Laws or regulations, which target risk factors for drowning, include laws requiring regular safety checks of transportation vessels, and laws on alcohol use while boating or swimming.

Individual and community education on drowning awareness, learning water survival skills and ensuring the presence of lifeguards at swimming areas are promising strategy to prevent drowning.

Falls

Globally, falls are a major public health problem. An estimated 424,000 fatal falls occur each year, making it the second leading cause of unintentional injury death, after road traffic injuries. Some of the risk factors include:

- Occupations at elevated heights or other hazardous working conditions
- Alcohol or substance use
- Socioeconomic factors including poverty, overcrowded housing and young maternal age

- Underlying medical conditions such as neurological, cardiac or other disabling conditions
- Side effects of medication, physical inactivity and loss of balance, particularly among older people
- Unsafe environment, particularly for those with poor balance and limited vision.

Prevention of Fall

For children, effective interventions include multifaceted community programs; engineering modifications of nursery furniture, playground equipment and other products; and legislation for the use of window guard.

For older individuals, fall prevention programs can include a number of components to identify and modify risk such as:

1. Screening within living environments for risks of falls.
2. Clinical interventions to identify risk factors such as medication review and modification, treatment of low blood pressure, vitamin D and calcium supplementation, treatment of correctable visual impairment.
3. Home assessment and environmental modification for those with known risk factors or a history of falling.
4. Prescription of appropriate assistive devices to address physical and sensory impairments.
5. Muscle strengthening and balance retraining prescribed by a trained health professional.

Burns

Burn is an injury to the skin or other organic tissue primarily caused by heat or due to radiation, radioactivity, electricity, friction or contact with chemicals. Thermal (heat) burns occur when some or all of the cells in the skin or other tissues are destroyed by:
- Hot liquids (scalds)
- Hot solids (contact burns)
- Flames (flame burns).

Burns are a global public health problem, accounting for an estimated 195,000 deaths annually. About 11 million people worldwide require medical attention due to severe burns. The majority of these occur in low- and middle-income countries and almost half occur in the South-East Asia region.

In many high-income countries, burn death rates have been decreasing and the rate of child deaths from burns is currently over seven times higher in low- and middle-income countries than in high-income countries.

Risk Factors of Burns

Gender
Females suffer burns more frequently than males. Women in the South-East Asia region have the highest rate of burns, accounting for 27% of global burn deaths and nearly 70% of burn deaths in the region. The high risk for females is associated with open fire cooking or inherently unsafe cookstoves, which can ignite loose clothing. Open flames used for heating and lighting are also important factors (although understudied).

Age
Along with adult women, children are particularly vulnerable to burns. These are the 11th leading cause of death of children aged 1–9 years and are also the fifth most common cause of non-fatal childhood injuries. While a major risk is improper adult supervision, a considerable number of burn injuries in children result from child maltreatment.

Socioeconomic factors
People living in low- and middle-income countries are at higher risk for burns than people living in high-income countries. Within the countries also, burn risk correlates with socioeconomic status.

Other Risk Factors

There are a number of other risk factors for burns, including:
- Occupations that increase exposure to fire
- Risk factors include poverty, overcrowding and lack of proper safety measures
- Placement of young girls in household roles such as cooking and care of small children
- Underlying medical conditions, including epilepsy, peripheral neuropathy, and physical and cognitive disabilities
- Alcohol abuse and smoking
- Easy access to chemicals used for assault (such as in acid violence attacks)
- Use of kerosene (paraffin) as a fuel source for non-electric domestic appliances
- Inadequate safety measures for liquefied petroleum gas and electricity.

Burns occur mainly in the home and workplace. Community surveys in Bangladesh and Ethiopia showed that 80–90% of burns occur at home. Children and women usually get burns in domestic kitchens, from upset receptacles containing hot liquids or flames, or from cookstove explosions. Men are more likely to get burns in the workplace due to fire, scalds, chemicals and electricity.

Prevention of Burns

Burns are preventable. High-income countries have made considerable progress in lowering rates of burn deaths, through a combination of prevention strategies and improvements in the care of people affected by burns. Most of these advances in prevention and care have been incompletely applied in low- and middle-income countries. Increased efforts to do so would likely lead to significant reduction in rates of burn-related death and disability.

Prevention strategies should address the hazards for specific burn injuries, education for vulnerable populations and training of communities in first aid. An effective burn prevention plan should be multisectoral. There are a number of specific recommendations for individuals, communities and public health officials to reduce burn risk.

First Aid for Burns

Do's

1. Stop the burning process by removing clothing and irrigating the burns.
2. Use cool running water to reduce the temperature of the burn.
3. Extinguish flames by allowing the person to roll on the ground, by applying a blanket, or by using water or other fire-extinguishing liquids.
4. In chemical burns, remove or dilute the chemical agent by irrigating with large volumes of water.
5. Wrap the patient in a clean cloth or sheet and transport to the nearest appropriate facility for medical care.

Don'ts

1. Do not start first aid before ensuring one's own safety (switch off electrical current, wear gloves for chemicals, etc.).
2. Do not apply paste, oil, haldi (turmeric) or raw cotton to the burn.
3. Do not apply ice because it deepens the injury.
4. Avoid prolonged cooling with water because it may lead to hypothermia.
5. Do not open blisters until topical antimicrobials is being applied by a healthcare provider.
6. Do not apply any material directly to the wound, as it might become infected.
7. Avoid application of topical medication until the patient has been placed under appropriate medical care.

Snake Bite

Snake bite is a neglected public health issue in many tropical and subtropical countries. About 5 million snake bites occur each year, resulting in up to 2.5 million envenomings (poisoning from snake bites) at least 100,000 deaths and around three times as many amputations and other permanent disabilities.

The outcome of snake bite depends on numerous factors, including the species of snake, the area of the body bitten, the amount of venom injected, and the health condition of the victim. Feelings of terror and panic are common after a snake bite, and can produce a characteristic set of symptoms mediated by the autonomic nervous system, such as a tachycardia and nausea. Bites from non-venomous snakes can also cause injury, often due to laceration. A bite may also trigger an anaphylactic reaction, which is potentially fatal. First aid recommendations for bite depend on the snakes inhabiting the region, as effective treatment for bite inflicted by some species can be ineffective for others.

The venom of poisonous snakes may be predominantly neurotoxic or predominantly cytolytic. Neurotoxins cause respiratory paralysis and cytolytic venoms cause tissue destruction by digestion and hemorrhage due to hemolysis, and destruction of the endothelial lining of the blood vessels. The manifestations of rattlesnake envenomation are mostly local pain, redness, swelling and extravasation of blood. Perioral tingling, metallic taste, nausea and vomiting, hypotension and coagulopathy may also occur. Neurotoxic envenomation may cause ptosis, dysphagia, diplopia, and respiratory failure. Venom emitted from some types of cobras, almost all vipers, cause necrosis of muscle tissue. Muscle tissues begin to die throughout the body and it results in accumulation of myoglobin in the renal tubules, which leads to acute renal failure. Early clues that a patient has severe envenoming, which include:

- Snake identified as a very dangerous one
- Rapid early extension of local swelling from the site of the bite
- Early tender enlargement of local lymph nodes, indicating spread of venom in the lymphatic system
- Early systemic symptoms: Collapse (hypotension, shock), nausea, vomiting, diarrhea, severe headache, heaviness of the eyelids, inappropriate (pathological) drowsiness or early ptosis/ophthalmoplegia
- Early spontaneous systemic bleeding
- Passage of dark brown/black urine.

First Aid

The Government of India developed a National Snakebite Protocol in 2007, which includes following advice:

1. Reassure the patient. About 70% of all snake bites are from non-venomous species. Only 50% of bites by venomous species actually envenomate the patient.

2. Immobilize in the same way as a fractured limb. Use bandages or cloth to hold the splints, not to block the blood supply or apply pressure. Do not apply any compression in the form of tight ligatures, they do not work and can be dangerous.
3. Do not give alcoholic beverages or stimulants. They are known as vasodilators and they speed up the absorption of venom.
4. Remove any items or clothing, which may constrict the bitten limb, if it swells (rings, bracelets, watches, footwear, etc.).
5. Do not incise or manipulate the bitten site. Do not apply ice.
6. Transport the patient to a medical faculty for definitive treatment.

Antivenom is injected into the person intravenously and works by binding to neutralizing venom enzymes. It cannot undo damage already caused by venom, so antivenom treatment should be sought as soon as possible. Modern antivenoms are usually polyvalent, making them effective against the venom of numerous snake species.

SUICIDE

Human beings are enlisted to the combination of unforeseen circumstances, which needs an immediate intervention. Emotional stress is inclined as a pathologic issue, which physically endangers the affected individual or others, or that significantly disrupts the fundamental equilibrium in his/her environment.

Meaning

The meaning of suicide ('sui' means 'self' and 'cide' means 'murder') is deliberating self-harm. So, it is the action of the individual killing his/her own life. It is the intentional taking of one's own life in a culturally not endorsed manner. Suicide is neither a sign of insanity nor a mark of genius.

Magnitude of Problem

At every 80 seconds, a person commits suicide in the world. The latest report of 1988 issued by the Government of India estimated as much as 25% of deaths due to suicide. Suicide rate is expressed as number of death/100,000 population in each state:
- Puducherry had the highest: 56.3
- Bengaluru: 25.6
- Kerala: 24.7
- Tripura: 21
- Tamil Nadu: 17.9
- West Bengal: 15.7.

Age

Suicide is more in the age group of 18–30 years (43.4%) and 30–50 years (29.9%); below 18 years (12.7%) and above 50 years (14%). The maximum suicides committed by the elderly are men than the women, the percentage in men is 58.7% and in women is 41.3%.

Methods of Suicide

- Organophosphorus or vegetable poison: 31.6%
- Hanging: 25%
- Drowning: 12.2%
- Fire: 9.3%.

Causes

Important causes for suicide in India are:
- Dreadful disease: 14.3%
- Quarrels with in-laws: 6.8%
- Quarrels with spouse: 6.2%
- Love affairs: 4.1 %
- Insanity: 3.4%
- Poverty: 1.6%
- Unemployment: 1.6%
- Dowry disputes: 1.6%
- Failure in examination: 1.4%
- Other unknown causes: 14.3%.

Theories of Suicide

There is no single solitary reason for a person to commit suicide. It is a spectrum of disruptions such as medical, psychosocial, social, cultural and philosophical reasons that are responsible for the tendency:
1. Psychiatric disorders:
    a. Affective disorders and substances abuse in adults.
    b. Conduct disorders and depression in young people.
    c. Alcoholism.
2. Personality disorders:
    a. Aggressive.
    b. Impulsivity.
    c. Hopelessness.
3. Psychosocial factors:
    a. Early parental loss.
    b. Negative life events.
    c. Decreased social support, etc.
4. Genetic factor: Suicide cluster in the families due to the genetic factor of suicide.

5. Biochemical factors:
   a. A deficiency in the neuron.
   b. Serotonin is associated with violent suicidal behavior across all psychiatric diagnosis.
6. Central nervous system:
   a. Epilepsy.
   b. Cerebral multiple sclerosis.
   c. Head injury.
   d. Spinal cord injury.
   e. Parkinson's disease, etc.
7. Gastrointestinal disorders:
   a. Ulcerative colitis.
   b. Infective hepatitis.
   c. Peptic ulcer.
8. Miscellaneous:
   a. Renal dialysis.
   b. Limb amputation.
   c. Drafter laryngectomy.
   d. End stage of cancer.

Assessing Suicide Risk

Person who will commit suicide always ask about thoughts and plans for suicide:
1. Pills hoarded.
2. A rope bought.
3. The procedure lived through in imagination and other preparations are:
   a. Bills paid.
   b. Wills made.
   c. Insurance arranged.
   d. Pets housed.
4. Assess for depression.
5. Living alone from the family setting.
6. Recent life events such as:
   a. Death of a spouse.
   b. Loss of status for the ambitions.
   c. Appearing in court in a sex charge by a married man.
   d. Impending marriage of a child for a lonely widow.
7. The persons who deliberate self-harm such as self-injecting with poison drugs, narcotics, sedatives, consuming overdose of analgesics, sedatives and psychotropic drugs.

Difficulties in Assessing Suicidal Patients

1. Varying degree of distress.
2. Pulse improvement.
3. Anger resentment in uncooperative difficult behavior.
4. False assumptions that openly admitted suicidal ideas are manipulative threats than serious indicators.

Prevention

Individual Methods

Accurate diagnosis and supportive treatment for associated psychiatric disorders. It includes:
- Psychotherapy
- Cognitive therapy by improving self-esteem, social skills and problem-solving ability
- Family therapy
- Group therapy, etc.

Community Methods

1. Improving the mental ability of the high-risk persons and particularly training medical and paramedical workers.
2. Reducing the availability of the means of suicide.
3. Provision for appropriate information and training to relevant organization groups and general public.
4. Provision of emergency telephone services and hot lines.
5. Provision of crisis intervention services to individuals and family counseling.
6. Targeted programs for schools, colleges and hospitals.

Suicidal Prevention in Hospitals

1. Environment.
2. The hospital personnel should have awareness about suicide risks as the principal care.
3. Staff education and attitude includes the basic issues of the suicidal tendencies, first aid and resuscitation. It is a challenge for the staff because of negative attitudes toward suicide.

Suicide calls for emergency intervention. More attention is needed in the community. There are very few of crisis intervention centers in India. Voluntary befriending hot line services are available only in Madras, Delhi and Hyderabad. These services are inadequate to tackle the whole population. There is an urgent necessity to have programs, which are appropriate to our country. This program should include the entire system, the individual, family, school, workplaces and other organizations as well as to the largest community context.

CONCLUSION

Accidents can occur in any age group. Accidents occur due to carelessness, thoughtlessness and overconfidence. According to WHO, accidents are unpremeditated events resulting in recognizable damage. Accidents are classified as roadside accidents, industrial accidents, domestic accidents, drowning, suicide and train accidents. These accidents can be controlled and prevented by eliminating the causative factors, legislative measures, breaking the chain of transmission, promotion of safety measures and health education.

Diabetes Mellitus

CHAPTER 42

INTRODUCTION

Diabetes mellitus (DM) is a disease resulting from a breakdown in the bodies to produce or to utilize insulin, i.e. insulin insufficiency characterized by the abnormalities of the endocrine secretions of the pancreas resulting in disordered metabolism of carbohydrates, fat and protein in the structural abnormalities in a variety of tissues.

A clinical syndrome of hyperglycemia with glycosuria either due to lack of insulin or its inefficient action is termed as DM. It is a metabolic disorder, which involves carbohydrates, fats, proteins and electrolytes, and produces a varied clinical picture. Diabetes is now seen as a heterogeneous group of disease characterized by a state of chronic hyperglycemia resulting from a diversity of etiologies, both environmental and genetic, acting jointly. Characteristically, diabetes is long-term disease with variable clinical manifestations and progression, chronic hyperglycemia, from whatever cause, leads to a number of complications such as cardiovascular, renal, neurological and other intermittent infections.

MAGNITUDE OF DIABETES MELLITUS

Diabetes is an 'iceberg' disease. Although increase in both the prevalence and incidence of type 2 diabetes have occurred globally, they have been especially dramatic in societies, in economic transition, in newly industrialized countries and in developing countries. Currently, the number of cases of diabetes worldwide is estimated to be around 347 million; of these more than 90% are type 2 diabetes. In 2008, an estimated 1.2 million people died from consequences of high blood sugar. More than 80% diabetes deaths occur in low- and middle-income countries.

The apparent prevalence of hyperglycemia depends on the diagnostic criteria used in epidemiological surveys. The global prevalence of diabetes in 2008 was estimated to be 10% in adults aged 25 years. The prevalence of diabetes was highest in the Eastern Mediterranean Region and the regions of the America (11% for both sexes) and lowest in the World Health Organization (WHO), and in European and Western Pacific Regions (9% for both sexes). The magnitude of diabetes and other abnormalities of glucose tolerance are considerably higher than the above estimates, if the categories of 'impaired fasting' and 'impaired glucose tolerance' are also included. The estimated prevalence of diabetes was relatively consistent across the income groupings of countries. Low-income countries showed the lowest prevalence (8% for both sexes) and the upper-middle-income countries showed the highest (10% for both sexes).

Unfavorable modification of lifestyle and dietary habits that are associated with urbanization are believed to be the most important factors for the development of diabetes. The prevalence of diabetes is approximately twice in urban areas than in rural population. The population in India has an increased susceptibility to DM. This propensity was demonstrated by multiple surveys of migrant Indians residing in Fiji and Singapore.

EPIDEMIOLOGY

Epidemiology is worldwide in distribution. Its prevalence rate is 1–2% and affects 120 million people worldwide. Its incidence is rising. It is estimated that it will affect 220 million by the year 2020. It is predicted that by the year 2025, India will be the capital of diabetes. The ratio between type 2 and type 1 is 3:1 in most countries; 50% patients of type 2 diabetes remain undetected till they seek medical advice for some ailments; hence, they mostly present with complications. November 14 is observed as the World Diabetic Day to create awareness amongst the people.

Type 2 DM is common in all population enjoying an affluent lifestyle and predominantly occurs in adults. It runs in families and increasing age, obesity and certain ethnic groups predispose to it. In poor countries, diabetes is a disease of the rich and in rich countries, it is a disease of the poor. The onset may be accelerated by pregnancy, drug treatment and intercurrent infection. The prevalence of type 2 DM is highest in Pacific Islands, India, China and United States of America (USA), and lowest in Russia. The increasing weight (obesity) in young and adolescents due to overeating and sedentary lifestyles is becoming a health hazard throughout the world and may lead to epidemic form of diabetes.

Epidemiological Features

Agent

1. Pancreatic disorders, e.g. inflammatory, neoplastic and other disorders such as cystic fibrosis.
2. Defects in the formation of insulin, e.g. synthesis of an abnormal biologically less active insulin molecules.
3. Destruction of beta (β) cells, e.g. viral infections and chemical agents.
4. Decreased insulin sensitivity due to decreased numbers of adipocyte and monocyte insulin receptors.
5. Genetic defects, e.g. mutation of insulin gene.
6. Autoimmunity.

Host

Age: Diabetes can occur at any age, surveys indicate that prevalence rises steeply with age, non-insulin-dependent diabetes mellitus (NIDDM) usually comes to light in the middle years of life and thereafter begins to rise. Malnutrition-related diabetes affects large numbers of young people.

Sex: In some countries, i.e. in United Kingdom (UK), the male and female suffer equally. In Asia, males are more prone than females.

Genetic factors: As follows:
1. Concordance for NIDDM was approximately 90%.
2. Insulin-dependent diabetes mellitus (IDDM) concordance was only 50%, it is not totally a genetic entity.

Immune mechanisms: Some evidence of both cell mediated and humoral activity against islet cells.

Obesity: It has long been accepted as a risk factor for NIDDM.

Environmental risk factors: Are as follows:
1. Sedentary lifestyle: This appeals to be an important risk factor for the development of NIDDM.
2. Diet: Studies indicated that the diet of diabetics did not appear to differ in any marked way from that of nondiabetics except in quantity.
3. Malnutrition: Protein-energy malnutrition (PEM) in early infancy and childhood may result in partial failure of β-cell function.
4. Viral infections: Viruses are rubella, mumps and human coxsackievirus.
5. Chemical agents: A number of chemical agents are known to be toxic to β cells, e.g. alloxan, streptozotocin, rodenticides, etc. High intake of cyanide-producing foods, e.g. cassava and certain beans also have toxic effects on β cells.
6. Stress: Surgery, trauma and stress of situations, internal or external may cause the disease.

Other factors: Include social factors such as occupation, nutritional status, religion, economic status, education, urbanization and changes in lifestyles, which are elements of what is broadly known as social class.

TYPES OF DIABETES MELLITUS

There are two types of DM:
1. Growth onset or juvenile diabetes.
2. Maturity onset.

Juvenile Diabetes

Juvenile diabetes is also known as IDDM. Persons with juvenile diabetes usually lack insulin because of primary derangement in the insulin-producing cells or in some other hormonal, or enzymatic activity necessary for regulating the secretion or the use of insulin and require exogenous insulin therapy.

Maturity Onset Diabetes

Maturity onset diabetes is also known as NIDDM. Those with maturity onset diabetes have insulin circulating in the blood and respond more satisfactorily to oral hypoglycemic drugs. Both types produce effects on the capillaries of every organ, system and on the peripheral nerves.

CLASSIFICATION

Basically, it is divided into two major categories, but other types of secondary diabetes have been taken from the recommendations by the National Diabetic Data Group. The primary diabetes is either type 1 or type 2, the course of which is not known. Type 1 diabetes implies IDDM patients require insulin for their management, otherwise they run the risk of developing ketoacidosis. Type 2 diabetes, though implies NIDDM, yet it does not mean that these patients do not require insulin. It simply means that patients can easily be controlled without insulin except in a few circumstances for example, type 2 diabetes with complications. These two types do not show an absolute distinction in the matter of age and requirement of insulin.

Maturity-onset diabetes of young (MODY) syndrome is an example of such an overlap. Secondary diabetes refers to those conditions where the cause of diabetes is detectable or is evident.

WHO Classification of Diabetes Mellitus

Primary Diabetes

1. Type 1 DM (IDDM):
   - Immune mediated (islet cell antibodies present)
   - Idiopathic.
2. Type 2 DM (NIDDM):
   - Obese
   - Nonobese.
3. Specific types of diabetes:
   - Genetic defects of antibody cell function, e.g. MODY 1 to MODY 6
   - Genetic defect in insulin action:
     - Type A insulin resistance.
   - Other genetic syndrome associated with DM are Klinefelter's syndrome, Down syndrome, Turner's syndrome, diabetes insipidus, optic atrophy and deafness (DIDMOAD) syndrome, and others.

Secondary Diabetes

1. Diseases of exocrine pancreas.
2. Pancreatitis, cystic fibrosis, hemochromatosis, Malnutrition-related diabetes mellitus (MRDM), neoplasm and pancreatectomy.
3. Endocrinopathies (hormonal): Symptoms such as Cushing's syndrome, acromegaly, pheochromocytoma, hypothyroidism and glucagonoma.
4. Viral infections (rubella, cytomegalovirus)
5. Drug-induced (thiazides, steroids, antiretroviral).
6. Other types or abnormalities such as:
   - Impaired glucose tolerance (IGT)
   - Gestational diabetes mellitus (GDM).

Type 1 diabetes or IDDM is the most common form of the disease. Its onset is typically abrupt and is usually seen in individuals less than 30 years of age. It is lethal unless promptly diagnosed and treated. This form of diabetes is immune mediated in over 90% of cases and idiopathic in less than 10% cases. The rate of destruction of pancreatic β cells is quite variable; rapid in some individuals and slow in others. Type 1 diabetes is usually associated with ketosis in its untreated state. It occurs mostly in children, the incidence is highest among 10–14 years old age group, but occasionally occurs in virtually absent, elevated plasma glucagon and when pancreatic β cells fail to respond to all insulinogenic stimuli. Exogenous insulin is therefore required to reverse the catabolic state, prevent ketosis, reduce the hyperglucagonemia and reduce blood glucose.

Type 2 diabetes is much more common than type 1 diabetes. It is often discovered by chance. It is typically gradual in onset and occurs mainly in the middle aged and elderly, frequently mild, slow to ketosis and is compatible with long survival, if given adequate treatment. Its clinical picture is usually complicated by the presence of other disease processes. Impaired glucose tolerance describes a state intermediate 'at-risk' group between DM and normality. It can only be defined by the oral glucose tolerance test.

ETIOLOGY

Genetic predisposition and environmental factors are implicated in the pathogenesis of DM. The pattern of inheritance and interactions between genetic and environmental factors differ in both type 1 and type 2.

Type 1 Diabetes Mellitus

Genetic Factors

Type 1 DM is not only genetically determined but also increases susceptibility to the disease, may be inherited. About 95% of patients with type 1 DM have *human leukocyte antigen (HLA)-DR_3* or *HLA-DR_4* genes, which are markers of susceptibility and predispose to increased risk of the disease.

Heredity does not play a major role in type 1 DM as concordance rate among identical twins is just 30–50%. A child with diabetic mother has 3% chance of inheriting it, while a child with diabetic father has 6% chance of inheriting it and if both parents are diabetic, then there is 12–25% chance of inheriting type 1 DM.

Environmental Factors

The rising incidence of type 1 DM suggests involvement of some environmental factors such as infection (rubella, coxsackie) and consumption of cow's milk. This theory is referred as hygiene hypothesis.

Autoimmunity and Immune Destruction

Human leukocyte antigen linkage, association with other autoimmune diseases, lymphocytic infiltration of β cells and use of immunosuppressive drugs suggest that type 1 DM is an autoimmune disease. Autoantibodies destroy the β-cell leaving behind intact alpha (α) cells.

Type 2 Diabetes Mellitus

Type 2 DM is neither HLA linked nor there any evidence of autoimmunity or virus playing a role. Various factors that play a role in its pathogenesis are detailed below.

Genetics

Concordance rate of 100% for monozygotic twins in type 2 only indicates that genetics influence is powerful in type 2 than type 1, but there is little information about 'what material is inherited'. Genetic and environmental factors combine to cause both the insulin inaction and β-cell failure.

Abnormal Insulin Secretion

Abnormal insulin secretion is primary and basic defect responsible for development of diabetes. This is genetically determined by chromosome 11.

Progressive β-cell Failure

The hyperinsulinemia and insulin resistance lead to β cell exhaustion.

Environmental Factors

Epidemiological data reveal that physical inactivity and obesity act as diabetogenic factors only in those patients who are genetically susceptible to develop type 2 diabetes.

Age

The occurrence of type 2 diabetes after 30 years of age indicates the age as an important risk factor.

Gestation

Diabetes may occur for the first time in pregnancy in women who are genetically predisposed to type 1 and type 2. This is due to relative lack of insulin. Although insulin levels are higher in pregnancy due to stimulating effect of placental lactogens on β cells, but these are still insufficient to cater the metabolic needs during pregnancy resulting in hyperglycemia and development of gestational diabetes. Therefore, pregnancy is also a factor for determination of diabetes in genetically predisposed women.

Insulin-resistance Syndrome (Syndrome X)

Insulin resistance is related not only to type 2 diabetes but also seen independently in obesity, hypertension and hyperlipidemia, i.e. different components of syndrome 'X' or metabolic syndrome. From these findings, it appears that type 2 is polygenic, each component being represented by a separate gene, which gets expressed during life at different stages with interactions of environmental factors or change in the lifestyles. Only presence of insulin resistance does not mean diabetes, therefore, abnormal insulin secretion is essential to produce diabetes. Secondly, it has been hypothesized that diabetes is due to a combination of major and minor genes affecting insulin secretion, action and obesity. Insulin secretion is under the influence of major genes, while other factors are governed by minor genes.

In obese patients with type 2 diabetes, the association of hyperglycemia, hyperinsulinemia, dyslipidemia and hypertension, which lead to coronary artery disease and stroke, may result from a genetic defect producing insulin resistance, with the latter being exaggerated by obesity. It has been proposed that insulin resistance predisposes to hyperglycemia, which results in hyperinsulinemia (which may or may not be of sufficient magnitude to correct the hyperglycemia), and this excessive insulin level then contributes to high levels of triglycerides and increased sodium retention by renal tubules, thus inducing hypertension. High levels of insulin can stimulate endothelial proliferation to initiate atherosclerosis.

PATHOPHYSIOLOGY

Insulin is a hormone, secreted by the β cells in the islets of Langerhans in pancreas. It promotes:
- The storage of glycogen in the liver
- The utilization of glucose in the muscles
- The storage of fat in adipose tissue by enhancing the transport of glucose across the cell wall.

Because of the nonproportion in the role of insulin released and the amount of glucose in the portal vein, the diabetes occurs. In the absence of sufficient insulin, the raised blood sugar may increase the transfer of glucose into the cells. Glucose in the blood comes from ingested carbohydrate and from the conversion of amino acids, and fatty acids to glucose by the liver.

Normally, the β cells in the pancreas stimulate or withhold insulin secretion minute by minute, according to changing blood glucose levels. The characteristic of diabetic state is the metabolization of fat and protein, when the muscles cannot utilize glucose, the liver forms acid substances called ketone bodies to supply energy to the muscles. The body compensates for the acidosis by hyperventilation and the loss of sodium, potassium, chloride and water in the urine. If the intake of these substances is insufficient, dehydration, electrolyte imbalance and uncompensated acidosis develop. If the concentration of glucose in the blood is about 150–200 mg/100 mL, the kidney does not reabsorb all of the filtered glucose, which then appears in the urine, the condition is called glycosuria.

Long-term diabetes is associated with atherosclerosis of large vessels of the brain, heart, kidneys and extremities, and thickening of the walls of the capillary in the eye muscles and skin. The damage to the peripheral nerves (neuropathy) is related to persistent hyperglycemia.

Type 1 DM

Type 1 DM is considered as an autoimmune disease in which there are antibodies against β cells that destroy the β-cell mass resulting in lack of production of insulin. The factors that govern pathophysiology of type 1 DM are:
- Insulin deficiency (no insulin)
- Increased counterregulatory hormones:
  - It includes unrestrained gluconeogenesis, lipolysis and ketogenesis
  - Peripheral utilization of glucose blocked.
- Ketonemia/Ketoacidosis
- Protein catabolism resulting in muscle wasting and negative nitrogen balance.

In type 1 DM, there is either absolute or relative deficiency of insulin, which results in significant abnormalities in the metabolism of carbohydrate, proteins and fat. There is increase in counterregulatory hormones, e.g. GlucaGen leading to hyperglucagonemia. The net result is gluconeogenesis, lipolysis and ketogenesis and underutilization of peripheral glucose (hyperglycemia). All these metabolic disturbances lead to clinical picture of polyuria (osmotic diuresis), wasting of muscles (protein catabolism), vulvitis (glycosuria) and ketoacidosis.

Type 2 DM

- Insulin resistance:
  - Hepatic and peripheral
  - Postprandial (insulin-mediated glucose uptake is impaired especially in skeletal muscles).
- Hyperglucagonemia:
  - Enhanced hepatic glucose output
  - Impaired peripheral utilization.
- Ketoacidosis rarely develops as insulin, whatsoever secreted is sufficient to prevent ketoacidosis.

Insulin resistance is a characteristic feature of type 2 DM that occurs both in obese and non-obese individuals. It is due to three factors:

1. Abnormal insulin molecule.
2. An excess of circulating insulin antagonists.
3. Target tissue defect either at receptor or postreceptor level. It is the common cause.

In type 2 diabetes, there is hyperinsulinemia and insulin resistance indicating β-cell stimulation. Later on stimulation is followed by β-cell exhaustion and there is reduction of pancreatic β-cell mass with reduction in insulin levels. The characteristic pathological change in islet cells (β cell) is amyloid deposition, which in fact, is not the cause of diabetes, but reflects pancreatic amyloidosis in type 2 diabetes.

When β cells are reduced by 20–30%, the uninvolved α cells produce glucagon and lead to hyperglycemia. Insulin resistance and inherited defect in type 2 diabetes tends to raise blood sugar by stimulating insulin secretion and thus results in hyperinsulinemia. When maximal insulin secretary capacity has been exceeded, any further rise in blood sugar causes decline in insulin secretion due to β-cell exhaustion or failure.

Hyperglycemia is a characteristic feature of both types of DM, whether it is due to lack of insulin or due to its inaction, results due to increased hepatic output of glucose as well as poor glucose utilization by peripheral tissues.

CLINICAL FEATURES

Juvenile Diabetes

In most of the cases, onset is abrupt with:
- Weight loss
- Weakness
- Polyuria
- Polydipsia
- Polyphagia.

Maturity Onset Diabetes

In case of maturity onset, the majority of patients are overweight. When the condition is discovered, the onset is insidious, symptoms may be mild:
- Early symptoms are:
  - Sweating
  - Fatigue
  - Irritability
  - Itching of the skin
  - Blurring of the vision
  - Muscle cramps
  - Postprandial drowsiness
  - Nocturia
  - Loss of weight
  - Delayed wound healing.

- Later symptoms are:
  - Polyuria
  - Polydipsia
  - Polyphagia.

  If untreated, it may lead to ketoacidosis and coma.

COMPLICATIONS

Complications of insulin treatment are:
- Hypoglycemia
- Diabetic ketoacidosis.

  Other complications include:
- Vascular complications
- Diabetic retinopathy
- Infections.

  Infections are more protracted and serious in diabetics for the following reasons:
- Hyperglycemia causes decreased leukocytes and phagocytosis
- Ketonemia causes decreased leukocyte migration.

PREVENTION

Preventive health care for DM may include primary, secondary, early detection and control of disease or tertiary control of complications.

Primary Prevention

Primary prevention is directed toward avoidance of obesity and weight reduction, if necessary to prevent the onset of NIDDM. Although hereditary or genetic factors have a role in development of IDDM and NIDDM, genetic counseling is still not recommended because of the unknown nature of the pattern of transmission. This does not deny family history as a risk factor particularly for NIDDM.

Secondary Prevention

Secondary prevention estimated that there are 4–6 million persons with undiagnosed DM. Although mass screening has been ruled out, many authorities believe that screening of high-risk persons is a better use of resources in the screening of the entire population. IDDM is not effectively identified with screening approach because of its agents onset. Screening programs can be carried out in health department, neighborhood clinics, hospital outpatient clinics, physicians, officers, industry and health workers and mobile health units offering screening programs for diabetes and other health problems. Follow-up of positive findings is essential. When diabetes is detected, it must be adequately treated. The aims of treatment are:
- To maintain blood glucose levels as close within normal limits
- To maintain ideal body weight
- Diet and oral antidiabetic drugs
- Diet and insulin, good control of the blood glucose protects against the development of complications.

  Proper management of the diabetics is most important to prevent complications. Routine checking of blood sugar of urine for proteins and ketones of blood pressure, visual activity and weight should be done periodically. The feet should be examined for any defective block circulation, loss of sensation and the health of the skin.

Self-care

A crucial element in secondary prevention is self-care, i.e. the diabetic person should take a major responsibility for his/her own care with medical guidance, for example, adherence to diet and drug regimens, examination of their own urine and if possible, blood glucose monitoring, self-administration of insulin, abstinence from alcohol, maintenance of optimum weight, attending periodic check-ups, recognition of symptoms associated with glycosuria and hypoglycemia, etc.

Home Blood Glucose Monitoring

Assessment of control has been greatly aided by the recent facilities of immediate, reasonably accurate capillary blood glucose measurements by any of the many devices now available. The patient should carry an identification card, showing his/her name, address, telephone number and the details of treatment they receive. In short, he/she must have a working knowledge of diabetes to optimize the effectiveness of primary healthcare services.

Tertiary Prevention

Diabetes is a major cause of disability through its complications, e.g. blindness, kidney failure, coronary thrombosis, gangrene of the lower extremities, etc. The main objective at the tertiary level is to organize a specialized clinics (diabetic clinics) and units capable of providing diagnostic and management skills of a high order. There is a great need to establish such clinics in large towns and cities. The tertiary level should also be involved in basic, clinical and epidemiological research. It has also been recommended that local and national registries for diabetics should be established.

NURSING MANAGEMENT

The goals of therapy irrespective of the type of diabetes are:
1. To achieve a normal metabolic state by bringing the blood glucose to normal or near normal levels without inducting hypoglycemic episodes.
2. To maintain ideal body weight.
3. To keep the patient symptoms free.
4. To allow the patients to lead a normal life.
5. To prevent or retard the onset of complications.

In type 2 DM, in addition to the goals of therapy mentioned above, there is need to control the associated conditions such as obesity, hypertension, dyslipidemia and coronary artery disease, etc.

Objectives of Nursing Management

1. To correct biochemical and metabolic abnormalities.
2. To attain and maintain optimal body weight.
3. Prevent complications.
4. To promote patients education.

These objectives can be achieved by following the guidelines below.

Psychological Considerations

The limitations impaired by a therapeutic diet, fear of continuous medication of therapeutic diet, fear of continuous medication of insulin or a hypoglycemic preparation and fear of complications (blindness, insulin shock and strokes of which they have heard). They must be reassured that although the disease cannot be cured, it can be controlled to live a reasonably normal life. Many centers have facilities for group discussions among diabetics, which prove helpful.

Diet

The purpose of dietary management is to achieve normal metabolism as far as possible by measures described below:
1. Diet and drug treatment should be matched, so as to avoid fluctuations in blood glucose. Daily diet intake should be kept constant as far as possible.
2. To keep ideal body weight, total energy intake should be specified.
3. Dietary constituents, i.e. carbohydrates, fats and proteins must be in adequate proportions.
4. Frequent small meals should be advised to prevent glycemic peaks and troughs.

Diet Formulations

Daily energy requirement for an individual is calculated according to age, weight, height and activity. On an average 36 kcal/kg for non-obese man and 34 kcal/kg for non-obese woman is reasonable as initial treatment; further adjustment may be done, if necessary to achieve the ideal body mass index (BMI) (BMI of 22 kg/m^2). The recommended allocation of calories to various dietary constituents include carbohydrate providing 50–50% of total calories, proteins 10–15% and fats 30–35% of total energy intake. The diet should be palatable and according to the taste of the patient.

Carbohydrates: All the carbohydrates prescribed should be taken in the form of starch and complex sugars. About 100–300 g of carbohydrates spread over three meals (60 g each) and three snacks (30 g each) with ½ liter of milk (30 g) are advised. The division of carbohydrates into frequent meals and snacks provides good matching between drug treatment and diet; lowers blood lipids and prevents hypoglycemia. Simple sugars, i.e. glucose and sucrose are avoided.

Fiber content of the diet should be high. Fiber-rich food (barley, oats, legumes, beans and peas) supplemented with soluble fibers (guar gum and pectin) improves glycemic control.

Proteins: Amino acids stimulate insulin secretion, hence proteins combined with carbohydrates in diet, lower the blood sugar effectively. Proteins stimulate appetite also. Daily intake of proteins should be 60–100 g (1.0–1.5 g/kg) divided between meals constituting 10–15% of total calories.

Fats: The fat intake should be adjusted to bring the total calories to the desired level. The amount varies from 50 to 150 g daily divided between meals. The fat should contain 10% as polyunsaturated fat.

Alcohol: It is prohibited, if a person is obese, hypertensive and hyperlipidemic. Otherwise, alcohol in moderation (30–60 mL) may be allowed, but caloric value of alcohol taken must be adjusted within the daily total caloric intake.

Salts: Normal salt intake of 6 g daily is allowed to diabetics. It is reduced to half, i.e. 3 g if the diabetic is hypertensive also.

Sweetening agents: Saccharin, cyclamate and non-nutritive sweeteners are allowed to diabetics on low-caloric diet.

Types of Diet

Low energy and weight reducing: It is for obese type 2 diabetes treated with insulin and oral hypoglycemic agent (OHA). These diets provide daily deficit of 500 kcal and induce a weekly loss of 0.5 kg of weight. Patients on this diet should omit snacks in between meals. Weight reduction restores insulin sensitivity.

Weight maintenance diet: It is prescribed to non-obese (normal BMI) type 2 diabetes. This diet is low in fat and

rich in carbohydrates. The fat consumed should be mostly monosaturated or polyunsaturated fat. Diet and weight control are the foundations of diabetics management, reasonable expectations for the nutritional management of the patient with diabetes are to:
1. Provide all the essential food constituents.
2. Supply enough calories for optimum growth.
3. Achieve and maintain ideal weight.
4. Enquire energy needs.
5. Achieve normal range blood glucose levels.
6. Lower blood lipid levels.

The meals should be measured and served at regular intervals and obesity is to be corrected as quickly as possible. The menu is varied with emphasis on the patient's likes and dislikes, lifestyles and to provide variety.

Calorie Requirement

The calorie intake should equal the energy output to avoid a positive balance with a resultant hyperglycemia and weight increase, or a negative balance that may lead to an excessive fat breakdown with the risk of ketoacidosis. The dietary prescription indicates the number of calories required each day and the proportions of these calories to be allocated to carbohydrate, protein and fat. The first step in preparing the meal plan is to determine the patient's basic calorie requirements, taking into consideration age, sex, body weight and degree of activity. The simple method to assess calorie needed is to multiply ideal weight by 30–35 cal/kg, for weight reduction, a 15–20 cal/kg ideal weight is suitable.

Lifestyle Modifications

Lifestyle modification is the mainstay of treatment of impaired glucose tolerance (IGT) and type 2 obese DM. It not only helps to reduce weight or BMI but also lowers insulin resistance as well as restores insulin sensitivity, therefore:
- Encourage healthy lifestyles for all individuals
- Prescribe lifestyle modifications for all patients with prediabetes and DM with the prehypertension and hypertension
- The components of lifestyle modifications are given in Table 42.1.

Exercise

A moderate amount of exercise is an important part of diabetic treatment. It promotes the use of glucose and may diminish the amount of insulin or oral hypoglycemic agents to control the blood sugar level. It also stimulates and improves the circulation, helps to maintain muscle tone, prevents obesity and promotes a sense of well-being. Regular physical exercise is an essential part of diabetic management. The benefits of exercise are:

Table 42.1: Lifestyle modification recommendation

Modifications	Recommendations
Weight reduction	Maintain normal body weight [body mass index (BMI) 18.5–24.9 kg/m^2]
Eating plan	Adopt a diet rich in fruits, vegetables and low-fat dairy products with reduced content of saturated and total fat
Dietary sodium restriction	Reduce dietary sodium intake to < 100 mmol/day (2.4 g sodium or 6 g sodium chloride)
Aerobic physical exercise	Regular aerobic physical activity, e.g. brisk walking at least 30 min/day, most day of the week or 90 min/twice a week or 150 min/week
Moderation of alcohol consumption	Men: Limit to < 2 drinks/day Women and lighter weight persons: Limit to < 1* drink/day

*1 drink = ½ or 15 mL ethanol (e.g. 12 oz beer, 5 oz wine, 1.5 oz 80 proof whiskey)

1. It contributes to weight loss and improves the insulin sensitivity.
2. Lowers blood sugar by increasing peripheral glucose utilization.
3. Improves lipid profile, lowers low-density lipoprotein (LDL) and increase high-density lipoprotein (HDL).
4. Improves circulation, cardiovascular fitness and sense of well-being.
5. Improves muscle strength and flexibility.

The risks of exercise in diabetes include precipitation of angina in patients with asymptomatic coronary artery disease, risk of hypoglycemia in patients receiving insulin and worsening of hyperglycemia, and long-term complications.

Nurse must keep benefits and risks of exercise in mind before prescribing regular exercise program. The exercise tips (Do's and Don'ts) are given in Table 42.2.

Table 42.2: Exercise tips (Do's and Don'ts)

Do's	Don'ts
Always consult the doctor before starting the exercise routine Start gradually, but regularly	Do not exercise on an empty stomach
Exercise at the same time everyday	Avoid exercise soon after injecting insulin

Contd...

Contd...

Do's	Don'ts
Participate in active sports such as jogging, swimming, etc.	Do not exercise if your blood sugar values are high and your diabetes is not under control
Keep sugar or something sweet handy to avoid low blood sugar levels	
Always have someone around who can detect symptoms of hypoglycemia	

All patients of diabetes must be assessed for cardiovascular status and existing long-term complications before advising them to take up an exercise program. A stress electrocardiography (ECG) should be done in all diabetics above the age of 30 years:

1. For most patients, the exercise program should include both aerobic and resistance exercises. Patient should begin with aerobic exercises. In the absence of contraindication, patients with diabetes should be encouraged to perform resistance exercise involving all the muscle groups. Diabetes Prevention Program (DPP) data showed that a 7% reduction in body weight with moderate exercise (150 min/week) resulted in 58% reduction in the incidence of diabetes.
2. The frequency of exercise should be three to five times a week.
3. Exercise session: Short bursts of physical exercise 30 min/day about four times a week is sufficient to get rid of fat and burn up glucose. Each session should include a warm up phase (5 minute), exercise period (10–20 minute) and cool down period (5 minute). The patient should gradually increase the exercise period.

Health Education

Explanations are made in simple lay terms and demonstrations are broken into steps, slowly repeated as often as necessary and sufficient opportunity is provided to the patient to practice illustrations. Films, written explanations and directions are used for clarification. Recording material (books, pamphlets) written for diabetes should be made available.

CONCLUSION

Diabetes mellitus can occur at any age. It occurs due to agent factors and other environmental factors such as lack of exercise, high intake of saturated fat, surgery and removal of pancreas. Its prevention and disease. Prevention and control is required to reduce the burden of disease. Prevention and control at primary level, secondary level and tertiary level is required.

Mental Illness

CHAPTER 43

INTRODUCTION

Health is a condition in which all functions of the body and mind are normally active. Health is a complete state of physical, mental, social and spiritual not merely absence of disease or infirmity. Accordingly mental health is said to be a mentally healthy, where the individual has a perfect state of balance with the surrounding world, having harmonious relationship with others, the intelligence, memory learning capacity, judgment are normal, not having any internal conflicts, accepts criticism sportively has got good self-emotional control, solve the problems intelligently, has full self-confidence, well-adjusted with others and is satisfied with what he/she has possessed; totally person in cheerful and calm.

Mental health is not mere absence of mental illness. A mentally healthy person has three main characteristics:

1. He/She feels comfortable about themselves, i.e. he/she feels reasonably secure and adequate. They neither underestimate nor overestimates their own ability. He/She accepts shortcomings and has self-respect.
2. The mentally healthy person feels right towards others. This means that he/she is able to be interested in others and to love them. Person has friendships that are satisfying and lasting. He/She is able to feel a part of a group without being submerged by it. They are able to like and trust others. He/She takes responsibility for their neighbors and fellow men.
3. The mentally healthy person is able to meet the demands of life. He/She does something about the problems as they arise. They are able to think for themself and to take their own decisions. He/She sets reasonable goals for themself. He/She shoulders their daily responsibilities. He/She is not bowled over by their own emotions of fear, anger, love or guilt.

DEFINITION

The opinion and the mental health community differ as to what mental health and mental illness are:

1. Mental health has been defined in many ways. This definition includes the ability to do the following:
   - Be flexible
   - Be successful
   - Form close relationships
   - Make appropriate judgment
   - Solve problems
   - Cope with daily stress
   - Have a positive sense of self.
2. Mental illness is defined as experiencing the following:
   - Impaired ability to think, feel, make sound judgment and to adapt
   - Difficulty in coping or inability to cope with reality
   - Difficulty in forming or inability to form strong personal relationships.

SIGNIFICANCE OF PROBLEM

Mental illness is a global problem. It causes considerable disability, imposing a heavy burden of suffering and economic loss. It constitutes 8% of global burden of all diseases measured in disability-adjusted life years (DALY).

The prevalence of mental illness is estimated to be about to per 1,000 populations. During the whole lifetime, about 25% of persons suffer from one or the other form of mental illness. About 25% of the patients attending hospital will have a psychological basis. The 80% of the mental illness are found in the developing countries, 30% of which occur among children below 15 years. Globally there are about 40 million cases of severe mental illness, 20 million cases of epilepsy and about 200 million cases with minor mental illness, and neurological conditions.

In India, the situation is as follows:
- Serious mental disorder: 10–20 per 1,000 (10–12 million)
- Minor mental disorder: 20–60 per 1,000
- Emotional problems: 200 per 1,000.

About 30% of the cases occur among children below 15 years, majority of those cases being mental retardation. In India, about 2.5 lakh new cases are added per year and this has been gradually increasing.

ETIOLOGY

Mental illness such as physical illness is due to multiple causes. There are many known factors of agent, host and environment in the natural histories of mental disorders. Among the known factors are detailed below. The etiology of mental health is very complex and not well understood. A large group of mental disorders are still called 'functional' because no pathological, biochemical or hormonal changes are discovered with the present investigative techniques. Various etiological factors are as follows:

1. Heredity: It may be an important factor in some cases. A child born to both the schizophrenia parents has 40 times higher risk of having schizophrenia than a child born to normal parents.
2. Physical factors (organic conditions): Conditions such as infections, toxins, tumors, vascular injury, nutritional deficiency, metabolic defects and degenerative and autoimmune processes, endocrine diseases and chronic diseases also result in various types of organic mental disease; senile dementia is Alzheimer's disease.

    Mental illnesses may have their origin in organic conditions such as cerebral arteriosclerosis, neoplasms, metabolic diseases, neurological diseases, endocrine diseases and chronic diseases such as tuberculosis, leprosy, epilepsy, etc.
3. Socioenvironmental factors: The social and environmental factors associated with mental ill health comprise such as worries, anxieties, emotional stress, tension, frustration, unhappy marriages, broken homes, poverty, economic insecurity, drug addiction, lack of cooperation during crises by the dear ones, sexual starvation, sexual assault, cruelty, industrialization, urbanization, changing family structure, population mobility, economic insecurity, cruelty, rejection, neglect and the like, etc. So to produce any disease, there must be a combination of genetic and environmental factors. The social environment not only determines the individual's attitudes but also provides the 'framework' within which mental health is formulated.

Environmental factors other than psychological ones capable of producing abnormal human behavior are:

1. Toxic substances: Carbon disulfide, mercury, manganese, tin, lead compounds, etc.
2. Psychotropic drugs: These are barbiturates, alcohol and griseofulvin.
3. Nutritional factors: Deficiency of thiamine, pyridoxine.
4. Minerals: Deficiency of iodine.
5. Infective agents: Infectious disease (e.g. measles, rubella) during the pre-, peri- and post-natal periods of life may have adverse effects on the brain's development and the integration of mental functions.
6. Traumatic factors: Road and occupational accidents.
7. Radiation: Nervous system is most sensitive to radiation during the period of neural development. In addition to the action, there are certain key points in the development of the human being, which are important from the point of view of mental health. These are:
    a. Prenatal period: Pregnancy is a stressful period for some women. They need help not only for their physical but also emotional needs.
    b. First 5 years of life: The roots of mental health are in early childhood. The infant and young child should experience a warm, intimate and continuous relationship with his/her mother and father. It is in this relationship where underlies the development of mental health. It follows that broken homes are likely to produce behavior disorders in children and this has been confirmed by several studies.
    c. School child: Everything that happens in the school affects the mental health of the child. The programs and practices of the school may satisfy or frustrate the emotional needs of the child. Children who have emotional problems may need child guidance clinic or psychiatric services. From the standpoint of the child's mental health and their effectiveness in learning, proper teacher-pupil relationship and climate of the classroom are very important.
    d. Adolescence: The transition from adolescence to manhood is often a stormy one and fraught with dangers to mental health, manifested in the form of mental ill health among the young and juvenile delinquents in particular. The basic needs of the adolescents are:
        - The need to be needed by others
        - The need for increasing independence
        - The need to achieve adequate adjustment to the opposite sex
        - The need to rethink the cherished beliefs of one's elders, the failure to recognize and understand these basic needs may prevent sound mental development.

CHAPTER 43 — Mental Illness

e. **Old age:** The mental health problems of the aged have received considerable attention in recent times in the developed countries. The causes of mental illness in the aged are organic conditions of the brain, economic insecurity, lack of a home, poor status and insecurity.

Thus, throughout his life, the needs of man are:
- Affection
- Belonging
- Independence
- Achievement
- Recognition or approval
- Sense of personal worth
- Self-actualization.

These needs only differ in degree and qualitative importance at various ages, but remain the same.

TYPES OF MENTAL HEALTH DISORDERS

Mental illness is a vast subject, broad in its limits and illnesses; the major and minor illnesses. The major illness is called psychoses. Here, the person is 'insane' and out of touch with reality. There are three major illnesses:

1. Schizophrenia (split personality) in which the patient lives in a dream world of his/her own.
2. Manic depressive psychosis in which the symptoms vary from heights of excitement to depths of depression.
3. Paranoia, which is associated with undue and extreme suspicion and a progressive tendency to regard the whole world in a framework of delusions. The minor illnesses are of two groups:
   a. **Neurosis or psychoneurosis:** In this, the patient is unable to react normally to life situations. He/She is not considered 'insane' by their associates, but nevertheless exhibits certain peculiar symptoms such as morbid fears, compulsions and obsessions.
   b. **Personality and character disorders:** This group of disorders is the legacy of unfortunate childhood experiences and perceptions.

Mental and behavioral disorders are understood as clinically significant conditions characterized by alteration in thinking, mood (emotions) or behavior associated with personal distress and/or impaired functioning. Any conditions where individuals may suffer from one or more disorders during one or more periods of their life are:

1. **Anxiety disorders:**
   a. **Phobia:** Irrational fear of object or situation.
   b. **Panic disorder:** Extreme fear, feeling of impending doom and palpitations.
   c. **Generalized anxiety disorder:** Worry, restlessness and palpitations.
   d. **Obsessive compulsive disorder:** Uncontrollable repetitive thoughts, urges or action.
   e. **Post-traumatic stress disorder:** Real threat of death or harm.
2. **Mood disorders (affective disorder):**
   a. **Unipolar (depression):** Depressed mood, weight changes, anhedonia, sleep disturbances and social withdrawal.
   b. **Bipolar (manic-depressive illness):** Signs and symptoms of depression cycling with euphoria, delusions and hallucinations.
3. **Somatoform (psychosomatic disorders):**
   a. For example, thyrotoxicosis, hypertension, coronary artery disease, duodenal ulcer, rheumatoid arthritis and conversion disorder.
4. **Schizophrenia:** The patient lives in a dream world of his/her own and shows:
   a. Disorganized speech and behavior.
   b. Ineffective thinking and decision-making.
   c. Trouble functioning at school and work, self-care deficit.
   d. Positive symptoms: Hallucination delusions.
   e. Negative symptoms: The symptoms such as apathy, flat affect and anhedonia are common.
5. **Substance abuse disorders:** The common signs and symptoms of drug, alcohol abuse and dependency are:
   a. Inability to fulfill obligations at work, school or home.
   b. Recurrent legal or interpersonal problems.
   c. Participation in physical hazardous situations, while impaired.
6. **Personality disorders.**
7. **Organic disorders:**
   a. Acute brain disorder, e.g. delirium, acute alcoholic intoxication.
   b. Chronic brain disorder: Cerebral syphilis, senile dementia (Alzheimer's disorders).

The International Classification of Diseases (ICD-10) classifies the mental and behavioral disorders as:

1. Organic including symptomatic, mental disorders, e.g. dementia in Alzheimer's diseases and delirium.
2. Mental and behavioral disorders due to psychoactive substance use, e.g. harmful use of alcohol and opioid dependence syndrome.
3. Schizophrenia, schizotypal a delusional disorder, e.g. paranoid schizophrenia, delusional disorders, acute and transient psychotic disorders.
4. Mood (affective) disorders, e.g. bipolar affective disorder and depressive episode.
5. Neurotic, stress-related and somatoform disorders, e.g. generalized anxiety disorders and obsessive compulsive disorders.

6. Behavioral syndromes associated with physiological disturbances and physical factors, e.g. eating disorders, non-organic sleep disorders.
7. Disorders of adult personality and behavior paranoid personality disorder, transsexualism.
8. Mental retardation.
9. Disorder of psychological development, e.g. specific reading disorders and childhood autism.
10. Behavioral and emotional disorders with onset usually occurring in childhood and adolescence, e.g. hyperkinetic disorders, conduct disorders and tic disorder.
11. Unspecified mental disorder.

PREVENTION AND CONTROL OF MENTAL ILLNESS

Prevention and control of mental illness can be described under three levels, i.e. primary, secondary and tertiary.

Primary Prevention

The aims of primary prevention are:
1. To reduce the incidence of new cases and the mental disorders.
2. To promote emotional robustness specially among the vulnerable high-risk groups (to avoid the onset of emotional disturbance).

The strategies of primary prevention are education at nutritional and social, as follows:
1. Universal iodization of common salt is the best method preventing cretinism and mental retardation. Industrial safety measures prevent lead encephalopathy and mercurial erethism.
2. Early diagnosis and treatment of conditions such as hypertension, syphilis, diabetes during pregnancy will prevent mental defects in the offspring.
3. Prevention of infections such as syphilis, rubella, encephalitis and human immunodeficiency virus (HIV).
4. Prevention of nutritional deficiencies such as pellagra, beriberi and anemia.
5. Early diagnosis and treatment of genetic diseases such as phenylketonuria (by diet low in phenylalanine), hypothyroidism (by maintenance of thyroxin level in the blood) and hydrocephalus (by ventriculostomy).
6. Other general measures, which can provide securing love and affection, specially among children are good housing, child-placement services (adoption, foster homes, orphanages, etc.). Other measures include welfare services for refugees, disaster survivors, etc.

Miscellaneous measures are:
1. Personality development measures such as disciplined environment both at home and at school. Scout, National Cadet Corps (NCC), air wing, etc. foster team spirit and good personality also helps in adjusting to adverse situations. School authorities are cautioned against overburdening the children with classes and homeworks. High school children are made aware of the dangers of alcohol, smoking and drug abuse.
2. Youth welfare services will save frustration and disappointment among youths, who are at the threshold of adult responsibilities.
3. Social welfare measures such as amelioration of poverty, ignorance and illiteracy, and provision of proper education and job opportunities will reduce mental tension and frustrations.
4. Avoiding late marriages and consanguineous marriages.
5. Legal measures such as prohibition of sale of uniodized salt, ban on the manufacture and sale of psychoactive drugs, etc. also constitute primary preventive measures.

So, primary prevention operates on a community basis. This consists of 'improving the social environment', and promotion of the social, emotional and physical well-being of all people. It includes working for better living conditions and improved health and welfare resources in the community.

Secondary Prevention

Secondary prevention consists of early diagnosis and treatment of mental illness through screening procedures specially among the susceptible and vulnerable groups of population in the schools, industries, antenatal clinics, etc. Family-based health services have a greater role. The family service agencies identify emotional problems and help family members to cope up with the family stress, mainly by counseling among those with marital conflicts.

Since secondary prevention consists of early diagnosis of mental illness and social and emotional disturbances through screening programs in schools, universities, industry, recreation centers, etc. and provision of treatment facilities and effective community resources. In this regard, 'family-based' health services have much role to play. The family service agencies identify emotional problems and early symptoms of mental illness, help family members to cope with overwhelming stress, treat problems of individual and social maladjustment when required and prepare individual family members for psychiatric care. 'Casework' or 'counseling' is the method most commonly employed by the family service, counseling service and help to families with marital conflict, disturbed parent-child relationships and strained interpersonal relationships. Family counseling is one method of treatment intervention for helping the mentally ill. Family counselors make an accurate psychosocial diagnosis.

Treatment is through specific drug therapy, general measures and electroconvulsive therapy. Drugs are diazepam for anxiety states, imipramine for depressive psychosis and lithium for manic state and chlorpromazine for schizophrenia. General measures include yoga and meditation therapy, relaxation therapy, social support therapy, etc.

Tertiary Prevention

Tertiary prevention seeks to reduce the duration of mental illness and thus reduce the stresses they create for the family and the community. In short, the goal at this level is to prevent further breakdown and disruption. The aim is to reduce the duration of mental illness, to minimize disability and to rehabilitate the patient as a useful member to the family and to the community at large. The different measures are detailed below.

Day Care Programs

Day care programs are for those patients, who have undergone hospital treatment. They spend their time in a structured way, which helps them to learn social skills for living.

Halfway Homes

Halfway homes are set up between the hospital and patient's family. Patients with unequivocal recovery are placed for few weeks to few months depending upon the case, where they live like a family with other patients. They manage their daily needs independently with some support from social workers. They are popular in the west. They are established in one or two cities in South India. It is a kind of social rehabilitation.

Self-help Groups

Self-help groups are the groups of parents having mentally retarded children. They share their problems among the coparents and resolve the problems by formation of welfare associations, special schools or training centers for mentally retarded children.

Family Service Programs

Family service programs are offered professional counseling services for the affected families. Not only they sort out problems within the family but also provide vocational training care for the chronically ill patients and the aged.

Industrial Therapy Centers

In industrial therapy centers, the patients are grouped according to their abilities and skills and are given specific work assignments with salary and prepared for open employment in the community. One of its kind functioning is in Chennai.

Vocational Training Centers

Vocational training center is a cost-effective method of rehabilitation of not only mentally handicapped persons but also for physically handicapped individuals.

Rehabilitation in Family

Rehabilitation in family constitutes the home care for the mentally ill persons, which is one of the most preferred way because the patient feels more comfortable. The joint family system provides a better opportunity than the nuclear family. But the family members need to be motivated for accepting these patients. It is also a very cost-effective method, specially for psychosocially disabled persons.

Rehabilitation of psychosocially disabled persons is neglected by the society and health planners. Therefore, there is a need to develop models of psychosocial rehabilitation, which are implementable, actionable and affordable.

Mental Health Services

Mental health services in a community are concerned not only with early diagnosis and treatment but also with the preservation and promotion of good mental health and prevention of mental illness. The mental health service comprises:
- Early diagnosis and treatment
- Rehabilitation
- Group and individual psychotherapy
- Mental health education
- Use of modern psychoactive drugs
- Aftercare services.

Comprehensive Mental Health Program

Since 95% of psychiatric cases can be treated with or without hospitalization close to their homes, the current trend is full integration of psychiatric services with other health service. The Community Mental Health Program includes all community facilities pertinent in any way to prevention, treatment and rehabilitation. The philosophy of Community Mental Health Program consists of the following essential elements:

- Inpatient services
- Outpatient services
- Partial hospitalization
- Emergency services
- Diagnostic services
- Precare and aftercare services including foster home placement and home visiting
- Education services
- Training
- Research and evaluation.

CONCLUSION

Mental health disorders interfere with the person's ability to perform the activities, learn and communicate in a proper way. The mental health disorders can be due to organic, genetic, psychosocial and environmental factors. Prevention and control of mental health disorders include early diagnosis, treatment, family-based health services, improve social environment, group and individual psychotherapy, and care during life cycle of human beings.

Epilepsy

CHAPTER 44

INTRODUCTION

Epilepsy is the group of disorders of cerebral function characterized by chronic, recurrent, paroxysmal and non-synchronous discharge of cerebral neurons:
- Seizures is defined as an episode of neurological dysfunction
- Convulsions are seizures accompanied by motor manifestation, i.e. limb jerking, incontinence, etc. seizures are need not be always convulsive.

The normal stability of the neuron cell membrane is impaired in individual with epilepsy. This inability allows for abnormal electrical discharges to occur. These discharges cause characteristics symptoms during seizures.

Epilepsy is the most common neurological disorder affecting 0.5–2% of the population. They can occur at any age. An isolated non-recurrent seizure occurring in an otherwise healthy individual for no obvious reasons should not be labeled as epilepsy. Epilepsy may be acquired or idiopathic causes of acquired epilepsy include traumatic brain injury and anoxic events. No cause has been identified for idiopathic epilepsy. The most common time for idiopathic epilepsy to begin is before age 20. New onset seizures after this age are most commonly caused by an underlying neurological disorder.

CLASSIFICATION

The seizures starting in localized area of brain are called partial or focal seizures. If they remain localized and awareness (consciousness) is preserved, then they are termed as simple partial seizures. If however the activity spreads and awareness is lost, they are termed as complex partial seizures. Further spread of these partial seizures must then generalize called secondary generalized seizures. Some seizures producing unconsciousness are termed as primary generalized seizures (Box 44.1).

Box 44.1: Classification of epilepsy

Primary partial or focal seizures
• Simple partial seizures (awareness preserved) depending on the concomitant signs, they are: – Motor   – Versive   – Sensory   – Psychomotor   – Visual   • Complex partial seizures (awareness lost) depending on the area involved due to spread, they are: – Temporal lobe   – Frontal lobe   – Partial seizure with secondary generalization
Primary generalized seizures
• Tonic-clonic (grand mal)   • Tonic   • Akinetic   • Absence (petit mal)   • Myoclonic
Unclassified seizures
• Seizures, which do not fit into above two categories: – Neonatal seizures   – Infantile spasms

ETIOLOGY

The common causes of epilepsy in adults are:
- Central nerves system (CNS) infection, e.g. encephalitis, meningitis and brain abscess
- Metabolic cause, e.g. hypoglycemia and hypocalemia
- Structural abnormalities, e.g. cerebral palsy, Sturge-Weber syndrome
- Head injury/Trauma
- Brain tumors and neurocysticercosis
- Cerebrovascular accident (CVA), hypertensive encephalopathy
- Drugs and alcohol withdrawal

- Arteriovenous (AV) malformations
- Idiopathic
- Familial.

The precipitating factors of epilepsy includes insomnia, physical or mental fatigue, drugs, flashes of bright light (photosensitivity), loud noise or mute, stress, pyrexia, infection, alcohol ingestion or withdrawal, reading or writing, display of colors, etc.

PATHOPHYSIOLOGY

Normally, neurons discharge synchronously under the influence of both inhibitory and excitatory systems. The inhibitory neurotransmitter, gamma-aminobutyric acid (GABA) plays an important role in limiting the synchronous discharge of neurons as well as amongst neighboring neurons by acting on recurrent and collateral inhibitory circuits. Drugs, which block GABA receptors provoke seizures. A diminution of GABA inhibition may also be involved in some form of chronic focal epilepsy. It has been postulated that some forms of generalized epilepsy could also be due to an abnormality in this GABA inhibitory system. There are also a large number of excitatory neurotransmitters of which acetylcholine and amino acids, glutamate and aspartate are some examples. It is likely that both reduction in inhibitory system and stimulation of excitatory system play a part in genesis of seizural activity.

Epilepsy is an altered physiological state in which there is a rhythmic and repetitive hypersynchronous discharge of many neurons in a localized area of the brain, which can be observed in the electroencephalogram (EEG). During the seizure, the EEG may display low-voltage fast activity or high-voltage spikes or spike-and-wave discharges throughout both hemispheres. Normally, EEG records α waves (9–13/sec) during relaxation with eyes closed. Thus, it follows that many kinds of metabolic abnormalities and anatomical lesions of brain can alter its electrical activity and reduce seizures.

CLINICAL MANIFESTATION

Symptoms of seizures activity correlated with the area of the brain where the seizure begins. Some patients experience an aura or sensation that warns than a seizure in about to occur. An aura may be a visual distortion on noxious odor or an unusual sound. Patients who experience an aura may have enough time to sit or lie down before the seizure starts, thereby minimizing the chance of injury.

Partial Seizure

Partial seizure can occur with many neurological manifestations as detailed below.

Motor

The focus of excitation lies in the motor area (precentral gyrus) of one of the cerebral hemisphere, hence, motor signs are limited to contralateral side (face, arm, trunk and legs). Seizures (fits) are characterized by rhythmical jerking or sustained contractions/spasms of the affected parts. The motor activity of partial seizures may remain limited to one part or may spread to involve the whole one side. Some attacks begin in one part, e.g. mouth, thumb, great toe and spread gradually, this form being called jacksonian epilepsy named after Jackson, who first described it. Attacks vary in duration from few seconds to several hours. More prolonged attacks may leave paresis of the involved limb for several hours after cessation of seizure. This is called *Todd's paralysis*. EEG shows regularly occurring spike discharge on the affected motor area of cortex.

Sensory

The focus of excitation lies in the sensory cortex (postcentral gyrus). Sensory partial seizures cause tingling sensation in the contralateral face and limbs. A spread of this discharge may also lead to sensory jacksonian seizures.

Versive

The focus lies in the frontal lobe and involves frontal eye fields. It is characterized by deviation of eyes to the opposite side. This type of attack may spread rapidly and become generalized (tonic-clonic seizure).

Visual

The focus is stated in the occipital lobe. The partial seizures are characterized by visual hallucinations such as balls of light or a pattern of colors. Formed visual hallucinations of faces or scenes may also be seen.

Psychomotor or Temporal Lobe

The site of focus is medial temporal lobe. Seizure causes alteration of psychic phenomena such as mood, memory and perception. This is a common type of epilepsy, which may manifest both partial (simple and complex) as well as generalized seizures. Simple partial seizures of temporal lobe cause false perception such as undue familiarity (Déjà vu phenomenon) or unreality (Jamais vu phenomenon), hallucinations of sound, vision, taste, emotional changes (fear and sexual arousal) or visceral sensation (nausea, epigastric discomfort). These phenomena may form an aura of complex partial seizures last for seconds or minutes and then awareness is lost. During this phase of complex partial seizures, patient may have staring look or may be unresponsive to questions. Automatic movements such as smacking of lips, protruding of tongue, undressing in public may occur at this stage. If the attack proceeds further, generalized tonic-clonic movements may occur.

Arising from the parental lobe may cause paresthesia on the side of the body opposite to the seizure focus. Visual disturbances are seen by the seizure originates and the occipital lobe. Involvement of the motor cortex results in individual movements of the opposite sides of the body. Typically movements begin in the arm and hand and may spread to legs and face.

Generalized Seizures

Affect the entire brain. Two types of generalized seizures are absence of seizures and tonic-clonic seizure. Absence of seizures referred as petit mal, occurs most often in children and manifested by a period of staring that lasts for several seconds. Tonic-clonic seizures are that most people envision when they think of seizures. They are sometimes called 'general oral seizures or convulsion'. Tonic-clonic seizures follow a typical progression. Aura and loss of consciousness may or may not occur. The tonic phase lasting for 30–60 seconds is characterized by rigidity, causing the patient to fall, if the patient temporarily stops breathing. The clonic phase is signaled by contraction and relaxation of all muscles in a jerky rhythmic fashion. The extremities may move forcefully causing injury, if the patient strikes with furniture or walls. The patient is often incontinent. Biting the lips or tongue may cause bleeding. The clinical features of grand mal fit/fits are as follows:

- The first occur in a coordinated fashion due to hypersynchronous discharge of neurons
- Stereotyped movements of limbs (tonic and clonic) occur
- Attacks can occur during any time of the day
- Patient may injure himself/herself during an attack
- These are unprovoked fits, there is no purpose behind these fits and these are true seizures
- There may be an aura before a fit; postictal phenomena are common
- There may be biting of tongue during seizure
- There is urine and fecal incontinence
- The seizures may be precipitated by some known factors
- Pattern of the fits is fixed
- The EEG is often abnormal
- Serum prolactin levels high during or after seizure.

The postictal period in the recovery period after a seizure following partial seizures. This phase may be no more than a few minutes of disorientation. Patient who experience generalized seizures may sleep deeply from 30 minutes to several hours. Following the deep sleep patient may report headache, confusion and fatigue; patient may realize than they had seizures, but not remember the event itself.

MANAGEMENT

Treatment of epilepsy is directed at the elimination of the cause of seizures, suppressing the expression of seizure and dealing with psychosocial consequences. The nature of epilepsy should be explained to the patient as well as to the parents or relatives. It should be clearly emphasized that this is a common disorder, which affects approximately 1% of the population and control of seizures can be expected in more than 80% of the patients with drug treatment. It should be made clear that treatment is to be taken regularly and for a long period. This will ensure better compliance.

First Aid Treatment of a Seizure

This type of first aid treatment of a seizure is needed, if a nurse happens to witness a patient with epilepsy on the roadside:

1. Move the patient to a safer place or side.
2. Loosen any tight clothing around the neck and move the public away from the scene so that the patient may breathe fresh air.
3. During a convulsion, do not allow the helpers to put the fingers inside the mouth. Try to prevent tongue biting by putting the tightly rolled handkerchief or a piece of cloth into the mouth.
4. After a convulsion ceases, turn the patient into semi-prone position and make the air passage clear.
5. Advise the patient to consult the doctor for medical advice. Summon the medical help, if convulsion continues for more than 5 minutes.

Drug Therapy

A single seizure is not an indication for drug therapy unless a second attack follows closely. Drug treatment should definitely be considered after two seizures and in some cases, some physicians start therapy in a single unprovoked seizure with abnormal EEG and positive family history. The goal of therapy is to prevent further attacks.

Use of Antiepileptic Drugs

Several effective drugs are available. These drugs suppress expression of seizures by stabilizing the neuronal membranes and by promoting the inhibitory activity of neurotransmitters. A singly drug is effective to control the seizures in more than 80% patients with epilepsy, if given in adequate doses. Drug therapy should be monitored by plasma levels of the drug. Drug regimen should be simple and multiple drugs or combinations of drugs should be discouraged unless or until it is absolutely necessary. The antiepileptic drugs, the dosage, uses and the side effects are detailed below.

Guidelines for Use of Antiepileptic Drugs

Main aim of treatment is to suppress seizures, hence:
1. Start treatment with a single drug.
2. Use small dose of those drugs, which have sedative effect, i.e. phenobarbital, primidone, clonazepam to start with, then gradually increase it over a period of 4–6 weeks.
3. Dose of the drug to be adjusted, so as to keep minimal therapeutic levels.
4. If seizures are not controlled, increase the dose of drug not exceeding the upper limit of therapeutic levels.
5. If seizures are not controlled still, then switch over to the other drug; control the seizure by increasing the dose of the drug. Once seizures are controlled, withdraw the older drug in gradual graded manner.
6. Try at least four single drugs before resorting to combination drug regimen. Some physicians prefer combination therapy if a single drug is not effective in maximum tolerated doses.
7. After a period of complete control of seizures for at least 3 years, withdrawal of medication is considered.

Precautions

The following precautions have to be observed by epileptics before a good control of seizures is achieved with drug therapy. Nurse should advise as follows:
1. Work or recreation near open fires or operation of dangerous machinery should be avoided.
2. Patients should not lock the bathroom doors. They should take shallow bath in a pond or a canal, that too in the presence of someone.
3. Cycling, swimming, mountaineering should be discouraged until at least 6 months seizure-free period has been achieved with treatment. Later on, these activities may be allowed in the company of someone.
4. Patient is allowed driving if he/she has not experienced any fit for the last 1 year (on or off medicines).

Interventions for Seizures

Seizure precautions in the hospital:
- Side rails pad of the hospital bed with commercial pads or bath blankets folded over and pinned in place
- Keep call light within reach
- Assists patient when ambulating
- Keep suction and oral airway at bedside.

  Nursing care during seizure includes the following:
- Stay with the patient
- Do not restrain patient
- Protect from injury (move nearly objects)
- Loosen tight clothing
- Turn to side when able to prevent occlusion of airway aspiration
- Suction of needed
- Monitor viral signs, when able
- Be prepared to assist with breathing, if necessary
- Observe and document progression of symptoms
- Refer patient for investigations and suitable treatment to hospital
- Advice patient or family for use of epileptic drugs, if previous accordingly
- Give nursing care after control of seizure, i.e. fluids, electrolytes, nutrients and skin care
- Advice the patient and family follows do not in epilepsy
- Use relaxation therapy and biofeedback system to reduce seizures
- Avoid alcohol intake, fatigue and insomnia
- Avoid precipitator and providing factors
- Educate the patient about first aid and treatment, and its importance
- Advice client to shift the patient to hospital, if status epilepticus develops
- Advice regular follow-up and biochemical terms
- Do regular phased exercise, do not stress or fatigue
- Take medication regularly, avoid alcohol and substance abuse
- Consult the doctor in case of problem
- Do not sit near the fire, do not crack fireworks
- Do regular follow-up
- Take all precaution to prevent seizures
- Do not take bath in a pond or bolted bathroom
- Do not engage in any activities that provoke seizure.

CHAPTER 44 — Epilepsy

CONCLUSION

Epilepsy is a disorder characterized by recurrent seizures of cerebral origin with or without loss of consciousness. The causes of epilepsy are head trauma, cerebrovascular diseases, brain tumors, multiple sclerosis and CNS infection. The risk factors associated with epilepsy are ingestion of alcohol, cerebral palsy and mental retardation. The prevention and control of epilepsy include diagnosis, treatment, food obstetrical care, prevention of CNS infections, trauma, stroke and health education, and fluorosis is the problem of excess fluoride.

Fluorosis

45 CHAPTER

INTRODUCTION

Fluorine is the most abundant element in nature. Being so highly reactive, it is never found in its elemental gaseous form but only in combined form. About 96% of the fluoride in the body is found in bones and teeth. Fluorine is essential for the normal mineralization of bones and formation of dental enamel. The principal sources of fluorine available to man are:

1. Drinking water: The major source of fluorine to man is drinking water. In most parts of India, the fluoride content of drinking water is about 0.5 mg/L, but in fluorosis-endemic areas, it may be as high as 3–12 mg/L.
2. Foods: Fluorides occur in traces in many foods, but some foods such as sea fish, cheese and tea are reported to be rich in fluorides.

Fluorine is often called two-edged sword. Prolonged ingestion of fluorides through drinking water in excess of the daily requirement is associated with dental and skeletal fluorosis, and inadequate intake with dental caries. The use of fluoride is recognized as the most effective means available for the prevention of dental caries.

Fluorosis is endemic in India. Fluorosis is disease caused by prolonged use of fluorine. In many parts of the world where drinking water contains excessive amounts of fluorine (3–5 mg^2) endemic fluorosis has been observed. It has been registered to be an important health problem in certain parts of the India, e.g. Andhra Pradesh (Nellore, Nalgonda and Prakasam districts), Punjab, Haryana, Karnataka and Tamil Nadu. The affected population is 25 million and at risk is 66 million.

Fluorosis is most abundant element in nature. It is never found in gaseous form because it is highly reactive. So it is always found in combined form. Fluorine is essential for mineralization of bones and formation of dental enamel. It prevents dental caries probably by reducing the solubility of the enamel in the acids produced by the bacteria of the mouth. The main sources of fluorosis are drinking water and foods. The other sources of fluoride are black tea, black salt, supari, tinned food and fruit juices. The recommended fluoride level in drinking water is 0.5–0.8 g/L. The foods rich in fluoride are sea fish, tea and cheese.

ETIOLOGY

As stated earlier, fluorine is often called 'double-edged sword' because neither it should be consumed in excess nor in deficiency prolonged ingression of fluoride through drinking water containing more than 1 mg^2 results in dental and skeletal fluorosis and inadequate intake results in dental caries, i.e. with fluoride level below 0.5 mg^2 of water. An indicator of dental caries in the community is the decayed, missing, filled (DMF) index.

The high-risk groups are children, elderly people, pregnant and lactating mothers, and patient with serial and cardiovascular diseases.

CLINICAL MANIFESTATION

The onset of fluorosis is marked by non-skeletal changes, which can easily be reversed by safe-drinking water and nutritional intervention. If left untreated, the disease progresses into non-curable dental and crippling skeletal fluorosis. The toxic manifestations of fluorosis comprise the following.

Dental Fluorosis

Fluorosis of dental enamel occurs when excess fluoride is ingested during the years of tooth classification particularly during first 7 years of life. It is characterized by mottling of dental enamel, which had been reported at levels above 1.5 mg^2 intakes. It is characterized by loss of shiny appearance of chalky white patches (mottling) over the teeth. Patches later became brownish/black. In severe cases, pitting occurs to give the teeth corroded appearance.

It is commonly seen in incisors and molars, and not seen in deciduous teeth. It becomes permanent feature. It is almost entirely confined to the permanent teeth and develops only during the period of formations.

Skeletal Fluorosis

Skeletal fluorosis is associated with lifetime daily intake of 3.0–6.0 mg/L or more. There is heavy fluoride deposition in the skeleton. When a concentration of 10 mg/L is exceeded, crippling fluorosis can ensure. It leads to permanent disability. The skeletal fluorosis characterized by the calcification of tendons and ligaments, and later pain and stiffness of back. Radiological changes include new bone formation (exostosis) and calcification of tendons and ligaments.

Genu Valgum

Genu valgum is a new form of fluorosis, i.e. in a manifestation of skeletal fluorosis is often seen in children, due to osteoporosis, as reported on Nalgonda (AP). Genu valgum is a syndrome was observed among people whose staple was sorghum (jowar). Studies showed that diet based on sorghum promoted higher retention of ingested fluoride than do diets based on rice.

Laboratory Examination

Laboratory examination shows that in high levels of fluoride in drinking water or urine and anemia with changes in red blood cell (RBC) structure and X-ray showing increased growth, thickness and density of bone. There are variety of methods of fluoride testing includes calorimetric, photometric and ion-selective method. The ion-selecting method is accurate.

PREVENTION AND CONTROL

The recommended level of fluorides in drinking water in India is accepted as 0.5–0.8 mg/L. In temperate countries where the water intake is low, the optimum level of fluorides in drinking water is accepted as 1–2 mg/L. Dental caries can be prevented by fluoridation of water supplies fluorosis can be prevented by defluoridation of water by Nalgonda technique recommends by National Environmental Engineering Research Institute (NEERI), Nagpur.

Change of Water Source

Change of water source is always better to prevention and control of fluorosis is to change the water source that is to find a new source of drinking water with lower fluoride consent (0.5–0.8 mg/L) and running surface water contain lower quantities of fluoride than groundwater sources such as wells.

Fluoridation of Water

As stated earlier, fluorine is one of the constituents naturally present in water supplies. In fact, the main source of fluorine is drinking water. Deficiency of fluorine in drinking water is associated with dental caries and excess of dental and skeletal fluorosis. Leading workers in India regard fluorine in concentration of 0.5–0.8 ppm in drinking water as optimum (a concentration of 1 ppm is regarded as optimum in temperate climates because the consumption of water is low). The WHO in 1969 recommended fluoridation of community water supplies in areas where the total intake of fluorides by the population is below the optimal levels for protection against dental caries. Fluoridation is now an accepted public health procedure in many developed countries.

The term fluoridation has been given to the process of supplementing the natural fluoride content of potable water to the point of optimum concentration leading workers in India regard fluorine in concentration of 0.5–0.8 ppm is regarded as optimum. Fluoridation needed for protecting persons from dental caries.

Defluoridation of Water

Defluoridation of water is by Nalgonda technique. This can be carried out in a bucket with a tap 3–5 cm above the bottom of the container. 40 L of raw water is taken in the bucket mixed slowly with adequate amount of alum (500 mg/L) followed by lime or sodium carbonate (300 mg/L) and bleaching powder (120 mg/40 L). Water is stirred slowly for 10–20 minutes and allowed to settle for nearly 1 hour. The settled sludge will be below the top level. The supernatant water becomes less in fluorine (i.e. permissible limit of fluoride) and is withdrawn through the tap for consumption. The settled sludge is discarded. Nalgonda technique involves the addition of two chemicals, i.e. lime and alum in sequence followed by flocculation sedimentation and filtration.

In some geographical areas, water may contain a high level of fluorides. In such communities, water is defluoridated by phosphate to reduce fluorides to optimum levels.

Other Measures

The reverse osmosis techniques retain not only fluoride but also nitrates and sulfates from the drinking water.

Domestic filters are also available based on activate aluminum technology.

Darkly requirement of fluoride is 0.5–0.8 mg/L of drinking water (i.e. 0.5–0.8 ppm). The use of fluoride toothpaste in areas of endemic fluorosis is not recommended for children up to 6 years of age.

CONCLUSION

The endemicity of fluorosis results from drinking water, which is having high fluorine. WHO guidelines have suggested the level of fluorine as 1.5 mg/L as desirable. Its prevention and control include provision of safe water, diagnosis, treatment and health education.

SECTION 6

Demography

- Demography
- Population and its Control

Demography

CHAPTER 46

INTRODUCTION

The word 'demo' means population and 'graphy' means study. Demography means study of population. Today it is the scientific study of population. So, now demography deals with the study of human population in a given area, usually a country, during a given year with reference to the size, composition, behavior and distribution. So, demography focuses its attention on readily observable human phenomenon, i.e. change in population size (growth decline), the composition of population and the distribution of population in space and behavior of population:

1. Size of the population means that total number of persons residing in the country, which can be determined or enumerated by 'census'. The size refers to the quantity of the population.
2. Composition of the population means breakdown of the population according to the age, sex, literacy level, occupation, income, marital status, language spoken, religion, etc. Thus composition refers to the quality of the population.
3. Behavior of the population means the growth of the population over a period of decade, i.e. positive growth, zero growth or negative growth. The behavior of the population or the trend can be estimated through population projection, i.e. growth rate of the population in the difference between the birth rate and the death rate. Growth rate when expressed as a number, it is called 'demographic gap'.
4. Distribution of the population means density of the population per square kilometer, rural population ratio and location of the dense or sparse pockets of the population.

DEMOGRAPHIC PROCESS

Demography deals with five demographic processes namely fertility, mortality, marriage, migration and social mobility. These five preverses are continuously at work within a population determining size, composition behavior and distribution. In other words the processes, which influence the size, composition, behavior and distribution of the population are marriages, births, deaths, migration and social mobilization, which are all continuously at work. The study of all the processes, which results in the mode of change in population is called 'population dynamics'. The study of all the components of the population and factors related to it called 'demographic statistics'. The term vital statistics refers to the study of viral events such as births, deaths, diseases, marriages and divorces.

Need for Demography in Nursing

Community health nursing is virtually concerned with population because health in the group depends upon the dynamic relationship between the numbers of people the space, which they occupy and the skill that they have acquired is providing their needs. The main sources of demographic statistics in India are population censuses, national sample surveys, registration of vital events and ad hoc demographic studies. Since, demography is the study of population including statistics about distribution by age and place of residence mortality (death) and morbidity (incidence of disease). From demographic data, needs of population for nursing services can be assessed, e.g. mortality and morbidity study revealed the presence of risk factors. Many of these risk factors, e.g. smoking are the major cause of death and disease that can be prevented through changes in lifestyle. The nurse role in assessing risk factors and helping clients make healthy lifestyle changes.

DEMOGRAPHIC CYCLE

The trend of the population growth in a country undergoes changes or variations in a stepwise manner. These variations are called stages of demographic cycle. In the history of world population since 1650 suggests that there is a demographic cycle of five stages through which a country passes—first stage (high stationary), second stage (early expanding), third stage (late expanding), fourth stage (low stationary) and fifth stage (declining). Brief descriptions of these stages are as follows:

1. **First stage (high stationary):** This stage characterized by a high birth rate and a high death rate, which cancel each other and the population remains stationary at high level. For example, in India before 1920 the birth rate was 49.2/1,000, the death rate was 48.6/1,000 and the growth rate was 00.6/1,000 (= 0.06%) (the growth rate was less than 1%).
2. **Second stage (early expanding):** In this stage, the death rate begins to decline, while the birth rate remains unchanged. The population grows slowly. This stage was experienced in India between 1921 and 1930. When birth rate was 49/1,000, death rate 36/1,000 and growth rate 13/1,000 (1.3%).
3. **Third stage (late expanding):** Here the death rate declines still further and birth rate tends to fall. The population continuous to grow because of birth exceeds death. Presently India in this stage, growth rate is about 2%, i.e. 20/1,000 population.
4. **Fourth stage (low stationary):** In this stage, birth rate falls rapidly and becomes equal to death rate. This stage characterized by a low birth and low death rate with the result that population remains stationary at low level growth rate is zero level, e.g. Australia, Denmark (1980) we expect India must enter this stage.
5. **Fifth stage (stage of decline):** Hence the population begins to decline because birth rate is lower than the death rate, so population goes on declining:
Growth rate > 0% ≤ 0% (−) death rate
For example, Germany and Hungary after effects of World War II.

Population growth in India has been mainly due to:
- High birth rate
- Decline in death rate
- Higher level of immigration than emigration.

Some causes of high birth rate in India are early marriage of women, universal marriage of women, joint family system, illiteracy, beliefs and superstitions regarding desire for getting a male child, limited acceptance of family planning, slow process of urbanization and poverty. Decline in death rate has been made possible by the advancements in public health services, control of communicable diseases, control of famines, economic development, etc.

Theory of demographic transition is the effect of economic development on the growth and size of the population of a country. According to this theory, every country passes through three stages of population growth:

- In the first stage, there is a slow and uneven growth of population with high birth rate and high death rate
- In the second stage, there is a population explosion with static birth rate and decline in death rate
- In the third stage, the birth rate and death rate decline.

DEMOGRAPHIC TRENDS IN THE WORLD

Nearly 2,000 years ago the world population was estimated to be around 250 million. It required all the human history up to the year 1800 for the world population to reach 1 billion, the 2 billion came in 130 years (around 1930), the 3 billion in 30 years (around 1960), the 4 billion in 15 years (in 1974), the 5 billion in 12 years (in 1987) and the 6 billion in 12 years (1999). It is expected to reach 8 billion by 2025. According to United Nation (UN) estimation, the world's population grew at an annual rate of 1.23% during 2000–2010. China registered a much lower annual growth rate of population (0.53%) as compared to India 1.64% (2000–2010). At present, India (17.5%), Indonesia (3.4%) and Bangladesh (2.4%) are among the most population 10 countries of the world. According the UN projection, India population will reach 1.53 billion by the year 2050 and will be highest population in the world.

Demographic characteristics provide an overview of its population size, composition, territorial distribution, changes therein and the components of changes such as nativity, mortality and social mobility. Demographic indicators have been divided into two parts such as population statistics and vital statistics. Population statistics include indicators that measure the population size, sex ratio, density and dependency ratio. Vital statistics include indicators such as birth rate, death rate, natural growth rate, life expectancy at birth, mortality and fertility rates.

These indicators help in identifying areas that need policy and programmed interventions, setting near and far-term goals and deciding priorities besides understanding them in an integrated structure. The consequences of population change in the agrarian's countries will include the following.

Rising Poverty and Retards Development

A rate of investment of 3–5% of national income is required to produce 1% increase in per capital income, whereas with population growing at 3% per year an investment between 10 and 12% of the national income is required. A poor country finds its extremely difficult to invest even 10% of its national.

CHAPTER 46 — Demography

Income in Economic Development, Youth Unemployment and Political Instability

When the mortality reduced rapidly in the age structure, the population gets more youthful, because the greater gain in saving lives are made in infancy and childhood. So, now most of countries in the world have more youths/youngest population. Further women are so burdened with constant childbearing, they cannot participate in economic production beyond traditional task. India agrarian economy failure to educate children, no schools deprives than their main chance of acquiring ideas and attitudes conducive to social change.

Pressure on Land and Migration

Land is fixed resource. It is a problem to get enough land to growing population in agrarian countries. With large family, childcare is a constant burden, the available land is even more inadequate the aspiration even more unreachable. The consequences of population change in the industrialized countries will include.

Cost of Goods and Services Become Costly

Overurbanization leads to problem of overcrowding the cost of gain is space is more expensive and there is the problems of utility services such as water, schools, parks, electricity, housing, etc.

Environment Degradation

Industrialization caused air pollution, water pollution, noise pollution, global warming and its consequence effects of disastrous.

Cost of All This Becomes Staggering

When the level of living in measures in per capital income or per capital gross national product (GNP), it is a summary index of all economic transaction, not an index of human welfare or satisfaction. Population concentration in urban area indicates natural imbalance problem of refugees due to anarchy, work natural calamities in certain countries. Population growth degrade the quality of life and problem of migration.

DEMOGRAPHIC TRENDS IN INDIA

India has about 2.4% of the world's land area and accommodates about 16.7% of the world's population. If the world's population were to stand in a line, every sixth person in the world would be an Indian. India has less than 1.2% of the world's income.

The size of the population in a country is determined in terms of the number of people. The population in India has risen from 23.84 crores in 1951, 102.27 crores in 2001 and was 119 crores in 2011. It is predicted that in March 2016, it will be 126.35 crores. After China, India's population ranks second in the world. According to the projections, India may overtake China in 2045 to become the most populous country in the world. The growth rate in India rose from 0.5 (1901–1911) to 21.34% (1991–2001) and 17.54% (2001–2011) per decade and currently India's population growth is 1.74%.

With regard to birth rate and death rate (birth rate refers to the number of births per 1,000 of population and death refers to number of deaths per 1,000 of population), the birth rate has declined from 39.9 (in 1951) to 20.97 (in 2011) and the death rate has declined from 27.4 (in 1951) to 7.48 (in 2011).

Density of population refers to the number of persons per square kilometer. It varies from state to state. Density of population has increased from 117 (in 1951) to 274 (in 1991), 324 (in 2001) and finally 382 (in 2011). Kerala, Bihar, West Bengal and Uttar Pradesh have population density higher than the national average. Industrially well-developed states have a higher density of population.

Sex ratio refers to the number of females to 1,000 males. This is also changing. Sex ratio has increased from 927 (in 1999) to 943 (in 2011). Kerala has a favorable sex ratio of 1,084 females per 1,000 males in 2011.

Because of the various public health measures and advancements in medical science, the life expectancy in India risen from 32% (in 1951) to 65.5% (in 2011).

Because of various policies, the literacy rate has also increased in India. Literacy rate refers to the numbers of literates as a percentage of the total population. Literacy rate in India rose from 16.7 (in 1951) to 73% (in 2011) literacy rate of males is 80.9% and females is 64.6%. At present, the literacy rate stands at 74.04%. Literacy rate is higher among the urban population. Kerala has a literacy rate of more than 90% (94% in 2011) taking it far above the national average.

Causes of Population Growth in India

The following are the causes for population growth in India.

Peaceful Conditions and Achievements in Medical Science

During in modern India, death rate was very low and all most peace was restored. Elimination of infectious disease, especially under the auspicious of international agencies such as World Health Organization (WHO), United Nation International Children's Emergency Fund (UNICEF), Food and Agriculture Organization (FAO) and independent India have been trying to eradicate diseases, e.g. malaria, yellow fever, cholera, plague, typhoid, smallpox, chickenpox, dysentery, etc. Insecticide, e.g. dichlorodiphenyltrichloroethane (DDT); antibiotics, e.g. penicillin; vaccines, e.g. bacille Calmette-Guérin (BCG); drugs, e.g. sulfanilamide; better instruments such as X-ray machine and rationalized public health companies by government and employing only a handful of specialist can save millions of lives at the cost of few thousands.

Widening Gap Between Birth and Death Rate

The average annual birth rate in India, which was 42% per 1,000 population in 1951 as come down to 26% per 1,000 population in 2001. The death rate in 1951 was 26.1% and decreased to 8.7% in 2001. Since, birth rate has shown a small decline and the death rate has gone down sharply, the widening gap has increased population rapidly (Table 46.1).

Universal and Low Age at Marriage

Marriage is almost obligatory and unavoidable for an average Indian. Life without marriage is almost unthinkable in this country and there is a social stigma attached to those who remain unmarried. There is a deep rooted, long-standing and widespread tradition in favor of marriage as a basic ritual.

Child marriages have been very common in the country. According to 1931 census, 72% marriages in India were performed before 15 years of age and 34% of marriages before 10 years of age. Since then, there has been a continuous increase in the mean age of marriage among both males and females.

The mean age at marriage of females increased from 17.6 (in 1981) to 18.4 (in 1991), against this mean age at marriage of males increased from 19.9 (in 1951), 22.6 (in 1981) to 22.9 (in 1991).

Thus, though the mean age of marriage has been increasing, yet a large number of girls even today marry at an age, which they are not ready for marriage either socially or emotionally and physically. The infant mortality and fertility rate is directly related to the age of women at marriage. As the age at marriage increases, the infant mortality rate and fertility decreases.

Table 46.1: Sex ratio and density of population

Year	Ratio	Density (km²)
1951	946	117
1961	941	142
1971	930	177
1981	934	216
1991	927	267
2001	933	324
2011	943	382

High Illiteracy and Poverty

High birth rate is correlated with ignorance and poverty. All these qualities are rampant in the Indian masses. Hence, no wonder large families are found amongst the poorer people in India (Table 46.2).

Table 46.2: Literacy rate

Year	Male	Female	National average
1951	27.16	8.36	18.33
1961	40.40	15.34	28.31
1971	45.95	21.97	34.45
1981	56.37	29.75	43.56
1991	64.13	39.29	52.21
2001	75.90	54.20	65.40
2011	74.04	82.14	65.46

Family planning has a direct link with female education and female education is directly linked with age at marriage, general status of women, their fertility and mortality rate and so forth. Education makes a person, liberal, broad minded, open to ideas and rationale. If both men and women are educated, they will easily understand the logic of planning their family. This is evident from the fact that Kerala, which has the overall literacy rate of 90.59% has lowest birth rate of 22.4 per 1,000 (female literacy rate in 2001 was 87.9%), while Rajasthan has lowest female education (female literacy in 2001 was 44.3%) and has highest birth rate (36.3%).

Development in Agriculture and Industry

Invention and spread of agriculture, animal husbandry and other agricultural allied industries immensely speeded up the rate of population growth. The industrial revolution with advances technology became worldwide and favored the growth of population. Absence of family planning facilities, promotion of widow remarriage, social stigma placed on women who are infertile, the desire to keep land in families, fatalistic attitude are other contributory factors to a high birth rate.

Persistency of Joint Family System

Joint family system serves as an incentive to high birth rate. It does not insist on the economic solvency of the husband and the division of responsibility for the care of large number of children creates a sense of irresponsibility among the parents. The conservative attitude of the elders toward birth control methods restricts their use.

Tropical Climatic Condition

The tropical climatic condition exerts an effect on the age of onset of ovulation and menstruation. According to age of consent committee, about 80% of Indian girls get their menstruation between the age of 12 and 15 and about 50% of them get married before they complete 15 years.

Religious Attitude Toward Family Planning

The religiously orthodox and conservative people are against the use of family planning measures. There are some women, who disfavor family planning on the plea that they cannot go against the wishes of God. There are some women, who argue that the purpose of women's life is to bear children. Indian Muslims have higher birth rate as well as fertility rate than the Hindus. Muslim women having rate of 4.4 as compared to 3.3 among Hindu women.

Lack of Recreational Facilities

Force the couple to involve in more sexual activities and lack of information or wrong information about, the effects of vasectomy, tubectomy and the loop. Many poor parents produce children not because they are ignorant, but because they need them. This is evident from the fact that there are some 35 million child workers in our country. If families stop these children from working their family funds will be ruined.

Demography is the statistical description and analysis of human population, demography has been defined as the study of statistical methods of human population involving primarily the measurements of the size, growth and diminution of the numbers of the people, the proportions of live born (wrong). Demography is considered as the study of human population. The population is studied in terms of size, structure and distribution. It also includes the changes, which are occurring over time and place. It studies both the aspects of human population, i.e. quantitative and qualitative:

1. The quantitative aspects of human population include composition, size, distribution, movement, density, structure and growth.
2. The qualitative aspects of human population include education, development, wealth, social class crime and nutrition.

So, demography is the study of all populations that can be applied to any kind of population that changes over time or space. It studies, the birth, death, age patterns and diseases in a community by which statistical information can be obtained. In other words, it is the study of population in terms of density and distribution such as age, gender, race, occupation, etc.

SCOPE OF DEMOGRAPHY

The scope of demography is broad as this is studied under various subjects related to community. Demography helps us in understanding the population in relation to age and sex composition, dependency and independency ratio, concentration of population, the size of population, education, occupation of people, age and duration of marriage and also about the distribution, i.e. whether the population is more in urban or rural. These types of data helps the planners to forecast health and education needs. By this the services required for elderly can be identified. Not only this, the policies related to birth control, social welfare, manpower and economy can be developed. Demography preserves the cultural minority group. Demography is oftenly regarded as a branch of anthropology, economics or sociology. The population processes are measured in formal demography, while the social demography analyses the relationships between economic, social, cultural and biological processes. Demography is taught in many universities across the world. Being studied in different disciplines such as geography, economy, sociology or epidemiology, demography provide a tool to approach a large range of population issues by combining a more technical quantitative approach. Demography represents the core of other disciplines. Researches on demography are conducted in universities in research institutes as well as in statistical departments.

Methods of Data Collection

Concepts of Data Collection

The data for any study can be collected either from primary source known as primary data or secondary source known as secondary data. Primary data are those which are collected afresh or for the first time, while secondary data are those which are collected from data already available from other sources such as institutional records, published reports or studies.

Data can be collected either by quantitative or by qualitative method. Quantitative methods are adopted to obtain information of descriptive type and will provide data for estimations. These may be either survey method or experimentation. Qualitative methods of data collection are for understanding underlying causes of occurrence of a phenomenon or a particular event. It will provide information to understand 'why' of an event. The method seeks to understand the behavioral patterns such as beliefs, actions or norms of subjects under study. Usually the method does not provide data for making estimations.

Quantitative methods of data collection should confirm to the following principles:
- Sample should be representative and preferably of large size
- Should adopt standardized individual questionnaires
- Only limited number of variables of interest is studied
- Information collected should be quantifiable and amenable to statistical procedures.

In contrast to above principles, in qualitative methods of data collection:
- Sample is purposive
- Methods adopted are interviews, either of individuals or groups, observations, case studies or group discussions
- Information obtained is extensive, descriptive and subjective, but may not be amenable to routine statistical analytical methods
- Relationship with the respondent is structured or semistructured
- Method tries to get the inside of the interviewee's world.

Quantitative methods of data collection

Important methods of collection of quantitative data are:
- Interview method
- Observation method
- Questionnaire method.

Selection of appropriate method depends on nature and scope of the study, availability of funds and availability of time and precision of estimates to be made from the data.

Interview method

Interview method is the most commonly used method in field studies. It involves presentation of oral-verbal stimuli and reply in terms of oral-verbal responses. The interviews may be personal interviews or telephonic interviews. Personal interviews are usually carried out in a structured way and are known as structured interviews. In this technique, predetermined questions are asked and recorded on a predesigned and pretested proforma. Unstructured interviews do not follow a system of predetermined order of questioning. However, unstructured interviews require deep knowledge on the subject.

The advantages of interview method of data collection are:
- More information in greater depth can be obtained
- Interviewer with his/her skill can overcome the resistance from the respondent
- Has greater flexibility and questions can be restructured as per situations
- Personal information can be obtained
- Samples can be covered completely with repeated visits
- Interviewer can capture lot of information
- Can also collect supplementary information
- Desired information can be collected at one point
- Provides accurate data for calculation of various rates or ratios.

However, the method is expensive and time consuming. Great care has to be taken to avoid interviewer's bias. This can be attained by careful selection and training of interviewers. The method involves establishment of good rapport with the interviewee.

Observation method

Observation method is a common method used in behavioral sciences or clinical case studies, where information is obtained by investigator's own observation. Before starting observation it is necessary to make a checklist of items to be observed as well as structuring the style of recording to facilitate easy analysis.

The advantages of this method are that subjective bias of both observer and respondent is eliminated since information pertains to what is happening. Further the observations are independent of respondent's willingness to answer questions. This method is useful especially when the respondents are not capable of answering verbal question.

However, the method is expensive, information provided is limited and sometimes unforeseen factors may interfere with observation. In some cases respondents may not be willing to be observed.

The observation may be participant's observation, where the observer shares the experiences, being a member of the group. It may be a non-participant observation when the observer is a detached emissary. It may also be disguised observation when the observations are made without people knowing that they are being observed.

Questionnaire method

In questionnaire method a predesigned and pretested questionnaire is circulated to the respondents, either in person or through mail, who will answer the questions by themselves. The answers to the questions may be structured or open ended. This method is less expensive compared to other methods since questionnaires can be circulated to large samples. However, the method has the disadvantage of loss of coverage since all the respondents may not return the questionnaires. Further all the questions may not be answered by all the respondents. Besides, there may be difficulty in understanding the questions by the respondents. This can be taken care of by adopting guided questionnaire method, where the groups of respondents are initially briefed about the questions.

Qualitative methods of data collection
Commonly used qualitative methods are:
- Case study method
- Focus group discussions.

Case study method
Case study method is a popular form of qualitative method of data collection and is a systematic research technique used extensively by sociologists, behavioral scientists and anthropologists, and even clinicians. The method involves complete and careful observation of a community, social unit, institution, family, individual or an episode or an event in the life of an individual. Usually an in-depth analysis of a limited number of variables and their interrelationships are carried out. The method is more for understanding the behavior patterns, cause and effect, and to formulate hypothesis, which can be tested through a detailed study to generalize the observations.

Major advantages of case study technique are that it helps to understand the behavioral patterns, collect personal data, trace the natural history of the event and their relationship with other factors, study intensively the social units and to provide a basis for formulation of further studies.

However, through case studies it may not be possible to arrive at generalizations since the data pertains only to the case under study, which may not be a representative sample.

Focus group discussions
The method is a semistructured discussion of a given topic with a homogeneous group of 6–10 individuals. In this method the discussions are not rigidly controlled as in the case of an interview using a standardized questionnaire, but are neither an unstructured conversation. The discussion is led by a trained facilitator, who uses a checklist of items to be discussed and encourages the participants to respond to open-ended questions and to come out with their responses.

Advantages of focus group discussions are that the group members can spontaneously express their ideas and they are not pressurized to answer questions. The flexible format allows the facilitator to explore the situations in an open manner. A wide range of information can be elicited in a less expensive manner.

However, the limitations of group discussions are that the information elicited may not be representative of the population and special statistical techniques are to be used for analysis. The analysis and interpretation of information elicited is more subjective.

Tools Preparation for Data Collection
Tools may be questionnaires or schedules, or proforma for field investigations through which the desired information is collected and recorded. They contain the variables in question form. The answers to the questions are recorded in either a prestructured or unstructured form. Prestructured refers to the answers in a predesigned form, while unstructured means open-ended answers. Tools developed should have validity and reliability. Validity refers to the collection of desired information in complete and true form, while reliability refers to obtaining same answers, when information is collected again for a particular question from the same respondent. While designing tools the following aspects are to be kept under consideration:

1. Objectives of the study are to be clearly stated.
2. Tools should be prepared keeping in mind type of respondents, nature of information and method of analysis to be adopted.
3. All the variables to be covered under the study are to be listed in advance.
4. Questions pertaining to the listed variables are framed in a simple and understandable form and are to be logically sequenced. Sometimes particular variable may require more than one question.
5. The tools designed are to be pretested through pilot studies for testing for validity and reliability. Pretesting will also help the investigator to understand other aspects such as time required for each interview and other practical aspects.
6. Tools are to be thoroughly edited on the basis of results of pretesting.
7. Questionnaires should not be lengthy and they are to be split into more number of simple ones.
8. Questions are to be well-framed in an understandable manner and should be simple and straight forward.
9. Subjective questions should have clear-cut definitions for their classifications to attain uniformity in answers.
10. In structured tools, the predesigned answers should be clearly defined to avoid subjectivity and to enable collection of information in a uniform pattern.
11. It would be advantageous for analysis, if computerized format is used for data collection.

Collection of Morbidity Data

There is no regular system for the collection of morbidity data either at state or national level. Still major health institutions compile the outpatient and inpatient records according to the names of the diseases. From these reports the Central Bureau of Health Intelligence attached to the Director General of Health Services publishes periodical reports after compiling and collating health data from various sources.

Periodical or ad hoc surveys are also undertaken by organizations such as Central Statistical Organization, National Sample Survey Wing of Cabinet Secretariat, Indian Council of Medical Research, etc. to obtain information on various morbidities.

Records and Reports

Further information regarding communicable diseases is compiled from the reports of infectious diseases. Morbidity information can also be obtained from:
- Hospital and dispensary records
- General practitioners records
- Records of health and welfare centers and educational institutions
- Recruitment and sickness records of armed forces
- Records of social security schemes such as Employees State Insurance Scheme, Contributory Health Service Scheme, Life Insurance, etc.
- Records of notifiable diseases
- Reports of routine and special sickness surveys
- Statistical abstracts of important diseases
- Statistical reports of important health institutions
- Reports of registries established for certain diseases such as cancer.

Observation

Observation is a method to record behavioral pattern of people in a systematic manner. Various methods such as structured, unstructured, natural, personal, mechanical, participant and nonparticipants are used to collect the data. Observation method provides the information what is actually observed, but bias can be there, as two observers has observed the behavioral pattern differently. Even the behavioral pattern will be different under different circumstances.

Diaries

Diaries are to record the data obtained from the individuals. The data from the people, which was expressed in depth can be recorded and utilized for research purposes.

Critical Incidents

The critical incidents are recorded.

Secondary Data

The data collected indirectly, i.e. not directly from individual, but from other sources such as hospital records census data, etc.

Sources of Demographic Data

- Census
- National survey
- Registration of vital events
- Demographic studies
- Records.

Census

Census is the direct method of collection of demographic data. It is conducted by the national government every 10 years. Census is an attempt to contact every member of the population in a country, which requires proper organization. Census not only provides information regarding number of people but also more than that. The data is collected about families as well as individuals in regard to age, sex, marital status, occupation, education and employment status, migration, language, religion, etc. So census covers social and economic aspects of population. It is conducted at the end of first quarter of the 1st year of each decade. The census commissioner for India guides, operates and directs the census.

Registration of Vital Events

Registration of events is the basis of vital statistics. Vital events mean live births, deaths, marriages, divorces and fetal deaths pertaining to statistics are registered in India. In 1873, Government of India passed the Births, Deaths and Marriage Registration Act. Indian states such as Karnataka, Tamil Nadu, etc. have passed their own acts related to registration of vital events. But the main drawback is that the act has the provision only for voluntary registration. So, the data is not accurate and complete as people do not voluntarily get the birth, death or marriages registered. The data tends to be unreliable and is grossly deficient in completeness. There are other reasons, which result in incompleteness of data such as illiteracy, ignorance, lack of concern, lack of motivation, lack of uniformity, multiple registration agencies, etc.

CHAPTER 46: Demography

In order to improve the civil registration system, Central Birth and Death Registration Act, was passed on 1st April 1970 by Government of India. Under this act, it is mandatory to register birth within 14 days and deaths within 1 day and in case of failure of doing so, a fine up to ₹50 will be imposed.

In some of countries births and deaths are recorded by the first time health workers such as village health guides. The countries, where vital events registration does not exist, there the alternative source used is demographic survey.

National Survey

National survey means survey conducted at central level to collect the information related to population from various states.

Demographic Studies

Studies conducted on demography also provide data about the population's education, occupation, etc. The demographic studies provide information about the latest demographic changes occurring from time to time.

Records

Records kept in the hospital constitute the basic and primary source of information about births and deaths due to specific diseases. Hospital data provides the numerator, i.e. cases, but not the denominator. For example, from hospital records, it can be found that how many women in the reproductive age has given birth, but the total population of women of reproductive age cannot be found from hospital data. Records in maternal and child health (MCH) centers, private and government hospital are the sources of demographic data, but lack denominator.

Analysis and Interpretation of Data

Analysis of Data

Data is collected directly or indirectly from population. The data collected directly from individuals by face-to-face survey is called primary data, e.g. data collected during census, data related to health from an individual data related to illness from an individual.

The data, which is collected from outside the source, i.e. indirectly data, is collected about individual from other sources than that individual such as records, e.g. data taken from hospital records and data taken from census.

The data collected needs to be arranged in tables, charts, diagrams, graphs, pictures and curves to stress important points. The data presented should be based on the principles designed to meet the criteria.

Tabulation

The tables whether simple or complex should be based on certain principles such as analysis of data, before the data is used for analysis or interpretation, it is presented by tables.

Table should contain the following:
- Title of each table: Brief and self-explanatory
- Number to the table such as table 1, etc.
- Clear and concise headings of columns or rows
- Tables should not be too large
- Present data: Chronologically, alphabetically or geographically.

Charts

The data collected can be presented in form of charts as they retain in the memory than statistical tables. The data presented should be in simple form by using various types of charts these are as follows.

Bar charts: These are easy to prepare and enable values to be compared at a glance. In bar charts, bars proportional to the magnitude are presented. These bars are presented in a set of numbers.

Histogram: It is pictorial diagram, which consists of series of blocks. If the midpoint of histograms blocks is joined then a line with fluctuation is seen, which is representing the frequency polygon. Thus, a frequency polygon is obtained by joining the midpoints of histogram blocks.

Line diagrams: These show the trend of events occurring over a passage of time in continuation such as rise or fall of diarrheal cases over a period of 5 years, i.e. during the year 1991, 1992, 1993, 1994 and 1995.

Pie charts: These are diagrammatically represented in circles with the radius 0 and at radius angle of 360°. The area of the circle in the form of segment, which depends upon the angle. These segments within the circle are comparable. The segments are indicated in percentages. To find out the angle at radius 0 from the data, which is given in percentage can be calculated by the formula as given below:

Degree to be presented = Given percentage/100 × 360

For example, suppose 75% of people are literate and 25% are illiterate and this is to be presented in a pie chart, then:

- Angle for literate = 75/100 × 360 = 270
- Angle for illiterate = 25/100 × 360 = 90.

It means an angle of 270° will be drawn to represent the literacy rate and 90° to represent the illiteracy rate. But keep in mind that the data will be presented in percentage as shown in pie chart.

Pictogram: In pictogram, small pictures or symbol are used to present the data.

Statistical map: These are used to present the data of different sizes and are presented in form of shaded maps or dot maps. In order to indicate the relationship of two variables, scattered diagrams are used. A linear relationship is evident if the dots are near or around a straight line.

Statistical averages and dispersion of measures of variations: Statistical average means the value in distribution around which other values are distributed such as mean, median and mode. These are commonly used averages, which provide information of about central value. The statistical formulas are used to calculate the statistical averages. Sometime there are individual variations, then to study the values, which vary from person to person or within the same subject, measures of variations are used, such as range, mean deviation and standard deviation.

Normal distribution curve: This is used to present the values for a very large number of people after creating narrow class intervals with frequency distribution. The shape of curve is based on mean and standard deviation. There is a mean value and the limits on either side of mean are the confidence limits from which the probability of a subject falling outside the confidence limit can be identified.

Chi square test, correlation and regression test: There are statistical methods, which are used to analyze the data. Chi square test is used to test the significance of difference between two proportions. A correlation test is to find out the association between two variables and regression test is used to find out the estimated value of one variable from value of another.

Interpretation of data: The data collected is analyzed and then interpreted, so that interpretations can be generalized to public. The values interpreted should be in simple way so as to make these understandable. While interpreting, the maximum and minimum values should be shown so as to have an estimation of in-between values.

The data interpreted should be in rate, ratio, percentage, mean, median, mode and normal curve. The demographic data can be analyzed and interpreted in forms of mainly rates and ratios such as fertility rate, net reproductive rate, crude birth rate, crude death rate and ratio such as child-woman ratio, abortion ratio, etc.

The other means of statistical method are used to study the demography in relation to other variables such as education level of people in relation to general health. These help to draw the conclusion, whether there is any relation of education in promotion of health. The demographic data can also be analyzed and interpreted by tables, charts, diagrams, pie charts, pictograms, etc.

DEMOGRAPHIC RATES AND RATIOS

Demographic data is represented in rates and ratio such as birth rate, death rate, fertility rate, marital fertility rate, net reproductive rate, etc.

Fertility rate: Fertility may be measured by a number of indicators as given below. Stillbirths, fetal deaths and abortions, however are not included in the measurement of fertility in a population.

Birth rate: It is the simplest indicator of fertility and is defined as 'the number of live births per 1,000 estimated midyear population, in a given year'. It is given by the formula:

$$\text{Birth rate} = \frac{\text{Number of live births during the year}}{\text{Estimated midyear population}} \times 1{,}000$$

The birth rate is an unsatisfactory measure of fertility because the total population is not exposed to childbearing. Therefore, it does not give a true idea of the fertility of a population.

General fertility rate: It is the number of live births per 1,000 women in the reproductive age group (15–44 or 49 year) in a given year:

$$\text{GFR} = \frac{\text{Number of live births in an area during the year}}{\text{Midyear female population age 15–44 (or 49) in the same area in same year}} \times 1{,}000$$

where,
GFR: General fertility rate.

General fertility rate is a better measure of fertility than the crude birth rate because the denominator is restricted to the number of women in the childbearing age, rather than the whole population. The major weakness of this rate is that not all women in the denominator are exposed to the risk of childbirth.

General marital fertility rate: It is the number of live births per 1,000 married women in the reproductive age group (15–44 or 49) in a given year.

Age-specific fertility rate: A more precise measure of fertility is age-specific fertility rate, defined as the 'number of live births in a year to 1,000 women in any specified age group'.

The age-specific fertility rates throw light on the fertility pattern. They are also sensitive indicators of family planning achievement.

Age-specific marital fertility rate: It is the number of live births in a year to 1,000 married women in any specified age group.

Total fertility rate (TFR): It represents the average number of children; a woman would have if she were to pass through her reproductive years bearing children at the same rates as the women now in each age group. It is computed by summing the age-specific fertility rates for all ages. If 5-year age groups are used, the sum of the rates is multiplied by 5. This measure gives the approximate magnitude of 'completed family size'.

Total marital fertility rate: Average number of children that would be born to a married woman. If she experiences the current fertility pattern throughout her reproductive span.

Gross reproduction rate: Average number of girls that would be born to a woman if she experiences the current fertility pattern throughout her reproductive span (15–44 or 49 years), assuming no mortality.

Net reproduction rate (NRR): It is defined as the number of daughters a newborn girl will bear during her lifetime assuming fixed age-specific fertility and mortality rates. NRR is a demographic indicator. The present level of NRR in India is 1.5 (1990). NRR of 1 is equivalent to attaining approximately the two-child norm. If the NRR is less than 1, then the reproductive performance of the population is said to be below replacement level.

The Government of India in 1983 adopted the policy of attaining a NRR of 1 by the year 1996 (now to be achieved by 2006). Demographers are of the view that the goal of NRR = 1 can be achieved only if at least 60% of the eligible couples are effectively practicing family planning.

Child-woman ratio: It is the number of children 0–4 years of age per 1,000 women of childbearing age, usually defined as 15–44 or 49 years of age. This ratio is used where birth registration statistics either do not exist or are inadequate. It is estimated through data derived from censuses.

Pregnancy rate: It is the ratio of number of pregnancies in a year to married women in the ages 15–44 (or 49) years. The 'number of pregnancies' includes all pregnancies, whether these had terminated as live births, stillbirths or abortions or had not yet terminated.

Abortion rate: The number of all types of abortions, usually per 1,000 women of childbearing age.

Abortion ratio: This is calculated by dividing the number of abortions performed during a particular time period by the number of live births over the same period.

Marriage rate: It is the number of marriages in the year per 1,000 population.

Crude marriage rate = Number of marriages in the year × 1,000

Midyear population: Demographers consider this a very unsatisfactory rate, because the denominator is comprised primarily of population that is not eligible to marry. A more sensitive rate is the general marriage rate:

$$GMR = \frac{\text{Number of marriages within 1 year}}{\text{Number of unmarried person's age 15-49}} \times 1,000$$

where,

GMR: General marriage rate.

This rate is more accurate, when computed for women than for men because more men than women marry at the older age.

Fertility Trends in India

Researches indicate that the level of fertility in India is beginning to decline. The crude birth rate, which was about 49 per 1,000 populations during 1901–1911 has declined to about 25.0 per 1,000 population in 2002 and 22.1 per 1,000 populations in 2010. The rural-urban differential had narrowed. However, the crude birth rate has continued to be higher in rural areas as compared to urban areas in the last three decades.

The TFR has declined from 306 (in 1991) to 2.6 (in 2008). The TFR in rural areas has declined from 5.4 (in 1971) to 2.9 (in 2008), whereas the corresponding decline in urban areas has been from 4.1 to 2.0 during the same period. There are considerable interstate variations in TFR, in bigger states it varies from 1.7 (in Kerala) to 3.8 (in Uttar Pradesh and Bihar).

Crude birth rate (2008) and TFR (2010) for major states: Recent estimates of the fertility indicators and age-specific fertility rates in India are given in Table 46.3.

Birth and Death Rates

The birth and death rates are important components of population growth. The birth and death rates in India are given in Table 46.4. The death rate has considerably declined from 27.4 (in 1951) to an estimated 7.2 per 1,000 populations (in 2010), the birth rate has declined niggardly from 39.9 (in 1951) to an estimated 22.1 per 1,000 (in 2010).

The objective of Fifth Five-year Plan (1974–1979) was to reduce the birth rate from 35 per 1,000 at the beginning of the plan to 30 per 1,000 by 1978–1979. During 1979–1984, the birth rate was stagnating around 33 per

1,000 with no obvious decline. During 1990, however, the birth rate showed a slight decline to an estimated 30.2, further declining to 26.4 by the year 1998. The current picture indicates that birth and death rates are both declining in India.

High Birth Rate

India like other developing countries is faced with the dilemma of a high birth rate and a declining death rate. This is a vicious circle, not easy to break. The causes of high birth rate are:

1. Universality of marriage: Marriages are universal and sacramental. Everyone, sooner or later (usually sooner) gets married and participates reproduction. The individual's economic security or emotions maturity are seldom a prerequisite to marriage.

Table 46.3: Fertility indicators of India 2010

Indicator	Age group	Total	Rural	Urban
Age-specific fertility rates	15–19	37.2	43.1	19.6
	20–24	198.6	218.5	147.3
	25–29	156.8	167.5	132.9
	30–34	66.0	70.1	56.2
	35–39	29.7	34.5	18.1
	40–44	9.3	11.6	3.8
	45–49	3.9	5.2	1.0
Age-specific marital fertility rates	15–19	37.2	268.7	233.9
	20–24	313.2	322.0	283.4
	25–29	179.4	186.4	162.1
	30–34	70.8	74.5	61.4
	35–39	32.0	37.1	19.7
	40–44	10.3	12.8	4.2
	45–49	4.5	6.0	1.1
Crude birth rate		22.1	23.7	18.0
General fertility rate		83.9	91.9	64.0
Total fertility rate		2.5	2.8	1.9
Gross reproduction rate		1.2	1.3	0.9
General marital fertility rate		117.3	126.6	93.0
Total marital fertility rate		4.4	4.5	3.8

Table 46.4: Birth and death rates in India

Year	Birth rate	Death rate
1941–1950	39.9	27.4
1951–1960	41.7	22.8
1961–1970	41.2	19.0
1971–1980	37.2	15.0
1981	33.9	12.5
1991	29.5	9.8
1995	28.3	9.0
1998	26.8	9.0
1999	26.1	8.7
2002	25.0	8.1
2004	24.1	7.5
2006	23.5	7.5
2008	22.8	7.4
2010	22.1	7.2

2. Early marriage: Marriages are performed early. Data indicate about 60% of the girls aged 15–19 years are already married.
3. Early puberty: Indian girls attain puberty early between 12 and 14 years.
4. Low standard of living: When standards of living are low, birth rates are high.
5. Low lead of literacy: The 2011 census showed that only 74.04% of the population was literate. The female literacy is still lower especially in the rural areas.
6. Traditional customs and habits: Customs dictate that every woman must marry and every man must have a son. Children are considered a gift of God and their birth should not be obstructed.
7. Absence of family planning habit: Family planning is of recent origin. It has not yet become part of the marital mores of the people.

Declining Death Rate

The declining death rate has been attributed to:
1. Absence of natural checks, e.g. famine and large scale epidemics.
2. Mass control of diseases, e.g. smallpox, plague, cholera, malaria, etc.
3. Advances in medical science, e.g. extensive use of chemotherapeutics, antibiotics and insecticides.
4. Better health facilities, e.g. establishment of primary health centers and more treatment centers.

5. Impact of national health programs.
6. Improvements food supply.
7. International aid in several directions.
8. Development of social consciousness among the masses demographers opine that further rapid decline in India, death rate may not continue in future.

The reason is that most of the 'easy' conquest of mortality has been accomplished through the widespread use of vaccines, antibiotics insecticides and other lifesaving measures. The tasks that remain now are the most difficult ones such as improvement in environmental sanitation and nutrition; and control of noncommunicable and genetic diseases.

Growth Rate

Prior to 1921, the population of India grew at a slow rate. This was due to the operation of natural check (e.g. famines and epidemics), which took a heavy toll on human life. After 1921, the 'great divide', the occurrence famines and epidemics was effectively controlled through better nutrition and improved healthcare services, with the result that the death rate declined more steeply than the birth rate. Consequently, there was a net gain in births over death leading to rapid growth in population, which rose from 1 to 2% (in 1951) to 1.96% (in 1961), 2.20% (in 1971), 2.22% (in 1981), 2.14% (in 1991), 1.93% (in 2001) and 1.64% (in 2011). India is now the second most populous country in the world, adding 16 million every year to 1,210 million at the time of 2011 census. However, the most recent data indicates a decline in India's population growth rate.

The national health goal was to attain a birth rate of 21 and a death rate of 9 per 1,000 by 2007. This would yield an annual growth rate 1.2%, which was considered essential for the stabilization of population of India over the next 50 years or so.

CONCLUSION

Demography is the study of human population in terms of size, structure and distribution. The study of demography can be applied to any kind of population that changes over time or space. Five stages of demographic cycle are high stationary, low stationary and declining. The countries are in various phases of demographic cycle. The scope of demography is broad. It is regarded as the branch of anthropology, economics or sociology. It is studied under various subjects related to community. As demography is studied in different disciplines such as geography, economy and epidemiology; it provides a tool to approach a large range of population issues by combining a more technical quantitative approach. Data is collected by interviews, observations, questionnaires, diaries and record of critical incidents. Various sources of demographic data are census national survey, registered vital events, records and demographic studies. Data collected is analyzed and interpreted by tables, charts, line diagrams, pictograms and statistical map. The statistical averages such as mean, median and mode, and statistical dispersion or measures of variations such as mean deviation, standard deviation and range. The other statistical methods such as chi-square, correlation and regression test are also used to analyze the data. Demographic data is represented in rates and ratio such as birth rate, death rate, fertility rate, marital fertility rate, net reproductive rate, etc.

Population and its Control

CHAPTER 47

INTRODUCTION

India is the second most populous country in the world today, next to China. The rate of growth of population increased after industrial revolution. The first census was estimated in India, 1881. When the population was about 20 crores, it was almost stationary between 1911 and 1921 about 24–25 crores. After 1921, there was sudden increase in the population. On the basis of growth rate (GR), the growth can be divided into three periods, i.e. up to 1921 it was stagnant period, from 1921 to 1951 was the moderate growth period (average growth rate 1.26% per year) and the rapid growth period of average GR 2.26% per year, since 1951 to present. The population of India was 68.5 crores in 1981, 84.65 crores in 1991, 102.70 crores in 2001 and 12.1 crores in 2011.

At the time of independence in 1947, the population was about 34 crores. Within the span of 34 years by 1981 it became 68 crores. Since then almost 1 crore of population is being added every year. By 2001 it crossed 100 crores (1 billion), thus it is observed that during 20th century first doubling took place after 60 years and next doubling work place in just 30 years. The time required for the population to get doubled is called 'doubling time'. Higher the GR of the population, shorter is the doubling time. Thus, the doubling time is determined by the growth rate.

The population of the world is growing at the rate of about 200 birth per month or 10,000 per hour or 2.5 lakhs per day or 10 crores per year. This growth of the population is the single greatest obstacle for the development and progress of the country.

PROBLEMS OF OVERPOPULATION IN INDIA

Overpopulation in India has had an impact on the following aspects:
1. Food production: In spite of increase in food production, per capita food supply has gone down to 1,200 calories as against the recommended average normal of 2,400 calories due to the increase in population.
2. Clothing: Against the per capita minimum of 25 meters per annum, the supply is only of 14 meters. So, there is scarcity of clothing due to population explosion.
3. Employment: More than 25 million people are unemployed today.
4. Education: We need more schools and teachers to meet the educational needs of children.
5. Shelter: With an ever-increasing population, shelter and healthy houses are not available to everyone.
6. Health: The demand for health programs increases with an increase in population. Existence facilities are not enough to cater to the present population. All these factors have an adverse effect on health.
7. Poverty: Since 1970s, India's economic GR has increased and social indicators have improved. Even then 28.6% of the Indian population currently lives below poverty line.
8. Inadequate freshwater: There is not enough clean water for use as drinking water, for sewage treatment as well as for effluent discharge.
9. Depletion of natural resources: The ever-increasing population has been a huge drain on the natural resources of the country such as coal and petroleum leading to dwindling reserves in a short span.
10. Pollution: Increased levels of air pollution, water pollution, soil contamination and noise pollution have resulted because of overpopulation. The atmospheric composition has changed, which is a major contributor to global warming.
11. Deforestation and loss of ecosystems: Increased demand for farmlands and housing has led to deforestation on a large scale. Industrialization has also had a toll on forests. About 8 million hectares of forest are lost every year. Due to loss of forests, many wild animals have been rendered homeless and are endangered.

The loss of forest cover means that the atmospheric oxygen and carbon dioxide balance is getting disturbed.

POPULATION EXPLOSION

It is observed that 2,000 years ago, the population of the world has hardly 250 million. It required 1,800 years to reach 1 billion. It required 130 years to reach 2 billion, then 30 years to reach 3 billion, then 15 years to reach 4 billion and then 12 years to reach 5 billion and another 12 years to reach 6 billion. At this GR, it is expected to reach 8 billion by 2025 AD.

An increase in the population in an area from 1 year to another is called 'population growth'. GR is computed by subtracting crude death rate (CDR) from crude birth rate (CBR). But in reality:

GR = (CBR − CDR) + Immigration − Emigration.

The current GR in India is 24.1−7.5 = 16.6; per 1,000 MYP = 1.6% (2005).

The difference between the birth rate and death rate in graph marked in 'demographic gap'.

As long as natural resources of the country such as water, soil, minerals, forests, etc. are able to support and sustain the population by providing basic needs, such as food, cloth, shelter, so long the increase in population is called 'population growth'. But when the growth of the population is so much that the natural resources are unable to support and provide the basic needs, it described as 'population explosion' or 'population bomb'. As stated earlier, world population is currently growing in the rate of 3 per second, 180 per minute, 10,800 per hour, 2,59,200 per day and 9.2 crores per year. As the growth increases, the doubling time becomes shorter. The rampant population growth is a greatest obstacle to the social and economic development of the country.

Reasons for Population Explosion

The main reasons for population explosion in previous century are advances in medicines, increasing birth rate in the postwar period, i.e. after 1945, economic growth, green revolution in the world, decrease in death rate as a result of improved obstetrical services, eradicates and control of epidemic diseases, invention of antibiotics, and progress of in sanitation and hygienic conditions. Among them high-birth rate and low-death rate are main reasons of population explosion.

Causes of High-birth Rate

1. Early onset of puberty (between 11 and 13 years among girls).
2. Universality of arrange, i.e. everyone must and should get marry and prove their fertility.
3. Early age at marriage, i.e. 60% of Indian girls get marry before 19 years of age, which results in early pregnancy, too many pregnancies and too frequent pregnancy.
4. High proportions of young adults are potential parents.
5. Sociocultural factors such as poverty, illiteracy, ignorance, poor standard of living, lack of knowledge about family planning, religious better against birth control, belief to have son, etc.

Causes of Low-death Rate

1. Decrease frequency of natural calamities such as earthquakes, floods, famines, epidemics and pandemics.
2. Advancement in medical science and technology.
3. Development of health consciousness among people.
4. Availability of better healthcare facilities.
5. Launching of various health programs.
6. International organization support for health care of human beings.

Evil Effects of Population Explosion

The rapid population increase poses a serious threat to development efforts of the overpopulated countries. The task of providing food, school, employment, health facilities, housing, etc. for the increasing number is staggering. Following are the effects of population explosion.

Pressure on Land

The distribution of population is quite uneven in the country though the average density of population is 324 in 2001. Yet there are areas, which are crowded with humanity such as Delhi 6,352; Kerala 749; Chandigarh 5,632 and less density in areas such as Arunachal Pradesh 10, Himachal Pradesh 93, Sikkim 57 and 129 in Rajasthan. With the increase in population, fragmentation of land holding into division and subdivision, and finally uneconomic land holders per capita land availability is also very.

Shortage of Food

In recent year, there has been a growing concern about the widening gap between population growth and food supply. As insufficient and ill-balanced diet giving only 2,380 calories per head per day as against the needed 3,000; food deficiencies have retarded physical and mental development of the young children, and has caused deficiency and diseases among the adults, which do not invariably cause actual death, but lead to general ill-health. Susceptibility to diseases, impair efficiency, which in turn affects productivity in different spheres and causes heavy deaths both among the infants, and the mother. Country has a whole 135th position in world Human Development Index (HDI), nearly 270 million people are living below poverty line.

Poor Levels of Health

Persistent high fertility causes important health problems. Married women aged 17–37 are characterized by continuous nutritional drain from repeated pregnancies and lactation, and increased risk of maternal mortality, with every pregnancy. Premature curtailment breastfeeding cause malnutrition.

India is the largest country in the world where large numbers of persons are defective, infirm, socially inadequate and diseased persons and feeble-minded person. India has ranked foremost among the countries with people infected with leprosy sharing about 58%. It is estimated that there are more than 12 million economically blind persons in India. It is estimated that there are 3–5 million human immunodeficiency virus (HIV) infected people in India, likely to be the largest number of infected people in the world. The sporadic outbreak of communicable disease such as malaria, plague, cholera and dengue are quite common. There are about 20 lakh cases of cancer and about 7 lakh new cases occur every year.

According to United Nation Development Program (UNDP) report, India invests only $14 (about ₹500) per person annually on health and education unlike other developing countries such as South Korea, Malaysia and Sri Lanka, which spend $150–160.

About 74% of the doctors are in urban areas and rest in rural areas. When it is remembered that 75% of people are living in villages the extent to which provision of skilled medical aid is lacking in the country as a whole becomes quite obvious.

Housing Shortage

The phenomenal swelling of both the urban and rural population has placed a heavy strain on the available housing space. Considerable majority of people live in single-roomed tenements with overcrowding ranging from two to six persons and in few cases 10–12 person. The bustees of Kolkata or the chawls of Mumbai and ahatas of Kanpur very well-reflect this fact.

These facts illustrate the congestion, which exists in urban areas. The acute shortage of housing has resulted in the soaring value of residential plots, rock renting, acute congestion, unhygienic living, adverse sex ratio, promiscuity, venereal diseases and alcoholism. The slums even become generation of frustration and other problems.

Unemployment and Economic Losses

There has been an alarming rise in unemployment in our country since independence. Most of social scientist are of the opinion that quite a large proportion of the working population is not regularly employed in our country. These unemployed and underemployed people, and their family members are dependent upon their family members or kin even for their basic necessities.

The growth of employment per annum is only 2%. Approximately, 3 million educated youth enter the labor market every year. Total 40 million unemployed in the country, the Government of India has to dole out 1,200,000 crores per year to spare for the unemployed alone.

This trend to tamper economic growth because of increasing investment required for providing transport, housing and other social services. Not only this but also the problem of drinking water, sewage disposal and sanitation will become more acute, and will require large investment.

Therefore, unless the rate of population growth is reduced economic progress is difficult. Without economic progress and higher per capita income population control is not easy. This vicious circle is not easy to break.

Health Hazards of Population Explosion

1. Physical hazards:
   - Housing (eruption of slums with poor living condition)
   - Environmental pollution (air, soil, water, etc.)
   - Vector problems.
2. Psychological hazards:
   - Behavioral hazards
   - Mental illness (neuroses and psychosis)
   - Anxiety (due to stress and strain)
   - Tension and worries.
3. Social hazards:
   - Alcoholism
   - Broken homes
   - Corruption
   - Divorces
   - Drug abuse
   - Gambling
   - Unemployment problem
   - Antisocial activities such as theft, murder, sex crime, rape, prostitution, robbery, child abuse and juvenile delinquency.
4. Miscellaneous hazards:

- Malnutrition
- Infections
- Sexually transmitted disease (STD) including acquired immune deficiency syndrome (AIDS)
- Accidents
- Epidemics
- Hypertension due to stress and strain
- Diabetic mellitus.

Thus, population explosion is not only health problem but also a social, economic, and demographic problem.

Impact of Population Explosion

In population explosion there is an overpopulation. The overpopulation refers to an increased numbers of people than they can live on earth in comfort happiness and health.

Environmental Impact

The impact of increased population towards environment is increased demand of energy, climate changes, degradation of natural resources and food scarcity. Overpopulation has serious consequence of sustainability and total environment. One simple model, which can be environmental impact, is:

$$I = P \times A \times T$$

where,

I: Environment impact
P: Number of people
A: Denotes affluence per person (conduction)
T: Denotes technologies effect on use of resources.

At present all are increasing, i.e. number of persons and use of resources thereby increasing environmental impact and thwarting sustainability.

Social Impact

Population explosion will lead to certain social problems these are due to economic problems such as poverty, unemployment and starvation. These problems will lead to several problems such as beggary, smuggling, trafficking and delinquent behaviors such as antisocial activities.

Economic Impact

Population explosion has its impact on economy of the individual, society and community. Increasing population causes illiteracy, unemployment, poverty and starvation. Illiteracy effect the earning capacity, poverty and starvation. Starvation will cause health problems. More health problem leads to more economic burden and burden of healthcare facilities of the country.

Increasing population leads to search for land, there will be deforestation, which in turn leads to environment pollution. The environmental pollution again causes health problems creates more economic burden.

Increasing population leads to unemployment, which may lead to more social crime and more socioeconomic burden for planning, and implementation of policies and program. Economic burden due to population explosion affects the group of country and there is need to have control of over increasing population to reduce the effects of population explosives.

People have to face so many consequences due to population are problems of land or space, housing, good supply, water supply, sewage disposal and sanitation, health care, education, employment, poverty and crimes. Traffic problems, fuel and energy problems, and also ecological problems such as deforestation, soil erosion, floods, pollutions, and excess use of fertilizer and pesticides.

POPULATION STABILIZATION

As these hazards stated above, there is an urgent need to control and stabilize the population. Since, it is not possible to reduce the population to preindependence level; at least it can be stabilized and kept stationary. Stabilization of population is a national priority. To stabilize the population either the birth rate has to be decreased or death rate has to be increased. Since death rate cannot be increased, the one and the only way to stabilize the population is by reducing the birth rate, and to bring it down to that of death rate, so that low-birth rate and low-death rate will cancel each other resulting in low stationary phase. India is in late expanding stage of the demographic cycle. It must enter low stationary stage.

Reduction of Birth Rate

There are two strategies:
- Non-birth control measures (social welfare measures)
- Birth control measures (family planning methods).

Non-birth Control Measures

Raising age at marriage
Under the Child Marriage Restraint Act, 1978, the minimum age at marriage has been fixed to 18 years for girls and 21 years for boys. Still this is not strictly implemented. There is a need for educating the people about the dangers of early marriage. Raising the age at marriage stabilizes the population by lengthening the generation gap and increasing the doubling time. If all girls get married at 15 years of age, the population doubles every 16 years, but if

they get marry at 25 years, it doubles once in 26 years, all other things being equal.

Eradicating illiteracy (raising the literacy level)
It has been observed that the fertility rates and family size are lower among literate women compared to illiterate women. Therefore, there is a need to increase the female literacy. Different measures undertaken to increase the literacy are:
1. Establishment of Anganwadi and Balwadi centers.
2. Enrollment of all children, specially female children for primary education retention of enrolled children [reducing the dropout rate from the schools by continuous promotion up to Secondary School Leaving Certificate (SSLC)].
3. Establishment of primary schools at the rate of one for every 200 children encouraging adult literacy.

Improvement of economic status
- By sanctioning loans (for education, for agricultural activities, for home industries, etc.)
- By encouraging self-employment programs
- By encouraging job-oriented training courses (Jawahar Rozgar Yojana).

Raising the housing standards
- By allotment of free sites to the poor
- By sanctioning of house loans (Indira Awaas Yojana).

Improving the status of women
- By giving equal opportunities and equal salary to women
- By information, education and communication (IEC) activities.

Adopting one-child norm (be it a boy or girl)
- By massive educational campaign
- Improving the quality of health services specially maternal and child health services.

If all these measures are taken to reduce infant mortality rate (IMR), child mortality rate to a very low level, people will be sure that their child does not die prematurely. Only then they will come forward to adopt one-child norm.

Birth Control Measures (Family Planning Methods)

Methods of fertility regulation (contraception)
The methods of fertility regulation or contraceptive methods are by definition, preventive methods to help women avoid unwanted pregnancies. These methods can be divided into appliance and non-appliance methods. The non-appliance methods will include total abstinence, periodic abstinence, temperature method and coitus interrupts, coitus reservatus and coitus interfemoris. The appliance methods are condom by the male and diaphragms, cervical caps, vimules, jellies, aerosol foams, etc. by the females. They can be used alone or in combination with the cervical cap, vimule or diaphragm by the female and the condom by the male and the female. These contraceptives can be divided as temporary methods (spacing) and permanent method (terminal), the different methods of family planning are shown in Figure 47.1.

Spacing methods
Non-appliance methods or non-hormonal contraceptives (natural methods) are methods of that contraception prevent pregnancy without the use of chemical agents or physical devices.

Total sexual abstinence
Total sexual abstinence is a practice of Brahmacharya. It costs nothing except self-denial on the part of the couple. It is absolutely reliable in that the failure rate is nil, if it can be followed successfully. It is however, difficult to practice and it is doubtful whether the modem couple will subscribe to it, except on health ground.

Periodic abstinence
Periodic abstinence is otherwise known as rhythm or calendar method, or safe period. This method is based on restricting the sex act to the infertile period of the female partner. That means, the avoidance of sexual intercourse during the period surrounding ovulation, i.e. 2–3 days before and after ovulation is deemed to have taken place. The release of egg or ovulation occurs about 12–14 days prior to the onset of the next menses and the egg is fertilizable for 24 hours after ovulation. The spermatozoa in the human semen retain the fertilizing ability for about 72 hours after ejaculation. Taking these facts into consideration and the length of menstrual cycle, calculation of the period is made for woman. As stated above, the ovum is usually released in the fallopian tube of the female, 14 days prior to the start of the next menses or 13th to 17th day after onset of present menses. The period about 3 days before and after the stoppage of menses may be considered as the safe period.

This method is based on the record of the woman's previous six menstrual cycles. The safe period may be calculated on the basis of the number of days in the shortest and longest cycle. The woman then calculates first unsafe day (the beginning of the fertile time) by subtracting 18 days from the shortest cycle. The last unsafe day is determined by subtracting 11 days from the longest cycle. An example of the calculation is given here:
- Shortest cycle: 25 days so, 25 – 18 = 7 days
- Longest cycle: 32 days so, 32 – 11 = 21 days.

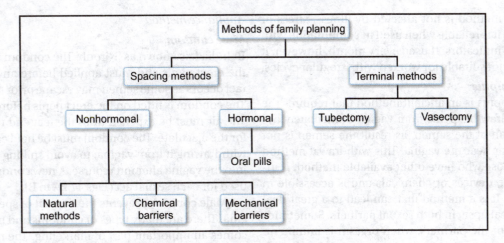

Figure 47.1: Methods of family planning

For the woman in this example, the fertile or unsafe period is calculated to be 14 days from days 7 through 21 of each of her cycle. Using this calendar month alone, this woman must abstain from sexual intercourse for longer than she may desire.

This rhythm method is only practicable in women who have regular menstrual periods. Even such women cannot predict when fertilization of the ovum will take place. In addition, it is known that ovulation in some women is stimulated by sexual intercourse, as in the rabbit. For these reasons the failure rate of this method of birth control is high.

Temperature method

This form of periodic abstinence is based on the prediction of the time of ovulation by taking the basal body temperature (BBT) daily and avoiding sexual intercourse around the time of ovulation, i.e. when there is a rise of 0.5°C BBT. The temperature is taken every day after the woman awakens and before any physical or emotional activity occurs. She uses a basal thermometer, which measures in 0.1 calibration rather than 0.2 increments so that small changes are easily noted. The rise in body temperature during menstrual cycle indicates the occurrence of ovulation. The rise is small, i.e. 0.3–0.50°C and may occur either abruptly or slowly. Before ovulation the BBT remains low. About 24 hours before ovulation the temperature dips lightly (0.10–0.20°F) and then rises sharply within 24 hours. The rise of 0.7–0.80°F is maintained during the life of the corpus luteum for about 12 days. The day before menstruation, it drops again to the previous level. This shift results from the thermogenic influences of progesterone, which is secreted in higher level after ovulation. Therefore, a temperature elevation lasting 3 days signifies an end to the abstinence, even if the calendar count has not ended.

This method is not a practicable method where there is a high level of illiteracy. The illiterate will not be able to read the thermometer or chart the temperature even if they know, which end of the thermometer is put in the mouth. For the educated it is a good method, but even the educated woman finds it a little bothersome. Needless to say, this method has proved difficult to teach and interpret and motivate to practice. And abstinence is necessary for the entire postovulatory period.

Billing method

The billing method relies on the changes in cervical mucus secretion also called mucus method. This method is based on the observation of changes in the characteristics of cervical mucus. After menstruation, the discharge appears yellowish and viscid, and is impenetrable to sperm. About 2–3 days before ovulation, the mucus changes to a clear, colorless liquid similar to an egg white. If this mucus was tested, the glucose levels would be found increased and the pH would be more alkaline. It resembles raw egg white and is smooth, slippery and profuse. After ovulation, under the influence of progesterone, the mucus thickens and lessens in quantity.

It is recommended to use a tissue paper to wipe the inside vagina to assess the quantity and characteristics of mucus. To practice, this method the woman should be able to distinguish between different types of mucus. This method requires a high degree of motivation than most other methods.

Symptothermal method

Symptothermal method combines the use of BBT with analysis of cervical mucus changes to make predictions more accurate. Individual change also may be noted. A urine test that detects the luteinizing hormone (LH) surge that occurs before ovulation may be used at home.

Because this method is not affected by illness, stress or activity levels it is reliable when used in combination with other fertility indicators. If used every month, however, it is costly. It is not suitable for women with irregular cycles.

Coitus interruptus

Coitus interruptus is an ancient method that requires the male to withdraw his penis from vagina immediately before ejaculation of the semen, as result the semen is not deposited in or near the vagina. This withdrawal method is useful to those who have other available method. It involves no cost, devices or chemicals and is accessible in any situation. It is a method that can lead to a great deal of psychological upset in both sexual partners. Sometimes it is difficult for the partners, when orgasm is imminent. It is extremely frustrating for both partners. Even though ejaculation may be held back, pre-ejaculatory fluid can escape before ejaculation.

A small drop contains millions of sperms. There is a possibility of sperm deposited near the external genitalia to reach ovum. Thus the method is unreliable. The method calls for a great deal of self-control on the part of both partners and requires a great deal of motivation for its continued use.

Coitus reservatus

In this method, penetration of the vagina takes place, but there is little or no motion and the man does not ejaculate into the vagina. It is not a good method.

Coitus interfemoris

The erect penis is placed between the thighs of the female, so ejaculation, if it occurs; does so outside the vagina.

Lactational amenorrhea method

It is believed that there is a high probability that the woman who is amenorrheal while breastfeeding, will be able to regulate her fertility in first 6 months postpartum even if she introduces supplementation in the baby's feedings. When a baby sucks from the mother's breast, there is reflex release of prolactin from the pituitary, which acts to prevent ovulation. However, the biological life of prolactin is very short and therefore, repeated suckling is necessary to maintain a high level of prolactin in blood. The key to the suppression of fertility is excellent breastfeeding skills, as long as amenorrhea continues. Once spotting or menses begins, other methods of contraception need to be implemented.

The above natural family planning methods demand discipline and understanding of sexuality. It is not meant for everybody. The educational component is more important with this approach than with other methods.

Appliance method

Male condom

In India it is known as 'Nirodh'. The condom is rolled on to the erect penis and must applied before any genital contact occurs as some semen may escape prior to ejaculation. The condom is fitted on the erect penis before intercourse. The air must be expelled from the teat end to make room for the ejaculate. The condom must be held carefully when withdrawing it from vagina; to avoid spilling seminal fluid into the vagina after intercourse. A new condom should be used for each sexual act (Figs 47.2A to E).

Male condom prevents the deposit of sperm in the vagina. There are many types of condoms and packaging becomes an important part of marketing. The male condom is a sheer rubber sheath used before intercourse.

Condom prevents the semen from being deposited in vagina. The effectiveness of condom may be increased by using it in conjunction with a spermicidal jelly inserted into vagina before intercourse. It serves as additional protection in the unlikely event that the condom should slip off or tear. The condom should not be used after the expiry date and should be stored away from extreme heat, light and damp.

Female condom

Consists of a polyurethane sheath that is inserted into vagina. The closed inner and is anchored in place by a polyurethane ring. Whilst the open outer edge lies flat against the vulva.

The female condom is a prelubricated transparent sheath that forms a second skin inside the vagina when inserted properly, shields the vaginal and urethral areas from contact with the penis, while capturing semen during intercourse.

General advantages of condoms include the easy availability, safe and inexpensive, easy to use, do not require medical supervision, light, compact and disposable, protects against pregnancy and also STD and HIV infections. Disadvantages includes, it may slip off or tear, during intercourse and interferes with sex sensations locally (Figs 47.3A to D).

Barrier method

Barrier methods of contraception have a long history. The ancient Egyptians used such methods, which consisted of honey-coated pessaries. The original reason for honey coating was probably sexual pleasure, but later honey coating was found to have a contraceptive effect. Honey is effective in killing sperms as well as bacteria. Now a variety of barriers or occlusive methods suitable for men and

CHAPTER 47   Population and its Control   745

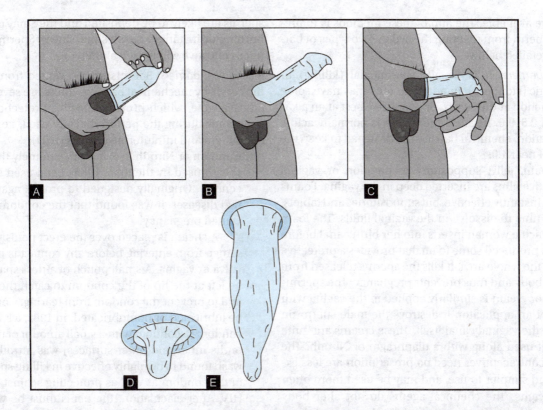

Figures 47.2A to E: Ways of using male condom. **A.** Application; **B.** Withdrawal; **C.** Removal and disposal; **D.** Rolled-up sheath; **E.** Unrolled sheath (condom).

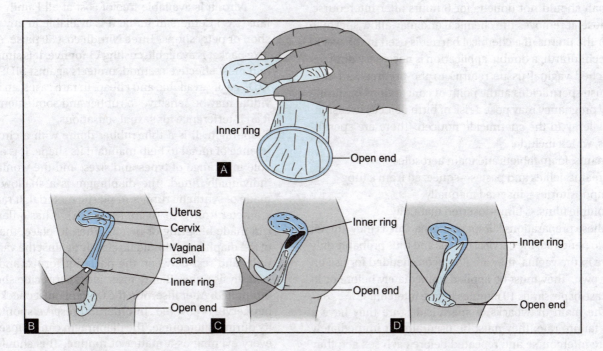

Figures 47.3A to D: Ways of using female condom. **A.** Squeeze inner ring of condom of inneration; **B to D.** Placement.

women are available. The aim of these methods is to prevent live sperm from meeting the ovum. Two types of barriers are detailed below.

Chemical barriers: It is usually spermicidal (killing) or spermistatic (stopping). In addition, they may have some blocking action at the cervix. Sperm thrive best at an alkaline pH of 8.5–9.0. Because the vagina is normally acidic until ovulation, chemical barriers are designed to keep the vaginal pH near 4.0.

The foam, jelly, suppository preparation or vaginal contraceptive films are inserted deep in the vagina. Foams and jellies instantly effective, but suppositories and tablets, films take time to dissolve in the vaginal fluids. The foam tablets, which a woman inserts into her birth canal before having sex produced some foam that provides a protective coating to the whole area. It kills the sperms released from the man's body and thus prevents pregnancy. The spermicidal jelly or cream is similarly applied in the vagina with the help of an applicator. It destroys the male sperm on contact in the vaginal canal itself. These creams are quite effective, if used along with a diaphragm or Nirodh. The chemical contraceptives need no prescription are less expensive and simpler to use, and may be used more often by adolescents. The chemical agents do not alter body physiology, but increase vaginal lubrication. Use of these creams also helps to protect against sudden infant death syndrome (SID), AIDS to some extent. By effectiveness woman should not douche for 6 hours after intercourse, because, it removes the chemical and may allow sperm to enter the uterus. If a chemical barrier is used in the weeks after childbirth, a double application is necessary until the stretched vaginal tissue returns to the prepregnant size. The use spermicides at the point of conceptions or during early pregnancy may pose a risk of birth defects, occasionally allergy to the spermicide noticed. There are spermicides, which include:

- Foams, foam tablets and foam aerosoles
- Creams, jellies and pastes—squeezed from a tube
- Suppositories—inserted manually
- Soluble films, C film—inserted manually.

These preparations kill spermatozoa, but as they are not able to penetrate the cervical mucus and thus probably only active in the vagina, they are not recommended for use on their own. They must be applied immediately before or in the case of pessaries 10 minutes before intercourse.

The main drawbacks of spermicides are they have a high failure rate; they must be used almost immediately before intercourse and repeated before each sex act; they must be introduced into those regions of the vagina where sperms are likely to be deposited and they may cause mild burning or irritation, besides messiness. Spermicides are not as effective when used alone.

Mechanical barriers: Sperms are prevented from entering the cervix by mechanical barriers. There are several methods available, which provide effective protection against pregnancy during the period they are used, i.e. condom, diaphragm and intrauterine devices (IUD):

1. Condom or Nirodh use: It is an extremely thin rubber sheath used by the man. It has been used since 14th century. Originally designed to protect against venereal diseases, it was found that the condom also prevented pregnancy.

    A sheath is placed over the erect penis to prevent semen from entering before any contact is made with vulva or vagina. A small pouch of airless space should be left at the tip of the condom to catch the ejaculate and to prevent the condom from tearing. Condom can be lubricated or nonlubricated. In 1982, a spermicidal condom (a condom with a small amount of nonoxynol on its inner and outer surfaces) was introduced and wash found to be highly effective in killing sperm within the condom as well as protecting against STDs and HIV. After ejaculation, the penis must be withdrawn from the vagina while still erect and care must be taken to prevent the condom from slipping off to prevent semen from entering the vagina (Figs 47.4A to E).

    Nirodh is available free of cost at all Family Welfare (FW) Centers in India. It is available in any drug shop or petty shops. Three Nirodh cost 50 paise. A deluxe packet is available costing ₹1 for five. It is simplest and most effective method, protects against SIDS and AIDS easily available and cheap. In rare cases, an individual may be sensitive to rubber and some men find it an interference for sexual sensations.

2. Diaphragm: It is a thin rubber dome with a circumference of metal to help maintain its shape. It is available in a range of types and sizes, and the woman is individually fitted. The diaphragm is a shallow cup made of synthetic rubber or plastic material. It ranges diameter from 5 to 10 cm (2–4 inch). It has a flexible rim made of spring or metal. When in place, the rim of the diaphragm should lie closely against the vaginal walls and rest between the posterior fornix, and the symphysis pubis. Before insertion, spermicide should be applied. After insertion the woman must check that her cervix is covered. In order to preserve spontaneity during intercourse. The diaphragm can be inserted every evening as a matter of routine. This should be done after bathing, if applicable rather before.

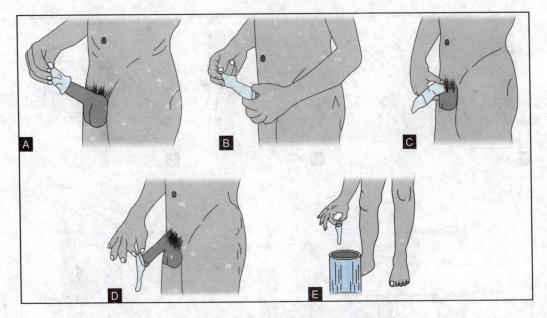

Figures 47.4A to E: Steps to use a male condom safely

The diaphragm is a barrier contraceptive that blocks sperm from entering the cervix. This palm-sized cup is easily inserted by hand or introducer, it is designed to be used with spermicidal cream or gel.

If intercourse occurs more than 3 hours after insertion, then additional spermicide is required. The diaphragm must be left in place for at least 6 hours after the last intercourse. On removal, the diaphragm should be washed with a mild soap, dried and inspected for any damage. A new diaphragm should be fitted annually and following any alteration in weight by more than 3 kg. In case of postpartum period, preferably new diaphragm should be used after assessing size of the same.

The diaphragm is a curved rubber dome enclosed by a flexible metal ring that rests in the vagina and covers the cervix. It was invented by a German physician in 1882, also known as 'Dutch cap'. It is introduced into the vagina to cover the mouth of the uterus to prevent the sperm entering into it. Cream or jelly may also be used with it. It is inserted before sexual intercourse and must remain in place for not less than 6 hours after coitus.

The woman should check for proper placement by feeling for cervix (which feels like a rounded knob or tip of the nose). The anterior rim can be felt resting against the symphysis pubis. Once in a place, the diaphragm should not be felt by either partner during intercourse (Figs 47.5A to E). Its use is less due to the difficult technique of application, high cost and lack of toilet facilities in areas. Sometimes, women may cause cystitis due pressure on urethra. Cervical cap is another device functional on diaphragm (Figs 47.6A to C). It blocks sperm from entering the cervical canal. It is a thimble-shaped cup. The cap is designed to its snugly over the cervix when correctly inserted.

3. Vaginal contraceptive sponge: It is a small, rounded one, size fits all polyurethane device that has a dimple on one side so that it fits snugly over the cervix, the other side of the sponge has a woven loop used for its removal from the vagina. The sponge is permeated with spermicide. Water is used to moisten the sponge for easier insertion. Once in place, it provides continuous protection for 24 hours. It should remain in place for at least 6 hours after intercourse. Sperm becomes trapped in the sponge and is then destroyed by the spermicide.

The availability of the sponge is a benefit for many women. It may be inserted 18 hours before intercourse. It is more convenient to use than some of the other vaginal contraceptives.

4. Intrauterine devices: The IUD is the devices, which are placed in the womb (Figs 47.7A to C). There are many types of IUDs, but the Lippes loop and the Copper-T (Cu-T) are the most commonly used in India (Figs 47.8A to D). The IUDs provide a method of conception control combining a high degree of effectiveness and safety with the advantages of easy insertion (Figs 47.9A and B) and removal:

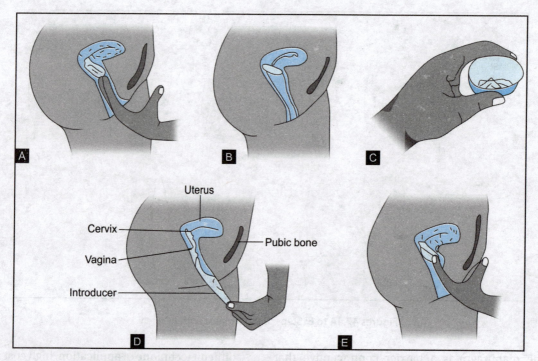

Figures 47.5A to E: Steps to use a diaphragm

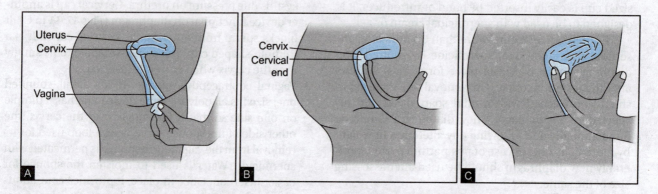

Figures 47.6A to C: Use of cervical cap. **A.** Insertion; **B** and **C.** Placement.

a. **Lippes loop:** The loop is a small double S-shaped device made of polythene and inert plastic material being produced in India. IUDs attached to one of the two ends in a fine plastic filament, which extends through the cervix to the vagina when the loop is inserted into the uterine cavity by plunger. It remains in the uterine cavity for years and does not interfere with sex life. As long as it remains in the uterus no conception can take place. In case the couple decides to have another child, the loop can be removed and conception can take place.

The mechanism of action of the IUD in women is still not clear in spite of its use for so many years. The most likely explanation of IUD action is the migration of white blood cells in the uterine cavity due to presence of the foreign body. These cells capture the ascending sperm during intercourse and probably alter, and destroys blastocysts in case these are formed.

Loop should not be used in the woman who had suspected pregnancy, pelvic infection, history of bleeding, suspicion of malignancy, acute cervicitis and erosion of cervix.

CHAPTER 47 — Population and its Control

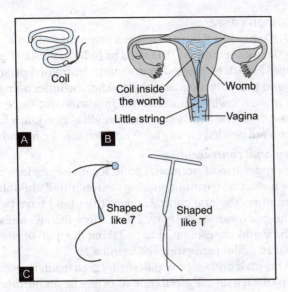

Figures 47.7A to C: Intrauterine contraceptive device and application. **A.** Coil, which is inserted in the womb; **B.** After application of the coil; **C.** Other shapes of coils.

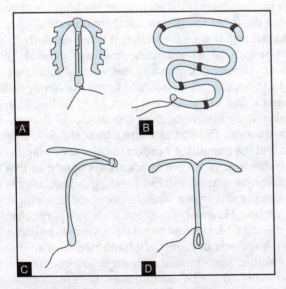

Figures 47.8A to D: Some intrauterine contraceptive devices. **A.** Multiload 375; **B.** Lippes loop; **C.** Copper-T; **D.** Nova-T.

The side effects of IUD will include bleeding, pain, vaginal discharge and pelvic infection (Fig. 47.10). An integral part of the information given to the woman with an IUD is the early IUD danger signals according to following acronym **PAINS** for easier client recall:
- **P:** Period of late pregnancy, suspected abnormal spotting or bleeding
- **A:** Abdominal pain or pain with intercourse
- **I:** Injection (abnormal vaginal discharge)
- **N:** Not feeling well, fever and chills
- **S:** Stirring lost, shorter or longer.

b. **Copper-T:** This brand of intrauterine copper contraceptive has now been found most effective. The Cu-T also made of plastic, but is wrapped with fine copper, which enhances its contraceptive effect. Its acceptance is higher than that of loop. The number of pregnancy expulsions and adverse reactions are less.

In this, a white thread with two strands is attached to the Cu-T, to check that it is in place. As stated earlier, it is a small plastic object, 'T' shaped with a copper wire wrapped around the stem of the Cu-T makes it more effective as IUD. It enhances the efficacy as it acts as a drug. Recent development of copper and hormonal systems are shown in Figures 47.11A and B.

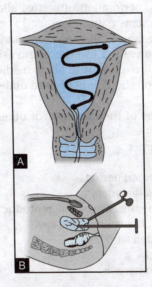

Figures 47.9A and B: Insertion of the intrauterine device

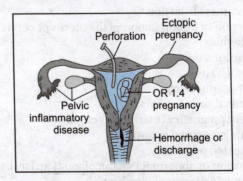

Figure 47.10: Complications of intrauterine devices (OR, odds ratio)

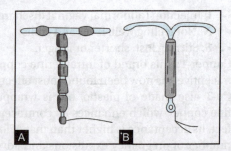

Figures 47.11A and B: Recent developments in copper and hormonal systems: The levonorgestrel intrauterine system of delivery in the Mirena intrauterine device. **A.** Copper 1220-C; **B.** Mirena.

Removal of Cu-T is easy, but no other person except the physician or surgeon should try to remove Cu-T.

There may be adverse reactions and side effects with Cu-T, which includes bleeding, painful period, painful intercourse, erosion of uterus and infection, pregnancy outside the uterus, perforation of uterus, allergic reactions, expulsion, backache, pain in legs, and vaginal discharge. The warning signals of these reactions may be taught to a woman undergone Cu-T insertions and ask her to report, when she finds them, and rush her to medical help.

Copper-T loop should not be used under the following conditions:

- Abnormalities of the uterus or of other reproductive organs
- Allergy to copper
- Anemia
- Bleeding between periods
- Blood clotting disorders
- Cancer or other diseases of the reproductive organs
- Cortisone or other steroid therapy
- Diabetes treated with insulin
- Fainting attacks
- Genital actinomycosis
- Heart disease
- Heart murmur
- Heavy menstrual flow
- Infection or inflammation of the uterus or cervix
- Leukemia
- Pelvic infection
- Prior IUD use
- Prior uterine surgery
- Recent abortion or miscarriage
- Recent pregnancy (uterine or ectopic)
- Severe menstrual cramps
- Suspected pregnancy
- Suspicion or abnormal Papanicolaou (Pap) test
- Unexplained vaginal bleeding
- Vaginal discharge or infection
- Venereal disease
- Wilson's disease
- IUD should not be inserted in a pregnant woman.

The most common IUD used in India is the Cu-T and Lippes loop. It is inserted in the uterus by trained personnel and prevents pregnancy by making the inner lining of the uterine cavity unsuitable for implantation. Once inserted, it can be kept 3–5 years. Periodical check-ups by a doctor are needed for any advice, which may be required.

Hormonal contraceptive

The proper use of hormonal contraceptives provides the best means of ensuring spacing between one childbirth to another. The oral contraceptives ('the pill') have been in the market since the early 1960s. More than 65 million in the world are estimated to be taking the 'pill' of which about 10 million are estimated in India.

One oral contraceptive pill is to be taken regularly everyday by the females. The pill consists of female sex hormone, synthesis of estrogen and progesterone. It is a combination of female hormones in various proportions. It suppresses ovulation, makes cervical mucus thick, making the passage for the sperms difficult to enter the uterine cavity and makes the inner lining unsuitable for implantation of the fertilized egg. It is very effective, if taken regularly. It corrects menstrual irregularities, improves general health and also prevents ovarian and endometrial cancer.

In India, the pill is available under the family welfare Program, free of charge in a pack of 28 tablets. One pill is taken daily beginning from the 5th day of the onset of menstruation. The first 21 white tablets are contraceptive pills and the remaining 7 brown in color are iron pills, it is advisable to keep an extra pack always handy, so that the cycle can be started without break. This regularity is the most important aspect, which ensures the high efficacy of the method. However, if a pill is missed on a particular day, the missed tablet should be taken as soon as possible, i.e. two tablets next day, one in the morning and another in the evening. Since missed on more than a couple of occasions it should not be discontinued, but another method of contraception such as condom should be used, along with it up to the date of next menstruation.

The pill is prescribed by the doctor after examination of the woman or by a trained nurse with the help of a checklist given in Table 47.1.

If all the above are answered in negative, the woman may be selected for oral contraceptives. If any of the above are answered in positive the woman must be seen by a physical before oral contraceptives are prescribed. The oral contraceptive pill should not be taken in case the woman is pregnant, has had jaundice, breast cancer or genital organs or is a nursing mother.

Population and its Control

Table 47.1: Checklist to prescribe a pill

Sl No.	Queries	Response
1.	Above 35 year	Yes/No
2.	Married for more than 2 years, has no children	Yes/No
3.	Poorly nourished	Yes/No
4.	Fat (overweight)	Yes/No
5.	Yellow color of skin and eyes for last 6 months	Yes/No
6.	Smoker	Yes/No
7.	History of diabetes	Yes/No
8.	Complaint of prolonged/recurrent headache	Yes/No
9.	Visual disturbances	Yes/No
10.	Fits	Yes/No
11.	Lump in the breasts	Yes/No
12.	Selling of arm and legs	Yes/No
13.	Palpitations	Yes/No
14.	Breathlessness on exertion	Yes/No
15.	Irregular vaginal bleeding	Yes/No
16.	History of swelling of feet and/or fits during pregnancy	Yes/No

The oral pill may produce side effects such as nausea, dizziness, abdominal pain, tender breast, weight gain and irregular bleeding. Reassurance may help to come out with side effects. In case, woman complains of pain in calf muscles with or without swelling, severe headache, skin rash, itching of the skin and yellow discoloration of eyes and skin, should be advised to seek further medical help by the doctor.

It should be remembered that woman with history of toxemia of pregnancy should not be put on pills and nulliparas should be put on pills only after they have been examined by a doctor. The pills are costly and requires daily use.

When prescribing oral contraceptives, the woman should be informed about the warning signals related to the oral pills as given below acronym '**ACHES**' to seek prompt medical attention. Is the woman:

- **A:** Abdominal pain severe (may mean gallbladder or liver problem)
- **C:** Chest pain, severe cough, shortness of breath (may mean a blood clot)
- **H:** Headache severe, dizziness, weakness and numbness (may mean hypertension or impending stroke)
- **E:** Eye problems, vision lesser, blurring, speech problem (may mean stroke)
- **S:** Severe pain in legs, calf or thighs (may mean blood clot).

Terminal methods

Sterilization has one major difference from other methods of contraception and this is mostly irreversible and permanent. The permanency of the method is an advantage from the population control point of view, but is a disadvantage for motivation and acceptance. However, surgical sterilization usually is a permanent measure and should be undertaken only after a great deal of consideration. It is important not to choose sterilization because there are side effects or difficulties with other methods. The person being sterilized must be absolutely sure that they cannot even think of any circumstances where they would wish to have another child.

Psychological implications accompany the loss of reproductive ability. Everyone choosing the option of sterilization needs to explore personal feelings reproductive process often is equated with the degree of maleness and femaleness a man or woman feels, and loss of reproductive ability may lower self-esteem. Most men and women who undergo surgical sterilization are however, not adversely affected. It is common to equate sterilization with castration and even those who realize that the two are different may still need reassurance. Men need reassurance of continuation of the libido and orgasm, and that the ejaculate comes mainly from the accessory glands, therefore no changes occur in the volume of the ejaculate after sterilization. Women may need information in regard to fate of ovulated eggs. The legal aspects of sterilization should be taken care of while counseling. It is always preferable to have a satisfied volunteer than those having regrets following sterilization.

Male sterilization

Harrison (1899) recommended vasectomy in men as a supposed cure for prostate enlargement. Vasectomy is a very simple method and no hospitalization is necessary. It is relatively quick, simple, effective and ideal for male (Fig. 47.12).

The word 'vasectomy' means cutting of the 'vas'. Before vasectomy is undertaken, the assessment of the health of

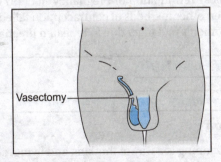

Figure 47.12: Vasectomy involves excision of a segment of the vas deferens

the individual is essential. Special attention is necessary for those having varicocele, hernia, cyst in the epididymis, etc. where major procedures may be necessary. A person with hemophilia or diabetes have the risk of bleeding or infection due to the operation.

The operative technique may vary depending upon the surgeon. After vasectomy, the person should get his semen tested before he continues his normal sexual life. There is no side effect.

Female sterilization

Tubal ligation or tubectomy: Lundgren (1881) performed the world's first tubal ligation in women. The principle of female sterilization is the blocking each of the fallopian tube, which carries eggs from the ovaries to the womb. A wide variety of surgical procedures to approach the tubes and more than 200 methods have been described. A number of occlusive mechanisms can be employed including ligation, use of a clip, a variety of surgical procedures or heat cauterization. The approaches to the fallopian tubes include conventional laparotomy, minilaparotomy, colpotomy (vaginal sterilization), culdoscopy, laparoscopy and hysteroscopy (Figs 47.13A to C).

The best time for a tubal ligation is within 24–48 hours after the woman has given birth, when the tubes have been displaced towards the anterior part of the abdomen and are easily visualized. If not, tubal ligation should usually be done 4–7 days after delivery, when the uterus is high, it can be done at any time. It requires hospitalization for 10–20 days or less depending upon the procedure. There is no effect on the sex life of the women. The menses continue as before the operation, there is no side effects. It can be reversed by recolonization.

In certain cases of unfortunate situation, e.g. death of children, the reversal operation is possible in the case of both males and females. But such operations are only done by expert surgeons in major hospitals where the required facilities are available.

Induced abortion: This has been legalized in India under the Medical Termination of Pregnancy Act (1971). This is used when other methods of contraception failed or when life of mother is in danger due to repeated pregnancy.

FAMILY PLANNING

Limiting Family Size: By Family Planning

Definition

Family planning is a way of thinking and living, i.e. adopted voluntarily upon the basis of knowledge, attitude and responsible decisions by individuals, and couples in order to promote the health and welfare of the family group; and thus contribute effectively to the social development of a country (WHO, 1971).

Objectives

Family planning refers to practices that help individuals or couples to attain certain objectives (WHO, 1971) given below:
- To avoid unwanted births
- To bring about wanted births
- To regulate the intervals between pregnancies
- To control the time at which birth occurs in relation to the age of the parents
- To determine the number of children in the family
  Services that make these practices possible include:
- Education and counseling on family planning
- The provisions of contraceptives

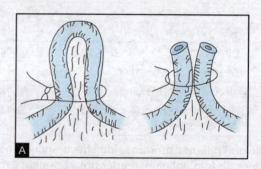

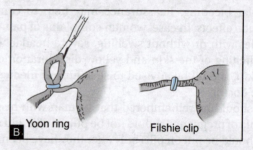

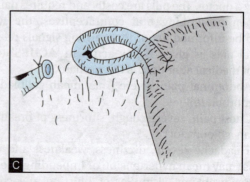

Figures 47.13A to C: Tubectomy. **A.** Sterilization by tubal ligation and excision; **B.** Sterilization by occlusion; **C.** Burial of stumps.

CHAPTER 47
Population and its Control

- The management of infertility
- Education about sex and parenthood
- Organizationally related activities such as genetic and marriage counseling, screening for malignancy, and adoption services.

Scope of Family Planning Services

Family planning is recognized as a basic human right (UNO, 1968). All couples and individuals have the basic human right to decide freely and responsibly on the number and spacing of their children, and to have the information, education and means to do so. The modern concept of family planning, not synonymous with birth control includes and extends the following:

1. The proper spacing and limitation of birth.
2. Advice on sterility.
3. Education for parenthood.
4. Sex education.
5. Screening for pathological conditions related to the reproductive system.
6. Genetic counseling.
7. Premarital consultation and examination.
8. Carrying out pregnancy tests.
9. Marriage counseling: The preparation of couples for the arrival of first child.
10. Providing services for unmarried mothers.
11. Teaching home economics and nutrition.
12. Providing adoption services.

Family Welfare Program

The family planning aims at small family, which will serve the welfare of the individual, the family and the community; it is also associated with numerous misconceptions. One of them is its strong association in the minds of people, with birth control. The recognition of welfare concept came only a decade and half after its inception, when it was named Family Welfare Program (1977). Although, the welfare components were already included in the programs earlier, the new connotation of the word 'welfare' gave more stress to these components.

Family planning is a family welfare program and its aim is to create a social welfare state. Family planning is the responsibility of man and woman, while population control is a government policy to reduce birth rate, motivated by social and economic interest with the help of community health. The Planning Commission of India has given top priority for stabilizing populations and has recommended:

1. Widespread education to create necessary social background for the success of family planning program.
2. Integration of family planning with the normal health services.
3. Provision of family planning services, even sterilization through medical and health centers.
4. To develop training program in teaching hospitals and medical college.
5. To stimulate and utilize the voluntary leadership.

Role of nurses in family welfare program

The nurses are in an excellent position to participate in family planning activities that is through the provision of daily care, those working in hospitals quickly gain the confidence of sick person. This confidence provides an effective base for preventive nursing care. Those employees in community health agencies, perhaps because of the comprehensive nature of the care they give are in a unique position for participation in family welfare program.

The role of the nurses in family welfare will be governed by the policy of the government and/or of the health institution employing them. Policies may vary from those that require nurses to participate in family welfare activities to those that forbid them to do so or that limit their participation to giving advice to high risk mothers eligible because of specific health reasons. The ethical aspects of nursing care are of extreme importance in program, which deals with human fertility, its promotion or its control. Because these programs involve social as well as sexual matters of an intimate nature, nurses are expected to use discretion and sensitivity in the use, and evaluation of any information provided by individuals or couples. The role of nurses in family welfare program will include in:

- Administrative role
- Supervisory role
- Functional role
- Educational role
- Role in research
- Role in evaluation.

Administrative role

Nurses who are in senior positions may be called upon to participate in the organization of family welfare programs at national, regional or community level and in the development of nursing activities within the framework of these programs. The nursing personnel have various functions and responsibilities at different levels with regard to family planning.

As nurse administrator

1. Maintains an up-to-date and relevant knowledge about family planning services in the country.
2. Makes sure that all her nursing staff is aware of family planning measures during their training or in-service education program.

3. Ensures that adequate educational material on family planning is available in the ward library and all the contraceptive methods for demonstration to patients are made available in the wards.
4. Formulates a policy on imparting knowledge on family welfare services to all patients before they are discharged from the hospital.
5. Establishes a good referral system between each ward of the hospital and the family planning department, so that each eligible client gets required contraceptives.
6. Incentivize nurses to make their best contributions to family planning services.
7. Supervises nurses, auxiliary nurse midwives (ANMs), anganwadi workers and multipurpose health workers in relation to activities on family planning.
8. Participates or conducts research on family planning.
9. Plans and conducts in-service education programs for nursing personnel.

Supervisory role

Nurses who are responsible for the practical experience supervision and in-service education of other health workers, professional and auxiliary nursing and midwifery personnel, new staff students and volunteers assisting in the activities of nursing understand the policy of family welfare. As a supervisor community health nurses should encourage their staff to watch carefully for indication that mother or couples would accept advice on how to space their children and so on.

Functional role

The primary function of nurse in family planning is case finding, i.e. finding eligible couples and making referral to adopt suitable family planning method. In addition that nurses will have routine clinical functions, which includes assisting doctor in prenatal, postnatal examination, and with vario to choose one of the more simple and/or suitable methods of contraception and follow-up services.

Educational role

Usually all nurses have an educational role to fulfill with their patients and the community. As a basis for counseling in family planning nurses must have sound knowledge of the biology of human reproduction, education for family life, the concept and principles underlying family planning, the factors which influence it of existing methods, regulating fertility, and the facilities and services available in this respect. Moreover, they must be able to transmit this knowledge effectively. The counseling on fertility can be held with their clients in hospital, health centers, schools, homes and community centers by using proper audiovisual aids.

As a nurse educator

- Integrates family planning component in nursing curriculum, while teaching
- Teaches family planning as a subject
- Selects and organizes learning experience both in theory, and practice for student nurses
- Coaches ANM, health visitors, multipurpose health workers and anganwadi workers regarding family planning
- Helps nurse administrators to organize in-service education programs for nurses
- Also clarifies doubts of patients regarding family planning, during her supervisory rounds
- Conducts or participates in nursing research on family planning.

Role in research

Nurses are essential members of the multidisciplinary research team and then nursing as a science or a practice must be systematically studies research mindedness gradually being introduced into the basic education of nurses is being reinforced in postbasic programs and increasingly being advocated as an approach to the solution of problems. Nurses know to keep careful records and reports relating to their nursing activities, and can now begin to keep systematic records and reports relating to family planning activities, i.e. methods of contraception used, their side effects and contraindications (if any), the consistency with which they are used, their efficacy and any other patient information. These provide valuable data upon which research may be based.

As a research worker

- Conducts surveys of eligible couples from different communities with varying socioeconomic data
- Studies the attitude of community toward family planning
- Organizes surveys on knowledge of family planning among patients in hospital setting
- Imparts sex education to adolescent
- Participates in conducts studies on family planning and other related topics.

Role of evaluation

Evaluation is an important part of planning for nursing services including those related to the regulation of fertility and should be built into the plan as it is being formulated.

When nurses asked to participate in the establishment of criteria whereby achievement may be evaluated, they should be responsible for criteria related to the nursing and midwifery component of the family welfare program.

The concern of nurses and midwives with individual family and community health has led to their increasing interest and involvement in health services related to family planning, human reproduction, and population dynamics. Contraception has become an integral part of life for many people. Every birth control method available for use today has risks and benefits associated with its use. Each method carries responsibilities on the part of the user to learn about the side effects, advantages and disadvantages. All education about family planning is based on firm understanding of the anatomy and physiology of reproduction. Using this knowledge, nurses can counsel and support individuals in their choices, and in health care.

As a clinical nurse in hospital/community

1. Identifies eligible couples: They can be identified at the time of hospital registration, while history taking, when giving nursing care, reviewing records, during visiting hours and also while giving home visits.
2. The nursing responsibility also involves evaluating patients according to their reproductive age group, number of children, those who are suffering from illness that is detrimental to pregnancy or childbirth and also those who express interest in spacing or limiting the family size. These couples may either come to hospital or community health centers (CHCs), or they may be identified in special clinics for tuberculosis (TB), cancer, etc.
3. Imparts information to the eligible couples: The eligible couples are informed about various methods of family planning. The information would include methods of contraception, their practicality, effectiveness, advantages, disadvantages, side effects and the health facilities to visit in case some complication arises. This information can be disseminated:
    a. Through individual and group teaching.
    b. Using films/video or other visual aids.
    c. Using literature on family planning in local languages.
    d. Motivates the couple to adopt family planning methods; the nurse tries to develop in them, a sense of responsibility and highlights the benefits of a small family, so that they accept 'small family' system.
    e. Counsels the couples to identify their problems due to a large family and take steps to solve those problems.
    f. Assists the doctor in surgical methods such as vasectomy and tubectomy.
    g. Maintains the stock book and ensures adequate supplies in the healthcare center.
    h. Manages referral services and follow-up care.
    i. Maintains proper documents and records of vital statistics, essential for eventual evaluation of the rate of implementation and success of the measures.

Small Family Norm Promotion and its Importance

Promotion of small family norms

Population control can be achieved by promoting small family norms. The difference in family size can make a tremendous difference in birth rate. The one child norm per family over decades has created a tremendous impact on the growth of population. The small family norms in the objective of family welfare program. This is to achieve control over country's population. The small family norms were promoted by the slogans 'do ya teen bus' in the year 1970, because of three child family model. In 1980s campaign was 'sons or daughters—two will do' or 'second child after 3 years'. These slogans were to achieve small family. Welfare program was to achieve a net reproduction rate of unity (NRR = 1) by the year 2006. The emphasis is still to adopt small family. Various ways can be adopted to achieve and promote small family norms:

- Family welfare programs
- Family planning methods
- Mass communication
- Information, education and communication
- Registration of eligible couples
- Target couple (who have two to three living children) to be directed towards family planning methods
- Cafeteria approach for adoption of family planning methods
- Involvement of health education institutions for promotion of small family
- Empowering women.

A significant achievement of the Family Welfare Program has been decline of fertility rate from 6.4 (in the 1950s) to 4.2 (in 1980s). The national target is to achieve a family size of 2.3 children by 2000. All the efforts are being made through mass communication that the concept of 'small family norms' is accepted, adopted and woven into lifestyle of the people. India adopted the goal of universalizing the two-child norm by the end of the century. The norm in relation to family size implies a pattern, which sets the limits of any community's fertility behavior. The achievement of the goal has consequences both at the micro level, i.e. for the nation as a whole.

The size of the family affects the quality of life of human beings. Family size affects the family in following spheres of life:

1. Basic human need: In any society, other things being equal, the larger the size of the family the relatively small per capita income share of basic needs (food, clothing, shelter, health care and education) for the

individuals and the family. Similarly, declining the size of the family results in bigger per capita share required for existence arid development.

2. **Income:** Thus, increase in family size lowers the per capita income. This lower per capita income leads to low domestic savings lesser resources for economic development, which further leads to small rate of economic development of family and the community.
3. **Nutrition:** An increase in family size results in decrease in per capita food, nutrition and improvement of the health standards. This in turn, exerts pressure on urban public systems, leading to poor social and economic development.
4. **Health:** According to certain studies large size families lead to higher morbidity and mortality amongst mothers and children. Early marriage followed by too early pregnancy, too many children till the advanced reproductive age of the mother affects the health of the mother as well as the child.
5. **Education:** Family size is seen to be related to education. Where the mother's education is high, the family size is usually smaller and infant mortality is also relatively lower. The level of the mother's education and its impact on family size are evident in the state of Kerala, where female literacy is the highest and it has the lowest birth rate, and the child mortality rate is also the lowest in the country.

Hazards of the Large and Unplanned Family

There are certain hazards of large and unplanned families, which are going to affect not only the mother and children but also the family as a whole, and subsequently the community and the nation.

Too early marriages (below 18 years for girls and 21 years for boys) lead to hazards, and pregnancy and childbirth, i.e. abortion, stillbirth, premature birth and increased chances to develop cancer of cervix. The early marriage may be the cause of discontinuation of education, which leads to lack of proper job opportunity.

Too early pregnancy leads to increased risk from pregnancy and childbirth, low-birth-weight (LBW) baby, sickness and ill health of mother (morbidity), increasing IMR and maternal mortality rate (MMR).

Too frequent pregnancies lead to LBW or sick baby, more chances of developing cervical cancer and may lead to economic hardship. Parent's attention is divided among children, devoting them of proper care.

Too many pregnancies lead to unhappiness and disharmony in the family, and may cause difficulty in providing proper education to children, and also increased risk of pregnancy and childbirth-related disorders.

The late age pregnancies may lose social status and leads to congenital abnormalities, e.g. the birth of a Mongoloid child.

Advantages for Adopting Small Family

A small planned family has many advantages and benefits. The planning for a family starts from marriage at the proper age. Keeping in view the legal and biological aspects, a girl should not be married before the completion of 18 years and a boy not before 21 years. The safest time for pregnancy for the health of both the mother and child is when the woman is between 20 and 30 years of age. For woman 20s are considered the optimal reproductive period. The reasonable gap between two children will give the mother sufficient time to replenish her body nutrients depleted due to the earlier pregnancy.

The other advantages of a small and planned family, to mother, child, father and community are given below.

Advantages to mother

1. In a small planned family, a mother can maintain her health by restricting the number of children and spacing pregnancy.
2. It creates loss of fear about unwanted pregnancy if any.
3. Mother will have less strain and worry due to limited number of children.
4. Mother will have more time and energy to give proper attention and love to her children.
5. Mother will have more time to participate in other fruitful activities such as education, vocational training, community projects, etc.
6. Mother can avail better job opportunities in a small family.
7. Mother can save child's health: There will be less chances of fetal death, birth defects, mortality during infancy and childhood.

Advantages for the child

1. The child will have conducive atmosphere for his/her proper physical and psychological growth and development.
2. Child gets proper nutrition, education, parental care and love.
3. Child can provide sound economic base for the family.

Advantages for the father

1. Father can provide children with better education, comfort, food, clothing, recreation, etc.
2. He will be more relaxed and enjoy good health.
3. He will have improved living standards, better health and more productive labor force.

Advantages for the community
1. Small family leads to conservation of natural resources and savings.
2. Small family norm helps the nation to have enough schools, hospitals and other basic services.
3. Small family norm yields more employment.
4. Small planned families would gradually bring happiness, peace, harmony and prosperity.

Practices for Small Family Norm

Small family norm has to become a way of life. For this purpose, organization of population, education in the school and colleges, for the out-of-school youth, the adult education programs would be most vital. For creating favorable atmosphere conducive to adoption of small family norm and acceptance, and practice of effective contraception the following means may be adopted:

1. For educating the community, the family and the couple, systematic and coordinated use of mass media, group orientation, and interpersonal communication would be important. The goal of the health worker would be:
   a. Supply necessary information for education and motivation.
   b. Assist the client to evaluate contraceptive information and services, and make an informed choice and decision about these.
   c. To encourage them for continued contraceptive use.
2. The health personnel should be properly trained with a view to strengthen their knowledge and skills in properly educating, and motivating the perspective users, to develop in themselves a proper attitude and faith in the program.
3. The service agency should be properly geared for effective implementation, monitoring and evaluation of contraceptive services; and the logistics for procurement and supply should ensure continued regular supply of contraceptives.
4. Effective delivery of contraceptive services at the doorsteps of the people is considered to be an important measure for promotion of small family norm.
5. For promoting acceptance of family planning, the IMR has to be brought down speedily and the chances of child survival have to be substantially improved.
6. Enforcement of universal primary education and prevention of dropouts would be an important step towards acceptance of small family norm special attention needs to be given to the girls and women.
7. Studies have shown that optimum age of the mothers for reproductive outcome is in her 20s. Therefore, enforcement of law on the minimum age of marriage as well as counseling of women not to bear any child before the age of 20 would be an important strategy.
8. Since, women have been found to be important instrument for social change, raising the social status of women and involving them in various welfare activities including family planning would be important.

Barriers of Small Family

The efforts are being made in two ways. First, by providing the necessary information and services to help people adopt the small family norm. Secondly, attempts are being made to change the associated environmental factors, i.e. increase in female literacy, raising the status of women and the age of marriage, improvements in general, social and economic conditions, which are often described as beyond family planning measures. While it may appear self-evident that two-child family is happy family, widespread acceptance of the two-child norm has not yet taken place in the country due to many existing barriers:

1. As per religious point everybody desires son for inheritance of property and performing rites after death.
2. Children are considered social security in old age.
3. There is an ethical uneasiness about medical termination of pregnancy (MTP).
4. Death rate of infants is very high.
5. Lack of recreation among the rural masses.

In order to remove barriers, the government and the people should take step to:

1. Provide recreation facilities and social security for old age.
2. Educate the poor, ignorant and illiterate people regarding small family norm, and its importance. It should be community oriented.
3. Voluntary maternity of woman must have proper place in formation of the family and its size.
4. Make family planning a people's program and way of life.
5. Ensure proper role of voluntary organizations.
6. Conditioning the mind and group pressure.

Thus concerted efforts, therefore, need to be made to provide the necessary information and education to the people, especially in rural areas and urban slums to motivate them to accept two-child family norm. It is indeed imperative on the part of each one of us to advocate and adopt the two-child family norm and constructively contribute our share in our own work settings. In the developmental efforts aimed at achieving the quality of life—physical, mental and socioeconomic well-being of the people, and the family and the community at large, and nation as a whole.

Family Planning and Women Empowerment

As stated earlier, family planning is a way of thinking and living that is adopted voluntary upon the basis of knowledge, attitude and responsible decisions by individuals and couple, in order to promote the health and welfare of the family group, and thus contribute effectively to the social development of the country. Family planning refers to practices that help individuals or couples to attain certain objective, which include:

- To avoid unwanted births
- To bring about wanted births
- To regulate the interval between pregnancies
- To control the time at which births occur in relation to the ages of the parent
- To determine the number of children in the family.

Some people feel that 'fertility regulations' is perhaps more acceptable than the word 'family planning'. As a rule, family planning conjures up in the minds of the people of developing countries, the idea of population control. Fertility regulation implies a situation where fertile couples space out their children and have the number of children they want. Infertile couples can be assisted to become fertile. Since, the word 'family planning' is widely accepted for a long time it has been continued to use.

Family planning is very necessary in communities where the birth rate is high and medical services, and financial resources are poor. Infant mortality rate is high because the parents cannot give proper care to the children on their limited resources. Moreover, involuntary parenthood creates emotional and social problems. Other indications for family planning are medical conditions such as cardiac disease, hypertension and chronic renal disease. Patients with these conditions cannot afford large families because of their impaired health. They also need to space out these pregnancies. Family planning is still a novelty to some people. As such the people need to be educated about it. They should be made to understand that family planning does not mean limiting one's family. It means judicious spacing children, so that their essential needs in life can be provided for by their parents. Family planning is becoming widely accepted in some developing countries including India.

Now people are thinking that the objective of family planning will be best achieved by women, i.e. population control can be achieved by overall development of women. It means, women need to be empowered and they should be developed socially, economically and educationally, so as to decide, and take appropriate measures to have small size family, which in turn reduces the population and achieve populations control.

Women empowerment means strengthening the capacity of women in order to identify understand and control their lives. Women due to lack of control have little to say in decisions, so they need to be empowered to achieve control and to participate in decision-making related to their health matters. According to women empowerment, the process by which women strengthens their capacity; and collectively to identify, understand and overcome gender discrimination, thus taking control of their lives.

Women empowerment can be achieved by changing policy and programs of actions in directing these policies, and programs that will improve women's access to secure livelihood and economic resources. Alleviating their extreme responsibility with regard to house work, remove legal impediments to their participation in public life and raising social awareness through effective programs of education and mass communication. Even improving the status of women also enhances the decision-making capacity at all levels in all spheres of life. The full participation of women is required in productive and reproductive life in order to achieve control over population, and to have development in the society.

The women need to be developed socially, educationally and economically in order to achieve empowerment among them:

1. Social development of women means raising the status of women in society. Women in male dominating society, i.e. patriarchal form of society do not get the same status as men especially in decision-making. As a result, they are facing threats to their lives, health and well-being. They are overburdened with work and lack of power, and influence. Some studies have shown that the disease reporting is less in women as compared to man in most parts of world. Social legislation has brought a change by developing the women socially. Nowadays, if women compared with the women of earlier ages, they are having more privileges. This is due to certain social legislations:
    a. In 1950s, new Constitutions of India accorded equal rights to women. All women now enjoy equal political rights with men. They have the right to vote and have right to hold public offices.
    b. In 1955, Hindu Marriage Act and Divorce Act has removed several disabilities. No Hindu can marry second time unless wife or husband is dead or divorced.
    c. In 1978, the Child Marriage Restraint Amendment Act has raised the marriage of girls from 15 to 18 years, for boys 18–21 years.
    d. In 1976, the Equal Remuneration Act provide for equal payment of remuneration to men and women workers.

All the legislative measures help in bringing awareness among women and removing social prejudices and inequalities; thereby bringing social development.
2. Educational development: Women need to be educationally developed. It has been seen that women receive less formal education than men and at the same time, women's own knowledge, abilities and coping mechanisms often go unrecognized. Education will help them in creating awareness regarding demerits and merits of large, and small family size as well as other aspects of health. If she is educated, then she can educate the whole family and can care the family by adopting appropriate measures.

Lack of education has been an obstacle in the development of women. So, there is need to take all special efforts to raise the literacy rate among women and girl's education. Government is making the efforts to raise the educational level of women. The central Government is providing financial assistance under the plan schemes to establish schools and colleges exclusively for girls in backward states. Special programs have been started for improving girl's education level. Other incentives are also provided such as clothing or free tuition.

The grants are provided by Central Social Welfare Board to voluntary organization to conduct courses of 2 or 3 years duration for having education. In order to achieve increased literacy rate, there is need to bring changes in policies and programs.
3. Educational development and social development: These will bring a change in economic condition of the women. Women can be empowered economically by:
   a. Implementing income-generating schemes: By these schemes, rural and poor women come together, and develop an understanding of their problems, and fulfill their need. Under these schemes:
      i. Technical information is imparted and strategies to plan action towards development, and against injustice.
      ii. Vocational courses for women.
      iii. Opening of women polytechnics.
      iv. Rehabilitation of women: By providing vocational training cum employment and residential care to old widows, and deserted women.
   b. To raise the economic level of women, women's development corporations are playing an important role in providing employment opportunities to women so that they will become economically dependent.
   c. It is essential for the sustainable development of community that the women should be empowered and developed socially, educationally, politically and economically. Experience shows that population and development programs are effective, if overall development occurs in women.
   d. In 2000, the Government of India adopted a national policy for the empowerment of women. This was to bring about gender justice. National Health Policy was under consideration in 2005 for implementation and it to be reviewed twice a year. The aims of the policy are:
      i. Women equality in power sharing and active participation in decision-making.
      ii. Comprehensive economic and social empowerment of women.
      iii. The advancement, development and empowerment of women in all spheres of life.
      iv. Strengthening and formation of relevant institutional mechanisms.
      v. Partnership with community-based programs.
      vi. Implementation of international, obligations and cooperation at international, regional and subregional levels.
      vii. More responsive judicial legal systems, i.e. sensitive to woman's need.

To review laws and legislation related to women, a task force for women headed by Deputy Chairperson of Planning commission has been constituted. The laws related to divorce, marriage and succession were amended to empower the women. National Commission on women has formulated a code of conduct for preventing sexual harassment at place of work. The 10th Five-year Plan (2002–2007) is concerned towards promotion of gender equality and empowering women, which include three strategies of empowering women. These are social empowerment, economic empowerment and gender injustice. Social empowerment means to create and develop environment through various policies and programs for development of women, and providing them easy access to basic minimum services. Economic empowerment ensures provision of training, employment and income generation activities to make women self-reliant and independent. Gender injustice eliminates all forms of gender discrimination.

Evolution of fertility regulating methods

Fertility control is not a new concept. The ancient religious leaders exorcized in favor of having few children. In Rigveda, 'A man with many children succumbs to miseries' is probably the oldest statement suggesting against a large family. In virtually every culture, which is of historical importance, as also in 'Hindu dharma', of India, there existed a desire for birth control by natural as well as artificial means. The written history of contraception and antifertility measures goes as far back as to the 'Atharvaveda', Urihadaranyapanishat and Kausika Sutra, there is reference to prayers, surgical measures such as crushing of testicle, vasectomy, hysterectomy and medicaments for producing sterility and infertility; both in the male and the female.

Some birth preventing and birth limiting measures practiced in Ancient Indian Society are as follows (Bhagawan Das, 1975):

1. There were restrictions in the Varnasrama that man has to marry only after the completion of their professional education and followed the principles of Brahmacharya Ashrama, which helps to delay marriages. Now this is one of the concepts emphasized today to delay marriages with so many reasons.
2. There was some prohibition of cohabitation on certain days, i.e. sexual intercourse was prohibited for the first 4 days after the appearance of the menstrual flow as well as on the 8th, 14th and 15th days of the dead parents, nights previous to the anniversaries and sankranthi (the passage of sun and other planetary bodies from one sign of the zodiac to another), in the day time, at midnight, and during eclipse among others.
3. They believed that certain seasons of the year, i.e. adanakala (time of absorption January to June) are said to be not conductive for sexual intercourse, as this may seriously affect the health of the individual.

In fact many methods have been used throughout history to prevent pregnancy. In ancient Egypt, women used domes or formed of hollowed lemon halves to cover the cervix. Other cultural groups have used tampons or followed elaborate rituals to prevent conceptions. In many countries a parturient woman is not allowed to go out until 40 days after delivery. Sexual intercourse is prohibited during the period of lactation, which in many developing countries lasts 2–3 years. In addition, after the mandatory 40 day period of rest, the woman usually goes to live with her parents-in-law until the infant is weaned. This segregation of the wife from the husband is a method of birth control by total abstinence. In addition to the above, men and women wore rings, amulets, etc. to protect themselves against an unwanted pregnancy.

In addition to the above practices, certain contraceptive devices were also being practiced in ancient India:

1. After stoppage of menstrual flow or during menstruation, the woman was asked to fumigated get her genital tract with smoke of margosa wood by burning it, to prevent conception [Yoga Ratnakara (1600 AD), Brihadyoga Tarangini (806 AD) and Tantrasara Sangraha].
2. A piece of rock salt smeared with til oil was used to be kept in the vaginal tract of female before and after coitus.

Today contraception means choosing and using a method to delay, prevent or space pregnancy. It affords many alternatives and choices during the reproductive years (Table 47.2). Contraception is an important factor in many women's lives, with needs varying according to

Table 47.2: Methods of contraception

Methods	Failure rate: Accidental pregnancy rate (typical use): First year (%)	Postpartum use	Risk and disadvantages	Benefits
Abstinence	0	Is the method of choice for first 4–6 week, especially for operative deliveries complications and lacerations	May be unacceptable to woman or partner; may cause relationship problems when there is disagreement	Promotes healing and involution
Oral contraceptives (two types) • Regular pill: Combined estrogen + progestin • Minipill: Progestin-only	3	May interfere with lactation by decreasing milk supply; if lactating, use minipill or wait until lactation is well established	Minor side effects are breast tenderness, nausea, irregular bleeding (especially with minipill); major risks are rare in women of aged 36 and younger who do not smoke; blood clots, liver tumor, cerebrovascular accident, myocardial infarction, gallbladder disease; requires regular monitoring by healthcare provider	May be acceptable for healthy women aged 36–50 year who do not smoke; menses are lighter and shorter and there are fewer cramps; may protect against breast, ovarian and uterine disease

Contd...

Contd...

Methods	Failure rate: Accidental pregnancy rate (typical use): First year (%)	Postpartum use	Risk and disadvantages	Benefits
Norplant	0.04	No studies are available of use during first 6 weeks, lactating concerns same as those for the birth control pill	Requires insertion and removal of implants in arm by trained healthcare provider; change in bleeding pattern common; risks similar to minipill; expensive	Contains progestin-only; circulating hormone level less than that with minipill; lasts 5 years, little monitoring required after insertion
Depo-Provera	0.04	Not recommended first 6 weeks, does not prevent lactation; can be passed to infant via breast milk; no known harmful effects on newborn	Must be given by healthcare provider; irregular menses common; risks similar to those of minipill	Injected intramuscularly every 12 weeks, lasts for 3 months
Intrauterine device (IUD)	3	Is not recommended during postpartum period	Must be inserted by healthcare provider; during menses has an increased risk of pelvic infection; may increase menstrual flow and cramps	Once in place, requires little monitoring by woman; for suitable candidate, may be inserted during first menses after childbirth
Cervical cap with spermicide	18	Same as diaphragm	Are same as for diaphragm, except may leave in place longer; may increase risk of cervical neoplasia; few healthcare providers fit caps	Not recommended during the postpartum period
Sponge	28	May cause irritation related to decreased levels of estrogen may increase risk of pelvic infection	Is difficult to remove; causes irritation and allergic reactions; linked to toxic shock syndrome	Is available over-the-counter; may be left in place longer than diaphragm; is disposable
Spermicide alone	21	May cause irritation because of decreased levels of estrogen	May cause allergic reactions; is messy; insert just before intercourse	Available over-the-counter, affords some protection against sexually transmitted diseases
Foams with condoms used together	3	Have no contraindications	Irritation and allergic reactions are rare; must be inserted/put on just before intercourse; is messy; may decrease sensation; protect against sexually transmitted diseases	As effective as the pill when used together; foam is lubricant; available over-the-counter; protect against sexually transmitted diseases
Condoms alone	12	Have no contraindications	Irritation and allergic reactions are rare; must be inserted/put on just before intercourse; is messy; may decrease sensation when used correctly	Available over-the-counter; used together; protect against sexually transmitted diseases

Contd...

Contd...

Methods	Failure rate: Accidental pregnancy rate (typical use): First year (%)	Postpartum use	Risk and disadvantages	Benefits
Natural family planning, fertility awareness, periodic abstinence	20	Are not recommended; requires signs and symptoms of hormone fluctuation during normal cycling; this cycling does not occur during the postpartum period, especially during lactation	No risks; require practice and education from trained professional; require self-monitoring and record keeping as well as varying periods of abstinence	Require no devices or chemicals; may be acceptable for couples who do not wish to use other methods because of religious or other reasons
Withdrawal	18	Have no contraindications	Requires interruption of sexual response cycle; fluid with sperm is often released before ejaculation	Requires no devices or chemicals
Vasectomy or male sterilization	0.15	Have no contraindications	Is permanent; may present surgical minor surgery	No further monitoring required after verification that all sperm in system have been ejaculated
Bilateral tubal ligation or female sterilization	0.4	May be performed during cesarean delivery or soon after vaginal delivery	Is permanent; may present surgical complications	Requires no further monitoring

the particular stage of life continuum, and should also be viewed in wider context of sexual and reproductive health. It has been argued that control of their own fertility is the largest single factor affecting the independence of women. The capacity to enjoy and control sexual and reproductive behavior is key element of sexual health. Unintended pregnancies can have long-lasting effects on the quality of life of parents and children.

Family planning or fertility regulation is not a new concept. The word fertility regulation is perhaps more acceptable than family planning. As a rule, family planning countries up in the minds of the people of developing countries, the ides of population control. Fertility regulation implies a situation where fertile couples space out their children and have the number of children they want. Infertile couples can be assisted to become fertile.

In fact, several methods have been used throughout the known history to prevent pregnancy and birth control measures have been initiated. Studies showed that in ancient times, Indians practiced limiting the size of the family. In those days, people rather wanted to have more children, due to certain social and religious obligations, as well as perhaps due to the high IMR. Even so, the ancient religious leaders exhorted in favor of having few children.

CONCLUSION

The population of India is growing after industrial revolution. The population of India has crossed 1 billion. On the basis of growth rate, the growth is divided into stagnant period, moderate growth period and rapid growth period. Increased population has caused overcrowding in cities, town and villages. The causes of increased population, i.e. overpopulation are advanced technology, education, improved standard of living and decreased death rate. Overpopulation has resulted in depletion of resources. It means overpopulation has consequences on social, economic and health. All these further increases burden on country, thereby hindering the development of country. Women need to empowered so as to take decision regarding family planning methods. Women need to be empowered socially, educationally and economically. The overall development helps in achieving the development of nation. Small family norm are vital to achieve population control. These small family norms are promoted by mass media to make people aware about the benefits of small family norms. People should be educated about various family planning methods. This awareness helps them in understanding and motivate them to take decision regarding adoption of small family norms.

Index

Page numbers followed by *f* refer to figure and *t* refer to table

A

Abdomen 218, 221
Abortion 750
   rate 735
Abscess
   brain 715
   scrotal 501
Abstinence 760
Acarus scabiei 235
Accidents 631, 690, 741
   causes 692
   domestic 691, 692, 694
   prevention of 693
   road 691, 692
   types of 690
Acid rain 103
Acid reflux 334
Acidemia 509
Acid-fast bacilli 439
Acquired heart disease 665, 666
Acquired immunodeficiency syndrome (AIDS) 206, 279, 363, 589, 610, 611, 620, 741
   control program 621
   in India 618
   infection 617
Acquired syphilis 611
Actinomyces 204
Acyanotic heart disease 665, 671
Adenovirus 206, 418, 478
Adult worm 493, 584, 585
Aedes aegypti 506, 543
Aedes africanus 542
Aedes albopictus 506
Aflatoxicosis 502
Agranulocytosis 607
Air pollution 97, 102-104
   causes of 97
   classification of 99
   control 104, 106, 198
   effects of 102*f*
   index 101, 104
   metallic 99
   prevention and control of 104, 105
   source of 97
Albendazole 588
Albuminuria 423
Alcohol 670
   consumption 317
   use of 297
Aldehyde test 528
Alimentary system 308
Alkaline hydrolysis 172
Allodermanyssus sanguineus 242
Aluminum phosphate 212
Alzheimer's disease 51, 315
Amanita muscaria 503
Amanita pantherina 503
Amanita phalloides 503
Amebiasis 487
American Cancer Society 661
American Nurses Association 18
Amoxicillin 571
Ancylostoma duodenale 495
Anemia 204, 571, 637, 647
   grading and treatment of 653*t*
   hemolytic 607
   nutritional 651, 652
Aneroid barometer 133*f*
Angina pectoris 667, 669
Angiomatous malformations 678
Animal bites 536
Anopheles
   culicifacies 517
   fluviatilis 517
   head of 218*f*
   larva 219*f*
   minimus 517
   philippinensis 517
   stephensi 220, 517
   subpictus 546
   sundaicus 517
   thorax of 219*f*
Antecedent viral infection 418
Anthrax 172, 271, 566, 568*t*
   bacilli 566*f*
   cutaneous 566
Antidiphtheria serum 211, 213
Anti-gas gangrene serum 213
Antileprosy drugs 604, 606
Antiphospholipid syndrome 678
Antirabies serum 538
Antirabies vaccine 211, 538, 539
   dose schedule 538*t*
Antisera 213, 424, 390
Anti-snake venom 213
Anti-tetanus serum 211, 213
Antitoxins 390
Antitubercular drugs 435
Antituberculosis treatment 441, 443*t*
Antityphoid vaccines 476
Antiviral therapy 416
Aorta, coarctation of 665, 671
Aortic incompetence, congenital 671
Aortic stenosis, congenital 671
Aplocheilus panchax 220
Arboviruses, classification of 541
Argemone mexicana 263
Arrhythmias, cardiac 667, 678, 679
Arsenic trioxide 572
Arteriovenous malformations 716
Arteritis, cerebral 678
Arthritis, monoarticular 501
Arthropod 215
   classes of 217
   classification of 215
   infestations 506
Ascaris lumbricoides 491, 491f, 492
   eggs of 492*f*

Ascites 668
Aspergillus flavus 502
Aspergillus parasiticus 502
Assmann psychrometer 139
Asthma 39, 631
    bronchial 103
Astrovirus 478
Atherosclerosis, progressive 679
Atmospheric pressure 132
Attention deficit hyperactivity disorder 326
Avian flu 449
Avian influenza 172
Avidin-biotin-peroxidase complex 539

B

Bacillary dysentery 483
    nursing management of 486
Bacille Calmette-Guérin (BCG) 210, 432, 435
Bacillus anthracis 566
Bacillus cereus 505
Backache 550, 577
Bacteria
    growth of 204
    structure of 204
Bacterial endocarditis, subacute 666
Bacterial food poisoning 503, 504t
Bacterial index 603
Bacterial pollution 95
Balantidium coli 81
Bandicota bengalensis 558
Barium carbonate 242, 244
Bartonella quintana 216
Beef tapeworm 582
Benzene hexachloride 529, 561, 591
Beriberi 637
Berkefeld filter 77, 77f
Biogas plant 161, 162f
    benefits of 161
Biopsy 603
Bird flu 449
Birth control measures 56
Birth rate 734, 735
    reduction of 741
Black fly 225, 226f
Bleaching powder 76
Blindness 631, 633
    nutritional 650
    problem of 594
Blood clotting disorders 750

Blood diseases 678
Blood pressure 670, 674, 675, 679
    classification of 674t
Blood urea nitrogen 509
Blotting paper method 470
Body mass index 295, 327, 328, 644, 658t, 658
Borderline lepromatous 605
Borderline leprosy 602
Borderline tuberculoid 605
Bordetella bronchiseptica 425
Bordetella parapertussis 425
Bordetella pertussis 425
Borrelia recurrentis 216, 230
Breastfeeding, failure of 418
Broca's method 658
Bronchiectasis 103
Bronchitis 100, 103, 415, 631
Bronchopneumonia 412, 427
Brucella abortus 205
Brucella melitensis 554
Brudziński's sign 431, 460
Brugia malayi 530
Brugia timori 530
Bubonic plague 560
Budd-Chiari syndrome 587
Burkitt's lymphoma 683
Burns 695
    prevention of 696

C

Cadmium 82, 100
Caisson's disease 133
Calcium
    bicarbonate 87
    sulfate 87
Calicivirus 478
Calymmatobacterium granulomatis 610
Campylobacter jejuni 478
Canadian Nurses Association 18
Cancer 261, 631, 633
    breast 689
    cells 684
    end stage of 698
    etiology of 682
    gallbladder 688
    lung 684
    oral 688
    prevention 685
    skin and lung 101
    uterine 684

Candida albicans 610, 627
Candy's filter 72
Carbohydrates 328
Carbon dioxide 100, 205
Carbon monoxides 99
Carcinogenesis, stages of 682
Cardiovascular diseases 69, 631, 632, 665
Cardiovascular disorders 39
Cardiovascular system 312
Carey Coombs' murmur 673
Cataract 594, 634
    mucosa 634
Cat-eye syndrome 54
Cellular fractions 211, 212
Centers for Disease Control and Prevention 453, 507
Central and State Pollution Control Boards 91, 199
Central Committee for Food Standards 267
Central Council of Health 180
Central Ground Water Board 90
Central nervous system 215, 314, 406, 458, 535, 570, 578, 585, 596, 698
Central Pollution Control Board 92
Cerebral edema, reduction of 679
Cerebrospinal fluid 460, 614
Cerebrovascular accidents 678, 715
Cerebrovascular disease 678
Cervical adenitis, 412
Cervical cap 761
    use of 748f
Cervicitis 610
Chancroid 610, 612
    phagedenic 613
Chemical oxygen demand 166
Chemoprophylaxis 213, 436, 522, 562, 573
Chemotherapy 435, 561, 593, 604, 615
    short-course of 435, 438
Chest pain 453, 580, 587
Cheyne-Stokes breathing 133, 134
Chi square test 734
Chick embryo cell vaccine 212
Chickenpox 401f, 403, 404, 404t
    nursing management of 404
    vaccine 211
Chikungunya 514
    fever 511
Child Survival and Safe Motherhood Program 287
Child Welfare Services 287

Index

Chipko movement 192
Chlamydia psittaci 613
Chlamydia trachomatis 610, 613
Chloramine 74
Chlorides 79
Chlorination, methods of 74
Chlorine
    gas 74
    solution 76
    tablets 77
Chocolate agar 614
Cholera 468
    nursing management of 471
Chorea 673
Chromium 82
Chromosomal aberrations 53
Chromosomal mutation 53
Chromosome 49
    functions of 51
    structure of 50f
Chrysanthemum cinerariaefolium 221
Cimex hemipterus 231
Cimex lectularius 231
Ciprofloxacin 568
Claviceps fusiformis 502
Claviceps purpurea 502
Clofazimine 604, 607
Clostridium botulinum 271, 422, 505
Clostridium histolyticum 626
Clostridium perfringens 81, 86, 505, 626
Clostridium septicum 626
Clostridium sporogenes 626
Clostridium tetani 205, 422, 595, 596, 596f
Clostridium welchii 205, 626
Cobalt therapy installation 686
Codex alimentarius 264
    commission 264
Cohort study 381
Coitus interfemoris 744
Coitus interruptus 744
Coitus reservatus 744
Colpotomy 752
Communication 176
    barriers of 178
    group 178
    non-verbal 177
    oral 177
    process 176
    types of 176
    verbal 177
Community
    characteristics of 5
    concepts of 3
    definitions of 3
    dimensions of 7
    environment hygiene 293
    functions of 5
    health programs 43
    health center 182, 439
    health nurse 175, 354
    nutritional education of 482
Condom 745f, 746, 761
    female 744, 745f
    male 744, 745f
Conjunctivitis, neonatal 610
Conn's syndrome 674
Constipation 295, 583
Consumer Protection Act 266
Contact lenses 306
Contraception 56, 742
    methods of 760t
Convulsions 427
Copper-T 749f
Corona virus 418
Corpulence index 658
Corticosteroid 568
Cortisone 750
Corynebacterium diphtheriae 421, 422, 422f
Cough 100, 415, 453, 587
    non-productive 580
    whooping 425
Councilman bodies 542
Cover garbage containers 578
Coxiella burnetii 233, 575, 579
Crab louse 229
Creutzfeldt-Jakob disease 172
Cri-du-chat syndrome 51
Crude birth rate 372, 735, 736
Crude death rate 372, 739
Cryptosporidium 620
Cubic space 114, 146
Culdoscopy 752
Culex fatigans 506
Culex vishnui 546
Cushing's syndrome 674, 702
Cyanide 82
Cyanogas fumigation 561
Cyanotic heart diseases 665, 671
Cyclops 70, 237, 238, 238f, 501
Cyst 488
    hydatid 586, 586f
Cystic fibrosis 702
Cysticercus cellulosae 584
Cytomegalovirus 620

D

Dapsone 604, 607
Dark ground illumination test 614
Daughter cysts, formation of 587
Day Care Programs 713
Dead bodies, disposal of 171
Deafness 120
Dehydration 261, 646
    moderate 503
    treatment of 480t
Dementia 631
Demography, scope of 729
Dengue
    fever 506, 507, 514, 571
    hemorrhagic fever 141f, 506, 507, 509
    shock syndrome 506, 507, 509
    viral fever 506
Dental fluorosis 720
Deoxyribonucleic acid 49, 50f, 52f, 206, 217, 360, 467, 617, 682
Deoxyribonucleoproteins 204
Dermacentor andersoni 231
Dermatitis, exfoliative 607
Dermatophagoides pteronyssinus 235
Dexamethasone 568
Diabetes 631, 632
    glomerulonephritis 674
    mellitus 204, 631, 670, 678, 700
        epidemiology 700
        gestational 702
        insulin-dependent 701
        introduction 700
        magnitude of 700
        non-insulin-dependent 701
        types 1 702, 704
        types 2 703, 704
        types of 701
    prevention program 708
    WHO classification of 702
Diaminodiphenyl sulfone 213, 604
Diaphragm 746, 748f
Diarrhea 415, 453, 550, 571, 580, 583
    nursing management of 482
Diarrheal disease 478
    Control Program 490
Dichlorodiphenyltrichloroethane 220, 243, 510, 558, 574, 589
Dideoxyinosine 623
Diethylcarbamazine 533
Diethylene triamine pentaacetic acid 131
Digestion 169

Diphtheria 213, 424, 425, 421
  antitoxin 424
  immunization 423
  nursing management of 424
  pertussis, tetanus 210, 389, 424, 464
Diphyllobothrium latum 238
Directly Observed Treatment Short Course (DOTS) 438
Disability-adjusted life years (DALY) 709
Disseminated intravascular coagulation 678
District Cancer Control Scheme 686
District Tuberculosis Control Program 437
Docosahexaenoic acid 676
Donovania granulomatis 614
Down syndrome 51, 53, 54, 671
Dowry 281
Doxycycline 568
Dracunculus medinensis 81, 238, 500
Droplet infection 387, 570
Drowsiness 460
Drug and Cosmetic Act 267
Drug resistant strains 436
Drug therapy 717
Drugs Technical Advisory Board 268
Dry bulb thermometer 134, 138*f*
Dry cough 447
Dust mite 235
Dutch cap 747
Dyspnea 587, 668

E

Ears, care of 306, 402, 412
Echinococcus granulosus 585, 586*f*
  life cycle of 587*f*
Echinococcus multilocularis 585
Echinococcus, egg of 586*f*
Ectocyst 586, 587
Edema 668
  pulmonary 668
Edward's syndrome 53, 54
Eisenmenger's complex 671
Electrocardiography 708
Electrolytes 646
  imbalances 509
Electromagnetic radiations 127
Emphysema 103, 631
Encephalitis 715
Endemic typhus, transmission of 227
Endocyst 586, 587
Endogamy 280
Entamoeba histolytica 81, 478, 488*f*
  life cycle of 489*f*
Enterobius vermicularis 493
  egg of 494*f*
  life cycle of 494*f*
Environment Friendly Product Scheme 195
Environment Protection Act 196
Environmental Control Programs 33, 43
Enzyme-linked immunosorbent assay (ELISA) 448, 509, 571, 583, 621
Epidemic typhus, transmission of 230
Epidermophyton 89
Epilepsy 698, 715
  classification 715
  clinical manifestation 716
  etiology 715
  management 717
  pathophysiology 716
Epstein-Barr virus 620, 682
Erythema marginatum 673
Erythema nodosum leprosum 607
Erythromycin lactobionate 568
Escherichia coli 81, 166, 205, 328, 419, 478
Ethionamide 604
Eugenics 49
  classification of 55
Euthenics 56
Exercise 38, 310, 557, 670, 707
  benefits of 312
  intensity of 311
  isometric 311
  isotonic 311
  types of 311
Exogamy 280
Eye, care of 298, 304, 402, 412

F

Fainting attacks 750
Family planning 752
  methods 742, 743*f*
  services, scope of 753
Family service programs 713
Family structure, definitions of 281
Family Welfare Program 753
Fasciola hepatica 271
Fecal streptococci 81
Fertility rate 372, 734, 736
  regulation, methods of 742
Fever 39, 453, 460, 577, 672
  breakbone 509
  hemorrhagic 571
  high 577, 578, 580
  paratyphoid 477
  rheumatic 666, 672, 673*t*
  sudden onset of 550
Fibrillation, atrial 678
Filaria survey 532
Filarial indices 532
Filariasis 529
  lymphatic 530
  vectors of 531
Flavivirus 206, 549
Flea 216
  alimentary canal of 226*f*
  borne diseases 241
  indices 559
  life cycle of 227*f*
Flies 216
Flocculation 73
Fluid loss 479
Fluid toxoid 598
Fluorescent antibody test 614
Fluorescent treponemal antibody test 614
Fluoroacetamide 572
Fluorosis 637, 720
  clinical manifestation 720
  etiology 720
  prevention and control 721
Folic acid 331
  deficiency 637
Follicular chancroid 613
Fomites 387
Food
  additives 246, 247*t*, 326
  adulteration 261
  allergy 272, 502
  classification of 266, 266*f*
  consumption 260, 639
  fortification 260
  poisoning 271, 502
    classification of 503
    non-bacterial 503
  preservation 249
    importance of 249
    methods of 250
    process of 249

Index

storage, principles of 257
transportation of 258
Foodborne diseases 241, 502, 503t
Foot arch 304
Forests maintain climate 190
Fumigation 243, 572

G

Gallstone 261
Gambusia affinis 220
Gamma-aminobutyric acid 316, 716
Gandhi Memorial Leprosy Foundation 608
Ganga action plan 196
Gas gangrene 213, 626
Gastrointestinal anthrax 566
Gastrointestinal disorders 698
Gastrointestinal system 312
Gastrointestinal tract 216, 458, 460
Genes
    functions of 52
    structure of 52f
Genital actinomycosis 750
Genital herpes 610
Genitalia
    female 613
    male 613f
Genitourinary malignancies 689
Genu valgum 721
German measles 411, 413
Ghon complex 434
Giardia lamblia 478
Giemsa stain 558
Glare, absence of 108, 109
Glaucoma 594, 634, 635
Global warming 103, 140
Globe thermometer 134, 135f
Glomerulonephritis 674
Glomerulosclerosis 674
Glucagonoma 702
Goiter 204, 637
    prevalence rate 654t, 655t
Gomez classification 639, 642, 642t
Gonorrhea 610, 612
    nursing management of 616
Gram stain 614
Granuloma inguinale 610, 614, 615
Great arteries, complete transposition of 671
Guillain-Barré syndrome 465, 466, 466t
Guinea worm eradication program 502

H

Haemaphysalis spinigera 231
Haemaphysalis tick, life cycle of 551
Haemophilus ducreyi 610, 612
Haemophilus influenzae 211, 391, 394, 418
Hair, care of 298, 301
Hands and feet, care of 303
Hard tick 550
    morphology 550f
Hazards
    chemical 69, 70, 340
    occupational 340
Head 218, 221
    drop sign 460
    injury 698, 715
    trauma 715
Headache 100, 415, 447, 460, 550, 577, 578, 580
Health dimensions of 15
Health education 38, 213, 335, 428, 436, 449, 471, 477, 510, 564, 572, 573, 594, 608, 663, 708
    contents of 335
    principles of 336
Health models of 14
Health promotion 21, 27, 32, 37, 44, 419, 648, 649, 673
    model 28, 29f
    programs, types of 42
Health protection 27, 40
Health restoration 21
Healthcare services 39
Heart 542
Heart block 415
Heart disease 750
    classification of 665
    congenital 665, 671
    coronary 34, 35t, 666
    ischemic 632, 667
    rheumatic 666, 632, 672, 673t
Heart failure, congestive 647, 668
Heart irregularities of 669
Heart murmur 750
Heat
    cramps 137
    exhaustion 137
    hyperpyrexia 137
    stroke 136
    syncope 137
Helicobacter pylori 682
Helminthic infections 70

Hemiplegia 676
Hemochromatosis 702
Hemoptysis 571, 587
Hemorrhage
    cerebral 676, 678
    pulmonary 557
    subarachnoid 678
    subconjunctival 427
Hemorrhagic fevers, viral 172
Hepatitis 571, 607
    A virus 467
    acute 610
    B 682
        immunoglobulin 213
        virus 467, 610
    C 172, 682
        virus 467
    E 468
        virus 467
    G 468
        virus 468
    infective 467, 467t, 698
    serum 467, 467t
    virus 206
Hereditary diseases 634
Hernia, inguinal 427
Herpes simplex virus 206, 610, 615, 620
Hexachlorocyclohexane 228
Histamine test 603
Home blood glucose monitoring 705
Hookworm 495f
    egg of 496f
    infestation 495
    life cycle of 496f
Hormones 209, 670
Host 206, 488, 492, 495, 554
Housefly 221, 221f
    control measures of 223
    life cycle of 223f
    thorax of 222f
    transmitting diseases 222
Human blood index 520
Human development index 740
Human diploid cell vaccines 212, 539
Human filarial infection 530t
Human immunodeficiency virus (HIV) 206, 290, 310, 365, 682, 712, 740
    infection 617
    structure of 619f
Human lice 216
    control measures 230
Human papilloma viruses 610
Human rabies immunoglobulin 213

Human salmonellosis 563
Human T-cell leukemia virus 682
Human tetanus immunoglobulin 213
Humidity 132, 138
Humoral immunity 209, 388
Huntington's chorea 57
Huntington's disease 57
Hydatid cyst, structure of 587f
Hydatid disease 585
Hydatid fluid 586
Hydrocele 501
Hydrochloric acid 602
Hydrotherapy 462
Hygiene 39
  oral 301
  types of 293
Hymenolepis diminuta 216, 240
Hymenolepis nana 227, 241
Hypercholesterolemia 633
Hyperlipidemia 678
Hyperpnea 668
Hypersomnia 318
Hypertension 632, 633, 667, 669, 674, 678, 741
  pregnancy induced 470
  prevention and control of 677
Hypertensive encephalopathy 715
Hypocalemia 715
Hypoglycemia 647, 705, 715
Hypotension 633
Hypothermia 647
Hypothesis, formulation of 377
Hysteroscopy 752

Immunity 208, 388, 541
  active 209, 388, 389
  artificial passive 210
  cell-mediated 599
  cellular 209, 388
  contact 210
  herd 210, 389
  natural passive 210
  passive 210, 388
  types of 210, 390
Immunization 432, 476, 538, 551
  active 210, 407, 427, 462, 598
  hazards of 213
Immunoglobulins 212, 389
Immunoprophylaxis 547, 562
Impaired glucose tolerance 702
In vitro fertilization 55

Inactivated polio vaccine, modified 464
Indian Academy of Pediatrics 391t
  classification 639, 642
Indian Council of Agriculture Research 153
Indian Forest Act 192
Indian Leprosy Association 608
Indian Medical Association 481
Indian Penal Code and Pollution 122, 201
Indian Standards Institution 264
Indian Tick Typhus 575, 578
Indigestion 583
Infant feeding, types of 332
Infectious disease 422
  transmission, dynamics of 390
Influenza 414
  nursing management of 416
  virus 418, 450f
    structure of 414f
Inoculation rate 520
Insomnia 318
Insulin-resistance syndrome 703
Integrated Child Development Service 649
  Scheme 287
International Council of Nurses 18
Intestinal infections 458
Intrauterine device (IUD) 747, 750f, 761
  complications of 749f
  insertion of 749f
Intraventricular septal defect 665
Iodine deficiency 637
  disorders 654
    prevention and control of 655
    spectrum of 654
Ionizing radiation
  health hazards of 128
  types of 129
Iron deficiency 652
  anemia, problem of 653
  cutoff points of 652t
Ischemic attack, transient 678
Itch mite 235

Jacobsen syndrome 53
Japanese encephalitis 141f, 544
  virus 541
Jaundice 101, 571
  epidemic 467
Jelliffe classification 639, 642

Joint family 283
Joint pain 577
Juvenile diabetes 701, 704

K

Kala-azar 224, 526-528, 588, 589
  prevention and control of 591
Kaposi's sarcoma 620, 682
Kata thermometer 135, 135f, 136
Katadyn filter 77
Kernig's sign 431, 460
Ketoacidosis, diabetic 705
Kidney 423, 542
  stones 261
Kiss knee test 460
Klebsiella aerogenes 81
Klebsiella pneumonia 419
Klinefelter's syndrome 51, 53, 54
Koplik's spot 408, 410f, 411
Korotkoff sound 674
Kwashiorkor 637, 639, 639t, 640, 641f, 642, 648
Kyasanur forest disease 233, 548, 551
  natural cycle of 552f
  vaccine 211
  virus 541

L

Lactational amenorrhea method 744
Lacunar infarct 678
Laparoscopy 752
Laparotomy, conventional 752
Larva 219, 551, 582
Laryngectomy 698
Laryngitis 100, 412
Laser radiations 127
Lassa fever virus 541
Lead 83, 100
Legionella 620
Leishmania braziliensis 224, 589
Leishmania donovani 224, 589, 589f, 590f
Leishmania tropica 224, 527, 589
Leishmaniasis 588
  cutaneous 526, 527, 528
  life cycle of 590f
Leishmanin test 529
Lepra reaction 602
Lepromatous leprosy 600f, 602, 602f
Lepromin test 603

Index

Leprosy 40, 599
   control, methods of 603
   division 605
   mission of 608
   multibacillary 604
   paucibacillary 604
   social aspect of 608
Leptospira 570f
   icterohaemorrhagiae 241
   interrogans 569
Leptospiral infection 70
Leptospirosis 569, 570, 572
Leptotrombidium akamushi 234, 234f, 576
Leptotrombidium deliense 234, 234f, 576
Leptotrombidium intermedia 234
Leptotrombidium pallidum 234
Lethargy 447
Leukemia 681, 750
Leukopenia 509, 549
Levonorgestrel intrauterine system 750f
Limb amputation 698
Limb pain 550
Liponyssoides sanguineus 242
Lippes loop 748, 749f
Live attenuated vaccine 389
Liver 542
   failure 571
Louse 228
   egg of 229
   life cycle of 230f
Low density lipoprotein, 669, 707
Low-death rate, causes of 739
Lower respiratory infection, acute 418
Lugol's iodine 656
Lumen 108
Luminous flux 110
Luminous intensity 110
Lutzomyia longipalpis 224f
Lymphogranuloma venereum 610, 613, 614
Lymphoma 681, 689
Lyssophobia 540

M

Macaca rhesus 543
Magnesium
   bicarbonate 87
   sulfate 87

Malaise 415
Malaria 515, 571, 577, 580
   cerebral 678
   measurement of 520
   nursing management of 525
   survey 520
   transmission of 517
   treatment of 522
   vectors of 517
Malarial parasite 516
   life cycle of 517f, 518f
Malnutrition 594, 637, 741
Mandie's solution, throat pain of 416
Man-made pollution sources, classification of 98
Mansonella ozzardi 530
Mansonia annulifera 531
Mansonia uniformis 531
Mantoux test 645
Marasmus 637, 639, 639t, 640f, 648
Marfan syndrome 671
Marital fertility rate 734, 736
   age-specific 735, 736
Marriage 280
   counseling 56
   group 280
   importance of 279
   rate 735
   restrictions 280
   system 278
   types of 279
   universality of 736
Mass chemoprophylaxis 431
Mass communication 178
Mass miniature radiography 434
Maternal mortality rate 372, 653
Maternal nutrition 481
Maternal-fetal transmission 620
Maturity-Onset Diabetes of Young (MODY) syndrome 702
McConkey's lactose 87
Measles 408, 411
   mumps, rubella 212, 389
      vaccine 211
   nursing management of 411
   vaccine 210
   virus 409f
Medical Termination of Pregnancy (MTP) 56, 757
Membrane filtration technique 87
Meningeal irritation, symptoms of 571

Meningitis 261, 571, 715
   meningococcal 429
   nursing management of 432
   plague 561
   viral 571
Meningococcal vaccine 211, 389
Meningoencephalitis 408, 415
Menstrual cramps, severe 750
Mental attitude 556
Mental dimension 16
Mental diseases 631
Mental disorders 631, 632
Mental health disorders, types of 711
Mental health disorders services 713
Mental illness 709
   etiology 710
   prevention and control of 712
Mesocyclops hyalinus 237
Mesocyclops leuckarti 237
Mesocyclops varicans 237
Microcyclops karvei 237
Micturition disturbances 460
Milk hygiene 269
Milk, pasteurization of 564
Milkborne disease 270
Mineral deficiency diseases 651
Minilaparotomy 752
Minocycline 606
Miscarriage 750
Mite 216
   control of 233
Mite-borne diseases 241
Mitral stenosis 666
Monogamy 279
Monounsaturated fatty acids 676
Montenegro test 529
Morphological index 603
Mortality rate
   infant 372, 653
   neonatal 372
   perinatal 373
   postnatal 373
Mosquito 216, 217
   control measures 220
   density 520
   mouthparts of 218f
   pupa of 219f
Mountain sickness, acute 134
Mouse-borne diseases 242
Mouth, care of 412
Mucocutaneous leishmaniasis 526, 528, 591

Multidrug therapy 604
  regimen 604
Multiple drug resistance 689
Multiple sclerosis, cerebral 698
Mumps 405
  nursing management of 407
Murine typhus 577
Murray valley encephalitis virus 541
Musca domestica 221
Muscle aches 453
Muscle cramps 704
Muscle fasciculation 460
Muscle pain 578
Muscular system 308
Musculoskeletal disorders 631
Musculoskeletal system 312
Mushroom poisoning 503
Myalgia 415, 447, 550, 573, 580
Mycobacterium leprae 599, 599f, 601
Mycobacterium tuberculosis 205, 360, 432, 433, 433f, 620
Myocardial infarction 669
Myocarditis 415, 423, 666
Myxovirus 406f

N

Nails, care of 304
Narcolepsy 318
Nasopharyngeal leishmaniasis 224
National Antimalaria Program 523
National Cancer Control Program 631, 686
  evolution of 686
National Cancer Registry Program 632, 633, 687
National Cardiovascular Disease Control Program 631
National Crime Records Bureau 632
National Diabetes Control Program 631
National Diarrheal Disease Control Program 482, 483
National Drug Policy, revised 522
National Environmental Campaign 195
National Environmental Engineering Research Institute 721
National Filaria Control Program 533
National Forest Policy 192
National Forestry Action Program 192
National Immunization Schedule 390t

National Institute of Communicable Diseases 532
National Iodine Deficiency Disorders Control Program 631
National Leprosy Eradication Program 604
National Malaria Control Program 523
National Malaria Education Program 522, 523, 589
National Mental Health Program 631
National Nutrition Monitoring Bureau 637
National Nutritional Anemia Prophylaxis Program 652
National Program for Control of Blindness 594, 631
National Tuberculosis Control Program 437
National Tuberculosis Institute 437
National Vitamin A Prophylaxis Program 650
National Water Supply and Sanitation Program 90, 490
Nausea 261, 415, 577, 580, 583
Necator americanus 495
Neisseria gonorhoeae 205, 610, 611
Neisseria meningitidis 205, 429
Nephritis 423
Nerve palsy, cranial 415
Nervous system 308
Neuritis, traumatic 465, 466
Neurocysticercosis 715
Niacin deficiency 637
Nicotinic acid 331
Night blindness 637
Nocturia 704
Nocturnal enuresis 318
Nodules, subcutaneous 673
Noise 119, 340, 670
Non-communicable disease 631, 633t
Non-Hodgkin's lymphoma 682
Non-steroidal anti-inflammatory drugs 514
Noroviruses 478
Nose, care of 306, 402, 412
Nucleic acid 49, 50f
Nursing care 456
  isolation 414
  purposes of 20
  standards of 22
Nursing management 420, 567

Nutrition 204, 209, 342, 668
  education 38, 649
Nutritional anemia, prevention and control of 652
Nutritional blindness, prevention and control of 649

O

Obesity 204, 295, 631, 637, 657, 659, 670
  classification of 658t
  phenotypes of 658f
Obstructive pulmonary disease, chronic 103, 207
Occupational diseases, classification of 343
Ofloxacin 606
Onchocerca volvulus 530
Oral Health Programs 631
Oral polio vaccine 210, 461, 463, 463t, 464
Oral rehydration
  salt 470, 480t, 481, 510
  therapy 479, 486
Orientia tsutsugamushi 575
Ornithodoros moubata 231
Orodental diseases 631
Orthomyxovirus 206
Orthotolidine-arsenite test 75, 78
Osmosis 251
Osteomalacia 637

P

Pain, abdominal 415, 571, 578, 580
Pallister-Killian syndrome 54
Palsy, cerebral 715
Pancreatitis 702
Papanicolaou test 684, 750
Papovavirus 206
Paramyxovirus 206
Parkinson disease 315, 698
Passive immunization 211, 428, 461, 465
Pasteur-Chamberland filter 77
Pasteurization 270
Patau syndrome 53, 54
Patent ductus arteriosus 666, 671
Paterson's chloronome 74
Paterson's filter 72
Pediculus humanus 228, 229

Index

Pellagra 637
Pelvic infection 750
Pericarditis 666
Persistent truncus arteriosus 671
Pertussis 425
    nursing management of 428
    vaccine 427
Pestis siderans 560
Peyer's patches 477
Pharyngitis 100
Phenylketonuria 56
Pheochromocytoma 674
Phlebotomine sandflies 224f
Phlebotomus argentipes 528, 590
Phlebotomus papatasi 528, 589
Phlebotomus sergenti 528
Phthirus pubis 228, 627
Picornavirus 206
Pig-borne diseases 241
Pinworm infestation 493
Pistia stratiotes 531
Plague 172, 558
    management of 562
    pneumonic 558, 560
    prevention and control of 561
    septicemic 560
    transmission of 227
Plasmodium falciparum 516, 525
Plasmodium malariae 516
Plasmodium ovale 516
Plasmodium vivax 516
Pneumocystis carinii 620
Pneumonia 415, 420, 578
    community acquired 418
    neonatal 419
    severe 420
Pneumothorax 427
Polio vaccine, inactivated 462, 463, 463t
Poliomyelitis 458, 465, 466, 466t
    abortive 461
    eradication of 465
    non-paralytic 461
    paralytic 461
Polyarthritis 672
    epidemic 511
Polycythemia 678
Polydipsia 705
Polygamy 279
Polymerase chain reaction 448, 453
Polynuclear aromatic hydrocarbons 83, 100
Polyphagia 705
Polyuria 705

Polyvinyl chloride 90
Population
    density of 728t
    explosion, health hazards of 740
    stabilization 741
Pork tapeworm 584
Post-kala-azar dermal leishmaniasis 591
Postmeasles encephalitis 413
Poxvirus 206, 399, 399f
Pre-exposure prophylaxis 537
Pregnancy, toxemia of 674
Prevention of Food Adulteration Act 265
Primary health care 482
Prophylaxis 427
Prosthetic eyes 306
Prostitution 610
Protein-energy malnutrition 204, 634, 637, 640f, 642, 642f, 642t, 643f, 646, 701
    classification of 646t
Prothionamide 604
Pseudohydrophobia 540
Psychiatric disorders 631
Psychosis 607
Pthirus pubis 228, 229
Pulex irritans 559

Q

Q fever 575
    transmission of 233
Quarantine 579
Quetelet index 644

R

Rabies 172, 213, 535, 540f
    nursing management of 539
    virus 536f
Radiation
    hazards, prevention and control of 130
    sources of 124
    types of 126, 128
Rapid eye movements 316
Rash 578
    allergic 607
    macular 577
Rat 240, 241
    bite fevers 241
    control of 242

    economic impact of 242
    flea 226
    trapping of 561
    types 240
Rattus norvegicus 240, 558
Rattus rattus 558, 559
Rectal swab method 470
Red blood cells 517, 672
Refuse disposal, methods of 151
Renal dialysis 698
Renal diseases 631
Renal failure 571
Renal insufficiency 578
Respiratory diseases, chronic 631
Respiratory distress syndrome 447, 448, 571
Respiratory infection 287, 399, 417, 460
Respiratory syncytial virus 418
Respiratory system 308, 312
Respiratory tract infection, upper 468
Reticular activity system 316
Retina, detachment of 427
Retinopathy, diabetic 705
Retrovirus 206
Revised National Tuberculosis Control Program 438, 441t-443t
Rhabdovirus 206
Rhadinomyia orientalis 576
Rhinorrhea 415
Rhinovirus 418
Riboflavin 331
Ribonucleic acid 49, 50f, 206, 408, 458, 535, 617, 619f
Rickets 637
Rickettsia akari 575, 579
Rickettsia burnetii 579
Rickettsia conorii 575, 578
Rickettsia mooseri 227
Rickettsia prowazekii 230, 574, 575
Rickettsia quintana 230, 575
Rickettsia rickettsii 575, 578
Rickettsia tsutsugamushi 577
Rickettsia typhi 575, 576
Rickettsial diseases, classification of 575t
Rickettsialpox 575, 579
Rochalimaea quintana 579
Rocky mountain spotted fever 575, 579
Rodents 240
    classification 240
    control of 573
    domestic 240
Rose bengal dye test 651

Rotavirus 478
Roundworm 70
    infestation 491
    life cycle of 493f
Rubella 411, 413
    vaccine 211

S

Sabin vaccine 464
Salmonella enteritidis 241
Salmonella paratyphi 476
Salmonella typhimurium 241, 563
Salmonellosis, nursing management of 564
Salpingitis 610
Sandfly 223, 225f
    control of 529
Sarcoptes scabiei 235, 236f, 237f
Scab mite 235
Schick test 423
School Health Promotion Programs 43
Scrub typhus 575, 576
Scurvy 637
Seizure, treatment of 717
Septal defect
    atrial 671
    ventricular 671
Serological test 549, 614, 624
Severe acute respiratory syndrome (SARS) 172, 363, 446, 446f, 446t, 448f
Sex chromosome
    abnormalities 54
    disorders 54
Sex specific death rate 373
Sexually transmitted diseases 40, 290, 297, 364, 592, 609, 610t, 741
Shigella dysenteriae 484
Shigella flexneri 484
Shigella sonnei 484
Sickle cell anemia 56
Simulium indicum 225
Skeletal fluorosis 721
Skene's ducts 614f
Skene's gland 613f
Skin
    care of 298
    itching of 704
Skinfold, thickness of 645
Sleep apnea 318
Sleep deprivation 318
    symptoms of 318t

Sleep disorders 318
Slim disease 617
Sling psychrometer 138, 139f
Smallpox 399, 400f, 400t, 404, 594, 634
    nursing management of 401
Smoke index 101, 104
Snake bite 696
Sodium 80
    carbonate 88
    fluoroacetate 572
Soft sore 610
Soiling index 101, 104
Solar radiation thermometer 136, 136f
Sore eye 305
Sore throat 415, 447, 453, 580
Spinal cord injury 698
Spirillum minus 241
Sporozoite rate 520
Sputum collection 440
Sputum disposal 557
Sputum transportation 440
Stable community 375
Stack-driven ventilation 115, 116f
Staphylococcus aureus 419, 505
State Tuberculosis Demonstration and Training Centers 438
Sterilization 56, 271
    female 752
    male 751
    vaginal 752
Streptobacillus moniliformis 241
Streptococcus agalactiae 419
Streptococcus pneumoniae 418
Streptococcus pyogenes 672
Stress 39, 701
Stroke 632, 678
    hemorrhagic 678
    ischemic 678
Strongyloides stercoralis 478
Sturge-Weber syndrome 715
Sudden infant death syndrome 746
Suicide 692, 697
    methods of 697
    theories of 697
Sulfur dioxide 99, 101
Summer encephalitis virus 541
Surveillance program, establishment of 621
Sushruta samhita 469
Swedish International Development Agency 525
Swollen lymph 578

Syphilis 610, 614
    congenital 611
    nursing management of 616
Systemic lupus erythematosus 674

T

Taenia echinococcus 497
Taenia saginata 497, 582, 583f, 584, 584t
Taenia solium 271, 497, 582, 584, 584t, 585f
Tapeworm
    infestation 271, 497
    life cycle of 499f
Teeth, care of 302
Tetanus 213, 595
    toxoid 424, 598
    types of 597
Tetracycline 568
Tetralogy of Fallot 665, 671
Tetrapetalonema perstans 530
Tetrapetalonema streptocerca 530
Thallium sulfate 572
Thermometer 135f
Thiamin 331
Thiamine deficiency 637
Thorax 218, 221
Threadworm 70
Throat, care of 412
Thrombocytopenia 509, 549
Thrombosis, cerebral 676, 678
Tick 231
    control of 233, 551
    life cycle of 233f, 551f
    morphology of 550
    typhus 578
Tissue anthropometry 645
Todd's paralysis 716
Togavirus 549f
Tonsillar diphtheria 425
Toxoids antitoxin floccules 424
Toxoplasma gondii 620
Tracheotomy 423
Trachoma 592, 594, 634, 635
Traditional birth attendants 337
Transmission, breaking channel of 543, 561, 591
Trench fever 575, 579
    transmission of 230
Treponema pallidum 204, 610, 611, 611f, 624f
    morphology of 611

Index

Treponema pertenue 623
Treponemal immunization test 614
Trichinella spiralis 241, 271
Trichomonas vaginalis 610, 627
Trichophyton 89
Tricuspid atresia 665, 671
Triple X syndrome 51, 54
Tripod sign 460
Trisomy 13 54
Trisomy 18 54
Trisomy 21 54
Trombicula mite
   life cycle of 235f
   morphology of 234f
Tsetse fly 224, 225f
Tubal ligation 752
Tubectomy 752, 752f
Tuberculosis 39, 40, 271, 290, 354, 432
   health visitor 442
   nursing management in 445
   prevention and control of 434
   pulmonary 410
Tumors
   brain 678, 715
   solid 681
Turner's syndrome 51, 53, 54, 671
Twenty point program 437
Typhoid
   fever 472, 571
      control of 475
      pathogenesis 474f
   nursing management of 477
   vaccine 211
Typhus
   endemic 576
   epidemic 574, 575

U

Ulcer 261
   peptic 698
Ulcerative colitis 698
Union Ministry of Health and Family Welfare 180
United Nations Development Program 740
United Nations International Children Emergency Fund (UNICEF) 408
Universal Immunization Program 437, 466
Urethritis 610
Urinary system 308, 312

V

Vaccines 211, 389, 390, 454
   preventable diseases 437
   types of 416
   vial monitor, stages of 465
Vaginal bleeding 750
Vaginal discharge 750
Vaginal infection 750
Vaginitis 610
Van Sanrakshan Samiti 192
Varicella zoster immunoglobulin 213, 404
Vasculitis 578
Vector-borne infection 387
Vehicle-borne transmission 387
Ventilation 114, 679
   artificial 116, 117
   exhaust 116
   mechanical 104
   natural 115
   standards of 114
   types of 115
   wind-driven 115
Vibrio 204
Vibrio cholerae 77, 173, 204, 205, 469
Vibrio parahaemolyticus 271, 505
Vibrio proteolyticus 271
Viral infections 701, 702
Virus 205, 620
   genetic sequence of 513
   isolation 621
   large number of 682
Visceral leishmaniasis 224, 526, 591
Vision
   blurring of 704
   loss 571
Vitamin 329, 646
   A 331
      deficiency 418, 637, 650
      prophylaxis 651t
   B12 331
      deficiency 637
   C deficiency 637
   D 331
   deficiencies 204
      diseases 649
Vomiting 261, 415, 571, 577

W

Waist circumference 659
Waist-to-hip ratio 659
Warts
   anal 610
   genital 610
Water pollution 68, 91
   sources of 69
Water-and food-borne diseases, control of 343
Waterlow classification 639, 643
Wayson stain 558
Weil's disease 70, 571
Wellcome classification 639, 641, 642
Wet-bulb thermometers 134, 138f
Wet-globe thermometer 135
Whipworm 70
White blood cell 447, 461
Wilson's disease 750
Wolf-Hirschhorn syndrome 53
Worksite Wellness Programs 43
World Health Organization 40, 58, 63
Wounds, classification of 538
Wuchereria bancrofti 530
   life cycle of 531f
   microfilaria of 530f

X

Xenopsylla astia 226
Xenopsylla braziliensis 226
Xenopsylla cheopis 226, 559, 576
Xerophthalmia 637, 649
XYY syndrome 54

Y

Yaws 623
Yellow fever 541
   nursing management of 544
   prevention of 543
   virus 541
Yersinia pestis 227, 558, 562

Z

Zidovudine 623
Ziehl-Neelsen method 599f, 602
Ziehl-Neelsen stained smear 433, 433f
Zinc 80
   phosphide 244, 572
Zoonoses
   bacterial 554
   parasitic 582
   rickettsial 574
   viral 535